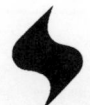

Stedman's

OB-GYN
& PEDIATRIC
WORDS

INCLUDES
NEONATOLOGY
Fifth Edition

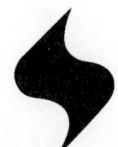

Stedman's

OB-GYN
&PEDIATRIC
WORDS

INCLUDES
NEONATOLOGY
Fifth Edition

 Wolters Kluwer | Lippincott Williams & Wilkins
Health

Philadelphia • Baltimore • New York • London
Buenos Aires • Hong Kong • Sydney • Tokyo

Publisher: Julie K. Stegman
Editorial Manager: Eric Branger
Associate Managing Editor: Erin M. Cosyn
Manufacturing Coordinator: Margie Orzech-Zeranko
Typesetter: Aptara, Inc.
Printer & Binder: Data Reproductions Corporation

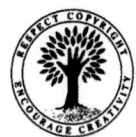
Printed in the United States of America

Fifth Edition, 2008

Library of Congress Cataloging-in-Publication Data

Stedman's OB-GYN & pediatrics words : includes neonatology. – 5th ed.
 p. ; cm. – (Stedman's word book series)
 Includes bibliographical references.
 ISBN 978-0-7817-7614-1
 1. Gynecology–Terminology. 2. Obstetrics–Terminology. 3. Pediatrics–Terminology.
4. Neonatology–Terminology. I. Stedman, Thomas Lathrop, 1853-1938. II. Title: OB-GYN
& pediatrics words. III. Title: Stedman's OB-GYN and pediatrics words. IV. Series:
Stedman's word books.
 [DNLM: 1. Obstetrics–Terminology–English. 2. Gynecology–Terminology–English.
3. Pediatrics–Terminology–English. WQ 15 S812 2008]
 RG47.S74 2008
 618.01′4–dc22   2008008839

                                                                          08 09 10 11
                                                                      1 2 3 4 5 6 7 8 9 10

Contents

Acknowledgments

An important part of our editorial process is the involvement of medical transcriptionists–as advisors, reviewers, and editors.

We extend special thanks to Jeanne Bock, CSR, MT and Nicole Peck, CMT for editing the manuscript, helping to resolve many difficult content questions, and contributing material for the appendix sections. We also extend special thanks to Helen Littrell, IMT, for performing the final prepublication review.

We are grateful, as well, to our MT Editorial Advisory Board members, including Sandra Alvarez, Cindy Brown, Jo-Ann Clarke, Robin Hall, Robin Koza, Heather A. Little, CMT, and Tracy Smith. These medical transcriptionists and medical language specialists served as important editors and advisors.

Other important contributors to this edition include Janet West, who focused on the appendix sections, and Shemah Fletcher; Rhonda Hase; Diane S. Heath, CMT; Robin Koza; Heather A. Little, CMT; Helen Littrell, IMT; Jenifer Walker, MA and Patricia Lee White, CMT. Kathy Cadle played an integral role in the process by reviewing the content files and updating the database.

As with all our *Stedman's* word references, this resource incorporates the suggestions and expertise of our many contacts in the medical transcriptionist community. Thanks to all of our advisory board participants, reviewers, and editors; AAMT meeting attendees; and others who have written us with requests and comments—keep talking, and we'll keep listening.

Editors' Preface

Life begins with the cry of a newborn entering the world after its mom has experienced 9 months of gestation, which have been accompanied by weight gain, morning sickness, charley horses, discomfort, heartburn, and more, followed by the ensuing hours of labor. But life really begins before that, when the sperm and embryo from two parents merge to begin the process of forming a new human being.

There are many factors that affect the growth of an embryo into a fetus and then into a newborn. Today we understand that genetic mutations, nutrition, sickness, disease, toxicities to which an unborn child's parents are exposed—such as chemicals in the environment, air quality, and drugs (legal and illegal)—all impact the health of the unborn child.

Then, once out in the world, there are additional factors that impact the growth of the baby as it matures into a child, into a teenager, and finally into an adult. We understand that genetics, environment, and social factors all have a profound impact on that developmental process.

There have been significant advances in technology for reproductive health in recent years. Disappearing are the days of standard black-and-white, 1-dimensional ultrasounds; they are being replaced by the technology of 3-dimensional images. Movies are made where we can actually see a fetus grow and develop in the womb.

Babies born prematurely now have a greater chance at survival than they did 50 years ago, or even 10 years ago. Testing for potentially life-changing diseases in a fetus while still inside the womb is now a reality, and in utero treatment of some of those very same diseases is now relatively commonplace.

With today's increased length of childbearing years for a woman and the viability of infants born extremely premature, the fact is that a large number of the medical specialties are now tightly interwoven with OB-GYN, pediatrics, and neonatology. Consequently, the matter of determining what terminology should be included in (or excluded from) this book was surprisingly more complex than we had anticipated. With that realization, we placed focused attention to the task of developing a reference that offers a comprehensive listing of terms most important to medical language specialists as they relate to conception, reproduction, birth, women's cyclical and general health, and pediatrics.

We extend thanks to the content researchers for this project, who reviewed textbooks, medical journals, and other sources to glean the most current terminology pertinent to this book. We would like to thank the Editorial Advisory Board for their input and insight. We also thank our managing editor, Erin Cosyn, for her excellent guidance and constant support during the editing process.

Jeanne Bock, CSR, MT
Nicole Peck, CMT

Publisher's Preface

Stedman's OB-GYN & Pediatric Words, Includes Neonatology, Fifth Edition offers an authoritative assurance of quality and exactness to the wordsmiths of the healthcare professions—medical transcriptionists, medical editors and copyeditors, health information management personnel, court reporters, and the many other users and producers of medical documentation.

We received many requests for updates to *Stedman's OB-GYN & Pediatric Words, Includes Neonatology, Fourth Edition.* As the requests continued to accumulate, we realized that medical language professionals needed a current, comprehensive reference for these specialties.

In *Stedman's OB-GYN & Pediatric Words, Includes Neonatology, Fifth Edition* users will find thousands of words related to gynecologic oncology, maternal-fetal medicine, endocrinology, infertility, ART, neonatology, and medical genetics. Users will also find terms for diagnostic and therapeutic procedures, new techniques, and lab tests, as well as equipment names and abbreviations with their expansions. The appendix sections provide anatomical illustrations with useful captions and labels; sample reports; common terms by procedure; and drugs listed by indication. This new edition also includes a listing and brief explanations of infertility studies and procedures, as well as a listing of routine antepartum tests. For quick reference, we have also included tables of genetics symbols, biophysical profile scores, and normal lab values.

This compilation of more than 65,000 entries, fully cross-indexed for quick access, was built from a base vocabulary of approximately 38,000 medical words, phrases, abbreviations and acronyms. The extensive A–Z list was developed from the database of *Stedman's Medical Dictionary, 28th Edition,* and supplemented by terminology found in current medical literature (please see list of References on page xvii).

We at Lippincott Williams & Wilkins strive to provide you with the most up-to-date and accurate word references available. Your use of this word book will prompt new editions, which we will publish as often as updates and revisions justify. We welcome your suggestions for improvements, changes, corrections, and additions—whatever will make this *Stedman's* product more useful to you. Please contact us through www.stedmans.com and send us your recommendations.

Explanatory Notes

Medical transcription is an art as well as a science. Both approaches are needed to correctly interpret the dictation of a physician, whose language is a product of education, training, and experience. This variety in medical language means that there are several acceptable ways to express certain terms, including jargon. *Stedman's OB-GYN & Pediatric Words, Includes Neonatology, Fifth Edition* provides variant spellings and phrasings for many terms. These elements, in addition to complete cross-indexing, make *Stedman's OB-GYN & Pediatric Words, Includes Neonatology, Fifth Edition* a valuable resource for determining the validity of terms as they are encountered.

Alphabetical Organization

Alphabetization of main entries is letter by letter as spelled, ignoring punctuation, spaces, prefixed numbers, or other special characters. For example:

4-chamber view
chameleon tongue

Terms beginning with Greek letters show the Greek letter spelled out and listed alphabetically. For example:

alpha, α

> a. helix
> interferon a. (IFN-alpha)
> interstitial positive-pressure interferon a.

In subentry alphabetization, the abbreviated singular form or the spelled-out plural form of the noun main entry word is ignored.

Format and Style

All main entries are in **boldface** to expedite locating a sought-after term, to enhance distinction between main entries and subentries, and to relieve the textual density of the pages.

Irregular plurals and variant spellings are shown on the same line as the singular or preferred form of the word. For example:

corona, pl. coronae
malacoplakia, malakoplakia

Hyphenation

As a rule of style, multiple eponyms (e.g., Dandy-Walker malformation) are hyphenated. Also, hyphens have been added between a manufacturer and one or more eponyms (e.g., Rochester-Ochsner forceps). Please note that in many cases, hyphenation is a question of style, not of accuracy, and thus is a matter of choice.

Possessives

Possessive forms have been dropped in this reference for the sake of consistency and conformance with the guidelines of the American Association for Medical Transcription (AAMT) and other groups. Please note, however, that in many cases, retaining the possessive, like hyphenating, is a question of style, not of accuracy, and thus is a matter of choice. To form the possessive of a word, simply add the apostrophe or apostrophe "s" to the end of the word.

Cross-indexing

The word list is in an index-like main entry-subentry format that contains two combined alphabetical listings:

(1) A *noun* main entry-subentry organization, which is typical of the A–Z section of medical dictionaries like *Stedman's*:

lamina	**test**
elastic l.	object assembly t.
l. lucida	t. of linkage disequilibrium

(2) An *adjective* main entry-subentry organization, which lists words and phrases as you hear them. The main entries are the adjectives or modifiers in a multiword term. The subentries are the nouns around which the terms are constructed and to which the adjectives or modifiers pertain:

familial
  f. tremor
  f. Turner syndrome

laparoscopic
  l. myomectomy
  l. oophorectomy

This format provides the user with more than one way to locate and identify a multiword term. For example:

abdominal
  a. crisis

crisis
  abdominal c.

female
  f. reproductive cycle

cycle
  female reproductive c.

It also allows the user to see together all terms that contain a particular descriptor, as well as all types, kinds, or variations of a noun entity. For example:

intensive
  i. care nursery (ICN)
  i. diabetes management (IDM)
  i. phototherapy

metabolism
  estrogen m.
  fat m.
  placental m.

Wherever possible, abbreviations are separately defined and cross-referenced. For example:

NICU
  neonatal intensive care unit

neonatal
  n. intensive care unit (NICU)

unit
  neonatal intensive care u. (NICU)

References

In addition to the manufacturers' literature we gather at various medical meetings, scientific reports from hospitals, and the lists created by our MT Editorial Advisory Board members from their daily transcription work, we used the following sources for new terms in *Stedman's OB-GYN & Pediatric Words, Includes Neonatology, Fifth Edition*:

Books

Berek JS, Adashi E, Hillard PA, eds. *Novak's Gynecology, Twelfth Edition*. Baltimore: Williams & Wilkins, 1996.

Gabbe SG, Niebyl JR, Simpson JL, eds. *Pocket Companion to Obstetrics: Normal & Problem Pregnancies, Third Edition*. Philadelphia: Churchill Livingstone, 1999.

Jacobs DS, DeMott WR, Grady HJ, Horvat RT, Huestis DW, Kasten BL, eds. *Laboratory Test Handbook, Fourth Edition*. Hudson, OH: Lexi-Comp, 1996.

Lambrou NC, Morse AN, Wallach EE, eds. *The Johns Hopkins Manual of Gynecology and Obstetrics*. Philadelphia: Lippincott Williams & Wilkins, 1999.

Lance LL. *2006 Quick Look Drug Book*. Baltimore: Lippincott Williams & Wilkins, 2006.

McKusick VA. *Mendelian Inheritance in Man: A Catalog of Human Genes and Genetic Disorders, Twelfth Edition*. Baltimore: The Johns Hopkins University Press, 1998.

Reece EA, Hobbins JC, eds. *Medicine of the Fetus and Mother, Second Edition*. Philadelphia: Lippincott-Raven Publishers, 1999.

Reiss HE, ed. *Reproductive Medicine: From A to Z*. Oxford: Oxford University Press, 1998.

Rivlin ME, Martin RW, eds. *Manual of Clinical Problems in Obstetrics and Gynecology, Fifth Edition*. Philadelphia: Lippincott Williams & Wilkins, 2000.

Scott JR, Di Saia PJ, Hammond CB, Spellacy WN, eds. *Danforth's Obstetrics and Gynecology, Eighth Edition*. Philadelphia: Lippincott Williams & Wilkins, 1999.

Stedman's Medical Dictionary, 28th Edition. Baltimore: Lippincott Williams & Wilkins, 2000.

Vera Pyle's Current Medical Terminology, Seventh Edition. Modesto, CA: Health Professions Institute, 1998.

CDs

Briggs GB, Freeman RK, Yaffe S, eds. *Drugs in Pregnancy and Lactation: A Reference Guide to Fetal and Neonatal Risk, on CD-ROM*. Philadelphia: Lippincott Williams & Wilkins, 1998.

Sciarra JJ, ed. *Gynecology and Obstetrics Looseleaf CD-ROM, Volumes 1–6.* Philadelphia: Lippincott Williams & Wilkins, 1999.

Journals

ADVANCE for Health Information Professionals. King of Prussia, PA: Merion, 1999.

American Journal of Human Genetics. Chicago: University of Chicago Press, 1995.

American Journal of Obstetrics and Gynecology. St. Louis: Mosby, 1999.

Clinical Dysmorphology. Philadelphia: Lippincott Williams & Wilkins, 1999–2000.

Contemporary OB/GYN. Montvale, NJ: Medical Economics, 1995–1997, 1999.

The Female Patient. Chatham, NJ: Quadrant HealthCom, 1999–2000.

Genetics in Medicine. Baltimore: Lippincott Williams & Wilkins/American College of Medical Genetics, 1998–1999.

Infertility and Reproductive Medicine Clinics of North America. Philadelphia: WB Saunders, 1995.

Internal Medicine. Montvale, NJ: Medical Economics, 1995–1997.

Journal of Reproductive Medicine. St. Louis: Journal of Reproductive Medicine, 1995.

The Latest Word. Philadelphia: WB Saunders, 1995.

OB-GYN Clinical Alert. Atlanta: American Health Consultants, 2000.

OB-GYN News. Morristown, NJ: International Medical News Group, 1995–1997, 1999–2000.

Obstetrical and Gynecological Survey. Baltimore: Lippincott Williams & Wilkins, 1995, 1997, 1999–2000.

Obstetrics and Gynecology. New York: Elsevier/The American College of Obstetricians and Gynecologists, 1995–1997, 1999–2000.

Stedman's WordWatcher. Baltimore: Lippincott Williams & Wilkins, 1995–2000.

Websites

http://asrm.abstracts.org/1997TOC.HTM

http://genomics.phrma.org

http://news.bmn.com/hmsbeagle

http://www.acog.com

http://www.ama-assn.org/insight/h_focus/wom_hlth/wom_hlth.htm

http://www.ama-assn.org/special/womh/womh.htm

http://www.amwa-doc.org
http://www.cdc.gov/genetics/update/current.htm
http://www.centerwatch.com/studies/LISTING.HTM
http://www.geneticalliance.org
http://www.hpisum.com
http://www.hum-molgen.de
http://www.mayohealth.org/mayo/0003/htm/hrt.htm
http://www.mtdesk.com
http://www.mtmonthly.com
http://www.nhgri.nih.gov
http://www.nlm.nih.gov/mesh/jablonski/syndrome_title.html
http://www.obgyn.net/medical.asp
http://www.sph.uth.tmc.edu/retnet/what-dis.htm
http://www.virtualdrugstore.com
http://www.womens-health.org

A
- abortus
- alveolar
  - A and D Ointment
  - A antigen

A1
- A1 diabetes mellitus

A2
- A2 diabetes mellitus

A4
- androstenedione

a-A
- arterial to alveolar

A-a
- alveolar-arterial
  - A-a gradient

AA
- acetabular anteversion
- acute appendicitis
- atlantoaxial
  - AA genotype

AAA
- achalasia-addisonianism-alacrimia
  - AAA syndrome

AABR
- automated auditory brainstem response
  - AABR hearing screening

AAC
- acute acalculous cholecystitis
- antibiotic-associated colitis
- augmentative and alternative communication

AACAP
- American Academy of Child and Adolescent Psychiatry

AAD
- antibiotic-associated diarrhea

AADH
- alopecia, anosmia, deafness, hypogonadism
  - AADH syndrome

Aagenaes syndrome

AAI
- axial acetabular index

AAMD
- American Association on Mental Deficiency
  - AAMD Adaptive Behavior Scale for Children and Adults

AAMR
- American Association on Mental Retardation

AAP
- American Academy of Pediatrics

AAPCC
- American Association of Poison Control Centers

Aarskog-Scott syndrome (ASS)
Aarskog syndrome
AAS
- abuse assessment screen
- acute abdominal series
- atypical absence seizure

Aase-Smith syndrome
Aase syndrome
AASH
- adrenal androgen-stimulating hormone

AAST
- American Association for the Surgery of Trauma
  - AAST organ injury scaling of vulva, vagina, bladder, urethral, rectal injury (grade I–V)

AAT
- animal-assisted therapy

A&B
- apnea and bradycardia
  - A&B spell

AB
- abdominal
- abortion
- abortus
- apnea and bradycardia
- asthmatic bronchitis

ABA
- applied behavior analysis

abacavir
ABAER
- automated brainstem auditory evoked response

abarelix
- a. depot-F
- a. depot-M

Abate
Abbe-McIndoe
- A.-M. total endoscopic vaginal reconstruction procedure
- A.-M. vaginal reconstruction

Abbe-McIndoe-Williams vaginoplasty procedure
Abbe vaginal construction
Abbe-Wharton-McIndoe vaginal reconstruction procedure
Abbokinase

Abbott
A. LCx Uriprobe assay
A. LifeCare PCA Plus II infusion
system
ABC
absolute band count
airway, breathing, circulation
argon beam coagulator
aspiration biopsy cytology
ABCDE
airway, breathing, circulation, disability,
exposure
ABCDE assessment
abdomen
acute a.
bloated a.
distended a.
milk lines of a.
pendulous a.
scaphoid a.
tympanitic a.
abdominal
a. actinomycosis
a. adhesion
a. approach
a. auscultation
a. ballottement
a. binder
a. breathing
a. bruit
a. cavity
a. circumference (AC)
a. coarctation
a. compartment syndrome
(ACS)
a. crisis
a. delivery
a. distention
a. dystocia
a. enlargement
a. epilepsy
a. examination
a. fetal echocardiography
a. fetal electrocardiography
a. free-fluid sign
a. girth
a. hernia
a. heterotaxy
a. hysterectomy (AH)
a. hysteropexy
a. hysterotomy
a. incision
a. irradiation
a. leak point pressure
(ALPP)
a. mass
a. metroplasty
a. migraine

a. muscle deficiency
a. muscle deficiency anomalad
a. muscle deficiency syndrome
a. muscular deficiency
a. musculature aplasia
syndrome
a. myomectomy
a. neurofibroma
a. ostium
a. pain
a. paravaginal repair
a. percussion
a. peritoneum
a. pregnancy
a. radiograph
a. rectopexy
a. rescue
a. retractor
a. sacral colpoperineopexy
a. sacral colpopexy (ASC)
a. sacrocolpopexy
a. sacropexy
a. sacrospinous ligament
colposuspension
a. salpingo-oophorectomy
a. salpingotomy
a. sheath
a. stria
a. strip radiotherapy
a. tenderness
a. trauma
a. tuberculosis
a. ultrasound
a. wall
abdominis
a. muscle
rectus a.
abdominocyesis
abdominocystic
abdominogenital
abdominohysterectomy
abdominohysterotomy
abdominopelvic
a. CT scan
a. irradiation
a. pain
a. procedure
a. scan
**abdominoperineal resection
(APR)**
abdominoscrotal hydrocele
abdominovaginal hysterectomy
abducens
a. facial paralysis
a. nerve
a. palsy
abducent palsy
abducted thumbs syndrome

abduction
> a. cast
> defective eye a.
> forefoot a.
> resisted a.
> a. splint

abductor lurch

Abelcet

abembryonic

Aberdeen knot

Aberfeld syndrome

aberrancy
> puberal a.

aberrant
> a. coronary artery
> a. course
> a. course of testicular descent
> a. regeneration
> a. right subclavian artery (ARSA)
> a. subclavian artery
> a. supraventricular tachycardia
> a. systemic feeding artery
> a. vitamin D metabolism

aberration
> chromosomal a. (CA)
> fetal growth a.
> G-banded cytogenetic a.
> genetic a.
> heterosomal a.
> newtonian a.
> a. of normal development and involution (ANDI)
> penta-X chromosomal a.
> sex chromosome a.
> steroidogenic a.
> tetra-X chromosomal a.
> triple-X chromosomal a.

abetalipoproteinemia (ABL)

ABG
> arterial blood gas

ABI
> ABI model 373 DNA sequencing system
> ABI model 377 DNA sequencing system
> ABI Prism dye terminator cycle sequencing ready reaction kit

ability
> cognitive a.
> Illinois Test of Psycholinguistic Abilities (ITPA)
> McCarthy Scales of Children's Abilities (MSCA)
> Revised Tests of Cognitive A.

Abiotrophia
> *A. defectiva*
> *A. elegans*

abiotrophy
> Leber a.

Abitrate

ABL
> abetalipoproteinemia

ablactation

ablation
> balloon endometrial a.
> endometrial a.
> endometrial resection and a. (ERA)
> hysteroscopic endometrial a.
> laparoscopic uterine nerve a. (LUNA)
> laparoscopic uterosacral nerve a.
> laser a.
> laser uterosacral nerve a. (LUNA)
> microwave endometrial a. (MEA)
> mucosal intact laser tonsillar a. (MILTA)
> Nd:YAG laser a.
> NovaSure endometrial a.
> outpatient endometrial resection and a. (OPERA)
> ovarian a. (OA)
> partial rollerball endometrial a.
> percutaneous transluminal coronary rotational a. (PTCRA)
> radioactive iodine a.
> radiofrequency a. (RFA)
> radiofrequency catheter a. (RFCA)
> rectoscopic endometrial a.
> rollerball endometrial a. (REA)
> rollerbar-loop-rollerbar a.
> stellate ganglion a.
> a. therapy
> thermal balloon a.
> transurethral a.
> uterosacral nerve a.
> valve a.

ablatio placentae

ablative
> a. procedure
> a. surgery
> a. therapy with bone marrow rescue

ablator
> endometrial a.

ablepharon-macrostomia syndrome (AMS)

ABM
> adult bone marrow

aBMD
> areal bone mineral density

abnormal

a. aortic valve attachment
a. cortical visual input
a. cortisol secretion
a. deceleration
a. dysfluency
a. embryo
a. face
a. facies
a. feedback signal
a. fetal development
a. gastric emptying
a. gene expression
a. gestational sac
a. glucosylceramide storage
a. head size
A. Involuntary Movement Scale (AIMS)
a. karyotype
a. labor
a. laxity of upper airway
a. lie
a. menstruation
a. mitochondrion
a. opacity
a. palate
a. palpebral fissure
a. penile curvature
a. phonation
a. placentation
a. puberty
a. respiratory pattern
a. response
a. thoracic conformity
a. transit
a. uterine bleeding (AUB)
a. vaginal bleeding (AVB)
a. vasculature flow pattern

abnormality

acral dysostosis with facial and genital abnormalities
cardiac a.
central serotonin a.
cervical a.
chromosomal structural a.
coagulation a.
congenital enamel a.
conotruncal a.
cord a.
cortical gyral a.
deflexion a.
dermatoglyphic a.
electrographic background a.
electroretinal a.
epithelial cell a.
extracardiac a.
Fairbank skeletal a.
fetal chromosome a.
fetal postural a.
fetal thoracic a.
fibrinogen a.
fishmouth a.
genetic a.
genitourinary a.
gestational a.
gyral a.
hemodynamic a.
histologic a.
hormonal a.
immune-mediated a.
intersex a.
intrapartum fetal heart rate a.
mammographic a.
metabolic a.
midbrain a.
MOMO a.
müllerian a.
müllerian duct aplasia, unilateral renalagenesis, and cervicothoracic somite abnormalities
müllerian, renal, cervicothoracic, somite abnormalities (MURCS)
multiple endocrine abnormalities (MEA)
neurobehavioral a.
neurologic a.
nonpalpable a.
oral-facial-digital syndrome with retinal abnormalities
ovarian a.
palpable bony a.
perisylvian a.
placental a.
placentation a.
platelet a.
possible migrational a.
posterior fossa malformations, hemangiomas, arterial anomalies, coarctation of aorta, cardiac defects, eye abnormalities (PHACE)
regional wall motion a.
reproductive tract a.
Ribbing skeletal a.
sex chromosome a.
single-gene a.
situs a.
skeletal a.
skeletal abnormalities, cutis laxa, craniostenosis, psychomotor retardation, facial abnormalities (SCARF)
soft tissue a.
spinal cord injury without radiographic a. (SCIWORA)
sporadic chromosome a.
ST and T-wave a.
ST-segment a.

tuberous breast a.
T-wave a.
umbilical artery waveform notching
a.
urinary tract a.
uterine a.
vaginal epithelial a.
X chromosome a.
**abnormally wide splitting of second
heart sound**
ABO
ABO antigen
ABO blood group system
ABO erythroblastosis
ABO hemolytic disease
ABO hemolytic disease of the
newborn
ABO incompatibility
aboral flow
abort
aborted ectopic pregnancy
aborter
habitual a.
abortient
abortifacient
abortigenic
abortion
accidental a.
ampullar a.
aneuploid a.
complete a.
a. complication
criminal a.
elective a. (EAB)
euploid a.
habitual a.
idiopathic a.
imminent a.
incipient a.
incomplete a. (IAB)
induced a. (IAB)
inevitable a.
infected a.
justifiable a.
labor induction a.
legal a.
medical a.
menstrual extraction a.
missed a.
recurrent a.
recurrent euploidic a.
recurrent spontaneous a.
(RSA)
repeated a.
saline a.
selective a.
septic a.
spontaneous a. (SAB)
surgical a.

surgically induced a.
therapeutic a. (TA, TAb, TAB)
threatened a.
tubal a.
abortionist
abortive poliomyelitis
abortus (A, AB)
trisomic a.
Aboulker stent
ABP
ambulatory blood pressure
arterial blood pressure
ABPA
allergic bronchopulmonary
aspergillosis
ABPM
ambulatory blood pressure monitoring
ABQ
attitude behavior questionnaire
ABR
auditory brainstem response
abrachia
abrachiocephalia
Abramson classification
abrasion
corneal a.
pleural a.
Abraxane
abrogated neonatal alveolization
abruption
placental a.
sinus a.
abruptio placentae (AP)
ABS
arterial blood sample
abscess
amebic hepatic a.
amebic liver a.
appendiceal a.
auricular a.
Bartholin gland a.
Bezold a.
biliary a.
brain a.
breast a.
Brodie a.
a. cavity
cold a.
cranial epidural a. (CEA)
crypt a.
dental a.
Douglas a.
Dubois a.
embolic a.
epidural a.
extradural a.
a. formation
intermuscular a.
intersphincteric a.

abscess (*continued*)
    intraabdominal a. (IAA)
    intramedullary spinal a.
    ischiorectal a.
    lung a.
    metastatic tuberculous a.
    milk a.
    myocardial a.
    neonatal scalp a.
    orbital subperiosteal a.
    otogenic brain a.
    ovarian a.
    parametritic a.
    parapharyngeal a.
    parauterine a.
    paravertebral a.
    parenchymal a.
    pelvic a.
    perianal a.
    periappendiceal a.
    perinephric a.
    perirectal a.
    perirenal a.
    peritonsillar a. (PTA)
    premammary a.
    psoas a.
    pyogenic a.
    retroesophageal a.
    retropharyngeal a.
    retrotonsillar a.
    spinal epidural a. (SEA)
    stitch a.
    subareolar a.
    subdural a.
    subperiosteal a. (SPA)
    subphrenic a.
    supralevator a.
    tuberculous a.
    tuboovarian a. (TOA)
    visceral a.

abscessus
    Mycobacterium a.

absence
    a. attack
    atypical a.
    congenital a.
    a. defect
    a. epilepsy
    myoclonic a.
    a. of abdominal muscle syndrome
    a. of branch pulmonary artery
    a. of rectal muscles
    protein-induced vitamin K a.
    a. seizure
    a. status
    a. status epilepticus
    testicular a.
    uterine a.
    vaginal a.

absent
    ankle reflexes a.
    a. antihelical fold
    a. cerebellum
    a. menses
    a. patella
    a. pulmonary valve syndrome
    a. radius
    a. splenium
    a. tears
    a. testis

Absolok endoscopic clip applicator
absolute
    a. band count (ABC)
    a. cardiac dullness
    a. CD4 count
    a. length gain
    a. lymphocyte count
    a. neutrophil count
    a. nucleated red blood cell
      (ANRBC)
    a. shunt
    a. sterility
    a. temperature
    a. weight gain

absorbable
    a. gelatin sponge
    a. ligature
    a. staple
    a. suture

absorbance, absorbancy, absorbency
    time-of-flight and a. (TOFA)
absorbancy (*var. of* absorbance)
absorbed
    rabies vaccine, a. (RVA)
absorbency (*var. of* absorbance)
absorbent gelling material (AGM)
Absorbine Jr. Antifungal
absorptiometer
    Hologic 1000 QDR dual-energy a.
    Lunar DPX dual-energy a.
absorptiometry
    dual-energy photon a.
    dual-energy x-ray a.
      (DEXA, DXA)
    dual-photon a.
    radiographic a.
    single-energy photon a.
    single-photon a.
    x-ray a.
absorption
    calcium a.
    coefficient of fat a.
    defective tryptophan a.
    fat a.
    a. fever
    fluorescent treponemal antibody a.
      (FTA-ABS)
absorptive hypercalciuria

ABSR
    auditory brainstem response
abstinence
    a. score
    a. syndrome
abstract thinking
ABT
    alternating breath test
    autologous blood transfusion
    autologous bone marrow transplantation
Abt-Letterer-Siwe syndrome
abuse
    adolescent sexual a.
    alcohol a.
    a. assessment screen
    CAGE test for alcohol a.
    child a. (CA)
    child physical a. (CPA)
    child sexual a. (CSA)
    domestic a.
    a. dwarfism syndrome
    emotional a.
    exit plan for a.
    maternal drug a.
    maternal substance a.
    partner a.
    physical a.
    physical-sexual a. (PSA)
    psychological a.
    sexual a.
    abuse, sexuality, safety assessment
    spousal a.
    substance a.
    verbal a.
abuser
    child of substance a. (COSA)
A$_{1c}$
    hemoglobin A$_{1c}$
AC
    abdominal circumference
    acromioclavicular
    anterior colporrhaphy
ACA
    anticentromere antibody
acalculous cholecystitis
acalvaria
Acanthamoeba
    A. castellani
    A. culbertsoni
    A. keratitis
    A. polyphagia
    A. rhysodes
acanthocyte
acanthocytosis
acantholysis bullosa
acanthosis
    a. nigricans
    paraductal a.
acarbose

acardia
acardiac
    a. fetus
    a. twinning
acardius
    acephalus a.
    fetus a.
Acarosan
ACAT
    automated computerized axial tomography
acatalasemia
acatalasia, acatalasemia
acathisia (*var. of* akathisia)
Acceava Trichomonas test kit
accelerate
accelerated
    a. atherosclerosis
    a. hypertension
    a. junctional ectopic tachycardia
    a. painless labor (APL)
    a. rejection
    a. skeletal maturation, Marshall-Smith type
    a. starvation
acceleration
    FHR a.
    a. injury
    a. phase
    a. phase of labor
acceleration-deceleration force
accelerator
    betatron electron a.
    linear a.
accentuation
    perifollicular a.
acceptance stage
access
    fetoplacental a.
    transcervical tubal a.
    uterine a.
accessoria
    mamma a.
accessory
    a. auricle
    BabyFace 3D surface rendering a.
    a. breast
    a. chromosome
    a. lobe of placenta
    a. müllerian funnel
    a. muscle
    a. muscle retraction
    a. navicular
    a. nerve
    a. nipple
    a. ovarian tissue
    a. ovary
    a. placenta
    a. protein

accessory (*continued*)
    a. sex gland
    a. soleus
    a. spleen
    a. tragus
    a. yolk
accident
    cerebrovascular a. (CVA)
    cord a.
    neonatal vascular a.
    obstetric a.
    umbilical cord a.
accidental
    a. abortion
    a. caustic ingestion
    a. dural puncture
    a. fetal injury
    a. hemorrhage
    a. penetration
    a. poisoning
    a. pregnancy
Accolate
accommodation
    gastric a.
accommodative esotropia
accompanying mood state
accouchement forće
accreta
    placenta a.
accretio cordis
accretion
    bone a.
    mass a.
    neural tissue a.
Accu-Chek
    A.-C. Easy glucose monitor
    A.-C. II Freedom blood glucose
     monitor
    A.-C. II glucometer
    A.-C. test
accumbens
    nucleus a.
accumulation
    dermatan sulfate a.
    glycogen a.
    heparan sulfate a.
    ketoacid a.
    lipid a.
Accupep HPF enteral formula
accuracy
    assay a.
    diagnostic a.
AccuSite injectable gel
AccuSpan tissue expander
AccuStat
    A. hCG pregnancy test
    A. Strep A assay
accustimulation
    electrical a.

Accutane
    A. dysmorphic syndrome
    A. effect
ACD
    alopecia, contracture, dwarfism
    area of cardiac dullness
     ACD level
     ACD mental retardation syndrome
ACE
    angiotensin-converting enzyme
    antegrade continence enema
     ACE genotype
     ACE inhibitor
     ACE procedure
acebutolol
Acel-Imune vaccine
acellular
    a. pertussis
    a. pertussis vaccine
acentric chromosome
acephalia (*var. of* acephalus)
acephalobrachia
acephalocardia
acephalochiria
acephalogastria
acephalopodia
acephalorrhachia
acephalostomia
acephalostomus
acephalothoracia
acephalothorus
acephalous
acephalus, acephalia
    a. acardius
Acephen
aceruloplasminemia
Aceta
acetabular
    a. anteversion (AA)
    a. dysplasia
    a. index (AI)
    a. labrum
    a. roof
acetabuli
    protrusio a. (PA)
acetabuloplasty
    Pemberton a.
acetamide
    modafinil a.
acetaminophen
    hydrocodone and a.
    oxycodone and a.
    propoxyphene and a.
    a. toxicity
    a. Uniserts
Acetasol HC otic
acetate
    aluminum a.
    calcium a.

cellulose a. (CA)
Cortone A.
cyproterone a.
depomedroxyprogesterone a. (DMPA)
desmopressin a. (DDAVP)
estradiol cypionate and
  medroxyprogesterone a.
estradiol/norethindrone a.
flecainide a.
Florinef A.
ganirelix a.
glatiramer a.
gonadorelin a.
goserelin a.
histrelin a.
leuprolide a.
leuprorelin a.
m-cresyl a.
medroxyprogesterone a. (MPA)
megestrol a.
methylprednisolone a.
nafarelin a.
norethindrone a.
octreotide a.
quingestanol a.
sermorelin a.
sodium a.
acetazolamide
acetic acid
acetoacetate
acetohexamide
acetone
acetonide
  fluocinolone a.
  triamcinolone a.
acetonuria
acetophenazine
acetophenetidin
acetophenide
  dihydroxyprogesterone a.
acetowhite
  a. epithelium
  a. lesion
  a. reaction
acetoxyprogesterone derivative
acetylcholine chloride
acetylcholinesterase (AChE, AchE,
  ACHE)
  a. assay
  a. histochemical stain
acetyl-CoA
  a.-CoA carboxylase
  a.-CoA dehydrogenase
acetylcysteine drug
acetyldigitoxin
acetylsalicylic acid (ASA)
ACF
  asymmetric crying facies
  ACF syndrome

achalasia
  familial a.
  infantile a.
achalasia-addisonianism-alacrimia (AAA)
achalasia-microcephaly syndrome
Achard syndrome
Achard-Thiers syndrome
ache
  stomach a.
AChE, AchE, ACHE
  acetylcholinesterase
acheilia
acheiria, achiria
acheiropody, achiropody
Achenbach
  A. Child Behavior Checklist
  A. questionnaire
achievable
  as low as reasonably a. (ALARA)
achievement
  Kaufman Test of Educational A.
  (K-TEA)
  Woodcock-Johnson Tests of A.
Achilles
  A. tendon
  A. tendon insertion
  A. tendon lengthening (ATL)
  A. tendon xanthoma
Achillis
  tendo A.
achiria (*var. of* acheiria)
achiropody (*var. of* acheiropody)
achlorhydria
acholic stool
achondrogenesis syndrome
achondroplasia
  homozygous a.
  a. syndrome
achondroplastic dwarfism
achromasia
achromia
achromians
  incontinentia pigmenti a.
achromic nevus
Achromobacter
  A. *lwoffii*
  A. *xylosoxidans*
Achromycin
  A. Ophthalmic
  A. Topical
  A. V
acid
  acetic a.
  acetylsalicylic a. (ASA)
  all-*trans*-retinoic a.
  alpha-aminoadipic a.
  alpha-ketoadipic a.
  alpha-linolenic a. (ALA)
  amino a.

acid (*continued*)

aminocaproic a.
5-aminosalicylic a.
amoxicillin-clavulanic a.
antideoxyribonucleic a. (anti-DNA)
arachidic a.
arachidonic a.
arginine-glycine-aspartic a.
  (arg-gly-asp)
argininosuccinic a.
arylalkanoic a.
arylcarboxylic a.
arylpropionic a.
ascorbic a.
aspartic a.
a. aspiration syndrome
bichloracetic a.
bicinchonic a. (BCA)
bile a.
boric a.
branched-chain amino a.
branched chain fatty a. (BCFA)
branched deoxyribonucleic a.
  (bDNA)
carbonic a.
a. ceramidase deficiency
9-cis-retinoic a.
citrate and citric a.
clavulanic a.
complementary deoxyribonucleic a.
  (cDNA)
conjugated linoleic a. (CLA)
C-palmitic a.
d-amino a.
deoxyadenylic a. (dAMP)
deoxycytidylic a. (dCMP)
deoxyguanylic a. (dGMP)
deoxyribonucleic a. (DNA)
deoxythymidylic a. (dTMP)
dibasic amino a.
dichloroacetic a.
diethylenetriaminepentaacetic a.
  (DTPA)
diisopropyl iminodiacetic a.
  (DISIDA)
dimercaptosuccinic a. (DMSA)
docosahexaenoic a. (DHA)
docosapentaenoic a.
eicosapentaenoic a.
elevated bile a.
a. elution test
epsilon aminocaproic a. (EACA)
erucic a.
essential amino a.
essential fatty a. (EFA)
ethacrynic a.
ethylenediaminetetraacetic a. (EDTA)
excitotoxic amino a. (EAA)
fatty a.

flufenamic a.
folic a.
folinic a.
formic a.
formiminoglutamic a. (FIGLU)
free fatty a.
fusaric a.
gamma aminobutyric a. (GABA)
glutamic a.
gossypol acetic a. (GAA)
homovanillic a. (HVA)
hydriodic a.
hydroxybenzoic a. (HABA)
hydroxyeicosatetraenoic a.
5-hydroxyindoleacetic a. (5-HIAA)
21-hydroxyindoleacetic a. (21-HIAA)
hypochlorous a.
iduronic a.
iocetamic a.
iopanoic a.
isobutyric a.
isovaleric a.
kinetoplast deoxyribonucleic a.
  (kDNA)
lactic a.
l-amino a.
linoleic a.
linolenic a.
a. lipase deficiency disease
lipid-associated sialic a.
lipoic a.
long-chain fatty a.
long-chain polyunsaturated fatty a.
  (LCPUFA)
lysergic a.
a. maltase
a. maltase deficiency (AMD)
mandelic a.
a. mantle
medium-chain fatty a. (MCFA)
mefenamic a.
messenger ribonucleic a. (mRNA)
methylmalonic a.
methylsuccinic a.
mitochondrial deoxyribonucleic a.
  (mtDNA)
mycophenolic a.
N-acetylaspartic a.
N-acetylneuraminic a. (NANA)
nalidixic a.
neuraminic a.
nicotinic a.
noncarbonic a.
nonessential amino a.
nonvolatile a.
nucleic a.
omega fatty a.
omega-3 fatty a.
orotic a.

palmitic a.
pantothenic a.
paraaminosalicylic a. (PAS)
a. peptic disease
phenylacetic a.
phenylpyruvic a.
a. phosphatase
phytanic a.
plasma linoleic a.
plasma very long chain fatty a.
polyglycolic a.
polyunsaturated fatty a. (PUFA)
pteroylglutamic a.
pyruvic a.
quinolinic a.
a. reflux
retinoic a.
ribonucleic a. (RNA)
salicylic a.
salicylsalicylic a.
serum amino a.
serum uric a.
short-chain fatty a. (SCFA)
short-chain polyunsaturated fatty a. (SCPUFA)
sialic a.
Slow Fe with folic a.
sodium citrate with citric a.
sulfur and salicylic a.
thioctic a.
ticarcillin/clavulanic a.
tolfenamic a.
tranexamic a.
trans fatty a. (tFA)
transfer ribonucleic a. (tRNA)
trichloroacetic a. (TCA)
2,4,5-trichlorophenoxyacetic a.
umbilical venous plasma amino a.
undecylenic a.
unsaturated linolenic a.
uric a.
urinary orotic a.
urine organic a.
urine vanillylmandelic a.
urocanic a.
ursodeoxycholic a.
valproic a.
vanillylmandelic a. (VMA)
very long chain fatty a. (VLCFA)
volatile a.
xanthurenic a.

acid-base
a.-b. balance
a.-b. disorder
a.-b. equilibrium
a.-b. measurement
a.-b. problem
a.-b. status
a.-b. value

acid-binding resin
acidemia
branched chain amino a.
fetal a.
glutaric a. (type I, II)
hyperpipecolic a.
isovaleric a.
lactic a.
metabolic a.
methylmalonic a.
mevalonic a.
mixed umbilical arterial a.
organic a.
orotic a.
pipecolic a.
propionic a.
pyroglutamic a.
trihydroxycoprostanic a.
acid-fast
a.-f. bacillus (AFB)
a.-f. sputum smear
a.-f. stain
acidic fibroblast growth factor (FGFa)
acidification
disordered renal a.
renal a.
vaginal a.
acidified serum lysis test
acidity
fecal a.
acid-loaded infant
acidophilus
Lactobacillus a.
acidosis
bicarbonate therapy in a.
chronic respiratory a.
congenital lactic a.
cord blood a.
diabetic a.
fetal a.
fetal respiratory a.
hyperchloremic metabolic a.
hyperchloremic renal a.
hyperchromic a.
hypokalemic a.
lactic a.
metabolic a.
nonanion gap metabolic a.
organic a.
perinatal a.
primary lactic a.
renal tubular a. (RTA)
respiratory a.
transient respiratory a.
uncompensated respiratory a.
acid-reacting substance
acid-Schiff
periodic a.-S. (PAS)
a.-S. staining

aciduria
- alpha-aminoadipic a.
- alpha-ketoadipic a.
- argininosuccinic a.
- beta-aminoisobutyric a.
- ethylmalonic-adipic a.
- glutaric a. (type I, II)
- hereditary orotic a.
- 3-hydroxy-3-methylglutaric a.
- isovaleric a.
- 3-methylglutaconic a.
- methylmalonic a. (MMA)
- mevalonic a.
- organic a.
- orotic a.
- paradoxical a.
- urocanic a.
- xanthurenic a.

Aci-Jel vaginal jelly
acinar artery
Acinetobacter
- A. *baumannii*
- A. *lwoffii*

acinic cell carcinoma
ACIP
- Advisory Committee on Immunization Practices

AcipHex
ACIS
- adenocarcinoma in situ

acitretin
aCL
- anticardiolipin
- anticardiolipin antibody

ACL
- anterior cruciate ligament

aclasis
- diaphysial a.

Aclovate Topical
ACLS
- advanced cardiac life support

acne
- acute febrile ulcerative a.
- a. conglobata
- cosmetic a.
- a. cyst
- drug-induced a.
- a. fulminans
- a. (grade I–IV)
- gram-negative a.
- halogen a.
- neonatal a.
- a. neonatorum (AN)
- nodular cystic a.
- occupational a.
- a. rosacea
- steroid a.
- toddler-age nodulocystic a.

- truncal a.
- a. vulgaris

acnes
- *Propionibacterium a.*

ACOG
- American College of Obstetricians and Gynecologists

acollis
- uterus a.

acorn cannula
Acosta endometriosis classification
acoustic
- a. admittance
- a. blink reflex
- a. enhancement
- a. impedance
- a. meningioma
- a. nerve
- a. neuroma
- a. reflectometry
- a. reflex test
- a. respiratory motion sensor (ARMS)
- a. schwannoma
- a. shadow
- a. stimulation study
- a. stimulation test (AST)
- a. trauma

acoustical interference
ACPS
- acrocephalopolysyndactyly

acquired
- a. abducens palsy
- a. agammaglobulinemia
- a. angioedema (type I, II)
- a. antithrombin III deficiency
- a. ascending undescended testis
- a. chylothorax
- a. C1 INH deficiency
- a. conjunctivitis
- a. cutis laxa
- a. epileptic aphasia
- a. growth hormone deficiency
- a. heart disease
- a. hemolytic anemia
- a. hemophilia
- a. hydrocephalus
- a. hypogammaglobulinemia
- a. hypothalamic lesion
- a. hypothyroidism
- a. immune deficiency syndrome (AIDS)
- a. immunodeficiency
- a. immunodeficiency syndrome (AIDS)
- a. immunodeficiency syndrome-related virus (ARV)
- a. inflammatory Brown syndrome

a. melanocytic nevus (AMN)
nosocomially a. (NA)
a. nystagmus
a. PAP
a. platelet disorder
a. pneumonia
a. protein C, S deficiency
a. sixth nerve palsy
a. thrombophilia
a. torticollis
a. urticaria
acquisita
epidermolysis bullosa a.
acquisition
intrauterine a.
multiple gated a. (MUGA)
acral
a. cyanosis
a. demineralization
a. dysostosis with facial and genital
abnormalities
a. keratotic papule
a. skin lesion
acral-renal-mandibular syndrome
acrania
acridine orange stain
acrid odor
acrivastine
acroblast
acrobrachycephaly
acrocallosal syndrome (ACS)
acrocentric chromosome
acrocephalia (*var. of* acrocephaly)
acrocephalopolysyndactyly (ACPS)
acrocephalosyndactyly (type I–V)
(ACS)
acrocephaly, acrocephalia
acrochordon
acrocraniofacial dysostosis
acrocyanosis
peripheral a.
acrodermatitis
a. chronica atrophicans
a. enteropathica (AE)
papular a.
papulovesicular a.
acrodynia
acrodysgenital syndrome
acrodysostosis syndrome
acrodysplasia
acrodysplasia-dysostosis syndrome
acrofacial
a. dysostosis (AFD)
a. dysostosis with postaxial defects
syndrome
acrofrontofacionasal (AFFN)
acrokeratosis paraneoplastica
acromastitis
acromegalia (*var. of* acromegaly)

acromegaloid-cutis verticis gyrata-leukoma
syndrome
acromegaloid facial appearance
(AFA)
acromegaly, acromegalia
acromelic
a. frontonasal dysplasia
a. shortening
acromesomelia
acromesomelic
a. dwarfism
a. dysplasia
acromial dimple
acromicric dysplasia
acromioclavicular (AC)
a. ligament
acromion
a. presentation
a. process
acroosteolysis
cranioskeletal dysplasia with a.
hereditary osteodysplasia with a.
a. syndrome
a. with osteoporosis and changes in
skull and mandible
acropectorovertebral dysplasia
acropustulosis
infantile a.
a. of infancy
acrorenal syndrome
acrorenomandibular syndrome
acrorenoocular syndrome
acrosin
acrosomal cap
acrosome
a. reaction
a. reaction with ionophore challenge
(ARIC)
acrosome-intact sperm
acrosphenosyndactyly
acrosyndactyly
acrotism
acrylic splint
ACS
abdominal compartment syndrome
acrocallosal syndrome
acrocephalosyndactyly (type I–V)
acute chest syndrome
American Cancer Society
anterior cricoid split
ACS procedure
act
Americans with Disabilities A.
(ADA)
Child Abuse Prevention and
Treatment A. (CAPTA)
Dietary Supplement Health and
Education A. (DSHEA)
Family Medical Leave A. (FMLA)

A

act (*continued*)
Individuals with Disabilities
Education A. (IDEA)
self-harming a.
Violence Against Women A.
ACT
activated clotting time
Actamin
ACTH
adrenocorticotropic hormone
ACTH deficiency
ACTH gel
ACTH insufficiency
ACTH stimulation
ACHT stimulation test
ACTH unresponsiveness
Acthar gel
ActHIB vaccine
Acticin Cream
Acticort Topical
Actidose-Aqua
Actidose with Sorbitol
Actifed Allergy Tablet
Actigall
actigraphy
limb a.
Actimmune
actin
muscle a.
actinic prurigo
actin-myosin interaction
Actinobacillus actinomycetemcomitans
Actinomadura madurae
Actinomyces
A. *georgiae*
A. *gerencseriae*
A. *israelii*
A. *meyeri*
A. *naeslundii*
A. *neuii*
A. *odontolyticus*
A. *pyogenes*
A. *viscosus*
actinomycetemcomitans
Actinobacillus a.
actinomycin D
actinomycosis
abdominal a.
cervicofacial a.
genital a.
pelvic a.
action
discoordinated uterine a.
excessive insulin a.
fetal heart a.
gene a.
law of mass a.
luteolytic a.
mediating a.

muscarinic a.
self-priming a.
uterine a.
ACTION
Adjuvant Chemotherapy in Ovarian
Neoplasia
Actiprofen
activated
a. charcoal
a. clotting factor X
a. clotting time (ACT)
a. estrogen receptor
a. partial thromboplastin time
(APTT)
a. partial thromboplastin time
coagulation test
a. protein C (APC)
a. protein C resistance
(APCR)
a. T cell
activation
egg a.
embryonic genome a.
endothelial cell a.
genome a.
polyclonal B cell a.
activator
gli family zinc-finger transcriptional
a.'s
lymphocyte a.
plasminogen a. (PA)
Platelin Plus A.
recombinant tissue type plasminogen
a. (rt-PA)
tissue plasminogen a. (TPA, t-PA)
urokinase plasminogen a. (u-PA)
active
a. and intense crying state
a. bowel sounds
Free A.
a. ignoring
a. immunization
Immunization Monitoring Program,
A. (IMPACT)
a. learner
a. phase
a. phase arrest
a. phase of labor
a. range of motion (AROM)
a. sleep
a. specific immunotherapy (ASI)
a. third-stage management
Activella
activin A
activity
antigen a.
antigravity a.
aspartoacylase hydrolytic a.
breech-born with delayed fetal a.

cause-and-effect a.
ceramidase a.
colony-stimulating a. (CSA)
conjugation a.
daily a.
elevated enzyme a.
endometrial cycling a.
enzyme a.
epileptiform a.
fetal cardiac a.
fetal heart a.
fetal somatic a.
functional brain a.
high-voltage slow a. (HVSA)
home life, education level, activities,
  drug use, sexual a. (HEADS)
low-voltage electrocortical a.
  (LVECoG, LV ECoG)
low-voltage fast a. (LVFA)
lupus anticoagulant a.
lymphotoxin antitumor a.
Manning score of fetal a.
mitogenic a.
nonweightbearing a.
activities of daily living
  (ADL)
opioid a.
ovarian a.
oxidative-reductase a.
peripheral androgen a.
phospholipase a.
PK a.
plasma renin a.
play a.
progestational a.
proline aminopeptidase a.
a., pulse, grimace, appearance,
  respiration
pulseless electrical a.
quantification of fetal a.
ristocetin cofactor a.
sexual a.
stool-withholding a.
tonic-clonic seizure a.
uterine a.
vagal a.
weightbearing a.
withdrawal-like a.
actometer
Actonel
Actron
actuarial survival
acuity
baseline visual a.
hearing a.
VEP a.
visual a.
Acular Ophthalmic
acuminata (*pl. of* acuminatum)

acuminate
a. papule
a. plaque
acuminatum, *pl.* **acuminata**
condyloma a.
giant anorectal condyloma a.
acupuncture for dysmenorrhea
Acuson
A. color Doppler
A. computed sonography
A. 128 Doppler ultrasound
A. 128XP-10 ultrasound
A. 128XP ultrasound machine
acuta
pityriasis lichenoides et varioliformis
  a. (PLEVA)
pustulosis vacciniformis a.
acute
a. abdomen
a. abdominal series
a. acalculous cholecystitis (AAC)
a. acquired neutrophilia
a. adrenal crisis
a. anaphylaxis
a. angle closure glaucoma
a. anterior uveitis
a. appendicitis (AA)
a. ascending radiculomyelitis
a. aseptic meningitis syndrome
a. atherosis
a. atrophic candidiasis
a. bacterial endocarditis
a. barotitis
a. bronchiolitis
a. cerebellar ataxia
a. cerebellar ataxia of unknown
  cause
a. cerebellitis
a. chagasic encephalitis
a. chemotherapy associated nausea
a. chest syndrome (ACS)
a. childhood ataxia
a. childhood ITP
a. circulatory collapse
a. coalescent mastoiditis
a. confusional migraine
acute, critical, unexpected, treatable,
  easily diagnosed
a. cystitis
a. dacryocystitis
a. disseminated encephalomyelitis
  (ADEM)
a. disseminated histiocytosis
a. disseminated histiocytosis X
a. epidemic conjunctivitis
a. epiglottitis
a. eruptive lichen planus
a. exudative tonsillitis
a. fatty liver

acute (*continued*)
a. fatty liver of pregnancy (AFLP)
a. febrile neurophilic dermatosis
a. febrile ulcerative acne
a. fibrinous pericarditis
a. flaccid paralysis
a. follicular tonsillitis
a. fulminant colitis
a. fulminant disease
a. glomerulonephritis
a. graft-versus-host disease (AGVHD)
a. headache
a. hemarthrosis
a. hematogenous osteomyelitis
a. hemorrhagic conjunctivitis
a. hemorrhagic edema of infancy (AHEI)
a. hemorrhagic pancreatitis
a. hepatitis
a. hydrocephalus
a. illness
A. Illness Observation Scale (AIOS)
a. infantile hemiplegia
a. infectious colitis
a. infectious polyneuritis
a. inflammatory demyelinating polyneuropathy (AIDP)
a. influenza A encephalitis
a. injury
a. insulin response
a. intermittent porphyria (AIP)
a. interpersonal loss
a. interstitial myocarditis
a. interstitial nephritis
a. interstitial pneumonia
a. intrapartum transfusion
a. iridocyclitis
a. iron poisoning
a. labyrinthitis
a. laryngotracheal bronchitis
a. life-threatening event (ALTE)
a. lower respiratory infection (ALRI)
a. lower respiratory tract infection (ALRTI)
a. lymphatic leukemia
a. lymphoblastic leukemia (ALL)
a. lymphocytic leukemia (ALL)
a. lymphonodular pharyngitis
a. mastoid osteitis
a. megakaryoblastic leukemia
a. meningoencephalitis syndrome
a. motor-axonal neuropathy (AMAN)
a. motor-sensory axonal neuropathy (AMSAN)
a. mountain sickness (AMS)
a. MS

a. myeloblastic leukemia (AML)
a. myelogenous leukemia (AML)
a. myeloid leukemia (AML)
a. myeloradiculitis
a. myocardial infarction (AMI)
a. necrotizing ulcerative gingivitis (ANUG)
a. neonatal herpes
a. neuritis
a. neuronopathic Gaucher disease
a. nonlymphoblastic leukemia (ANLL)
a. nonlymphocytic leukemia
a. oliguric renal failure (AORF)
a. otitis media (AOM)
a. pancarditis
a. parotitis
a. pericoronitis
a. perinatal conjunctivitis
a. perinatal transfusion
A. Physiology and Chronic Health Evaluation (APACHE)
a. pneumonitis
a. postinfectious glomerulonephritis (APGN)
a. postinfectious nephritis
a. poststreptococcal glomerulonephritis (APSGN)
a. progressive glomerulonephritis
a. pseudomembranous candidiasis
a. purulent conjunctivitis
a. pyelonephritis
a. radiation syndrome
a. recurrent ataxia
a. rejection
a. renal failure (ARF)
a. renal parenchymal inflammation
a. respiratory alkalosis
a. respiratory disease (ARD)
a. respiratory distress syndrome (ARDS)
a. respiratory failure (ARF)
a. respiratory infection (ARI)
a. retroviral syndrome
a. rheumatic carditis
a. rheumatic fever
a. schistosomiasis
a. scombroid intoxication
a. secondary localized peritonitis
a. sera
a. sinusitis
a. spasmodic laryngitis
a. spastic paraparesis
a. splenic sequestration
a. splenic sequestration crisis
a. streptococcal gangrene
a. stress disorder (ASD)
a. subdural hematoma
a. subglottic stenosis

a. suppurative cervical
lymphadenopathy
a. suppurative otitis media
a. suppurative thyroiditis
A. Surgical and Scientific
Instruments
a. surgical mastoiditis
a. syphilitic leptomeningitis
a. tocolysis
a. torticollis
a. total asphyxia
a. tracheitis
a. transfusion reaction
a. transverse myelitis
a. traumatic compartment syndrome
a. tubular necrosis (ATN)
a. urethral syndrome
a. urticaria
a. uterine inversion
a. vaginal bleeding
acute-on-chronic
a.-o.-c. SCFE
a.-o.-c. tissue hypoxemia
acute-phase
a.-p. attrition
a.-p. reactant
a.-p. serum study
AcuTrainer device
Acutrim
A. II
A. Late Day
A. Precision Release
acutum
ulcus vulvae a.
ACV
assist-control ventilation
acyanotic
a. cardiac anomaly
a. congenital cardiac defect
a. congenital heart disease
a. lesion
a. tetralogy of Fallot
acyclicity
acyclic pelvic pain
acyclovir
acyesis
acylcarnitine
a. analysis
a. profile
acystia
A-D
antidiarrheal
Imodium A-D
ad
a. lib feeding
a. libitum diet
AD
Asperger disorder
autistic disorder

ADA
adenosine deaminase
American Diabetes Association
Americans with Disabilities Act
ADA diet
Adacel
adactylia, adactyly
adactyly (*var. of* adactylia)
Adagen
Adair-Dighton syndrome
Adair-Veress needle
Adalat CC
Adam
A. complex
A. position
adamantinoma
Adamkiewicz
artery of A.
Adams
A. advancement
A. advancement of round
ligaments
A. forward-bending test
A. test for scoliosis
Adams-Oliver syndrome
Adams-Stokes syndrome
adapalene
Adapin
adaptability
poor a.
adaptation
bowel a.
immediate extrauterine a.
maternal ocular a.
uterine artery hemodynamic a.
adapter, adaptor
Briggs T a.
side-port a.
adaptive
a. behavior
a. chair
a. delay
a. development
a. domain
a. immunity
a. landscape
a. peak
a. radiation
a. surface
a. switch
a. value
adaptor (*var. of* adapter)
ADB
anti-DNase B
ADB antibody
ADB titer
ADC
AIDS dementia complex
ADC Medicut shears

ADCC
   antibody-dependent cell-mediated cytotoxicity
Adcon-L anti-adhesion barrier
ADD
   attention deficit disorder
add-back
   a.-b. regimen
   a.-b. therapy
   a.-b. treatment
Adderall
ADDES
   Attention Deficit Disorders Evaluation Scale
addict
   sex a.
addiction
   alcohol a.
   cocaine a.
   drug a.
   opioid a.
   sexual a.
Addison
   A. disease
   A. disease-cerebral sclerosis syndrome
   A. disease-spastic paraplegia syndrome
addisonian
   a. crisis
   a. pernicious anemia
   a. syndrome
Addison-Schilder syndrome
additive genetic variance
additivity
adducted
   a. great toe
   a. thumb-clubfoot syndrome
   a. thumbs-mental retardation syndrome
   a. thumbs syndrome
adduction
   a. deformity
   eye retraction with a.
   forefoot a.
adductor
   a. angle
   a. interosseous compartment
   a. spasm
adductus
   a. clubfoot
   congenital metatarsus a.
   forefoot a.
   metatarsus a. (MA)
   simple metatarsus a.
adefovir dipivoxil
adelomorphous

ADEM
   acute disseminated encephalomyelitis
   recurrent ADEM
adenine
   a. arabinoside
   a. nucleotide
   a. phosphoribosyltransferase
adenitis
   bacterial cervical a.
   cervical a.
   inguinal a.
   mesenteric a.
   periodic fever, aphthous stomatitis, pharyngitis, cervical a. (PFAPA)
   salivary a.
   sclerosing a.
   tuberculous a.
   vestibular a.
adenoacanthoma
   endometrial a.
   lymph node endometriotic a.
adenocarcinoma
   cervical clear cell a.
   ciliated cell endometrial a.
   clear cell a.
   endometrial clear cell a.
   endometrial secretory a.
   a. in situ (ACIS, AIS)
   mesonephric a.
   metastatic a.
   microinvasive a.
   minimal deviation a.
   mucinous a.
   a. of infantile testis
   ovarian clear cell a.
   papillary a.
   secretory a.
   serous a.
   vaginal clear cell a.
   vulvar adenocystic a.
   vulvar adenoid cystic a.
Adenocard
adenocystic carcinoma
adenofibroma
adenofibromyoma
adenofibrosis
adenohypophysis
adenohypophysitis
   lymphocytic a.
adenoidal
   a. face
   a. hypertrophy
adenoid cystic carcinoma
adenoidectomy
   tonsillectomy and a. (T&A)
adenoiditis
adenoleiomyofibroma

adenoma, *pl.* **adenomas, adenomata**
  apocrine a.
  benign hepatic a.
  beta-cell a.
  chromophobic a.
  ductal a.
  eosinophilic a.
  growth hormone-secreting a.
  islet cell a.
  lactating a.
  a. malignum
  a. of nipple
  ovarian tubular a.
  parathyroid a.
  pituitary a.
  prolactin-producing a.
  prolactin-secreting a.
  a. sebaceum
  suspected pituitary a.
  testosterone-secreting adrenal a.
  thyrotropin-secreting pituitary a.
  virilizing a.
adenomas (*pl. of* adenoma)
adenomata (*pl. of* adenoma)
adenomatoid
  a. malformation
  a. oviduct tumor
adenomatosis
  beta-cell a.
  familial multiple endocrine a.
  fibrosing a.
  islet cell a.
  multiple endocrine a. (MEA)
adenomatous
  a. colonic polyposis
  a. endometrial hyperplasia
  a. hyperplasia (AH)
  a. polyp
adenomegaly
adenomere
adenomyoma
adenomyomatosis
adenomyosis
  stromal a.
  a. uteri
adenopathy
  axillary a.
  cervical a.
  inguinal a.
  phenytoin-associated a.
  postinflammatory a.
  preauricular a.
  reactive a.
adenosalpingitis
adenosarcoma
  müllerian a.
adenosine
  a. deaminase (ADA)
  a. deaminase deficiency

  a. monophosphate (AMP)
  a. phosphate
  a. triphosphatase (ATPase)
  a. triphosphate (ATP)
adenosis
  blunt duct a.
  congenital vaginal a.
  fibrosing a.
  mammary sclerosing a.
  microglandular a.
  sclerosing a.
  a. vaginae
  vaginal a.
adenosquamous
  a. carcinoma
  a. sarcoma
adenosylcobalamin
adenosyltransferase
  cobalamin a.
adenotomy
adenotonsillar hypertrophy
adenotonsillectomy
adenotonsillitis
adenoviral
  a. pneumonia
  a. tonsillitis
adenovirus
  a. 7
  enteric a.
  epidemic keratoconjunctivitis a.
  a. infection
  a. type 3
adenylate cyclase
adenyl cyclase
adenylosuccinate
  a. deficiency
  a. lyase deficiency (ASLD)
adequate caliber of anus
adermia
adermogenesis
ADH
  antidiuretic hormone
  atypical ductal hyperplasia
adhalin gene
ADHD
  attention deficit hyperactivity disorder
  Girls, Ritalin LA, and ADHD
    (GRACE)
adherens
  fascia a.
  zonula a.
adherent
  a. placenta
  a. pseudomembrane
  a. vaginal discharge
adhesiolysis
adhesion
  abdominal a.
  amniotic a.

adhesion (*continued*)
    banjo-string a.
    cell-extracellular matrix a.
    dense a.
    endometrial a.
    fiddle-string a.
    filmy a.
    fimbrial a.
    intracervical a.
    intrauterine a.
    labial a.
    lysis of a.'s
    a. molecule
    omental a.
    paraovarian a.
    pelvic a.
    peritubal a.
    piano-wire a.
    platelet a.
    A. Scoring Group (ASG)
    serosal a.
    sperm-egg a.
    tongue-lip a.
    vaginal cuff a.
adhesiotherapy
adhesiva
    vaginitis a.
adhesive
    a. band
    Biobrane a.
    a. disease
    a. endometriosis
    a. otitis
    Testoderm with A.
    a. vaginitis
    a. vulvitis
Adhibit adhesion prevention gel
ADI
    atlantodens interval
    Autism Diagnostic Interview
adiabatic effect
adiadochokinesia
A/4-6-diamidino-2-phenylindole
    distamycin A/4-6-d.-2-p.
Adie
    A. chronic pupillary syndrome
    A. pupil
Adipex-P
adipocyte
adiponecrosis subcutanea neonatorum
adipose tissue
adiposity
adiposogenital syndrome
adipsia, adipsy
adipsy (*var. of* adipsia)
ADI-R
    Autism Diagnostic Interview-Revised
aditus ad antrum

adjunctive
    a. radiation therapy
    a. treatment
adjusted gestational age
adjustment
    a. disorder
    psychosocial a.
adjuvant
    a. chemoradiation therapy
    a. chemotherapy
    A. Chemotherapy in Ovarian Neoplasia (ACTION)
    Freund a.
    a. medication
    a. radiotherapy
ADL
    activities of daily living
    Amsterdam Depression List
ADMCKD
    autosomal dominant medullary cystic kidney disease
administration
    exogenous estrogen a.
    Food and Drug A. (FDA)
    Health Care Financing A. (HCFA)
    oral a.
    oxytocin a.
    parenteral a.
    pulsatile GnRH a.
    rectal a.
    RSV immunoglobulin for intravenous a.
    sequential a.
    silver nitrate a.
    surfactant a.
    transdermal a.
    transnasal a.
    vaginal a.
admission
    antenatal a.
admittance
    acoustic a.
    peak a.
    static a.
adnata
    alopecia a.
adnatum
    filiform a.
adnexa (*pl. of* adnexum)
adnexal
    a. adhesion classification system
    a. cyst
    a. infection
    a. involvement
    a. mass
    a. metastasis
    a. torsion
    a. tumor
adnexectomy

adnexitis
adnexopexy
adnexum, *pl.* **adnexa**
ADOD
    arthrodentoosteodysplasia
adolescence
    early a.
    late a.
    middle a.
adolescent
    A. and Pediatric Pain Tool (APPT)
    a. breast
    a. bunion
    Computerized Diagnostic Interview
      for Children and A.'s (cDICA)
    Functional Impairment Scale for
      Children and A.'s (FISCA)
    a. gynecology
    a. idiopathic scoliosis (AIS)
    Interview Schedule for Children and
      A.'s (ISCA)
    a. medicine
    a. obesity
    Pictorial Instrument for Children
      and A.'s (PICA)
    a. pregnancy
    a. scoliosis
    a. seborrhea
    Service Assessment for Children
      and A.'s (SACA)
    a. sexual abuse
    a. sterility
    a. stretch syncope
    a. tibia vara
    a. vulvovaginitis
adolescentis
    Bifidobacterium a.
adolescent-onset patient
adoptive
    a. immunotherapy
    a. nursing
ADOS
    Autism Diagnostic Observation
      Schedule
    autosomal dominant Opitz syndrome
ADPKD
    autosomal dominant polycystic kidney
    disease
ADR
    adverse drug reaction
    ataxia-deafness-retardation
    ADR syndrome
    ADR syndrome with ketoaciduria
adrenal
    a. androgen
    a. androgen secretion
    a. androgen-stimulating hormone
      (AASH)
    a. axis dysfunction

    a. calcification
    a. cell rest tumor
    a. cortex
    a. cortical carcinoma
    a. cortical deficiency
    a. cortical hyperfunction
    a. crisis
    a. excess
    a. gland
    a. gland morphology
    a. hematoma
    a. hemorrhage
    a. hyperandrogenism
    a. hyperandrogenism marker
    a. hyperplasia
    a. hypofunction
    a. hypoplasia
    a. hypoplasia congenita (AHC)
    a. insufficiency
    a. leukodystrophy
    Marchand a.'s
    a. maturation
    a. medulla
    a. morphologic consideration
    a. neoplasm
    a. reticularis
    a. steroid
    a. steroidogenesis
    a. suppression
    a. virilism
    a. virilizing syndrome
adrenalectomy
Adrenalin Chloride
adrenaline injection
adrenalitis
    autoimmune a.
    necrotizing a.
adrenarche
    idiopathic premature a.
    precocious a.
    premature a.
adrenergic
    alpha a.
    a. blocker
    a. drug
    a. receptor
    a. stimulator
adrenocortical
    a. atrophy-cerebral sclerosis
      syndrome
    a. function
    a. hormone
    a. hyperplasia
    a. insufficiency
    a. steroid
    a. steroidogenesis
    a. stress
adrenocorticotrophic (*var. of*
    adrenocorticotropic)

adrenocorticotropic, adrenocorticotrophic
   a. hormone (ACTH)
   a. hormone deficiency
   a. hormone insufficiency
adrenocorticotropin
   chorionic a.
adrenogenital syndrome (AGS)
adrenoleukodystrophy (ALD)
   neonatal a. (NALD)
   X-linked a.
adrenoleukomyeloneuropathy (ALMN)
adrenomedullary
adrenomegaly
adrenomyeloneuropathy (AMN)
adrenomyodystrophy
Adriamycin
   A., fluorouracil, methotrexate
   (AFM)
   A. PFS
   A. RDF
adRP
   autosomal dominant retinitis
   pigmentosa
Adrucil Injection
ADS
   anonymous donor sperm
Adson
   A. forceps
   A. ganglion scissors
   A. pickups
adult
   AAMD Adaptive Behavior Scale for
   Children and A.'s
   a. bone marrow (ABM)
   a. generalized gangliosidosis
   a. granulosa cell tumor (AGCT)
   a. NCL
   a. onset adrenal hyperplasia
   (AOAH)
   a. polycystic disease
   a. progeria
   a. pseudohypertrophic muscular
   dystrophy
   a. Refsum disease
   a. respiratory distress syndrome
   (ARDS)
   a. T-cell leukemia/lymphoma
   (ATLL)
adult-directed instruction
adult-onset
   a.-o. congenital adrenal hyperplasia
   a.-o. diabetes mellitus (AODM)
   a.-o. hypogammaglobulinemia
   a.-o. polycystic kidney disease
   a.-o. polyglandular syndrome
   a.-o. spinocerebellar ataxia
adultorum
   scleredema a.
adult-type hypolactasia

Advair Diskus
advance
   a. directive
   A. formula
advanced
   a. carcinoma
   a. cardiac life support (ACLS)
   A. Collection breast pump
   a. epithelial ovarian cancer
   Imodium A.
   a. life support (ALS)
   a. maternal age (AMA)
   a. oxidation protein product
   a. pediatric life support (APLS)
   a. trauma life support (ATLS)
advanced-stage disease
advancement
   Adams a.
   mandibular a.
   maxillary a.
   vaginal a.
Advantage
   A. 24 bioadhesive contraceptive
   gel
   A. mesh
   A. midurethral sling
   A. ultrasound
adventitia
adventitious
   a. breath sounds
   a. choreiform movement
   a. deafness
Advera formula
adverse
   a. drug reaction (ADR)
   a. food reaction
   a. maternal effect
   a. outcome
Advil Cold & Sinus Caplet
Advisory Committee on Immunization
  Practices (ACIP)
advocacy
   protection and a. (P&A)
advocate
adynamia episodica hereditaria
adynamic ileus
adysplasia
   hereditary renal a.
   hereditary urogenital a.
AE
   acrodermatitis enteropathica
AEA
   antiendomysium antibody
AEC
   ankyloblepharon, ectodermal dysplasia,
   clefting
     AEC syndrome
AED
   antiepileptic drug

Aedes triseriatus
aEEG
    amplitude-integrated
        electroencephalogram
Aegis sonography management system
AENNS
    Albert Einstein Neonatal
        Developmental Scale
AEP
    auditory evoked potential
Aequitron 9200 apnea monitor
AER
    aldosterone excretion rate
    auditory evoked response
aeration
        lung a.
        unequal a.
aeroallergen
aerobe
aerobic metabolism
aerobics
        digital auditory a. (DAA)
        water a.
AeroBid-M Oral aerosol inhaler
AeroBid Oral aerosol inhaler
AeroChamber spacer device
aerocolpos
aerodigestive tract
Aerolate
        A. III
        A. JR
        A. SR S
Aeromonas hydrophila
Aeroneb nebulizer
aerophagia, aerophagy
aerophagy (*var. of* aerophagia)
aerophore
Aeroseb-Dex Topical Aerosol
Aeroseb-HC Topical
aerosol
        Aeroseb-Dex Topical A.
        Breezee Mist A.
        Bronkometer A.
        cromolyn sodium inhalation a.
        Dexacort Phosphate Turbinaire
            Intranasal A.
        Nasalide Nasal A.
        a. therapy
        Tilade Inhalation A.
        Virazole A.
aerosolization
aerosolized
        a. amphotericin B
        a. medication
        a. racemic epinephrine
        a. ribavirin
aerotitis
aeruginosa
        Pseudomonas a.

aestivale
        hydroa a.
AF
    amniotic fluid
    anterior fontanelle
        SSD AF
AFA
    acromegaloid facial appearance
        AFA syndrome
AFAFP
    amniotic fluid alpha-fetoprotein
AFB
    acid-fast bacillus
AFDC
    Aid to Families with Dependent
        Children
AFE
    amniotic fluid embolism
afebrile
        a. bacteremia
        a. convulsion
        a. pneumonia syndrome
        a. seizure
afetal
affect
        a. attunement
        Eating Disorders Inventory Score for
            Interoceptive Awareness A.
        flat a.
affective
        a. disorder
        a. storm
affectivity
        negative a.
afferent
        somatic a.
        a. vessel
        visceral a.
Affinity bed
Affirm
        A. VPIII test
        A. VP microbial identification
            system
AFFN
    acrofrontofacionasal
        AFFN dysostosis
        syndrome 1
affricate
Affymetrix GeneChip system
AFI
    amaurotic familial idiocy
    amniotic fluid index
afibrinogenemia
        congenital a.
Afipia felis
Afko-Lube
aflatoxin poisoning
AFLP
        acute fatty liver of pregnancy

AFM
  Adriamycin, fluorouracil, methotrexate
AFO
  ankle-foot orthosis
AFP, aFP
  alpha-fetoprotein
    AFP X-tra
AFP-EIA
  alpha-fetoprotein enzyme immunoassay
AFRAX
  autism-fragile X syndrome
africae
    Rickettsia a.
African
    A. American variant galactosemia
    A. Burkitt lymphoma
    A. tick bite fever
    A. trypanosomiasis
africanum
    Mycobacterium a.
Afrin
Afrinol
AFS
  American Fertility Society
    AFS adhesion scoring system
    AFS Revised Classification of
    Endometriosis
Aftate Antifungal
afterbirth pain
after-coming head
afterload
    a. applicator
    a. colpostat
    LV a.
    a. reduction therapy
    ventricular a.
afterpain
after-pains
AFUD
  American Foundation for Urologic
  Diseases
    AFUD classification
AFV
  amniotic fluid volume
afzelii
    Borrelia a.
A/G
  albumin-globulin
AGA
  antigliadin antibody
  appropriate for gestational age
  aspartylglucosamine
  average for gestational age
    AGA deficiency
    postterm AGA
    term AGA
agalactia, agalactosis
agalactiae
    Streptococcus a.

agalactorrhea
agalactosis
agalactous
agammaglobulinemia
  acquired a.
  Bruton a.
  X-linked a. (XLA)
aganglionic
  a. bowel
  a. colon
  a. megacolon
  a. rectum
  a. sphincter
aganglionosis
  colonic a.
  congenital intestinal a. (CIA)
  intestinal a.
  long-segment a.
  total colonic a.
  zonal a.
agar
  BiGGY a.
  blood a.
  charcoal a.
  chocolate a.
  a. gel precipitation technique
  Hektoen a.
  a. immunoprecipitin technique
  MacConkey II a.
  nalidixic acid a.
  Novy-McNeal-Nicolle biphasic
    blood a.
  a. plate
  Ryan a.
  Thayer-Martin a.
  xylose lysine deaminase a.
AGC
  atypical glandular cell
AGCT
  adult granulosa cell tumor
AGCUS
  atypical glandular cells of uncertain
    significance
  atypical glandular cells of
    undetermined significance
age
  adjusted gestational a.
  advanced maternal a. (AMA)
  Ages and Stages Questionnaire
    (ASQ)
  appropriate for gestational a.
    (AGA)
  average for gestational a. (AGA)
  birth weight for gestational a.
    (BWGA)
  bone a.
  childbearing a.
  chronological a.
  coital a.

conception a.
corrected gestational a. (CGA)
delayed bone a.
developmental a. (DA)
Dubowitz/Ballard Exam for
  Gestational A.
estimated gestational a. (EGA)
estimation of gestational a.
fertilization a.
fetal a. (FA)
functional a.
gestation-adjusted a.
gestational a. (GA)
Greulich and Pyle bone a.
growth-adjusted sonographic a.
  (GASA)
hand-wrist bone a.
a. index
large for gestational a.
  (LGA)
maternal a. (MA)
mean a.
menstrual a. (MA)
mental a. (MA)
ovulatory a.
paternal a.
postconceptional a. (PCA)
postnatal a.
postovulatory a.
premenarchal a.
reproductive a.
small for gestational a.
  (SGA)
weight for a. (WFA)

age-adjusted obesity
agency
child protective a.
lead a.
local education a. (LEA)
protective service a.

Agenerase
agenesia corticalis
agenesis
anorectal a.
bilateral facial a.
bilateral renal a.
callosal a.
caudal a.
cerebellar vermis a.
cervical a.
corpus callosum partial a.
cortical a.
diaphragmatic a.
gonadal a.
hereditary renal a.
lumbosacral a.
müllerian a.
nuclear a.
a. of cerebellar vermis

a. of corpus callosum
a. of corpus callosum-mental
  retardation-osseous lesions
  syndrome
a. of corpus callosum with
  stenogyria
a. of lung
a. of septa pellucida
ovarian a.
pancreatic a.
partial a.
penile a.
pulmonary a.
renal a.
sacral a.
septum pellucidum a.
thymic a.
thyroid and pituitary a.
unilateral a.
unilateral renal a.
uterine a.
vaginal a.

agenitalism
agent
alkylating a.
alpha-adrenergic a.
AngioMark MRI contrast a.
anthelminthic a.
antianxiety a.
anticancer a.
anticholinergic a.
antidysrhythmic a.
antifibrinolytic a.
antifolic a.
antiinflammatory a.
antimicrobial a.
antineoplastic a.
antiplatelet a.
antiprostaglandin a.
antistaphylococcal a.
anxiolytic a.
beta-2 adrenergic a.
beta-adrenergic a.
betamimetic a.
beta-sympathomimetic a.
butenafine antifungal a.
cervical-priming a.
chemotactic a.
chemotherapeutic a.
Combidex MRI contrast a.
cycle-nonspecific a.
cycle-specific a.
cytoprotective a.
cytotoxic a.
delta a.
emetic a.
fertility a.
fibrinolytic a.
Hawaii a.

agent (*continued*)
    hyperosmotic a.
    immunosuppressive a.
    infertility a.
    inotropic a.
    intraluminal a.
    intravaginal a.
    myelosuppressive a.
    neuromuscular blocking a.
    nonalkylating a.
    nondepolarizing paralyzing a.
    Norwalk a.
    A. Orange
    osmotic a.
    pressor a.
    progestational a.
    prokinetic a.
    satumomab pendetide imaging a.
    sclerosing a.
    Snow Mountain a.
    teratogenic a.
    tocolytic a.
    TWAR a.
    uterine contractile a.

age-related
    a.-r. pharmacodynamic response
    a.-r. risk

age-to-dose pattern
agglomeration schedule
agglutination
    a. assay
    febrile antigen a. (FAA)
    a. inhibition
    a. inhibition test
    labial a.
    latex a. (LA)
    latex particle a. (LPA)
    pediatric labial a.
    rickettsial a.

agglutinin
    cold a.
    Lens culinaris a.

aggregated mucopolysaccharide
Aggregate Neurobehavioral Student Health & Education Review System
aggregation
    defective primary platelet a.
    platelet a.

aggression
    inattention-overactivity with a. (IOWA)

aggressive
    a. behavior
    a. conduct disorder
    a. management

aging
    a. gamete
    premature a.

agitated depression

agitation
aglossia-adactylia syndrome
aglossia congenita
aglossostomia
AGM
    absorbent gelling material
agminated lentigo
agnathia
agnogenic myeloid metaplasia (AMM)
agnosia
    auditory a.
    finger a.
    verbal-auditory a. (VAA)
agonadal
agonadism, mental retardation, short stature, retarded bone age syndrome
agonal respirations
agonist
    beta-2 a.
    beta adrenergic a.
    beta-receptor a.
    beta-sympathomimetic a.
    calcium a.
    cholinergic a.
    dopamine receptor a.
    dopaminergic a.
    estrogen a.
    GnRH a. (GNRHa)
    gonadotropin-releasing hormone a. (GnRHa)
    inhaled beta-2 a.
    motilin receptor a.
agoraphobia
agouti protein
AGR
    aniridia, ambiguous genitalia, mental retardation
    AGR syndrome
    AGR triad
agranulocytosis
    congenital a.
    infantile a.
    Kostmann infantile a.
AGS
    adrenogenital syndrome
AGT
    aminoglutethimide
AGU
    aspartylglucosaminuria
AGUS
    atypical glandular cells of undetermined significance
AGVHD
    acute graft-versus-host disease
agyria
agyria-pachygyria
    a.-p. band
    a.-p. cortical dysplasia
    a.-p. syndrome

AH
>abdominal hysterectomy
>adenomatous hyperplasia
>assisted hatching
>>AH antibody
>>AH titer

AHC
>adrenal hypoplasia congenita
>alternating hemiplegia of childhood

AHD
>arteriohepatic dysplasia

AHDS
>Allan-Herndon-Dudley syndrome

AHEI
>acute hemorrhagic edema of
>infancy

AHF
>antihemophilic factor

Ahlfeld sign (I, II)

AHO
>Albright hereditary osteodystrophy

A-hydroCort Injection

AI
>acetabular index
>anal index
>artificial insemination

AIA
>allergen-induced asthma

Aicardi-Goutières syndrome

Aicardi syndrome

aid
>>BD Sensability breast
>>self-examination a.
>>communication a.
>>Compoz Nighttime Sleep A.
>>crawling a.
>>electronic communication a.
>>Foille Medicated First A.
>>hearing a.
>>low vision a.
>>mobility a.
>>Sensability breast self-examination a.
>>Swim-Ear water drying a.
>>A. to Families with Dependent
>>Children (AFDC)
>>vibrotactile hearing a.

AID
>artificial insemination by donor
>artificial insemination donor

AIDP
>acute inflammatory demyelinating
>polyneuropathy

AIDS
>acquired immune deficiency syndrome
>acquired immunodeficiency syndrome
>>AIDS Clinical Trials Group
>>AIDS Clinical Trials Group
>>protocol
>>AIDS dementia complex (ADC)

>>AIDS encephalopathy
>>AIDS gastropathy
>>transfusion-related AIDS (TRAIDS)

AIDS-related
>>AIDS-r. complex (ARC)
>>AIDS-r. lymphoma

AIE
>autoimmune enteropathy

AIF
>antiinflammatory

AIH
>artificial insemination by husband

AIHA
>autoimmune hemolytic anemia

AIM
>area of interest magnification

AIMS
>Abnormal Involuntary Movement Scale
>Alberta Infant Motor Scale

AIN
>anal intraepithelial neoplasia
>autoimmune neutropenia

AIOS
>Acute Illness Observation Scale

AIP
>acute intermittent porphyria

air
>>a. arthrogram
>>a. bronchogram
>>a. embolism
>>a. embolus
>>a. enema
>>a. evacuation
>>extrapulmonary extravasation of a.
>>free peritoneal a.
>>high-efficiency particulate a.
>>(HEPA)
>>humidified a.
>>a. hunger
>>a. leak
>>a. leak syndrome
>>a. leak test
>>a. pollution
>>a. reduction
>>reflux of a.
>>room a. (RA)
>>A. Shields incubator
>>subdiaphragmatic a.
>>a. swallowing
>>a. trapping

airbag injury
airborne allergen
air-contrast barium enema
AIRE
>autoimmune regulator
>>AIRE gene
>>AIRE promoter

Airet
air-filled heart

airflow
    laminar a.
    turbulent a.
air-fluid level
Airlift balloon retractor
AirPacks backpack
airplane glue
Airshields
    A. isolette
    A. jaundice meter
airspace
Airtec ergonomic backpack
airway
    abnormal laxity of upper a.
    a. and cervical spine precautions
    a. branching
    airway, breathing, circulation
      (ABC)
    airway, breathing, circulation,
      disability, exposure (ABCDE)
    a. compromise
    a. conductance
    a. control
    double-lumen a.
    a. epithelium
    extrinsic compression of a.
    a. fluoroscopy
    laryngeal mask a. (LMA)
    a. malformation
    a. management
    a. obstruction
    a. obstruction syndrome
    a. occlusion
    a. opening pressure (P_{ao})
    a. protection
    reactive a.
    a. reactivity testing
    a. resistance (RAW)
    reversible obstructive a.
    a. smooth muscle
    a. suction
    a. transmural pressure
AIS
    adenocarcinoma in situ
    adolescent idiopathic scoliosis
AI 5200 S Open Color Doppler imaging
  system
AIT
    auditory integration thinking
    auditory integration training
AITP
    autoimmune thrombocytopenic purpura
AIUM
    American Institute of Ultrasound in
      Medicine
akari
    Rickettsia a.
Akarpine Ophthalmic
akathisia, acathisia

AK-Con Ophthalmic
akinesia algera
akinesic (*var.* of akinetic)
akinetic, akinesic
    a. mutism
    a. seizure
Akineton
akiyami
AK-Mycin
AK-NaCl
Akne-Mycin
AK-Pentolate
AK-Sulf
ala, *pl.* alae
    nasal a.
    a. nasi
ALA
    alpha lactalbumin
    alpha-linolenic acid
Ala-Cort Topical
alacrima
    a., achalasia, adrenal insufficiency
    a. congenita
Aladdin Infant Flow System
alae (*pl. of* ala)
Alagille
    A. arteriohepatic dysplasia
    A. syndrome
Alagille-Watson syndrome (AWS)
Alajouanine syndrome
Alamast ophthalmic solution
alanine
    a. aminotransferase (ALT)
    a. transaminase (ALT)
alaninuria
ALARA
    as low as reasonably achievable
    ALARA principle
alar flaring
alarm
    Nite Train-r A.
    Sioux a.
Ala-Scalp Topical
Alateen
alba, *pl.* albae
    cutis marmorata a.
    linea a.
    lochia a.
    pityriasis a.
    pneumonia a.
albae (*pl. of* alba)
Albalon Liquifilm Ophthalmic
albendazole
Albers-Schönberg
    A.-S. disease
    A.-S. syndrome
Alberta Infant Motor Scale (AIMS)
Albert Einstein Neonatal Developmental
  Scale (AENNS)

Albert-Smith pessary
albescens
    retinopathy punctata a.
albicans
    Candida a.
albicantes
    lineae a.
Albini nodule
albinism
    cutaneous a.
    Forsius-Eriksson type ocular a.
    generalized a.
    localized a.
    Nettleship-Falls ocular a.
    ocular a. (OA)
    oculocutaneous a. (OCA)
    partial oculocutaneous a.
    tyrosinase-negative oculocutaneous a.
    tyrosinase-positive oculocutaneous a.
albinism-deafness syndrome
albinismus circumscriptus
albipunctatus
    fundus a.
albopapuloid
    a. epidermolysis bullosa variant
    a. Pasini form of dominant
      dystrophic epidermolysis bullosa
Albright
    A. disease
    A. hereditary osteodystrophy (AHO)
    A. syndrome
albuginea
    tunica a.
albumin
    a. gradient
    plasma a.
    serum a.
Albuminar
albumin-bound toxin
albumin-globulin (A/G)
albuminocytologic dissociation
albuminorrhea (*var. of* albuminuria)
albuminuria, albuminorrhea
Albutein
albuterol
    sustained-release a.
Alcaine
Alcaligenes xylosoxidans
ALCAPA
    anomalous left coronary artery from
      pulmonary artery
      ALCAPA syndrome
alcaptonuria, alkaptonuria, alkaptonuria
Alcare formula
alclometasone
Alcock canal
alcohol
    a. abuse
    a. addiction

    a. and other drugs (AOD)
    benzyl a.
    blood a.
    cetyl a.
    ethyl a. (EtOH, ETOH)
    fetal effects of a.
    a. ingestion
    isopropyl a.
    nicotinyl a.
    a. related (AR)
    alcohol, tobacco, and other drugs
      (ATOD)
    A. Use Disorders Identification Test
      (AUDIT)
alcoholic
    children of a. (COA)
    a. embryopathy
    a. tincture
    a. tincture of opium
alcoholism
    maternal a.
alcohol-related neurodevelopmental
  disorder (ARND)
ALD
    adrenoleukodystrophy
Aldactazide
Aldactone
Aldara cream
Alder anomaly
Alder-Reilly anomaly
aldolase
Aldomet
Aldoril
aldosterone
    a. deficiency
    a. excretion rate (AER)
    a. replacement therapy
aldosteronism
    juvenile a.
aldosteronism-normal blood pressure
  syndrome
Aldred syndrome
Aldrich
    hypoganglionic segment of A.
    A. syndrome
Aldridge
    A. rectus fascia sling
    A. tubal ligation
    A. urethral sling procedure
Aldridge-Studdefort urethral suspension
ALEC
    artificial lung-expanding compound
alendronate sodium
alert inactivity
alertness
    quiet a.
    a., response to voice, response to
      pain, unresponsive (AVPU)
    state of a.

Alesse
aleukia
    congenital a.
Aleve
Alexander
    A. anomaly
    A. aplasia
    A. disease
    A. operation
    A. syndrome
    A. unit
Alexander-Adams
    A.-A. hysteropexy
    A.-A. uterine suspension
alexandrite laser
alexithymia
alfa
    alglucosidase a.
    choriogonadotropin a.
    dornase a.
    epoetin a.
    a. interferon
    poractant a.
alfa-2a
    interferon a.-2a
alfa-2b
    interferon a.-2b
alfa-N1
    interferon a.-N1
alfa-N2
    interferon a.-N2
alfa-N3
    interferon a.-N3
alfa-NL
    interferon a.-NL
Alfenta
alfentanil
Alferon N
AL 110 formula
ALFW
    anterolateral free wall
algae
    blue-green a.
algal oil
algera
    akinesia a.
algesimeter (*var. of* algesiometer)
algesiometer, algesimeter, algometer
    vulvar a.
alginate
    calcium a.
    a. wound dressing
AlgiSite dressing
alglucerase
alglucosidase alfa
algodystrophy
algomenorrhea
algometer (*var. of*
  algesiometer)

Algo newborn hearing screener
algorithm
    atypical a.
algorithmic approach
Algosteril dressing
Alice in Wonderland syndrome
alignment
    body a.
    ocular a.
    torsional a.
alimentary
alimentation
    intravenous a.
    parenteral a.
Alimentum
    A. Advance formula
    A. feeding
    A. formula
aliphatic hydrocarbon
aliquot
Alitraq formula
Alkaban-AQ
Alka-Butazolidin
alkalemia
alkalemic
alkali
    a. burn
    a. infusion
    a. therapy
    a. toxicity
alkaline
    a. diuresis
    a. phosphatase (ALP)
    a. reflux
alkalinization
alkaloid
    levorotatory a.
    plant a.
    Veratrum a.
    Vinca a.
alkalosis
    acute respiratory a.
    cerebral lactic a.
    chronic respiratory a.
    diet-induced hypochloremic
      metabolic a.
    hypochloremic metabolic a.
    hypokalemic a.
    maternal respiratory a.
    metabolic a.
    respiratory a.
Alka-Mints
alkaptonuria
Alka-Seltzer Plus Children's Cold
  Medicine
Alkeran
alkylating
    a. agent
    a. chemotherapy

ALL
    acute lymphoblastic leukemia
    acute lymphocytic leukemia
**Allan-Herndon-Dudley syndrome
(AHDS)**
Allan-Herndon syndrome
allantoic
    a. artery
    a. cyst
    a. duct
    a. sac
    a. stalk
allantoidoangiopagus
allantois
Allegra
Allegra-D
allele
    fixed a.
    a. frequency
    multiple a.'s
    mutant a.
    papG a.
    premutation a.
    recessive a.
    silent a.
    a. specific associated primer
    a. specific oligo
    wild-type a.
    Z a.
allele-specific
    a.-s. oligonucleotide
      hybridization
    a.-s. PCR
allelic
    a. exclusion
    a. gene
    a. heterogeneity
allelism
Allemann syndrome
Allen
    A. and Capute neonatal
      neurodevelopmental examination
    A. chart
    A. fetal stethoscope
    A. Kindergarten Picture Card
    A. laparoscopic stirrups
    A. picture test
Allen-Doisy test
Allen-Masters syndrome
Allerest
    A. Children's Tablets
    A. Headache Strength
    A. Maximum Strength
allergen
    airborne a.
    contact a.
    food a.
    a. immunotherapy
allergenic

allergen-induced asthma (AIA)
allergic
    a. anlage
    a. bowel disease
    a. bronchopulmonary aspergillosis
      (ABPA)
    a. colitis
    a. conjunctivitis
    a. contact dermatitis
    a. coryza
    a. crease
    a. diaper rash
    a. encephalitis
    a. encephalomyelitis
    a. enterocolitis
    a. eosinophilic gastroenteritis
    a. esophagitis
    a. gape
    a. gastroenteropathy
    a. inflammatory response
    a. polyp
    a. rhinitis
    a. rhinitis perennial
    a. rhinoconjunctivitis
    a. salute
    a. shiner
    a. sinusitis
    a. triad
    a. vulvitis
allergy
    barley a.
    cow's milk a. (CMA)
    cow's milk protein a.
    fire ant a.
    gluten a.
    honeybee a.
    latex a.
    milk a.
    milk-protein a.
    milk/soy-protein a.
    non-IgE-mediated food a.
    pollen a.
    soy-protein a.
    sperm a.
    stinging insect a.
    a. treatment
    vespid a.
    wasp a.
    yellow jacket a.
AllerMax Oral
Allerphed
Allevyn dressing
all-fours
    a.-f. maneuver
    a.-f. maneuver for shoulder
      dystocia
Allgrove syndrome
alliance
    Sudden Infant Death Syndrome A.

alligator
> a. forceps
> a. skin

Allis
> A. clamp
> A. forceps

Allis-Abramson
> A.-A. breast biopsy
> A.-A. breast biopsy forceps

alloantibody
alloantigen
allodiploid
allodynia
alloenzyme
allogeneic (*var. of* allogenic)
allogenic, allogeneic
> a. antigen
> a. BMT
> a. bone marrow transplantation
> a. disease
> a. fetal graft
> a. stem cell transplantation

allogenicity
allograft
> composite a.
> cryopreserved valved a.
> dura mater a.
> fascia lata a.
> a. membrane
> a. rejection
> a. survival

alloimmune
> a. disease
> a. factor
> a. mechanism
> a. neonatal neutropenia
>   (ANN)
> a. neonatal thrombocytopenic
>   purpura
> a. thrombocytopenia

alloimmunity
alloimmunization
> antepartum a.
> Kell a.

alloimmunize
Alloiococcus otitis
alloisoleucine
alloploidy
allopolyploidy
allopurinol
all-or-none phenomenon
allosome
> paired a.

allosyndesis
allotetraploidy
allothreonine
allotropism, allotropy
allotropy (*var. of* allotropism)
allotype

allowance
> recommended daily a. (RDA)
> recommended dietary a. (RDA)

allozygote
Allport retractor
all-progestin contraceptive
all-*trans*-retinoic acid
allylamine
ALMN
> adrenoleukomyeloneuropathy

Almora
alobar holoprosencephaly
Alocril
Aloka
> A. 650 CL ultrasound
> A. OB/GYN ultrasound
> A. 650 scanner
> A. SD ultrasound system
> A. SSD-720 real-time scanner

Alomide
alopecia
> a. adnata
> androgenic a.
> a., anosmia, deafness, hypogonadism
>   (AADH)
> a. areata
> cicatricial a.
> a. congenitalis
> a., contracture, dwarfism (ACD)
> generalized a.
> a. hereditaria
> marginal a.
> pyoderma a.
> secondary a.
> a. totalis congenita
> toxic a.
> traction a.
> traumatic a.
> a. universalis
> a. universalis totalis
> a. universalis with mental
>   retardation

alopecia-mental retardation (AMR)
Alora
> A. Transdermal
> A. transdermal patch

ALP
> alkaline phosphatase
> bone ALP

AlPase
> alkaline phosphatase

Alpern-Boll Developmental Profile
Alpers
> A. disease
> A. syndrome

alpha, α
> a. adrenergic
> a. antitrypsin level
> Curosurf poractant a.

a. error
estrogen receptor a. (Er alpha)
F2 a.
follitropin a.
a. helix
interferon a.
interstitial positive-pressure interferon
a.
A. Keri soap
a. lactalbumin (ALA)
macrophage inflammatory protein-1
a. (MIP-1 alpha)
a. particle
prostaglandin F2 a.
a. Proteobacteria
recombinant human MIP-1 a.
a. thalassemia
transforming growth factor a. (TGF
alpha)
tumor necrosis factor a.
alpha-1
a.-1 antitrypsin
a.-1 antitrypsin deficiency
a.-1 PI
a.-1 protease inhibitor
a.-1 proteinase inhibitor (A1PI)
a.-1 thymosin product
alpha-2
a.-2 antiplasmin
a.-2 antiplasmin coagulation inhibitor
a.-2 antiplasmin level
a.-2 antitrypsin inhibitor
a.-2 macroglobulin
a.-2 macroglobulin coagulation
inhibitor
alpha-2a
interferon a.-2a
17-alpha-acetoxyprogesterone derivative
alpha-adrenergic
a.-a. agent
a.-a. blocker
a.-a. receptor
a.-a. stimulator
alpha-aminoadipic
a.-a. acid
a.-a. aciduria
3-alpha-androstanediol glucuronide
alpha-antilysin deficiency
alpha-1-antitrypsin disease
alpha-2AP coagulation inhibitor
alpha-2AT coagulation inhibitor
alpha-2b
interferon a.-2b
alphabet
manual a.
alpha-chain disorder
alpha-chemokine receptor
Alphaderm
5-alpha-dihydroprogesterone

17-alpha-ethinyl testosterone
alpha-fetoprotein (aFP, AFP)
amniotic fluid a.-f.
a.-f. elevation
a.-f. enzyme immunoassay (AFP-EIA)
maternal serum a.-f.
alpha-glucosidase
a.-g. deficiency
a.-g. inhibitor
alpha-granule
giant platelet a.-g.
17-alpha-hydroxypregnenolone
17-alpha-hydroxyprogesterone
alpha-ketoadipic
a.-k. acid
a.-k. aciduria
alpha-L-fucosidase (FUCA)
alpha-L-iduronidase (IDA, IDUA)
alpha-linolenic acid (ALA)
alpha-lipoprotein deficiency
alpha-mannosidosis (type I, II)
alpha-2M coagulation inhibitor
**alpha-melanocyte-stimulating hormone
(alpha-MSH)**
alpha-melanotrophin
**alpha-methylcrotonyl-coenzyme A
carboxylase**
alpha-methyl-para-tyrosine (AMPT)
alpha-methyl-*p*-tyrosine
alpha-MSH
alpha-melanocyte-stimulating hormone
alpha-N-acetylgalactosaminidase deficiency
Alphanate
AlphaNine SD
alphaprodine
alpha-recombinant interferon
5-alpha reductase
alpha-reductase deficiency
Alpha-Tamoxifen
alpha-thalassemia
alpha-thalassemia/mental
a.-t/m. retardation
a.-t/m. retardation syndrome, deletion
type
a.-t/m. retardation syndrome,
nondeletion type
alpha-tocopherol concentration
Alphatrex Topical
alphavirus
Alport
A. syndrome
A. syndrome-like nephritis
ALPP
abdominal leak point pressure
alprazolam
alprostadil
ALPS
autoimmune lymphoproliferative
syndrome

ALRI
 acute lower respiratory infection
ALRTI
 acute lower respiratory tract
 infection
ALS
 advanced life support
 amyotrophic lateral sclerosis
Alsoy 1, 2 formula
Alström
 A. sign
 A. syndrome
Alström-Hallgren syndrome
ALT
 alanine aminotransferase
 alanine transaminase
ALTE
 acute life-threatening event
 apparent life-threatening event
Altemeier
 A. operation
 A. perineal rectal pullthrough
 procedure
 A. perineal rectosigmoidectomy
alteration
 a. of lipoprotein metabolism
 uterine activity a.
altered
 a. gastric motility
 a. sensorium
 a. state of consciousness
alternans
 electrical a.
 pulsus a.
 strabismus convergens a.
Alternaria
alternate-cover test
alternating
 a. breath test (ABT)
 a. hemiplegia
 a. hemiplegia of childhood
 (AHC)
alternative
 a. birthing position
 a. communication device
 a. hypothesis
 a. pathway defect
 a. reproductive option
 a. system
 a. therapy
Alteromonas putrefaciens
altretamine
altruism
Aludrine
aluminum
 a. acetate
 a. acetate solution
 a. chloride
 a. hydroxide

 a. intoxication
 a. toxicity
Alupent
Alurate
alveolar (A)
 arterial to a. (a-A)
 a. capillary dysplasia
 a. consolidation
 a. cyst
 a. development
 a. echinococcosis
 a. fibrinous exudate
 a. hydatidosis
 a. hypoxia
 a. lavage
 a. lumen of breast
 a. lymphangioma
 a. myofibroblast differentiation
 a. notch
 a. osteitis
 a. partial pressure (PA)
 a. period
 a. proteinosis
 a. recruitment
 a. ridge
 a. RMS
 a. saccule formation
 a. sarcoid
 a. soft part sarcoma
 a. stage
 a. stage of lung development
 a. ventilation
alveolar-arterial (A-a)
 a.-a. oxygen diffusing capacity
 a.-a. oxygen gradient
 a.-a. pressure gradient
alveoli (*pl. of* alveolus)
alveolitis
 cryptogenic fibrosing a.
 extrinsic alveolar a.
alveolization
 abrogated neonatal a.
alveolus, *pl.* **alveoli**
 functional a.
 pulmonary a.
alymphocytosis
alymphoplasia
 thymic a.
Alzate catheter
Alzheimer
 A. disease
AM
 anovular menstruation
AMA
 advanced maternal age
amalonaticus
 Citrobacter a.
AMAN
 acute motor-axonal neuropathy

Amanita
    A. *mushroom*
    A. *phalloides*
amantadine
amastia
amaurosis
    a. congenita
    a. fugax
    Leber congenital a. (LCA)
    Leber congenital retinal a.
    recessive Leber congenital a.
amaurotic familial idiocy (AFI)
amazia
Amazon thorax
AmB
    amphotericin B
AmBd
    amphotericin B deoxycholate
ambenonium
Ambien
ambient
    a. light
    a. oxygen concentration
    a. sound
    a. temperature
ambiguity
    frank a.
    genital a.
    sexual a.
ambiguous
    a. external genitalia
    a. reference
ambiguus
    situs a.
AmBisome
amblyogenic stimulus
Amblyomma americanum
amblyopia
    ametropic a.
    anisometropic a.
    deprivation a.
    disuse a.
    image-degradation a.
    isoametropic a.
    occlusion a.
    strabismic a.
    transient a.
amblyopic eye
amboceptor
ambosexual area
Ambras syndrome
Ambu
    A. bag
    A. infant resuscitator
    A. respirator
ambulate
ambulation
ambulatory
    a. antibiotic treatment

    a. anticoagulation
    a. anticoagulation therapy
    a. blood pressure (ABP)
    a. blood pressure monitoring
    (ABPM)
    a. monitoring
    a. obstetric care
    a. obstetrics
    a. polysomnography
    a. testing
    a. urodynamic monitoring (AUM)
    a. uterine contraction test
AMC
    arthrogryposis multiplex congenita
    ataxia-microcephaly-cataract
    AMC syndrome
Amcill
amcinonide
AMD
    acid maltase deficiency
AME
    apparent mineralocorticoid excess
    congenital AME
amebiasis
    cerebral a.
    hepatic a.
amebic
    a. colitis
    a. dysentery
    a. hepatic abscess
    a. liver abscess
    a. meningoencephalitis
    a. vaginitis
amelia
    upper limb a.
ameliorate
amelioration
ameloblastoma
amelogenesis imperfecta
ameloonychohypohidrotic syndrome
amenia
amenorrhea
    athletic a.
    ballet dancer's secondary a.
    dietary a.
    emotional a.
    eugonadal a.
    eugonadotropic a.
    exercise-induced a.
    hypergonadotropic a.
    hyperprolactinemic a.
    hypogonadotropic a.
    hypophysial a.
    hypothalamic a.
    hypothalamic-pituitary a.
    jogger's a.
    lactation a.
    ovarian a.
    pathologic a.

amenorrhea (*continued*)
    physiologic a.
    postmenopausal a.
    postpartum a.
    postpill a.
    primary a.
    secondary a.
    traumatic a.
amenorrhea-galactorrhea syndrome
amenorrheal, amenorrheic
    a. patient
    a. woman
amenorrheic (*var. of* amenorrheal)
amentia
    nevoid a.
Amerge
America
    Human Milk Banking Association of North A.
    Pharmaceutical Research and Manufacturers of A.
    Pharmaceutical Research and Manufacturers of A. (PhRMA)
Americaine
American
    A. Academy of Child and Adolescent Psychiatry (AACAP)
    A. Academy of Pediatrics (AAP)
    A. Association for the Surgery of Trauma (AAST)
    A. Association of Gynecologic Laparoscopists
    A. Association of Poison Control Centers (AAPCC)
    A. Association on Mental Deficiency (AAMD)
    A. Association on Mental Retardation (AAMR)
    A. Board of Obstetrics and Gynecology
    A. Board of Pediatrics
    A. Burkitt lymphoma
    A. Cancer Society (ACS)
    A. Cancer Society procedure
    A. College of Nurse Midwives
    A. College of Obstetricians and Gynecologists (ACOG)
    A. College of Obstetrics Gynecology network
    A. College of Radiology (ACR)
    A. College of Surgeons (ACS)
    A. Diabetes Association (ADA)
    A. Diabetes Association diet
    A. Fertility Society (AFS)
    A. Fertility Society Revised Classification of Endometriosis
    A. Foundation for Urologic Diseases (AFUD)
    A. Foundation of Urologic Disease Consensus Panel
    A. Foundation of Urologic Diseases classification
    A. Institute of Ultrasound in Medicine (AIUM)
    A. Medical staging system
    A. Medical Systems (AMS)
    A. Medical Women's Association
    A. Pediatric Society/Society for Pediatric Research
    A. Sign Language (Ameslan, ASL)
    A. Sleep Disorders Association (ASDA)
    A. Society for Colposcopy and Cervical Pathology (ASCCP)
    A. Society for Parenteral and Enteral Nutrition (ASPEN)
    A. Society for Reproductive Medicine
    A. Society of Anesthesiologists (ASA)
    A. Society of Anesthesiologists classification
    A. Society of Clinical Oncology (ASCO)
    A. Society of Hematology (ASH)
    A. trypanosomiasis
    A. Urogynecologic Society
    A.'s with Disabilities Act (ADA)
americanum
    Amblyomma a.
americanus
    Ancylostoma a.
    Necator a.
Ameslan
    American Sign Language
A-methaPred Injection
amethocaine gel
amethopterin
Ametop gel
ametria
ametropic amblyopia
AMF
    autocrine motility factor
AMH
    antimüllerian hormone
AMI
    acute myocardial infarction
    amitriptyline
    non-Q-wave AMI
Amicar
amicrobic pyuria
Amiel-Tison test
amifostine
amikacin sulfate
Amikin
amiloride

amine
- a. odor
- primary a.
- secondary a.
- sympathomimetic a.
- tertiary a.
- a. test

Amines test card

amino
- a. acid
- a. acid analyzer
- a. acid chromatography
- a. acid metabolism
- a. acid screening
- a. acid transport defect

aminoacetic analog
aminoacidemia
aminoacidopathy
aminoaciduria
- dibasic a.
- generalized a.
- renal a.

aminocaproic acid
Amino-Cerv pH 5.5 cervical cream
aminoglutethimide (AGT)
aminoglycoside
- antimicrobial a.
- a. nephrotoxicity

aminogram
- plasma a.

aminoguanidine
Amino-Opti-E
aminopenicillin
aminopeptidase
- leucine a.

aminophospholipid
Aminophyllin
aminophylline
aminopterin
- a. embryopathy syndrome
- a. syndrome sine aminopterin (ASSA)

aminopterin-like embryopathy syndrome
aminopyrine
5-aminosalicylic acid
Aminosyn-PF supplement
amino-terminal peptide
aminotransferase
- alanine a. (ALT)
- aspartate a. (AST)
- branched chain a.
- serum a.
- tyrosine a. (TAT)

amiodarone
Amipaque
AMIS
- antibody-mediated immune suppression

Amish brittle hair syndrome
amisulpride

Amitid
Amitone
Amitril
amitriptyline
AML
- acute myeloblastic leukemia
- acute myelogenous leukemia
- acute myeloid leukemia

AMLA
- antimyolemmal antibody

AMM
- agnogenic myeloid metaplasia

Ammon
- A. fissure
- A. horn sclerosis

ammonemia, ammoniemia, hyperammonemia
ammonia
- a. metabolism
- plasma a.
- serum a.

ammoniac
ammoniemia (var. of ammonemia)
ammonium
- a. bromide
- a. chloride
- a. lactate

AMN
- acquired melanocytic nevus
- adrenomyeloneuropathy

amnesia
- hysteric a.
- posttraumatic a.
- retrograde a.

amnesic, amnestic
- a. response
- a. shellfish poisoning

amnestic (var. of amnesic)
amnii
- liquor a.

amniocentesis
- early a. (EA)
- genetic a.
- second-trimester a.

amniochorion
amniocyte
amniogenesis
amniogenic cell
amniogram
amniography in hydatidiform mole
Amniohook
amnioinfusion
- a. therapy
- transabdominal a.

amnioma
amnion
- inner a.
- a. nodosum
- a. ring

amnion (*continued*)
    a. rupture
    squamous metaplasia of a.
amnion-chorion separation
amnionic (*var. of* amniotic)
amnionicity
amnionitis
    silent a.
amniopatch
amnioreduction
amniorrhea
amniorrhexis
amnioscope
amnioscopy
AmnioStat-FLM
    A.-FLM maturity screening
    A.-FLM screening test
amniotic, amnionic
    a. adhesion
    a. band anomalad
    a. band disruption sequence
    a. band limb amputation
    a. band syndrome
    a. caruncle
    a. cavity
    a. constriction band
    a. debris
    a. fluid (AF)
    a. fluid alpha-fetoprotein (AFAFP)
    a. fluid aspiration
    a. fluid assessment
    a. fluid bilirubin
    a. fluid cell culture
    a. fluid embolism (AFE)
    a. fluid embolism syndrome
    a. fluid embolus
    a. fluid embolus syndrome
    a. fluid fluorescence polarization
    a. fluid index (AFI)
    a. fluid infection
    a. fluid level
    a. fluid liquor
    a. fluid pocket
    a. fluid pool
    a. fluid quantitation
    a. fluid supernatant
    a. fluid volume (AFV)
    a. fluid volume disorder
    a. fluid white blood cell count
    a. infection syndrome (AIS)
    a. infection syndrome of Blane
    a. membrane
    a. sheet
amniotic-chorionic surface
amniotome
    Baylor a.
amniotomy plus oxytocin method
AmniSure test

amobarbital
A-mode
    A-m. echocardiography
    A-m. ultrasound
amorphous
    a. breast calcification
    a. fetus
    a. inspissation
amorphus
    fetus a.
amotio placentae
amotivational syndrome
amoxapine
amoxicillin
amoxicillin-clavulanate treatment
amoxicillin-clavulanic acid
Amoxil
AMP
    adenosine monophosphate
    assisted medical procreation
AmpErase electrocautery
amphetamine
    a. aspartate
    a. sulfate
amphidiploidy
amphigonous inheritance
amphimixis
Amphojel
Amphotec
amphotericin, amphotericin B
    a. B
    a. B cholesteryl sulfate complex
    a. B deoxycholate (AmBd)
    a. B lipid complex
ampicillin
    a. and sulbactam
    a. rash
    a. resistant
    a. sodium/sulbactam sodium
    a. trihydrate
ampicillin-resistant Escherichia coli
ampicillin/sulbactam
Ampicin
Amplatz catheter
Amplatzer
    A. device
    A. septal occluder
Amplicor
    A. Chlamydia assay
    A. HBV monitor test
    A. HIV-1 test kit
    A. PCR diagnostics
    A. PCR kit
    A. typing kit
amplification
    DNA a.
    gene a.
    nucleic acid a. (NAA)

nucleic acid sequence-based a.
(NASBA)
transcription-mediated a. (TMA)
Y-specific DNA a.
amplified fragment length polymorphism
AmpliTaq DNA polymerase FS
amplitude
oscillation a.
amplitude-integrated
a.-i. EEG
a.-i. electroencephalogram (aEEG)
amprenavir
AMPT
alpha-methyl-para-tyrosine
ampulla, *pl.* **ampullae**
a. of oviduct
a. of Vater
ampullae (*pl. of* ampulla)
ampullar
a. abortion
a. pregnancy
amputation
amniotic band limb a.
birth a.
cervical a.
congenital a.
intrauterine a.
Jaboulay a.
spontaneous a.
Syme a.
traumatic a.
AMR
alopecia-mental retardation
AMR syndrome
Amreich vaginal extirpation
amrinone lactate
AMS
ablepharon-macrostomia syndrome
acute mountain sickness
American Medical Systems
AMS Apogee vault suspension
AMS 800 artificial urethral
sphincter
amsacrine
AMSAN
acute motor-sensory axonal neuropathy
Amsel criteria
amstelodamensis
typus degenerativus a.
Amsterdam
A. Depression List (ADL)
A. dwarfism
A. infant ventilator
A. type
amyelencephalia
amyelencephalic, amyelencephalous
amyelencephalous (*var. of* amyelencephalic)

amyelia
amyeloic (*var. of* amyelous)
amyeloid leukemia
amyelous, amyeloic
amygdala, *pl.* **amygdalae**
amygdalae (*pl. of* amygdala)
amygdalin
amygdalohippocampectomy
Amyl
A. Nitrate Vaporole
A. Nitrite Aspirols
amylase
human pancreatic a. (HPA)
salivary a.
serum a.
amylobarbitone
amyloidosis
paraneoplastic a.
secondary a.
amylopectinosis
branching enzyme deficiency a.
amylophagia
amyopathic
a. JDM
a. juvenile dermatomyositis
amyoplasia
bimelic a.
a. congenita
oculomelic a.
segmental a.
amyotonia congenita
amyotrophia (*var. of* amyotrophy)
amyotrophic
a. lateral sclerosis (ALS)
a. lateral sclerosis-Parkinson-dementia
complex
amyotrophy, amyotrophia
Amytal
A/N
Pen A/N
AN
acne neonatorum
anorexia nervosa
ANA
antinuclear antibody
ANA seropositive
anabolic androgenic steroid
Anabolin
anabolism
anacatadidymus, anakatadidymus
Anacin
anaclitic
a. depression
a. depression of infancy
anadidymus
anadysplasia
metaphysial a.
anaemicus (*var. of* anemicus)
anaerobe

anaerobic, anaerobiotic
- a. bacteria
- a. cellulitis
- a. environment
- a. glycolysis
- a. streptococcus
- a. vaginosis

anaerobiotic (*var. of* anaerobic)
anaerobius
- *Peptococcus a.*

Anafranil
anagen effluvium
anagenesis
anakatadidymus (*var. of* anacatadidymus)
Ana-Kit
anal
- a. atresia
- a. canal
- a. cancer
- a. condyloma
- a. dimple
- a. EMG PerryMeter sensor
- a. fissure
- a. incontinence
- a. index (AI)
- a. intercourse
- a. intraepithelial neoplasia (AIN)
- a. manometry
- a. margin
- a. Pap smear
- a. penetration
- a. pruritus
- a. sphincter
- a. sphincter cinedefecography
- a. sphincter disruption
- a. sphincter dysplasia
- a. sphincter electromyography
- a. sphincter laceration
- a. sphincter oscillation
- a. sphincter paralysis
- a. sphincter tone
- a. squamous intraepithelial lesion (ASIL)
- a. stenosis
- a. thrombosis
- a. verge
- a. wink
- a. wink reflex

analbuminemic patient
anal-ear-renal-radial malfunction syndrome
analeptic
analgesia
- caudal a.
- conduction a.
- congenital a.
- continuous epidural a.
- epidural a.
- labor a.

narcotic a.
obstetric a.
patient-controlled a. (PCA)
peridural a.
perineal a.
procedural sedation and a. (PSA)
regional a.
segmental epidural a.
spinal a.
subarachnoid a.

analgesic, analgetic
narcotic a.

analgesic-rebound headache
analgetic (*var. of* analgesic)
analog (*var. of* analogue)
- aminoacetic a.
- gonadotropin-releasing hormone a. (GnRHa)
- LH-RH a.
- luteinizing hormone-releasing hormone a.
- nucleoside a.
- oxytocin a.
- prostaglandin E a.
- tetracycline a.
- vasopressin a.

analogue, analog
analyses (*pl. of* analysis)
analysis (anal.), *pl.* **analyses**
- acylcarnitine a.
- applied behavior a. (ABA)
- aqueous a.
- automated multiple a.
- base sequence a.
- bioelectrical impedance a. (BIA)
- bioimpedance a.
- blood chromosome a.
- blood component a.
- blood gas a.
- bulked segregant a.
- capillary electrophoresis/frontal a. (CE/FA)
- cell block a.
- chorionic villus haplotype a.
- chromosomal a.
- chromosome a.
- clinicopathological a.
- computer-assisted semen a. (CASA)
- cytogenetic a.
- cytologic a.
- deoxyribonucleic acid a.
- DNA a.
- endonuclease a.
- fat a.
- fetal chromosome a.
- FISH a.
- flow cytometric a.
- fluorescence depolarization a.
- fragile X a.

genetic bit a.
genetic linkage a.
hair cotinine a.
heart rate power spectral a. (HRSA)
heteroduplex a.
induced sputum a. (ISA)
karyotype a.
latent class a. (LCA)
linkage a.
M-mode a.
molecular genetic a.
oligonucleotide probe a.
pedigree a.
photometric a.
pleural fluid a.
postoperative symptom a.
power spectral a. (PSA)
prenatal cytogenetic a.
restriction endonuclease a.
RFLP a.
risk-benefit a.
saturation a.
semen a.
seminal fluid a. (SFA)
sequential multiple a. (SMA)
spectophotometrical a.
spectral power a.
synovial fluid a.
toxicologic a.
transgenerational a.
Trauma Score and Injury Severity Score A.
white blood cell lysosomal enzyme a.

analyte
serum a.

analyzer, analyzor
amino acid a.
AVL 9110 pH a.
Bayer DCA2000 a.
BiliChek bilirubin a.
BiliChek noninvasive bilirubin a.
Clinitek 50 urine chemistry a.
Cobas fast centrifugal a.
computer-assisted semen a. (CASA)
cooximeter a.
CO-Stat end tidal breath a.
Coulter Channelyzer cell a.
Elecsys 1010 a.
HemoCue blood glucose a.
HemoCue blood hemoglobin a.
LeadCare handheld blood lead a.
multichannel discrete a. (MDA)
NE-8000 a.
Osteomeasure computer-assisted image a.
Serono SR1 FSH a.
Sonoclot coagulation a.

SRI automated immunoassay a.
STA a.

analyzor (*var. of* analyzer)
AnaMantle HC cream
anamnestic immune response
Anandron
ANA-negative lupus
anaphase
a. I, II
a. lag
anaphylactic
a. purpura
a. reaction
a. shock
anaphylactoid
a. purpura
a. reaction
a. shock
a. syndrome of pregnancy
anaphylatoxin, anaphylotoxin
anaphylaxis
acute a.
biphasic a.
cold a.
drug-related a.
gastrointestinal a.
recurrent a.
spontaneous a.
anaphylotoxin (*var. of* anaphylatoxin)
anaplasia
anaplasma phagocytophilia
anaplastic
a. carcinoma
a. large cell lymphoma
a. oligodendroglioma
a. pathology
a. pilocytic astrocytoma
Anaprox-DS
anarthria
anasarca
fetal a.
fetoplacental a.
anaspadias
Anaspaz
anastomoses (*pl. of* anastomosis)
anastomosis, *pl.* **anastomoses**
arteriovenous a.
bidirectional Glenn a.
circular end-to-end a. (CEEA)
Clado a.
colorectal a.
cornual a.
Damus-Kaye-Stansel a.
descending aorta a.
end-to-side a. (ESA)
esophageal a.
extended end-to-end a.
extracardiac conduit cavopulmonary a.

anastomosis (*continued*)
    gastrointestinal a. (GIA)
    Glenn a.
    ileal pouch-anal a. (IPAA)
    ileoanal a. (IAA)
    ileoileal a.
    intrarenal a.
    intrauterine laser ablation of
      vascular anastomoses
    jejunojejunal a.
    LAT cavopulmonary a.
    microsurgical tubocornual a.
    onlay patch a.
    placental vascular a.
    primary a.
    Roux-en-Y a.
    side-to-end a.
    staple a.
    total cavopulmonary a.
    tubocornual a.
    ureterotubal a.
    ureteroureteral a.
    Waterston aortopulmonary a.
anastrozole
anatomic, anatomical
    a. asplenia
    a. conjugate
    a. profile (AP)
    a. shunt
    a. support defect
anatomical (*var. of* anatomic)
anatomy
    fetal intracranial a.
    immune system a.
    intracranial a.
    pelvic a.
Anavar
Anbesol Maximum Strength
AN-BP
    anorexia nervosa with binging and
      purging
ANCA
    antineutrophil cytoplasmic antibody
    ANCA titer
Ancef
ancestor
    leading a.
anchor
    bone a.
    Mainstay urologic soft tissue a.
    Mitex GII mini a.
    press-in bone a.
anchoring
    a. fibril
    a. villus
Ancobon
Ancotil
Ancylostoma, Ankylostoma
    A. americanus

    A. braziliense
    A. caninum
    A. ceylanicum
    A. duodenale
ancylostomiasis
AND
    axillary node dissection
Andermann syndrome
Andernach ossicle
Andersen
    A. deficiency
    A. disease
    A. syndrome
Anderson-Fabry disease
andersoni
    Dermacentor a.
ANDI
    aberration of normal development and
      involution
Andogsky syndrome
Andrews infant laryngoscope
androblastoma
Androcur Depot
Andro-Cyp
Androderm Transdermal System
Andro/Fem
androgen
    adrenal a.
    a. antagonist
    a. assay
    attenuated a.
    a. binding
    a. dynamics
    excess a.
    a. excess
    a. excess disorder
    a. insensitivity
    a. insensitivity syndrome
    a. interaction
    a. metabolism
    a. receptor
    a. replacement therapy
    a. resistance
    a. resistance syndrome
    a. secretion
    a. synthesis defect
androgen-dependent carcinoma
androgenesis
androgenic
    a. alopecia
    a. steroid
androgenicity
androgenized woman
androgenous
androgen-producing
    a.-p. adrenal tumor
    a.-p. ovarian tumor
    a.-p. tumor
androgynism

androgynous
androgyny
android
  a. obesity
  a. pattern
  a. pelvis
Android-F
andrology
Androlone 50
Androlone-D
Andronate
Andropository-200
androstane
androstenediol
androstenedione (A$_4$)
androsterone glucuronide
Androvite
anechoic
  a. space
  a. tissue
anectasis
Anectine Chloride
anejaculation
anembryonic
  a. gestation
  a. pregnancy
anemia
  acquired hemolytic a.
  addisonian pernicious a.
  angiopathic hemolytic a.
  anti-Kell a.
  aplastic a.
  aregenerative a.
  autoimmune acquired hemolytic a.
  autoimmune hemolytic a. (AIHA)
  Benjamin a.
  Blackfan-Diamond a.
  blood-loss a.
  B$_6$-responsive a.
  cardiac hemolytic a.
  chronic nonspherocytic hemolytic a.
  congenital aplastic a.
  congenital dyserythropoietic a.
   (CDA)
  congenital Heinz body a.
  congenital hypoplastic a. (CHA)
  congenital nonregenerative a.
  congenital nonspherocytic
   hemolytic a.
  congenital pernicious a.
  congenital sideroblastic a.
  Cooley a.
  Coombs-negative autoimmune
   hemolytic a.
  Coombs-positive isoimmune
   hemolytic a.
  copper deficiency a.
  crescent cell a.
  Czerny a.

Diamond-Blackfan a. (DBA)
Diamond-Blackfan congenital
  hypoplastic a.
Diamond-Blackfan juvenile
  pernicious a.
dilutional a.
drug-induced hemolytic a.
elliptocytic a.
erythroblastic a.
familial erythroblastic a. (FEA)
Fanconi a. (FA)
Fanconi aplastic a.
fetal a.
folate-deficiency a.
functional a.
globe cell a.
Heinz body hemolytic a.
hemolytic a.
hereditary hemolytic a.
hereditary nonspherocytic a.
Herrick a.
homozygous sickle cell a.
hypochromic microcytic a.
hypoplastic a.
hypoproliferative a.
iatrogenic a.
idiopathic acquired sideroblastic a.
  (IASA)
iron deficiency a. (IDA)
isoimmune a.
Jaksch a.
juvenile pernicious a.
Larzel a.
macrocytic megaloblastic a.
Mediterranean a.
megaloblastic a.
microangiopathic hemolytic a.
microcytic a.
mild a.
mitochondrial myopathy and
  sideroblastic a. (MLASA)
mixed iron and folate deficiency a.
myopathy, lactic acidosis,
  sideroblastic a.
neonatal isoimmune hemolytic a.
a. neonatorum
nonspherocytic a.
normochromic a.
normocytic a.
a. of CRF
a. of prematurity
ovalocytary a.
pernicious a. (PA)
PGK hereditary nonspherocytic a.
physiologic a.
posthepatic aplastic a.
pregnancy-associated hypoplastic a.
a. pseudoleukemica infantum
pyridoxine-refractory sideroblastic a.

anemia (*continued*)
    pyridoxine-responsive a.
    refractory dyserythropoietic a.
    Runeberg a.
    schistocytic hemolytic a.
    severe megaloblastic a.
    sickle cell a.
    sideroblastic a.
    a. syndrome
    thiamin-response sideroblastic a.
    von Jaksch a.
    X-linked pyridoxine-responsive
      sideroblastic a.
anemic effect
anemicus, anaemicus
    nevus a.
anencephalia (*var. of* anencephaly)
anencephalic, anencephalous
anencephalous (*var. of* anencephalic)
anencephaly, anencephalia
anergy
aneroid sphygmomanometer
Anestacon Topical Solution
anesthesia
    a. bag
    caudal a.
    conduction a.
    CSE a.
    epidural a.
    extradural a.
    general endotracheal a.
    hypotensive a.
    inhalation a.
    local a.
    lumbar epidural a. (LEA)
    mask inhalation a.
    maternal a.
    neuraxial a.
    nonpharmacologic a.
    obstetric a.
    office laparoscopy under local a.
      (OLULA)
    paracervical a.
    peridural a.
    perineal a.
    pudendal a.
    regional block a.
    saddle block a.
    spinal a.
    systemic a.
anesthesia-related maternal mortality
anesthesiologist
    American Society of A.'s (ASA)
    pediatric a.
anesthetic
    eutectic mixture of local a.'s
      (EMLA)
    gas a.
    a. gas exposure

    local a.
    a. skin lesion
    volatile a.
    walking epidural a.
anesthetist
    certified registered nurse a. (CRNA)
anestrous
anetoderma of prematurity
aneugamy
aneuploid abortion
aneuploidy
    atypical a.
    fetal a.
    a. infant
    mosaic a.
    Pallister mosaic a.
    recurrent a.
    segmental a.
    X chromosome a.
    XXXXY a.
aneurysm
    aortic a.
    arterial a.
    berry a.
    cerebral artery a.
    circle of Willis a.
    cirsoid a.
    CNS a.
    congenital cerebral a.
    coronary a.
    coronary artery a. (CAA)
    dissecting aortic a.
    fusiform a.
    giant coronary artery a.
    intracerebral a.
    intracranial arterial a.
    intrauterine cirsoid a.
    left ventricular apical a.
    mycotic a.
    a. of vein of Galen
    ruptured cerebral a.
    ruptured sinus of Valsalva a.
    saccular a.
    splenic artery a.
    vein of Galen a.
    ventricular a.
aneurysmal bone cyst
AneuVysion Assay prenatal genetic test
Anexsia
ANF
    atrial natriuretic factor
Angeliq
Angelman syndrome
angel-shaped phalangoepiphysial dysplasia
  (ASPED)
angel's kiss
anger
    A. Expression Scale
    a. stage

angiectatic skin rash
angiitic luminal compromise
angiitis, angitis
    granulomatous a.
    hypersensitivity a.
    leukoclastic a.
    leukocytoclastic a.
    lupus a.
angina
    bowel a.
    Ludwig a.
    nocturnal a.
    Vincent a.
angiocardiogram
    Elema a.
Angiocath catheter
angiocatheter
angiodysplasia
angioedema
    acquired a. (type I, II)
    episodic a.
    hereditary a. (type I)
    recurrent a.
angiofibroma
    juvenile nasopharyngeal a. (JNA)
angiofollicular lymph node hyperplasia
angiogenesis
    placental adaptive a.
angiogenic growth factor
angiogram
    superior mesenteric a.
angiographic embolization
angiography
    catheter a.
    cerebral a.
    digital subtraction a.
    fluorescein fundus a.
    magnetic resonance a. (MRA)
    pulmonary a.
    radioisotope a.
    selective a.
angiokeratoma
    a. circumscriptum
    a. corporis diffusum
    Mibelli a.
    a. of Mibelli
    vulvar a.
angiolysis
angioma, *pl.* **angiomas, angiomata**
    a. capillare et venosum calcificans
    capillary a.
    cavernous venous a.
    cerebral a.
    cutaneocerebral a.
    cutaneous a.
    dural spinal a.
    facial a.
    intradural spinal a.
    leptomeningeal a.

    port-wine stained a.
    retinal a.
    spider a.
    spinal a.
    subependymal cryptic a.
    venous a.
AngioMark MRI contrast agent
angiomas (*pl. of* angioma)
angiomata (*pl. of* angioma)
angiomatoid tumor
angiomatosis
    bacillary a. (BA)
    cerebrocutaneous a.
    cutaneomeningospinal a.
    encephalocraniofacial a.
    encephalofacial a.
    a. encephalofacialis
    encephalotrigeminal a.
    leptomeningeal a.
    meningeal capillary a.
    meningooculofacial a.
    a. meningoulofacialis
    neurooculocutaneous a.
    Sturge-Weber a.
angiomatosis-oculo-orbito-thalamo-encephalic syndrome
angiomatous involuting nevus
angiomyofibroblastoma
angiomyolipoma rupture
angiomyoma of oviduct
angiomyxoma
angioneurotic edema
angioosteohypertrophy syndrome
angiopathic hemolytic anemia
angiopathy
    vulvar congenital dysplastic a.
angioplasty
    percutaneous transluminal a. (PTA)
    pulmonary artery a.
angiosarcoma
    uterine a.
angiosonography
angiostrongyliasis
Angiostrongylus cantonensis
angiotensin-converting
    a.-c. enzyme (ACE)
    a.-c. enzyme inhibitor
angiotensin (I, II, III)
angiotensinogen
angitis (*var. of* angiitis)
angle
    adductor a.
    anterior chamber a.
    calcaneotibial a.
    center edge a.
    A. classification
    A. classification of occlusion
    corneoscleral a.

angle (*continued*)
    costovertebral a. (CVA)
    decreased talocalcaneal a.
    femoral-tibial a.
    foot-progression a. (FPA)
    hip-knee-ankle a.
    knee a.
    metaphysial-diaphysial a.
    neck-shaft a. (NSA)
    a. of His
    popliteal a.
    Q a.
    talar to first metatarsal a.
    talocalcaneal a. (TCA)
    thigh-foot a. (TFA)
    thigh-leg a. (TLA)
    transmalleolar axis a. (TMA)
    urethral a.
    urethrovesical a. (UVA)
angular (ang)
    a. cheilitis
    a. cheilosis
    a. deformity
    a. movement
    a. stomatitis
angulation
    congenital anterolateral tibial a.
    congenital posteromedial tibial a.
    flow a.
    metaphysis a.
    volar a.
anhedonia
anhidrosis, anidrosis
    ipsilateral a.
    neuropathic a.
anhidrotic
    a. ectodermal dysplasia
    a. sweating
anhydramnion
anhydremia
anhydrohydroxyprogesterone
Anhydron
anhydrous (anh)
    betaine a.
    a. magnesium sulfate
ani (*pl. of* anus)
ANI
    autoimmune neutropenia of infancy
anicteric
    a. hepatitis
    a. leptospirosis
anideus
    embryonic a.
anidrosis (*var. of* anhidrosis)
anileridine
aniline dye
animal
    a. antisera
    a. bite
    a. dander
    a. scabies
animal-assisted therapy (AAT)
anion
    competing a.
    a. gap
aniridia
    aniridia, ambiguous genitalia, mental retardation (AGR)
    aniridia, cerebellar ataxia-oligophrenia syndrome
    nonfamilial a.
    sporadic a.
    a., Wilms tumor association (AWTA)
    a., Wilms tumor association syndrome
    a., Wilms tumor, gonadoblastoma syndrome
anisindione
anismus
anisocoria
    ipsilateral a.
    simple central a.
anisocytosis
anisodactyly
anisomastia
anisomelia
anisometropia
anisometropic amblyopia
anisotropic
anisotropine
ankle
    a. clonus
    dancer's a.
    a. equinus
    jogger's a.
    a. reflexes absent
    a. stability
    a. stirrup splint
ankle-foot orthosis (AFO)
ankyloblepharon
    a., ectodermal dysplasia, clefting (AEC)
    a., ectodermal dysplasia, clefting syndrome
ankylocheilia
ankylocolpos
ankylodactylia (*var. of* ankylodactyly)
ankylodactyly, ankylodactylia
ankyloglossia superior syndrome
ankyloproctia
ankylosing
    a. spondylitis
    a. spondyloarthropathy
ankylosis
    artificial a.
    interbody a.
Ankylostoma (*var. of* Ancylostoma)

ankyrin
anlage, *pl.* **anlagen**
    allergic a.
    anlagen of auditory ossicle
    fibrous a.
    ventral pancreatic a.
anlagen (*pl. of* anlage)
ANLL
    acute nonlymphoblastic
    leukemia
ANN
    alloimmune neonatal neutropenia
Ann Arbor staging system
anneal
annexectomy
annexin
annexitis
annexopexy
annual
    a. goal
    a. review
annular (*var. of* anular)
annulare
    granuloma a.
    perforating granuloma a.
    subcutaneous granuloma a.
annulati (*var. of* anulati)
annuloaortic ectasia
annuloplasty
    De Vega tricuspid a.
annulus (*var. of* anulus)
ano
    fissure in a.
anococcygeal raphe
anocutaneous reflex
anodontia
anogenital
    a. region
    a. tract
    a. wart
anomalad
    abdominal muscle
      deficiency a.
    amniotic band a.
    facioauriculovertebral a.
    holoprosencephaly a.
    Poland a.
    Robin a.
    Sturge-Weber a.
anomalies (*pl. of* anomaly)
anomalous
    a. coronary artery
    a. fetus
    a. left coronary artery from
      pulmonary artery (ALCAPA)
    a. left pulmonary artery
    a. pulmonary vein
    a. pulmonary venous connection
    a. pulmonary venous drainage

    a. right pulmonary vein
      dextroposition
    a. uterus
anomaly, *pl.* **anomalies**
    acyanotic cardiac a.
    Alder a.
    Alder-Reilly a.
    Alexander a.
    aortic arch a.
    Arnold-Chiari a.
    arthrogryposis-like hand a.
    Axenfeld a.
    Axenfeld-Rieger a.
    birth a.
    body stalk a.
    branchial cleft a.
    cardiac a.
    cervical a.
    Chédiak-Higashi a.
    Chiari a.
    chromosomal a.
    cloacal plate a.
    congenital a. (CA)
    conotruncal facial a.
    craniofacial a.
    DiGeorge a.
    Duane a.
    duplication a.
    ear a.
    Ebstein a.
    extracardiac a.
    facial a.
    fetal skeletal a.
    fetal vascular a.
    gastrointestinal a.
    genetic a.
    Greig cephalopolysyndactyly a.
    gyral a.
    immunodeficiency, centromeric
      instability, facial anomalies (ICF)
    imperforate anus, hand, and foot
      anomalies
    intracranial dural vascular a.
    intraspinous vascular a.
    iridogoniodysgenesis with somatic
      anomalies
    Klippel-Feil a.
    May-Hegglin a.
    Michel a.
    microcephaly-cervical spine fusion
      anomalies
    microphthalmia or anophthalmos
      with associated anomalies (MAA)
    Möbius a.
    Mondini a.
    morning glory disc a.
    müllerian duct a.
    multiple congenital anomalies
    Nager a.

anomaly (*continued*)
    orthopedic a.
    pancreaticobiliary a.
    partial DiGeorge a.
    Pelger-Huet a.
    Peters a.
    Poland a.
    Rieger a.
    Scheibe a.
    sex chromosomal a.
    Shone a.
    skeletal a.
    sling a.
    Sprengel a.
    structural a.
    Taussig-Bing a.
    thymic hypoplasia a.
    Uhl a.
    umbilical cord a.
    Undritz a.
    urinary tract a.
    urogenital congenital a.
    uterine a.
    vaginal a.
    valvuloplasty and angioplasty of
      congenital anomalies (VACA)
    vascular a.
    vertebral anomalies, anal atresia,
      cardiac defects, tracheoesophageal
      fistula, renal anomalies, limb
      anomalies (VACTERL)
    X-linked mental-retardation-bilateral
      clasp thumb a.
    X-linked mental retardation/multiple
      congenital a. (XLMR/MCA)
    XO chromosome a.
anomaly-striated-metaphyses
    spondylar changes-nasal a.-s.-m.
anomeric
anonychia, anonychosis
anonychia-ectrodactyly
anonychia-onychodystrophy
anonychosis (*var. of* anonychia)
anonymous donor sperm (ADS)
anophthalmia, anophthalmos
    a., hand-foot defects, mental
      retardation syndrome
anophthalmia-limb anomalies syndrome
anophthalmia-syndactyly syndrome
anophthalmia-Waardenburg syndrome
anophthalmos (*var. of* anophthalmia)
anoplasty
anorchia
anorchism, anorchia
anorectal
    a. agenesis
    a. canal
    a. incontinence
    a. perfusion manometry

    a. plug
    a. stenosis
    a. syndrome
anorectic, anoretic, anorexic
    a. reaction
anorectoplasty
    anterior sagittal a.
    laparoscopically assisted a.
    Pena midsagittal a.
    posterior sagittal a.
anorectum
anoretic (*var. of* anorectic)
Anorex
anorexia
    a. athletica
    infantile a.
    a. nervosa (AN)
    a. nervosa with binging and
      purging (AN-BP)
anorexic (*var. of* anorectic)
anorgasmia, anorgasmy
anorgasmic
anorgasmy (*var. of* anorgasmia)
anosmia
    congenital a.
anotia
anovular menstruation (AM)
anovulation
    chronic a. (CA)
    hyperandrogenic a. (HA)
    hyperandrogenic chronic a.
    normogonadotropic a.
    persistent a.
anovulatory
    a. bleeding
    a. infertility
    a. patient
anoxia
    cerebral a.
    fetal a.
    a. neonatorum
    tissue a.
anoxic-ischemic
    a.-i. encephalopathy
    a.-i. injury
anoxic seizure
ANP
    atrial natriuretic peptide
ANRBC
    absolute nucleated red blood cell
ANS
    antenatal corticosteroid treatment
    autonomic nervous system
Ansaid Oral
ANSD
    autonomic nervous system
      dysfunction
anserinus
    pes a.

Anspor
Answer Plus
Antabuse
antacid
antagonism
antagonist
    androgen a.
    bradykinin a.
    calcium channel a.
    coactivated a.'s
    estrogen a.
    folate a.
    folic acid a.
    FSH a.
    gonadotropin-releasing hormone a.
    GRH a.
    leukotriene receptor a. (LTRA)
    narcotic a.
    opioid receptor a.
    progesterone a.
    proton pump a.
    serotonin receptor a.
antagonistic muscle
antagonist-induced gonadotropin deprivation
antalgic
    a. gait
    a. limp
antecedent
    cerebral palsy a.
    plasma thromboplastin a. (PTA)
antecedent-behavior-consequence relationship
antecubital
    a. space
    a. vein
anteflexed
    anteverted and a. (AV/AF)
anteflexion
antegrade
    a. continence enema (ACE)
    a. continence enema procedure
antenatal
    a. admission
    a. anti-D immunoglobulin
    a. assessment
    a. complication
    a. corticosteroid
    a. corticosteroid therapy
    a. corticosteroid treatment (ANS)
    a. diagnosis
    a. disease process
    a. fetofetal transfusion
    a. management
    a. morbidity
    a. patient
    a. phenobarbital treatment
    a. record
    a. screening

    a. steroid
    a. testing
    a. testing unit
    a. thyrotropin releasing hormone
    a. ultrasound
antepartum
    a. alloimmunization
    a. asphyxia
    a. bed rest
    a. bleeding
    a. care
    a. complication
    a. dosage
    a. fetal assessment
    a. fetal BPP
    a. fetal CST
    a. fetal NST
    a. fetal surveillance
    a. fetal testing
    a. hemorrhage (APH)
    a. home care
    a. hospital bed rest
    a. hospitalization
    a. management
    a. monitor (APM)
    a. period
    a. pyelonephritis
    a. Rh isoimmunization
    a. steroid therapy
    a. stress
    a. support group
    a. surveillance program
    a. testing
    a. unit
anteposition
anterior
    a. abdominal wall
    a. and posterior (A&P)
    a. and posterior repair
    a. apical vault defect
    a. asynclitism
    a. chamber
    a. chamber angle
    a. chamber cleavage syndrome
    a. chamber dysgenesis syndrome
    a. colporrhaphy
    a. commissure
    a. cord syndrome
    a. cricoid split (ACS)
    a. cricoid split procedure
    a. cruciate ligament (ACL)
    a. drawer test
    duplicitas a.
    dysgenesis mesostromalis a.
    a. enterocele
    a. ethmoidal sinusitis
    a. exenteration
    a. fontanelle (AF)
    a. head cap

anterior *(continued)*
    a. horn cell degeneration
    a. horn cell disease
    a. hypospadias
    a. labial arteries of vulva
    a. labial nerves
    a. lenticonus
    a. lie
    a. lip of cervix
    a. microphthalmia
    a. nasal packing
    a. nasal septum
    a. neural tube closure
    a. neural tube defect
    occiput a. (OA)
    a. pectoral node
    a. pelvic exenteration
    a. pituitary disorder
    a. pituitary-like hormone
    a. rectoperineal fistula
    a. rectus sheath
    a. resection rectopexy
    a. retrosternal hernia of
      Morgagni
    a. sagittal anorectoplasty
    a. sling rectopexy
    a. spinal fusion
    a. spinal instrumentation
    a. superior iliac spine
    a. synechia
    a. talofibular ligament (ATFL)
    a. thoracic wall
    a. tibial bowing
    a. tibialis transfer
    a. translation
    a. translation of knee
    a. urethritis
    a. vagina
    a. vaginotomy
    a. wall defect
anteriorly displaced anus
anterolateral
    a. fontanelle
    a. free wall (ALFW)
    a. tibial bowing
anteroposterior (AP)
    a. colporrhaphy
    a. diameter (APD, A-PD)
    a. diameter of the pelvic
      inlet
    a. laxity
    a. view
antetorsion
    femoral a.
anteversion
    acetabular a. (AA)
    bilateral increased femoral a.
    femoral a. (FA)
    increased femoral a.

anteverted
    a. and anteflexed (AV/AF)
    a. naris
    a. nostril
    a. pinna
anthelix
anthelminthic, anthelmintic
    a. agent
    a. drug
anthelmintic *(var. of* anthelminthic)
anthracycline
anthrax
    cutaneous a.
    pulmonary a.
anthropi
    Ochrobactrum a.
anthropoid pelvis
anthropometric
    a. measure
    a. measurement
anthropometry
anthropomorphic measurement
anti-ACh antibody
antiadrenal antibody
anti-A isohemagglutinin
antiandrogen receptor blocker
antiangiogenic therapy
antiannexin V antibody
antianxiety
    a. agent
    a. drug
antiarrhythmic
antiasthmatic
antibacterial
    a. drug
    a. therapy
antibasement membrane antibody
antibiotic
    antitumor a.
    beta-lactam a.
    beta-lactamase-resistant
      antistaphylococcal a.
    broad-spectrum a.
    a. drug
    a. infusion therapy
    intravenous a.
    a. irrigation
    A. Otic
    preventive a.
    prophylactic a.
    a. prophylaxis
    a. resistance
    a. treatment
antibiotic-associated
    a.-a. colitis
    a.-a. diarrhea (AAD)
**antibiotic-resistant gram-negative
  organism (ARGNO)**
anti-B isohemagglutinin

antibody

ADB a.
AH a.
anti-ACh a.
antiadrenal a.
antiannexin V a.
antibasement membrane a.
anticardiolipin a.
anticentromere a. (ACA)
anticholera toxin a.
anti-CMV a.
anticytomegalovirus a.
anti-D a.
anti-DNase B a.
antidrug IgE a.
anti-EBNA a.
antiendomysium a. (AEA)
anti-Epstein-Barr nuclear antigen a.
antiferritin a.
anti-GBM a.
antigliadin a. (AGA)
antihistone a.
anti-Histoplasma a.
anti-HIV a.
antihyaluronidase a.
anti-I a.
antiidiotype a.
antiinsulin a.
anti-Kell a.
anti-La a.
anti-Lewis a.
anti-M a.
antimitochondrial a.
antimyolemmal a. (AMLA)
antineutrophil a.
antineutrophil cytoplasmic a.
   (ANCA)
antinuclear a. (ANA)
antiovarian a.
antipaternal antileukocytotoxic a.
antiphospholipid a. (aPL)
antiplatelet IgG a.
antireticulin a.
antiribosomal P a.
anti-Ro a.
anti-*Saccharomyces cerevisiae* a.
anti-smooth-muscle a.
antisperm a.
anti-SS-A a.
anti-SS-B a.
antithyroid a.
anti-TNF a.
antitoxocaral a.
ASO a.
blood group a.
celiac a.
circulating platelet a.
cold a.
complement-fixing serum a.

conjugated antichlamydial
   monoclonal a.
Coombs a.
cytophilic a.
a. deficiency
direct fluorescent a. (DFA)
endomysium a. (EMA)
fluorescent antimembrane a. (FAMA)
fluorescent treponemal a. (FTA)
Frei a.
genus-specific monoclonal a.
glutamic acid decarboxylase a.
hantavirus immunoglobulin M a.
hemagglutination inhibition a. (HIA)
hepatitis B core a. (HBcAb)
hepatitis B early a. (HBeAb)
hepatitis B surface a. (HBsAb)
heterophil a. (HA)
HI a.
HPV type 16 capsid a.
humoral a.
IgA antiendomysium a.
IgA antireticulin a.
IgD a.
IgE a.
IgG a.
IgM a.
immunofluorescent a. (IFA)
immunoglobulin a.
immunoglobulin M fluorescent
   treponemal a.
indirect fluorescent a. (IFA)
indirect hemagglutination a. (IHA)
a. induction therapy
InSite HER2/neu monoclonal a.
intrathecal anti-HIV a.
islet cell a. (ICA, ICAb)
Jo-1 a.
Kell a.
Ki67 a.
Kveim a.
link a.
lupus anticoagulant a.
maternal antibodies
maternal antiplatelet a.
maternal antithyroid a.
maternal-fetal transmission of a.
maternal IgG a.
maternal sperm a.
monoclonal a. (MAb)
monoclonal antiendotoxin a.
monoclonal anti-IgE a.
mycoplasmal a.
natural a.
neurofilament a.
OncoScint CR103 monoclonal a.
oregovomab murine monoclonal a.
ovarian a.
parietal cell a.

A

51

antibody (*continued*)
    perinuclear antineutrophil cytoplasmic a. (pANCA)
    phospholipid a.
    platelet-associated a.
    polyclonal antiendotoxin anticore a.
    polyclonal-monoclonal a.
    a. production assay
    a. reaction site
    a. replacement therapy
    a. response
    Rh a.
    rhesus a.
    Rh-negative a.
    Rh-positive a.
    RSV monoclonal a.
    S-100 a.
    a. screening
    serum a.
    serum antienterocyte a.
    species-specific a.
    sperm surface a.
    streptococcal a.
    tissue-specific a.
    titer of anti-ragweed IgE a.
    a. to hepatitis A virus (anti-HAV)
    a. to hepatitis B core antigen (anti-HBcAg)
    a. to hepatitis B surface antigen (anti-HBs, anti-HBsAg, HBsAb)
    transglutaminase a.
    transplacental maternal a.
    a. transplacental transfer
    Treponema pallidum a.
    vibriocidal a.
    virus-neutralizing a. (VNA)
    VZV-specific IgM a.
    warm a.
    xenogeneic a.
antibody-dependent cell-mediated cytotoxicity (ADCC)
antibody-mediated
    a.-m. hemolysis
    a.-m. immune suppression (AMIS)
antibody-positive
    anticardiolipin a.-p.
antibody-secreting cell (ASC)
anticancer agent
anticardiolipin (aCL)
    a. antibody
    a. antibody-positive
anticentromere antibody (ACA)
antichlamydial antibody titer
anticholera toxin antibody
anticholinergic
    a. agent
    a. drug
    a. plant
    a. poisoning

anticholinesterase medication
anticipated
    a. behavioral milestone
    a. developmental milestone
anticipation
    evidence of a.
anticipatory
    a. anxiety
    a. chemotherapy associated nausea
    a. grief
anti-CMV antibody
anticoagulant
    circulating a.
    lupus a. (LAC)
anticoagulation
    ambulatory a.
    outpatient a.
    peripartal heparin a.
    prophylactic a.
    therapeutic a.
    a. therapy
anticodon
anticonvulsant
    a. drug
    a. hypersensitivity syndrome
    a. intoxication
    a. treatment
anticus
    saccus a.
anticysticercal therapy
anticytomegalovirus antibody
anti-D
    a.-D antibody
    a.-D autoantibody
    a.-D globulin treatment
    a.-D immunoglobulin
    a.-D therapy
antideoxyribonucleic acid (anti-DNA)
antidepressant
    a. drug
    heterocyclic a.
    a. poisoning
    a. therapy
    tricyclic a. (TCA)
antidiarrheal (A-D), antidiarrhetic
antidiarrhetic (*var. of* antidiarrheal)
antidiuresis
antidiuretic hormone (ADH)
anti-DNA
    antideoxyribonucleic acid
    anti-DNA antitopoisomerase 1
anti-DNase
    a.-DNase B (ADB)
    a.-DNase B antibody
    a.-DNase B titer
antidromic conduction
antidrug IgE antibody

anti-ds DNA antibody titer
antidysrhythmic agent
anti-EBNA antibody
antiembolism stocking
antiemetic
    a. medication
    a. therapy
antiendometriotic effect
antiendomysial
    IgA a.
antiendomysium antibody (AEA)
antiepileptic drug (AED)
anti-Epstein-Barr nuclear antigen
  antibody
antiestrogen effect
antiestrogenic effect
antiferritin antibody
antifibrinolytic agent
antifolic agent
antifungal
    Absorbine Jr. A.
    Aftate A.
    a. azole
    a. drug
    a. drug therapy
antigalactagogue
antigalactic
Anti-Gas
    Maalox A.-G.
anti-GBM antibody
antigen
    A a.
    ABO a.
    a. activity
    allogenic a.
    antibody to hepatitis B core a.
      (anti-HBcAg)
    antibody to hepatitis B surface a.
      (anti-HBsAg)
    antigen-specific a.
    antiproliferating cell nuclear a.
      (anti-PCNA)
    anular erythema a.
    Australia a.
    a. binding site
    CA 125 a.
    cancer a. 125 (CA-125, CA 125)
    carcinoembryonic a. (CEA)
    carcinoma a.
    cell surface a.
    chorioembryonic a.
    cryptococcal a.
    DD a.
    a. detection test
    a. determinant
    direct fluorescent a. (DFA)
    Duffy a.
    E a.
    epithelial membrane a. (EMA)

    Epstein-Barr nuclear a. (EBNA)
    fetal histocompatibility a.
    fluorescent antibody to membrane a.
      (FAMA)
    Forssman a.
    glomerular basement membrane a.
    hepatitis B a. (HBAg)
    hepatitis B surface a. (HBsAg)
    heterophil a.
    histocompatibility locus a. (HLA)
    histone a.
    HIV-1 p24 a.
    HLA-B27 a.
    human leukocyte a.
    human platelet a. (HPA)
    H-Y a.
    incompatible blood group a.
    Kell a.
    La/SSB a.
    leukocyte integrin lymphocyte
      function-associated a. 1
    Lewis a.
    lipoglycan a.
    lymphocyte function-associated a. 1
    M a.
    major histocompatibility a.
    melanoma specific a.
    MHC a.
    nuclear a.
    O a.
    oncofetal a.
    ovarian carcinoma a.
    pancreatic oncofetal a. (POA)
    platelet a.
    Pm-Scl a.
    polysaccharide group-specific a.
    RBC P a.
    red blood cell a.
    respiratory syncytial virus a.
    Rh a.
    rhesus a.
    ribonucleoprotein a.
    Ro/SSA a.
    RSV a.
    sclerodermatomyositis a.
    a. screen
    sialylated Lewis A a.
    sialyl Tn a.
    Sm a.
    surface a.
    Thomsen-Friedenreich a.
    thymic lymphocyte a. (TL)
    T-independent a.
    a. tolerance
    Toxoplasma a.
    transplantation a.
    Treponema pallidum a.
    tumor a.
    tumor-associated a. (TAA)

antigen (*continued*)
    tumor-specific transplantation a.
      (TSTA)
    viral capsid a. (VCA)
    von Willebrand factor a.
    vWF a.
antigen-antibody complex
antigenemia
antigenic
    a. mimicry
    a. modulation
    a. paralysis
    a. stimulus
antigenicity
    tumor a.
antigen-presenting cell
 (APC)
antigen-sensitive cell
antigen-specific antigen
antigenuria
antigliadin
    a. antibody (AGA)
    IgA a.
antiglobulin test
antiglomerular basement membrane
 antibody disease
antigonadotropin
antigravity
    a. activity
    a. position
anti-HAV
    antibody to hepatitis A virus
    IgG a.-HAV
anti-HBcAg
    antibody to hepatitis B core antigen
anti-HBsAg
    antibody to hepatitis B surface antigen
    anti-HBsAg concentration
antihelical fold
antihelix, anthelix
antihelminthic therapy
antihemophilic factor (AHF)
antihistamine
    a. drug
    histamine 1 a.
Antihist-D
antihistone antibody
anti-*Histoplasma* antibody
anti-HIV antibody
antihyaluronidase
    a. antibody
    a. titer
antihypertensive
    a. drug
    a. therapy
anti-I antibody
antiidiotype antibody
anti-IgE therapy
antiimmunoglobulin reagent

antiincontinence
antiinflammatory
    a. agent
    a. effect
    a. intervention
    a. therapy
    a. treatment
antiinhibitor coagulant complex
antiinsulin antibody
anti-Jo1
anti-Kell
    a.-K. anemia
    a.-K. antibody
    a.-K. sensitization
anti-La antibody
antileukemic therapy
anti-Lewis antibody
antilewisite
antilipolysis
antiluteogenic
antilymphocyte
    a. globulin
    a. sera
antimalarial
    a. drug
    a. poisoning
antimanic treatment
anti-M antibody
antimesenteric surface
antimetabolite
antimicrobial
    a. agent
    a. aminoglycoside
    beta-lactam a.
    a. prophylaxis
    a. susceptibility testing
    a. therapy
    a. treatment
antimicrosomal
antimitochondrial antibody
antimongolism
antimongoloid
    a. deformity
    a. eye slant
    a. obliquity
    a. palpebral fissure
antimüllerian hormone (AMH)
antimycobacterial
antimycoplasma titer
antimyolemmal antibody (AMLA)
antinauseant poisoning
antineoplastic
    a. agent
    a. drug
antineutrophil
    a. antibody
    a. cytoplasmic antibody
     (ANCA)
antinuclear antibody (ANA)

A

anti-O-specific polysaccharide
antiovarian antibody
antioxidant
    chain-breaking a.
    a. enzyme
    preventive a.
    a. release
    a. release
    a. therapy
antiparasitic drug therapy
antipaternal antileukocytotoxic antibody
anti-PCNA
    antiproliferating cell nuclear antigen
antiperistaltic intestinal interposition
antiphospholipid
    a. antibody (aPL)
    a. antibody syndrome (APAS)
    a. syndrome (APS)
antiplasmin (AP)
    alpha-2 a.
    a. deficiency
antiplatelet
    a. agent
    a. IgG antibody
    a. therapy
antipregnancy
    a. immunization
    a. vaccine
antiprogesterone
antiprogestin
antiprogestogen
antiproliferating cell nuclear antigen (anti-PCNA)
antiprostaglandin agent
antipruritic medication
antipsychotic
    a. drug
    a. poisoning
antipyretic therapy
antipyrine and benzocaine
antirabies serum
antireceptor
antireticulin antibody
antiretroviral
    a. drug
    a. medication
    a. resistance
    a. therapy
anti-Rh gamma globulin
anti-Rho(D)
    a.-R. globulin
    a.-R. titer
antiribosomal P antibody
anti-Ro antibody
anti-RSV
anti-Saccharomyces cerevisiae antibody
anti-Scl-70 autoantibody
antisense
    a. nucleotide

    a. oligodeoxynucleotide
    a. oligonucleotide
    a. strand
antiseptic
    Avagard instant hand a.
antiserum
    animal antisera
    SB-6 a.
    tetanus a.
antishock trousers
antisialagogue
antisiphon device
anti-smooth-muscle antibody
antisocial
    a. behavior
    a. personality disorder (ASPD)
Antispas Injection
antispasmodic poisoning
antispastic
    a. drug
    a. medication
antisperm antibody
anti-SS-A antibody
anti-SS-B antibody
anti-ssDNA
antistaphylococcal
    a. agent
    a. IgE
    a. penicillin
antistreptolysin O (ASO)
antithrombin (AT)
    a. III (AT3)
    a. III coagulation inhibitor
    a. III deficiency
    a. I, II, III
    protein S a.
antithymocyte globulin
antithyroglobulin
antithyroid
    a. antibody
    a. drug
    a. drug therapy
anti-TNF antibody
antitopoisomerase
    anti-DNA a. 1
antitoxin
    botulinum a. (type A, B, E)
    diphtheria a.
    equine a.
    scarlatina a.
    tetanus a. (TAT)
antitoxocaral antibody
anti-*Toxoplasma*
    serum immunoglobulin G a.-*T.*
antitragus
antitreponemal test
antitrypsin
    alpha-1 a.
antituberculosis chemotherapy

antituberculous therapy
antitumor antibiotic
antitussive medication
antivenin polyvalent
antivenom
Antivert
antiviral therapy
Antizol
Antley-Bixler syndrome
Antopol disease
antral
    a. choanal polyp
    a. follicle
    a. gastritis
    a. lavage
    a. stenosis
    a. washout
Antrizine
antrum
    aditus ad a.
    nasal a.
anucleate fragment
ANUG
    acute necrotizing ulcerative
    gingivitis
anular, annular
    a. band
    a. erythema antigen
    a. lesion
    a. pancreas
    a. placenta
    a. stenosis
    a. testis
    a. tubule
anular-array transducer
anulati, annulati
    pili a.
    pseudopili a.
anuli (*pl. of* anulus)
anulus, annulus, *pl.* anuli
Anumed
anuria
anuric
anus, *pl.* ani
    adequate caliber of a.
    anteriorly displaced a.
    arcus tendineus levator ani
    ectopic a.
    high imperforate a.
    imperforate a.
    levator ani
    low imperforate a.
    a. of Rusconi
    Paget disease of a.
    patent a.
    pruritus ani
    spastic levator ani
    supralevator imperforate a.
    translevator imperforate a.

    vaginal ectopic a.
    vestibular a.
    vulvovaginal a.
anus-hand-ear syndrome
Anusol
    A. HC-1 Topical
    A. HC-2.5% Topical
Anusol-HC Suppository
anxiety
    anticipatory a.
    childhood a.
    a. depression
    a. disorder
    A. Disorder Interview for Children
    a. management
    a. rating for children (ARC)
    a. sensitivity index (ASI)
    separation a.
    stranger a.
anxiety-withdrawal scale
anxiogenic
anxiolytic
    a. agent
    a. drug
    a. medication
Anzemet
AO
    arthroophthalmopathy
AOAH
    adult onset adrenal hyperplasia
AOD
    alcohol and other drugs
    arterial occlusive disease
AODM
    adult-onset diabetes mellitus
AOI
    apnea of infancy
AOM
    acute otitis media
    arthroophthalmopathy
AOP
    apnea of prematurity
AORF
    acute oliguric renal failure
aorta, *pl.* aortae
    coarctation of a.
    descending a.
    a. dilation
    fetal a.
    hypoplastic a. (HA)
    overriding a.
    primitive a.
    traumatic rupture of thoracic a.
      (TRA)
aortae (*pl. of* aorta)
aortic
    a. aneurysm
    a. arch
    a. arch anomaly

a. arch anomaly, peculiar facies, mental retardation syndrome
a. arch coarctation (CoA)
a. arch malformation
a. arch rupture
a. bifurcation
a. blood flow velocity waveform
a. blood pressure
a. bruit
a. bud
a. coarctation
a. cusp prolapse
a. dissection
a. ejection click
a. ejection murmur
a. knob
a. laceration
a. node
a. node metastasis
a. oxygen content
a. regurgitation
a. root
a. root diameter
a. runoff
a. sac
a. stenosis, corneal clouding, growth and mental retardation syndrome
a. valve
a. valve atresia
a. valve disease
a. valve insufficiency
a. valve stenosis
a. valvotomy
aorticopulmonary, aortopulmonary
a. septation
a. window defect
aortic-to-pulmonary shunt
aortitis
aortogram
thoracic a.
aortography
aortopexy
aortoplasty
prosthetic patch a.
subclavian flap a. (SFA)
aortopulmonary, aorticopulmonary
a. collateral coil embolization
a. septum
a. shunt
a. transposition
a. window
A&P
anterior and posterior
A&P repair
AP
abruptio placentae
anatomic profile
anteroposterior

antiplasmin
appendiceal perforation
AP diameter
Apacet
APACHE
Acute Physiology and Chronic Health Evaluation
apareunia
APAS
antiphospholipid antibody syndrome
apathy
APC
activated protein C
antigen-presenting cell
atrial premature contraction
APCR
activated protein C resistance
A-PD
anteroposterior diameter
APECED
autoimmune polyendocrinopathy, candidiasis, ectodermal dystrophy
ape hand
Apert
A. disease
A. syndrome
aperta
spina bifida a.
Apert-Crouzon
A.-C. disease
A.-C. syndrome
aperture
supraglottic a.
apex, *pl.* **apices**
a. linguae
a. of intussusception
a. of vagina
prolapsing a.
vaginal a.
Apgar
A. rating
A. scale
A. score
A. scoring system
A. timer
activity, pulse, grimace, appearance, respiration
APGN
acute postinfectious glomerulonephritis
APH
antepartum hemorrhage
aphakia
pediatric a.
aphasia
acquired epileptic a.
Broca a.
expressive a.
global a.
infantile acquired a.

aphasia (*continued*)
    migraine with a.
    receptive a.
    thymic a.
    Wernicke a.
apheresis
    LDL a.
aphonia
aphrodisiac
aphrophilus
    Haemophilus a.
aphtha, *pl.* **aphthae**
    Bednar aphthae
aphthae (*pl. of* aphtha)
aphthosis
    perianal a.
aphthous
    a. stomatitis
    a. ulcer
    a. ulceration
A1PI
    alpha-1 proteinase inhibitor
APIB
    Assessment of Preterm Infants'
    Behavior
apical
    a. 4-chamber view
    a. ectodermal ridge
    a. heave
    a. impulse
    a. pleural stripping
    a. presystolic murmur
    a. pulse
    a. vertebra
apices (*pl. of* **apex**)
apista
    Pandoraea a.
aPL
    antiphospholipid
    antiphospholipid antibody
APL
    accelerated painless labor
aplasia
    Alexander a.
    a. axialis extracorticalis
      congenita
    bone marrow a.
    cerebellar vermis a.
    complete cerebellar a.
    complete radial a.
    congenital cutis a.
    congenital RBC a.
    congenital skin a.
    congenital vaginal a.
    a. cutis
    a. cutis congenita
    extracortical axial a.
    gonadal a.
    heminasal a.

    hereditary retinal a.
    idiosyncratic marrow a.
    Leydig cell a.
    Michel a.
    Mondini a.
    nuclear a.
    optic nerve a.
    ovarian a.
    parvovirus B19-induced red blood
      cell a.
    parvovirus B19 red blood cell a.
    pulmonary acinar a.
    pure red blood cell a.
    radial ray a.
    retinal a.
    Scheibe a.
    selective a.
    thymic a.
    thymic-parathyroid a.
    thyroid a.
    vas deferens a.
aplastic
    a. abdominal muscle syndrome
    a. anemia
    a. crisis
    a. leukemia
    a. pancytopenia
    a. patella
Apley compression test
APLS
    advanced pediatric life support
    APLS model
APM
    antepartum monitor
apnea
    a. alarm mattress
    a. and bradycardia (A&B)
    central sleep a.
    expiratory a.
    hyperreflexic a.
    idiopathic a.
    infantile sleep a.
    initial a.
    late a.
    mixed sleep a.
    a. monitor
    neonatal a.
    a. neonatorum
    obstructive a.
    obstructive sleep a. (OSA)
    a. of infancy (AOI)
    a. of prematurity (AOP)
    pathologic a.
    postanesthetic a.
    postoperative a.
    posttussive a.
    prolonged expiratory a.
    secondary a.
    sleep a.

unrecognized a.
vasovagal reflex a.
apnea-bradycardia
apnea-hypopnea combination
apnea/hypoventilation
obstructive sleep a./h (OSA/H)
apneic
a. event
a. seizure
APO
apolipoprotein
Apo-Amoxi
Apo-Ampi
apoB
apobetalipoprotein
apobetalipoprotein (apoB)
Apo-Bromocriptine
Apo-Cephalex
Apo-Cimetidine
Apo-Cloxi
apocrine
a. adenoma
a. cell
a. chromhidrosis
a. cyst
a. cystadenoma
a. duct
a. gland of Moll
a. hydrocystoma
a. metaplasia
a. miliaria
a. sweat gland
apodia
Apo-Diazepam
Apo-Diclo
Apo-Diflunisal
Apo-Doxy Tabs
apoenzyme deficiency
apoferritin
Apo-Flurbiprofen
apogamy
Apogee
A. mesh
A. 800 ultrasound system
A. vaginal vault prolapse repair system
A. vaginal vault suspension
apolipoprotein
serum a.
apomorphine sexual dysfunction
Apo-Naproxen
aponeurosis
epicranial a.
gastrocnemius a.
Apo-Pen VK
apophysary (*var. of* apophysial)
apophyseal (*var. of* apophysial)
apophysial, apophyseal, apophysary
a. space

apophysis
apophysitis
calcaneal a.
iliac crest a.
olecranon a.
traction a.
Apo-Piroxicam
apoplectic
apoplexy
parturient a.
uteroplacental a. (UPA)
apoprotein
ApopTag Plus kit
apoptosis
neutrophil a.
postasphyxial a.
spinal a.
spontaneous a.
apoptotic cell death
Apo-Ranitidine
Apo-Sulfamethoxazole
Apo-Sulfatrim
Apo-Tamox
Apo-Terfenadine
Apo-Tetra
apotransferrin infusion
Apo-Zidovudine
apparatus, *pl.* **apparatus**
Barcroft/Haldane a.
figure-of-8 a.
Golgi a.
Heyns abdominal decompression a.
vestibular a.
apparent
a. exophthalmos
a. life-threatening event (ALTE)
a. mineralocorticoid excess (AME)
a. paresis
appearance
acromegaloid facial a. (AFA)
apple-peel a.
bag of worms a.
bat wing a.
bird's beak a.
bread-and-butter a.
bull's eye sonographic a.
cobblestone a.
copper-wire a.
corkscrew a.
cottage cheese a.
cushingoid a.
drooping lily a.
Erlenmeyer flask a.
ground-glass a.
hair-on-end a.
hatchet face a.
honeycombed a.
Hurler-like facial a.
lamellated a.

appearance (*continued*)
    meconium ileus a.
    onion-skin a.
    peau d'orange a.
    powder-burn visual a.
    puppetlike a.
    salt-and-pepper a.
    silver-wire a.
    slapped cheek a.
    snowstorm a.
    soap-bubble a.
    sporotrichoid a.
    stacked coin a.
    strawberry a.
    sunburst a.
    toxic a.
    water bottle a.
    wing-beating a.
    worried facial a.

appendage
    testicular a.
    a. torsion

appendectomy, appendicectomy
    inversion-ligation a.

appendical (*var. of* appendiceal)

appendiceal, appendical
    a. abscess
    a. fecalith
    a. intussusception
    a. inversion
    a. lumen
    a. perforation (AP)
    a. structure
    a. stump

appendicectomy (*var. of* appendectomy)

appendices (*pl. of* **appendix**)

appendicitis
    acute a. (AA)
    gangrenous a.
    pelvic a.
    perforated a.
    ruptured a.
    suppurative a.

appendicolith
    calcified a.

appendicostomy

appendicovesicostomy
    Mitrofanoff a.

appendicular artery

artery

appendix, *pl.* **appendices**
    a. epididymis
    ligation of a.
    obstruction of a.
    a. testis
    a. testis torsion
    torsion of a.
    vascularized a.
    vermiform a.

apperception

appetite
    decreased a.

apple
    A. Medical bipolar forceps
    a. pattern

apple-peel
    a.-p. appearance
    a.-p. atresia

appliance
    dental speech a.
    lingual a.
    orthodontic a.
    orthopedic a.
    ThumbGuard a.

application
    bioelectromagnetic a.
    nonionizing nonthermal a.
    silicone band a.
    spring clip a.
    topical iodine a.

applicator
    Absolok endoscopic clip a.
    afterload a.
    benzoin a.
    Bloedorn a.
    cotton-tipped a.
    Falope ring a.
    Filshie clip a.
    Fletcher-Suit a.
    radioactive a.
    ring a.

applied behavior analysis (ABA)

applier
    LDS clip a.
    vascular clip a.

appointment
    prenatal a.

appositional ossification

apposition of skull suture

apprehension
    a. sign
    a. test

approach
    abdominal a.
    algorithmic a.
    family-centered a.
    hysteroscopic a.
    Kahn a.
    opt-in a.
    opt-out a.
    staircase a.
    transrectal a.

appropriate
    a. blood pressure cuff size
    a. for gestational age (AGA)
    a. learning experience

APPT
    Adolescent and Pediatric Pain Tool

APR
  abdominoperineal resection
apractic (*var. of* apraxic)
apraxia
  ataxia-oculomotor a.
  buccolingual a.
  congenital ocular motor a.
    (COMA)
  gait a.
  oculomotor a.
  sensory a.
apraxia-ataxia-mental deficiency syndrome
apraxia-oculomotor contracture-muscle atrophy syndrome
apraxic, apractic
Apresoline
  A. Injection
  A. Oral
Apri
aprobarbital
aproctia
Aprodine
apron
  Hottentot a.
  perineal surgical a.
  pudendal a.
aprosencephaly-atelencephaly syndrome
aprosencephaly syndrome
aprosopia
aprotinin
APS
  antiphospholipid syndrome
APSGN
  acute poststreptococcal
    glomerulonephritis
APT-Downey test
Aptima Combo 2 assay
aptitude
  Detroit Test of Learning A. 2
APTT
  activated partial thromboplastin time
  APTT coagulation test
Apt test
AQ
  Beconase AQ
  Nasacort AQ
  Vancenase AQ
Aqua
  A. Glycolic
  A. Tar
Aquacel dressing
Aquachloral Supprettes
Aquacort
Aquaflex ultrasound gel pad
Aquagel lubricating gel
AquaMEPHYTON Injection
Aquaphor
  A. gauze
  A. healing ointment

AquaSens FMS 1000 fluid monitoring system
Aquasol
  A. A
  A. E
  A. E Oral
Aquasonic 100 ultrasound transmission gel
Aquasorb dressing
Aquaspirillum itersonii
Aquatensen
aqueduct
  cochlear a.
  a. of Sylvius
aqueductal
  a. forking
  a. gliosis
  a. stenosis
aqueous
  a. analysis
  A. AVP
  a. beclomethasone
  a. crystalline penicillin
  a. crystalline penicillin G
  a. humor
  a. penicillin sodium
  a. phase
arabinoside
  adenine a.
  cytosine a.
arabinosylcytosine (araC, Ara-C)
Ara-C, araC
  arabinosylcytosine
arachidic
  a. acid
  a. bronchitis
arachidonic
  a. acid
  a. acid level
  a. acid metabolite
arachnid envenomation
arachnidism
  necrotic a.
arachnodactyly
  congenital contractural a. (CCA)
arachnoid
  a. cyst
  a. granulation
  a. villus
arachnoiditis
  chronic adhesive a.
  obliterative a.
  posterior fossa a.
  spinal a.
  tuberculous spinal a.
aragonite precipitation
Arakawa syndrome
Aralen
Aramine

Aran-Duchenne
  A.-D. disease
  A.-D. muscular dystrophy
araneus
  nevus a.
ARAS
  ascending reticular activating system
arbitrarily
  a. primed polymerase chain reaction
  a. primer
arborization
  dendritic a.
  pulmonary a.
  vaginal fluid a.
arborvirus (*var. of* arbovirus)
arbor vitae
arboviral encephalitis
arbovirus, arborvirus
arc
  xenon a.
ARC
  AIDS-related complex
  anxiety rating for children
  Association for Retarded Citizens
arcade
  mitral a.
Arcanobacterium haemolyticum
arch
  aortic a.
  bifid spinal a.
  branchial a.
  double aortic a. (DAA)
  hypoplastic zygomatic a.
  a. insole pad
  interrupted aortic a. (type A, B)
  medial longitudinal a.
  narrow pubic a.
  neural a.
  pubic a.
  right aortic a. (RAA)
  tendinous a.
  vertebral laminar a.
  zygomatic a.
archencephalon
archenteron
archenteronoma
archiblast
archigastrula
architectural disturbance
architecture
  breast a.
  cortical a.
  crypt-villus a.
  dysplastic cortical a.
  histologic a.
  lobular a.
  mixed cystic/solid a.
  pelvic a.
  sleep a.

arciform lesion
arcing spring diaphragm
Arcoxia
ARCS
  azoospermia, renal anomaly,
  cervicothoracic spine dysplasia
arcuate
  a. artery
  a. ligament of pubis
  a. line
  a. nucleus
  a. uterus
arcuatus
  uterus a.
arcus
  a. juvenilis
  a. tendineus
  a. tendineus fasciae pelvis
  a. tendineus fascia rectovaginalis
  a. tendineus levator ani
ARD
  acute respiratory disease
ARDS
  acute respiratory distress syndrome
  adult respiratory distress syndrome
area
  ambosexual a.
  body surface a. (BSA)
  Broca a.
  delivery a.
  developmental a.
  echolucent a.
  flexural a.
  frontal pole a.
  hypoechogenic a.
  infraclavicular a.
  inguinal a.
  intertriginous a.
  Kiesselbach a.
  Little a.
  a. of cardiac dullness (ACD)
  a. of interest magnification (AIM)
  paracervical a.
  placental surface a.
  pudendal a.
  skip a.
  social-emotional developmental a.
  subpannicular a.
  subpulmonic a.
  total body surface a. (TBSA)
  Wernicke a.
areal bone mineral density (aBMD)
areata, areatus
  alopecia a.
areatus (*var. of* areata)
Aredia
areflexia
areflexic paraparesis
aregenerative anemia

Arenavirus
areola, *pl.* **areolae**
    nevoid hyperkeratosis of nipple
      and a.
    ptotic a.
    a. umbilicus
areolae (*pl. of* areola)
areolar enlargement
Arey rule
ARF
    acute renal failure
    acute respiratory failure
    acute rheumatic fever
      ARF excimer laser
      nonoliguric ARF
      oliguric ARF
      postrenal ARF
      prerenal ARF
Arfonad Injection
Argentine hemorrhagic fever
Argesic-SA
arg-gly-asp
    arginine-glycine-aspartic acid
arginase deficiency
arginate
    heme a.
arginine
    a. glutamate
    a. hydrochloride
    plasma a.
    a. tolerance test (ATT)
    a. vasopressin (AVP)
    a. vasopressin regulation
    a. vasotocin
**arginine-glycine-aspartic acid
(arg-gly-asp)**
arginine-insulin
    a.-i. stimulation test
    a.-i. tolerance test
argininemia
argininosuccinic
    a. acid
    a. acid synthetase deficiency
    a. aciduria
argininosuccinicacidemia
argininosuccinicaciduria
ARGNO
    antibiotic-resistant gram-negative
      organism
argon
    a. beam coagulation
    a. beam coagulator
      (ABC)
    a. diode
    a. laser
Argonz-Del Castillo syndrome
Argyle arterial catheter
Argyll Robertson pupil
argyrophilic granule

**arhinencephaly, arrhinencephalia,
arrhinencephaly**
arhinia, arrhinia
    a., choanal atresia, microphthalmia
      syndrome
ARI
    acute respiratory infection
Arias-Stella
    A.-S. effect
    A.-S. phenomenon
ariboflavinosis
ARIC
    acrosome reaction with ionophore
      challenge
Aries-Pitanguy procedure
Arimidex
Aristocort
    A. A Topical
    A. Forte Injection
    A. intralesional injection
    A. Oral
    A. Topical
Aristospan
    A. intraarticular injection
    A. intralesional injection
arithmetic method
Arkless-Graham syndrome
arm
    a. board
    a. circumference
    a. dysfunction
    nuchal a.
    a. of chromosome
    parallel study a.
    a. position
    a. presentation
    a. recoil
    sling a.
    a. span
armamentarium
armboard (*var. of* arm board)
ARMS
    acoustic respiratory motion sensor
Army-Navy retractor
ARND
    alcohol-related neurodevelopmental
      disorder
Arnold-Chiari
    A.-C. anomaly
    A.-C. deformity
    A.-C. malformation
    A.-C. syndrome
AROM
    active range of motion
    artificial rupture of membranes
Aromasin
aromatase inhibitor
aromatherapy
aromatization

arousal
    a. center
    confusional a.
    a. disorder
    a. level
    sexual a.
ARPKD
    autosomal recessive polycystic kidney disease
ARPTH
    autosomal recessive renal proximal tubulopathy and hypercalciuria
array
    density spectral a.
    superficial linear a. (SLA)
arrayed library
arrest
    active phase a.
    cardiac a.
    circulatory a.
    deep hypothermia and total circulatory a. (DHCA)
    deep hypothermic circulatory a.
    deep transverse a.
    a. disorder
    follicular development a.
    growth a.
    midplane a.
    a. of labor
    physial a.
    preterm labor a.
    puberal a.
    respiratory a.
    secondary a.
    sinus a.
    transverse a.
arrest/akinetic fit
arrested
    a. development
    a. hydrocephalus
arrhenoblastoma
arrhinencephalia (*var. of* arhinencephaly)
arrhinencephaly (*var. of* arhinencephaly)
arrhinia (*var. of* arhinia)
arrhythmia
    cardiac a.
    clinically significant a. (CSA)
    digitalis-induced a.
    fetal a.
    late a.
    malignant a.
    nonspecific a. (NSA)
    primary cardiac a.
    respiratory sinus a.
    sinus a.
    Xylocaine HCl I.V. Injection for Cardiac A.'s
arrhythmic twitching
arrhythmogenesis

arrhythmogenic
    a. right ventricular dysplasia (ARVD)
    a. syncope
arrival
    born on a. (BOA)
Arrow catheter
ARSA
    aberrant right subclavian artery
arsenic
    a. nickel silicon
    a. poisoning
arsenical
    organic a.
ART
    assisted reproductive technology
    automated reagin test
    ART treatment
Artane
artefact (*var. of* artifact)
Artemisinin
arterenol
arteria (*var. of* artery)
arterial
    a. aneurysm
    a. banding
    a. blood gas (ABG)
    a. blood pressure (ABP)
    a. blood sample (ABS)
    a. calcification
    a. cannulation
    a. catheter
    a. ectasia
    a. embolization
    a. fibrosing sclerosis
    a. lactate
    a. ligation
    a. linear density
    a. line flush solution
    a. obstruction
    a. occlusive disease (AOD)
    a. oxygen delivery (DO_2)
    a. partial pressure (Pa)
    a. pressure
    a. puncture
    a. retransposition
    a. rupture
    a. spasm
    a. stick
    a. supply
    a. switch operation
    a. switch procedure
    a. thrombosis
    a. to alveolar (a-A)
    a. to alveolar oxygen tension ratio
    a. transposition
    a. vascular bed
    a. vascular disease
    a. waveform

arterial-ascitic fluid pH gradient
arterialized blood
arteriogram
    pelvic a.
    pulmonary a.
arteriography
    selective pulmonary a.
arteriohepatic dysplasia (AHD)
arteriola (*var. of* arteriole)
arteriolar occlusion
arteriole, arteriola
    pulmonary a.
arteriolitis
    necrotizing a.
arteriolopathy
    decidual a.
arteriomesenteric duodenal compression syndrome
arteriopathy
arterioplasty
arterioportal fistula
arteriosclerosis
    infantile a.
arteriosus
    ductus a. (DA)
    machinery murmur in patent ductus a.
    patent ductus a. (PDA)
    right ductus a. (RDA)
    truncus a.
    Van Praagh classification of truncus a.
arteriovenous (AV)
    a. anastomosis
    a. canal defect
    a. fistula
    a. fistula malformation (AVFM)
    a. malformation (AVM)
    a. oxygen difference
    a. shunt
arteritis
    familial granulomatous a.
    giant cell a.
    inflammatory a.
    necrotizing a.
    Takayasu a. (TA)
    a. umbilicalis
artery, arteria
    aberrant coronary a.
    aberrant right subclavian a. (ARSA)
    aberrant subclavian a.
    aberrant systemic feeding a.
    absence of branch pulmonary a.
    acinar a.
    allantoic a.
    anomalous coronary a.
    anomalous left coronary artery from pulmonary a. (ALCAPA)
    anomalous left pulmonary a.

appendicular a.
arcuate a.
basal a.
brachial a.
caliber-persistent a.
carotid a.
celiac a.
central retinal a.
cervical a.
circumflex a.
coiled a.
colic a.
complete transposition of great arteries
deep circumflex iliac a.
discordant umbilical arteries
D-transposition of great arteries (D-TGA)
endometrial spiral a.
epigastric a.
external iliac a.
femoral circumflex a.
fetal cranial a.
a. forceps
gastroepiploic a. (GEA)
great arteries
hemorrhoidal a.
hypogastric a.
ileocolic a.
iliac a.
iliofemoral a.
inferior epigastric a.
inferior mesenteric a.
innominate a.
intercostal perforating a.
interior epigastric a.
internal iliac a.
internal mammary a.
internal pudendal a.
Kugel a.
lateral thoracic a.
left main coronary a.
L-transposition of great arteries (L-TGA)
lumbar a.
major aortopulmonary collateral a. (MAPCA)
mesenteric a.
middle cerebral a. (MCA)
middle sacral a.
obliterated umbilical a.
obturator a.
a. of Adamkiewicz
a. of Sampson
omphalomesenteric a.
ovarian a.
Parrot a.
pelvic a.
perineal a.

artery (*continued*)
    posterior inferior cerebellar a. (PICA)
    posterior labial arteries
    proximal pulmonary a.
    pudendal a.
    pulmonary a. (PA)
    radial a.
    right common carotid a. (RCCA)
    right femoral a. (RFA)
    sinuatrial node a.
    spiral endometrial a.
    subclavian a.
    superficial circumflex iliac a.
    superficial epigastric a.
    superficial external pudendal a. (SEPA)
    superior epigastric a.
    superior mesenteric a.
    thalamostriatal a.
    thoracoacromial a.
    thoracodorsal a.
    transposition of great arteries (TGA)
    umbilical a. (UA)
    uterine a.
    vaginal a.
    vertebral a.

arthralgia
    psychogenic a.

arthritides (*pl. of* **arthritis**)

arthritis, *pl.* **arthritides**
    candidal a.
    chronic juvenile a.
    degenerative a.
    gonococcal a.
    gouty a.
    hematogenous septic a.
    idiopathic chronic a.
    infectious a.
    juvenile a. (JA)
    juvenile chronic a. (JCA)
    juvenile idiopathic a. (JIA)
    juvenile idiopathic polyarticular a.
    juvenile psoriatic a.
    juvenile rheumatoid a. (JRA)
    juvenile rheumatoid a. (type I, II) (JRA)
    Lyme a.
    migratory peripheral a.
    monarticular a.
    mumps a.
    neonatal septic a.
    a. of rheumatic fever
    oligoarticular a.
    pauciarticular juvenile chronic a.
    pauciarticular-onset juvenile a.
    peripheral a.
    polyarticular juvenile chronic a.
    postdysenteric a.
    postenteritis a.
    postinfectious a.
    poststreptococcal reactive a.
    Pseudomonas septic a.
    psoriasis-associated a.
    psoriatic a.
    purulent a.
    pyogenic a.
    reactive a.
    rheumatoid a. (RA)
    septic a.
    spondylitis, enthesitis, a. (SEA)
    suppurative a.
    systemic juvenile chronic a.
    systemic-onset juvenile rheumatoid a.
    viral a.
    Yersinia a.

arthritis-dermatitis syndrome
Arthrobacter globiformis
arthrocentesis
arthrochalasis multiplex congenita
arthrodentoosteodysplasia (ADOD)
arthrodesis
    Dennyson-Fulford extraarticular subtalar a.
    triple a.

arthrogram
    air a.

arthrography
arthrogryposis
    distal a. (type I, II)
    a., ectodermal dysplasia, cleft lip/palate developmental delay syndrome
    fetal a.
    a. multiplex
    a. multiplex congenita (AMC)
    skeletal a.

arthrogryposis-like hand anomaly
arthrogrypotic clubfoot
arthroophthalmopathy (AO, AOM)
    hereditary progressive a.

Arthropan
arthropathy
    hemophilic a.
    human parvovirus a.
    sensory a.
    seronegativity, enthesopathy, a. (SEA)

arthropod-borne virus
arthropod-induced blister
arthrosis
Arthus reaction
articular
articulate
articulation
    calcaneonavicular a.
    compensatory a.
    cricoarytenoid a.
    a. disorder

artifact, artefact
    cultural a.
    deodorant a.
    point-spread a.
    technical a.
artificial
    a. anal sphincter
    a. ankylosis
    a. chromosome
    a. erection
    a. fever
    a. insemination (AI)
    a. insemination by donor (AID)
    a. insemination by husband (AIH)
    a. insemination donor (AID)
    a. insemination with donor sperm
    a. intravaginal insemination
    a. lung-expanding compound
      (ALEC)
    a. pacemaker
    a. respiration
    a. rupture of membranes (AROM)
    a. spermatocele
    a. sphincter implantation
    a. temperature
    a. urethral sphincter (AUS)
    a. urinary sphincter
    a. vagina
    a. vaginal epithelium
Arts syndrome
ARV
  acquired immunodeficiency
  syndrome-related virus
ARVD
  arrhythmogenic right ventricular
  dysplasia
Arvee Medical model 2400 infant apnea monitor
aryepiglottic fold, arytenoepiglottidean fold
arylalkanoic acid
arylcarboxylic acid
arylpropionic acid
arylsulfatase
arylsulfatase-activator deficiency
arytenoepiglottidean fold
arytenoid
arytenoidopexy
    King a.
arzoxifene
as
    a. low as reasonably achievable
      (ALARA)
ASA
  acetylsalicylic acid
  American Society of Anesthesiologists
    MSD Enteric Coated ASA
asaccharolyticus
    Peptococcus a.

Asacol Oral
AS
  Asperger syndrome
  Duracillin AS
ASB
  asymptomatic bacteriuria
  ASB syndrome
ASC
  abdominal sacral colpopexy
  altered state of consciousness
  antibody-secreting cell
  asthma symptom checklist
  atypical squamous cell
A-scan
ascariasis, ascaridiasis, ascaridosis, ascariosis
    pulmonary a.
ascaridiasis (*var. of* ascariasis)
ascaridosis (*var. of* ascariasis)
ascariosis (*var. of* ascariasis)
Ascaris lumbricoides
ASCCP
  American Society for Colposcopy and
    Cervical Pathology
ascending
    a. cholangiopathy
    a. cholangitis
    a. colon
    a. intrauterine infection
    a. radiculomyelitis
    a. reticular activating system
      (ARAS)
    a. venography
ascensus
ascertainment
    total a.
ASC-H
  atypical squamous cells-cannot exclude
    high-grade lesion
  high-grade squamous intraepithelial
    lesion
Ascher syndrome
Aschheim-Zondek (AZ)
    A.-Z. test
aschistodactylia
Aschoff
    A. body
    A. nodule
ascites
    biliary a.
    chylous a.
    congenital neonatal a.
    culture-negative neutrocytic a.
    eosinophilic a.
    exudative a.
    fetal a.
    lues a.
    massive a.
    refractory a.

ascites (*continued*)
    tense a.
    tumor a.
ascitic fluid
ASCO
    American Society of Clinical
    Oncology
ascorbate
ascorbic
    a. acid
    a. acid deficiency
Ascriptin A/D
ASCUS
    atypical squamous cells of
    undetermined significance
    ASCUS smear
ASCUS/LSIL Triage Study
ASD
    acute stress disorder
    atrial septal defect
    autism spectrum disorder
    autistic spectrum disorder
    canal type ASD
    ostium primum ASD
    ostium secundum ASD
    ostium venosus ASD
ASDA
    American Sleep Disorders
    Association
aseptic
    a. fever
    a. meningitis
    a. meningitis syndrome
    a. meningoencephalitis
    a. necrosis
    a. necrosis of bone
    a. preparation
    a. temperature
Asepto syringe
asexual dwarfism
ASG
    Adhesion Scoring Group
    ASG system
A-200 Shampoo
Asherman syndrome
Ashkenazi
    A. Jew
    A. Jewish cancer susceptibility
    mutation
    A. Jewish heritage
ash-leaf
    a.-l. macule
    a.-l. spot
Ashworth
    A. score
    A. score of spasticity
ASI
    active specific immunotherapy
    anxiety sensitivity index

ASIL
    anal squamous intraepithelial lesion
Askanazy cell
Askin tumor
Ask-Upmark kidney
ASL
    American Sign Language
Aslan
    A. endoscopic scissors
    A. 2-mm minilaparoscope
ASLD
    adenylosuccinate lyase deficiency
ASO
    antistreptolysin O
    ASO antibody
    ASO assay
asoma
asoprisnil
asparaginase
asparagine
aspartate
    a. aminotransferase (AST)
    amphetamine a.
    a. transaminase (AST)
aspartic acid
aspartoacylase hydrolytic activity
aspartylglucosamine (AGA)
aspartylglucosaminidase
aspartylglucosaminuria (AGU)
A-Spas S/L
ASPD
    antisocial personality disorder
ASPED
    angel-shaped phalangoepiphysial
    dysplasia
aspen
    A. laparoscopy electrode
    A. ultrasound platform
ASPEN
    American Society for Parenteral and
    Enteral Nutrition
Asperger
    A. disorder
    A. syndrome (AS)
aspergilloma
aspergillosis
    allergic bronchopulmonary a.
    (ABPA)
    bronchopulmonary a.
    cerebral a.
    fatal cutaneous a.
    ocular a.
    pulmonary a.
Aspergillus
    A. *flavus*
    A. *fumigatus*
    A. *nidulans*
    A. *niger*
    A. *terreus*

Aspergum
aspermatogenesis
aspermia
asphyctic infant
asphyxia
    acute total a.
    antepartum a.
    autoerotic a.
    birth a.
    blue a.
    fetal a.
    intrapartum a.
    intrauterine a.
    a. livida
    neonatal a.
    a. neonatorum
    a. pallida
    perinatal a.
    prenatal a.
    prolonged partial a.
    sexual a.
asphyxial
    a. birth injury
    a. brain injury
    a. event
asphyxiating
    a. thoracic chondrodystrophy
    a. thoracic dysplasia
    a. thoracic dysplasia syndrome
    a. thoracic dystrophy (ATD)
    a. thoracic dystrophy syndrome
asphyxiation
    intrapartum a.
aspiny interneuron
aspirate
    blood-flecked gastric a.
    bone marrow a. (BMA)
    bubo a.
    nasogastric a.
    nasopharyngeal a. (NPA)
    surveillance tracheal a.
    tracheal a.
    tracheobronchial a.
aspiration
    amniotic fluid a.
    a. biopsy
    a. biopsy cytology (ABC)
    bone marrow a.
    caustic a.
    chronic a.
    cyst a.
    electric vacuum a. (EVA)
    epididymal sperm a. (ESA)
    fine-needle a. (FNA)
    foreign body a.
    gastric fluid a.
    manual vacuum a. (MVA)
    maxillary sinus a.
    meconium a.

    menstrual a.
    metaphysial a.
    microsurgical epididymal sperm a.
      (MESA)
    needle a.
    a. of gastric contents
    a. of mature oocyte
    percutaneous cyst a.
    percutaneous epididymal sperm a.
      (PESA)
    a. pneumonia
    a. pneumonitis
    a. prophylaxis
    pulmonary a.
    rete testis a. (RETA)
    sperm a.
    subperiosteal a.
    suction a.
    suprapubic bladder a.
    a. syndrome
    testicular sperm a. (TESA)
    transtracheal a.
    Vabra a.
    vacuum a.
aspiration-tulip device
aspirator
    Aspirette endocervical a.
    BBG nasal a.
    blunt a.
    Cavitron ultrasonic surgical a.
      (CUSA)
    Cook a.
    electric vacuum a.
    Endo-Assist sponge a.
    endocervical a.
    endometrial a.
    GynoSampler endometrial a.
    manual vacuum a.
    mucus a.
    nasal a.
    Nezhat-Dorsey a.
    Sharplan USA ultrasonic
      surgical a.
    Vabra cervical a.
    vacuum a.
Aspirette endocervical aspirator
aspirin
    Bayer A.
    buffered a.
    oxycodone and a.
    a. triad
Aspirols
    Amyl Nitrite A.
asplenia
    anatomic a.
    congenital a.
    functional a.
    surgical a.
    a. syndrome

asplenic
ASQ
Ages and Stages Questionnaire
ASS
Aarskog-Scott syndrome
Asthma Severity Score
ASSA
aminopterin syndrome sine aminopterin
assault
sexual a.
a. victim
assaultive
verbally a.
assay
Abbott LCx Uriprobe a.
a. accuracy
AccuStat Strep A a.
acetylcholinesterase a.
agglutination a.
Amplicor Chlamydia a.
androgen a.
antibody production a.
Aptima Combo 2 a.
ASO a.
BCA protein a.
Bethesda a.
biologic a.
CA 125 a.
CH_{50} a.
Chiron branched DNA a.
Clinitest a.
clonogenic a.
Coat-A-Count a.
C1q a.
cytomegalovirus total
immunoglobulin a.
Detect HIV-1 a.
Digene HPV A.
DNA hybridization a.
dot immunobinding a. (DIA)
electrophoretic mobility shift a.
(EMSA)
ELISpot a.
enzyme a.
enzyme immunosorbent a.
(EIA)
enzyme-linked immunofiltration a.
(ELIFA)
enzyme-linked immunosorbent a.
(ELISA)
estradiol a.
factor Xa inhibition a.
FAMA a.
fetal fibronectin a.
FSH MAIAclone immunoradiometric
a.
genotypic a.
Gen-Probe amplified CT a.
hamster egg penetration a.

hemagglutinin enzyme-linked
immunosorbent a. (H(c)ELISA)
hemizona a. (HZA)
HemoQuant a.
Heptest Xa a.
HerpeSelect-1 ELISA IgG a.
HerpeSelect-2 ELISA IgG a.
HerpeSelect-1 Immunoblot IgG a.
HerpeSelect-2 Immunoblot IgG a.
HIV-1 RNA PCR a.
hormone a.
Hybrid Capture DNA A.
5-hydroxyindoleacetic a.
IIF a.
immunoblot a.
immunochemiluminometric insulin a.
immunofluorescent a. (IFA)
immunofunctional a.
immunologic a.
immunoradiometric a. (IRMA)
immunosorbent agglutination a.
(ISAGA)
IMx Estradiol A.
IVAP a.
latex agglutination a.
LCR a.
ligase chain reaction a.
limulus amebocyte lysate a.
luciferase a.
lysosomal hydrolase enzyme a.
a. marker
measles virus enzyme-linked
immunosorbent a. (MV(c)ELISA)
microhemagglutination a. (MHA)
NucliSens a.
PCR a.
PIVKA-II a.
prostacyclin a.
Pyrilinks-D a.
quantitative Bethesda a.
quantitative serum drug a.
radioantigen-binding a. (RABA)
radioimmunoprecipitation a. (RIPA)
radioreceptor a.
Raji cell a.
receptor a.
Recombigen a.
recombinant immunosorbent a.
(RIBA)
respiratory burst a.
ristocetin cofactor a.
Roche Amplicor Monitor a.
salivary cortisol a.
sandwich a.
a. sensitivity
serum a.
serum hexosaminidase a.
solid-phase enzyme-linked
immunospot a.

a. specificity
sperm penetration a. (SPA)
stem cell a.
tetrazolium dye a.
Thomsen-Friedenreich antigen a.
thyroid-stimulating hormone a.
TMA a.
transcription-mediated amplification a.
tumor-cloning a.
TUNEL a.
ultrasensitive a.
Vidas varicella zoster a.
ViraType HPV DNA typing a.
virologic a.

assembly
brush border a.
infant nasal cannula a.
  (INCA)

assertive

assessment
ABCDE a.
abuse, sexuality, safety a.
amniotic fluid a.
antenatal a.
antepartum fetal a.
Ballard gestational a.
behavioral a.
burn a.
child and adolescent burden a.
  (CABA)
Child and Adolescent Psychiatric A.
  (CAPA)
Child and Adolescent Services A.
  (CASA)
clinical risk a. (CRA)
developmental a.
Dubowitz Neurological A.
Erhardt developmental prehension a.
fetal movement a.
gestational age a.
high-risk pregnancy a.
HRQOL a.
A. in Infancy Ordinal Scales of
  Psychological Development
lipid profile a.
Lund and Browder chart for
  burn a.
maternal a.
morphologic a.
neonatal a.
neurodevelopmental a.
neuromuscular maturity a.
nutritional a.
A. of Preterm Infants' Behavior
  (APIB)
ovulation a.
perinatal a.
periodic patient a.
phallometric a.

preconception risk a.
preschool-age psychiatric a. (PAPA)
projective a.
psychometric a.
4-quadrant a.
quadrant a.
qualitative developmental a.
risk a.
rubella titer a.
Scanlon A.
school, home, activities,
  depression/self-esteem, substance
  abuse, sexuality, safety a.
serial fetal a.
social a.
sonographic a.
TOVA ADD/ADHD a.
ultrasonographic a.
ultrasound a.
young adult psychiatric a. (YAPA)

ASSI bipolar coagulating forceps

assignment
gender a.
sex a.

assimilation
atlas a.
a. pelvis

assistant
Carter Tubal A.

assist-control ventilation

assisted
a. breech
a. breech delivery
a. cephalic delivery
a. conception
a. fertilization
a. hatching (AH)
a. medical procreation (AMP)
a. reproduction
a. reproductive technology (ART)
a. spontaneous vaginal delivery
a. ventilation (AV)
a. zona hatching (AZH)

assistive technology (AT)

association
American Diabetes A. (ADA)
American Medical Women's A.
American Sleep Disorders A.
  (ASDA)
aniridia, Wilms tumor a. (AWTA)
CHARGE a.
a. constant
Endometriosis A.
A. for Retarded Citizens (ARC)
Harry Benjamin International
  Dysphoria A. (HBIGDA)
New York Heart A. (NYHA)
A. of Women's Health, Obstetrics,
  and Neonatal Nursing (AWHONN)

association (*continued*)
    a. reaction
    VACTERL a.
assortative mating
ASSQ
    autism spectrum screening questionnaire
assurance
    National Committee for Quality A. (NCQA)
AST
    acoustic stimulation test
    aspartate aminotransferase
    aspartate transaminase
astasia-abasia
astatic seizure
asteatotic eczema
Astech Peak Flow Meter
Astelin Nasal Spray
astemizole
asterixis
asteroid body
asteroides
    Nocardia a.
asthenia
asthenospermia
asthenozoospermia
asthma
    A. Action Plan
    allergen-induced a. (AIA)
    atopic a.
    bronchial a.
    cardiac a.
    chronic a.
    cold-induced a.
    a. exacerbation
    exercise-induced a. (EIA)
    gestational a.
    infantile a.
    intrinsic a.
    labile a.
    maternal a.
    a. morbidity
    nocturnal a.
    perennial a.
    seasonal a.
    A. Severity Score (ASS)
    a. symptom checklist (ASC)
    thymic a.
    a. with vasculitis
asthmatic
    a. bronchitis (AB)
    a. response
asthmaticus
    status a.
astigmatism
Astler-Coller modification of Dukes classification
astomia

astragalus
Astramorph
    A. PF
    A. PF injection
Astrand 30-beat stopwatch method
astrocyte
    fibrinoid degeneration of a.'s
    a. footplate
astrocytic gliosis
astrocytoma
    anaplastic pilocytic a.
    chiasmatic pilocytic a.
    diffuse a.
    fibrillary a.
    a. (grade I–IV)
    juvenile pilocytic a.
    low-grade diffuse a.
    low-grade fibrillary a.
    malignant pilocytic a.
    pilocytic fibrillary a.
Astroglide personal lubricant
astrogliosis
astrovirus infection
Astrup blood gas value
asymbolia for pain
asymmetric, asymmetrical
    a. crying facies (ACF)
    a. growth restriction
    a. hyperopia
    a. IUGR
    a. muscle imbalance
    a. nystagmus
    a. palatal paresis
    a. short stature syndrome
    a. small foramen magnum
    a. tonic neck reflex (ATNR)
asymmetrical (*var. of* asymmetric)
    a. conjoined twins
asymmetrically
asymmetros
    syncephalus a.
asymmetrus
    janiceps a.
asymmetry
    facial a.
    left/right a.
    nasolabial fold a.
    a. of face
    truncal a.
asymptomatic
    a. bacteriuria (ASB)
    a. dehiscence
    a. infection
    a. infertility
    a. mild endometriosis
    a. myoma
    a. urinary tract infection (AUTI)
    a. viral shedding
asynapsis

asynchronous
  a. birth
  a. intermittent mandatory
    ventilation
  a. multifetal delivery
  a. puberty
**asynchronously shedding
  endometrium**
asynchrony
  marked a.
asynclitic
  a. position
  a. position of fetus
asynclitism
  anterior a.
  posterior a.
asynergia
  cerebellar a.
asystole, asystolia
asystolia (*var. of* asystole)
AT3
  antithrombin III
  AT3 coagulation inhibitor
  AT3 deficiency (types I, II)
atactic (*var. of* ataxic)
atactica
  heredopathia a.
Atad Ripener device
Atarax
ataxia, ataxy
  acute cerebellar a.
  acute childhood a.
  acute recurrent a.
  adult-onset spinocerebellar a.
  cerebellar a.
  chronic progressive a.
  congenital a.
  dominant recurrent a.
  episodic a. (1, 2)
  Friedreich a.
  gait a.
  hereditary paroxysmal a.
  infantile-onset spinocerebellar a.
  Machado-Joseph a.
  myoclonic a.
  a., myoclonic encephalopathy,
    macular degeneration, recurrent
    infections syndrome
  spastic a.
  spinocerebellar a. (type 1–7)
  a. telangiectasia
  transient cerebellar a.
  truncal a.
  a. with isolated vitamin E
    deficiency
  X-linked cerebellar a. (CLA)
ataxia-deafness-retardation (ADR)
  a.-d.-r. syndrome with ketoaciduria
ataxia-deafness syndrome

ataxia-microcephaly-cataract (AMC)
ataxia-oculomotor apraxia
ataxia-telangiectasia (AT)
  a.-t. syndrome
ataxic, atactic
  a. cerebral palsy
  a. gait
ataxy (*var. of* ataxia)
atazanavir
ATD
  antithyroid drug
  asphyxiating thoracic dystrophy
  ATD gel
atelectasis
  congenital a.
  linear a.
  massive a.
  obstructive a.
  plate-like a.
  primary a.
  resorption a.
  secondary a.
  subsegmental a.
atelectatic
atelectrauma
atelencephalia, atelencephaly
atelencephalic syndrome
atelencephaly (*var. of* atelencephalia)
atelia
ateliosis, atelia
ateliotic dwarfism
atelocardia
atelocephaly
atelocheiria
ateloglossia
atelognathia
atelomyelia
atelopodia
atelosteogenesis
atelostomia
atenolol
ATFL
  anterior talofibular ligament
Atgam
athelia
atherectomy
  directional coronary a. (DCA)
atherogenesis
atherogenic
atherosclerosis
  accelerated a.
atherosis
  acute a.
  decidual arteriolar a.
athetoid
  a. cerebral palsy
  a. movement
athetosis
  congenital a.

athetotic
  a. movement disorder
  a. posturing
athlete's foot
athletica
  anorexia a.
athletic amenorrhea
at-home activity restriction
athyrea (*var. of* athyroidism)
athyreotic (*var. of* athyrotic)
athyroid
athyroidism, athyrea
athyrotic, athyreotic
  a. cretinism
  a. hypothyroidism
  a. neonate
Ativan
Atkin-Flaitz-Patil syndrome
Atkin-Flaitz syndrome
Atkins diet
ATL
  Achilles tendon lengthening
  ATL HDI 3000 ultrasound system
  A.TL Ultramark 4,8,9 ultrasound
Atlanta Scottish Rite Hospital orthosis
atlantoaxial (AA)
  a. dislocation
  a. instability
  a. rotary subluxation
atlantodens interval (ADI)
atlantodidymus
atlantooccipital dislocation
atlas
  a. assimilation
  Greulich and Pyle radiographic a.
ATLL
  adult T-cell leukemia/lymphoma
ATLS
  advanced trauma life support
ATN
  acute tubular necrosis
ATNR
  asymmetric tonic neck reflex
ATOD
  alcohol, tobacco, and other drugs
atomic
  a. absorption spectrometer
  a. absorption spectrophotometry
  a. absorption spectroscopy
  a. milk
Atomlab 200 dose calibrator
atomoxetine
atonia (*var. of* atony)
atonic
  a. astatic diplegia
  a. cerebral palsy
  a. seizure
atony, atonia
  bowel a.

  diaphragmatic a.
  gastric a.
  uterine a.
atopic
  a. asthma
  a. child
  a. dermatitis
  a. diaper rash
  a. eczema
  a. erythroderma
  a. triad
atopy
atosiban
atovaquone
ATP
  adenosine triphosphate
  deoxy ATP
ATPase
  adenosine triphosphatase
atra
  Stachybotrys a.
atracurium besylate
atransferrinemia
  congenital a.
atraumatic forceps
AT1 receptor
AT2 receptor
atresia
  anal a.
  aortic valve a.
  apple-peel a.
  aural a.
  bilateral a.
  biliary a. (BA)
  bronchial a.
  cervical a.
  a. choanae
  choanal a.
  congenital aural a.
  congenital duodenal a.
  de la Cruz classification of
    congenital aural a.
  distal esophageal a.
  duodenal a.
  esophageal a. (EA)
  extrahepatic biliary a.
  a. folliculi
  functional pulmonary a.
  gastrointestinal a.
  ileal a.
  intestinal a.
  intrahepatic biliary a.
  jejunal a.
  jejunoileal a.
  laryngeal a.
  mitral valve a.
  a. of foramina of Luschka and
    Magendie
  a. of larynx

oocyte a.
primary repair of esophageal a.
pulmonary artery a.
pure esophageal a.
pyloric a.
Schuknecht classification of
  congenital aural a. (type A–D)
small bowel a.
tracheal a.
tracheoesophageal a.
tricuspid a.
urethral a.
vaginal a.

atretic
a. cervix
a. extrahepatic bile duct resection
a. follicle
a. gallbladder
a. ureter
a. vagina
atretocormus
atretocystia
atretogastria
atria (*pl. of* atrium)
atrial
a. bigeminy
a. contraction
a. fibrillation
a. flutter
a. hypertrophy
a. inversion procedure
a. natriuretic factor (ANF)
a. natriuretic hormone
a. natriuretic peptide (ANP)
a. premature contraction (APC)
a. premature depolarization
a. septal defect (ASD)
a. septectomy
a. septoplasty procedure
a. septostomy
a. septostomy procedure
a. septostomy via balloon
a. septum excision
a. shunt
a. switch operation
a. switch procedure
a. tachyarrhythmia
a. tachycardia
atriodigital dysplasia
atriotomy
atrioventricular (AV)
a. block
a. canal
a. canal defect
a. conduction delay
a. discordance
a. dissociation
a. nodal reentrant tachycardia
  (AVNRT)

a. node
a. node function
a. reciprocating tachycardia (AVRT)
a. septal defect
a. septum
a. shunt
a. valve
at-risk
a.-r. infant
a.-r. pregnancy
atrium, *pl.* **atria**
common a.
left a.
ventricles to a.
atrophia (*var. of* atrophy)
a. bulborum hereditaria
atrophic
a. change
a. endometrium
a. patch
a. urethritis
a. vaginal mucosa
a. vaginitis
a. vulvitis
atrophicae
lineae a.
striae a.
atrophicans
acrodermatitis chronica a.
atrophicus
lichen sclerosus et a. (LS)
atrophy, atrophia
Behr optic a.
brain a.
central a.
cerebral a.
congenital microvillus a.
cortical a.
corticosteroid-induced a.
cutaneous a.
Dejerine-Sottas a.
dentatorubral a.
dentatorubral-pallidoluysian a.
  (DRPLA)
diabetes insipidus, diabetes mellitus,
  optic a. (DIDMO)
disuse muscular a.
endometrial a.
epithelial a.
familial muscular a.
familial olivopontocerebellar a.
Fazio-Londe a.
focal a.
frontotemporal cortical a.
gastric a.
generalized gray matter a.
generalized white matter a.
genitourinary a.
gyral a.

atrophy (*continued*)
    gyrate a.
    hereditary optic neuron a.
    hereditary spinal muscular a.
    infantile cerebellooptic a.
    infantile progressive spinal muscular
      a. (type I–III)
    infantile spinal muscular a. (ISMA)
    intestinal villous a.
    juvenile spinal muscular a. (JSMA)
    Kjer-type dominant optic a.
    Leber hereditary a.
    leg a.
    Leydig cell a.
    limb girdle muscular weakness
      and a.
    linear a.
    macular a.
    microvillus a. (MVA)
    muscle a.
    muscular a.
    neurogenic a.
    olivopontocerebellar a. (OPCA)
    optic nerve a.
    Parrot a.
    partial villus a.
    perifascicular a.
    peroneal muscular a.
    postmenopausal a.
    primary macular a.
    progressive encephalopathy, edema,
      hypsarrhythmia, optic a. (PEHO)
    secondary macular a.
    skin a.
    spinal muscle a.
    spinal muscular a. (SMA)
    Sudeck a.
    syndrome of cerebral a.
    testicular a.
    total villous a.
    traction a.
    tubular a.
    urogenital a. (UGA)
    vaginal a.
    villous a.
    vulvar a.
    vulvovaginal a.
    Werdnig-Hoffmann muscular a.
atropine
    a. cromolyn
    diphenoxylate and a.
    a. sulfate
Atropine-Care Ophthalmic
Atropisol Ophthalmic
Atrovent
    A. Aerosol Inhalation
    A. Inhalation Solution
    A. Nasal Spray
ATRX syndrome

A/T/S Topical
ATT
    arginine tolerance test
attaching process
attachment
    abnormal aortic valve a.
    dismissing a.
    a. disorder
    disturbance of a.
    gubernacular a.
    maternal-infant a.
    nonautonomous a.
    a. parenting
    prosthetic a.
    secure a.
    testicular a.
attack
    absence a.
    cataplectic a.
    drop a.
    grand mal a.
    lightning a.
    migrainous a.
    narcoleptic a.
    panic a.
    paroxysmal hypercyanotic a.
    petit mal a.
    shuddering a.
    sleep a.
    Stokes-Adams a.
    transient ischemic a. (TIA)
attapulgite
attempted suicide
attending skill
attention
    a. deficit
    a. deficit disorder (ADD)
    A. Deficit Disorders Evaluation
      Scale
    a. deficit hyperactivity disorder
      (ADHD)
    joint a.
    a. span
    Test of Variables of A.
      (TOVA)
attentional difficulty
attention-distractibility problem
attenuated
    a. androgen
    live a.
    a. pyloric canal
attenuating tissue
attenuation
Attenuvax
Attia score
attitude
    a. behavior questionnaire (ABQ)
    fetal a.
    postpartum a.

attorney
    durable power of a.
attrition
    acute-phase a.
    follicular a.
    a. rate scale
    sperm a.
attunement
    affect a.
Attwood staining method
atypia
    bowenoid a.
    cervical a.
    cytologic a.
    glandular a.
    koilocytic a.
    koilocytotic a.
    nuclear a.
    vulvar a.
atypica
    Veillonella a.
atypical
    a. absence
    a. absence seizure
    a. adenomatous hyperplasia
    a. algorithm
    a. aneuploidy
    a. antipsychotic drug
    a. chondrodystrophy
    a. depression
    a. ductal hyperplasia (ADH)
    a. endosalpingiosis
    a. epithelium
    a. febrile seizure
    a. glandular cell
    a. glandular cells of uncertain significance (AGCUS)
    a. glandular cells of undetermined significance (AGCUS, AGUS)
    a. hemolytic uremia syndrome
    a. hyperplasia
    a. interest
    a. karyotype
    a. Kawasaki disease
    a. lobular hyperplasia
    a. measles
    a. melanocytic nevus
    a. mycobacteria
    a. petit mal seizure
    a. squamous cell (ASC)
    a. squamous cells-cannot exclude high-grade lesion (ASC-H)
    a. squamous cells of undetermined significance (ASCUS)
    a. squamous cells of undetermined significance/atypical glandular cells of undetermined significance
    a. teratoid/rhabdoid tumor
    a. teratoid tumor
    a. teratoma
    a. vasculature
    a. vessel colposcopic pattern
^{198}Au
    gold-198
AUB
    abnormal uterine bleeding
Auchincloss modified radical mastectomy
audible stridor
Audio Doppler D920
audiogram
audiological testing
audiologist
audiology
audiometer
    Pilot a.
audiometric
    a. evaluation
    a. examination
    a. testing
audiometry
    behavioral a.
    behavioral observation a. (BOA)
    brainstem evoked response a. (BSERA)
    conditioned play a.
    evoked response a. (ERA)
    impedance a.
    visual reinforcement a. (VRA)
    visual response a. (VRA)
AudioScope
    Welch Allyn A.
AUDIT
    Alcohol Use Disorders Identification Test
auditory
    a. agnosia
    a. brainstem response (ABR, ABSR)
    a. canal
    a. discrimination
    a. dysfunction
    a. evoked potential (AEP)
    a. evoked response (AER)
    a. impairment
    integrated visual and a. (IVA)
    a. integration thinking (AIT)
    a. integration training (AIT)
    a. learner
    a. meatus
    a. nerve
    a. ossicles
    a. response cradle
    a. response to bell
    a. training
audouinii
    Microsporum a.
Auerbach plexus
Aufricht nasal retractor

augmentation
    bladder a.
    colocecal bladder a.
    a. cystoplasty
    intestinal bladder a.
    labor a.
    a. mammaplasty
    oxytocin a.
    Pitocin a.
    submucosal urethral a.
    transumbilical breast a. (TUBA)
    a. ureterocystoplasty
    Wise areola mastopexy breast a.
    (WAMBA)
augmentative
    a. and alternative communication
    (AAC)
    a. communication device
augmented breast
Augmentin ES
augnathus
AUM
    ambulatory urodynamic
    monitoring
aura
    epileptic a.
    migraine with a.
    migraine without a.
    somatosensory a.
    viscerosensory a.
    visual a.
aural
    a. atresia
    a. atresia and microtia
    a. polyp
    a. temperature
Auralgan
auramine
auramine-rhodamine stain
auranofin
aureus
    borderline-resistant *Staphylococcus a.*
    (BRSA)
    community-acquired
    methicillin-resistant *Staphylococcus*
    a. (CAMRSA)
    methicillin-resistant *Staphylococcus a.*
    (MRSA)
    Staphylococcus a.
    Streptococcus a.
    vancomycin intermediate-resistant
    Staphylococcus a. (VISA)
    vancomycin-resistant *Staphylococcus*
    a. (VRSA)
AUR-7 flexible ureteroscope
auricle
    accessory a.
auricular
    a. abscess

    a. hematoma
    a. seroma
auriculoosteodysplasia
Auro ear drops
Aurolate
Aurora MR breast imaging system
aurothioglucose
Auroto
AUS
    artificial urethral sphincter
auscultation
    abdominal a.
    chest percussion and a.
    obstetric a.
    periodic a.
Auspitz sign
Austin
    A. Flint murmur
    A. syndrome
Australia antigen
australis
    Rickettsia a.
authority
    Human Fertilization and Embryology
    A. (HFEA)
AUTI
    asymptomatic urinary tract infection
autism
    a., dementia, ataxia, loss of
    purposeful hand use syndrome
    A. Diagnostic Interview (ADI)
    A. Diagnostic Interview-Revised
    (ADI-R)
    A. Diagnostic Observation Schedule
    (ADOS)
    early infantile a.
    high-functioning a. (HFA)
    infantile a. (IA)
    a. spectrum disorder (ASD)
    a. spectrum screening questionnaire
autism-fragile X syndrome (AFRAX)
autistic
    a. behavior
    a. disorder
    a. enterocolitis
    a. spectrum disorder (ASD)
    a. syndrome
autistic-like behavior
auto
    A. Suture ABBI system
    A. Suture Multifire Endo GIA
    stapler
    A. Syringe
autoamputate
autoamputation of ovary
autoantibody
    anti-D a.
    anti-Scl-70 a.
    E a.

Kell a.
thyroid a.
typhoid a.
warm a.
autoantigen
La (SS-B) a.
Ro/SSA a.
autoaugmentation
laparoscopic laser-assisted a.
autobiographical memory
auto-brewery syndrome
autochthonous tumor
autoclave
autocrine
a. communication
a. motility factor (AMF)
autocrine-acting growth factor
autocrine/paracrine-acting growth factor
AutoCyte System
AutoDELFIA
A. PRL molecule kit
A. unconjugated E3 kit
autodilation
autoeczematization
autoerotic asphyxia
autofluorescent
autogamy
autogenous vaccine
autograft
free tracheal a.
autohemolysis
autoimmune
a. acquired hemolytic anemia
a. adrenalitis
a. chronic acute hepatitis
a. cytopenia
a. disease
a. disease of vulva
a. enteropathy (AIE)
a. factor
a. glomerulonephritis
a. hemolytic anemia (AIHA)
a. interstitial nephritis
a. lymphoproliferative syndrome (ALPS)
a. mechanism
a. myasthenia gravis
a. neutropenia (AIN)
a. neutropenia of infancy (ANI)
a. oophoritis
a. polyendocrine syndrome
a. polyendocrinopathy, candidiasis, ectodermal dystrophy (APECED)
a. polyglandular syndrome
a. regulator (AIRE)
a. regulator gene
a. thrombocytopenia
a. thrombocytopenic purpura (AITP)
a. thyroiditis

autoimmune-associated congenital heart block
autoimmunity
autoinfarction
Auto-Injector
autoinoculation
autologous
a. blood donation
a. blood transfusion
a. BMT
a. bone marrow reinfusion
a. bone marrow transplantation
a. cord blood
a. ovarian transplant
a. reconstruction
a. stem cell transplantation
autolysis
automated
a. auditory brainstem response (AABR)
a. brainstem auditory evoked response (ABAER)
a. computerized axial tomography (ACAT)
a. hematocrit
a. multiple analysis
a. radiometric technique
a. reagin test (ART)
automatic
a. atrial tachycardia
a. karyotype system database
a. movement reaction
a. reflex
a. walking
automaticity
automatism
motor a.
autonomic
a. crisis
a. dysregulation
a. innervation
a. nerve tumor
a. nervous system (ANS)
a. nervous system dysfunction (ANSD)
a. neuropathy
a. seizure
a. walking reflex
autonomous
a. ovarian follicular cyst
a. replication sequence
autonomy
AutoPap
A. 300
A. automated screening device
A. 300 QC system
A. reader
A. Screening System

auto-PEEP
    auto-positive end-expiratory pressure
Autoplex T
autopolyploid
autopolyploidy
auto-positive end-expiratory pressure (auto-PEEP)
autoprothrombin (I, II, IIA, III)
autopsy
autoradiograph
autoradiography
autoreaction
Autoread centrifuge hematology system
autoregulation
autosite
autosomal
    a. chromosome disorder
    a. congenital tubular dysgenesis
    a. deletion
    a.-dominant
    a. dominant dystrophy
    a. dominant genetic disorder
    a. dominant inheritance
    a. dominant macrocephaly syndrome
    a. dominant medullary cystic kidney disease (ADMCKD)
    a. dominant nonsyndromic hearing loss (DFNA3)
    a. dominant Opitz syndrome (ADOS)
    a. dominant polycystic disease
    a. dominant polycystic kidney disease (ADPKD)
    a. dominant retinitis pigmentosa (adRP)
    a. dominant trait
    a. gene
    a. heredity
    a. monosomy
    a. recessive (AR)
    a. recessive disorder
    a. recessive inheritance
    a. recessive muscular dystrophy
    a. recessive mutation
    a.-recessive nonsyndromic hearing loss (DFNB1)
    a. recessive ocular Ehlers-Danlos syndrome
    a. recessive polycystic kidney disease (ARPKD)
    a. recessive renal proximal tubulopathy and hypercalciuria (ARPTH)
    a. recessive trait
    a. trisomy
autosome
    balanced rearrangement of a.
    group C a.
    a. translocation

autosplenectomized
autosplenectomy
autostapling device
autotransfusion
Auvard speculum
auxiliary orthotopic liver transplantation
auxometry
auxotyping
AV
    AV malformation
    AV nodal reentry tachycardia
    AV node dysfunction
    AV node
AV/AF
    anteverted and anteflexed
    AV/AF uterus
Avagard instant hand antiseptic
avascular
    a. necrosis (AVN)
    a. space of Graves
avascularity
    periungual a.
AVB
    abnormal vaginal bleeding
AVC
    AVC Cream
    AVC suppository
A-V dissociation
Aveeno Cleansing Bar
Aventyl Hydrochloride
average
    a. blood loss
    a. for gestational age (AGA)
    pure-tone a. (PTA)
    a. radiation dose
aversive
AVFM
    arteriovenous fistula malformation
Aviane
Aviane-28 tablet
Avicidin
Avirax
Avita
Avitene hemostatic material
avium
    Mycobacterium a.
avium-intracellulare
    Mycobacterium a.-i. (MAI)
Aviva mammography system
AVL 9110 pH analyzer
AVM
    arteriovenous malformation
AVN
    avascular necrosis
AVNRT
    atrioventricular nodal reentrant tachycardia
avoidance
    a. behavior

phobic a.
school a.
avoidant disorder
Avonex
AVP
arginine vasopressin
Aqueous AVP
AVPU
alertness, response to voice, response
to pain, unresponsive
AVRT
atrioventricular reciprocating
tachycardia
avulse
avulsion
dental a.
a. fracture
a. injury
avuncular relationship
awake and active state
awareness
inadequate body a.
phonemic a.
AWHONN
Association of Women's Health,
Obstetrics, and Neonatal
Nursing
AWS
Alagille-Watson syndrome
AWTA
aniridia, Wilms tumor association
AWTA syndrome
Axenfeld
A. anomaly
A. syndrome
Axenfeld-Rieger
A.-R. anomaly
A.-R. syndrome
axes (*pl. of* axis)
axetil
cefuroxime a. (CAE)
axial
a. acetabular index (AAI)
a. hypertonia
a. load
a. mesodermal dysplasia complex
a. resolution
a. traction
Axid AR Acid Reducer
axilla, *pl.* **axillae**
axillae (*pl. of* axilla)
axillary
a. adenopathy
a. freckling
a. hair
a. hair development
a. hematoma
a. irradiation
a. irradiation therapy

a. lymphadenopathy
a. lymph node
a. node dissection (AND)
a. node sampling
a. skin lesion
a. tail
a. tail of Spence
a. temperature
a. vein
a. vein insertion site
a. view
axiom
Jackson a.
axis, *pl.* **axes**
celiac a.
conjugate a.
a. deviation
embryonic a.
gonadal a.
HPA a.
HPO a.
hypothalamic-hypophysial-ovarian-
endometrial a.
hypothalamic-pituitary a. (HPA)
hypothalamic-pituitary-gonadal a.
hypothalamic-pituitary-ovarian a.
(HPOA)
long a.
neural a.
a. of pelvis
pelvic a.
pituitary a.
P-wave a.
reproductive a.
short a.
thigh-foot a.
a. traction
transmalleolar a.
T-wave a.
axis-traction forceps
axonal
a. degeneration
a. injury
a. retraction ball
a. type
axonotmesis
axon reflex
axon-reflex function
Axotal
Ayercillin
Aygestin
Ayr
A. Nasal
A. saline drops
A. saline nasal mist
Ayre
A. spatula
A. spatula-Zelsmyr Cytobrush
technique

ayurvedic diagnosis
AZ
  Aschheim-Zondek
Azactam
5-azacytidine
azar
  kala a.
azasteroid
azatadine
azathioprine
azelastine
AZF
  azoospermia factor
AZFa region of Yq
AZFb region of Yq
AZFc region of Yq
AZH
  assisted zona hatching
azidothymidine (AZT)
azithromycin dihydrate
azlocillin
Azmacort Oral Inhaler
azo dye
Azo-Gamazole
Azo-Gantrisin
azole
  antifungal a.
  a. therapy
azoospermatism (*var. of* azoospermia)

azoospermia, azoospermatism
  deleted in a. (DAZ)
  a. factor (AZF)
  obstructive a.
  azoospermia, renal anomaly,
    cervicothoracic spine dysplasia
    (ARCS)
azoospermic man
Azorean disease
Azo-Standard
azotemia
  prerenal a.
azotemic osteodystrophy
AZT
  azidothymidine
Aztec
  A. ear
  A. idiocy
aztreonam
Azulfidine EN-tabs
azygos
  a. artery of vagina
  a. continuation of inferior vena
    cava
  a. fissure
  a. lobe of lung
  a. lobe of right lung
  a. vein
azygous

B

B cell
B chromosome
B complex vitamin
B lymphocyte
B symptoms

B$_{12}$

vitamin B$_{12}$

B19

parvovirus B19
HPV B19
parvovirus B19 (B19)

B$_6$

B$_6$ deficiency
vitamin B$_6$

BA

bacillary angiomatosis
biliary atresia

Babcock

B. clamp
B. forceps

babe

B. OB ultrasound reporting system
B. ultrasound
B. ultrasound report software

Babee Teething

Babesia

B. divergens
B. microti
B. WA1 type

babesiosis

Babinski

B. reflex
B. response
B. sign

Babinski-Fröhlich syndrome

Babkin reflex

Babson chart

baby

B. Air mesh netting
blue b.
blueberry muffin b.
boarder b.
bottle-fed b.
b. bottle syndrome
breast-fed b.
breech b.
bronze b.
B. CareLink system
Clinical Risk Index for Babies (CRIB)
cocaine b.
collodion b.
crack b.
B. Doe regulations

B. Dopplex 4000
B. Dopplex 3000 antepartum fetal monitor
drug b.
febrile b.
giant b.
gray b.
B. Halo cushioned head support
jittery b.
juice b.
nipple-fed b.
B. Sense monitor
sling b.
b. teeth
test-tube b.
b. Tischler biopsy punch
well-hydrated b.
well-oxygenated b.
well-perfused b.

BABYbird

B. II ventilator
B. respirator

BabyFace 3D surface rendering accessory

babygram

Babylog

B. 8000 oscillator
B. 8000 respirator

baby's day diary

Babytherm IC

BAC

bacterial artificial chromosome
blood alcohol concentration

bacampicillin

Bacid

Baciguent Topical

Baci-IM Injection

bacillary

b. angiomatosis (BA)
b. dysentery
enteric gram-negative b. (EGNB)
b. meningitis
b. peliosis (BP)
b. peliosis hepatis

bacille

b. Calmette-Guérin (BCG)
b. Calmette-Gúerin vaccine

bacilli (*pl. of* bacillus)

bacilliformis

Bartonella b.

bacillus

b.
acid-fast b. (AFB)
b. Calmette-Gúerin vaccine
B. cereus

bacillus (*continued*)
    Döderlein b.
    Ducrey b.
    gram-negative b.
    gram-positive b.
    B. megaterium
    B. subtilis
bacitracin
    b. and polymyxin B
    neomycin, polymyxin B, b.
back
    b. board
    b. clamp
    flat b.
    b. pain
backache
backcross mating
background
    dirty b.
Backhaus
    B. clamp
    B. towel forceps
back-knee deformity
backpack
    AirPacks b.
    Airtec ergonomic b.
backscatter
    dipyridamole stress integrated b.
back-selected T cell
back-up
    b.-u. position
    b.-u. transverse lie
backward chaining
backwardness
    general reading b. (GRB)
backwash ileitis
baclofen
Bacon-Babcock operation
Bactec blood-culturing system
bacteremia, bacteriemia
    afebrile b.
    catheter-associated b. (CAB)
    clostridial b.
    coagulase-negative b.
    CoNS b.
    occult b.
    polymicrobial b.
    streptococcal b.
bacteremia-associated pneumococcal pneumonia (BAPP)
bacteremic shock
bacteria (*pl. of* bacterium)
bacterial
    b. artificial chromosome (BAC)
    b. artificial chromosome probe
    b. cervical adenitis
    b. conjunctivitis
    b. contamination
    b. count

    b. cystitis
    b. endocarditis
    b. endomyometritis
    b. enteritis
    b. exanthema
    b. growth
    b. homeostasis
    b. infection
    b. inhibition assay method of Guthrie
    b. keratitis
    b. labyrinthitis
    b. laryngotracheobronchitis
    b. mastitis
    b. meningitis
    b. meningoencephalitis
    b. overgrowth syndrome
    b. parotitis
    b. pericarditis
    b. peritonitis
    b. pharyngitis
    b. plaque
    b. pneumonia
    b. recovery
    b. rhinosinusitis
    b. sepsis
    b. sinusitis
    b. soilage
    b. toxin
    b. tracheitis
    b. translocation
    b. vaginitis (BV)
    b. vaginosis (BV)
bactericidal, bacteriocidal
    b. drug
bactericidal/permeability-increasing protein (BPI)
bacteriemia (*var. of* bacteremia)
bacteriocidal (*var. of* bactericidal)
bacteriologic, bacteriological
bacteriological (*var. of* bacteriologic)
bacteriology
bacteriophage
bacteriostatic drug
bacteriotoxic endometritis
bacterium, *pl.* **bacteria**
    anaerobic bacteria
    coccobacillary bacteria
    coliform bacteria
    gas-forming bacteria
    gram-negative bacteria
    gram-positive bacteria
    intracerebral seeding of bacteria
    occasional bacteria
    pathogenic bacteria
    pyogenic bacteria
    Salmonella b.
    Shigella b.
    Streptococcus b.

bacteriuria
    asymptomatic b. (ASB)
    rapid filter testing for b.
bacteroide
Bacteroides
    B. capillosus
    B. corrodens
    B. distasonis
    B. fragilis
    B. gingivalis
    B. melaninogenicus
    B. ovatus
    B. thetaiotaomicron
bacteroidosis
Bactine Hydrocortisone
BactoShield
Bactrim DS
Bactroban cream
Badenoch urethroplasty
BADS
    black locks with albinism and
     deafness syndrome
BAEP
    brainstem auditory evoked potential
BAER
    brainstem auditory evoked response
    BAER cavity
    BAER test
bag
    Ambu b.
    b. and mask
    b. and mask resuscitation
    b. and mask ventilation
    anesthesia b.
    B. Balm
    Barnes b.
    Cardiff resuscitation b.
    Champetier de Ribes b.
    Douglas b.
    Endopouch Pro specimen-retrieval b.
    Hope resuscitation b.
    intestinal b.
    manual ventilation b. (MVB)
    b. of waters (BOW)
    b. of worms appearance
    passenger air b. (PAB)
    Rusch b.
    sterile isolation b.
    bag, valve, mask (BVM)
    Vi-Drape bowel b.
    Void-Ease urine collection b.
    Voorhees b.
    zinc-free plastic b.
bagged urinalysis
Baggish hysteroscope
Bagshawe protocol
Bailey Physical Development Index
Bailey-Williamson forceps
Baird forceps

Bair
    B. Hugger patient warming system
    B. Hugger warming blanket
Bakelite cystoscopy sheath
Baker
    B. cyst
    B. punch
baker's leg
baking soda sitz bath
BAL
    blood alcohol level
    bronchoalveolar lavage
    BAL fluid
    BAL in Oil
Balamuthia
    B. mandrillaris
    B. meningoencephalitis
balance
    acid-base b.
    electrolyte b.
    fetal acid-base b.
    macronutrient b.
    negative b.
    b. reaction
    sodium b.
    transcapillary fluid b.
balanced
    b. chromosome rearrangement
    b. parental chromosome
     rearrangement
    b. rearrangement of autosome
    b. reciprocal translocation
    b. solution
    b. translocation
balancing
    soft tissue b.
balanic hypospadias
balanitis
    b. circinata
    circinate b.
    b. circumscripta plasmacellularis
    b. of Zoon
    plasma cell b.
balanoposthitis
Balantidium coli
balding
    temporal b.
baldness
    frontal b.
Baldy operation
Baldy-Webster
    B.-W. uterine displacement repair
     procedure
    B.-W. uterine suspension
Balfour
    B. bladder blade
    B. retractor
ball
    axonal retraction b.

ball (*continued*)
    Bichat fat b.
    birthing b.
    cauterizing b.
    b. electrode
    fungal b.
    fungus b.
    B. operation
    B. pelvimetry technique
    renal fungus b.
    TheraGym exercise b.
    tissue link floating b.
Ballantine clamp
Ballantyne-Runge syndrome
Ballantyne-Smith syndrome
Ballard
    B. Assessment Score (BAS)
    B. chart
    B. examination
    B. gestational assessment
    B. score
    B. test
Ball-Burch procedure
Baller-Gerold syndrome (BGS)
ballet dancer's secondary amenorrhea
8-ball hyphema
Ballinger-Wallace syndrome
ballism (*var. of* ballismus)
ballismus, ballism
balloon
    b. atrial septostomy (BAS)
    atrial septostomy via b.
    b. catheter technique
    electrode b.
    b. endometrial ablation
    24-French Foley b.
    gastric b.
    b. heating therapy
    Origin b.
    pediatric b.
    b. pulmonary valvoplasty
    Rashkind b.
    b. retractor
    Rigiflex b.
    b. septostomy
    b. septostomy catheter
    Soft-Wand atraumatic tissue manipulator b.
    SOS Bakri tamponade b.
    b. tamponade
    B. Therapy System
    b. thermoplasty
    transurethral self-detachable b.
    b. tuboplasty
    b. valvotomy
    b. valvulotomy
ballooning
balloon-tipped catheter
ballottable

ballottement
    abdominal b.
    uterine b.
ball-valve effect
balm
    Bag B.
    Butt B.
    lemon b.
Balmex cream
Balminil decongestant
Baló disease
balsalazide
balsa vaginal form
BALT
    bronchus-associated lymphoid tissue
Balthazar Scales of Adaptive Behavior (BSAB)
Baltic myoclonus
Bamberger fluid
bamboo
    b. hair
    b. spine
bambooing of digit
Bamforth syndrome
BAMO
    behavioral, anxiety, mood, and other types of disorders
    BAMO scale
banana
    Kanana B.
    b.'s, rice, applesauce, tea, toast (BRATT)
    b.'s, rice cereal, applesauce, toast (BRAT)
    b. sign
Bancap HC
band
    adhesive b.
    agyria-pachygyria b.
    amniotic constriction b.
    anular b.
    BB b.
    C b.
    b. cell
    chorioamnionic b.
    congenital intestinal b.
    congenital peritoneal b.
    cytological b.
    dense b.
    b. form neutrophil
    G b.
    b. heterotopia
    hymenal b.
    iliotibial b.
    b. keratopathy
    Ladd b.
    limbic b.
    lucent b.
    MM b.

myocardial b. (MB)
oligoclonal b.
pelvic b.
Q b.
R b.
silastic b.
b. stage
Streeter b.
T b.
vitreous b.
Z b.

bandage
Kerlix gauze b.
Kling b.
b. scissors
Tubigrip b.
tumescent absorbent b.
Velpeau b.
Webril b.

bandaging
elastic b.

Band-Aid operation

bandemia

banding
arterial b.
centromeric b.
chromosome b.
Giemsa b.
high-resolution b.
low-resolution b.
b. pattern
proximal pulmonary artery b.
pulmonary arterial b.
pulmonary artery b.
quinacrine b.
reverse b.
tubal b.

Bandl
pathologic retraction ring of B.
B. ring

banging
head b.

banjo curette

banjo-string adhesion

bank
clone b.
cord blood b.
milk b.
sperm b.
umbilical cord blood b.

Bankart lesion

banked breast milk (BBM)

banking

Banki syndrome

Bannayan-Riley-Ruvalcaba syndrome (BRRS)

Bannayan syndrome

Bannayan-Zonana syndrome (BZS)

Bannwarth syndrome

Banthine

Banti syndrome

BAP
bone alkaline phosphatase

BAPP
bacteremia-associated pneumococcal pneumonia

bar
Aveeno Cleansing B.
bilateral b.'s
Bill traction b.
calcaneonavicular b.
Denis Browne b.
Ensure Healthy Mom snack b.
Fostex B.
hyoid b.
Mercier b.
PanOxyl B.
pectus b.
stabilizing b.
syndet cleaning b.
talocalcaneal b.
unilateral b.

Baraitser-Burn syndrome

Baraitser-Winter syndrome

barbae
sycosis b.

Barbero-Marcial
B.-M. classification
B.-M. procedure

barber pole small intestine

Barber-Say syndrome

Barbilixir

barbiturate
b. intoxication
b. poisoning

barbotage

Barcroft/Haldane apparatus

Bard
B. Biopty cut needle
B. Biopty gun
B. Cap Sure Continence Shield
B. cervical cannula
B. PDA Umbrella

Bardet-Biedl syndrome (BBS)

Bard-Parker blade

bare lymphocyte syndrome

bargaining stage

Baridium

barium
b. contrast
b. enema
b. esophagography
b. esophagram
b. study
b. swallow

barium-impregnated plastic intrauterine device

Barkan infant lens

B

Barker low birth weight hypothesis
barking cough
barley
    b. allergy
    b. malt
Barlow
    B. and Ortolani test
    B. disease
    B. hip dysplasia test
    B. maneuver
    B. mitral regurgitation repair
      technique
    B. sign
    B. syndrome
Barnes
    B. Akathisia Scale (BAS)
    B. bag
    B. cerclage
    B. curve
    B. zone
baroceptor (*var. of* baroreceptor)
baromacrometer
Barophen
baroreceptor, baroceptor
baroreflex response
barotitis
    acute b.
barotrauma
barovolutrauma
Barr body
barrel
    b. cervix
    b. chest
    b. chest deformity
barrel-shaped
    b.-s. cervix
    b.-s. chest
    b.-s. lesion
    b.-s. upper central incisor
barren
Barré sign
Barrett esophagus
barrier
    Adcon-L anti-adhesion b.
    blood-brain b. (BBB)
    blood-testis b.
    b. contraception
    b. contraceptive
    ferric hyaluronate adhesion b.
    b. gown
    Interceed TC7 absorbable adhesion
      b.
    b. laparoscopy drape
    b. method
    b. method of contraception
    b. pack
    placental b.
    Sil-K OB b.
    TC7 adhesion b.

Barron pump
Barrow solution soak
Bart
    hemoglobin B.
    B. syndrome
Bartholin
    B. cystectomy
    B. duct
    B. duct cyst
    B. gland
    B. gland abscess
    B. gland carcinoma
    B. gland cyst
    Bartholin, urethral, Skene (BUS)
bartholinitis
Bartholin-Patau syndrome
Bartholomew rule of fourths
Barth syndrome
Bartonella
    B. bacilliformis
    B. henselae
    *B. henselae*infection
    B. quintana
Barton forceps
Bartsocas-Papas syndrome
Bartter syndrome (BS)
barymazia
BAS
    Ballard Assessment Score
    balloon atrial septostomy
    Barnes Akathisia Scale
basal
    b. arterial occlusion
    b. artery
    b. body temperature (BBT)
    b. body thermometer
    b. cell carcinoma
    b. cell epithelioma
    b. cell hyperplasia
    b. cell nevus syndrome
      (BCNS)
    b. cistern
    b. ganglion
    b. ganglion calcification
    b. ganglion disorder
    b. ganglion disorder-mental
      retardation (BGMR)
    b. ganglion necrosis
    b. lamina
    b. membrane (BM)
    b. metabolic rate (BMR)
    b. perivillous fibrin
    b. plate
    b. skull fracture
basale
    stratum b.
basalis
    decidua b.
    zona b.

BASC
> Behavioral Assessment Scale for
> Children
> BASC monitor

base
> broad nasal b.
> b. deficit
> b. excess
> hydrocortisone b.
> b. medication
> methylprednisolone b.
> nitrogenous b.
> b. pair
> b. sequence
> b. sequence analysis
> thickened b.

baseball
> b. finger
> b. stitch

baseline
> b. fetal bradycardia
> b. fetal heart rate
> b. fetal tachycardia
> FHR b.
> b. tonus
> b. value
> b. variability of fetal heart rate
> b. visual acuity
> zero-voltage b.

basement
> b. membrane
> b. membrane zone (BMZ)

bas-fond
basic
> b. fibroblast growth factor (bFGF)
> b. life support (BLS)
> b. skill

basicaryoplastin
basichromatin
basicranial flexure
basicranium
basilar, basilaris
> b. artery migraine
> b. consolidation
> b. impression (BI)
> b. invagination
> b. meningitis
> b. skull fracture

basilaris (*var. of* basilar)
basilemma
basis
> B. breast pump
> b. pontis
> B. soap

basket cell
basolateral membrane transport system
basophil, basophile
basophile (*var. of* basophil)
basophilia

basophilic, basophil
> b. leukemia
> b. stippling

basophilocytic leukemia
Bassen-Kornzweig
> B.-K. disease
> B.-K. syndrome

Basset radical vulvectomy
bassinet
Basson model of female sexual response
bastard
bat
> b. ear
> b. wing appearance

bath
> baking soda sitz b.
> belly b.
> colloidal oatmeal b.
> hexachlorophene b.
> pHisoHex b.
> B. respirator
> b. seat
> sitz b.
> sponge b.

bathing trunk nevus
bathrocephaly
batrachian position
Battelle Developmental Inventory (BDI)
Batten-Bielschowsky
> B.-B. type
> B.-B. type of late infantile and
> juvenile amaurotic idiocy

Batten disease
Batten-Mayou disease
Batten-Turner congenital myopathy
battered
> b. buttock syndrome
> b. child syndrome (BCS)
> b. fetus syndrome
> b. wife syndrome
> b. woman

battering cycle
battery
> MacArthur Story Stem B. (MSSB)
> Vulpe Assessment B.
> Woodcock-Johnson Psychoeducational
> B. (WJPB)

battery-operated breast pump
battledore
> b. cord
> b. placenta

Battle sign
Baudelocque
> B. diameter
> B. operation
> B. uterine circle

baumannii
> *Acinetobacter b.*

Baxa oral dispenser

B

Bayer
> B. Aspirin
> B. DCA2000 analyzer
> B. Timed-Release Arthritic Pain Formula

bayesian hypothesis

Bayley
> B. and Pinneau height-predicting method
> B. cognitive outcome
> B. Mental Developmental Index
> B. Mental Scale
> B. Motor Score
> B. Psychomotor Developmental Index
> B. Scales of Infant Development (BSID)
> B. Scales of Infant Development-II (BSID-II)
> B. Scales of Infant Development-Motor, 2nd Edition

Bayley-Pinneau table

Baylisascaris procyonis

Baylor
> B. amniotic perforator
> B. amniotome

Bayne Pap Brush

bayonet
> b. forceps
> b. leg

bazedoxifine

Bazett formula

Bazex-Dupré-Christol syndrome

Bazex syndrome

Bazin
> erythema induration of B. (EIB)

BBB
> blood-brain barrier
> bundle branch block
> BBB syndrome

BBD
> benign breast disease

BBG nasal aspirator

BBM
> banked breast milk

BBS
> Bardet-Biedl syndrome

BBT
> basal body temperature
> BBT chart

BC
> birth control
> breast cancer
> BC Cold Powder Non-Drowsy Formula

BCA
> bicinchonic acid
> BCA protein assay

BCAVD
> bilateral congenital absence of vas deferens

BCC
> benign cellular change

BCD
> blepharocheilodontic
> BCD syndrome

BCDDP
> Breast Cancer Detection Demonstration Project

BCDL
> Brachmann-Cornelia de Lange

BCDLS
> Brachmann-Cornelia de Lange syndrome

BCE
> benign childhood epilepsy
> bone collagen equivalent unit

B-cell
> B-c. dysfunction
> B-c. lineage
> B-c. lymphoma
> maternal B-c.

BCFA
> branched chain fatty acid

BCG
> bacille Calmette-Guérin
> BCG live
> Tice BCG
> BCG vaccine

BCI
> blunt cardiac injury

Bcl-2
> Bcl-2 oncogene
> Bcl-2 protein

BCNS
> basal cell nevus syndrome

BCNU
> bis-chloroethylnitrosourea

BCOT
> benign cystic ovarian teratoma

BCP
> birth control pill

BCPT
> breast cancer prevention trial

bcr
> breakpoint cluster region

BCS
> battered child syndrome

BCT
> benign cystic teratoma
> breast conservation therapy
> breast-conserving therapy

BD
> Becton-Dickinson
> BD Sensability breast self-examination

BD Sensability breast
self-examination aid
BD syndrome
BD test
BDD
body dysmorphic disorder
B₆-dependent convulsion
B_6**-dependent convulsion**
BDI
Battelle Developmental Inventory
BDI score
bDNA
branched deoxyribonucleic acid
BDNF
brain-derived neurotrophic
factor
BDProbeTec ET system
bead
Chelex b.
DEAE b.
Durasphere carbon b.
medical worry b.'s
beading
beak
medial metaphysial b.
beaked
b. nose
b. pelvis
beaking
BEAM
brain electrical activity map
brain electrical activity mapping
bean
cassava b.
castor b.
fava b.
b. gum
jelly b.
bear
B. Cub infant ventilator
InterMed B.
KidO's aerosol and oxygen
therapy b.
B. respirator
b. tracks
b. walk
bearclaw ulcer
beard ringworm
**Beare-Stevenson cutis gyrata
syndrome**
Beare syndrome
bearing down
bearing-down pain
beat
dropped b.
escape beats
left ventricular paced b.
b.'s per minute (bpm)
Beath pin
Beatson ovariotomy

beat-to-beat
b.-t.-b. continuous blood pressure
monitoring
b.-t.-b. variability
b.-t.-b. variability of fetal heart rate
Beau line
beaveri
Brugia b.
Beben
Because vaginal foam
Beccaria sign
Beck
B. Depression Inventory (BDI)
B. disease
B. triad
Becker
B. breast prosthesis
B. disease
B. melanosis
B. muscular dystrophy (BMD)
B. nevus
B. pseudohypertrophic muscular
dystrophy
B. tissue expander
B. type progressive muscular
dystrophy
Becker-Kiener muscular dystrophy
Becker-type tardive muscular dystrophy
Beckwith syndrome
Beckwith-Wiedemann syndrome (BWS)
Béclard nucleus
Becloforte
beclomethasone
aqueous b.
b. dipropionate
b. propionate
Beconase
B. AQ
B. AQ Nasal Inhaler
Becton-Dickinson (BD)
bed
Affinity b.
arterial vascular b.
bumper b.
hypoplastic pulmonary vascular b.
Ohio b.
oversewing placental b.
placental b.
pulmonary vascular b.
b. rest
b. rest checklist
B. Rest Helpline
b. rest support program
vascular b.
BED
binge eating disorder
Bednar aphthae
bedwetting
beef insulin

Beemer-Langer syndrome
Beemer lethal malformation syndrome
Beesix
bee sting challenge
Begeer syndrome
Béguez César disease
behavior
    adaptive b.
    aggressive b.
    antisocial b.
    Assessment of Preterm Infants' B.
     (APIB)
    B. Assessment System for Children
     monitor
    autistic b.
    autistic-like b.
    avoidance b.
    Balthazar Scales of Adaptive B.
     (BSAB)
    catatonic b.
    cognitive b.
    b. contract
    b. contract system
    defiant b.
    disorganized b.
    dysregulated b.
    externalizing b.
    fire-setting b.
    functional b.
    heterosexual high-risk b.
    hypersexual b.
    immature social b.
    b. modification (Bmod)
    b. modification program
    neuropsychiatric b.
    obsessive-compulsive b. (OCB)
    oppositional b.
    b. pattern
    B. Problem Inventory (BPI)
    B. Rating Scale (BRS)
    risk b.
    risk-taking b.
    risky b.
    self-comforting b.
    self-injurious b. (SIB)
    self-mutilating b.
    sexual b.
    social b.
    stereotypic b.
    withdrawn b.
behavioral
    B. and Emotional Rating Scale
     (BERS)
    behavioral, anxiety, mood, and other
     types of disorders (BAMO)
    b. assessment
    B. Assessment Scale for Children
     (BASC)
    b. audiometry

    b. disturbance
    b. family systems therapy
     (BFST)
    b. genetics
    b. inhibition
    b. intervention
    b. management
    b. milestone
    b. observation audiometry (BOA)
    b. pediatrics
    b. rebound
    b. state
    b. stress
    b. therapy (BT)
Behçet
    B. disease
    B. syndrome
Behr
    B. disease
    B. optic atrophy
    B. syndrome
BEI
    bioelectrical impedance
beigelii
    Trichosporon b.
Beighton criteria
bejel
belching
Belgian type mental retardation
bell
    auditory response to b.
    Gomco b.
    B. palsy
    B. staging criteria
    b. stethoscope
belladonna
Bell-Buettner hysterectomy
bell-clapper deformity
Bellergal
belli
    Isospora b.
Bellucci alligator forceps
belly
    b. bath
    b. bath therapy
    b. cleft
    b. crawl
    prune b.
Bel-Phen-Ergot S
belt
    b. mark
    Marsupial b.
belt-position booster seat
Benadryl
    B. decongestant allergy tablet
    B. injection
    B. Oral
    B. Topical
Bence Jones protein

bend
    deep-knee b.
    b. deformity
    b. fracture
Bendectin
Bender Visual Motor Gestalt Test
Bendopa
bendroflumethiazide
beneficence
BeneFix
Benelli mastopexy
benign
    b. breast disease (BBD)
    b. breast examination
    b. breast mass
    b. cellular change (BCC)
    b. childhood epilepsy (BCE)
    b. congenital hypotonia
    b. cystic ovarian teratoma
      (BCOT)
    b. cystic teratoma (BCT)
    b. cystic tumor
    b. epilepsy of childhood
    b. external hydrocephalus
    b. familial chronic pemphigus
    b. familial hematuria (BFH)
    b. familial macrocephaly (BFM)
    b. familial megalencephaly
    b. familial neonatal convulsion
      (BFNC)
    b. familial neonatal seizure
    b. familial recurrent cholestasis
    b. focal epilepsy
    b. fructosuria
    b. hepatic adenoma
    b. hyperphenylalaninemia
    b. idiopathic neonatal convulsion
      (BINC)
    b. implant
    b. infantile familial convulsion
      (BIFC)
    b. infantile hypotonia
    b. intracranial hypertension (BIH)
    b. jaundice
    b. juvenile melanoma
    b. lesion
    b. lymphoid hyperplasia
    b. mass
    b. maturation delay
    b. mesothelioma of genital tract
    b. migratory glossitis
    b. mucinous cystadenoma
    b. myoclonic epilepsy
    b. myoclonus of infancy
    b. nasopharyngeal fibroma
    b. neonatal epilepsy
    b. neonatal myoclonus
    b. neonatal sleep myoclonus
    b. neutropenia

    b. nevus
    b. nonprogressive familial chorea
    b. nonprolapsed uterus
    b. ovarian neoplasm
    b. papillomatosis
    b. papillomavirus infection
    b. paroxysmal torticollis
    b. paroxysmal torticollis of infancy
    b. paroxysmal vertigo (BPV)
    b. partial epilepsy
    b. partial epilepsy with
      centrotemporal spike (BPEC)
    b. pineal cyst
    b. recurrent hematuria
    b. rolandic epilepsy (BRE)
    b. transient gynecomastia
    b. transient optic disc edema
    b. tumor
    b. vascular neoplasm
    b. venous hum
    b. X-linked recessive muscular
      dystrophy
Benisone
Benjamin
    B. anemia
    B. syndrome
Bennett
    B. PR-2 ventilator
    B. respirator
Benoxyl
Benson baby pylorus separator
bent finger
Benton Visual Retention Test
Bentyl
    B. Hydrochloride Injection
    B. Hydrochloride Oral
Benylin
    B. Expectorant
    B. Pediatric
Benzac
    B. AC
    B. AC Gel
    B. W Gel
    B. W Wash
BenzaClin topical gel
5-Benzagel
10-Benzagel
Benzamycin
benzathine
    b. benzylpenicillin
    b. penicillin
    b. penicillin G (BPG)
    penicillin G b.
Benzedrine
benzene
benzimidazole
benzoate
    benzyl b.
    sodium phenylacetate and sodium b.

B

benzocaine
    antipyrine and b.
    b. lozenge
Benzodent
benzodiazepine
benzoin applicator
benzothiophene-derived selective estrogen
  receptor modulator
benzoyl peroxide
benzthiazide
benztropine mesylate
benzyl
    b. alcohol
    b. benzoate
benzylpenicillin, benzyl penicillin
    benzathine b.
benzylpenicilloyl-polylysine
BEP
    bleomycin, etoposide, Platinol
    BEP therapy
bepridil
beractant surfactant
Berardinelli-Seip-Lawrence syndrome
Berardinelli-Seip syndrome
Berardinelli syndrome
Berdon syndrome
Berens 3-character test
Berger
    B. paresthesia
    B. renal disease
bergeriae
    Gemella b.
Bergia syndrome
Bergmeister papilla
beriberi, beri beri
    infantile b.
    Shoshin b.
Berkeley
    B. suction curette
    B. suction machine
    B. Vacurette
Berkeley-Bonney retractor
Berkow formula for burns
Berkson-Gage
    B.-G. calculation
    B.-G. test/assay
Berlin
    B. breakage syndrome
    B. edema
    B. score
Bernard-Soulier syndrome
  (BSS)
Berne criteria
Bernoulli trial
Bernstein test
berry
    b. aneurysm
    B. syndrome
Berry-Kravis and Israel syndrome

Berry-Treacher Collins syndrome
BERS
    Behavioral and Emotional Rating
    Scale
Bertini syndrome
Besnier prurigo of pregnancy
best
    B. disease
    b. interests standards
bestiality
besylate
    atracurium b.
    mesoridazine b.
beta (β)
    b. adrenergic agonist
    b. carotene
    b. chain
    b. error
    estrogen receptor b. (Er beta)
    b. FGF-stimulated cell
      proliferation
    follitropin b.
    interferon b.
    b. interferon
    b. lactamase
    b. mimetic therapy
    b. phase
    b. ray
    b. receptor
    b. subunit
    b. thalassemia
    transforming growth factor b. (TGF
      beta)
beta-2
    b.-2 adrenergic agent
    b.-2 agonist
    b.-2 integrin
    b.-2 microglobulin
    b.-2 sympathomimetic terbutaline
beta-1a
    interferon b.-1a
beta-adrenergic
    b.-a. agent
    b.-a. blockade
    b.-a. drug
    b.-a. receptor
beta-aminoisobutyric aciduria
beta-1b
    interferon b.-1b
beta-blocker
beta-cell
    b.-c. adenoma
    b.-c. adenomatosis
beta-chemokine receptor
Betacort
Betaderm
Betadine PrepStick Plus
beta-endorphin
17-beta-estradiol dehydrogenase

B

17-beta-E2 transdermal drug-delivery system
beta-galactosidase
beta-galactosidase-1 (GLB-1)
   b.-g.-1 deficiency
beta-glucuronidase (GUSB)
   b.-g. deficiency
      mucopolysaccharidosis
beta-hCG
   beta-human chorionic gonadotropin
   beta-hCG discriminatory zone
beta-hemolytic
   b.-h. streptococcal coinfection
   b.-h. streptococcus (BHS)
3-betaHSD
   3-beta-hydroxysteroid dehydrogenase
11-beta-HSD2 deficiency
beta-human chorionic gonadotropin (beta-hCG, beta-HCG)
3-beta-hydroxysteroid dehydrogenase (3-betaHSD)
11-beta-hydroxysteroid dehydrogenase type 2 deficiency
betaine
   b. anhydrous
   b. hydrochloride
beta-1 integrin
beta-lactam
   b.-l. antibiotic
   b.-l. antimicrobial
beta-lactamase-resistant antistaphylococcal antibiotic
beta-lactamase-stable drug
beta-lipotropin
Betaloc
betamethasone
   b. dipropionate
   b. valerate
betamimetic agent
17-beta-ol-dehydrogenase
5-beta-pregnane-3,20-dione
beta-receptor agonist
beta-recombinant
   interferon b.-r.
Betasept
Betaseron
beta-spectrin
beta-sympathomimetic
   b.-s. agent
   b.-s. agonist
betasympathomimetic
beta-synthase
   cystathionine b.-s. (CBS)
beta-thalassemia
   HbE b.-t.
   sickle b.-t.
Betatrex Topical
betatron electron accelerator
bethanechol chloride

Bethesda
   B. assay
   B. 2001 cervical cytology classification
   B. classification system
   B. II system
   B. System guidelines
   B. System Pap smear classification
   B. unit
Bethlem myopathy
Betke-Kleihauer test
Betke stain
Betnesol
Betnovate
Betz cell
Beuren syndrome
Bevan incision
Beverly-Douglas lip-tongue adhesion technique
BeWo cell
bexarotene
Bexophene
Bextra tablet
bezafibrate
bezoar
Bezold abscess
Bezold-Jarisch reflex
bFGF
   basic fibroblast growth factor
BFH
   benign familial hematuria
BFL
   Börjeson-Forssman-Lehmann
BFLUTS
   Bristol Female Lower Urinary Tract Symptoms
      BFLUTS questionnaire
BFM
   benign familial macrocephaly
BFNC
   benign familial neonatal convulsion
BFST
   behavioral family systems therapy
BF-STS
   biologic false-positive serologic test for syphilis
BFU-E
   burst-forming units-erythroid
bG
   blood glucose
   Chemstrip bG
BGMR
   basal ganglion disorder-mental retardation
      BGMR syndrome
BGS
   Baller-Gerold syndrome
BH4
   tetrahydrobiopterin cofactor

BH₄ loading test
BHS
    Bogalusa Heart Study
BIA
    bioelectrical impedance analysis
Biafine
biallelic marker
Bianchine-Lewis syndrome
biatriatum
    cor triloculare b.
Biaxin
bibasilar
BICAP
    bipolar circumactive probe
    BICAP cautery
bicarbonate (HCO₃)
    b. concentration
    b. infusion
    plasma b. (PHCO₃)
    sodium b. (NaHCO₃)
    b. therapy in acidosis
    b. wasting
bicarbonate-carbonic acid
  system
bicarbonaturia
bicephalus
biceps
    b. femoris muscle
    b. reflex
Bichat fat ball
bichloracetic acid
Bicillin
    B. C-R
    B. C-R 900/300
    B. L-A
bicinchonic acid
bicipital tuberosity
Bicitra
Bickers-Adams syndrome
BiCOAG forceps
biconcave vertebra
bicornate (*var. of* bicornuate)
bicornis
    uterus b.
bicornous (*var. of* bicornuate)
bicornuate, bicornate, bicornous
    b. uterus
bicuculline-induced seizure
bicuspid
    b. aortic valve
    first b.
    second b.
bicycle ergometer
bicycling movement
bidet
bidirectional
    b. Glenn anastomosis
    b. Glenn procedure
    b. Glenn shunt

    b. PDA
    b. shunting
bidiscoidal placenta
BIDS
    brittle hair, intellectual impairment,
    decreased fertility, short stature
    BIDS syndrome
Biederman sign
Bielschowsky-Jansky disease
Bielschowsky syndrome
Biemond syndrome 1, 2
bieneusi
    Enterocytozoon b.
Bierer
    B. ovum forceps
    B. tenaculum
Bieri scale
bifascicular block
BIFC
    benign infantile familial convulsion
bifenestratus
    hymen b.
bifid
    b. cervix
    b. clitoris
    b. earlobe
    b. exencephalia
    b. nose
    b. pelvis
    b. scrotum
    b. spinal arch
    b. spinal cord
    b. uterus
    b. uvula
    b. xiphoid
bifida
    closed spina b.
    open spina b.
    spina b.
Bifidobacterium
    B. adolescentis
    B. bifidum
    B. breve
    B. catenulatum
    B. infantis
    B. longum
bifidum
    Bifidobacterium b.
    cranium b.
bifidus
    b. factor
    Lactobacillus b.
    uterus b.
biforate uterus
biforis
    hymen b.
    uterus b.
bifurcate, bifurcated
bifurcated (*var. of* bifurcate)

bifurcation
    aortic b.
bigeminal pregnancy
bigeminy
    atrial b.
Biggers medium
BiGGY
    bismuth sulfite, glucose, glycine, yeast
      BiGGY agar
biguanide
    polyhexamethyl b. (PHMB)
BIH
    benign intracranial hypertension
biischial diameter
bikini cut incision
bilabial
    b. closure
    b. speech sound
bilaminar blastoderm
BiLAP
    bipolar laparoscopic probe
bilateral
    b. acoustic neurofibromatosis
    b. acoustic neuromas
    b. atresia
    b. atresia of external auditory meatus
    b. bars
    b. breast pump
    b. cephalhematomas
    b. cerebral ventriculomegaly
    b. choreoathetosis
    b. choroid plexus cyst
    b. club feet
    b. congenital absence of vas deferens (BCAVD)
    b. congenital ptosis
    b. conjunctivitis
    b. corticobulbar disruption
    b. cryptorchidism
    b. ductus
    b. ectopic pregnancy
    b. facial agenesis
    b. flank masses
    b. gonadal failure
    b. hearing impairment
    b. increased femoral anteversion
    b. left-sidedness
    b. lung hypoplasia
    b. mediolateral episiotomies
    b. myocutaneous graft
    b. myringotomy tubes (BMT)
    b. optic nerve hypoplasia
    b. optic nerve sheath fenestration
    b. optic neuritis
    b. otitis media with effusion (BOME)
    b. ovarian neoplasm
    b. PC-IOL implantation

    b. periventricular nodular heterotopia
    b. pyramidal tract signs
    b. renal agenesis
    b. retinoblastomas
    b. salpingo-oophorectomy (BSO)
    b. schizencephalic clefts
    b. simultaneous tubal pregnancies
    b. slowing
    b. spasticity
    b. stocking hypesthesia
    b. subcostal incisions
    b. tubal ligation (BTL)
    b. ureteral diversion
    b. ureteral obstruction (BUO)
    b. uropathy
    b. uterine artery ligation
bile
    b. acid
    b. acid defect syndrome
    b. acid flux
    b. acid malabsorption
    b. acid sequestration
    b. acid synthesis
    b. chenodeoxycholic acid level
    b. duct
    b. duct catheter
    b. duct paucity
    b. duct resection
    b. duct stenosis
    b. ductule
    inspissated b.
    milk of calcium b.
    b. peritonitis
    b. pigment
    b. plug syndrome
    b. salt
    b. salt-stimulated lipase (BSSL)
    b. stasis
    supersaturation of b.
bile-stained emesis
bilevel positive airway pressure (BiPAP)
bili
    bilirubin
    Bili mask phototherapy eye cover
biliary
    b. abscess
    b. ascites
    b. atresia (BA)
    b. cirrhosis
    b. colic
    b. hypoplasia
    b. lithiasis
    b. microhamartoma
    b. microlithiasis
    b. neonatal hepatitis
    b. perforation
    b. tract
Bili-Bassinet
BiliBed phototherapy unit

BiliBlanket Plus phototherapy system
BiliBottoms
BiliChek
    B. bilirubin analyzer
    B. noninvasive bilirubin analyzer
bilineal category
bilingual
biliopancreatic diversion
bilious
    b. emesis
    b. vomiting
bilirubin
    amniotic fluid b.
    b. blanket
    conjugated b.
    cord blood b.
    direct b.
    direct-reacting b.
    elevated conjugated b.
    b. encephalopathy
    free b.
    hour-specific total serum b.
    indirect b.
    b. infarction
    b. light
    serum b.
    total b.
    total serum b. (TSB)
    transcutaneous b. (TcB)
    unconjugated b.
bilirubin-albumin binding
bilirubin-induced neurologic dysfunction
  (BIND)
bilirubinometer
    BiliTest transcutaneous b.
bilirubinometry
BiliTest transcutaneous bilirubinometer
Bili-Timer
Bill
    B. maneuver
    B. traction bar
    B. traction handle forceps
Billings method
Billroth tumor forceps
biloba
    Ginkgo b.
    placenta b.
bilobate placenta
bilobed placenta
biloculare
    cor b.
bilocularis
    uterus b.
biloma
Bilopaque
Biloptin
Biltricide
bimanual
    b. massage

    b. pelvic examination
    b. version
bimelic amyoplasia
bimodal pattern
binary process
binasal prongs
BINC
    benign idiopathic neonatal convulsion
BIND
    bilirubin-induced neurologic dysfunction
    BIND score
binder
    abdominal b.
    breast b.
    Dale abdominal b.
    obstetric b.
    Scultetus b.
    B. syndrome
binding
    androgen b.
    bilirubin-albumin b.
    breast b.
    C1q b.
    fragment antigen b. (Fab)
    ligand b.
    protein b.
    b. protein
    b. protein-2 insulinlike growth factor
    b. protein-3 insulinlike growth factor
    b. site
    sperm-zona pellucida b.
binge
    b. drinking
    b. eating
    b. eating disorder (BED)
    b. eating syndrome
bingeing (*var. of* binging)
binging, bingeing
binocular
    b. function
    b. vision
binomial
binovular twins
bioactive hormone
bioactivity
bioassay
BioBands bracelet
biobehavioral shift
Biobrane adhesive
Biobrane/HF dressing
Biocef
Biocell RTV saline-filled breast implant
Biocept-G pregnancy test
Biocept-5 pregnancy test
biochemical
    b. defect
    b. genetics
    b. pregnancy
    b. study

B

biochemistry
Bioclate
biocompatibility
Bio-E-Gel
bioelectrical
    b. impedance (BEI)
    b. impedance analysis (BIA)
bioelectromagnetic application
biofeedback
    b. technique
    b. therapy
biofield therapeutics
biofilm
bioflavonoid
Biogel
    B. Reveal glove
    B. Reveal puncture indication
      system
bioidentical hormone
bioimpedance analysis
bioinformatics
bioinjectable
Biojector 2000
biokit HSV-2 rapid test kit
biologic, biological
    b. assay
    b. factor
    b. false-positive serologic test for
      syphilis (BF-STS)
    b. response modifier (BRM)
    b. risk
    b. sampling
    b. satiation curve
    b. therapy
    b. treatment
biological (*var. of* biologic)
biologically plastic femora
biomanipulation
biomedical factor
BioMerieux Vitek system
biometric profile
biometry
    fetal b.
biomicroscopy
    slit-lamp b.
Biopatch dressing
biophysical
    b. profile (BPP)
    b. profile score
biopsy
    Allis-Abramson breast b.
    aspiration b.
    bone marrow b.
    cervical cone b.
    chorionic villus b. (CVB)
    ciliary b.
    coin b.
    cold cup b.
    cold knife b.

cold knife cone b.
cone b.
core b.
core needle b. (CNB)
cul-de-sac b.
b. dating
directed b.
embryo b.
endometrial b. (EMB)
endomyocardial b.
excisional b.
fetal tissue b.
fine-needle aspiration b.
  (FNAB)
b. forceps
frozen b.
full-thickness bowel b.
full-thickness intestinal b.
hot b.
image-guided breast b.
jejunal b.
Kevorkian punch b.
Keyes punch b.
kidney b.
laparoscopic full-thickness
  intestinal b.
liver b.
lymph node b.
mirror image breast b.
mucosal b.
muscle b.
needle localization breast b.
negative punch b.
omental b.
open b.
open lung b. (OLB)
out-of-phase endometrial b.
percutaneous renal b.
peritoneal b.
Pipelle b.
pleural b.
b. probe
punch b.
punch skin b.
quadriceps femoris muscle b.
renal b.
sentinel lymph node b. (SLNB)
single cell b.
skeletal muscle b.
skin b.
skinny-needle b.
small bowel b.
stereotactic breast b.
stereotactic core needle b.
sural nerve b.
synovial b.
timed endometrial b.
transanal rectal b.
transvaginal fine-needle b.

biopsy (*continued*)
>TriMark marker system for breast b.
>trophectoderm b.
>vulvar b.

biopsychosocial syndrome
biopterin
Biopty cut needle
biosampler
Bioself fertility indicator
BioStar
>B. Flu OIA
>B. Flu optical immunoassay
>B. Strep A OIA test

biostatistics
biosynthesis
>inborn error of bile acid b.
>prostaglandin b.
>steroid b.

biosynthetic defect
biotechnology
biotin
>b. factor
>B. Forte
>B. Forte Extra Strength

biotinidase deficiency
biotinylated
Biotirmone
biotyping
BiPAP
>bilevel positive airway pressure
>BiPAP machine

biparental inheritance
biparietal
>b. bulge
>b. diameter (BPD)
>b. diameter level

bipartita
>placenta b.

bipartite
>b. patella
>b. uterus

bipartitum
>ovarium b.

bipartitus
>uterus b.

bipedal
>b. lymphangiography
>b. posture

biperiden
biphasic
>b. anaphylactic reaction
>b. anaphylaxis
>b. fever
>b. response
>b. stridor
>b. temperature pattern

biphenyl
>polychlorinated b.

biplane
>b. cineangiocardiography
>b. cineangiography
>b. intracavitary probe
>b. seriography

bipolar
>b. cautery
>b. circumactive probe (BICAP)
>b. cutting loop
>b. depression
>b. diathermy coagulation
>b. disorder (type 1, 2) (BPD)
>b. electrocautery
>b. electrode
>b. laparoscopic forceps
>b. laparoscopic probe (BiLAP)
>b. taxis
>b. urological loop
>b. vaporization
>b. version

bipolarity
>prepuberal-onset b.

bipotential
bipotentiality
Bipp paste
BIRADS
>Breast Imaging Reporting and Data System

Birbeck
>B. granule
>B. granule-positive cell

birch tree pollen
bird
>B. Mark 8 respirator
>B. OP cup
>B. vacuum extractor

bird-beak jaw
bird-headed
>b.-h. dwarfism
>b.-h. dwarf of Seckel
>b.-h. dwarf syndrome

birdlike
>b. face syndrome
>b. facies

bird's beak appearance
Birnberg bow
birth
>b. amputation
>b. anomaly
>b. asphyxia
>asynchronous b.
>breech b.
>b. canal
>b. canal laceration
>b. care center
>b. certificate
>b. control (BC)
>b. control pill (BCP)
>b. cushion

date of b. (DOB)
b. defect
dry b.
b. fracture
gravida, para, multiple births, abortions, live b.'s (GPMAL)
head b.
higher-order b.
home b.
b. injury
b. length
live b.
multiple b.'s
b. paralysis
premature b.
preterm b.
b. rate
spontaneous preterm b. (SPTB)
b. trauma
b. trauma theory
twin b.
b. weight (BW)
b. weight discordance
b. weight for gestational age (BWGA)
b. weight Z score
wrongful b.
year of b. (YOB)
birthing
    b. ball
    b. chair
    b. position
    b. process
    b. process plan
    b. room
birthmark
    vascular b.
BIS
    budesonide inhalation suspension
Bisac-Evac
bisacodyl
    b. suppository
    b. tablet
    b. Uniserts
bis-chloroethylnitrosourea
biscoumacetate
    ethyl b.
Bi-Set catheter
bisexual
    gay, lesbian, b. (GLB)
    b. relationship
bisexuality
bisferiens
    pulsus b.
bishop
    B. pelvic scoring system
    B. Prelabor Scoring System
    B. score
    B. score of cervical ripening

Bishop-Harmon forceps
Bishop-Koop
    B.-K. ileostomy
    B.-K. procedure
bishydroxycoumarin
Bismatrol
bismuth
    b. subsalicylate
    b. sulfite, glucose, glycine, yeast (BiGGY)
    b. toxicity
bisphosphonate therapy
bis(piareloyloxymethyl) (bis-POM)
bis-POM
    bis(piareloyloxymethyl)
bitartrate
    dihydrocodeine b.
    metaraminol b.
bite
    animal b.
    black widow spider b.
    cat b.
    b. cell
    chigger b.
    closed b.
    dog b.
    human b.
    insect b.
    interrupted b.'s
    open b.
    b. reflex
    spider b.
    stork b.
    tick b.
bitemporal
    b. aplasia cutis congenita
    b. diameter
    b. forceps marks syndrome
    b. hemianopia
bithionol
biting
    tongue b.
bitolterol
Bitot spot
bitterling pregnancy test
bivalent chromosome
bivalved cast
bivalve speculum
bivalving of uterus
bivariate
biventricular hypertrophy
bivia
    Prevotella b.
Bixler
    B. hypertelorism
    B. syndrome
Björnstad syndrome
BK
    human papovavirus BK

black
- b. cohosh
- b. dot
- b. dot ringworm
- B. Draught
- b. hairy tongue
- b. jaundice
- b. line
- b. locks with albinism and deafness syndrome (BADS)
- b. measles
- b. pigmentation
- b. spot
- b. widow spider
- b. widow spider bite

blackened speculum

Blackfan-Diamond
- B.-D. anemia
- B.-D. syndrome

blackhead

blackout
- weight-lifter b.

blackwater fever

bladder
- b. augmentation
- b. blade
- b. bubble
- b. capacity
- b. catheter
- b. catheterization
- Christmas tree b.
- b. control
- defunctionalized b.
- b. diary
- b. diverticulum
- b. drill
- b. dysfunction
- b. emptying
- b. exstrophy
- exstrophy of the b.
- fetal b.
- b. filling
- b. flap
- b. function
- b. habit
- b. hypotonia
- hypotonic b.
- iatrogenic b.
- b. injury
- b. instability
- b. installation therapy
- b. instrumentation
- in utero drainage of fetal b.
- kidneys, ureters, b. (KUB)
- b. laceration
- low pressure b.
- b. muscle stress test
- b. neck
- b. neck elevation test
- b. neck mobility
- b. neck obstruction (BNO)
- b. neck stenosis
- b. neck surgery
- b. neck suspension
- neurogenic b.
- neuropathic b.
- nonneurogenic neurogenic b.
- occult neurogenic b.
- b. outlet syndrome
- overactive b. (OAB)
- b. pain
- b. pillar
- b. pressure
- psychological nonneuropathic b.
- radiolucent circular shadow in b.
- b. reflection
- b. retractor
- b. retraining
- b. retraining drill (BRD)
- b. spasm
- b. sphincter paralysis
- stammering b.
- b. stretching
- b. tap
- b. training
- b. tumor (BT)
- uninhibited b.
- unstable b.
- urinary b.
- b. wall
- walnut-shaped b.

BladderManager portable ultrasound scanner

BladderScan BVI2500

bladder-stretching exercise

blade
- Balfour bladder b.
- Bard-Parker b.
- bladder b.
- E-Mac laryngoscope b.
- Endo-Assist retractable b.
- laryngoscope b.
- Miller b. (#0, #1)
- Orbit b.

Blair-Brown procedure

Blaivas
- B. classification
- B. classification of urinary incontinence

Blake closure of peritoneum

Blalock-Hanlon
- B.-H. atrial septostomy procedure
- B.-H. operation

Blalock-Park procedure

Blalock-Taussig
- B.-T. operation
- B.-T. shunt
- B.-T. shunt procedure

B

blanch
blanching
    cutaneous b.
    episodic b.
    laser b.
    b. macule
    b. pallor
    b. wheal and flare lesion
bland cytology
Bland-Garland-White syndrome
Blane
    amniotic infection syndrome of B.
blanket
    Bair Hugger warming b.
    bilirubin b.
    cooling b.
    forced-air b.
    plastic b.
    space b.
    b. swinging
Blaschko line
blast
    b. crisis
    leukemic b.
blastema
    metanephric b.
    renal b.
blastemic
blastocele, blastocoele
blastocoele (var. of blastocele)
blastocyst
    b. hatching
    b. implantation
    b. splitting
    b. transfer
Blastocystis hominis
blastocyte
blastoderm, blastoderma
    bilaminar b.
    embryonic b.
    trilaminar b.
blastoderma (var. of blastoderm)
blastodisc
blastogenesis
blastogenic period
blastolysis
blastoma
    nodular renal b.
    pleuropulmonary b. (PPB)
    primitive b.
blastomere
    b. cell
    b. separation
Blastomyces dermatitidis
blastomycosis
    Brazilian b.
    Lutz-Splendore-Almeida b.
    South American b.
blastomycosis-like pyoderma

blastotomy
blastula
bleb
    pulmonary b.
    subpleural b.
    venous b.
bleed
    brain b.
    extraembryonic b.
    fetomaternal b.
    herald b.
    intraparenchymal b.
    intraventricular b.
    joint b.
    physiologic neonatal withdrawal b.
bleed-back valve
bleeding, bleed
    abnormal uterine b. (AUB)
    abnormal vaginal b. (AVB)
    acute vaginal b.
    anovulatory b.
    antepartum b.
    breakthrough b. (BTB)
    catastrophic b.
    cyclic uterine b.
    b. diathesis
    dysfunctional uterine b. (DUB)
    estrogen breakthrough b.
    estrogen-progesterone withdrawal b.
    estrogen withdrawal b. (EWB)
    GI b.
    gum b.
    implantation b.
    intermenstrual b. (IMB)
    intracranial b.
    intractable uterine b.
    mucocutaneous b.
    mucosal b.
    pelvic b.
    placental b.
    postcoital b.
    postdouching b.
    postmenarchal b.
    postmenopausal b. (PMB)
    preadolescent vaginal b.
    premenopausal b.
    prepubertal vaginal b.
    progesterone breakthrough b.
    progesterone withdrawal b.
    b. scan
    self-limited b.
    severe gastrointestinal b. (SGIB)
    b. site
    b. site ligation
    space of Retzius b.
    subependymal b.
    third-trimester b. (TTB)
    b. time
    transplacental fetal b.

bleeding (*continued*)
    uterine withdrawal b.
    vaginal b.
    withdrawal b.
Bleier clip
blennorrhagia
blennorrhagic
blennorrhagicum
    keratoderma b.
blennorrhea, blennorrhagia
blennorrheal, blennorrhagic
Blenoxane
bleomycin
    cisplatin, vinblastine, and b.
    b., Eldisine, mitomycin, Platinol
    (BEMP)
    b., etoposide, Platinol (BEP)
    b., ifosfamide, Platinol (BIP)
    b. sulfate
Bleph-10
blepharitis
    seborrheic b.
    simple squamous b.
    staphylococcal b.
    ulcerative b.
blepharochalasis
blepharocheilodontic (BCD)
    b. syndrome
blepharoconjunctivitis
blepharonasofacial malformation
syndrome
blepharophimosis
    b., ptosis, epicanthus inversus
    (BPEI)
    b., ptosis, epicanthus inversus,
    primary amenorrhea syndrome
    b., ptosis, epicanthus inversus
    syndrome (BPEIS)
    b., ptosis, epicanthus inversus,
    telecanthus complex
    b., ptosis, syndactyly, short stature
    syndrome
    b. sequence
blepharoptosis, blepharophimosis,
epicanthus inversus, telecanthus
syndrome
blepharospasm, blepharospasmus
blepharospasmus (*var. of* blepharospasm)
blepharostenosis
BLES
    bovine lavage extract surfactant
Blessig groove
blighted ovum
blind
    legally b.
    b. loop syndrome
    b. trachea
    b. vagina
    b. vaginal pouch

blinded challenge
blind-ending vagina
blindness
    congenital retinitis b. (CRB)
    congenital stationary night b.
    cortical b.
    Episkopi b.
    gonococcal b.
    night b.
    transient cortical b.
blinking
    paroxysmal b.
    rapid b.
blink reflex
BLIS
    breast leakage inhibitor system
blister
    arthropod-induced b.
    b. cell
    fever b.
    intraepidermal b.
    recurrent b.
    rosettelike b.
    subepidermal b.
    sucking b.
    suprabasal b.
    tense b.
BlisterFilm dressing
blistering
    b. disease
    b. distal dactylitis
    b. sunburn
Blistik
Blizzard syndrome
BLL
    blood lead level
        capillary BLL
BLM
    borderline malignancy
bloat, bloating
    gas b.
bloated abdomen
bloating (*var. of* bloat)
bloc
    en b.
Bloch-Siemens syndrome
Bloch-Sulzberger
    B.-S. melanoblastoma
    B.-S. syndrome
block
    atrioventricular b.
    autoimmune-associated congenital
    heart b.
    bifascicular b.
    bundle branch b. (BBB)
    Cerrobend b.
    complete atrioventricular b.
    complete fetal heart b.
    congenital atrioventricular b.

congenital complete AV b.
congenital complete heart b.
  (CCHB)
congenital heart b. (CHB)
b. design test
dorsal penile nerve b. (DPNB)
enzymatic b.
extradural b.
field b.
first-degree AV b.
fixed-ratio atrioventricular b.
heart b.
iatrogenic complete heart b.
intramuscular b.
lead b.
left bundle branch b.
local b.
Mobitz (I, II) b.
motor b.
nerve b.
paracervical b.
peripheral nerve b.
pudendal b.
radial nerve b.
regional nerve b.
right bundle branch b. (RBBB)
saddle b.
second-degree heart b.
sinuatrial b.
somatic nerve b.
spinal subarachnoid b.
subarachnoid b.
supraorbital nerve b.
third-degree AV b.
ulnar nerve b.
b. vertebra
Wenckebach b.

blockade
beta-adrenergic b.
neuromuscular b.
paracervical b.
serotonergic reuptake b.
serotonin receptor b.
spinal b.
sympathetic b.

blockage
epiglottal b.
neuromuscular b.
proximal tubal b.
shunt b.

blocked
b. duct
b. premature atrial complex

blocker
adrenergic b.
alpha-adrenergic b.
antiandrogen receptor b.
calcium channel b.
cyproheptadine receptor b.

ganglionic b.
H_2 b.
serotonin reuptake b.
blocking factor
Block-Sulzberger incontinentia pigmenti
Bloedorn applicator
Blomdahl medical ear piercing system
blood
b. agar
b. alcohol
b. alcohol concentration (BAC)
b. alcohol level (BAL)
b. ammonia level
arterialized b.
autologous cord b.
b. cell indices
b. chimerism
b. chromosome analysis
b. clot
b. component
b. component analysis
b. component therapy
cord b.
b. count
b. culture
designated donor b.
donor-specific b.
b. dyscrasia
b. ethanol
b. extravasation
fetal cord b.
b. flow
b. gas
b. gas analysis
b. gas determination
b. glucose (bG)
b. glycine
b. group
b. group antibody
b. group D variant equivalent to
  Rh-negative (Du)
b. group immunization
b. group incompatibility
b. grouping
b. group isoimmunization
b. group system
intervillous b.
b. lactate
b. lead
b. lead level (BLL)
b. loss
maternal peripheral b.
menstrual b.
b. mole
occult b.
oxygenated fetal b.
b. patch
peripheral b.
b. PHE

B

105

blood (*continued*)
- b. pigment stain
- b. pressure (BP)
- b. pressure cuff size
- b. pressure gradient
- b. pressure measurement
- b. pressure monitor
- b. pressure transducer
- b. product
- b. relationship
- b. relative
- b. sample
- b. sampling
- b. smear
- b. spot
- b. substitute
- b. sugar
- b. sugar monitoring
- swallowed maternal b.
- b. transfusion
- b. type A, AB, B, O
- b. typing
- b. urea nitrogen (BUN)
- b. vessel
- b. vessel elasticity
- b. vessel formation
- b. vessel transillumination
- b. volume
- whole b.

blood-borne
- b.-b. metastasis
- b.-b. pathogen

blood-brain barrier (BBB)
blood-flecked gastric aspirate
Bloodgood
- B. disease
- B. syndrome

blood-loss anemia
bloodstream infection (BSI)
blood-testis barrier
blood-type test
bloody
- b. CSF
- b. diarrhea
- b. show

Bloom syndrome
blot
- Eastern b.
- enzyme-linked immunotransfer b. (EITB)
- Northern b.
- serum enzyme-linked immunoelectrotransfer b.
- Southern b.
- Western b.

blotting
Blount
- B. disease
- B. syndrome

blow-by
- b.-b. oxygen
- b.-b. through tubing

blowing decrescendo diastolic murmur
blowout
- b. fracture
- b. injury
- orbital b.

BLS
- basic life support

Bluboro powder
blue
- b. asphyxia
- b. baby
- b. baby syndrome
- b. Chux pad
- b. cone monochromatism
- b. diaper syndrome
- b. dome cyst
- b. dome syndrome
- b. dot sign
- b. histiocyte syndrome
- maternity b.'s
- methylene b.
- b. navel
- b. papule
- postpartum b.'s
- b. ring pessary
- b. rubber bleb nevus (BRBN)
- b. rubber bleb nevus syndrome (BRBNS)
- b. sclera
- b. scleral hue
- b. spell
- b. spot
- toluidine b.

blueberry
- b. muffin baby
- b. muffin nodule
- b. muffin rash
- b. muffin skin lesion
- b. muffin spot
- b. muffin syndrome

blue-cell sarcoma
blue-green algae
bluish-black macule
bluish discoloration of flank
Blumberg sign
Blumer shelf
blunt
- b. and sharp dissection
- b. aspirator
- b. cardiac injury (BCI)
- b. cardiac trauma
- b. chest trauma
- b. curettage
- b. duct adenosis
- b. probe
- b. trauma

Bluntport disposable trocar
blurred vision
blurring of left psoas margin
blush
    ciliary b.
    erythematous b.
    terminal b.
    tumor b.
B-Lynch
    B-L. technique
    B-L. uterine compression
    suture
BM
    basal membrane
    breast milk
BMA
    bone marrow aspirate
BMC
    bone mineral content
BMD
    Becker muscular dystrophy
    bone mineral density
BMI
    body mass index
    BMI Z-score
BMJ
    breast milk jaundice
BMM
    bone mineral mass
B-mode ultrasound
BMR
    basal metabolic rate
BMT
    bilateral myringotomy tubes
    bone marrow transplant
    bone marrow transplantation
    allogenic BMT
    autologous BMT
BMZ
    basement membrane zone
BN
    bulimia nervosa
BNBAS
    Brazelton Neonatal Behavioral
    Assessment Scale
BN-NP
    bulimia nervosa nonpurging
BNO
    bladder neck obstruction
BOA
    behavioral observation audiometry
    born on arrival
board
    arm b.
    back b.
    communication b.
    papoose b.
    prone b.
    recumbent infant b.

    scooter b.
    vestibular b.
boarder baby
Boari flap
Bobath
    B. physical therapy
    B. response
bobbing
    head b.
    ocular b.
bobble-head doll syndrome
Bochdalek
    congenital diaphragmatic hernia of
    B.
    B. hernia
Bockhart impetigo
BOD
    borderline
    brachymorphism, onychodysplasia,
    dysphalangism
    BOD syndrome
body
    b. alignment
    Aschoff b.
    asteroid b.
    Barr b.
    Call-Exner b.
    b. coils of cord
    b. composition
    b. conscious
    Cowdry types A, B inclusion b.
    Creola b.
    cytoid b.
    dense b.
    Döhle b.
    Donovan b.
    b. dysmorphic disorder (BDD)
    esophageal foreign b.
    extracranial foreign b.
    b. fat
    b. fluid
    foreign b.
    Golgi b.
    b. habitus
    Heinz b.
    b. homeostasis
    Howell-Jolly b.
    hyaline b.
    b. image
    inclusion b.
    intracranial foreign b.
    intranuclear inclusion b.
    b. jacket
    ketone b.
    Lafora b.
    lamellar b. (LB)
    lamellar inclusion b.
    b. language
    lateral geniculate b.

body (*continued*)
 b. lead burden
 loose b.
 Lostorfer b.
 b. louse
 b. mass index (BMI)
 b. mass index nomogram
 b. morphometrics
 Negri b.
 Nissl bodies
 osmiophilic b.
 owl's eye inclusion b.
 perineal b.
 b. phenotype
 pineal b.
 polar b.
 b. proportion measurement
 psammoma b.
 refractile b.
 retained foreign b. (RFB)
 b. ringworm
 b. rocking
 Schaumann b.
 Schiller-Duvall b.
 b. shell
 b. size
 b. stalk
 b. stalk anomaly
 b. stalk malformation
 striate b.
 b. surface area (BSA)
 b. surface area calculation
 b. temperature
 uterine b.
 vaginal foreign b.
 vertebral b.
 vitreous b.
 Weibel-Palade b.
 b. weight
 Winkler b.
 wolffian b.
 zebra b.
bodybuilding
body-image distortion
bodywork
BOF
 branchiooculofacial
BOFS
 branchiooculofacial syndrome
Bogalusa Heart Study (BHS)
boggy
 b. synovial effusion
 b. uterus
Bogros space
Bohn
 B. epithelial pearl
 B. nodule
Bohr effect
Bohring syndrome

Boix-Ochoa
 B.-O. GER score (BOS)
 B.-O. procedure
Bolivian hemorrhagic fever
bolster
bolt
 subarachnoid b.
bolus
 b. dose
 fecal b.
 fluid b.
 b. fluid therapy
 isotonic b.
 b. tube feeding
Bombay erythrocyte phenotype
BOME
 bilateral otitis media with effusion
Bonamine
Bonanno catheter
bond
 hydrogen b.
bonding
 maternal-child b.
 maternal-infant b.
 mother-infant b.
bone
 b. accretion
 b. age
 b. age determination
 b. age standard of Greulich and Pyle
 b. alkaline phosphatase (BAP)
 b. ALP
 b. anchor
 b. anchor support
 aseptic necrosis of b.
 b. attenuation coefficient
 b. avascular necrosis
 brittle b.'s
 capitate b.
 b. collagen equivalent unit (BCE)
 cortical b.
 craniobasal b.
 cuneiform b.
 b. demineralization
 b. densitometry
 b. density
 b. density measurement
 b. density study
 dwarfism and cortical thickening of tubular b.'s
 b. dysplasia
 ethmoid b.
 fiber b.
 flat frontal b.
 b. formation
 fragmentation of necrotic b.
 b. graft
 b. hemangioma

high frontal b.
hyoid b.
b. infection
innominate b.
ivory b.'s
lacrimal b.
lamellar b.
long b.
b. loss
marble b.'s
b. marrow
b. marrow aplasia
b. marrow aspirate (BMA)
b. marrow aspiration
b. marrow biopsy
b. marrow cytogenetics
b. marrow dysfunction
b. marrow failure
b. marrow hypoplasia
b. marrow infiltration
b. marrow puncture
b. marrow relapse
b. marrow stem cell
b. marrow suppression
b. marrow toxicity
b. marrow transplant (BMT)
b. marrow transplantation
  (BMT)
b. mass
b. matrix
maxillary b.
b. metastasis (BM)
b. mineral
b. mineral content (BMC)
b. mineral density (BMD)
b. mineral mass (BMM)
b. mineral measurement
b. mineral metabolism
b. mineral uptake
nasal b.
navicular b.
omovertebral b.
b. pain
parietal b.
b. quantitative ultrasound velocity
b. remodeling
b. resorption
round iliac b.
b. scan
b. sclerosis
short metacarpal b.
small maxillary b.
sphenoid b.
b. stippling
b. strength measurement
b. tissue mineralization
tubular b.
b. tumor
turbinate b.

b. turnover
weightbearing b.
wormian b.'s
woven b.
zygomatic b.
bone-age determination method
bone-specific alkaline phosphatase
Bonine
Boniva
**Bonnaire femoral neck screw fixation
  method**
Bonneau syndrome
Bonnet-Dechaume-Blanc syndrome
Bonnevie-Ullrich syndrome
Bonney
    B. abdominal hysterectomy
    B. blue stress incontinence test
Bontril
bony
    b. dysplasia
    b. enlargement
    b. erosion
    b. metastasis
    b. projection
    b. spur
Bookwalter retractor
boomerang
    b. dysplasia
    b. syndrome
Boom syndrome
BOOP
    bronchiolitis obliterans organizing
      pneumonia
boost
    B. nutritional drink
    B. nutritional supplement
booster
    b. dose
    tetanus toxoid b.
Boostrix
boot-shaped heart
BOR
    branchiootorenal
    BOR dysplasia
    BOR syndrome
borborygmi (*pl. of* borborygmus)
borborygmus, *pl.* **borborygmi**
border
    serpiginous b.
    shaggy heart b.
    smudged b.
borderline
    b. amniotic fluid index
    Child Version of the Retrospective
      Diagnostic Interview for B.'s
    b. diabetes
    b. epithelial ovarian carcinoma
    b. epithelial ovarian neoplasm
    b. epithelial ovarian tumor

borderline (*continued*)
 b. hypertension
 b. intelligence
 b. lepromatous leprosy
 b. malignancy (BLM)
 b. malignant epithelial neoplasm
 b. personality disorder
 b. tuberculoid
 b. tuberculoid leprosy
borderline-resistant *Staphylococcus aureus* **(BRSA)**
Bordetella
 B. bronchiseptica
 B. parapertussis
 B. pertussis
Bordet-Gengoi medium
boredom
Borg
 B. Perceived Exertion Scale
 B. Physical Activity Scale
boric
 b. acid
 b. acid capsule
Börjeson-Forssman-Lehmann (BFL)
 B.-F.-L. syndrome
Börjeson syndrome
born on arrival (BOA)
Borna disease virus
borne
Bornholm disease
boron (B)
Boropak
Borrelia
 B. afzelii
 B. burgdorferi
 B. burgdorferi sensu lato
 B. burgdorferi sensu stricto
 B. garinii
 B. recurrentis
borreliosis
Borsieri sign
BOS
 Boix-Ochoa GER score
Bosma Henkin Christiansen syndrome
bosselated
bossing
 frontal b.
 occipital b.
Boston
 B. exanthema
 B. Naming Test
 B. orthosis
Boston-type craniosynostosis
Botox
Botox
 botulinum toxin

botryoid
 b. pseudosarcoma
 sarcoma b.
 b. sarcoma
botryoides
Botryomycosis
bottle
 disposable b.
 b. fed
 b. feed
 Mead Johnson b.
 Nursette prefilled disposable b.
 prefilled disposable b.
 b. propping
 b. tooth decay
 transgrow b.
bottle-fed baby
botulinum
 b. antitoxin (type A, B, E)
 Clostridium b.
 b. immunoglobulin
 b. toxin
 b. toxin A (BTA)
botulinus
 b. intoxication
 b. neurotoxin
botulism
 Clostridium b.
 infantile b. (IB)
 b. toxin
 wound b.
Bouchut respiration
Boudreaux's Butt Paste
bougie
 b. dilator
 Holinger infant b.
bougienage
Bouin solution
boulardii
 Saccharomyces b.
boulimia (*var. of* bulimia)
bouncing
bound
 b. estradiol
 b. testosterone
bounding pulse
Bourneville
 B. disease
 B. syndrome
Bourneville-Brissaud disease
Bourneville-Pringle syndrome
Bourns infant respirator
boutonneuse fever
boutonnière
 b. finger
 b. incision
Bovie
 B. cauterization

B. cautery
B. unit
bovina
   facies b.
bovine
   b. dermal collagen
   b. face
   b. facies
   b. lavage extract surfactant (BLES)
   b. mucus penetration test
   pegademase b.
   b. pericardium patch
   b. spongiform encephalopathy (BSE)
   b. surfactant
   b. tuberculosis
bovis
   Mycobacterium b.
   Streptococcus b.
bow
   Birnberg b.
   Cupid's b.
   posteromedial b.
BOW
   bag of waters
bowel
   b. adaptation
   aganglionic b.
   b. angina
   b. atony
   b. clean-out
   b. duplication
   echogenic fetal b.
   b. function
   b. habit
   hyperechoic b.
   impacted b.
   b. infarction
   b. injury
   invaginated b.
   b. irrigation
   b. lengthening procedure
   b. loop resection
   malrotation of b.
   neurogenic b.
   b. obstruction
   perforated b.
   b. preparation
   proximal b.
   b. segment resection
   b. sounds (BS)
   b. stasis
Bowen
   B. disease
   B. double-bladed scalpel
   B. Hutterite syndrome
Bowen-Conradi syndrome
bowenoid
   b. atypia
   b. dysplasia
   b. papulosis
   b. vulvar intraepithelial neoplasia
bowing
   anterior tibial b.
   anterolateral tibial b.
   congenital posteromedial b.
   b. deformity
   b. fracture
   lateral tibial b.
   posteromedial tibial b.
   b. reflex
   tibial b.
   traumatic b.
bow-leg (*var. of* bowleg)
bowleg, bow-leg
   physiologic b.
bowleggedness
bowl of pelvis
Bowman
   B. capsule
   B. layer
   B. space
bowstringing of tendon
box
   head b.
   Hogness b.
   negative-pressure b.
   paired b.
   Pribnow b.
boxer's fracture
boydii
   Pseudallescheria b.
Boyle uterine elevator
Bozeman
   B. operation
   B. position
   B. uterine dressing forceps
Bozeman-Fritsch catheter
BP
   blood pressure
   breech presentation
BPD
   biparietal diameter
   bipolar disorder (type 1, 2)
   bronchopulmonary dysplasia
BPEC
   benign partial epilepsy with centrotemporal spike
BPEI
   blepharophimosis, ptosis, epicanthus inversus
BPEIS
   blepharophimosis, ptosis, epicanthus inversus syndrome
BPF
   bronchopulmonary fistula
BPG
   benzathine penicillin G

BPI
    bactericidal/permeability-increasing
      protein
    Behavior Problem Inventory
    brachial plexus injury
bpm
    beats per minute
    breaths per minute
BPP
    biophysical profile
      antepartum fetal BPP
      fetal BPP
      modified BPP
      BPP score
BPS
    bronchopulmonary sequestration
BPV
    benign paroxysmal vertigo
bra
    lead b.
    Veronique b.
braakii
    Citrobacter b.
BRACA
    multisite BRACA
    BRACA mutation test
    single site BRACA
brace
    cast boot b.
    Charleston b.
    Cruiser hip abduction b.
    Friedman Splint b.
    b. management
    Milwaukee b.
    Rhino Triangle b.
    Risser b.
    b. treatment
bracelet
    BioBands b.
    MedicAlert b.
brachial
    b. artery
    b. birth palsy
    b. plexopathy
    b. plexus
    b. plexus injury (BPI)
    b. plexus palsy
    b. plexus stretching
brachiocephalic vessel
brachioradialis reflex
brachioskeletogenital (BSG)
Brachmann-Cornelia
    B.-C. de Lange (BCDL)
    B.-C. de Lange syndrome (BCDLS)
Bracht maneuver
brachycephalic configuration
**brachycephaly, deafness, cataract,
  microstomia, mental retardation
  syndrome**

brachydactylia (*var. of* brachydactyly)
brachydactyly, brachydactylia
    b., dwarfism, hearing loss,
      microcephaly, mental retardation
      syndrome
    b., mesomelia, mental retardation,
      aortic dilation, mitral valve
      prolapse, characteristic facies
      syndrome
    b., nystagmus, cerebellar ataxia
      syndrome
    Pitt-Williams b.
    Sugarman b.
**brachydactyly-distal symphalangism
  syndrome**
brachydactyly-ectrodactyly
brachygnathia
brachymelia
    rhizomelic b.
brachymesomelia-renal syndrome
brachymesophalangism (*var. of*
  brachymesophalangy)
**brachymesophalangy,
  brachymesophalangism**
brachymetacarpalia, brachymetacarpalism
    b., cataract, mesiodens syndrome
brachymetacarpalism (*var. of*
  brachymetacarpalia)
brachymetacarpy
brachymetatarsus IV
brachymorphism
    b., onychodysplasia, dysphalangism
      (BOD)
    b., onychodysplasia, dysphalangism
      syndrome
brachyolmia
brachypellic (*var. of* brachypelvic)
brachypelvic, brachypellic
brachysyndactyly
brachytelephalangy
brachytherapy
    interstitial b.
    intracavitary b.
    remote afterloading b. (RAB)
Bradley
    B. childbirth education
    B. method
    B. method of prepared childbirth
bradyarrhythmia
bradycardia
    apnea and b. (A&B)
    baseline fetal b.
    feeding b.
    fetal b.
    post cordocentesis b.
    prolonged b.
    sinus b.
    vagotonic b.
bradycardiac, bradycardic

bradycardia-tachycardia syndrome
bradycardic (*var. of* bradycardiac)
bradygenesis
bradykinin
    b. antagonist
    lysyl b.
bradylexia
bradymenorrhea
bradyspermatism
brady-tachy syndrome
bradytocia
Bragg-Paul respirator
Bragg peak
Brailsford
    B. disease
    B. syndrome
brain
    b. abscess
    b. atrophy
    b. bleed
    butterfly b.
    coning of b.
    b. damage
    b. death
    b. death syndrome
    b. disorder
    b. dysfunction
    b. edema
    b. electrical activity map (BEAM)
    b. electrical activity mapping
      (BEAM)
    fetal b.
    b. function
    b. herniation
    b. imaging technique
    b. injury
    b. lesion
    b. mapping
    b. metabolism
    b. metastasis
    b. peptide
    b. sparing
    b. swelling
    b. tumor
    b. vesicle
    b. wart
    water on b.
    b. wave
brain-derived neurotrophic factor
(BDNF)
brain-sparing effect
brainstem, brain stem
    b. auditory evoked potential (BAEP)
    b. auditory evoked response (BAER,
      BSAER)
    b. auditory tract
    b. compression
    b. encephalitis
    b. evoked response (BSER)

    b. evoked response audiometry
      (BSERA)
    b. function
    b. glioma
    b. herniation
    b. lesion
branched
    branched-chain amino acid
    b. chain amino acidemia
    b. chain aminotransferase
    b. chain fatty acid (BCFA)
    b. chain ketoacid
    b. chain ketoaciduria
    b. chain ketonuria
    b. deoxyribonucleic acid (bDNA)
    b. DNA
brancher deficiency
branchial
    b. arch
    b. arch syndrome
    b. cleft
    b. cleft anomaly
    b. cleft cyst
    b. cleft fistula
    b. cleft remnant
    b. cleft sinus
    b. clefts-lip pseudocleft syndrome
    b. duct
    b. plexus
    b. pouch
branching
    airway b.
    b. enzyme deficiency
    b. enzyme deficiency
      amylopectinosis
    fetal capillary b.
    b. morphogenesis
    b. pattern
    b. snowflake test
branchiomere
branchiooculofacial (BOF)
    b. syndrome (BOFS)
branchiootic syndrome
branchiootorenal (BOR)
Brandt-Andrews maneuver
Brandt syndrome
Branhamella catarrhalis
brash
    weaning b.
brasiliensis
    Nocardia b.
    Paracoccidioides b.
brassy cough
BRAT
    bananas, rice cereal, applesauce, toast
    BRAT diet
BRATT
    bananas, rice, applesauce, tea, toast
    BRATT diet

B

Bratton-Marshall test
Braun
      B. episiotomy scissors
      B. tympanic thermometer
Braune canal
Braun-Schroeder single-tooth tenaculum
Bravelle
brawny
      b. dermatitis
      b. edema
      b. hyperpigmentation
      b. scaling
Braxton
      B. Hicks contraction
      B. Hicks sign
      B. Hicks version
Brazelton Neonatal Behavioral
  Assessment Scale (BNAS, BNBAS)
Brazilian blastomycosis
braziliense
      Ancylostoma b.
braziliensis
      Leishmania b.
BRBN
    blue rubber bleb nevus
BRBNS
    blue rubber bleb nevus syndrome
BRCA1
    breast cancer gene 1
      BRCA1 gene mutation
BRCA2
    breast cancer gene 2
      BRCA2 gene mutation
BRE
    benign rolandic epilepsy
bread-and-butter appearance
breakage
      catheter b.
      chromosome b.
Breakaway wound dressing
breakdown
      endometrial b.
      germinal vesicle b. (GVBD)
      skin b.
      wound b.
breakpoint cluster region (bcr)
breakthrough
      b. bleeding (BTB)
      b. varicella
breast
      b. abscess
      accessory b.
      adolescent b.
      alveolar lumen of b.
      b. architecture
      augmented b.
      b. binder
      b. binding
      B. Biopsy Guard

b. biopsy tissue
b. bud
caked b.
b. cancer (BC)
B. Cancer Detection Demonstration
  Project (BCDDP)
B. Cancer Detection Project
b. cancer gene 1
b. cancer gene 2
b. cancer prevention trial (BCPT)
b. cancer screening
B. Cancer System 2100
b. carcinoma
b. care
b. change
childhood b.
b. conservation
b. conservation therapy (BCT)
Contour Profile anatomically shaped
  silicone b.
Cooper irritable b.
b. cyst
cystic disease of the b.
cystic hyperplasia of the b.
b. development
b. disease
b. embryology
engorged b.
b. engorgement
b. enlargement
fibrocystic b.
b. flush
B. Imaging Reporting and Data
  System (BIRADS)
b. implant
irritable b.
keeled b.
lactating b.
b. leakage inhibitor system
lumpy b.
b. macrocalcification
b. malignancy
b. milk
b. milk jaundice (BMJ)
nonlactating b.
Paget disease of b.
peau d'orange appearance of b.
pendulous b.
pigeon b.
b. plate
proemial b.
b. prosthesis
b. pump
sclerosing adenosis of b.
b. secretion
b. self-examination (BSE)
shotty b.
b. stimulation contraction test
  (BSCT)

supernumerary b.
Trilucent b.
true accessory b.
BreastAlert differential temperature sensor
BreastCheck
breast-conserving therapy (BCT)
BreastExam
breast-fed, breastfed
b.-f. baby
breastfed (*var. of* breast-fed)
breast-feed, breastfeed
breastfeed (*var. of* breast-feed)
breast-feeding, breastfeeding
exclusive b.-f.
failed b.
b.-f. jaundice
breastfeeding (*var. of* breast-feeding)
breast/ovarian familial cancer syndrome
breast-preserving therapy
breaststroker's knee
breath
fetid b.
b. holding
b. H$_2$ test
b. hydrogen excretion test
b. hydrogen study
malodorous b.
b.'s per minute (bpm)
b. sounds (BS)
strep b.
b. testing
B. Tracker
uriniferous b.
breath-by-breath
b.-b.-b. method
b.-b.-b. method of gas collection
Breathe
B. Easy foam pad
B. Free
B. Right
breath-holding spell
breath-hold MR cholangiography
breathing
abdominal b.
fetal b.
intermittent positive pressure b. (IPPB)
mouth b.
mouth-to-mask b.
paradoxical b.
b. pattern
patterned b.
periodic b.
rescue b.
seesaw b.
sleep-disordered b.
spontaneous periodic b.
stridulous b.

synchronous b.
tidal b.
tubular b.
upper airway sleep-disordered b.
work of b. (WOB)
breathing-related sleep disorder
Breathmobile mobile asthma testing lab
Brecht feeder
breech
assisted b.
b. baby
b. birth
b. deformation sequence
b. extraction
frank b.
b. head
b. location
b. location out of pelvis
midfoot b.
nonfrank b.
b. position
b. presentation (BP)
b. singleton
spontaneous b.
b. transverse lie
b. type
b. vaginal delivery
breech-born with delayed fetal activity
breech-first twin
breed
breeding
cross b.
b. line
breeze
B. respirator
B. ventilator
Breezee Mist Aerosol
bregma
bregmatodymia
bregmocardiac reflex
Breisky-Navratil vaginal retractor
Brennen biosynthetic surgical mesh
Brenner
B. cell
B. cell tumor
B. tumor
brephoplastic
brequinar
Breslow-Day test
Breslow microstaging system
B$_6$-responsive anemia
Brethine
Brett
B. epileptogenic encephalopathy
B. syndrome
bretylium tosylate
Breuer-Hering inflation reflex

Breus mole
breve
    Bifidobacterium b.
Brevibloc
Brevicon
Brevi-Kath epidural catheter
brevis
    Demodex b.
Brevital Sodium
Brevoxyl-4
Brevoxyl-8
Brewster retractor
Briard-Evans syndrome
Bricker
    B. ileoureterostomy procedure
    B. ureteroileostomy
bridge
    B. extra-support over-the-wire renal stent system
    flat nasal b.
    low nasal b.
    membrane b.
    nasal b.
    physial b.
    B. Reading Program
bridging
    b. cross
    b. flap
    b. physis
    b. vein
brief
    b. reactive psychosis
    b., small, abundant motor-unit action potential (BSAP)
    b. tonic seizure
Brigance Diagnostic Inventory of Early Development
Briggs T adapter
bright
    b. thalamus syndrome
    b. white light therapy for postpartum depression
Brill disease
Brill-Zinsser disease
brim
    pelvic b.
    b. sign
brine flotation method
Brissaud
    B. dwarfism
    B. infantilism
    B. syndrome
Bristol Female Lower Urinary Tract Symptoms (BFLUTS)
British Society of Hematology
brittle
    b. bones
    b. diabetes
    b. hair

    b. hair, intellectual impairment, decreased fertility, short stature (BIDS)
    b. hair-mental deficit syndrome
    b. nail
brittle-bone disease
BRM
    biologic response modifier
broad
    b. A-band myopathy
    b. débridement
    b. flat nose
    b. forehead
    b. ligament
    b. ligament fold
    b. ligament hernia
    b. ligament pregnancy
    b. ligament tear syndrome
    b. nasal base
    b. nasal root
    b. physis
    b. thumb
    b. thumb-hallux syndrome
    b. thumb-mental retardation syndrome
    b. toe
broad-band scale
broad-based gait
broad-spectrum
    b.-s. antibiotic
    b.-s. antibiotic therapy
    b.-s. white light
Broca
    B. aphasia
    B. area
    B. pouch
Brockenbrough transseptal catheterization technique
Broders index
Brodie abscess
Brodie-Trendelenburg test
Brofed Elixir
Bromaline Elixir
Bromanate Elixir
Bromatapp
bromelin method
Bromfed
    B. Syrup
    B. tablet
Bromfenex PD
bromhidrosis, bromidrosis
    eccrine b.
    plantar eccrine b.
bromide
    ammonium b.
    calcium b.
    cyanogen b. (CNBr)
    decamethonium b.
    diphenyl tetrazolium b.

distigmine b.
ipratropium b.
mepenzolate b.
methantheline b.
oxyphenonium b.
pancuronium b.
Peacock b.
potassium b.
propantheline b.
pyridostigmine b.
sodium b.
strontium b.
triple b.
vecuronium b.
bromidrosis (*var. of* bromhidrosis)
bromium
bromocriptine
injectable b.
b. mesylate
b. prolactinoma
b. rebound
b. resistance
b. therapy
bromocriptine-resistant prolactinoma
bromodeoxyuridine (BUdR)
bromodiphenhydramine
bromomenorrhea
**bromopheniramine and
phenylpropanolamine**
bromsulfophthalein (BSP)
Bronalide
bronchi (*pl. of* bronchus)
bronchia (*pl. of* bronchium)
bronchial
b. asthma
b. atresia
b. breath sounds
b. bud
b. challenge test
b. hyperactivity
b. mucous cast
b. provocation
b. provocation challenge
b. provocation testing
b. tree
b. tube
b. wall thickening
bronchiectasis
congenital b.
bronchiolar thickening
bronchiole
ruptured b.
terminal b.
bronchiolectasia
bronchiolitis
acute b.
b. obliterans
b. obliterans organizing pneumonia
(BOOP)

obliterative fibroproliferative b.
respiratory syncytial virus b.
(RSVB)
RSV b.
viral necrotizing b.
bronchiseptica
Bordetella b.
bronchitis
acute laryngotracheal b.
arachidic b.
asthmatic b. (AB)
chronic obstructive b.
epidemic capillary b.
follicular b.
obliterative b.
plastic b.
wheezy b.
bronchium, pl. bronchia
bronchoalveolar
b. fluid
b. lavage (BAL)
bronchobiliary fistula
bronchoconstriction
bronchodilatation (*var. of*
bronchodilation)
bronchodilation, bronchodilatation
bronchodilator
b. drug
inhaled b.
oral b.
short-acting beta-2 agonist b.
bronchoesophageal fistula
bronchogenic cyst
bronchogram
air b.
bronchomalacia
bronchomotor tone
bronchophony
bronchopleural fistula
bronchopneumonia
bronchopulmonary
b. aspergillosis
b. dysplasia (BPD)
b. fistula (BPF)
b. lavage
b. malformation
b. sequestration (BPS)
bronchorrhea
bronchoscope
Holinger infant b.
infant b.
Storz infant b.
bronchoscopy
fiberoptic b.
flexible fiberoptic b.
open-tube b.
pediatric b.
rigid b.
virtual b.

B

bronchospasm
cold-induced b.
exercise-induced b. (EIB)
bronchospastic cough
bronchovesicular breath sounds
bronchus, *pl.* **bronchi**
elastic recoil of b.
main b.
bronchus-associated lymphoid tissue (BALT)
Bronkaid
Bronkometer Aerosol
Bronson chewable prenatal vitamin
Brontex
bronze
b. baby
b. baby syndrome
b. diabetes
b. Schilder disease
bronzed disease
Brooks syndrome
Brooks-Wisniewski-Brown syndrome
Broselow
B. chart
B. tape
broth
b. culture
Lim b.
Todd-Hewitt b.
Broviac catheter
brow
olympian b.
b. position
b. presentation
brow-anterior position
brow-down
b.-d. position
b.-d. presentation
brown
B. and Harris interview
b. baby syndrome
b. fat nonshivering thermogenesis
B. nodule
b. recluse spider
b. skin lesion
B. superior oblique tendon sheath syndrome
B. uvula retractor
B. vertical retraction syndrome
Brown-Adson tissue forceps
Browne
testis within superficial inguinal pouch of Denis B.
Brown-Hopp tissue Gram stain
Brown-Séquard syndrome
Brown-Symmers disease
Brown-Vialetto-van Laere syndrome

Brown-Wickham urethral pressure profilometry technique
brow-posterior position
brow-up position
Broxidine
broxuridine
Brozek body fat percentage formula
BRRS
Bannayan-Riley-Ruvalcaba syndrome
BRS
Behavior Rating Scale
BRSA
borderline-resistant Staphylococcus aureus
brucei
Trypanosoma b.
Brucella
B. agar plate
B. canis
B. melitensis
B. suis
brucellosis
Bruck-de Lange syndrome
Bruckner pupillary light reflex test
Brudzinski sign
Brugada syndrome
Brugia
B. beaveri
B. lepori
Bruhat
B. laser fimbrioplasty
B. neosalpingostomy technique
Bruininks-Oseretsky
B.-O. test
B.-O. Test of Motor Proficiency
bruisability
bruisabilty
easy b.
bruit
abdominal b.
aortic b.
carotid b.
cranial b.
b. placentaire
placental b.
Brun
layer of B.
Brunner
B. gland
B. syndrome
Brusa-Torricelli syndrome
brush
Bayne Pap B.
b. border assembly
cytology b.
b. cytology
endocervical sampling b.
FoamCare double scrub b.

Brushfield spot
Brushfield-Wyatt syndrome
brushing
 colposcopically directed b.
Bruton
 B. agammaglobulinemia
 B. disease
Bruton/B-cell tyrosine kinase gene
bruxism
 sleep b.
Bryan-Leishman stain
Bryant traction
Bryce-Teacher ovum
BS
 Bartter syndrome
 bowel sounds
 breath sounds
BSA
 body surface area
BSAB
 Balthazar Scales of Adaptive
 Behavior
BSAER
 brainstem auditory evoked response
BSAP
 brief, small, abundant motor-unit
 action potential
B-scanner
 real-time B-s.
 static B-s.
BSCT
 breast stimulation contraction test
BSE
 bovine spongiform encephalopathy
 breast self-examination
BSER
 brainstem evoked response
 BSER audiometry
BSERA
 brainstem evoked response audiometry
BSG
 brachioskeletogenital
 BSG syndrome
BSI
 bloodstream infection
BSID
 Bayley Scales of Infant Development
BSID-II
 Bayley Scales of Infant
 Development-II
BSO
 bilateral salpingo-oophorectomy
BSP
 bromsulfophthalein
B19-specific IgG
BSS
 Bernard-Soulier syndrome
BSSL
 bile salt-stimulated lipase

BT
 behavioral therapy
 bladder tumor
BTA
 botulinum toxin A
 BTA STAT test
BTB
 breakthrough bleeding
BTL
 bilateral tubal ligation
bubble
 bladder b.
 b. boy disease
 extraluminal gas b.
 gastric b.
 b. gum cytoplasm
 b. isolation unit
 b. isolette
 b. stability test
 stomach b.
bubbler humidifier
Bubbli-Pred
bubbly
 b. crackle
 b. lungs
 b. lung syndrome
bubo
 b. aspirate
 bullet b.
 chancroidal b.
 climatic b.
 primary b.
 tropical b.
 venereal b.
 virulent b.
bubonic
bucca, *pl.* **buccae**
buccae (*pl. of* bucca)
buccal
 b. cellulitis
 b. fat pad
 b. feeding technique
 b. mucosa
 b. mucosa graft
 Nitrogard B.
buccolingual apraxia
buccomandibular dystonia
bucket-handle fracture
buckle fracture
buckshot calcification
buclizine
bucrylate
bud
 aortic b.
 breast b.
 bronchial b.
 distal tongue b.
 end b.
 epithelial b.

bud (*continued*)
    hair b.
    limb b.
    liver b.
    metanephric b.
    pulmonary b.
    syncytial b.
    tail b.
    taste b.
    tooth b.
    ureteric b.
Budd-Chiari syndrome
Buddhalike habitus
Buddha stance
budding
buddy taping
budesonide
    controlled ileal release b.
    b. inhalation suspension (BIS)
    b. therapy
    b. Turbuhaler
Budin rule
BUdR
    bromodeoxyuridine
Buenos Aires type mental retardation
buffalo hump
Buffaprin
buffer
buffered
    b. aspirin
    b. lidocaine
Bufferin
Buffinol
buffy
    b. coat
    b. coat component
    b. coat examination
    b. coat layer
Bugbee electrode
Buhl disease
Buist intraabdominal pressure measurement method
bulb
    femoral b.
    b. of vestibule of vagina
    phototherapy b.
    Rouget b.
    sinovaginal b.
    b. suction
    b. suctioning
    b. syringe
    vaginal b.
    vestibular b.
    vestibulovaginal b.
bulbar
    b. conjunctiva
    b. conjunctival injection
    b. hereditary motor neuropathy (type I, II)

    b. palsy
    b. paralysis
    b. polioencephalitis
    b. poliomyelitis
bulbi (*pl. of* bulbus)
bulbitis
bulbocavernosus
    b. fat flap
    b. muscle
    b. reflex
bulbospinal poliomyelitis
bulbospongiosus muscle
bulbourethral gland
bulbous nasal tip
bulboventricular foramen
bulbus, *pl.* **bulbi**
    b. cordis
    b. penis
    b. pili
    b. urethrae
    b. vestibuli vaginae
bulgaricus
    Lactobacillus b.
bulge
    biparietal b.
    parietal b.
    precordial b.
bulging
    b. flank
    b. fontanelle
bulimia, boulimia
    b. nervosa (BN)
    b. nervosa nonpurging (BN-NP)
bulimorexia
bulk
    b. flow
    Modane B.
    muscle b.
    b. selection
bulked segregant analysis
bulk-forming laxative
bulky carcinoma
bulla, *pl.* **bullae**
    sausage-shaped b.
    scaling b.
    transparent b.
bullae (*pl. of* bulla)
bulldog syndrome
bullet bubo
bullosa
    acantholysis b.
    albopapuloid Pasini form of dominant dystrophic epidermolysis b.
    Cockayne-Touraine variant of dominant dystrophic epidermolysis b.
    concha b.
    dermolysis b.
    dominant dystrophic epidermolysis b.

dystrophic epidermolysis b.
epidermolysis b. (EB)
generalized atrophic benign
  epidermolysis b. (GABEB)
hereditary macular epidermolysis b.
junctional epidermolysis b.
recessive dystrophic epidermolysis b.
  (RDEB)
varicella b.

bullous
b. congenital ichthyosiform
  erythroderma
b. dermatosis
b. drug eruption
b. erythema multiforme
b. impetigo
b. mastocytosis
b. myringitis
b. pemphigoid
b. reaction
b. varicella

bull's eye sonographic appearance
bumetanide
Bumex
Buminate
Bumm curette
bump
Bumpa Bed crib bumper pad
bumper bed
BUN
blood urea nitrogen

bundle
b. branch block (BBB)
hypertrophic b.
b. of His
b. of Probst
papillomacular b.

bungarotoxin
bunion
adolescent b.
dorsal b.

bunionette deformity
bunny hopping
Bunostomum phlebotomum
Bunyaviridae
Bunyavirus
BUO
bilateral ureteral obstruction

Buphenyl
buphthalmia, buphthalmus, buphthalmos
buphthalmos (*var. of* buphthalmia)
buphthalmus (*var. of* buphthalmia)
bupivacaine collagen sponge
buprenorphine
bupropion hydrochloride
Burch
B. colposuspension
B. colpourethropexy
B. modification

B. procedure
B. retropubic urethropexy

burden
body lead b.
genetic b.
b. of care interview for
  children
tumor b.

burgdorferi
Borrelia b.

Burger triangle
buried
b. penis
b. suture
b. vaginal island procedure

Burkholderia
B. cepacia
B. cepacia genomovar (III)
B. gladioli
B. mallei
B. multivorans
B. multivorans genomovar (II)
B. norimbergensis
B. pickettii
B. pseudomallei
B. vietnamiensis

Burkitt
B. lymphoma (BL)
B. sarcoma
B. tumor cell

burn
alkali b.
b. assessment
Berkow formula for b.'s
circumferential b.
deep partial-thickness b.
dry chemical b.
electrical b.
b. encephalopathy
first-degree b.
flame b.
fourth-degree b.
full-thickness b.
immersion b.
b. management
partial-thickness b.
second-degree b.
splash b.
TBSA b.
thermal b.
third-degree b.

Burnet acquired immunity
burnetii
Coxiella b.

burning
b. vulva syndrome
vulvovaginal b.

burnlike dermatitis
Burn-McKeown syndrome

B

burnout
    mother b.
Burow solution
burp
    wet b.
burping
burrow
    pus b.
burr-shaped erythrocyte
bursa, *pl.* **bursae**
    gastrocnemius-semimembranosus b.
    greater trochanteric b.
    iliopectineal b.
    b. of Fabricius
bursa-dependent system
bursae (*pl. of* bursa)
bursitis
    pes anserina b.
    prepatellar b.
    septic b.
    suppurative b.
burst
    suppression b.
burst-forming units-erythroid (BFU-E)
bursting fracture
burst-suppression pattern
Burton gum lead line
Burt Word Reading Test
BUS
    Bartholin, urethral, Skene
    BUS glands
Busacca iris nodule
Buschke
    scleredema of B.
Buschke-Ollendorf syndrome
buserelin stimulation test
BuSpar
buspirone hydrochloride
busulfan, busulphan
busulphan (*var. of* busulfan)
butabarbital
Butalan
butalbital
butaperazine
Butazolidin
Butazone
butenafine antifungal agent
butoconazole
    b. 2% cream
    b. nitrate
butorphanol
    b. tartrate
    b. tartrate nasal spray
butoxide
    piperonyl b.
    pyrethrins and piperonyl b.
butriptyline hydrochloride
Butschli granule
Butt

    B. Balm
    B. Paste
butterbur
butterfly
    b. brain
    b. distribution
    b. drain
    b. flap
    b. rash
    b. scalp vein needle
    b. vertebrae
button
    gastrostomy b.
    peritoneal b.
buttonhole incision
buttonholing
buttonpexy fixation
buttress
    facial b.
    mechanical b.
    b. response
butyrate
    hydrocortisone b.
    b. therapy
butyrophenone
Buxton clamp
BV
    bacterial vaginitis
    bacterial vaginosis
BVBLUE test
BVI2500
    BladderScan BVI2500
BVM
    bag, valve, mask
    BVM device
    BVM ventilation
BW
    birth weight
BWGA
    birth weight for gestational age
BWS
    Beckwith-Wiedemann syndrome
Byers hypospadias flap
Byler
    B. disease
    B. syndrome
by-mouth feeding
bypass
    cardiopulmonary b.
    b. continence mechanism
    gastric b.
    jejunoileal b.
    low-flow cardiopulmonary b.
    b. surgery
    ventricular b.
bystander effect
by way of rectum (p.r.)
BZS
    Bannayan-Zonana syndrome

3C
craniocerebellocardiac
3C dysplasia
3C syndrome
C
C band
C syndrome
C1
C1 esterase inhibitor
C1 esterase inhibitor deficiency
C$_4$
leukotriene C$_4$ (LTC$_4$)
C21
C$_{21}$ progestin
C$_{21}$ progestogen
C-500
Optimox C-500
CA
CA 15-3
CA 125 antigen
CA 125 assay
CA 15-3 breast cancer marker
CA 125 endometrial cancer marker
CA monitor
CA 549 tumor marker
CA126 level
Ca
calcium
cancer
carcinoma
CA-125
cancer antigen 125
CAA
coronary artery aneurysm
CAB
catheter-associated bacteremia
CABA
child and adolescent burden assessment
cabbage leaves
cabergoline
CaBF
carotid blood flow
cable
twister c.
Cabot
C. cannula
C. trocar
cachectic infantilism
cachectin
cachexia
cancer c.
cacogenesis
cacomelia

Ca/Cr
calcium-creatinine ratio
Ca/Cr ratio
CAD
computer-aided diagnosis
cadaveric donor
CADD-Prizm pain control system
cadence
CAE
cefuroxime axetil
childhood absence epilepsy
caecum (*var. of* cecum)
caerulea (*var. of* cerulea)
caeruleus
locus c.
CAF
cell adhesion factor
coronary artery fistula
CAFAS
Child and Adolescent Functional Assessment Scale
Cafatine
Cafcit
café
c. au lait (CAL)
c. au lait macule (CALMs)
c. au lait spot
Cafergot
caffeine
c. citrate
citrated c.
c. terbutaline
c. therapy
caffeinism
Caffey
C. disease
C. pseudo-Hurler syndrome
Caffey-Kenny disease
Caffey-Silverman syndrome
CAFMHS
child, adolescent, and family mental health service
cage
manual splinting of thoracic c.
CAGE
cutting, annoyance, guilt, eye-opener
CAGE test
CAGE test for alcohol abuse
CAG expansion
CAH
congenital adrenal hyperplasia
CAHMR
cataract, hypertrichosis, mental retardation
CAHMR syndrome

CAHV
    central alveolar hypoventilation
CAIS
    complete androgen insensitivity
       syndrome
Caisson disease
Caitlin mark
CAIV
    cold-adapted influenza vaccine
CAIV-T
    trivalent live cold-adapted influenza
       vaccine
Cajal-Retzius neuron
cake
        omental c.
caked breast
CAL
    café au lait
    coronary artery lesion
Calabro syndrome
Caladryl for Kids
calamine lotion
Calan SR
calcaneal, calcanean
    c. apophysitis
    c. compartment
    c. fracture
    c. prominence
    c. tendon
    c. view
calcanean (*var. of* calcaneal)
calcanei (*pl. of* calcaneus)
calcaneocuboid ligament (CCL)
calcaneofibular ligament (CFL)
calcaneonavicular (CN)
    c. articulation
    c. bar
    c. coalition
    c. fusion
calcaneotibial angle
calcaneovalgus
    c. deformity
    c. flatfoot
    c. foot
    talipes c.
calcaneovarus
    talipes c.
calcaneum (*var. of* calcaneus)
calcaneus, calcaneum, *pl.* **calcanei**
    talipes c.
Cal Carb-HD
Calci-Chew
calcidiol
calcifediol
calciferol
calcificans
    angioma capillare et venosum c.
    chondrodystrophia fetalis c.
    liponecrosis microcystica c.

calcification
    adrenal c.
    amorphous breast c.
    arterial c.
    basal ganglion c.
    buckshot c.
    cardiovascular c.
    cervical disc space c.
    coarse c.
    dystrophic c.
    granulomatous c.
    hepatic capsular c.
    intervertebral disc c. (IDC)
    intracranial c.
    malignant c.
    perivascular c.
    popcorn-like c.
    provisional c.
    secretory c.
    skin c.
    subcutaneous c.
    sutural c.
    vascular c.
    zone of preparatory c. (ZPC)
calcific vasopathy
calcified
    c. appendicolith
    c. bacterial plaque
    c. exostosis
    c. fecalith
    c. fetus
    c. mass
    c. matrix
    c. myoma
    c. outline of cyst
    c. phlebolith
    c. phleboliths in pelvis
    c. uterine fibroid
calcifying epithelioma
Calcijex
Calci-Mix
calcineurin inhibitor
calcinosis
    c., Raynaud phenomenon, esophageal
       dysmotility, sclerodactyly,
       telangiectasia (CREST)
    c., Raynaud phenomenon,
       sclerodactyly, telangiectasia (CRST)
calciotropic hormone
Calciparine
calcipotriene
calcitonin
    c. receptor
    c. salmon
calcitriol
calcium (Ca)
    c. absorption
    c. acetate
    c. agonist

c. alginate
c. alginate swab
c. bromide
c. carbonate
c. channel antagonist
c. channel blocker
c. chloride
c. citrate
c. crystal
c. cyclamate
death by c.
c. deficiency
C. Disodium Versenate
docusate c.
fenoprofen c.
c. glubionate
c. gluconate
c. heparin
c. indicator rhod-2
intracellular c.
c. ion
ionized c. (iCa)
c. leukovorin
c. pantothenate
c. phosphate
c. polycarbophil
c. rich
c. salt
serum c.
c. supplement
c. supplementation
calcium-creatinine ratio
calcivirus
calcofluor white stain
calculation
Berkson-Gage c.
body surface area c.
free water c.
water deficit c.
calculi (*pl. of* calculus)
calculus, *pl.* **calculi**
indinavir calculi
lacteal c.
mammary c.
renal c.
urate c.
urinary c.
uterine c.
Caldecort
C. Anti-Itch Topical Spray
C. Topical
Calderol
Caldesene Topical
Caldwell-Moloy
C.-M. classification
C.-M. pelvis type
Caldwell view
Calendar of Premenstrual Syndrome Experience

calf
c. compression unit
c. lung surfactant extract (CLSE)
calfactant
Calgiswab
caliber-persistent artery
calibrator
Atomlab 200 dose c.
calicectasis (*var. of* caliectasis)
calices (*var. of* calyces)
calicivirus
human c. (HuCV)
C. infection
caliectasis, pyelocaliectasis, calicectasis
California
C. encephalitis
C. Verbal Learning Test-Children's Version
californium-252 (^{252}Cf)
calipers
Harpenden c.
Tenzel c.
calix (*var. of* calyx)
Calkins sign
Call-Exner body
callosal
c. agenesis
c. inhibition
callosum
agenesis of corpus c.
corpus c.
hereditary agenesis of corpus c.
X-linked mental retardation-seizures-acquired microcephaly-agenesis of corpus c.
callus
exuberant c.
Calmers
Robitussin Cough C.
Sucrets Cough C.
Calmette-Guérin
bacille C.-G. (BCG)
calmodulin
Calmol 4
Calmoseptine ointment
CALMs
café au lait macule
Calm-X Oral
calomel
caloric
c. challenge
c. insufficiency
c. intake
c. method
calorie (cal), calory
c. per ounce (cal/oz)
20-calorie formula
24-calorie formula

calorimeter
    Deltatrac II indirect c.
calorimetry
    indirect c.
    infrared thermographic c. (ITC)
    resting c.
calory (*var. of* calorie)
cal/oz
    calorie per ounce
calpainopathy
calprotectin
    fecal c.
    median fecal c.
Caltrate 600
calusterone
calvarial
    c. hyperostosis
    c. osteomyelitis
calvarium
Calvé-Legg-Perthes syndrome
Calvé-Perthes disease
calyces (*pl. of* calyx)
Calymmatobacterium granulomatis
calyx, calix, *pl.* **calyces**
    obstructed c.
    renal c.
CAM
    cell adhesion molecule
    child-adult mist
    chorioallantoic membrane
    complementary and alternative
      medicine
    cystic adenomatoid malformation
    cystic adenomatous malformation
      CAM tent
CAMAK
    cataract, microcephaly, arthrogryposis,
      kyphosis
      CAMAK syndrome
Cameco
    C. syringe holder
    C. syringe pistol aspiration device
Cameron-Myers vaginoscope
Camey
    C. ileocystoplasty
    C. reservoir
CAMFAK
    cataract, microcephaly, failure to
      thrive, kyphoscoliosis
      CAMFAK syndrome
Camino monitor
camomile (*var. of* chamomile)
cAMP
    cyclic adenosine monophosphate
      cAMP test
CAMP
    Childhood Asthma Management
      Program
Campbell Soup kid facies

Camper
    C. fascia
    C. fascia of vulva
campesterol
camphor
camphorated oil
camplodactyly (*var. of* camptodactyly)
**CAMP-specific phosphodiesterase
  inhibitor**
camptobrachydactyly
camptodactylia (*var. of* camptodactyly)
camptodactylism (*var. of* camptodactyly)
**camptodactyly, camptodactylia,
  camplodactyly, camptodactylism,
  streblodactyly**
camptomelia
camptomelic
    c. dwarfism
    c. dysplasia
    c. syndrome
Camptosar
Campylobacter
    C. coli
    C. concisus
    C. cryaerophilia
    C. enteritis
    C. fetus
    C. fetus intestinalis
    C. fetus jejuni
    C. gastroenteritis
    C. gracilis
    C. hyointestinalis
    C. infection
    C. jejuni
    C. jejuni doylei
    C. lari
    C. mucosalis
    C. pylori
    C. sputorum
    C. upsaliensis
CAMRSA
    community-acquired methicillin-resistant
      Staphylococcus aureus
camsylate
    trimethaphan c.
Camurati-Engelmann syndrome
Canadian
    C. Acute Respiratory Illness and
      Flu Scale (CARIFS)
    C. Crohn Relapse Prevention Trial
canal
    Alcock c.
    anal c.
    anorectal c.
    atrioventricular c.
    attenuated pyloric c.
    auditory c.
    birth c.
    Braune c.

cervical c.
complete atrioventricular c.
ear c.
elastic c.
endocervical c.
external auditory c. (EAC)
Hunter c.
inguinal c.
Kohn c.
Kovalevsky c.
medullary c.
neurenteric c.
Nuck c.
obstetric c.
c. of Nuck
c. of Nuck cyst
omphalomesenteric c.
parturient c.
Petit canals
plane of pelvic c.
pudendal c.
rectal c.
Schlemm c.
semicircular c.
Steiner c.
c. type ASD
uterovaginal c.
vesicourethral c.

canalicular
c. period
c. stage
c. stage of lung development
c. testis
canaliculi (*pl. of* **canaliculus**)
canaliculus, *pl.* **canaliculi**
pili trianguli et canaliculi
Canavan disease
Canavan-van Bogaert-Bertrand disease
Cancell
cancer
advanced epithelial ovarian c.
anal c.
c. and steroid hormone (CASH)
c. antigen 125 (CA-125, CA 125)
c. antigen 125 test
breast c.
c. cachexia
cervical stump c.
c. chemotherapy
clear cell vaginal c.
Collaborative Group on Hormonal
Factors in Breast C.
colorectal c.
C. Committee of College of
American Pathologists
endometrial c.
epithelial ovarian c. (stage I–IV)
familial ovarian c.
c. family syndrome

c. genetics
gynecologic c.
hereditary nonpolyposis c. (HNPCC)
hereditary nonpolyposis colon c.
(HNPCC)
hereditary nonpolyposis colorectal c.
(HNPCC)
hereditary ovarian c.
inflammatory breast c. (IBC)
International Union Against C.
(UICC)
intraductal c.
intraepithelial endometrial c.
invasive c. (IC)
invasive cervical c. (ICC)
lung c.
microinvasive cervical c. (MICA)
morphology of breast c.
mucinous c.
National Institutes of Health
Consensus Conference on
Ovarian C.
c. nest
occult c.
ovarian c.
ovarian epithelial c. (OEC)
persistent c.
c. predisposition syndrome
premenopausal breast c.
RECAF blood test for breast c.
rectal c.
recurrent cervical c.
SGO classification of c.
site-specific familial ovarian c.
testicular c.
c. therapy
thyroid c.
tubular c.
vaginal c.
Wolfe classification of breast c.
cancericidal dose
Candela laser
candicidin
Candida
C. albicans
C. albicans vaginitis
C. colonization
C. diaper dermatitis
C. dubliniensis
C. glabrata
C. glabrata vaginitis
C. infection
C. krusei
C. meningitis
C. parapsilosis
C. paratropicalis
C. pseudotropicalis
recurrent *C.*
C. skin test

C

Candida (*continued*)
   C. stellatoides
   C. tropicalis
   C. tropicalis vaginitis
candidal
   c. arthritis
   c. diaper dermatitis
   c. diaper rash
   c. glossitis
   c. onychomycosis
   c. paronychia
   c. vaginitis
   c. vulvovaginitis
candidasis
   congenital cutaneous c.
   interdigital c.
candidemia
   transient c.
candidiasis, candidosis
   acute atrophic c.
   acute pseudomembranous c.
   chronic mucocutaneous c.
   congenital c.
   cutaneous c.
   disseminated c.
   esophageal c.
   hepatosplenic c.
   intertriginous c.
   invasive c.
   mucocutaneous c.
   neonatal c.
   oral c.
   oropharyngeal c. (OPC)
   perianal c.
   recurrent vulvovaginal c.
    (RVVC)
   renal c.
   systemic c.
   vaginal c.
   vulvovaginal c. (VVC)
candidosis (*var. of* candidiasis)
   intertriginous c.
   vaginal c.
candiduria
Candistatin
candle
   cesium c.
   c. dripping
   urethral c.
   vaginal c.
candlestick sign
candy-cane stirrups
Canesten
   C. Topical
   C. Vaginal
canicola
   Leptospira c.
canimorsus
   Capnocytophaga c.

canine
   c. distemper
   c. scabies
   c. tooth
caninum
   Ancylostoma c.
canis
   Brucella c.
   Microsporum c.
   Pasteurella c.
   Toxocara c.
canker sore
Cannabis sativa
cannonball lesion
cannula, canula, *pl.* **cannulas, cannulae**
   acorn c.
   Bard cervical c.
   Cabot c.
   cervical c.
   Circon-ACMI c.
   Cohen uterine c.
   Core Dynamics disposable c.
   Dexide disposable c.
   disposable c.
   endometrial c.
   Ethicon disposable c.
   flexible MVA c.
   Genitor mini-intrauterine
    insemination c.
   Gesco c.
   Hasson c.
   high-flow nasal c.
   Hunt-Reich c.
   indwelling c.
   intrauterine balloon-type c.
   intrauterine insemination c.
   IUI disposable c.
   Jacobs c.
   Jarit disposable c.
   Kahn c.
   Karman c.
   LaparoSAC single-use obturator
    and c.
   Lübke uterine vacuum c.
   Marlow disposable c.
   nasal c.
   Olympus disposable c.
   Rubin c.
   Scott c.
   Semm uterine vacuum c.
   Solos disposable c.
   stable access c.
   stepdown c.
   Storz disposable c.
   trumpet c.
   Vabra c.
   vacuum c.
   Vancaillie uterine c.
   Weck disposable c.

Wisap disposable c.
Wolf disposable c.
cannulae (*pl. of* cannula)
cannulas (*pl. of* cannula)
cannulate
cannulated screw
cannulation, cannulization
arterial c.
jugular venous c.
peripheral arterial c.
posterior tibial artery c.
venoarterial c.
venovenous c.
cannulization (*var. of* cannulation)
canopy
surgical overhead c. (SOC)
cantharidin
cantharis
canthi (*pl. of* canthus)
canthomeatal line
canthorum
dystopia c.
canthus, *pl.* **canthi**
heterochromia of inner c.
inner c.
lateral displacement of inner c.
outer c.
Cantil
cantonensis
Angiostrongylus c.
Cantor tube
Cantrell
pentalogy of C.
C. syndrome
Cantú syndrome
Cantwell-Ransley repair
canula (*var. of* cannula)
cap
acrosomal c.
anterior head c.
cervical c.
Compoz Gel C.'s
cradle c.
Dutch cap
Oves Cervical C.
Oves conception c.
ProtectaCap c.
stockinette cap
Universal reducer c.
urethral c.
vault c.
CAPA
Child and Adolescent Psychiatric
Assessment
capacitation
sperm c.
capacitive
capacity
alveolar-arterial oxygen diffusing c.

bladder c.
closing c. (CC)
corticosteroid-binding globulin-binding
c. (CB-GBC)
cystometric c.
diffusing c.
fetal blood oxygen-carrying c.
forced vital c. (FVC)
functional residual c. (FRC)
inspiratory c. (IC)
iron-binding c. (IBC)
lung c.
maximum breathing c.
opsonic c.
oxygen-diffusing c.
plasma iron-binding c.
pulmonary diffusing c.
reduced bladder c.
renal reserve filtration c.
(RRFC)
serum bilirubin-binding c.
total iron-binding c. (TIBC)
total lung c. (TLC)
urinary concentrating c.
vital c. (VC)
Capasee diagnostic ultrasound system
CAPD
central auditory processing disorder
continuous ambulatory peritoneal
dialysis
capillariasis
hepatic c.
capillary
c. angioma
c. BLL
c. blood gas (CBG)
c. blood gas sampling
dilated c.
distended c.
c. dropout
c. electrophoresis
c. electrophoresis/frontal analysis
(CE/FA)
c. end loop
c. erection
c. filling time
c. hemangioma
c. isoelectric focusing technique
c. leak
c. leak injury
c. leak syndrome (CLS)
nail-fold c.
c. pattern
c. refill
c. refill time
tortuous c.
capillosus
Bacteroides c.
capita (*pl. of* caput)

capital
c. femoral epiphysis
c. femoral epiphysis slip
capitate bone
capitellar
c. epiphysis
c. osteochondritis
capitellum
displaced c.
osteochondritis of c.
capitis (*gen. of* caput)
caplet
Advil Cold Sinus C.
Dristan Sinus c.
Miles Nervine c.
Sinumist-SR c.
TripTone c.
Capnocytophaga canimorsus
capnograph
Microstream c.
capnography
low-flow sidestream c.
capnometry
Capoten
capped uterus
capreomycin
caproate
hydroxyprogesterone c.
17-alpha-hydroxyprogesterone c.
17-hydroxyprogesterone c.
Caprosyn monofilament suture
capsaicin
capsicum
Capsin
capsularis
decidua c.
capsular stripping
capsulatum
Histoplasma c.
capsule
boric acid c.
Bowman c.
contraceptive suppository c.
Crosby c.
Crosby-Kugler pediatric c.
Dexedrine Spansule c.
Glisson c.
Heyman c.
joint c.
Kadian sustained-release morphine c.
Norvir c.
ruptured c.
Uro-Mag c.
Virilon c.
Watson c.
CapSure continence shield
CAPTA
Child Abuse Prevention and Treatment Act

captopril
capture
ovum c.
caput, *gen.* **capitis,** *pl.* **capita**
c. medusae
pediculosis capitis
Pediculus humanus capitis
c. quadratum
c. succedaneum
tinea capitis
Capute scale
car
c. seat for newborn
c. sickness
Carafate
caramel test
carateum
Treponema c.
carbachol
Isopto C.
carbamazepine (CBZ)
carbamide peroxide
carbamoyl phosphate synthetase (CPS)
carbamoyltransferase
ornithine c. (OCT)
carbapenem
carbarsone
carbazole
carbenicillin
carbergoline
carbetocin
Carb-HD
Cal C.-HD
carbimazole
carbinoxamine
c. and pseudoephedrine
c. maleate
carbogen
carbohydrate
c. counting
c. deficient glycoprotein (CDG)
c. homeostasis
c. homeostasis transporter
c. intolerance
c. malabsorption
c. metabolism
c. overloading
c. tolerance
carbohydrate-deficient glycoprotein syndrome (type I, II)
carbohydrate-free
Ross c.-f. (RCF)
Carbolith
carbon
c. dioxide (CO_2)
c. dioxide gas
c. dioxide laser
c. dioxide laser beam conization
c. dioxide laser vaporization

c. dioxide retention
c. monoxide (CO)
c. monoxide poisoning
c. monoxide toxicity
c. tetrachloride
carbonaceous sputum
carbonate
   calcium c.
   lithium c.
carbonic
   c. acid
   c. anhydrase inhibitor
carbon-14 test
carbon-13 urea breath test
carbonyl iron
carboplatin
carboplatin/docetaxel
carboprost tromethamine
carboxamide
   dimethyl-triazeno-imidazole c.
   (DTIC)
carboxyhemoglobin (COHb)
carboxykinase
   phosphoenolpyruvate c. (PEPCK)
carboxylase
   acetyl-CoA c.
   alpha-methylcrotonyl-coenzyme A c.
   c. deficiency
   deficiency of pyruvate c.
carboxylation
carboxyl terminal peptide (CTP)
carboxypeptidase E
carboxyterminal
   c. propeptide
   c. propeptide of type 1 procollagen
   (PICP)
carbuncle
Carcassonne ligament
carcinoembryonic antigen (CEA)
carcinogen
   chemical c.
carcinogenesis
   pediatric thyroid c.
   radiation c.
carcinogenic
carcinoid
   nonappendiceal c.
   c. syndrome
   c. tumor
carcinoma (CA), *pl.* **carcinomas,**
carcinomata
   acinic cell c.
   adenocystic c.
   adenoid cystic c.
   adenosquamous c.
   adrenal cortical c.
   advanced c.
   anaplastic c.
   androgen-dependent c.

c. antigen
Bartholin gland c.
basal cell c.
borderline epithelial ovarian c.
breast c.
bulky c.
cecal c.
cervical c.
childhood thyroid c.
choroid plexus c. (CPC)
clear cell endometrial c.
colloid c.
colon c.
contralateral synchronous c.
ductal c.
embryonal cell c. (ECC)
endometrial c.
endometrioid c.
epithelial cell ovarian c.
esophageal c.
estrogen-dependent endometrial c.
estrogen-independent endometrial c.
FAB staging of c.
fallopian tube c.
fibrolamellar hepatocellular c.
  (FL-HCC)
focal lobular c.
gastric c.
glassy cell c.
gynecologic c.
hepatocellular c. (HCC)
infantile embryonal c.
infiltrating ductal c. (IDC)
infiltrating lobular c. (ILC)
infiltrating small cell lobular c.
inflammatory c.
c. in situ (CIS)
intracystic papillary c.
intraductal papillary c. (IPC)
invasive duct c.
invasive squamous cell c. (ISCC)
juvenile c.
keratinizing nasopharyngeal c.
lobular c.
lung c.
medullary thyroid c.
Merkel cell c.
mesometanephric c.
mesonephric c.
mesonephroid clear cell c.
metaplastic c.
metastatic c.
microinvasive c. (MICA)
mucinous c.
mucoepidermoid c.
multicentric c.
multiple nevoid-basal cell c.
  (MNBCC)
nasopharyngeal c.

carcinoma (*continued*)
    nevoid basal cell c. (NBCC)
    oat cell c.
    c. of cervix
    ovarian small cell c.
    papillary endometrial c.
    papillary serous cervical c.
    papillary squamous cell c.
    peritoneal c.
    peritoneal serous papillary c.
    Post Operative Radiation Therapy in Endometrial C. (PORTEC)
    preclinical c.
    primary hepatocellular c. (PHC)
    primary peritoneal c. (PPC)
    rectosigmoid c.
    recurrent c.
    renal cell c. (RCC)
    renal medullary c.
    scirrhous c.
    secretory c.
    serous c.
    signet ring cell c.
    small cell c.
    sporadic nonfamilial clear cell c.
    squamous cell c. (SCC, SCCA)
    thyroid c.
    tubular c.
    uterine corpus c.
    uterine papillary serous c. (UPSC)
    vaginal c.
    verrucous c.
    villoglandular endometrial c.
    vulvar adenosquamous c.
    vulvovaginal c.
    well-circumscribed c.
    wolffian duct c.
    yolk sac c.
carcinomas (*pl. of* carcinoma)
carcinomata (*pl. of* carcinoma)
carcinomatosis
    meningeal c.
carcinosarcoma
    uterine c.
card
    Allen Kindergarten Picture C.
    Amines test c.
    Guthrie c.
    neonatal Guthrie c.
    Peabody Developmental Motor Activity C.
    Sheridan-Gardiner visual acuity c.
    Sonksen-Silver visual acuity c.
    Sonogram fetal ultrasound image c.
cardiac
    c., abnormal facies, thymic hypoplasia, cleft palate, hypocalcemia syndrome
    c. abnormality
    c. abnormality, abnormal facies, thymic hypoplasia, cleft palate, hypocalcemia (CATCH, CATCH 22)
    c. abnormality, T-cell deficit, clefting, hypocalcemia phenotype
    c. anomaly
    c. arrest
    c. arrhythmia
    c. asthma
    c. autonomic modulation
    c. catheter
    c. catheterization
    c. compression
    c. cyanosis
    c. dysrhythmia
    c. ejection fraction
    c. event monitor
    c. failure
    c. flow
    c. function
    c. glycoside
    c. hemangioma
    c. hemolytic anemia
    c. index (CI)
    c. lesion
    c. looping
    c. malformation
    c. malposition
    c. massage
    c. monitoring
    c. murmur
    c. output
    c. rhabdomyoma
    c. rhythm disorder
    c. rupture
    c. septal defect
    c. septation
    c. silhouette
    c. size
    c. standstill
    c. stun
    c. syncope
    c. tamponade
    c. transplantation
    c. trauma
    c. troponin T
    c. twinning
    c. width
cardiac-apnea (CA)
    c.-a. monitor
cardiac-limb syndrome
Cardiff
    C. Count-to-Ten chart
    C. resuscitation bag
Cardilate

cardinal
    c. ligament
    c. movement
    c. movements of labor
    c. point
    c. vein
cardinal-uterosacral
    c.-u. ligament
    c.-u. ligament complex
Cardiobacterium hominis
cardiocranial syndrome
cardioesophageal junction
cardiofacial syndrome
cardiofaciocutaneous (CFC)
cardiogenesis
cardiogenic
    c. pulmonary edema
    c. shock (CGS)
cardiogenital syndrome
cardiogram
    impedance c.
cardioinhibitory syncope
cardiomegaly
cardiomyocyte
cardiomyopathy
    chronic chagasic c.
    congestive c.
    diabetic c.
    dilated c.
    fetal c.
    histiocytoid c.
    hypertrophic c.
    idiopathic dilated c.
    ipecac c.
    maternally inherited myopathy and
      c. (MIMyCA)
    neonatal c.
    peripartum c.
    postpartum c. (PPCM)
    restrictive c. (RCM)
    Sengers c.
    subaortic hypertrophic c.
    ventricular noncompaction c.
    X-linked c. (XLCM)
    X-linked dilated c. (XLCM)
cardioplegia
    cold potassium c.
cardioplegic solution
cardiopneumograph
cardioprotective effect
cardiopulmonary
    c. bypass
    c. collapse
    c. disorder
    c. dysfunction
    c. resuscitation (CPR)
cardiorespiratory
    c. function
    c. homeostasis

    c. monitor
    c. syndrome of obesity in child
cardiorespirogram (CR-gram)
CardioSeal device
cardioskeletal
    c. myopathy
    c. neutropenia
cardiospasm
cardiotachometer
cardiothoracic ratio
cardiothymic shadow
cardiotocogram
    terminal c.
cardiotocograph
cardiotocography (CTG)
    fetal c.
    intrapartum c.
cardiotoxicity
cardiovascular (CV)
    c. calcification
    c. collapse
    c. complication
    c. depression
    c. development
    c. effect
    c. injury
    c. malformation (CVM)
    c. manifestation
    c. performance
    c. pertubation
    c. sequela
    c. shock
    c. stabilization
    c. system (CVS)
cardiovascular/central nervous system syndrome
cardioversion
    synchronized DC c.
cardiovertebral syndrome
carditis
    acute rheumatic c.
    indolent c.
    rheumatic c.
Cardizem
    C. CD
    C. Injectable
    C. SR
care
    ambulatory obstetric c.
    antepartum c.
    antepartum home c.
    breast c.
    critical c.
    custodial c.
    followup c.
    foster c.
    hospice c.
    in-hospital postpartum c.
    kangaroo c.

care (*continued*)
   maternal c.
   monitored anesthesia c. (MAC)
   newborn intensive c. (NBIC, NIC)
   obstetric c.
   obstetric-gynecologic c.
   outpatient postpartum c.
   palliative c.
   pediatric neurocritical c.
   postoperative c.
   postpartum c.
   preconception c.
   prenatal c.
   prepregnancy c.
   respite c.
   routine postoperative c.
   skin-to-skin c.
   specialized prenatal c.
   substitute c.
   supportive c.
   well-child c. (WCC)
caregiver
   primary c.
caregiver-child interaction
caretaker
   primary c.
Carey-Fineman-Ziter syndrome
Carey Temperament Scale
caries
   dental c.
   early childhood c. (ECC)
   milk-bottle teeth c.
CARIFS
   Canadian Acute Respiratory Illness
   and Flu Scale
carina, *pl.* **carinae**
carinae (*pl. of* carina)
carinatum
   pectus c.
carinii
   Pneumocystis c.
C-arm
carmine
   indigo c.
Carmi syndrome
Carmol
Carmol-HC Topical
carmustine
Carnation
   C. Follow-Up
   C. Follow-Up soy formula
   C. Good Start formula
Carnegie stage
carneous
   c. degeneration
   c. mole
Carnett
   C. sign
   C. test

Carnevale syndrome
Carney syndrome
carnitine
   c. acylcarnitine translocase
      deficiency
   c. palmitoyltransferase (CPT)
   c. palmitoyltransferase I (CPT I)
   c. palmitoyltransferase II (CPT II)
   c. transferase enzyme disorder
Carnitor
carnivore
Carnoy fixative
carob
   c. gum
   c. seed flour
Caroli
   C. disease
   C. syndrome
**Carolina Curriculum for Infants and
Toddlers with Special Needs**
carotene
   beta c.
carotid
   c. artery
   c. artery-cavernous sinus fistula
   c. artery dissection
   c. blood flow (CaBF)
   c. bruit
   left common c.
   right common c.
   c. sinus pressure
carotid-cavernous fistula
carotin
carpal
   c. navicular
   c. tunnel syndrome
carpectomy
   proximal row c.
Carpenter syndrome
carphenazine maleate
carpi (*pl. of* carpus)
Carpine
   Isopto C.
carp-like mouth
carp mouth
carpopedal spasm
carpus, *pl.* **carpi**
Carrasyn Hydrogel dressing
carrier
   embryo c.
   Endo-Assist endoscopic ligature c.
   factor V Leiden c.
   fragile X c.
   gene c.
   gestational c.
   heterozygous c.
   latent c.
   linear in-line ligature c.
   Miya hook ligature c.

obligate c.
c. protein
c. screening
silent c.
c. testing
translocation c.

CARS
Childhood Autism Rating Scale

cart
SensorMedics Horizon metabolic c.

Carter Tubal Assistant

Cartesian theory

cartilage
costal c.
fetal c.
c. interposition
c. oligomeric matrix protein (COMP)
c. piercing

cartilage-hair hypoplasia (CHH)

cartilaginous coalition

cartridge
serum pregnancy assay c.

Cartwright blood group

caruncle
amniotic c.
myrtiform c.
c. of labium
urethral c.

caruncula
c. hymenalis
c. myrtiformis

Carus
C. circle
C. curve

Carvajal formula

carvedilol

CAS
central anticholinergic syndrome
child assessment schedule

CASA
Child and Adolescent Services Assessment
computer-assisted semen analysis
computer-assisted semen analyzer

Casal necklace

casanthranol
docusate and c.

cascade
coagulation c.
cytokine c.
inflammatory c.
toxic c.

cascara sagrada

case
index c.
c. manager

caseating necrosis

caseation

Casec
C. formula
C. powder

casein
c. hydrolysate
c. hydrolysate formula
powdered c.

caseosa
vernix c.

caseous node

caseum

CASG
Collaborative Antiviral Study Group

CASH
cancer and steroid hormone
classic abdominal Semm hysterectomy
cortical androgen-stimulating hormone
CASH study

Casodex

cassava bean

casseliflavus
Enterococcus c.

Casser fontanelle

casserian fontanelle

cast
abduction c.
bivalved c.
c. boot brace
bronchial mucous c.
cellular c.
clubfoot c.
cylinder c.
decidual c.
dense c.
Hexalite c.
hip spica c.
hyaline c.
hypereosinophilic mucoid c.
long leg c.
Petri c.
polysiloxane c.
red blood cell c.
Risser localizer c.
short leg walking c.
spica c.
C. syndrome
thumb spica c.
urinary c.
uterine c.

CAST
childhood accidental spiral tibial
Children of Alcoholics Screening Test

Castaneda tetralogy of Fallot repair procedure

castellani
Acanthamoeba c.

casting
> Cerrobend c.
> inhibitive c.
> serial c.

Castleman disease
castor
> c. bean
> c. bean poisoning
> c. oil

castrated
castration
Castroviejo fixation forceps
casual plasma glucose
cat
> c. bite
> c. dander

CAT
> Clinical Adaptive Test
> computed axial tomography
> CAT scan
> CAT scanning

catabolism
> tissue c.
> unregulated c.

catadidymus
Cataflam
catalase negative
catalytic
catamenia
catamenial
> c. hemoptysis
> c. pneumothorax

catamenialis
> iritis c.

catamenogenic
Catania-type acrofacial dysostosis
cataplectic attack
cataplexis (*var. of* cataplexy)
cataplexy, cataplexis
cataract
> cerulean c.
> congenital bilateral c.'s
> developmental c.
> c. formation
> c., hypertrichosis, mental retardation (CAHMR)
> infantile c.
> juvenile c.
> lenticular c.
> c., microcephaly, arthrogryposis, kyphosis (CAMAK)
> c., microcephaly, failure to thrive, kyphoscoliosis (CAMFAK)
> pediatric c.
> sunflower c.
> zonular c.

cataract-dental syndrome
cataractogenic
cataract-oligophrenia syndrome

catarrhalis
> *Branhamella* c.
> *Moraxella* c.

catarrhal jaundice
catastrophic
> c. bleeding
> c. hemorrhage
> c. injury

catatonia
> lethal c.

catatoniac (*var. of* catatonic)
catatonic, catatoniac, catatoniac
> c. behavior
> c. syndrome

catch
> midstream c.

CATCH
> cardiac abnormality, abnormal facies, thymic hypoplasia, cleft palate, hypocalcemia
> CATCH 22 phenotype
> CATCH 22 syndrome

CATCH-22
> cardiac abnormality, abnormal facies, thymic hypoplasia, cleft palate, hypocalcemia

catch-up growth
CAT/CLAMS
> Clinical Adaptive Test/Clinical Linguistic and Auditory Milestone Scale

cat-cry syndrome
catechol
> c. estrogen
> c. oxidase

catecholamine
> endogenous c.

categorical placement
category
> bilineal c.

Catel-Manzke syndrome
catenulatum
> *Bifidobacterium* c.

catgut suture
cathartic
> c. colon
> magnesium-containing c.
> saline c.

cathepsin D
catherized urine specimen
catheter
> Alzate c.
> Amplatz c.
> Angiocath c.
> c. angiography
> Argyle arterial c.
> Arrow c.
> arterial c.
> balloon septostomy c.

balloon-tipped c.
bile duct c.
Bi-Set c.
bladder c.
Bonanno c.
Bozeman-Fritsch c.
c. breakage
Brevi-Kath epidural c.
Broviac c.
cardiac c.
Caud-A-Kath epidural c.
central venous c. (CVC)
central venous pressure c.
Chemo-Port c.
Chronoflex c.
CliniCath peripherally inserted c.
Conceptus Soft Torque uterine c.
Conceptus VS c.
Cook c.
Corcath c.
coudé c.
Cystocath c.
Dacron sleeve c.
Davis bladder c.
DeLee suction c.
de Pezzer c.
Dobbhoff c.
Dorros infusion and probing c.
double-balloon c.
double-lumen c.
Drew-Smythe c.
Du Pen epidural c.
c. dysfunction
EASI c.
EchoMark salpingography c.
Ehrlich c.
elastomer c.
c. embolization
Embryon GIFT c.
Embryon HSG c.
Evert-O-Cath drug delivery c.
EZ-HSG c.
FAE c.
femoral artery c.
flexible Teflon c.
Fogarty arterial embolectomy c.
Fogarty atrioseptostomy c.
Foley c.
French Gesco c.
Gesco c.
Groshong c.
Haas intrauterine insemination c.
Hickman c.
Hohn c.
HUMI c.
Hurwitz c.
hysterosalpingography c.
indwelling c.
indwelling arterial c. (IAC)

indwelling venous c. (IVC)
Infuse-A-Port c.
c. insertion
intrauterine pressure c. (IUPC)
Johnson transtracheal oxygen c.
Judkins c.
jugular bulb c.
Kendall double-lumen c.
Kish urethral illuminating c.
Koala intrauterine pressure c.
Labcath c.
Labotect c.
Landmark c.
large-bore c.
L-Cath peripherally inserted neonatal c.
Leonard c.
LeRoy ventricular c.
Malecot c.
malpositioned c.
MediPort c.
Mentor c.
microendoscopic optical c.
Microtip c.
Micro-Transducer c.
Millar microtransducer urethral c.
Neo-Sert umbilical vessel c.
On-Command c.
Opti-Flow c.
over-the-needle c.
percutaneous central venous c. (PCVC)
percutaneous femoral venous c.
percutaneously inserted central line c. (PICC)
percutaneous nephrostomy c.
peripheral arterial c.
peripheral intravenous c.
peripherally inserted c. (PIC)
peripherally inserted central c. (PICC)
peritoneal c.
PermCath c.
Per-Q-Cath c.
Pezzer c.
pigtail c.
PIV c.
Pleur-evac chest c.
polyethylene c.
polyurethane c.
Port-A-Cath c.
PRO infusion c.
c. pullback
pulmonary thermodilution c.
Quinton dual-lumen c.
Raaf c.
radial arterial c.
radial artery c.
Raimondi c.

catheter (*continued*)
- red rubber c.
- Release c.
- Reliance urinary control insert c.
- Replogle suction c.
- c. reservoir
- scalp vein c.
- c. sepsis
- c. septostomy
- shearing of c.
- silastic c.
- silicone c.
- silicon rubber c.
- Soft-Cell c.
- soft seal c.
- Soft Torque uterine c.
- Sones c.
- Soules intrauterine insemination c.
- c. specimen
- Spectranetics c.
- split sheath c.
- Stamey c.
- Stamey-Malecot c.
- suction c.
- support c.
- suprapubic c.
- Swan-Ganz c.
- Tenckhoff c.
- tethered c.
- c. tip placement
- c. toe
- tracheal c.
- transcervical Foley c.
- transcervical tubal access c. (T-TAC)
- transducer-tipped c.
- transtracheal c.
- transurethral c.
- triple-lumen c.
- tunneled c.
- Tygon c.
- umbilical artery c. (UAC)
- umbilical vein c. (UVC)
- umbilical venous c. (UVC)
- umbilical vessel c.
- urinary c. (UC)
- uterine cornual access c. (UCAC)
- uterine ostial access c. (UOAC)
- Vabra c.
- Vas-Cath c.
- V-Cath c.
- venous c.
- ventricular c.
- Wallace c.
- water-perfused manometry c.
- whistle-tip c.
- Wholey balloon occlusion c.
- Word Bartholin gland c.
- Word bladder c.
- Yankauer c.

catheter-associated bacteremia (CAB)
catheterization
- bladder c.
- cardiac c.
- central venous c.
- clean intermittent c. (CIC)
- femoral artery c.
- fetal bladder c.
- intraoperative ureteral c.
- jugular bulb c.
- percutaneous central venous c.
- peripheral venous c.
- pulmonary artery c.
- radial artery c.
- scalp vein c.
- transvaginal tubal c.
- umbilical artery c.
- umbilical vein c.
- urethral c. (UC)
- urinary c.

catheter-over-needle technique
catheter-over-wire technique
catheter-within-a-catheter
cathode ray oscilloscope (CRO)
cati
- *Toxocara c.*

cat's
- c. cry
- c. cry syndrome
- c. eye pupil
- c. eye reflex
- c. eye syndrome (CES)
- c. urine syndrome

CATS
- Child Abuse Trauma Scale

cat-scratch
- c.-s. disease (CSD)
- c.-s. fever

Cattell
- C. Infant Intelligence Scale (CIIS)
- C. Infant Intelligence Test

Catterall classification (grade 1–4)
cauda
- c. equina
- c. equina syndrome

caudad
Caud-A-Kath epidural catheter
caudal
- c. agenesis
- c. analgesia
- c. anesthesia
- c. chordamesoderm
- c. direction
- c. duplication
- c. dysplasia
- c. dysplasia syndrome
- c. neuropore
- c. pole
- c. regression syndrome (CRS)

caudate
- c. hypometabolism
- c. nucleus

caudocranial

caul, cowl

causal
- c. embryology
- c. independence
- c. inference

causalgia

causation

cause
- acute cerebellar ataxia of unknown c.

cause-and-effect activity

caustic
- c. aspiration
- c. ingestion
- c. injury

cauterization
- Bovie c.
- nasal c.

cauterizing ball

cautery
- BICAP c.
- bipolar c.
- Bovie c.
- chemical c.
- c. conization
- Endoclip c.
- endoscopic c.
- laparoscopic c.
- L-shaped c.
- monopolar c.
- ovarian c.
- Oxycel c.

cava
- azygos continuation of inferior vena c.
- inferior vena c. (IVC)
- superior vena c. (SVC)
- vena c.

CAVD
- congenital absence of vas deferens

cave
- Meckel c.

Caverject

cavernosal
- c. artery thrombosis
- c. fibrosis
- c. infarction

cavernosum
- corpus c.

cavernous
- c. hemangioma
- c. lymphangioma
- c. plexus
- c. sinus
- c. sinusitis

- c. sinus syndrome
- c. sinus thrombosis
- c. venous angioma

CAVH
- continuous arteriovenous hemofiltration

caviae
- *Nocardia c.*

cavitary
- c. lung disease
- c. tuberculosis
- c. white-matter lesion

cavitation

Cavitron ultrasonic surgical aspirator (CUSA)

cavity
- abdominal c.
- abscess c.
- amniotic c.
- Baer c.
- celomic c.
- chorionic c.
- endometrial c.
- exocelomic c.
- intrauterine c.
- oral c.
- pelvic c.
- peritoneal c.
- pseudomonoamniotic c.
- syringomyelic c.
- thoracic c.
- uterine c.
- ventricles to peritoneal c.

CAVM
- cerebral arteriovenous malformation

cavovalgus
- talipes c.

cavovarus
- c. deformity
- c. foot

cavum
- c. septum pellucidum
- c. septum pellucidum, cavum vergae, macrocephaly, seizures, mental retardation syndrome
- c. vergae

cavus
- c. foot
- pathologic c.
- pes c.
- physiologic c.
- talipes c.

cayetanensis
- *Cyclospora c.*

Cayler cardiofacial syndrome

CBAVD
- congenital bilateral absence of vas deferens

CBC
- complete blood count

139

CBCL
Child Behavior Checklist
CBDC
chronic bullous disease of childhood
CBE
clinical breast examination
CBF
cerebral blood flow
CBFV
cerebral blood flow velocity
CBG
capillary blood gas
cord blood gas
corticosteroid-binding globulin
CB-GBC
corticosteroid-binding globulin-binding
capacity
CBN
chronic benign neutropenia
CBP
complete breech presentation
CBR
cord blood registry
CBRF
child behavior rating form
CBS
child behavioral study
cystathionine beta-synthase
CBS deficiency
CBT
cognitive behavioral therapy
cord blood transplantation
CBV
cerebral blood volume
CBZ
carbamazepine
cc
cubic centimeter
CC
clomiphene citrate
closing capacity
Adalat CC
hemoglobin CC
CCA
congenital contractural arachnodactyly
CCAI
Clinical Colitis Activity Index
CCAM
congenital cystic adenomatoid
malformation
cystic congenital adenomatoid
malformation
CCAM (type 1–3)
CCC
craniocerebellocardiac
CCC dysplasia
CCC syndrome
CCCT
clomiphene citrate challenge test

C2–C9 deficiency
CCG
Children's Cancer Group
CCH
chronic cryptogenic hepatitis
CCHB
congenital complete heart block
CCHD
cyanotic congenital heart disease
cc/hr
cubic centimeter per hour
CCHS
congenital central hypoventilation
syndrome
CCK
cholecystokinin
CCL
calcaneocuboid ligament
CCLO
child-centered literary orientation
CCM
cerebrocostomandibular
chronic cystic mastitis
CCMS
cerebrocostomandibular syndrome
CCNU
cyclohexylchloroethylnitrosurea
CCPD
continuous cyclic peritoneal dialysis
CCR
cumulative conception rate
CCS
Crippled Children's Services
CCSC
Children's Coping Strategies Checklist
CCSG
Children's Cancer Study Group
CCSS
Childhood Cancer Survivor Study
CCUP
colpocystourethropexy
CCVM
congenital cardiovascular malformation
CD
celiac disease
cesarean delivery
conduct disorder
Cardizem CD
Ceclor CD
CD4
CD4 cell count
CD4 marker
CD4 T cell
CD4+
CD4+ cell
CD4+ level
CD8
CD8 cell count
CD8 T cell

CDA
congenital dyserythropoietic anemia
CDAD
Clostridium difficile-associated diarrhea
CDAP
continuous distending airway pressure
CDC
Centers for Disease Control and
Prevention
Communicable Disease Center
CD4/CD8 ratio
CDD
childhood disintegrative disorder
CDE
color Doppler energy
CDE blood group system
CDFI
color Doppler flow imaging
CDG
carbohydrate deficient glycoprotein
CDH
congenital diaphragmatic hernia
congenital dislocated hip
congenital dislocation of hip
CDH repair
CDH-ECMO
congenital diaphragmatic
hernia-extracorporeal membrane
oxygenation
CD34 hematopoietic progenitor cell
CDHNF
Children's Digestive Health and
Nutrition Foundation
CDI
Children's Depression Inventory
communicative development inventory
Cotrel-Dubousset instrumentation
cDICA
Computerized Diagnostic Interview for
Children and Adolescents
CDIS
continuous distention irrigation
system
CDL
Cornelia de Lange
CDLS
Cornelia de Lange syndrome
cDNA
complementary deoxyribonucleic acid
complementary DNA
cDNA library
CDP
continuous distending pressure
CDRS-R
Children's Depression Rating
Scale-Revised
CDS
Children's Depression Scale
color Doppler sonography

CDU
color Doppler ultrasonography
CE
conductive education
conjugated estrogen
rhesus gene CE
(RhCE)
CEA
carcinoembryonic antigen
cranial epidural abscess
cebocephalus
cebocephaly
ceca (*pl. of* cecum)
cecal
c. carcinoma
c. pouch
cecocolic intussusception
Cecon
cecostomy
cecum, caecum, *pl.* **ceca**
exstrophic c.
CED
cranioectodermal dysplasia
Cedax
Cedilanid
Cedocard-SR
CEE
conjugated equine estrogens
CEEA
circular end-to-end anastomosis
CeeNU
CE/FA
capillary electrophoresis/frontal
analysis
cefaclor
cefadroxil monohydrate
Cefadyl
cefamandole
cefazolin sodium
cefdinir (CFDN)
cefepime HCl
cefixime
Cefizox
cefmetazole
Cefobid
cefonicid
cefoperazone sodium
ceforanide
Cefotan
cefotaxime sodium
cefotetan disodium
cefoxitin sodium
cefpodoxime proxetil
cefprozil
ceftazidime
ceftibuten
Ceftin Oral
ceftizoxime
ceftriaxone sodium

cefuroxime
    c. axetil (CAE)
    c. sodium
Cefzil
celery stalking
Celestoderm-EV/2
Celestoderm-V
Celestone
    C. Oral
    C. Phosphate injection
    C. Soluspan
celiac, coeliac
    c. antibody
    c. artery
    c. axis
    c. disease (CD)
    c. infantilism
    c. sprue
    c. syndrome
celibacy
celibate
celiohysterectomy
celiohysterotomy
celiomyomectomy
celiomyomotomy
celioparacentesis
celiosalpingectomy
celiosalpingotomy
celioscopy
celiotomy
    exploratory c.
    vaginal c.
cell
    absolute nucleated red blood c. (ANRBC)
    activated T c.
    c. adhesion factor (CAF)
    c. adhesion molecule (CAM)
    amniogenic c.
    c. and flare
    antibody-secreting c. (ASC)
    antigen-presenting c. (APC)
    antigen-sensitive c.
    apocrine c.
    Askanazy c.
    atypical glandular c. (AGC)
    atypical squamous c. (ASC)
    B c.
    back-selected T c.
    band c.
    basket c.
    Betz c.
    BeWo c.
    Birbeck granule-positive c.
    bite c.
    blastomere c.
    blister c.
    c. block analysis
    bone marrow stem c.

Brenner c.
Burkitt tumor c.
CD4+ c.
CD4 T c.
CD8 T c.
CD34 hematopoietic progenitor c.
cell-salvaged packed c.
choroid plexus c.
ciliated c.
circulating fetal c.
clue c.
c. collector
committed c.
corona radiata c.
crenated red blood c.
crypt c.
CTL c.
c. culture
cumulus c.
c. cycle
c. cycle-nonspecific drug
c. cycle-specific drug
c. cycling in chemotherapy
cytotoxic memory T c.
daughter c.
decidual c.
dendritic c.
desquamated epithelial c.
c. determination
diploid spermatogonial stem c.
c. division
dome c.
donor T c.
double c.
ductal c.
dysplastic c.
early embryonic c.
effector c.
egg c.
embryonic renomedullary interstitial c.
embryonic stem c. (ESC)
encephalitogenic c.
endodermal c.
endothelial c.
enterochromaffin c.
epithelial c.
epithelioid c.
erythroid progenitor c.
eukaryotic c.
exfoliated squamous c.
extragonadal germ c.
fetal nucleated c.
fetal red blood c.
foam c.
frozen red blood c.
ganglion c.
Gaucher c.
c. generation time

germ c.
giant c.
glandular c.
granulosa lutein c.
c. growth inhibitor
Haller c.
haploid c.
HeLa cells
helper T c.
hemopoietic stem c. (HSC)
HLA-identical haploidentical bone
 marrow stem c.
hobnail c.
Hofbauer c.
HuCNS-SC stem c.
human endothelial c. (HEC)
human umbilical vein endothelial c.
 (HUVEC)
Hürthle c.
hyperplasia of beta c.
immunocompetent c.
inclusion c. (I-cell)
c. interaction gene
interstitial c.
Ito c.
K c.
c. kill
killer c.
c. kinetics
koilocytotic c.
Kupffer c.
lack of natural killer c.'s
Langerhans c.
Langhans giant c.
leukemic c.
Leydig c.
lipid c.
luteal c.
lutein c.
lymphoblastoid c.
lymphoid c.
lymphokine-activated killer c.
 (LAKC)
c. lysate
mast c.
mastoid air c.
maturation of c.
MCF-7 breast cancer c.
memory c.
Merkel c.
mesenchymal c.
metamyelocyte c.
monster c.
multinucleated giant c.
mutant c.
myeloblast c.
myelocyte c.
myoepithelial c.
natural killer c. (NKC)

natural killer T c.
neural crest c.
neuroblastoma c.
neuroid c.
Niemann-Pick c.
nonencephalitogenic c.
normoblast c.
nuclear factor of activated T c.
 (NFAT)
nucleated red blood c.
Opalski c.
osteoblast-like c.
owl's eye c.
packed red blood c.'s (PRBC)
pancreatic islet c.
parabasal c.
peripheral blood mononuclear c.
 (PBMC, PBMNC)
peripheral blood stem c.
 (PBSC)
pituitary c.
placental-derived stem c.
 (PDSC)
placental giant c.
plasma c.
pneumatic c.
c. precursor
pregnancy c.
pregranulosa c.
primary embryonic c.
primordial germ c. (PGC)
primordial pluripotent stem c.
promyelocyte c.
pronormoblast c.
Purkinje c.
pyknotic c.
Raji c.
C. Recovery System (CRS)
red blood c. (RBC)
Reed-Sternberg c.
renal tubular epithelial c.
reticuloendothelial c.
Rh null c.
C. Saver
Schwann c.
senescent red c.
Sertoli c.
Sertoli-Leydig c.
sex c.
sickle c.
silver c.
smooth muscle c.
somatic c.
c. sorting
spherocytic red blood c.
spiculated red blood c.
spindle c.
squamous c.
stellate c.

cell (*continued*)
    stem c.
    steroid c.
    stromal c.
    suppressor T c.
    c. surface antigen
    syncytial c.
    syncytiotrophoblastic tumor giant c.
    syngeneic stem c.
    T c.
    target c.
    T-cell-depleted haploidentical bone marrow stem c.
    T cytotoxic c.
    technetium-labeled red blood c.
    thecal interstitial c.
    theca lutein c.
    T-helper c.
    totipotent c.
    totipotential c.
    triphasic pattern blastemal c.
    trophoblastic c.
    tuboendometrial c.
    vaginal smear intermediate c.
    vaginal smear parabasal c.
    vaginal smear superficial c.
    Vero c.
    viable endometrial c.
    Vignal c.
    white blood c. (WBC)
    whole c.
    WI-38 c.
    WISH c.
    yolk c.
2-cell
    2-c. embryo
    2-c. mechanism
    2-c. zygote
CellCept
cell-cycle actions of chemotherapy
4-cell embryo
8-cell embryo
cell-extracellular matrix adhesion
cell-mediated
    c.-m. immunity (CMI)
    c.-m. immunodeficiency
Cellolite patty
cell-salvaged packed cell
cellular
    c. and molecular regulation of lung development
    c. blue nevus
    c. cast
    c. cytotoxic mechanism
    c. debris
    c. desmoplastic stroma
    c. division
    c. edema
    c. hyperplasia

    c. hypertrophy
    c. hypoxia
    c. immunity
    c. immunodeficiency
    c. infiltrate
    c. leiomyoma
    c. migration
    c. proteolysis
    c. regulation
    c. viral
cellulicidal
cellulitic phlegmasia
cellulitis
    anaerobic c.
    buccal c.
    cuff c.
    Haemophilus influenzae c.
    incisional c.
    incisional c.
    orbital c.
    pelvic c.
    periorbital skin c.
    peritonsillar c.
    pneumococcal facial c.
    postoperative cuff c.
    postseptal c.
    preseptal c.
    retropharyngeal c.
    streptococcal c.
    vaginal cuff c.
cellulosae
    Cysticercus c.
cellulose acetate (CA)
Cell-VU disposable semen analysis chamber
celom, celoma
celoma (*var. of* celom)
celomic, coelomic
    c. cavity
    c. epithelium
    c. metaplasia
Celontin
celosomia
celosomy
Cel-U-Jec Injection
CEM
    cytosine arabinoside, etoposide, methotrexate
cementum
    dental c.
Cemill
cenadelphus
Cenafed Plus
Cena-K
Cenani-Lenz syndactyly
Cenestin
    C. synthetic conjugated estrogens
    C. tablet
Centany ointment

center
American Association of Poison
Control C.'s (AAPCC)
arousal c.
birth care c.
Children's National Medical C.
Communicable Disease C. (CDC)
c. edge angle
c. edge angle of Wiberg
electrophilic c.
epiphysial ossification c.
C.'s for Disease Control and
Prevention (CDC)
C. for Epidemiological Studies
Depression Scale for Children
germinal c.
Hopkins Lupus Pregnancy C.
hotline c.
hypothalamic thermoregulating c.
lower limb ossification c.
malleolar ossification c.
pneumotaxic c.
Poison Control C. (PCC)
regional perinatal intensive care c.
(RPICC)
school-based health c. (SBHC)
tertiary care c.
X inactivation c. (XIC)
centigray (cGy)
centimeter (cm)
cubic c. (cc)
c. of water (cmH_2O)
centimorgan (cM)
**Centocor CA 125 radioimmunoassay
kit**
central
c. alveolar hypoventilation
c. anticholinergic syndrome
(CAS)
c. atrophy
c. auditory processing disorder
(CAPD)
c. axis depth dose
c. cord lesion
c. cord syndrome
c. core disease
c. core myopathy
c. cyanosis
c. defect
c. dogma
c. fat distribution pattern
c. gliotic tuft
c. hepatic hematoma
c. hyperalimentation
c. hypothyroidism
c. hypoventilation syndrome
c. incisor
c. jaundice
c. monitoring

c. nervous system (CNS)
c. nervous system/cardiovascular
syndrome
c. nervous system differentiation
c. nervous system disease
c. nervous system lymphoma
c. nervous system trauma
c. neuroblastoma
c. neurogenic hyperventilation
c. placenta previa
c. pontine myelinolysis
c. porencephaly
c. precocious puberty (CPP)
c. primitive neuroectodermal tumor
(cPNET)
c. Recklinghausen disease (type I,
II)
c. respiratory drive
c. retinal artery
c. serotonergic hyperactivity
c. serotonin abnormality
c. shunt
c. sleep apnea
c. syndrome of rostrocaudal
deterioration
c. tendon of perineum
c. type neurofibromatosis
c. venous access device (CVAD)
c. venous catheter (CVC)
c. venous catheterization
c. venous catheter placement
c. venous line (CVL)
c. venous nutrition (CVN)
c. venous pressure (CVP)
c. venous pressure catheter
c. visual field
central-anterior
centralis
neurinomatosis c.
placenta previa c.
centralization
fetal circulatory c.
centralopathic epilepsy
centrencephalic
c. epilepsy
c. system
centric fusion translocation
centrifugation
Ficoll-Hypaque c.
centrifuge
centrifugum
leukoderma acquisitum c.
centrilobular necrosis
centripetal spread
centrizonal
c. hypoxia
c. sinusoidal distention
centrolobal sclerosis
centromere interference

centromeric
    c. banding
    c. instability-immunodeficiency
    syndrome
    c. region of chromosome
    c. signal
centronuclear myopathy (CNM)
centrotemporal
    c. epilepsy
    c. spike
CEP
    congenital erythropoietic porphyria
cepacia
    Burkholderia c.
    Pseudomonas c.
Cēpacol Anesthetic Troche
CEPH
    CEPH family
    CEPH pedigree
cephalad
cephalexin
cephalhematoma, cephalohematoma
    bilateral c.'s
    c. deformans
cephalhydrocele
cephalic
    c. cry
    c. delivery
    c. forceps
    c. pole
    c. presentation (CP)
    c. prominence
    c. replacement
    c. tetanus
    c. vein
    c. version
cephalization
    primordial c.
cephalocaudad (*var. of* cephalocaudal)
cephalocaudal, cephalocaudad
    c. film-screen mammogram
    c. sequence
    c. sequence of development
cephalocele
cephalocentesis
cephalodactyly
    Vogt c.
cephalodiprosopus
cephalohematoma (*var. of*
  cephalhematoma)
cephalomelus
cephalometric radiograph
cephalometry
    ultrasonic c.
cephalonia
cephalopagus
cephalopelvic disproportion (CPD)
cephalopelvimetry
cephalopolysyndactyly syndrome

cephalosporin
    first-generation c.
cephalosporin-resistant pneumococcus
cephalostat
cephalothin sodium
cephalothoracopagus
cephalotome
cephalotomy
cephalotribe
cephapirin
cephazolin
cephradine
Ceporacin
Ceptaz
CeraLyte drink mix
ceramidase activity
ceramide
    c. trihexose
    c. trihexoside alpha galactosidase
ceramidosis
c-erb
    c-*erb* B-2 oncogene
    c-*erb* B-2 oncoprotein
    c-*erb* B-2 protooncogene
cercaria
cercarial
    c. dermatitis
    c. skin penetration
cerclage
    Barnes c.
    cervical c.
    Mann isthmic c.
    McDonald cervical c.
    modified Shirodkar c.
    c. placement
    prophylactic c.
    rescue cervical c.
    Shirodkar cervical c.
    transabdominal cervicoisthmic c.
    web c.
cerebellar
    c. asynergia
    c. ataxia
    c. cerebral palsy
    c. degeneration
    c. dysfunction
    c. dysplasia
    c. encephalitis
    c. folium
    c. hemangioblastoma
    c. hematoma
    c. hemisphere compression
    c. hemorrhage
    c. hypertrophy
    c. mutism
    c. neoplasm
    c. nucleus
    c. tonsil
    c. tumor

c. vermis
c. vermis agenesis
c. vermis aplasia
c. vermis hypogenesis
c. vermis hypoplasia
c. vermis hypoplasia, oligophrenia,
   congenital ataxia, ocular coloboma,
   hepatic fibrosis (COACH)
cerebellar-vestibular system
cerebelli
   folia c.
   vermis c.
cerebellitis
   acute c.
   postinfectious c.
   viral c.
cerebelloparenchymal disorder (I–IV)
cerebellotrigeminal and focal dermal
  dysplasia
cerebellum
   absent c.
   dysplastic gangliocytoma of c.
   folia of c.
   inverse c.
cerebral
   c. amebiasis
   c. angiography
   c. angioma
   c. anoxia
   c. arteriovenous malformation
    (CAVM)
   c. artery aneurysm
   c. artery occlusion
   c. aspergillosis
   c. atrophy
   c. blood flow (CBF)
   c. blood flow velocity (CBFV)
   c. blood volume (CBV)
   c. compression
   c. contusion
   c. cortex
   c. cortical necrosis
   c. disturbance
   c. dysfunction
   c. dysfunction syndrome
   c. dysgenesis
   c. edema
   c. embolism
   c. falx
   c. function monitor (CFM)
   c. gigantism
   c. glucose metabolism
   c. GM1 gangliosidosis
   c. hematoma
   c. hemisphere
   c. herniation
   c. holosphere
   c. hypoperfusion
   c. hypothermia

c. infarction
c. injury
c. ischemia
c. laceration
c. lactic alkalosis
c. leukodystrophy
c. leukomalacia
c. malaria
c. metabolic rate
c. metastasis
c., ocular, dental, auricular, skeletal
  (CODAS)
c. oximetry
c. oxygen consumption
c. palsy (CP)
c. palsy antecedent
c. paragonimiasis
c. peduncle
c. perfusion pressure (CPP)
c. resuscitation
c. salt wasting (CSW)
c. schistosomiasis
c. sclerosis
c. swelling
c. syncope
c. thrombosis
c. trypanosomiasis
c. vasospasm
c. ventriculomegaly
cerebrale
   cranium c.
cerebral-placental ratio
cerebri
   pseudotumor c.
cerebriform
cerebritis
   lupus c.
cerebroarthrodigital syndrome
cerebroatrophic hyperammonemia
cerebrocostomandibular (CCM)
   c. syndrome (CCMS)
cerebrocutaneous angiomatosis
cerebrofacioarticular (CFA)
cerebrofaciothoracic syndrome or
  dysplasia
cerebrohepatorenal syndrome (CHRS)
cerebromacular degeneration
cerebroocular
   c. dentoauriculoskeletal (CODAS)
   c. dysgenesis (COD)
   c. dysgenesis-muscular dystrophy
    (COD-MD)
   c. dysplasia-muscular dystrophy
   c. muscular dystrophy
cerebrooculofacial-skeletal (COFS)
cerebrooculomuscular syndrome (COMS)
cerebrooculonasal syndrome
cerebroosteonephrodysplasia (COND)
   Hutterite c.

C

cerebroprotective mechanism
cerebroside lipidosis
cerebrospinal
    c. fluid (CSF)
    c. fluid leak
    c. fluid procalcitonin
    c. fluid sampling
cerebrospinalis
    liquor c.
cerebrotendinous xanthomatosis
cerebrovascular
    c. accident (CVA)
    c. disease
cerebrovasculosa
cerebrum
Cerebyx
Ceredase
cereus
    Bacillus c.
cerevisiae
    Saccharomyces c.
Cerezyme
ceroid lipofuscinosis
Cerose-DM
Cerrobend
    C. block
    C. casting
certificate
    birth c.
certified
    c. nurse-midwife (CNM)
    c. registered nurse anesthetist (CRNA)
Certiva vaccine
Cerubidine
cerulea, caerulea
    macula c.
cerulean cataract
ceruleus
    noradrenergic locus c.
ceruloplasmin
    c. deficiency
    c. level
cerumen
Cerumenex Otic
Cervex-Brush cervical cell sampler
cervical
    c. abnormality
    c. adenitis
    c. adenopathy
    c. agenesis
    c. amputation
    c. anomaly
    c. artery
    c. atresia
    c. atypia
    c. block kit
    c. canal
    c. cannula

c. cap
c. carcinoma
c. carcinoma stimulation
c. cerclage
c. clamp
c. clear cell adenocarcinoma
c. cockscomb
c. collar
c. combing
c. competence
c. condyloma
c. cone biopsy
c. conization
c. cord tumor
c. culture
c. cytology
c. dilation
c. disc space calcification
c. dysplasia
c. dystocia
c. ectopic pregnancy
c. ectopy
c. ectropion
c. effacement
c. epithelial neoplasia
c. epithelium
c. erosion
c. esophagostomy
c. esophagus
c. eversion
c. examination
c. factor
c. funneling
c. GIFT
c. hemorrhage
c. herpes
c. incision
c. incompetence (CI)
c. incompetence prevention randomized cerclage trial (CIPRACT)
c. infection
c. insemination
c. intraepithelial neoplasia (CIN)
c. isthmus
c. laceration
c. leiomyoma
c. length
c. lesion
c. lymphadenitis
c. lymphadenopathy
c. mass
c. motion tenderness (CMT)
c. mucorrhea
c. mucosa
c. mucus
c. mucus evaluation
c. myoma
c. os

c. polyp
c. position
c. pregnancy
c. priming
c. prolapse
c. rib
c. ripener
c. ripening
c. sap
c. sarcoma
c. score
c. sinus
c. smear
c. spinal cord injury
c. spine immobilization
c. spine injury
c. spine subluxation
c. stenosis
c. stenosis obstruction
c. stroma
c. stump
c. stump cancer
c. stump tumor
c. tenaculum
c. teratoma
c. tissue impedance range
topographic c.
c. transformation zone
c. venous hum
c. vertebral fusion
cervical-priming agent
cervicectomy
cervices (*pl. of* cervix)
cervicitis
chlamydial c.
chronic c.
gonorrheal c.
mucopurulent c.
nongonococcal c.
cervicofacial actinomycosis
cervicography
cervicomedullary
c. brainstem glioma
c. compression
c. junction
cervicoplasty
cervicothoracic spine dysplasia
cervicotomy
cervicovaginal
c. fetal fibronectin
c. fistula
c. infection
c. junction
c. ridge
c. secretion
Cervidil
C. ripening
C. vaginal insert
Cer-View lateral vaginal retractor

cervigram
Cervilaxin
Cerviprost gel
CerviSoft cytology collection device
cervix, *pl.* **cervices**
anterior lip of c.
atretic c.
barrel c.
barrel-shaped c.
bifid c.
carcinoma of c.
cockscomb c.
collared c.
cone biopsy of c.
congenital atresia of uterine c.
conization of c.
dilation of c.
effacement of c.
fishmouth c.
friable c.
incompetent c.
international classification of cancer of c.
malignant tumor of c.
multiple c.
c. neoplasm
short c.
shortened c.
strawberry c.
unfavorable c.
uninducible c.
CES
cat's eye syndrome
cauda equina syndrome
cranial electrical stimulation
cesarean
c. delivery (CD)
extraperitoneal c.
c. hysterectomy
Kerr c.
Latzko c.
low cervical c.
lower segment c. (LSCS)
low transverse c. (LTC)
c. operation
salvage c.
c. section (CS, C-section)
transperitoneal c.
trial of labor after c. (TOLAC)
vaginal birth after c. (VBAC)
CESD
cholesterol ester storage disease
cesium
c. candle
c. cylinder
c. implant
c. iodide (CsI)

cesium (*continued*)
    c. irradiation
    c. source
cesium-137 (^{137}Cs)
cessation
    c. of progress
    smoking c.
Cetacaine
Cetacort Topical
Cetamide
    Isopto C.
Cetaphil
cetirizine hydrochloride
Cetrorelix for injection
Cetrotide
cetyl alcohol
cetylpyridinium
Cevi-Bid
Ce-Vi-Sol
ceylanicum
    Ancylostoma c.
^{252}**Cf**
    californium-252
CF
    clavicular fracture
    clubfoot
    cystic fibrosis
        CF test
CFA
    cerebrofacioarticular
        CFA syndrome
CFC
    cardiofaciocutaneous
        CFC syndrome
CFD
    craniofacial dysostosis
CFL
    calcaneofibular ligament
CFM
    cerebral function monitor
c-fms protooncogene
CFND
    craniofrontonasal dysostosis
    craniofrontonasal dysplasia
CFNS
    craniofrontonasal syndrome
CFR
    coronary flow reserve
CFS
    chronic fatigue syndrome
CFTR
    cystic fibrosis transmembrane
     regulator
CFU
    colony-forming unit
CFUC
    colony-forming unit in culture
CFU-E
    colony-forming unit erythroid

CG
    chorionic gonadotropin
CGA
    corrected gestational age
CGAS
    Children's Global Assessment
    Scale
CGAT
    Constitutional Genetic Array Test
CGD
    chronic granulomatous disease
    continuous gastric drip
CGG
    cytosine-guanine-guanine
        CGG expansion
CGH
    chorionic gonadotropic hormone
    comparative genomic
     hybridization
CGI
    Clinical Global Impressions
    clinical global index
        CGI scale
cGMP
    cyclic guanosine monophosphate
cGMP-specific
    cGMP-s. phosphodiesterase
    cGMP-s. phosphodiesterase 5
CGS
    corrected gestational age
CGT
    chorionic gonadotropin
cGy
    centigray
CH
    congenital hypothyroidism
CH50
    hemolytic complement
CHA
    congenital hypoplastic anemia
CHADD
    children and adults with attention
    deficit disorder
Chadwick sign
chaffeensis
    Ehrlichia c.
Chagas disease
chagasic encephalitis
chagoma
chain
        beta c.
        c. cystourethrography
        globin c.
        heavy c.
        kappa c.
        light c.
        c. reaction
        sympathetic c.
chain-breaking antioxidant

chaining
    backward c.
    forward c.
chair
    adaptive c.
    birthing c.
    child's c.
    circumcision c.
    corner c.
chalasia, chalasis
chalasis (*var. of* chalasia)
chalaza (*var. of* chalazion)
chalazia (*pl. of* chalazion)
chalazion, chalaza, *pl.* **chalazia**
challenge
    acrosome reaction with ionophore c. (ARIC)
    bee sting c.
    blinded c.
    bronchial provocation c.
    caloric c.
    cow's milk c.
    diuretic c.
    double-blind placebo challenge food c.
    exercise bronchial c.
    gluten c.
    graded c.
    1-hour glucose c.
    intravenous glucose c.
    ionophore c.
    methacholine c.
    progestational c.
chamber
    anterior c.
    Cell-VU disposable semen analysis c.
    Enhanced Metabolic Testing Activity C. (EMTAC)
    face c.
    holding c.
    hyperbaric c.
    infundibular c.
    Makler reusable semen analysis c.
    Neubauer c.
    respiratory c.
    vitreous c.
Chamberlain line
Chamberlen forceps
4-chamber view
chameleon tongue
chamomile, camomile
Champetier de Ribes bag
Chanarin-Dorfman syndrome
Chance fracture
chancre
    hunterian c.
    trypanosomal c.
    tuberculous c.

chancroidal bubo
chancroid ulcer
chandelier sign
change
    atrophic c.
    benign cellular c. (BCC)
    breast c.
    concomitant c.
    dietary c.
    dysplastic c.
    dystrophic c.
    failed physiologic c.
    fibrocystic breast c.
    focal c.
    glomerular c.
    harlequin color c.
    hematological c.
    hormonal balance c.
    hormone-stimulated endometrial c.
    hydatidiform c.
    immunohistochemical c.
    immunologic c.
    libidinal c.
    lumbosacral skin pigment c.
    nonproliferative fibrocystic c.
    c. of life
    ovarian cycle c.
    papulosquamous skin c.
    personality c.
    physiologic c.
    polyneuropathy, organomegaly, endocrinopathy, M protein, skin c.'s (POEMS)
    postasphyxial c.
    postpartum hemodynamic c.
    proliferative c.
    puberal c.
    pupillary c.
    rachitic c.
    retinal c.
    sensorineural c.
    ST c.
    structural airway c.
    visual c.
    wave c.
change-point regression
channel
    common c.
    exposed large venous c.
    sinusoidal c.
    surface epithelium vascular c.
    vascular c.
    voltage-dependent calcium c.
channelopathy
    chloride c.
    sodium c.
2-channel pneumogram
Chantix

CHAOS
    congenital high airway obstruction
    syndrome
chaotic
    c. atrial tachycardia
    c. eye movement
character
    classifiable c.
    denumerable c.
    discrete c.
    Y-linked c.
characteristic
    c. electroencephalogram pattern
    c. emotional response
    epidemiologic c.
    isosexual sexual c.
    morphological c.
    organoleptic c.
    receiver operating c. (ROC)
    secondary sex c.
characterization
    immunohistochemical stromal
    leukocyte c.
charcoal
    activated c.
    c. agar
    multidose activated c. (MDAC)
    c. polyp
charcoal-blood medium
Charcot
    C. disease
    C. joint
    C. triad
Charcot-Leyden crystal
Charcot-Marie-Tooth
    C.-M.-T. disease
    C.-M.-T. disorder
    C.-M.-T. syndrome (CMTS)
    C.-M.-T. syndrome X-linked
    recessive type II
    C.-M.-T. syndrome, X-linked type II
    with deafness and mental
    retardation
Charcot-Marie-Tooth-Hoffmann
 syndrome
CHARGE
    coloboma, heart disease, atresia
    choanae, retarded growth and
    development, and/or CNS anomalies,
    genital hypoplasia, ear anomalies
    and/or deafness
    CHARGE association
    CHARGE syndrome
Charing Cross experience
Charleston brace
Charlevois-Saguenay syndrome
Charlevoix disease
Charlson comorbidity index
Char syndrome

chart
    Allen c.
    Babson c.
    Ballard c.
    BBT c.
    Broselow c.
    Cardiff Count-to-Ten c.
    Colorado Intrauterine Growth C.
    Denver Developmental c.
    Down syndrome growth c.
    Genentech growth c.
    growth c.
    letter c.
    Liley 3-zone c.
    pedigree c.
    pictorial blood loss assessment c.
     (PBAC)
    picture c.
    Ross growth c.
    sex-specific CDC growth c.
    Snellen acuity c.
    star c.
    Swedish national growth c.
    tumbling E c.
    Walker c.
    Welch Allyn SureSight eye c.
chartarum
    Stachybotrys c.
chaser
    Scot-Tussin DM Dough C.'s
Chassar
    C. Moir pubovaginal sling procedure
    C. Moir-Sims urinary fistula repair
    procedure
CH$_{50}$ assay
chaste
chasteberry
chastity
chat
    cri du c.
chatter
    cocktail c.
CHB
    congenital heart block
CHD
    congenital heart defect
    coronary heart disease
Cheadle
    C. disease
    C. syndrome
Chealamide
ChEAT
    Children's Eating Attitudes Test
check
    developmental c.
    c. valve obstruction
checklist
    Achenbach Child Behavior C.
    asthma symptom c. (ASC)

bed rest c.
Child Behavior C. (CBCL)
Children's Coping Strategies C. (CCSC)
Developmental Behaviour C.
Hopkins symptom c.
life events c. (LEC)
Pediatric Symptom C. (PSC)
Self-Injury and Self-Restraint c. (SISRC)
Wing Autistic Disorder Interview C. (WADIC)

checklist-revised
Noncommunicating Children's Pain C.-R. (NCCPC-R)

Chédiak-Higashi
C.-H. anomaly
C.-H. deficiency
C.-H. syndrome

cheek
chipmunk c.'s

cheese-wiring

cheesy
c. discharge
c. exudate

cheilitis, chilitis
angular c.

cheilognathopalatoschisis
cheilognathoprosoposchisis
cheilognathoschisis
cheilognathouranoschisis
cheiloschisis
cheilosis, chilosis
angular c.

cheiroarthropathy
diabetic c.

chelated gadolinium
chelation
iron c.
c. therapy

chelator
iron c.

Chelex bead
chelonae
Mycobacterium c.

Chemet
chemical
c. carcinogen
c. cautery
c. conjunctivitis
c. dependency
c. diabetes
c. peritonitis
c. pleurodesis
c. pneumonia
c. pneumonitis
c. pregnancy
c. sampling
c. shift imaging (CSI)

c. trauma
c. vaginitis
c. vulvovaginitis

chemically
c. exposed
c. exposed child

chemiluminescence, chemoluminescence
chemiluminescent
c. illumination
c. immunoassay (CIA)

chemiotaxis (*var. of* chemotaxis)
Chemke syndrome
chemoattractant
chemoceptor (*var. of* chemoreceptor)
chemoembolization
chemoimmunotherapy
chemokine
chemoluminescence (*var. of* chemiluminescence)
Chemo-Port catheter
chemoprevention
hormone c.

chemoprophylactic
chemoprophylaxis
intrapartum c.
selective intrapartum c. (SIC)

chemoradiation
chemoreceptor, chemoceptor
c. sensitivity
c. trigger zone (CTZ)

chemoreflex
laryngeal c.

chemosensitive reflex
chemosis
chemotactic
c. agent
c. factor

chemotaxis, chemiotaxis
positive c.
negative c.

chemotherapeutic
c. agent
c. retroconversion

chemotherapy
adjuvant c.
alkylating c.
antituberculosis c.
cancer c.
cell-cycle actions of c.
cell cycling in c.
CHOP c.
combination c.
high-dose c. (HDC)
induction c.
intraarterial c.
intraperitoneal c.
marrow-ablative c.
metabolism in intraperitoneal c.
multidrug c.

C

chemotherapy (*continued*)
near-myeloablative c.
neoadjuvant c.
c. phase trial
postoperative c.
prophylactic c.
c. protocol
salvage c.
second-line c.
chemotherapy-related neutropenia
Chemstrip
C. bG
Micral C.
Cheney syndrome
Cheracol D
Cherney incision
cherry-red
c.-r. macular spot
c.-r. macule
c.-r. spot myoclonus
syndrome
cherubism, gingival fibromatosis, epilepsy, mental deficiency syndrome
cherub sign
Chesapeake
hemoglobin C.
Cheshire cat smile
chessboard pattern
chest
barrel c.
barrel-shaped c.
c. compression
c. examination
flail c.
funnel c.
keel c.
c. mount
c. pain
c. percussion
c. percussion and auscultation
c. physical therapy (CPT)
c. physiotherapy (CPT)
c. radiograph
c. radiography
c. roentgenography
shield-shaped c.
c. suctioning
c. syndrome
c. trauma
c. tube
c. tube drainage
c. wall motion
c. wall radiation therapy
c. wall rigidity
c. wall weight
c. width
c. x-ray (CXR)
chewable
E.E.S. C.

chewing
rotary c.
Cheyne-Stokes respiration
CHF
congenital hepatic fibrosis
congestive heart failure
CHH
cartilage-hair hypoplasia
CHI
closed head injury
Chiari
C. anomaly
C. crisis
C. deformity
C. malformation (type I–IV)
C. net
C. procedure
Chiari-Arnold syndrome
Chiari-Frommel syndrome
chiasmal glioma
chiasmatic
c. cistern
c. pilocytic astrocytoma
chiasmatic-hypothalamic glioma
Chiba needle
CHIC
Coping Health Inventory for Children
Chicago human chromosome classification
Chicco breast pump
chicken ovalbumin upstream promoter transcription factor II (COUP)
chickenpox
gestational c.
c. pneumonia
c. vaccine
c. virus
Chid breast pump
chigger bite
Chiggertox
chikungunya virus
Chilaiditi syndrome
chilblain
child, *pl.* **children**
c. abuse (CA)
c. abuse and neglect (CAN)
c. abuse dwarfism
C. Abuse Prevention and Treatment Act (CAPTA)
C. Abuse Trauma Scale (CATS)
c., adolescent, and family mental health service (CAFMHS)
Aid to Families with Dependent Children (AFDC)
c. and adolescent burden assessment (CABA)
c. and adolescent forensic psychiatry
C. and Adolescent Functional Assessment Scale (CAFAS)

C. and Adolescent Psychiatric Assessment (CAPA)
c. and adolescent psychiatrist
C. and Adolescent Services Assessment (CASA)
children and adults with attention deficit disorder (CHADD)
Anxiety Disorder Interview for Children
anxiety rating for children (ARC)
c. assessment schedule (CAS)
atopic c.
Behavioral Assessment Scale for Children (BASC)
c. behavioral study (CBS)
C. Behavior Checklist (CBCL)
c. behavior rating form (CBRF)
burden of care interview for children
cardiorespiratory syndrome of obesity in c.
Center for Epidemiological Studies Depression Scale for Children
chemically exposed c.
CMV-shedding c.
Coping Health Inventory for Children (CHIC)
Developmental Programming for Infants and Young Children
Diagnostic Interview Schedule for Children (DISC)
Down syndrome c. (DSC)
emergency medical services for children (EMS-C)
C. Find
Functional Independence Measure for Children (WeeFIM)
C. Health and Illness Profile, Adolescent Edition (CHIP-AE)
c. health questionnaire (CHQ)
HIV Classification for Children (P0, P1, P2)
Hospital for Sick Children (HSC)
human immunodeficiency virus infected children
immune-competent c.
immunocompromised c.
International Study of Kidney Disease in Children
Kaufman Assessment Battery for Children (KABC)
KlaasKids Foundation for Children
living children (LC)
Lower Anchorages and Tethers for children (LATCH)
Neurologic Examination for Children (NEC)
children of alcoholic (COA)

Children of Alcoholics Screening Test (CAST)
c. of substance abuser (COSA)
parent c.
Personality Inventory for Children (PIC)
c. physical abuse (CPA)
c. protective agency
C. Protective Services (CPS)
puppet children
c. restraint
Schedule for Affective Disorders and Schizophrenia for School-Age Children (K-SADS)
c. sexual abuse (CSA)
C. Sexual Behavior Inventory (CSBI)
Silverman and Nelles Anxiety Disorders Interview Schedule for Children
Social Support Scale for Children (SSSC)
Stanford-Binet Intelligence Scale for Children
State-Trait Anxiety Inventory for Children (STAIC)
St. Joseph Aspirin-Free Cold Tablets for Children
C. syndrome
term birth, living c. (TBLC)
term infants, premature infants, abortions, living children (TPAL)
Trauma Symptom Checklist for Children (TSCC)
traumatic aortic injuries in children
treatment and education of autistic and related communications handicapped children (TEACCH)
unborn c.
C. Version of the Retrospective Diagnostic Interview for Borderlines
very low birth weight c.
Wechsler Intelligence Scale for Children (WISC)
Children with Special Health Care Needs (CWSN)
Women, Infants, Children (WIC)

CHILD
congenital hemidysplasia with ichthyosiform erythroderma and limb defects

child-adult mist (CAM)
childbearing
c. age
deferred c.
childbed fever
childbirth
Bradley method of prepared c.
Gamper method of c.

childbirth (*continued*)
    Grantley Dick-Read method of c.
    Kitzinger method of c.
    natural c. (NCB)
    physiologic c.
childbirth-related
    c.-r. medical condition
    c.-r. morbidity
child-centered literary orientation (CCLO)
child-directed instruction
childhood
    c. absence epilepsy (CAE)
    c. accidental spiral tibial (CAST)
    alternating hemiplegia of c. (AHC)
    c. anxiety
    C. Asthma Management Program (CAMP)
    C. Autism Rating Scale (CARS)
    benign epilepsy of c.
    c. breast
    C. Cancer Survivor Study (CCSS)
    chronic benign neutropenia of c.
    chronic bullous dermatosis of c.
    chronic bullous disease of c. (CBDC)
    chronic idiopathic arthritides of c. (CIAC)
    c. cicatricial pemphigoid
    c. conjunctivitis
    c. disintegrative disorder (CDD)
    c. epileptic encephalopathy
    erythroblastic anemia of c.
    c. fibromyalgia
    c. genital trauma
    c. idiopathic thrombocytopenic purpura
    irritable colon of c.
    limb pain of c.
    localized vulvar pemphigoid of c. (LVPC)
    overanxious disorder of c.
    papular acrodermatitis of c. (PAC)
    progressive bulbar paralysis of c.
    progressive muscular dystrophy of c.
    c. progressive systemic sclerosis
    c. pseudohypertrophic muscular dystrophy
    reactive attachment disorder of infancy or early c.
    recurrent abdominal pain of c.
    recurring digital fibroma of c. (RDFC)
    c. schizophrenia
    c. severity of psychiatric illness (CSPI)
    small round blue cell tumor of c.
    c. thyroid carcinoma
    transient erythroblastopenia of c. (TEC)
    c. trauma questionnaire (CTQ)
    universal nose of c.
    unstable bladder of c.
    vasculitis of c.
childhood-onset schizophrenia (COS)
childlessness
children (*pl. of* child)
children-revised
    Diagnostic Interview Schedule for C.-R. (DISC-R)
    Wechsler Intelligence Scale for C.-R. (WISC-R)
children's
    C. Cancer Group (CCG)
    C. Cancer Study Group (CCSG)
    C. Coping Strategies Checklist (CCSC)
    C. Depression Inventory (CDI)
    C. Depression Inventory Test
    C. Depression Rating Scale-Revised (CDRS-R)
    C. Depression Scale (CDS)
    C. Digestive Health and Nutrition Foundation (CDHNF)
    C. Eating Attitudes Test (ChEAT)
    C. Global Assessment Scale (CGAS)
    C. Health Insurance Program (CHIP)
    C. Interview for Psychiatric Disorders (ChIPS)
    C. Manifest Anxiety Scale (CMAS)
    C. Motrin
    C. Motrin Suspension
    C. National Medical Center
    C. Pepto
    c. service
    C. Silfedrine
    Tylenol Cold, C.
    C. Tylenol with Flavor Creator
child's chair
1-child sterility
chilitis (*var. of* cheilitis)
chill
    fever and c.'s (F&C)
chilosis (*var. of* cheilosis)
CHIME
    Collaborative Home Infant Monitoring Evaluation
    coloboma, heart defects, ichthyosiform dermatosis, mental retardation, ear defects
    CHIME syndrome
chimera
chimeric
    c. gene
    c. protein
chimerism
    blood c.

chin
  cleft c.
  c. dimple
  galoche c.
  c. lift
  c. position
  c. quivering
  underdeveloped c.
Chinese
  C. medicine
  C. restaurant syndrome
chip
  gene c.
CHIP
  Children's Health Insurance Program
  Coping Health Inventory for
  Parents
CHIP-AE
  Child Health and Illness Profile,
  Adolescent Edition
chipmunk cheeks
ChIPS
  Children's Interview for Psychiatric
  Disorders
Chiron branched DNA assay
chiropractic
CHL
  crown-heel length
chlamydia
  C. *pecorum*
  C. *pneumoniae*
  C. *psittaci*
  C. *sepsis*
  C. *trachomatis*
  C. *trachomatis* ligase chain reaction
  C. *trachomatis* pneumonia
  C. *trachomatis* tubal infertility
chlamydial
  c. cervicitis
  c. conjunctivitis
  c. infection
  c. pneumonia
  c. urethritis
  c. vaginitis
Chlamydiazyme
  C. immunoassay
  C. test
chloasma
Chlor-100
chloracne, chlorine acne
chloral
  c. hydrate
  c. hydrate sedation
chlorambucil
chloramphenicol
chloramphenicol-resistant isolate
chlorcyclizine hydrochloride
chlordecone
chlordiazepoxide

chlorhexidine
  c. gluconate
  c. solution
chloride
  acetylcholine c.
  Adrenalin C.
  aluminum c.
  ammonium c.
  Anectine C.
  bethanechol c.
  calcium c.)
  c. channelopathy
  doxacurium c.
  edrophonium c.
  ethyl c.
  ferrous c.
  Gebauer ethyl c.
  hexamethonium c.
  isotonic sodium c.
  magnesium c.
  mercuric c.
  methylbenzethonium c.
  obidoxime c.
  oxybutynin c.
  polyvinyl c.
  potassium c. (KCl)
  pralidoxime c.
  sodium c. (NaCl)
  sweat c.
  tridihexethyl c.
  tubocurarine c.
  vinyl c.
chloride-losing diarrhea
chloridometer
chloridorrhea
  congenital c.
chlorine acne
Chlor-Niramine
Chlorohist-LA
chloroma
Chloromycetin Injection
chlorophyllin copper complex
chloroplast DNA
chloroquine phosphate
chloroquine-resistant
  c.-r. malaria
  c.-r. *Plasmodium falciparum* (CRPF)
chloroquine-sensitive *Plasmodium falciparum*
chlorosis
chlorothiazide
chlorotrianisene
chlorpheniramine
Chlorpromanyl
chlorpromazine
chlorpropamide
chlorprothixene
chlortetracycline fluorescence test
chlorthalidone

C

Chlor-Trimeton
  C.-T. Injection
  C.-T. Oral
Chlor-Tripolon
chlorzoxazone
CHN
  congenital hypomyelinating
  neuropathy
choanae
  atresia c.
choanal
  c. atresia
  c. stenosis
chocolate
  c. agar
  c. agar plate
  c. cyst
choice
  forced c.
choked disc
choke mark
Cholac
cholangeitis (*var. of* cholangitis)
cholangiogram
  T-tube c.
cholangiography
  breath-hold MR c.
  magnetic resonance c. (MRC)
  non-breath-hold MR c.
  percutaneous c.
  single-film c.
cholangiopancreatography
  endoscopic retrograde c. (ERCP)
  magnetic resonance c. (MRCP)
cholangiopathy
  ascending c.
  infantile obstructive c.
  progressive obliterative c.
cholangitis, cholangeitis
  ascending c.
  primary sclerosing c.
  recurrent c.
  sclerosing c.
  suppurative c.
Cholebrine
cholecalciferol
  deficient hydroxylation of c.
cholecystectomy
  laparoscopic c. (LC)
cholecystitis
  acalculous c.
  acute acalculous c. (AAC)
  hydrops-like c.
cholecystokinin (CCK)
  fasting plasma c.
  postprandial plasma c.
choledochal
  c. cyst
  c. cyst-induced pancreatitis

choledochojejunostomy
  Roux-en-Y c.
choledocholithiasis
choledochus
  ductus c.
  terminal c.
cholelithiasis, chololithiasis
  cholesterol c.
cholera
  c. infantum
  c. vaccine
cholerae
  Vibrio c.
choleraesuis
  Salmonella c.
cholestasis
  benign familial recurrent c.
  familial intrahepatic c.
  hyperalimentation-associated c.
  intrahepatic c.
  maternal c.
  neonatal c.
  progressive familial intrahepatic c.
  (PFIC)
  total parenteral nutrition-associated c.
cholestasis-peripheral pulmonary stenosis
cholestatic
  c. hepatosis of pregnancy
  c. jaundice
  c. liver disease
  c. syndrome
cholesteatoma
  congenital c.
cholesterol
  c. cholelithiasis
  c. 20, 22 desmolase
  c. ester
  c. ester storage disease (CESD)
  c. gallstone
  c. granuloma
  LDL c.
  c. oxidase
  plasma c.
  c. stone
  c. synthesis
cholesterolemia
  familial c.
cholestyramine resin
choline
  free c.
  c. magnesium trisalicylate
  c. salicylate
  c. theophyllinate
cholinergic
  c. agonist
  c. crisis
  c. drug
  c. sympathetic function
  c. urticaria

cholinesterase inhibitor
chololithiasis (*var. of* cholelithiasis)
chondrification
chondroblastic osteosarcoma
chondroblastoma
chondrocyte
chondrodysplasia
    giant cell c.
    Grebe c.
    hereditary c.
    Jansen metaphysial c.
    c. punctata
    rhizomelic c.
chondrodysplasia-pseudohermaphrodism
  syndrome
chondrodystrophia
    c. calcificans congenita
    c. congenita punctata
    c. congenita tarda
    c. fetalis calcificans
    c. myotonica
chondrodystrophica
    myotonia c.
chondrodystrophic myotonia
chondrodystrophy, chondrodystrophia
    asphyxiating thoracic c.
    atypical c.
    hereditary deforming c.
    myotonic c.
    primary c.
chondroectodermal
    c. dysplasia
    c. dysplasia-like syndrome
chondroitin sulfate
chondrolysis
chondromalacia
    c. fetalis
    c. patella
chondromere
chondromyxoid fibroma, chondromyxoma
chondromyxoma (*var. of* chondromyxoid
  fibroma)
chondroosteodystrophy
chondroplastic dwarfism
chondrosarcoma
    uterine c.
Chooz
CHOP
    cyclophosphamide, hydroxydaunorubicin,
    methotrexate, prednisone
    CHOP chemotherapy
choramphenicol
chorda, *pl.* **chordae**
    chordae tendinea
    c. tympani
    c. umbilicalis
chordae (*pl. of* chorda)
chordamesoderm
    caudal c.

chordate
chordee
    c. correction
    dorsal c.
    penile c.
chordoid sarcoma
chordoma
chorea
    benign nonprogressive familial c.
    c. gravidarum
    hereditary benign c.
    Huntington c.
    c. magna
    c. minor
    Sydenham c.
chorea-acanthocytosis
choreic
    c. hand
    c. movement
choreiform movement
choreoathetoid
    c. cerebral palsy
    c. movement
choreoathetosis
    bilateral c.
    familial inverted c.
    paroxysmal kinesigenic c.
choreoathetotic
    c. movement
    c. movement disorder
Chorex
chorioadenoma destruens
chorioallantoic
    c. membrane (CAM)
    c. placenta
    c. vessel
chorioamnionic, chorioamniotic
    c. band
    c. infection
    c. placenta
chorioamnionitis (CA)
    Gardnerella vaginalis c.
    histologic c.
chorioamniotic (*var. of* chorioamnionic)
chorioangioma
chorioangiomatosis
chorioangiopagi parasiticus
chorioangiopagus placental vessel
chorioangiosis
chorioblastoma
choriocarcinoma
    nongestational c.
choriodecidual tissue
chorioembryonic antigen
chorioepithelioma
choriogenesis
choriogonadotropin
    c. alfa
    c. alfa for injection

C

choriomeningitis
  experimental lymphocytic c.
  lymphocytic c.
chorion
  c. frondosum
  c. laeve
  outer c.
  c. sampling
  smooth c.
  villous c.
chorionic
  c. adrenocorticotropin
  c. cavity
  c. cyst
  c. gonadotropic hormone (CGH)
  c. gonadotropin (CG, CGT)
  c. growth hormone
  c. human recombinant gonadotropin
  c. plate
  c. sac
  c. thyrotropin
  c. vascularization
  c. vesicle
  c. vessel thrombus
  c. villus biopsy (CVB)
  c. villus haplotype analysis
  c. villus infarction
  c. villus ischemia
  c. villus sampling (CVS)
chorionicity
chorioretinitis
  toxoplasmic c.
choriovitelline placenta
choroid
  c. plexus
  c. plexus carcinoma (CPC)
  c. plexus cell
  c. plexus cyst (CPC)
  c. plexus papillocarcinoma
  c. plexus papilloma (CPP)
  c. plexus primordia
  c. plexus pulse effect
  c. tubercle
choroiditis
Chotzen syndrome
CHQ
  child health questionnaire
Christchurch chromosome
**Christian-Andrews-Conneally-Muller
  syndrome**
Christian-Opitz syndrome
Christian syndrome (1, 2)
Christmas
  C. disease
  C. factor (CF)
  C. tree bladder
  C. tree distribution
  C. tree distribution eruption
  C. tree pattern

Christ-Siemens-Touraine syndrome
chromaffinoma
Chroma-Pak
chromatid
  sister c.
chromatin
  sex c.
  X c.
  Y c.
chromatinolysis (*var. of* chromatolysis)
chromatofocusing pH range
chromatography
  amino acid c.
  denaturing high-performance
    liquid c.
  gas c.
  high-performance liquid c.
    (HPLC)
  high-power liquid c. (HPLC)
  high-pressure liquid c. (HPLC)
  thin-layer c. (TLC)
chromatolysis, chromatinolysis
chromatophore nevus of Naegeli
chromhidrosis, chromidrosis
  apocrine c.
chromic
  c. gut pelviscopic loop ligature
  c. phosphate
chromidrosis (*var. of* chromhidrosis)
chromium
chromogen
chromohydrotubation
chromomere
chromoneme
chromopertubation
chromophobe
chromophobic adenoma
chromophore
chromosomal
  c. aberration (CA)
  c. analysis
  c. anomaly
  c. breakage-immunodeficiency
    syndrome
  c. defect
  c. deletion
  c. disorder
  c. dysfunction
  c. inversion
  c. karyotype
  c. marker
  c. mosaicism
  c. nondisjunction
  c. pattern
  c. segment
  c. sex
  c. structural abnormality
  c. study
  c. translocation

chromosome
  c. 1–23
  accessory c.
  acentric c.
  acrocentric c.
  c. analysis
  arm of c.
  artificial c.
  B c.
  bacterial artificial c. (BAC)
  c. banding
  bivalent c.
  c. breakage
  c. breakage test
  centromeric region of c.
  Christchurch c.
  c. complement
  contiguous gene syndrome of c. 13
  daughter c.
  c. deletion
  deletion of c.
  del(5p) c.
  derivative c.
  dicentric c.
  c. diploid/tetraploid mixoploidy
    syndrome
  expansion of c.
  founder c.
  fractured c.
  fragile X c.
  gametic c.
  giant c.
  c. GI deletion syndrome
  heterotropic c.
  heterotypical c.
  homologous c.
  human artificial c. (HAC)
  inactivated X c.
  insertion of c.
  inversion of c.'s
  c. 9 inversion syndrome
  c. 15 inverted duplication
  inverted duplication of c. 15
  inverted X c.
  iso-X c.
  c. jumping
  c. knob
  lampbrush c.
  late replicating c.
  long arm of c. (q)
  long arm of Y c.
  c. map
  c. mapping
  marker X c.
  metacentric c.
  metaphase c.
  c. microdeletion
  mitochondrial c.
  mitotic c.

  c. 1–22 monosomy syndrome
  c. 17 mutation
  nonhomologous c.
  nucleolar c.
  odd c.
  4p+ c.
  c. paint
  c. pair
  c. pairing
  parental inversion of c.'s
  c. 9p disorder
  Philadelphia c. (Ph1)
  c. 8p mosaic tetrasomy
  polytene c.
  c. 1p–22p deletion syndrome
  c. 1p–22p monosomy
  c. 1p–22p trisomy
  c. 1q–22q deletion syndrome
  c. 1q–22q duplication syndrome
  c. 1q–22q monosomy
  c. 1q–22q tetrasomy syndrome
  c. 1q–22q triplication syndrome
  c. 1q–22q trisomy
  c. 8 recombinant syndrome
  c. reduction
  c. 1–22 ring syndrome
  c. sequencing
  sex c.
  sex-linked c.
  short arm of c. (p)
  small c.
  somatic c.
  submetacentric c.
  supernumerary c.
  supernumerary marker c. (SMC)
  c. 22 supernumerary marker
    (SMG22)
  telocentric c.
  c. tetraploidy syndrome
  translocation of c. 22
  c. triploidy syndrome
  c. 1–22 trisomy
  c. 1–22 trisomy syndrome
  Turner syndrome in female with X
    c.
  c. 14 uniparental disomy syndrome
  unpaired c.
  W c.
  c. walking
  45,X c.
  X c.
  c. XA
  c. X autosome translocation
    syndrome
  c. X fragility syndrome
  c. X inversion syndrome
  X-linked recessive c.
  XO c.
  c. XO syndrome

C

chromosome (*continued*)
   c. Xp21 deletion syndrome
   c. Xp22 deletion syndrome
   c. X pentasomy
   c. Xp21 monosomy
   c. Xq deletion syndrome
   c. Xq duplication syndrome
   c. Xq monosomy
   c. Xq trisomy
   XX c.
   c. XXX syndrome
   c. 47,XXX syndrome
   c. XXXXX syndrome
   c. XXXXY syndrome
   c. XXY syndrome
   Y c.
   yeast artificial c. (YAC)
   c. Y;18 translocation syndrome
chromotubation
chronic
   c. active hepatitis
   c. adhesive arachnoiditis
   c. adrenal insufficiency
   c. anovulation (CA)
   c. aspiration
   c. aspiration syndrome
   c. asthma
   c. atrophic vulvitis
   c. behavior problem
   c. benign neutropenia (CBN)
   c. benign neutropenia of childhood
   c. biopsychosocial syndrome
   c. bullous dermatitis
   c. bullous dermatosis of childhood
   c. bullous disease of childhood (CBDC)
   c. cervicitis
   c. chagasic cardiomyopathy
   c. compartment syndrome
   c. conjunctival infection
   c. constipation
   c. cryptogenic hepatitis (CCH)
   c. cyanide toxicity
   c. cystic mastitis (CCM)
   c. eczematoid dermatitis
   c. fatigue syndrome (CFS)
   c. focal encephalitis
   c. Gaucher disease
   c. glomerulonephritis
   c. granulomatous amebic encephalitis
   c. granulomatous disease (CGD)
   c. headache
   c. hepatitis
   c. hydrocephalus
   c. hyperreninemia
   c. hypertension
   c. hypertransfusion program
   c. hypertrophic gastritis
   c. hypertrophic vulvitis

   c. hypervitaminosis A
   c. idiopathic arthritides of childhood (CIAC)
   c. idiopathic intestinal pseudoobstruction (CIIP)
   c. idiopathic neutropenia
   c. idiopathic urticaria
   c. illness
   c. inflammatory demyelinating polyneuropathy (CIDP)
   c. inflammatory demyelinating polyradiculoneuropathy (CIDP)
   c. interstitial fibrosis
   c. interstitial salpingitis
   c. intertrigo
   c. intestinal pseudoobstruction
   c. intravascular hemolysis
   c. iridocyclitis
   c. ITP
   c. juvenile arthritis
   c. lung disease (CLD)
   c. lung disease of maturity
   c. lymphocytic leukemia (CLL)
   c. lymphocytic meningitis
   c. lymphocytic thyroiditis
   c. mastoiditis
   c. maternal disease
   c. meningococcemia
   c. meningoradiculomyelitis
   c. mitral insufficiency
   c. motor tic disorder
   c. mucocutaneous candidiasis
   c. mumps encephalitis
   c. myelocytic leukemia
   c. myelogenous leukemia (CML)
   c. neuromuscular disease
   c. neuronopathic Gaucher disease
   c. non-A-E hepatitis
   c. nonspecific diarrhea
   c. nonspecific diarrhea of infancy
   c. nonspherocytic hemolytic anemia
   c. obstructive bronchitis
   c. osteomyelitis
   c. otitis media (COM)
   c. pain state
   c. pancreatitis
   c. papilledema
   c. parvoviral infection
   c. pelvic infection
   c. pelvic pain (CPP)
   c. peripheral neuropathy
   c. pneumonitis of infancy (CPI)
   c. progressive ataxia
   c. progressive encephalitis
   c. progressive external ophthalmoplegia (CPEO)
   c. pulmonary disease
   c. pulmonary histoplasmosis
   c. pulmonary insufficiency

c. pupillary syndrome
c. pyogenic lymphadenitis
c. recurrent multifocal osteomyelitis (CRMO)
c. rejection
c. relapsing polyradiculoneuropathy
c. renal failure (CRF)
c. renal insufficiency
c. respiratory acidosis
c. respiratory alkalosis
c. rhinosinusitis
c. SCFE
c. schistosomiasis
c. scrotal hypothermia
c. sickle cell lung disease
c. sinusitis
c. spongiform encephalopathy
c. subglottic stenosis
c. suppurative otitis media (CSOM)
c. synovial inflammation
c. syphilitic meningitis
c. tic
c. tic disorder (CTD)
c. tonsillar herniation
c. transfusion
c. unremitting polyradiculoneuropathy
c. urinary tract infection
c. vascular disease
c. vitamin A intoxication
chronica
pityriasis lichenoides c. (PLC)
chronicus
lichen simplex c. (LSC)
Chronoflex catheter
chronograph
chronological age
chronotherapy
phase delay c.
chronotropic
c. effect
c. response
chronotropy
CHRS
cerebrohepatorenal syndrome
congenital hereditary retinoschisis
Chryseobacterium
Chrysosporium
CHT
closed head trauma
combined hormone therapy
congenital hypothyroidism
contralateral head turning
CHTN
Cooperative Human Tissue Network
Chudley-Lowry-Hoar syndrome
Chudley syndrome (1, 2)
Churg-Strauss
C.-S. syndrome
C.-S. vasculitis

Chux pad
Chvostek sign
chyle
chyliform
chylomicron
c. formation
c. retention disease
chylomicronemia syndrome
chylopericardium
chylosus
chylothorax
acquired c.
congenital c.
chylous
c. ascites
c. liquid
c. pleural effusion
chyluria
chymopapain
CI
cardiac index
cervical incompetence
Colour Index
cord insertion
Ci
curie
CIA
chemiluminescent immunoassay
congenital intestinal aganglionosis
CIAC
chronic idiopathic arthritides of childhood
Cianchetti syndrome
CIC
clean intermittent catheterization
cicatrices (*pl. of* cicatrix)
cicatricial
c. alopecia
c. lesion
c. pemphigoid
c. retinal disease
cicatrix, *pl.* **cicatrices**
ciclopirox
CID
combined immunodeficiency
cytomegalic inclusion disease
Cidex soak
cidofovir topical gel
Cidomycin
CIDP
chronic inflammatory demyelinating polyneuropathy
chronic inflammatory demyelinating polyradiculoneuropathy
CIE
congenital ichthyosiform erythroderma
counterimmunoelectrophoresis
Ciel
Kay C.

cigarette-paper skin
ciguatera
    c. fish poisoning
    c. intoxication
CIIP
    chronic idiopathic intestinal
    pseudoobstruction
CIIS
    Cattell Infant Intelligence
    Scale
cilastatin
    imipenem and c.
ciliaris
    tylosis c.
ciliary
    c. biopsy
    c. blush
    c. dyskinesia
    c. dysmotility
    c. flush
    c. function
    c. function study
    c. muscle
    c. nerve
    c. neurotrophic factor (CNTF)
    c. paralysis
    c. spasm
ciliated
    c. cell
    c. cell endometrial adenocarcinoma
    c. columnar epithelium
    c. metaplasia
Ciloxan
cimetidine
CIN
    cervical intraepithelial neoplasia
cineangiocardiography
    biplane c.
cineangiogram
    continuous c.
cineangiography
    biplane c.
    radionuclide c.
cinedefecography
    anal sphincter c.
cine loop
Cineloop
    C. image review ultrasound
    system
    C. Ultrasound
cineradiography
cingulate gyrus
C1INH coagulation inhibitor
cinnarizine
Cinobac
cinoxacin
Cin-Quin
CIPA
    congenital insensitivity to pain

CIPRACT
    cervical incompetence prevention
    randomized cerclage trial
Cipro
    C. HC Otic
    C. Injection
    C. Oral
Ciprodex otic suspension
ciprofloxacin hydrochloride
circadian
    c. cycle
    c. rhythm
    c. rhythm dyssomnia
circinata
    balanitis c.
circinate balanitis
circle
    Baudelocque uterine c.
    Carus c.
    Huguier c.
    c. of Willis
    c. of Willis aneurysm
circling disease
Circon-ACMI
    C.-ACMI cannula
    C.-ACMI hysteroscope
    C.-ACMI trocar
CircPlus compression wrap/dressing
circuit
    failed Fontan c.
circular
    c. end-to-end anastomosis
    (CEEA)
    c. reaction
circulating
    c. anticoagulant
    c. estrogen
    c. fetal cell
    c. hormone
    c. neutrophils
    c. platelet antibody
    c. testosterone
circulation
    airway, breathing, c. (ABC)
    collateral c.
    duct-dependent pulmonary c.
    duct-dependent systemic c.
    enteromammary c.
    extracorporeal c. (ECC)
    fetal c.
    fetal cardiovascular c.
    fetal-placental c.
    fetal pulmonary c.
    fetoplacental c.
    hypophysial portal c.
    hypothalamic-hypophysial portal c.
    intrauterine c.
    parallel c.
    persistence of fetal c.

persistent fetal c. (PFC)
pituitary-hypothalamic c.
c. time
umbilical cardiovascular c.
uteroovarian c.
uteroplacental c.
circulation-cavopulmonary connection
circulatory
  c. arrest
  c. collapse
  c. crossover
  c. system
circumcise
circumcision
  c. chair
  c. clamp
  female c.
  Mogen c.
  pharaonic c.
  c. status
  Sunna c.
circumduction
  c. gait
  c. movement
circumference
  abdominal c. (AC)
  arm c.
  fetal abdominal c. (FAC)
  head c. (HC)
  head circumference/abdominal c.
   (HC/AC)
  mean arm muscle c. (MAMC)
  midarm c. (MAC)
  midarm muscle c. (MAMC)
  occipitofrontal c. (OFC)
  sonographic abdominal c.
circumferential
  c. burn
  c. eversion
  c. eversion of urethral epithelium
  c. examination
  c. ringed crease of limb
  c. skin crease of limb
  c. skin creases-psychomotor
   retardation syndrome
circumflexa
  ichthyosis linearis c.
circumflex artery
circummarginate placenta
circumoral pallor
circumscribed
  c. mass
  c. neurodermatitis
  well c.
circumscripta
  myositis ossificans c.
circumscriptum
  angiokeratoma c.
  lymphangioma c.

circumscriptus
  albinismus c.
Circumstraint
circumvallata
  placenta c.
circumvallate placenta
cirrhonosus
cirrhosis
  biliary c.
  compensated c.
  cryptogenic c.
  decompensated c.
  endemic Tyrolean infantile c.
  end-stage c.
  hepatic c.
  hypertrophic c.
  Indian childhood c. (ICC)
  liver c.
  macronodular c.
  micronodular liver c.
  c. of liver
  postnecrotic c.
  primary biliary c. (PBC)
  progressive biliary c.
  pseudolobular c.
cirsoid aneurysm
cirsomphalos
CIS
  carcinoma in situ
cisapride
cis-**atracurium**
cis-**diamminedichloroplatinum**
  cis-diamminedichloroplatinum II
cisplatin
  intraperitoneal c.
  c., methotrexate, vinblastine (CMV)
  c., vinblastine, and bleomycin
9-*cis*-retinoic acid
cistern
  basal c.
  chiasmatic c.
  prominent quadrigeminal plate c.
cisternal puncture
cisterna magna
cisternography
  isotope c.
  radioisotope c.
cistron
citalopram
citizen
  Association for Retarded C.'s (ARC)
Citracal Prenatal + DHA
citrate
  c. and citric acid
  c. blood sample
  caffeine c.
  calcium c.
  clomiphene c. (CC)
  cyclofenil c.

C

citrate *(continued)*
    diphenhydramine c.
    ethoheptazine c.
    fentanyl c.
    lithium c.
    magnesium c.
    oral transmucosal fentanyl c.
      (OTFC)
    potassium c.
    sildenafil c.
    sufentanil c.
    tamoxifen c.
    toremifene c.
    c. toxicity
citrated caffeine
citric acid cycle
Citrobacter
    C. amalonaticus
    C. braakii
    C. diversus
    C. farmeri
    C. freundii
    C. koseri
    C. sedlakii
    C. werkmanii
    C. youngae
citrovorum factor
citrulline
    plasma c.
citrullinemia
citrullinuria
C-IV
    Pemoline C-IV
CJD
    Creutzfeldt-Jakob disease
    iatrogenic CJD
    new variant CJD
CK
    creatine kinase
CKC
    cold knife conization
CK-MB
    myocardial muscle creatine kinase
    isoenzyme
CL
    cleft lip
    compliance of lung
    corpus luteum
CLA
    conjugated linoleic acid
    X-linked cerebellar ataxia
Clado anastomosis
cladogenesis
Cladosporium herbarum
cladribine
Claforan
clamp
    Allis c.
    Babcock c.

    back c.
    Backhaus c.
    Ballantine c.
    Buxton c.
    cervical c.
    circumcision c.
    DeBakey aortic c.
    extracutaneous vas fixation c.
    Gomco circumcision c.
    Heaney-Ballantine hysterectomy c.
    Heaney hysterectomy c.
    Hoffmann c.
    hysterectomy c.
    ICSI Massachusetts c.
    Kelly c.
    Kocher c.
    Lahey c.
    Masterson c.
    Mogen c.
    Péan c.
    pediatric bulldog c.
    pediatric vascular c.
    pedicle c.
    Pennington c.
    Phaneuf c.
    thoracic c.
    thyroid Lahey c.
    umbilical c.
    vulsellum c.
    Willett c.
    Winston cervical c.
    Yellen c.
    Zeppelin c.
clamped down
clamping
    cord c.
CLAMS
    Clinical Linguistic and Auditory
    Milestone Scale
clamshell-type catheter occlusion device
Clara cell 16 protein
Clarion hearing implant
Claripex
clarithromycin
Claritin
    C. RediTab
    C. syrup
Claritin-D 24-Hour
Clark
    C. classification of vulvar
    melanoma
    C. mechanistic classification
    C. microstaging system
Clarke
    C. column
    C. ligator scissor forceps
Clarke-Hadfield syndrome
Clarus model 5169 peristaltic pump

CLAS
  congenital localized absence of
    skin
**clasped thumbs-mental retardation
  syndrome**
clasp-knife
    c.-k. phenomenon
    c.-k. response
classic
    c. abdominal Semm hysterectomy
      (CASH)
    c. celiac disease
    c. incision
    c. medulloblastoma
    c. migraine
    c. migraine headache
    c. plaque psoriasis
    c. X-linked recessive muscular
      dystrophy
classical
    c. cesarean section
    c. galactosemia
    c. genetics
    c. incision extension
    c. lissencephaly
    c. migraine
    c. pathway defect
    c. transverse incision
    c. uterine incision
classifiable character
classification
    Abramson c.
    Acosta endometriosis c.
    AFUD c.
    American Foundation of Urologic
      Diseases c.
    American Society of
      Anesthesiologists c.
    Angle c.
    Astler-Coller modification of
      Dukes c.
    Barbero-Marcial c.
    Bethesda 2001 cervical cytology c.
    Bethesda System Pap smear c.
    Blaivas c.
    Caldwell-Moloy c.
    Catterall c. (grade 1–4)
    Chicago human chromosome c.
    Clark mechanistic c.
    Cori glycogen storage disease c.
    de la Cruz c.
    Delbet fracture c. (type I–IV)
    Denver c.
    Dukes c.
    EULAR c.
    FAB c.
    histologic c.
    HIV c.
    ILAR peripheral arthritis c.

    Jansky c.
    Jewett c.
    Kajava supernumerary breast
      tissue c.
    King c.
    microinvasive carcinoma c.
    Milch fracture c.
    Moss c.
    Neer c.
    PAAS c.
    Pulec and Freedman congenital ear
      abnormality c.
    Reese-Ellsworth c.
    Risser c.
    Rye c.
    Salter-Harris c.
    Schuknecht age-related hearing
      loss c.
    Tanner c. (1–5)
    TNM c.
    Wassel c.
    White c.
    White diabetes mellitus in
      pregnancy c.
    Zero to Three children's mental
      health diagnostic c.
clastic lesion
clastogenic stress
clathrin
clavicle
    congenital pseudoarthrosis of c.
claviclectomy
    distal c.
clavicular
    c. fracture (CF)
    c. injury
    c. pseudarthrosis
    c. shaft
claviculectomy
clavulanate
    c. potassium
    ticarcillin c.
clavulanic acid
Clavulin
claw
clawfoot, claw foot
clawhand, claw hand
    c. deformity repair
clawing
clay
    green c.
CLD
    chronic lung disease
    cytoplasmic lipid droplet
CLE
    congenital lobar emphysema
clean
    c. intermittent catheterization (CIC)
    c. intermittent self-catheterization

clean-catch
c.-c. midstream urine sample
c.-c. technique
c.-c. urinalysis
c.-c. urine specimen
cleaner
Sklar aseptic germicidal c.
clean-out
bowel c.-o.
cleanser
Dey-Wash skin wound c.
cleansing solution
clear
c. cell adenocarcinoma
c. cell endometrial carcinoma
c. cell hidradenoma
c. cell sarcoma
c. cell tumor
c. cell vaginal cancer
C. Eyes
c. mucoid sputum
clearance
creatinine c.
immune c.
mucociliary c.
c. of fetal product
ultrafiltration virus c.
urate c.
urea c.
virus c.
xenon c.
Clearblue
C. Easy
C. Improved
clearing
throat c.
ClearPlan
C. Easy
C. Easy fertility monitor
C. Easy ovulation predictor
ClearSite hydrogauze dressing
clearview
C. hCG pregnancy test
C. uterine manipulator
cleavage
embryonic c.
manual c.
c. plan
c. stage
c. syndrome
cleaved
c. amplified polymorphic sequence
c. embryo
cleft
belly c.
bilateral schizencephalic c.'s
branchial c.
c. chin
complete c.

c. face
genital c.
c. hand
hyobranchial c.
incomplete c.
intergluteal c.
c. jaw
Lanterman c.
laryngeal c.
laryngotracheoesophageal c.
c. lip (CL)
c. lip and palate (CLP)
c. lip-nasal reconstruction
nasal alar cartilage c.
c. nasal deformity correction
natal c.
orofacial c.
c. palate (CP)
c. palate-lateral synechia (CPLS)
c. palate repair
postalveolar c.
c. premaxillary process
schizencephalic c.
c. spine
Stillman c.
submucous c.
syndromic c.
c. vertebrae
visceral c.
clefting
ankyloblepharon, ectodermal
dysplasia, c. (AEC)
ectrodactyly, ectodermal dysplasia, c.
(EEC)
hypertelorism, microtia, c. (HMC)
cleidocranial
c. digital dysostosis
c. dysplasia
c. dysplasia syndrome
cleidocranialis
dysostosis c.
dysplasia c.
cleidocraniodigitalis
dysostosis c.
cleidocraniopelvina
dysostosis c.
cleidofacialis
dysplasia c.
cleidorhizomelic syndrome
cleidorrhexis
cleidotomy
clemastine
clenched
c. fist and pleural effusion
c. fist injury
c. fists
Cleocin
C. HCl
C. HCl Oral

C. Pediatric Oral
C. Phosphate
C. T
C. vaginal cream
C. Vaginal Ovules
Clevedon positive pressure respirator
click
aortic ejection c.
ejection c.
hip c.
midsystolic c.
Ortolani c.
pulmonary ejection c.
c. stimulus
systolic c.
clidinium
clidocranial dysplasia
clidoic
Clifford syndrome
climacteric, climacterium
grand c.
c. history
c. psychosis
c. syndrome
climacterium
Climara
C. estradiol transdermal system
C. estradiol transdermal system patch
climatic bubo
clinch knot
clindamycin
c. phosphate
c. phosphate topical solution
Clindoxyl
clinic
National Fertility C.
Teen-Tot C.
clinical
C. Adaptive Test (CAT)
C. Adaptive Test/Clinical Linguistic and Auditory Milestone Scale (CAT/CLAMS)
c. assessment in neuropsychology
c. breast examination (CBE)
c. cohort study
C. Colitis Activity Index (CCAI)
c. crib
c. dating
C. Evaluation of Language Fundamentals-Preschool
C. Evaluation of Language Fundamentals, 3rd Edition
c. finding
C. Global Impressions (CGI)
c. global index (CGI)
c. grouping
C. Linguistic and Auditory Milestone Scale (CLAMS)

c. pelvimetry
c. pregnancy
c. prognosis
c. response
c. risk assessment (CRA)
C. Risk Index for Babies (CRIB)
c. staging
c. test strip
c. type
clinically significant arrhythmia (CSA)
CliniCath peripherally inserted catheter
clinicopathologic, clinicopathological
clinicopathological (*var. of* clinicopathologic)
c. analysis
Clinistix
Clinitek 50 urine chemistry analyzer
Clinitest assay
clinocephaly
clinodactyly
fifth finger c.
Clinoril
clioquinol
clip
Bleier c.
Fetendo c.
Filshie c.
Hulka c.
Hulka-Clemens c.
c. technique
towel c.
clitoral
c. engorgement
c. hood
c. hypertrophy
c. ischemia
c. length
c. nerve
c. neurofibroma
c. sensitivity
c. strangulation
c. therapy device (CTD)
clitoridectomy
clitorides (*pl. of* clitoris)
clitoridis
fascia c.
phimosis c.
smegma c.
clitoriditis, clitoritis
clitoris, *pl.* **clitorides**
bifid c.
c. crisis
c. enlargement
frenulum of c.
glans c.
suspensory ligament of c.
c. tourniquet syndrome (CTS)
clitorism
clitoritis (*var. of* clitoriditis)

clitoromegaly
clitoroplasty
clivus
    inferior c.
CLL
    chronic lymphocytic leukemia
CLO
    congenital lobar overinflation
cloaca
    congenital c.
    primitive c.
cloacae
    Enterobacter c.
cloacal
    c. duct
    c. exstrophy
    c. extrophy
    c. malformation
    c. membrane
    c. plate anomaly
cloaking
    periosteal c.
clobetasol propionate
Clocort Maximum Strength
clocortolone
Cloderm Topical
clodronate
clofazimine
clofibrate
Clomid
clomiphene
    c. citrate (CC)
    c. citrate challenge test (CCCT, C3T)
    c. fetal malformation
clomiphene-resistant polycystic ovary syndrome
clomipramine hydrochloride
clomocycline
clonality
clonal selection theory
clonazepam
clone
    c. bank
    DNA c.
    molecular c.
    overlapping c.'s
    recombinant c.
clonic
    c. movement
    c. seizure
clonidine hydrochloride
cloning
    DNA c.
    embryo c.
    functional c.
    gene c.
    positional c.
    c. vector

clonogenic
    c. assay
    c. technique
clonorchiasis, clonorchiosis
clonorchiosis (*var. of* clonorchiasis)
Clonorchis sinensis
clonus
    ankle c.
    sustained c.
clopamide
Cloquet node
clorazepate
closed
    c. bite
    c. chest massage
    c. comedo
    c. drainage
    c. endotracheal tube suctioning
    c. fist injury
    c. head injury (CHI)
    c. head trauma (CHT)
    c. loop obstruction
    c. loop system passing electrode
    c. neural tube defect
    c. spina bifida
    c. thoracotomy
closed-circuit video recording
closing
    c. capacity (CC)
    c. coagulum
    c. ring of Winkler-Waldeyer
clostridial
    c. bacteremia
    c. myonecrosis
    c. otitis media
    c. toxin
clostridium
    C. botulinum
    C. botulinum type A toxin
    C. botulism
    C. difficile
    C. difficile-associated diarrhea (CDAC, CDAD)
    C. freundii
    C. perfringens
    C. ramosum
    clostridia septicemia
    C. septicum
    C. spiroforme
    C. tetani
closure
    anterior neural tube c.
    bilabial c.
    ClozeX wound c.
    delayed primary c.
    ductus c.
    early midsystolic c.
    epiphysial c.

Gestalt c.
hysteric glottic c.
incision c.
laryngeal c.
lip c.
neural tube c.
neurosurgical c.
nonlocking c.
palatal fistula c.
percutaneous patent ductus
  arteriosus c.
physial c.
posterior neural tube c.
premature airway c.
premature ductus arteriosus c.
primary c.
secondary c.
Steri-Strip skin c.
tertiary c.
Tom Jones c.
transcatheter c. (TCC)
ventricular septal defect patch c.
wound c.

clot
blood c.
c. formation
friable c.
hold c.
intraluminal c.
organized blood c.
c. resolution
retroplacental c.
c. sectioning
Clotrimaderm
clotrimazole
c. troche
c. vaginal cream 2%
clotting
c. factor
c. time
clouding
corneal c.
infantile corneal c.
mental c.
c. of sensorium
cloudy
c. cornea
c. discharge
c. nipple discharge
c. sputum
Clouston syndrome
cloven spine
clover
red c.
C. syndrome
cloverleaf
c. skull
c. skull deformity
c. skull syndrome

cloxacillin
clozapine
ClozeX wound closure
CLP
cleft lip and palate
CLS
capillary leak syndrome
CLSE
calf lung surfactant extract
CLTM
continuous long-term monitoring
club
clubbing
digital c.
hereditary c.
c. of fingers and toes
c. of nails
clubfoot, club foot
c. (CF)
adductus c.
arthrogrypotic c.
c. cast
congenital c.
c. deformity
c. dysplasia
equinus c.
idiopathic c.
medial rotation c.
neurogenic c.
positional c.
rigid c.
c. splint
Turco posteromedial release of c.
varus c.
clubhand, club hand
radial c.
ulnar c.
clue cell
clumsiness
clumsy child syndrome
clunk
hip c.
cluster
c. B disorder
DAZ gene c.
c. headache
cluster-stratified sampling method
cluttering
Clutton joints
cm
centimeter
cM
centimorgan
CMA
cow's milk allergy
CMAP
compound muscle action potential
CMAS
Children's Manifest Anxiety Scale

C

CMD
congenital muscular dystrophy
Fukuyama CMD
CMF
chondromyxoid fibroma
CMFTD
congenital muscle fiber-type
disproportion
CMG
cystometrogram
cmH$_2$O
centimeter of water
CMI
cell-mediated immunity
CMI vacuum extractor
CMI-Mityvac cup
CMI-O'Neil cup
CML
chronic myelogenous leukemia
CMP
cow's milk protein
CMT
cervical motion tenderness
CMTS
Charcot-Marie-Tooth syndrome
CMV
cisplatin, methotrexate, vinblastine
controlled mechanical ventilation
cytomegalovirus
disseminated CMV
CMV enteritis
CMV retinitis
CMV-IGIV
cytomegalovirus immune globulin
intravenous
CMV-seronegative transplant patient
CMV-shedding child
c-*myc* oncogene
CN
calcaneonavicular
CNAP
continuous negative airway pressure
CNB
core needle biopsy
CNBr
cyanogen bromide
CNBr activated Sepharose
CNEP
continuous negative extrathoracic
pressure
CNFS
craniofrontonasal syndrome
CNLDO
congenital nasolacrimal duct obstruction
CNM
centronuclear myopathy
certified nurse-midwife
CNMD
chronic neuromuscular disease

CNPAS
congenital nasal pyriform aperture
stenosis
CNS
central nervous system
CNS aneurysm
CNS development
CNS dysfunction
CNS hemorrhage
CNS infarction
CNS leukemia
CNS malignancy
primary angiitis of CNS (PACNS)
CNS tumor
CNTF
ciliary neurotrophic factor
^{60}Co
cobalt-60
CO
carbon monoxide
end-tidal CO
CO$_2$
carbon dioxide
end-tidal CO$_2$
CO$_2$ laser
pressure of CO$_2$ (PCO$_2$)
COA
children of alcoholic
CoA
aortic arch coarctation
coenzyme A
COACH
cerebellar vermis hypoplasia,
oligophrenia, congenital ataxia, ocular
coloboma, hepatic fibrosis
COACH syndrome
coach's finger
coactivated antagonists
coagula (*pl. of* coagulum)
coagulase
coagulase-negative
c.-n. bacteremia
c.-n. *Staphylococcus*
coagulase-positive *Staphylococcus*
coagulation
c. abnormality
argon beam c.
bipolar diathermy c.
c. cascade
cold c.
c. defect
c. disorder
disseminated intravascular c. (DIC)
c. disturbance
c. factor
c. factor zymogen
c. forceps
localized intravascular c.
c. necrosis

c. profile
c. study
c. test
tubal c.
coagulative myocytolysis
coagulator
argon beam c. (ABC)
cold c.
Elmed BC 50 M/M digital bipolar c.
Malis CMC-II bipolar c.
coagulopathy
consumption c.
consumptive c.
disseminated intravascular c. (DIC)
hereditary c.
heritable c.
incipient c.
inherited c.
maternal c.
coagulum, *pl.* **coagula**
closing c.
necrotic c.
coalescent mastoiditis
coalition
calcaneonavicular c.
cartilaginous c.
congenital tarsal c.
fibrinous c.
osseous c.
tarsal c.
coal tar
Coanda effect
coaptation
c. bipolar forceps
urethral c.
coarctation
abdominal c.
aortic c.
aortic arch c. (CoA)
complex c.
juxtaductal aortic c.
c. of aorta
postductal c.
preductal c.
recurrent c.
residual c.
simple c.
coarse
c. calcification
c. facial features
c. rale
c. tremor
coast
c. of California café au lait spot
c. of Maine café au lait spot
coat
buffy c.
lipopolysaccharide c.

Coat-A-Count
C.-A-C. assay
C.-A-C. neonatal 17 hydroxyprogesterone kit
coated Vicryl Rapide suture
Coats disease
coaxial
c. flow
c. position
c. sheath cut-biopsy needle
cobalamin
c. adenosyltransferase
c. reductase deficiency
cobalt
c. megavoltage machine
c. poisoning
radioactive c.
cobalt-60 (^{60}Co)
c.-6. moving strip technique
Coban dressing
Cobas fast centrifugal analyzer
Cobb
C. measurement technique
C. method
C. syndrome
cobblestone
c. appearance
c. sessile polyp
cobblestoning of conjunctiva
Cobb-Ragde needle
co-bedding
Coblation-Channeling surgical procedure
COC
combination oral contraceptive
combined oral contraceptive
coca
Erythroxylum c.
cocaine
c. addiction
c. baby
crack c.
freebase c.
c. hydrochloride powder
liquified powder c.
c. test
tetracaine, adrenaline, c. (TAC)
tetracaine, epinephrine, c. (TEC)
cocci (*pl. of* coccus)
coccidioidal
c. granuloma
c. placentitis
Coccidioides immitis
coccidioidin reaction
coccidioidomycosis
disseminated c.
c. meningitis
coccobacillary
c. bacteria
c. form

C

coccobacillus
  HACEK c.
coccus, *pl.* **cocci**
  gram-negative cocci
  gram-positive cocci
coccydynia
coccygeal
  c. fracture
  c. muscle
coccygeus muscle
coccygodynia
coccyx
cochlea
cochlear
  c. aqueduct
  c. implant
cochleopalpebral reflex
cochleosaccular degeneration
cochleovestibular paresis
Cochran Database of Systemic Reviews
Cochrane
  C. Incontinence Group
  C. Pregnancy and Childbirth
  Database
Cockayne syndrome A, B
Cockayne-Touraine variant of dominant dystrophic epidermolysis bullosa
cock-robin
  c.-r. position
  c.-r. sign
cockscomb
  cervical c.
  c. cervix
cocktail
  c. chatter
  GI c.
  lytic c.
  c. party patter
  c. party syndrome
  pediatric c.
COD
  cerebrooccular dysgenesis
CODAS
  cerebral, ocular, dental, auricular, skeletal
  cerebrooccular dentoauriculoskeletal
  CODAS syndrome
code
  genetic c.
codeine
  Fioricet With C.
  guaifenesin and c.
  Guiatussin With C.
  Mallergan-VC With C.
  promethazine, phenylephrine, c.
codfish vertebra
coding
  phonological c.
cod liver oil

Codman triangle
COD-MD
  cerebrooccular dysgenesis-muscular dystrophy
  COD-MD syndrome
codominance
codominant
  c. gene
  c. inheritance
codon
  termination c.
Codoxy
coefficient
  bone attenuation c.
  inbreeding c.
  intraclass correlation c.
  kappa c.
  c. of fat absorption
  c. of inbreeding
  c. of parentage
coeliac (*var.* of celiac)
coelomic (*var.* of celomic)
coenzyme
  c. A (CoA)
  c. Q_{10} (CoQ_{10})
coercive feeding
coeur en sabot
coexistent fetus
coexisting fracture
cofactor
  c. deficiency
  molybdenum c.
  ristocetin c.
  tetrahydrobiopterin c. (BH$_4$)
coffee-grounds
  c.-g. drainage
  c.-g. emesis
  c.-g. hematemesis
  c.-g. material
Coffey suspension
Coffin-Lowry syndrome
Coffin-Siris
  C.-S. defect
  C.-S. fifth digit syndrome
Coffin-Siris-Wegienka syndrome
Coffin syndrome 1, 2
COFS
  cerebrooculofacial-skeletal
  COFS syndrome
Cogan syndrome
Cogentin
Co-Gesic
cognition
  spatial c.
cognitive
  c. ability
  c. behavior
  c. behavioral psychotherapy

c. behavioral therapy (CBT)
c. deficiency
c. delay
c. developmental milestone
c. disability
c. domain
c. dysfunction
c. impairment
c. therapy
c. toxicity
cognitive-diathesis model
cognitive-stress diathesis
CO₂Guard
COH
    controlled ovarian hyperstimulation
cohabitation
COHb
    carboxyhemoglobin
Cohen
    C. criteria
    C. procedure
    C. syndrome
    C. transtrigonal technique
    C. uterine cannula
cohesion
    lexical c.
    referential c.
cohort
    Dunedin birth c.
    c. study
cohosh
    black c.
coil
    Dacron fiber-coated c.
    DuctOcclud c.
    Gianturco c.
    metal c.
    MRCP using HASTE with a phased array c.
    c. occlusion
    c. spring diaphragm
coiled artery
coiling
coin
    c. biopsy
    esophageal c.
    c. ingestion
    c. lesion
coincident pregnancy
coinfection
    beta-hemolytic streptococcal c.
coining
coital
    c. age
    c. contact
    c. dependence
    c. factor
    c. position
    c. timing

coitarche
coition
coitus
    c. incompletus
    c. interruptus
    c. reservatus
Coke-colored urine
Colace
cola-colored
    c.-c. neonate
    c.-c. urine
COL7A1 gene
Colaris genetic susceptibility test
Co-Lav
Colax
Colazal
Colcher-Sussman x-ray pelvimetry technique
colchicine
cold
    c. abscess
    c. agglutinin
    c. agglutinin disease
    c. anaphylaxis
    c. antibody
    c. biopsy forceps
    c. coagulation
    c. coagulator
    common c.
    c. cup biopsy
    c. hemagglutinin disease
    c. intolerance
    c. knife biopsy
    c. knife cervical conization
    c. knife cone
    c. knife cone biopsy
    c. knife conization (CKC)
    c. knife method
    c. nodule
    c. panniculitis
    c. potassium cardioplegia
    c. reactive
    c. stress
    c. urticaria
    c. water near drowning
cold-adapted
    c.-a. influenza vaccine (CAIV)
    c.-a. intranasal influenza vaccine
Cold-Eeze
cold-induced
    c.-i. asthma
    c.-i. bronchospasm
    c.-i. myotonia
Cole
    C. endotracheal tube
    C. intubation procedure
    C. orotracheal tube
    C. syndrome
Cole-Carpenter syndrome

colectomy
Cole-Hughes macrocephaly-mental retardation syndrome
coleocele
coleotomy
Cole-Rauschkolb-Toomey syndrome
colfosceril palmitate
coli
    ampicillin-resistant *Escherichia c.*
    Balantidium c.
    Campylobacter c.
    enterohemorrhagic *Escherichia c.* (EHEC)
    enteropathogenic *Escherichia c.* (EPEC)
    enterotoxigenic *Escherichia c.* (ETEC)
    Escherichia c.
    familial adenomatous polyposis c.
    hemorrhagic *Escherichia c.*
    Shiga toxin-producing *Escherichia c.* (STEC)
Colibri forceps
colic
    c. artery
    biliary c.
    infantile c.
    c. intussusception
    meconial c.
    menstrual c.
    Monday morning c.
    non-Wessel c.
    ovarian c.
    renal c.
    tubal c.
    uterine c.
    Wessel c.
colica
colicky abdominal pain
coliform
    c. bacteria
    c. organism
colistimethate sodium
colistin
colitides (*pl. of* colitis)
colitis, *pl.* colitides
    acute fulminant c.
    acute infectious c.
    allergic c.
    amebic c.
    antibiotic-associated c.
    Crohn c.
    eosinophilic allergic c.
    fulminant ulcerative c.
    granulomatous c.
    hemorrhagic c.
    Hirschsprung c.
    infectious c.
    inflammatory c.

    lymphoplasmacytic c.
    mild ulcerative c.
    moderate ulcerative c.
    necrotizing c.
    protein-induced eosinophilic c. (PEC)
    pseudomembranous c. (PMC)
    steroid-dependent c.
    tuberculous c.
    ulcerative c.
colla (*pl. of* collum)
collaborative
    C. Antiviral Study Group (CASG)
    C. Group on Hormonal Factors in Breast Cancer
    C. Home Infant Monitoring Evaluation (CHIME)
    C. Perinatal Study (CPS)
    C. Review of Sterilization (CREST)
CollaCote dressing
collagen
    bovine dermal c.
    C-terminal propeptide of type I c.
    GAX c.
    c. I, III, IV, V, X
    c. matrix
    microfibrillar c.
    c. vascular disease
    c. vascular disorder
    c. weakness
collagenase
    human neutrophil c.
collagenization
collagenosis
    mediastinal c.
    perforating c.
    reactive perforating c. (RPC)
collapse
    acute circulatory c.
    cardiopulmonary c.
    cardiovascular c.
    circulatory c.
collapse-consolidation lesion
collapsed subpectoral implant
collar
    cervical c.
    c. of pearls
    c. of Venus
    Philadelphia c.
    sebaceous c.
    venereal c.
collared cervix
collarette of rash
Collastat
collateral
    c. blood flow
    c. circulation
    c. ligament stability
    venous c.

collateralization
> coronary c.

collection
> breath-by-breath method of gas c.
> extravascular fluid c.
> first-morning urine c.
> gas c.
> 72-hour stool c.
> 24-hour urine c.
> oocyte c.
> subphrenic gas c.

collector
> cell c.
> Cytobrush cell c.
> Cytobrush Plus cell c.
> Endocell endometrial cell c.
> Flexi-Seal fecal c.
> Leukotrap red cell c.
> Papette cervical c.
> Uterobrush endometrial sample c.
> Wallach Papette disposable cervical cell c.

Colles
> C. fascia
> C. fracture

colli
> pterygium c.

colliculi (*pl. of* colliculus)
colliculus, *pl.* **colliculi**
> inferior c.

collimation
> pinhole c.

collimator
collinearity
Collins
> C. law
> C. test

collodion, collodium
> c. baby
> c. skin

collodium (*var. of* collodion)
colloid
> c. carcinoma
> c. cyst
> c. infusion
> c. oncotic pressure
> c. osmotic pressure (COP)
> radioactive c.
> c. solution
> c. therapy

colloidal oatmeal bath
collum, *pl.* **colla**
Collyrium Fresh Ophthalmic
coloboma
> congenital iris c.
> c., heart defects, ichthyosiform dermatosis, mental retardation, ear defects (CHIME)
> c., heart disease, atresia choanae, retarded growth and development, and/or CNS anomalies, genital hypoplasia, ear anomalies and/or deafness (CHARGE)
> ocular c.

coloboma-anal atresia syndrome
coloboma-hepatic fibrosis
colobomatous defect
colocecal bladder augmentation
colocolic intussusception
colocolponeopoiesis
colocolpopoiesis
colon
> aganglionic c.
> ascending c.
> c. carcinoma
> cathartic c.
> descending c.
> giant c.
> nervous c.
> c. pouch
> rectosigmoid c.
> sigmoid c.
> spastic c.
> transverse c.

colonic
> c. aganglionosis
> c. B-cell lymphoma
> c. conduit diversion
> c. diversion
> c. dysmotility
> c. interposition
> c. obstruction
> c. plug
> c. polyp
> c. polyposis
> c. stasis
> c. stricture
> c. transit study

colonization
> Candida c.
> oropharyngeal c.
> stool c.
> vaginal c.

colonopathy, colopathy
> fibrosing c.

colonoscopic release
colonoscopy, coloscopy
> surveillance c.

colony count
colony-forming
> c.-f. unit (CFU)
> c.-f. unit erythroid (CFU-E)
> c.-f. unit in culture (CFUC)

colony-stimulating
> c.-s. activity (CSA)
> c.-s. factor (CSF)

colopathy (*var. of* colonopathy)

C

color
c. analog scale
c. Doppler energy (CDE)
c. Doppler flow imaging (CDFI)
c. Doppler sonography (CDS)
c. Doppler ultrasonography (CDU)
c. echocardiogram
flight of c.
C. Power Angio imaging
C. Trails Test
c. vision
Colorado
C. Intrauterine Growth Chart
C. tick fever
color-coded duplex Doppler
colorectal
c. anastomosis
c. cancer
c. disease
c. tumor
colorectal-anal distress inventory (CRADI)
color-flow Doppler
colorimetric reverse dot blot hybridization
3-color immunofluorescence
ColorMate TLc BiliTest System
ColorpHast Indicator Strips
coloscope
ZM-1 c.
coloscopy (*var. of* colonoscopy)
colostomy
diverting c.
double-barrel c.
fecal diversion c.
c. formation
protective c.
temporary diverting c.
transverse loop c.
colostration
colostric
colostrorrhea
colostrous
colostrum
c. corpuscle
premature c.
Colour Index (CI, C.I.)
Colovage
colovaginal fistula
colpatresia
colpectasia (*var. of* colpectasis)
colpectasis, colpectasia
colpectomy
partial c.
skinning c.
total c.
Colpexin sphere intravaginal device
colpitis mycotica
colpocele

colpocleisis
Latzko c.
Le Fort partial c.
partial c.
colpocystitis
colpocystocele
colpocystoplasty
colpocystotomy
colpocystoureterotomy
colpocystourethropexy (CCUP)
colpodynia
colpohyperplasia
c. cystica
c. emphysematosa
colpohysterectomy
colpohysteropexy
colpohysterotomy
colpomicroscopy
colpomycosis
colpomyomectomy
colpopathy
colpoperineopexy
abdominal sacral c.
colpoperineoplasty
colpoperineorrhaphy
posterior c.
colpopexy
abdominal sacral c. (ASC)
sacral c.
sacrospinous c.
transvaginal sacrospinous c.
colpoplasty
colpopoiesis
colpoptosia (*var. of* colpoptosis)
colpoptosis, colpoptosia
colporectopexy
colporrhagia
colporrhaphy
anterior c.
anteroposterior c.
Goffe c.
posterior c.
colporrhexis
colposcope
Cooper Surgical overhead c.
Leisegang c.
Zeiss c.
colposcopic
c. diagnosis
c. examination
c. grading of cervical dysplasia
c. screening
colposcopically
c. directed brushing
c. directed laser therapy
colposcopist
colposcopy
digital imaging c.
endocervical canal c.

estrogen-assisted c.
    vulvar c.
colposcopy-trained
colpospasm
colpostat
    afterload c.
    Henschke c.
colpostenosis
colpostenotomy
colposuspension
    abdominal sacrospinous ligament c.
    Burch c.
    laparoscopic retropubic c.
    MMK c.
colpotomy incision
colpoureterotomy
colpourethrocystopexy
    retropubic c.
colpourethropexy
    Burch c.
    modified Burch c.
colpoxerosis
Columbia Impairment Scale
column
    Clarke c.
    spinal c.
    vertebral c.
columnar
    c. epithelium
    c. epithelium papilla
Coly-Mycin
    C.-M. M
    C.-M. S Otic drop
Colyte-Flavored Combitube
COM
    chronic otitis media
coma
    diabetic c.
    hepatic c.
    hyperammonemic hepatic c.
    hyperosmolar nonketotic c.
    myxedema c.
    nonketotic hyperosmolar c.
      (NKHC)
    pentobarbital c.
COMA
    congenital ocular motor apraxia
comatose
combat crawl
Combidex MRI contrast agent
combination
    apnea-hypopnea c.
    c. chemotherapy
    consonant-vowel c.
    c. estrogen-progestin contraceptive
    estrogen-progestogen c.
    norgestrel/ethinyl estradiol c.
    c. oral contraceptive (COC)
    xanthan/guar c.

combined
    c. birth control pill
    c. estrogen and progesterone
      injection
    c. estrogen and progesterone vaginal
      ring
    c. hormone therapy (CHT)
    c. immunodeficiency (CID)
    c. injectable contraceptive
    c. nevus
    c. oral contraceptive (COC)
    c. pregnancy
    c. spinal-epidural (CSE)
    c. transdermal hormonal
      contraceptive
    c. version
combing
    cervical c.
CombiPatch
Combitube
    Colyte-Flavored C.
Combivir
comedo
    closed c.
    c. extractor
    open c.
comedocarcinoma
comedomastitis
comedonicus
    nevus c.
Comfort personal lubricant gel
ComfortScan imaging system
Comhist LA
comitant strabismus
commando crawl
comma-shaped organism
commensal flora
comminuted fracture
commission
    physician payment review c.
      (PPRC)
commissioning couple
commissural
    c. lip pit
    c. separation
commissure
    anterior c.
    labial c.
    posterior c.
commissurotomy
    mitral c.
committed cell
committee
    Institute of Medical Safety Review
      C.
    National Vaccine Advisory C.
      (NVAC)
    C. on Infectious Diseases of the
      American Academy of Pediatrics

C

common
    c. atrium
    c. blue nevus
    c. channel
    c. cold
    c. hepatic duct
    c. migraine
    c. migraine headache
    c. sheath reimplant
    c. variable hypogammaglobulinemia
    c. variable immunodeficiency (CVI, CVID)
    c. wart
common-inlet single right ventricle
commotio
    c. cordis
    c. retinae
communal traumatic experiences inventory (CTEI)
communicable
    c. disease
    C. Disease Center (CDC)
    c. illness
communicating
    c. hydrocephalus
    c. uterus
communication
    c. aid
    augmentative and alternative c. (AAC)
    autocrine c.
    c. board
    c. disorder
    c. domain
    facilitated c. (F/C)
    fetal-maternal c.
    fistulous vascular c.
    interatrial c. (IAC)
    nonverbal c.
    paracrine c.
    total c.
    vascular c.
communicative development inventory (CDI)
communis
    macula c.
    truncus arteriosus c. (TAC)
community-acquired (CA)
    c.-a. methicillin-resistant *Staphylococcus aureus* (CAMRSA)
community medicine
comorbid anxiety disorder
comorbidity
    psychological c.
COMP
    cartilage oligomeric matrix protein
    COMP drug regimen

compacta
    decidua c.
    zona c.
compactum
    stratum c.
Companion 318 nasal CPAP system
comparative
    c. embryology
    c. genomic hybridization (CGH)
    c. mapping
comparison view
compartment
    adductor interosseous c.
    calcaneal c.
    extracellular fluid c.
    lateral c.
    medial c.
    superficial c.
    c. syndrome
compartmentalization
compassionate use
compatibility
    maternal-fetal HLA c.
Compazine
compensated
    c. cirrhosis
    c. hydrocephalus
    c. shock
compensatory
    c. antiinflammatory syndrome
    c. articulation
    c. erythropoiesis
    c. gliosis
    c. hyperinsulinemia
    c. movement
    c. scoliosis
competence
    cervical c.
    cultural c.
competing anion
complaint
    psychosomatic c.
    somatic c.
Compleat
    C. Modified formula
    C. Pediatric formula
complement
    c. chemotactic factor
    chromosome c.
    c. C3 level
    c. deficiency
    c. deficiency disorder
    c. deposition
    fetal chromosome c.
    c. fixation
    c. fixation test
    hemolytic c. (CH_{50})
    c. receptor
    serum c.

c. system component
c. test
total hemolytic c.
unbalanced parental chromosome c.
c. value
complemental inheritance
complementary
c. and alternative medicine
(CAM)
c. deoxyribonucleic acid (cDNA)
c. DNA (cDNA)
c. gene
c. RNA
c. sequence
complementation test
complement-fixing serum antibody
complete
c. abortion
c. androgen insensitivity syndrome
(CAIS)
c. androgen resistance syndrome
c. atrioventricular block
c. atrioventricular canal
c. blood count (CBC)
c. breech presentation (CBP)
c. cerebellar aplasia
c. cleft
c. cord transection
c. DiGeorge syndrome
c. feminizing testes syndrome
c. fetal heart block
Flintstones C.
c. fracture
c. hernia
c. hydatidiform mole
c. isosexual precocity
c. linkage
Pepcid C.
c. placenta previa
c. precocious puberty
c. radial aplasia
c. rectal prolapse
c. remission
c. subtalar release (CSTR)
c. suppression pattern
c. syndactyly
c. testicular feminization
c. transposition
c. transposition of great arteries
c. transposition of great vessels
c. vulvar duplication
complete/complete/+ station
complex
Adam c.
c. adnexal endometrioma
AIDS dementia c. (ADC)
AIDS-related c. (ARC)
amphotericin B cholesteryl sulfate c.
amphotericin B lipid c.

amyotrophic lateral
sclerosis-Parkinson-dementia c.
antigen-antibody c.
antiinhibitor coagulant c.
axial mesodermal dysplasia c.
blepharophimosis, ptosis, epicanthus
inversus, telecanthus c.
blocked premature atrial c.
cardinal-uterosacral ligament c.
chlorophyllin copper c.
c. coarctation
c. congenital heart disease
C. 15 cream
del 11/aniridia c.
Diana c.
disseminated *Mycobacterium avium*
c. (DMAC)
dystrophin-associated gene c.
early amnion vascular disruption c.
Eisenmenger c.
Electra c.
c. enteral feeding
epispadias-exstrophy c.
facioauriculovertebral malformation c.
Fallot c.
c. febrile seizure
gene c.
generalized bilaterally synchronous
sharp-wave and slow-wave
complexes
Ghon c.
Gollop-Wolfgang c.
c. heart defect
human factor IX c.
c. hyperplasia
immune c. (IC)
iron dextran c.
Jocasta c.
lap-belt c.
lateral collateral ligament c.
Lear c.
limb-body wall c. (LBWC)
major histocompatibility c. (MHC)
c. mass
membrane attack c.
c. motor tic
Mycobacterium avium complex
(MAC)
Mycobacterium avium-intracellulare
c. (MAC)
Mycobacterium fortuitum c.
c. myoclonic epilepsy
nipple-areola c. (NAC)
Oedipus c.
ostiomeatal c.
c. partial epilepsy
c. partial seizure (CPS)
c. partial status epilepticus
Phaedra c.

complex (*continued*)
    polyaluminum hydroxide c.
    pyruvate dehydrogenase c. (PDC, PDHC)
    QS c.
    c. regional pain syndrome (CRPS)
    Rh c.
    sicca c.
    spermatic venous c.
    spike and wave c.
    synaptonemal c.
    c. syndactyly
    triangular fibrocartilaginous c. (TFCC)
    tuberous sclerosis c. (TSC)
    tuboovarian c. (TOC)
    c. unroofed coronary sinus (CUCS)
    uterosacral c.
    VATER c.
    vitamin B c.
    c. vocal tic
    von Meyenburg c.
complexion
    florid c.
    pallid c.
compliance
    c. of lung (CL)
    pulmonary c.
    tympanic membrane c.
complicated
    c. gastroesophageal reflux
    c. meconium ileus
    c. migraine
    c. migraine headache
complication
    abortion c.
    antenatal c.
    antepartum c.
    cardiovascular c.
    diabetes-associated maternal c.
    end-organ c.
    fetal c.'s
    intraoperative c.
    intrapartum c.
    late c.
    maternal c.'s
    microvascular c.
    neurodevelopmental c.
    neurologic c.
    obstetric c.
    operative site c.
    postoperative c.
    pregnancy c.
    pulmonary c.
    respiratory c.
    thromboembolic c.
    vascular c.
component
    blood c.

    buffy coat c.
    complement system c.
    diastolic c.
    extensive intraductal c. (EIC)
    extracellular matrix c.
    systolic c.
    terminal complement c.
5-component vaccine
composite allograft
composition
    body c.
    milk c.
compound
    artificial lung-expanding c. (ALEC)
    c. heterozygote
    c. muscle action potential (CMAP)
    c. nevus
    nitroimidazole c.
    c. pregnancy
    c. presentation
    progestational c.
    pteridine ring c.
    C. W
compounding pharmacy
Compoz
    C. Gel Caps
    C. Nighttime Sleep Aid
Comprecin
compressed air-driven nebulizer
compressibility
compression
    brainstem c.
    cardiac c.
    cerebellar hemisphere c.
    cerebral c.
    cervicomedullary c.
    chest c.
    cord c.
    esophageal c.
    external pneumatic calf c. (EPC)
    c. force
    c. fracture
    head c.
    c. injury
    intermittent pneumatic c.
    intrauterine c.
    joint c.
    mechanical c.
    c. myelopathy
    pneumatic c.
    spinal cord c.
    spot c.
    c. stocking
    c. suture
    thorax c.
    tracheal c.
    tracheobronchial c.
    c. ultrasonography
    umbilical cord c.

uterine c.
vascular c.
vein c.
vertebral artery c.
compression-rarefaction strain
compressive dressing
compressor
Pari Proneb Turbo c.
c. urethra
compressus
fetus c.
compromise
airway c.
angiitic luminal c.
fetal c.
microcirculatory c.
neurovascular c.
respiratory c.
severe respiratory c.
compromised
c. fetus
c. host defense
Compton effect
compulsion
compulsive
c. echolalia
c. self-mutilation
computed
c. axial tomography
(CAT)
c. tomography (CT)
c. tomography laser mammography
(CTLM)
computer-aided diagnosis (CAD)
computer-assisted
c.-a. semen analysis (CASA)
c.-a. semen analyzer (CASA)
computerized
C. Diagnostic Interview for Children
and Adolescents (cDICA)
c. tomography (CT)
COMS
cerebrooculomuscular syndrome
Comtrex Cough Formula
Comvax vaccine
conal muscle
concave temporalis muscle
concavity
concealed
c. hemorrhage
c. penis
c. rectal prolapse
conceive
C. ovulation predictor
PreCare C.
concentrate
factor c.
platelet c.
protein C c.

concentrated
c. oral sucrose
c. urine
concentration
alpha-tocopherol c.
ambient oxygen c.
anti-HBsAg c.
bicarbonate c.
blood alcohol c. (BAC)
cord blood leptin c.
cortisol c.
elevated sweat chloride c.
fetal leptin c.
fetal steroid c.
fetal thrombopoietin c.
glucose c.
hemoglobin c.
hepatic iron c. (HIC)
hydrogen ion c. (pH)
inhibin c.
intracellular hydrogen ion c. (pHi)
lipoprotein c.
maternal steroid c.
mean cell hemoglobin c. (MCHC)
mean corpuscular hemoglobin c.
(MCHC)
mean hemoglobin c.
mean plasma iron c.
minimal bacterial c. (MBC)
minimal effective analgesic c.
(MEAC)
minimal inhibitory c. (MIC)
minimum inhibitory c. (MIC)
plasma amino acid c.
plasma bilirubin c. (PBC)
plasma histamine c.
plasma iron c.
plasma phosphate c.
plasma retinol c.
plasma theophylline c.
plasma vitamin A c.
platelet c.
pulmonary tissue c. (PTC)
serum albumin c.
serum amino acid c.
serum ferritin c.
serum lactate dehydrogenase c.
serum lithium c.
serum melatonin c.
serum protein c.
steroid c.
sweat chloride c.
concentrica
encephalitis periaxialis c.
concentric sclerosis
conception
c. age
assisted c.
estimated date of c. (EDC)

C

conception (*continued*)
    evacuation of retained products of
      c. (ERPC)
    natural c.
    products of c. (POC)
    retained products of c. (RPC)
    wrongful c.
Conceptrol
conceptus
    C. fallopian tube catheterization
    system
    C. Soft Torque uterine catheter
    C. VS catheter
Concerta
concha bullosa
Concise Plus hCG urine test
concisus
    Campylobacter c.
concomitant change
concordance
concordant twins
concrete pelvis
concurrent ultrasound guidance
concussion
    labyrinthine c.
    spinal c.
    c. syndrome
COND
    cerebroosteonephrodysplasia
condition
    childbirth-related medical c.
    fetal c.
    intersex c.
    local ovarian c.
    maternal systemic c.
    neonatal c.
    neurologic c.
    nonangiitic vasculopathic c.
    nonvertiginous c.
    orthopedic c.
    preexisting maternal medical c.
    Questionnaire for Identifying
      Children with Chronic C.'s
      (QuICCC)
    vertiginous c.
    X-linked dominant c.
    X-linked recessive c.
conditional probability
conditioned
    c. orientation reflex (COR)
    c. play audiometry
conditioning regimen
condom
    female c.
    intravaginal c.
    male c.
    c. negotiation
    Ramses C.
    Reality c.

    The Female C.
    vaginal c.
    Women's Choice c.
conductance
    airway c.
conduct disorder (CD)
conduction
    c. analgesia
    c. anesthesia
    antidromic c.
    c. defect
    orthodromic c.
conductive
    c. education (CE)
    c. hearing impairment
    c. hearing loss
    c. tissue
conductivity
conduit
    fetal vascular c.
    homograft c.
    ileal c.
    intestinal c.
    urinary c.
conduplicato corpore
condyle
    lateral c.
    medial c.
condyloma, *pl.* **condylomas,**
  condylomata
    c. acuminatum (CA)
    anal c.
    cervical c.
    c. latum
    recalcitrant c.
    resistant c.
    vulvar c.
condylomas (*pl. of* condyloma)
condylomata (*pl. of* condyloma)
condylomatous
Condylox solution
cone
    c. biopsy
    c. biopsy of cervix
    cold knife c.
    conference PARQ c.
    ectoplacental c.
    transvaginal c.
    vaginal c.
    weighted vaginal c.
conference
    PARQ c.
    c. PARQ cone
confetti lesion
Confide HIV test kit
configuration
    brachycephalic c.
    hourglass c.
    villoglandular c.

confinement
    estimated date of c. (EDC)
    expected date of c. (EDC)
    postpartum c.
confirmation
    microscopic c.
    tissue c.
conflict
confluent
    c. eyebrows
    c. plaque
Conformant dressing
conformity
    abnormal thoracic c.
confusion
    postictal c.
confusional
    c. arousal
    c. migraine
congenita
    adrenal hypoplasia c. (AHC)
    aglossia c.
    alacrima c.
    alopecia totalis c.
    amaurosis c.
    amyoplasia c.
    amyotonia c.
    aplasia axialis extracorticalis c.
    aplasia cutis c.
    arthrochalasis multiplex c.
    arthrogryposis multiplex c. (AMC)
    bitemporal aplasia cutis c.
    chondrodystrophia calcificans c.
    cutis marmorata telangiectatica c.
    dyskeratosis c.
    erythropoietic porphyria c.
    hypertrichosis universalis c.
    ichthyosis c.
    macrosomia adiposa c.
    myotonia c.
    pachyonychia c.
    paramyotonia c.
    pseudoglioma c.
    pterygoarthromyodysplasia c.
    spondyloepiphysial dysplasia c.
    syngnathia c.
    Thomsen myotonia c.
    X-linked dyskeratosis c.
congenital
    c. abducens facial paralysis
    c. absence
    c. absence of iron-binding protein
    c. absence of lactase
    c. absence of vas deferens (CAVD)
    c. acromicria syndrome
    c. adrenal hyperplasia (CAH)
    c. adrenal hypoplasia
    c. adrenal lipoid hyperplasia
    c. afibrinogenemia

    c. aganglionic megacolon
    c. agranulocytosis
    c. aleukia
    c. alveolar dysplasia
    c. alveolar proteinosis
    c. amaurosis of retinal origin
    c. amblyogenic stimulus
    c. AME
    c. amegakaryocytic thrombocytopenia
    c. amputation
    c. analgesia
    c. anemia of newborn
    c. anemia syndrome
    c. anomaly (CA)
    c. anosmia
    c. anosmia-hypogonadotropic hypogonadism syndrome
    c. anterolateral tibial angulation
    c. aortic stenosis
    c. aplastic anemia
    c. arthromyodysplastic syndrome
    c. articular rigidity
    c. asplenia
    c. ataxia
    c. atelectasis
    c. athetosis
    c. atransferrinemia
    c. atresia of bile duct
    c. atresia of uterine cervix
    c. atrioventricular block
    c. aural atresia
    c. bilateral absence of vas deferens (CBAVD)
    c. bilateral cataracts
    c. bone marrow failure syndrome
    c. bronchiectasis
    c. bronchopulmonary malformation
    c. bullous urticaria pigmentosa
    c. candidiasis
    c. carbohydrate malabsorption
    c. cardiac defect
    c. cardiac disease
    c. cardiovascular malformation (CCVM)
    c. cataracts, sensorineural deafness, Down syndrome facial appearance, short stature, mental retardation syndrome
    c. central hypoventilation
    c. central hypoventilation syndrome (CCHS)
    c. cerebral aneurysm
    c. chloridorrhea
    c. choledochal dilation
    c. cholesteatoma
    c. chylothorax
    c. clasped thumbs
    c. clasped thumbs-mental retardation syndrome

C

congenital (*continued*)
c. cloaca
c. clubfoot
c. complete AV block
c. complete heart block (CCHB)
c. condylar deformity
c. contractural arachnodactyly (CCA)
c. contracture of extremity
c. cutaneous candidasis
c. cutis aplasia
c. cystic adenomatoid malformation (CCAM)
c. cystic adenomatoid malfunction
c. cytomegalovirus
c. defect of phosphofructokinase
c. dermal melanocytosis
c. diaphragmatic hernia (CDH)
c. diaphragmatic hernia-extracorporeal membrane oxygenation (CDH-ECMO)
c. diaphragmatic hernia of Bochdalek
c. dislocated hip (CDH)
c. dislocation
c. dislocation of hip (CDH)
c. dislocation of patella
c. diverticulum
c. double pylorus
c. duodenal atresia
c. dyserythropoietic anemia (CDA)
c. dyskeratosis
c. ectodermal dysplasia of face
c. ectodermic scalp defect
c. ectropion
c. elephantiasis
c. elevation of scapula
c. emphysema, cryptorchidism, penoscrotal web, deafness, mental retardation syndrome
c. enamel abnormality
c. encephalo-ophthalmic dysplasia
c. endothelial corneal dystrophy (CECD)
c. epulis of newborn
c. erythropoietic porphyria (CEP)
c. esophageal stenosis
c. esotropia
c. eventration
c. extremity lymphedema
c. facial diplegia
c. familial lymphedema with ocular findings
c. fiber-type disproportion
c. fibrosarcoma
c. fibular hemimelia
c. folate malabsorption
c. gastrointestinal obstruction
c. generalized lipodystrophy
c. generalized phlebectasia

c. glaucoma
c. glenoid dysplasia
c. goitrous hypothyroidism
c. granulocytopenia
c. growth hormone deficiency
c. Guillain-Barré syndrome
c. hairy nevus
c. hearing loss
c. heart block (CHB)
c. heart defect (CHD)
c. heart defect syndrome
c. heart disease (CHD)
c. Heinz body anemia
c. hemidysplasia with ichthyosiform erythroderma and limb defects (CHILD)
c. hemiparesis
c. hemiplegia
c. hemolytic anemia with aplastic crisis
c. hemolytic jaundice
c. hepatic fibrosis (CHF)
c. hereditary hematuria
c. hereditary retinoschisis (CHRS)
c. herpes
c. heterochromia
c. high airway obstruction syndrome (CHAOS)
c. hip disease
c. hip dislocation (CHD)
c. hip disorder
c. hip dysplasia (CHD)
c. hydantoin syndrome
c. hydronephrosis
c. hypertrichosis-osteochondrodysplasia-cardiomegaly syndrome
c. hypertrophic pyloric stenosis
c. hypoaldosteronism
c. hypocupremia syndrome
c. hypofibrinogenemia
c. hypogammaglobulinemia
c. hypogonadotropic hypogonadism
c. hypomagnesemia
c. hypomyelinating neuropathy (CHN)
c. hypomyelination
c. hypopituitarism
c. hypoplastic anemia (CHA)
c. hypothalamic hamartoblastoma
c. hypothyroidism (CH, CHT)
c. hypothyroidism syndrome
c. hypotonia
c. ichthyosiform
c. ichthyosiform erythroderma (CIE)
c. ichthyosis
c. ichthyosis-mental retardation-spasticity syndrome

c. ichthyosis-trichodystrophy syndrome
c. infection
c. injury
c. insensitivity
c. insensitivity to pain (CIPA)
c. intestinal aganglionosis (CIA)
c. intestinal band
c. intrauterine infection
c. intrinsic factor deficiency
c. iris coloboma
c. jerky nystagmus
c. kyphosis
c. lacrimal duct obstruction
c. lactase deficiency
c. lactic acidosis
c. laryngeal stridor
c. laxity of ligament
c. LCMV syndrome
c. lesion
c. lethal hypophosphatasia
c. leukemia
c. lipase/colipase deficiency
c. lipoatrophic diabetes
c. lip pit
c. listeriosis
c. lobar emphysema (CLE)
c. lobar overinflation (CLO)
c. localized absence of skin (CLAS)
c. longitudinal deficiency
c. longitudinal deficiency of fibula
c. longitudinal deficiency of tibia
c. long QT syndrome
c. lung malformation
c. macular degeneration
c. manifestation
c. megakaryocytic hypoplasia
c. melanocytic nevus
c. mesoblastic nephroma
c. metatarsus adductus
c. metatarsus varus
c. microcephaly, hiatus hernia, nephrotic syndrome
c. microvillus atrophy
c. miosis
c. multiple myofibromatosis
c. muscle fiber-type disproportion (CMFTD)
c. muscular dystrophy (CMD)
c. muscular dystrophy with central nervous system involvement
c. muscular hypertrophy-cerebral syndrome
c. muscular torticollis
c. myasthenia
c. myasthenia gravis
c. mydriasis

c. myopathy
c. myotonic dystrophy
c. nasal pyriform aperture stenosis (CNPAS)
c. nasolacrimal duct obstruction (CNLDO)
c. neonatal ascites
c. nephrosis
c. nephrotic syndrome
c. nerve deafness
c. neutropenia
c. nevomelanocytic nevus
c. nevus
c. nonhemolytic jaundice
c. nonhemolytic unconjugated hyperbilirubinemia
c. nonregenerative anemia
c. nonspherocytic hemolytic anemia
c. obliterative jaundice
c. obstruction of nasolacrimal duct
c. obstructive mullerian malformation
c. ocular motor apraxia (COMA)
c. oculofacial paralysis
c. osteopetrosis
c. palatopharyngeal incompetence (CPI)
c. paretic neurosyphilis
c. paroxysmal atrial tachycardia
c. pendular nystagmus
c. perilymphatic fistula
c. peritoneal band
c. pernicious anemia
c. photosensitive porphyria
c. pigmental nevus
c. pneumonia
c. portosystemic venous shunt
c. posteromedial bowing
c. posteromedial tibial angulation
c. postural deformity
c. progressive muscular dystrophy with mental retardation
c. progressive oculoacousticocerebral degeneration
c. pseudarthrosis
c. pseudoarthrosis of clavicle
c. pseudoarthrosis of tibia
c. pseudohydrocephalic progeroid syndrome
c. pterygium
c. ptosis
c. pulmonary lymphangiectasia
c. quantitative disorder
c. RBC aplasia
c. retinitis blindness (CRB)
c. retinitis pigmentosa
c. rocker-bottom foot
c. rubella
c. rubella infection (CRI)
c. rubella syndrome (CRS)

C

congenital · conjugation

congenital (*continued*)
c. sensory neuropathy
c. sideroblastic anemia
c. sixth nerve palsy
c. skin aplasia
c. sodium diarrhea
c. spastic paraplegia
c. spherocytosis
c. stationary night blindness
c. stippled epiphysis
c. STORCH infection
c. structural defect
c. suprabulbar paresis
c. supraspinous fossa
c. syphilis (CS)
c. syphilitic infection
c. tarsal coalition
c. TC II deficiency
c. tendo Achillis contracture
c. tertiary neurosyphilis
c. thoracic scoliosis
c. thrombocytopenia, Robin sequence, agenesis of corpus callosum, distinctive facies, developmental delay syndrome
c. thyroid deficiency
c. thyroid deficiency with muscular hypertrophy
c. tibial hemimelia
c. toxoplasmosis
c. tracheal stenosis
c. transport defect
c. trypsinogen deficiency
c. tuberculosis
c. tubular stenosis
c. unilateral lower lip paralysis
c. universal muscular hypoplasia
c. upper airway malformation
c. urinary tract obstruction
c. vaginal adenosis
c. vaginal aplasia
c. varicella syndrome
c. vertical talus
c. warfarin syndrome
congenitale
poikiloderma c.
congenitalis
alopecia c.
heredoretinopathia c.
Congest
congestion
passive venous c.
pelvic vein c.
pulmonary vascular c.
vascular c.
congestive
c. cardiomyopathy
c. cardiomyopathy-hypergonadotropic hypogonadism syndrome

c. gastropathy
c. heart disease (CHD)
c. heart failure (CHF)
conglobata
acne c.
conglutination
Congo virus
conical teeth
conidial forest
conidium
coning of brain
conization
carbon dioxide laser beam c.
cautery c.
cervical c.
cold knife c. (CKC)
cold knife cervical c.
hot knife c.
laser cervical c.
laser excisional c.
loop diathermy cervical c.
c. of cervix
conjoined
c. tendon
c. twins
conjugata
c. anatomic pelvis
c. diagonalis pelvis
c. externa pelvis
c. vera pelvis
conjugate
anatomic c.
c. axis
diagonal c.
c. diameter (CD)
c. diameter of pelvic inlet
effective c.
external c.
false c.
internal c.
meningococcal c.
obstetric c.
c. of inlet
c. of pelvic outlet
c. pneumococcal vaccine
c. pupil
true c.
c. upward gaze
urinary steroid c.
conjugated
c. antichlamydial monoclonal antibody
c. bilirubin
c. equine estrogens (CEE)
c. estrogen (CE)
c. estrogen and meprobamate
c. hyperbilirubinemia
c. linoleic acid (CLA)
conjugation activity

conjunctiva, *pl.* **conjunctivae**
bulbar c.
cobblestoning of c.
palpebral c.
xerosis c.
conjunctivae (*pl. of* conjunctiva)
conjunctival
c. hyperemia
c. infection
c. injection
c. nevus
c. scraping
c. suffusion
c. telangiectasis
conjunctivitis
acquired c.
acute epidemic c.
acute hemorrhagic c.
acute perinatal c.
acute purulent c.
allergic c.
bacterial c.
bilateral c.
chemical c.
childhood c.
chlamydial c.
exudative c.
follicular c.
gonococcal c.
herpes simplex viral c.
inclusion body of chlamydial c.
infantile purulent c.
membranous c.
neonatal c.
palpebral c.
pediatric gonococcal c.
pseudomembranous c.
purulent c.
shipyard c.
silver nitrate c.
trachoma inclusion c. (TRIC)
vernal c.
viral c.
conjunctivitis-otitis syndrome
Conmed electrosurgical pencil
connatal form
connection
anomalous pulmonary venous c.
circulation-cavopulmonary c.
decidua-macrophage c.
total anomalous pulmonary venous c. (TAPVC)
total cavopulmonary c.
connective
c. tissue
c. tissue disease
c. tissue disorder
c. tissue nevus
connector

domino c.
T c.
tube c.
Y c.
Conners
C. Abbreviated Parent Questionnaire
C. continuous performance test
C. Hyperactivity indices
C. Rating Scale (CRS)
connexin
Conn syndrome
conorii
Rickettsia c.
conotruncal
c. abnormality
c. anomaly face syndrome (CTAF)
c. cardiac defect, abnormal face, thymic hypoplasia, cleft palate (CATCH 22)
c. cardiac malformation
c. facial anomaly
c. facial syndrome
c. heart defects
c. septum
conotruncus
conoventricular
Conradi
C. disease
C. syndrome
Conradi-Hünermann syndrome
consanguineous
c. mating
c. parents
consanguinity
parental c.
CoNS bacteremia
conscious
body c.
c. pain mapping
c. sedation
consciousness
altered state of c. (ASC)
level of c. (LOC)
loss of c.
consecutive loss
consensus sequence
consent
informed c.
written c.
conservation
breast c.
conservative
c. drug use
c. management
c. surgery
c. therapy
conserved
evolutionarily c.
c. sequence

consideration
    adrenal morphologic c.
consolability
    face, legs, activity, cry, c.
        (FLACC)
consolidation
    alveolar c.
    basilar c.
    lobar c.
    lung c.
    pneumonic c.
consonant
    glide c.
    nasal c.
consonant-vowel combination
consort
    high-risk c.
constancy
    object c.
constant
    association c.
    dissociation c.
    c. exotropia
    c. flow end-inspiratory airway
        occlusion
    Michaelis-Menten dissociation c.
    c. positive airway pressure
    pulmonary time c.
    c. strabismus
    c. tidal volume
constellates
    Streptococcus c.
Constilac
constipation
    chronic c.
    functional c.
    idiopathic c.
constituent
constitution
    genetic c.
constitutional
    c. delay of puberty
    c. dwarfism
    c. eugonadism
    C. Genetic Array Test (CGAT)
    c. growth delay
    c. hirsutism
    c. precocious puberty
    c. short stature
constitutionally large fetus
constraint-induced movement therapy
constriction
    c. band syndrome
    fetal ductus arteriosus c.
    ring c.
    c. ring
constrictive
    c. pericarditis
    c. pericarditis-dwarfism syndrome

construct
    solid rod segmental c.
construction
    Abbe vaginal c.
    Davydov vagina c.
    Frank vaginal c.
Constulose
consultant
    lactation c. (LC)
    PID c.
consumption
    cerebral oxygen c.
    c. coagulopathy
    maternal alcohol c.
    oxygen c. ($V\dot{I}SO_2$)
consumptive
    c. coagulopathy
    c. thrombocytopenia
contact
    c. allergen
    coital c.
    c. dermatitis
    c. factor
    heater probe thermal c.
    kangaroo c.
    c. sensitization
    sexual c.
    skin-to-skin c.
    sperm-cervical mucus c.
        (SCMC)
    c. urticaria
    c. vulvovaginitis
contagion
    c. factor
    symptom c.
contagiosa
    impetigo c.
contagiosum
    molluscum c.
contagious
containment
    surgical c.
contaminant
contaminate
contamination
    bacterial c.
content
    aortic oxygen c.
    aspiration of gastric c.'s
    bone mineral c. (BMC)
    evacuation of uterine c.'s
    fatty acid c.
    mixed venous oxygen c.
    poverty of c.
    pulmonary arterial oxygen c.
    pulmonary venous oxygen c.
    quantitative analysis of fat c.
    total body iron c.
Contiform incontinence device

Contigen
- C. Bard collagen implant
- C. glutaraldehyde cross-linked collagen implant

contiguous
- c. gene deletion syndrome
- c. gene syndrome of chromosome 13
- c. pigmentation

Contin
- MS C.

continence
- c. ring
- c. tampon

continent
- c. ileostomy
- c. supravesical bowel urinary diversion
- c. urinary pouch

contingency table

contingent
- c. reinforcement
- c. vestibular stimulation

continuant

continuous
- c. ambulatory peritoneal dialysis (CAPD)
- c. arteriovenous hemofiltration (CAVH)
- c. blood gas monitoring
- c. cineangiogram
- c. cyclic peritoneal dialysis (CCPD)
- c. distending airway pressure (CDAP)
- c. distending pressure (CDP)
- c. distention irrigation system (CDIS)
- c. epidural analgesia
- c. fetal heart monitoring
- c. gastric drip (CGD)
- c. glucose infusion
- c. intravenous oxytocin drip
- c. long-term monitoring (CLTM)
- c. milk infusion
- c. negative airway pressure (CNAP)
- c. negative extrathoracic pressure (CNEP)
- C. Performance Task
- c. performance test (CPT)
- c. positive airway pressure (CPAP)
- c. running monofilament suture
- c. shunt murmur
- c. subcutaneous infusion (CSQI)
- c. subcutaneous insulin infusion
- c. subcutaneous insulin injection
- c. tracheal gas insufflation
- c. tube feeding
- c. variation
- c. venovenous hemodialysis (CVVHD)
- c. venovenous hemofiltration (CVVH)
- c. wave Doppler
- c. wave Doppler interrogation

continuous/combined treatment

continuous-dose combined oral contraceptive

continuous-wave ultrasound imaging

continuum
- epilepsia partialis continua
- infantile Refsum disease c.

contour
- cranial c.
- C. Profile anatomically shaped silicone breast
- C. Profile Bechert 35 expander/implant

contoured tilting compression mammography

contraception
- barrier c.
- barrier method of c.
- emergency c. (EC)
- hormonal emergency c.
- lactational amenorrhea method of c.
- long-acting c.
- morning-after c.
- oral c.
- postcoital c. (PCC)
- rhythm method of c.
- symptothermal method of c.
- vaginal ring c.
- Yuzpe regimen of combined oral contraceptives for emergency c.

contraceptive
- all-progestin c.
- barrier c.
- combination estrogen-progestin c.
- combination oral c. (COC)
- combined injectable c.
- combined oral c. (COC)
- combined transdermal hormonal c.
- continuous-dose combined oral c.
- c. device
- c. diaphragm
- c. effectiveness
- estrogen-progestin c.
- Estrostep oral c.
- c. failure
- c. failure rate
- c. film
- c. foam
- Genora 0.5/35 c.
- Genora 1/35 c.
- c. history
- hormonal c.
- c. implant

contraceptive (*continued*)
    implantable hormonal c.
    injectable hormonal c.
    intravaginal c.
    c. jelly
    Lea's shield female barrier c.
    long-acting c.
    low-dose oral c.
    low steroid content combined oral
      c.
    c. method
    monophasic oral c.
    oral c. (OC)
    oral steroid c.
    ParaGard T380A intrauterine
      copper c.
    c. patch
    Plan B emergency c.
    progestin-only injectable c.
    progestin-only oral c.
    progestin oral c.
    c. ring
    Seasonale oral c.
    sequential oral c.
    c. sponge
    steroid c.
    c. suppository capsule
    c. technique
    triphasic oral c.
    vaginal c.
contract
    behavior c.
contracted pelvis
contractile
contractility
    detrusor hyperactivity with
      incomplete c. (DHIC)
    LV c.
    uterine c.
contraction
    atrial c.
    atrial premature c. (APC)
    Braxton Hicks c.
    detrusor c.
    c. monitoring
    myometrial c.
    c. pattern
    pelvic c.
    premature atrial c.
    premature ventricular c.
      (PVC)
    smooth muscle c.
    c. stress test (CST)
    tetanic uterine c.
    uninhibited detrusor c.
    uterine c. (UC)
    ventricular premature c. (VPC)
    volume c.
    Z degree of c.

    Z' degree of c.
    Z'' degree of c.
contractural
    c. arachnodactyly disease
    c. arachnodactyly syndrome
contracture
    congenital tendo Achillis c.
    flaccid c.
    flexion c.
    gastrocnemius c.
    general triceps c.
    heel-cord c.
    joint c. (JC)
    multiple articular c.
    contracture, muscle atrophy,
      oculomotor apraxia syndrome
    Volkmann ischemic c.
contraindication
contralateral
    c. head turning (CHT)
    c. hernia
    c. hypertrophy
    c. hypertrophy of testes
    c. ovary
    c. ovulation
    c. reflux
    c. synchronous carcinoma
contrasexual precocity
contrast
    barium c.
    Echovist c.
    c. esophagram
    c. venography
contrecoup injury
Contrelle continence tampon
control
    airway c.
    birth c. (BC)
    bladder c.
    fertility c.
    glycemic c.
    head c.
    intrapartum glucose c.
    motor c.
    poor head c.
    seizure c.
    trunk c.
    waitlist c.
controlled
    c. bronchoprovocation challenge
      study
    c. ileal release budesonide
    c. intubation
    c. mechanical ventilation (CMV)
    c. ovarian hyperstimulation (COH)
    c. vaginal delivery
controller
    Pepcid AC Acid C.
controversial

controversy
transfusion c.
contused tissue
contusion
cerebral c.
iliac crest c.
myocardial c.
pulmonary c.
conundrum
conus
c. medullaris syndrome
subaortic c.
convalescent serum
convection-warmed incubator
convergence
poor c.
convergent
c. nystagmus
c. sidewalls
c. squint
c. strabismus
conversion
c. disorder
extraglandular c.
c. reaction
skin test c.
convex probe
convoluted tubule
convolution
convulsion
afebrile c.
B_6-dependent c.
benign familial neonatal c.
(BFNC)
benign idiopathic neonatal c.
(BINC)
benign infantile familial c.
(BIFC)
epileptic c.
febrile c.
focal c.
gelastic c.
generalized c.
hysteric c.
multifocal clonic c.
myoclonic c.
neonatal c.
puerperal c.
salaam c.
tonic-clonic c.
convulsive
c. seizure
c. status epilepticus
cooing
Cook
C. aspirator
C. balloon-inflated continence ring
C. catheter
C. tubal ligation

Cooke-Medley Hostility Scale
Cookie Insert
Cooks syndrome
Cooley anemia
cooling blanket
cool-mist
c.-m. humidifier
c.-m. vaporizer
cool shock
Coombs
C. antibody
C. positive
C. test
Coombs-negative autoimmune hemolytic anemia
Coombs-positive isoimmune hemolytic anemia
Cooper
C. fascia
C. irritable breast
C. Surgical overhead colposcope
suspensory ligaments of C.
C. syndrome
cooperative
C. Human Tissue Network (CHTN)
c. study of sickle cell disease (CSSCD)
cooperativity
theca-granulosa cell c.
Coopernail sign
coordination
eye-hand c.
hand-eye c.
poor c.
visual-motor c.
coordinator
service c.
cooximeter analyzer
COP
colloid osmotic pressure
Copaxone
COPE
Calendar of Premenstrual Syndrome Experience
Copeland
C. fetal scalp electrode
C. Symptom Checklist for Attention Deficit Disorders
coping
C. Health Inventory for Children (CHIC)
C. Health Inventory for Parents (CHIP)
c. self-statement
copious
c. antibiotic irrigation
c. discharge

C

copper
    c. deficiency
    c. deficiency anemia
    c. deposition
    hepatic c.
    c. homeostasis
    c. metabolism
    serum c.
    c. sulfate ingestion
    c. T-380A IUD
    C. T intrauterine device
    C. T-380 nonhormonal IUD
    c. toxicosis
    c. transport disease
    urinary c.
copper-histidine
copper-induced rhabdomyolysis
copper-releasing IUD
copper-wire appearance
coprolalia
coproporphyria
    hereditary c. (HCP)
coproporphyrin
    c. excretion
    urinary c.
copropraxia
copulation plug
copy
    DNA c.
    large single c.
    small single c.
CoQ10
    coenzyme Q_{10}
cor
    c. biloculare
    c. pulmonale
    c. triatriatum
    c. triatriatum dexter
    c. triloculare biatriatum
coracoclavicular ligament
Corcath catheter
cord
    c. abnormality
    c. accident
    battledore c.
    bifid spinal c.
    c. blood
    c. blood acidosis
    c. blood bank
    c. blood bilirubin
    c. blood erythropoietin level
    c. blood gas (CBG)
    c. blood hemoglobin
    c. blood hemoglobinopathy screening test
    c. blood leptin concentration
    c. blood pH
    c. blood registry (CBR)
    c. blood sample

    c. blood specimen
    c. blood transplantation (CBT)
    body coils of c.
    c. clamping
    c. compression
    c. entanglement
    false knot of umbilical c.
    false vocal c.
    furcate insertion of c.
    genital c.
    heel c.
    hemisection of c.
    c. IgG level
    c. insertion (CI)
    kinked c.
    c. lipoma
    medullary c.
    milking of umbilical c.
    nephrogenic c.
    noncoiled c.
    nuchal c.
    omphalomesenteric c.
    palpable c.
    c. pH
    c. plasma leptin
    presentation of c.
    primary sex c.
    c. prolapse
    prolapsed c.
    prolapse of umbilical c.
    rete c.
    c. serum level
    sex c.
    spermatic c.
    spinal c.
    c. stem cell marrow transplantation
    tethered spinal c.
    tight heel c.
    c. torsion
    c. transection
    umbilical c. (UC)
    velamentous insertion of c.
    2-vessel c.
    3-vessel c.
    c. vessel identification
    vitelline c.
    vocal c.
Cordarone
cordate pelvis, cordiform pelvis
Cordguard
    C. II
    C. umbilical cord sampler
cordiform uterus
cordiformis
    uterus c.
cordis
    accretio c.
    bulbus c.

commotio c.
ectopia c.
thoracoabdominal ectopia c.
Cordis-Hakim shunt
cordocentesis
cordotomy
Cordran SP
core
c. biopsy
C. Dynamics disposable cannula
C. Dynamics disposable trocar
c. needle biopsy (CNB)
c. temperature
corectopia
Corey ovum forceps
Corgard
Cori
C. disease
C. enzyme deficiency
C. glycogen storage disease
classification
Coricidin-D Tablet
Coricidin Tablet
Cori-Forbes disease
coring
c. biopsy gun
intramyometrial c.
myometrial c.
uterine c.
corkscrew
c. appearance
c. conjunctival blood
vessel
c. maneuver
Cormax ointment
cornea
cloudy c.
c. verticillata
xerosis c.
corneal
c. abrasion
c. clouding
c. damage
c. dystrophy
c. edema
c. enlargement
c. haze
c. hypoesthesia
c. leukoma
c. light reflection
c. light reflex test
c. opacification
c. opacity
c. scarring
c. staining
c. stippling
c. trauma
c. ulcer
c. ulceration

Cornelia
C. de Lange (CDL)
C. de Lange syndrome
(CDLS)
corneocyte
corneoscleral angle
corner
c. chair
c. fracture
c. suture
Corner-Allen test
corneum
stratum c.
cornification
cornified
Corning method
Cornoy solution
cornu
c. uteri
uterine c.
cornual
c. anastomosis
c. gestation
c. pregnancy
c. resection
Corometrics
C. fetal monitor
C. Gold Quik Connect Spiral
electrode tip
C. 118 maternal/fetal monitor
C. Model 900SC in-office
mammography
corona, *pl.* **coronae**
c. of penis
c. radiata
c. radiata cell
coronae (*pl. of* corona)
coronal
c. craniosynostosis
c. sulcus
c. suture (CS)
c. suture line
c. suture line of skull
c. synostosis
coronary
c. aneurysm
c. arteriovenous fistula
c. artery aneurysm (CAA)
c. artery disease
c. artery fistula (CAF)
c. artery lesion (CAL)
c. collateralization
c. flow reserve (CFR)
c. heart disease (CHD)
c. sinus
c. sinusoid
c. thrombosis
c. vasospasm
coronary-cameral fistula

coronavirus
corpora (*pl. of* corpus)
corporal
    c. cavernosal patch
    c. punishment
corpore
    conduplicato c.
corpus, *pl.* corpora
    c. albicans cyst
    c. callosum
    c. callosum hypoplasia, retardation, adducted thumbs, spastic paraparesis, hydrocephalus (CRASH)
    c. callosum partial agenesis
    corpora cavernosa to spongiosa shunt
    c. cavernosum
    c. fibrosum
    c. hemorrhagicum
    corpora lutea
    c. luteum (CL)
    c. luteum cyst
    c. luteum deficiency syndrome
    c. luteum dysfunction
    c. luteum function
    c. luteum insufficiency
    c. luteum size
    c. luteum spurium
    c. luteum verum
    c. of uterus
    pediculosis c.
    pediculosis corporis
    Pediculus humanus corporis
    corpora quadrigemina
    c. spongiosum
    c. subthalamicum
    tinea c.
    uterine c.
corpuscle
    colostrum c.
    genital c.
    Hassall c.
    meconium c.
    Meissner c.
    pacinian c.
corpus-to-cervix ratio
correctable lesion
corrected gestational age (CGA)
correction
    chordee c.
    cleft nasal deformity c.
    Dwyer c.
    endoscopic c.
    loss of c.
    spectacle c.
    surgical c.
corrective surgery

correct-revised
    Percentage of Consonants C.-R. (PCC-R)
correlate
correlation
    mean intercriterion c.
Corrigan sign
corrodens
    Bacteroides c.
    Eikenella c.
CorrTest method
corrupting
Corsi block tapping test
Corson myoma grasping forceps
CortaGel Topical
Cortaid
    C. Maximum Strength Topical
    C. with Aloe Topical
Cortamed
Cortate
Cort-Dome
    C.-D. High Potency Suppository
    C.-D. Topical
Cortef
    C. Feminine Itch Topical
    C. Oral
Cortenema enema
cortex, *pl.* cortices
    adrenal c.
    cerebral c.
    double c.
    fetal zone of adrenal c.
    frontoparietal sensorimotor c.
    irregular c.
    mastoid c.
    metaphysial c.
    motor c.
    nociferous c.
    ovarian c.
    renal c.
    visual c.
cortical
    c. agenesis
    c. androgen-stimulating hormone (CASH)
    c. architecture
    c. atrophy
    c. blindness
    c. bone
    c. dysgenesis
    c. dysplasia
    c. granule
    c. granule exocytosis
    c. gyral abnormality
    c. hemorrhage
    c. hyperostosis
    c. implantation
    c. mantle
    c. mass

c. necrosis
c. nephron
c. reaction
c. reflex myoclonus
c. scintigraphy
c. spreading depression
c. supremacy stage
c. thrombophlebitis
c. thumbing
c. tuber
c. vision
c. visual impairment (CVI)
corticalis
agenesia c.
cortices (*pl. of* cortex)
corticography
corticoid
corticomedullary
c. differentiation
c. junction
corticospinal tract dysfunction
corticosteroid
antenatal c.
fluorinated c.
inhaled c. (ICS)
c. therapy
c. treatment
corticosteroid-binding
c.-b. globulin (CBG)
c.-b. globulin-binding capacity
(CB-GBC)
corticosteroid-induced
c.-i. atrophy
c.-i. osteoporosis
corticosterone
corticostriatal
corticotrope
corticotropin
**corticotropin-like intermediate lobe
peptide**
corticotropin-releasing
c.-r. factor
c.-r. hormone (CRH)
c.-r. inhibitor
Corticreme
Cortiment
cortin
double c.
cortisol
c. concentration
c. deficiency
24-hour urinary free c.
c. level
plasma c.
c. replacement
c. response
salivary c.
urinary free c.
cortisol-binding globulin

cortisol-cortisone shuttle
cortisone
Cortisporin
C. Ophthalmic Suspension
C. Otic
C. Otic Suspension
Cortisporin-TC
C.-TC otic
C.-TC otic suspension
Cortizone-5 Topical
Cortizone-10 Topical
Cortoderm
Cortone Acetate
Cortrosyn stimulation test
corynebacteria
Corynebacterium
C. diphtheriae
C. haemolyticum
C. minutissimum
C. parvum
C. vaginalis
C. vaginitis
coryza
allergic c.
coryzal croup
COS
childhood-onset schizophrenia
COSA
child of substance abuser
co-segregation
co-sleeping
Cosmegen
cosmetic acne
cost
response c.
costal
c. cartilage
c. cartilage interposition
c. margin
CO-Stat end tidal breath analyzer
Costello syndrome
costochondral junction
costochondritis
costovertebral
c. angle (CVA)
c. angle tenderness (CVAT)
c. angle tenderness to
percussion
c. dysplasia
cosyntropin stimulation test
cot
finger c.
Cotazym
Cotazym-S
cotinine level
co-transporter-1
sodium/glucose c.-t.-1
Cotrel-Dubousset instrumentation (CDI)
cotrimoxazole trimethoprim

cottage cheese appearance
Cotte operation
Cottle-Neivert retractor
cotton
    c. pledget
    c. swab method
    c. swab test
cotton-ball exudate
cotton-tipped
    c.-t. applicator
    c.-t. swab
cotton-wool spot (CWS)
cotunii
    liquor c.
co-twin
    death of c.-t.
cotyledon
    fetal c.
    maternal c.
    c. perfusion system
    placental c.
cotyledonary placenta
coudé catheter
cough
    barking c.
    brassy c.
    bronchospastic c.
    croupy c.
    Diphen C.
    habit c.
    harassing c.
    Pedituss C.
    c. pressure transmission ratio
    psychogenic c.
    c. receptor
    rhonchorous c.
    seal-like c.
    Silphen C.
    staccato c.
    staccato-like c.
    c. syncope
    c. test
    c. tic
    uterine c.
    whooping c.
cough-cold
    PediaCare C.-C.
coughing
    paroxysmal c.
    voluntary c.
Cough-X lozenge
Coulter
    C. Channelyzer cell analyzer
    C. counter
Coumadin
coumadinization
coumarin
    c. derivative
    c. syndrome

council
    Interagency Coordinating C.
    (ICC)
counseling
    family cancer genetic c.
    genetic c.
    nondirective c.
    preabortion c.
    preconception c.
    prenatal genetic c.
Counsellor-Davis artificial vagina
  operation
Counsellor-Flor modification of McIndoe
  vaginoplasty technique
Counsellor vaginal mold
counselor
    genetic c.
    National Society of Genetic C.'s
    (NSGC)
count
    absolute band c. (ABC)
    absolute CD4 c.
    absolute lymphocyte c.
    absolute neutrophil c.
    amniotic fluid white blood cell c.
    bacterial c.
    blood c.
    CD4 cell c.
    CD8 cell c.
    colony c.
    complete blood c. (CBC)
    differential cell c.
    erythrocyte c.
    fetal kick c.
    fetal movement c. (FMC)
    granulocyte c.
    Guthrie c.
    hemolysis, elevated liver enzymes,
     low platelet c. (HELLP)
    kick c.
    lamellar body c. (LBC)
    lap c.
    leukocyte c.
    platelet c.
    red blood c. (RBC)
    reticulated platelet c.
    reticulocyte c. (retic ct)
    sperm c.
    white blood cell c.
counter
    Coulter c.
    c. stab wound incision
    Sysmex NE8000 cell c.
counterimmunoelectrophoresis
  (CIE)
counterpulsation
    intraaortic balloon c.
counterregulatory hormone release
counterrotation

counting
    carbohydrate c.
    fetal movement c.
coup injury
couple
    commissioning c.
    c. testing
coupler
couplet
coupling
    c. defect
    receptor c.
course
    aberrant c.
    long c.
    short c.
    ureteral c.
court-ordered obstetrical intervention
couvade
Couvelaire uterus
cover
    Bili mask phototherapy eye c.
    Sheathes ultrasound probe c.
    c. test
coverage
    polymicrobial c.
Covera-HS
covering
    epidermal c.
Coverlet dressing
Covermark
Cover-Roll gauze
Cover-Strip wound closure strip
covert loss
cover-uncover eye test
Cowchock-Fischbeck syndrome
Cowchock syndrome
Cowden
    C. disease
    C. syndrome
Cowdry types A, B inclusion body
cowl (*var. of* caul)
cowlick
Cowper gland
cowperian duct
cow's
    c. milk allergy (CMA)
    c. milk challenge
    c. milk intolerance
    c. milk protein (CMP)
    c. milk protein allergy
COX
    cyclooxygenase
      COX pathway
      COX proportional hazard
      COX proportional hazard model
COX-1
    cyclooxygenase-1

COX-2
    cyclooxygenase-2
      COX-2 inhibitor
coxa, *pl.* **coxae**
    c. magna
    c. plana
    c. valga
    c. vara
    c. vara deformity
coxae (*pl. of* coxa)
coxarthrosis
Coxiella burnetii
coxoauricular syndrome
coxsackie virus
coxsackievirus, coxsackie virus
    C. A (1–22, 24)
    C. A16 infection
    C. B (1–6)
    C. B enterovirus infection
CP
    cephalic presentation
    cerebral palsy
    cleft palate
CPA
    child physical abuse
C-palmitic acid
CPAP
    continuous positive airway pressure
      CPAP machine
      nasal CPAP
      CPAP ventilator
CPC
    choroid plexus carcinoma
    choroid plexus cyst
CPD
    cephalopelvic disproportion
    chronic pulmonary disease
CPE
    cryopreserved embryo
    cytopathic effect
CPEDO
    cryopreserved embryo from donor oocyte
CPEO
    chronic progressive external ophthalmoplegia
C-peptide level
CPI
    chronic pneumonitis of infancy
    congenital palatopharyngeal incompetence
CPK
    creatine phosphokinase
CPLS
    cleft palate-lateral synechia
      CPLS syndrome
cPNET
    central primitive neuroectodermal tumor

C

CPP
central precocious puberty
cerebral perfusion pressure
choroid plexus papilloma
chronic pelvic pain
CPR
cardiopulmonary resuscitation
CPS
carbamoyl phosphate synthetase
Child Protective Services
Collaborative Perinatal Study
complex partial seizure
CPS deficiency
CPS ID chromogenic medium
CPT
carnitine palmitoyltransferase
chest physical therapy
chest physiotherapy
continuous performance test
CPT I, II deficiency
cPVL
cystic periventricular
leukomalacia
C1q
C1q assay
C1q binding
deficiency of C1q
C-R
Bicillin C-R
CR
Norpace CR
CRA
clinical risk assessment
crab louse
crack
c. baby
c. cocaine
cracked mucous membrane
cracked-pot
c.-p. head
c.-p. sign
c.-p. sound
crackle
bubbly c.
fine inspiratory c.
crackling rale
CRADI
colorectal-anal distress
inventory
cradle
auditory response c.
c. cap
Criss Cross C.
cradleboard
cramp
leg c.
menstrual c.
menstrual-like c.
nocturnal leg c.

cramping
uterine c.
cranberry
Crandall ectodermal dysplasia syndrome
Crane-Heise syndrome
cranial
c. bruit
c. contour
c. duplication
c. echoencephalography
c. electrical stimulation (CES)
c. encephalocele
c. epidural abscess (CEA)
c. fasciitis
c. hypothermia
c. meningocele
c. molding helmet
c. nerve defect
c. nerve (II–XII)
c. nerve nucleus
c. nerve palsy
c. nerve testing
c. neuritis
c. orthosis
c. sclerosis
c. sclerosis with striated bone disease
c. sign
c. space
c. suture
c. synostosis
c. ultrasonography
c. ultrasound
craniectomy
endoscopic strip c.
suboccipital c.
cranioacrofacial syndrome
craniobasal bone
CranioCap cranial orthosis
craniocarpotarsal
c. dystrophy
c. syndrome
craniocaudal view
craniocerebellocardiac (3C, CCC)
c. syndrome
craniocerebral trauma
craniocervical
c. dystonia
c. junction
c. myelopathy
cranioclasia, cranioclasis
cranioclasis (*var. of* cranioclasia)
cranioclast
craniocleidodysostosis
craniodiaphyseal (*var. of* craniodiaphysial)
craniodiaphysial, craniodiaphyseal
c. dysplasia
craniodidymus
cranioectodermal dysplasia (CED)

craniofacial
- c. anomaly
- c. disproportion
- c. dissociation
- c. dysmorphism-polysyndactyly syndrome
- c. dysmorphology
- c. dysostosis (CFD)
- c. tumor

craniofacies
craniofenestria
craniofrontal dysplasia
craniofrontonasal
- c. dysostosis (CFND)
- c. dysplasia (CFND)
- c. syndrome (CFNS)

craniolacunia
craniomalacia
craniomeningocele
craniometaphyseal (*var. of* craniometaphysial)
craniometaphysial, craniometaphyseal
- c. dysplasia

cranioorodigital syndrome
craniopagus
craniopathy
craniopharyngioma
cranioplasty
craniorachischisis
craniorhiny
cranioschisis
cranioskeletal dysplasia with acroosteolysis
craniospinal rachischisis
craniostenosis
craniostosis
craniosynostosis
- Boston-type c.
- coronal c.
- metopic c.
- primary c.
- sagittal c.
- secondary c.
- single-suture c.
- syndromic c.

craniosynostosis-lid anomalies syndrome
craniosynostosis-marfanoid habitus
craniosynostosis-radial aplasia syndrome
craniosynostotic syndrome
craniotabes
craniothoracopagus syncephalus
craniotome
craniotomy
craniotubular dysplasia
cranium
- c. bifidum
- c. bifidum cysticum
- c. bifidum occultum
- c. cerebrale

- visceral c.
- c. viscerale

crankshaft phenomenon
Cranley Maternal-Fetal Attachment Scale
CRASH
- corpus callosum hypoplasia, retardation, adducted thumbs, spastic paraparesis, hydrocephalus
- CRASH syndrome

craving
- dietary c.
- food c.
- pica c.
- salt c.

crawl
- belly c.
- combat c.
- commando c.

crawling aid
CRB
- congenital retinitis blindness

CRCT
- creamatocrit

C1r deficiency
C-reactive protein (CRP)
cream
- Acticin C.
- Aldara c.
- Amino-Cerv pH 5.5 cervical c.
- AnaMantle HC c.
- AVC C.
- Bactroban c.
- Balmex c.
- butoconazole 2% c.
- Cleocin vaginal c.
- clotrimazole vaginal c. 2%
- Complex 15 c.
- Cutivate c.
- Decadron Phosphate C.
- dihydrotestosterone c.
- Elimite C.
- EMLA c.
- emollient c.
- Estrace vaginal c.
- estradiol vaginal c.
- Eucerin Plus C.
- Exact C.
- Fungoid C.
- gentamicin c.
- Gynazole-1 vaginal c.
- imiquimod c.
- intravaginal c.
- Lamisil C.
- LCD c.
- lidocaine-prilocaine c.
- Masse Breast C.
- miconazole nitrate vaginal c.
- MimyX c.
- Monistat 3 vaginal c.

C

cream (*continued*)
Mother2Be breast nourishing c.
Mother2Be nipple restoration c.
Neosporin C.
Nivea c.
Nupercainal c.
Nutraderm c.
nystatin and triamcinolone c.
penciclovir c.
Pen Kera moisturizing c.
permethrin 5% c.
pimecrolimus c.
Preparation-H
  hydrocortisone c.
progesterone c.
Purpose c.
RVPaque c.
silver sulfadiazine c.
Sklar c.
SSD c.
stearin-lanolin c.
Stelactiv diaper rash c.
Stelatopia moisturizing c.
steroid c.
Sulfamylon c.
Sween C.
Terazol 3 vaginal c.
Terazol 7 vaginal c.
testosterone propionate c.
Topicort c.
triple sulfa c.
Trivagizole 3 vaginal c.
U-Cort c.
vaginal c.
vasodilator c.
Vite E C.
wild yam c.
yam c.
Zonalon Topical C.
creamatocrit (CRCT)
creamy vulvitis
crease
allergic c.
earlobe c. (ELC)
flexural c.
palmar c.
plantar c.
simian c.
single transverse palmar c.
sole c.
Sydney c.
transversal nasal c.
crease/pit
ear c./p.
creatine
c. deficiency
c. kinase (CK)
c. kinase MB
c. phosphokinase (CPK)

creatinine
c. clearance
c. phosphokinase
Creator
Children's Tylenol with
  Flavor C.
Credé
C. maneuver of eyes
C. maneuver of uterus
C. placental removal maneuver
C. prophylaxis
creep
creeping eruption
Cre/loxP system
cremasteric
c. fascia
c. reflex
c. response
cremnocele
crenated red blood cell
crenation sign
Creola body
Creon 10, 20
Creo-Terpin
crepitant rale
crepitation
crepitus
crescendo murmur
crescent
c. cell anemia
c. formation
C. pillow
crescentic
c. fashion
c. glomerulonephritis
c. lesion
crest
iliac c.
neural c.
posterior iliac c.
superior iliac c.
C. syndrome
CREST
calcinosis, Raynaud phenomenon,
  esophageal dysmotility, sclerodactyly,
  telangiectasia
Collaborative Review of Sterilization
Cresylate
creta
placenta c.
placenta previa c.
cretin dwarfism
cretinism
athyrotic c.
endemic c.
c. idiocy
**cretinism-muscular hypertrophy
syndrome**
cretinoid dysplasia

Creutzfeldt-Jakob
  C.-J. disease (CJD)
  C.-J. syndrome
CRF
  chronic renal failure
  anemia of CRF
CR-gram
  cardiorespirogram
CRH
  corticotropin-releasing hormone
cri du chat
CRI
  congenital rubella infection
crib
  clinical c.
  c. death
  open c.
  C. score
  tongue c.
CRIB
  Clinical Risk Index for Babies
Crib-O-Gram
cribriform
  c. fracture
  c. hymen
  c. plate
cribrosa
  lamina c.
  macula c.
cricoarytenoid
  c. articulation
  c. joint
cricoid
  c. pressure
  c. split
  c. split procedure
cricopharyngeal incoordination of infancy
cricothyroidectomy
cricothyroid membrane
cricothyroidotomy, cricothyrotomy
  needle c.
cricothyrotomy, cricothyroidotomy
  needle c.
  surgical c.
cri-du-chat syndrome, cri du chat syndrome, cat-cry syndrome
CRIES
  crying, requires oxygen, increased vital signs, expression, sleepless
  CRIES postoperative pain scale
Crigler-Najjar
  C.-N. disease (type I, II)
  C.-N. syndrome (type I, II)
Crile
  C. forceps
  C. hemostat
Crile-Wood needle holder
Crimean-Congo hemorrhagic fever

criminal abortion
criminology
Crinone bioadhesive progesterone gel
Crippled Children's Services (CCS)
crises (*pl. of* crisis)
crisis, *pl.* **crises**
  abdominal c.
  acute adrenal c.
  acute splenic sequestration c.
  addisonian c.
  adrenal c.
  aplastic c.
  autonomic c.
  blast c.
  Chiari c.
  cholinergic c.
  clitoris c.
  congenital hemolytic anemia with aplastic c.
  developmental c.
  encephalopathic c.
  Fabry c.
  hematologic c.
  hemolytic c.
  hepatic c.
  hypercalcemic c.
  hypertensive c.
  infectious c.
  c. intervention
  intrahepatic vasoocclusive c.
  lupus c.
  megaloblastic c.
  oculogyric c.
  pain c.
  scleroderma renal c.
  sequestration c.
  sickle cell c.
  sickling c.
  splenic sequestration c.
  thyroid c.
  thyrotoxic c.
  transient aplastic c. (TAC)
  vasoocclusive c.
Crisponi syndrome
Criss Cross Cradle
crisscross heart
crista, *pl.* **cristae**
  c. dividens
  c. supraventricularis
cristae (*pl. of* crista)
cristata
  Lepiota c.
criteria (*pl. of* criterion)
criterion, *pl.* **criteria**
  Amsel criteria
  Beighton criteria
  Bell staging criteria
  Berne criteria
  Cohen criteria

criterion (*continued*)
    death by neurological criteria
    DSM-IV criteria
    family history research diagnostic criteria (FH-RDC)
    GOS criteria
    ICSD criteria
    Jones rheumatic fever diagnostic criteria
    Joshi criteria
    Kass criteria
    Lorber criteria
    modified Beighton criteria
    Nugent criteria
    c. overlap
    Oxford diagnostic criteria
    Ranson criteria
    revised Jones criteria
    Rochester criteria
    Rubin criteria
    Shimada criteria
    Spiegel criteria
    Spiegelberg criteria
    Sydenham chorea criteria
    Waterlow criteria
criterion-referenced test
critical
    c. aortic stenosis
    c. body weight
    c. care
    c. care monitoring
    c. illness neuromuscular disease
    c. pulmonic stenosis
    c. temperature
    c. weight hypothesis
Criticare H formula
Crixivan
CRL
    crown-rump length
CRMO
    chronic recurrent multifocal osteomyelitis
CRNA
    certified registered nurse anesthetist
CRO
    cathode ray oscilloscope
crocodile
    c. skin
    c. tongue
Crohn
    C. colitis
    C. disease
    C. disease of vulva
Crolom
Crome syndrome

cromoglycate
    disodium c.
    PMS-Sodium C.
    sodium c.
cromolyn
    atropine c.
    c. sodium
    c. sodium inhalation aerosol
Cronkhite-Canada syndrome
crooked fingers syndrome
crop
    c. of macules
    c. of papules
    rash c.
Crosby capsule
Crosby-Kugler pediatric capsule
cross
    c. breeding
    bridging c.
    dihybrid c.
    monohybrid c.
    reciprocal c.
    C. syndrome
    c. table
crossbite
cross-brain oxygen extraction
cross-cradle position
Crosse
    La C.
crossed
    c. adductor reflex
    c. extension reflex
    c. fused ectopia
    c. polysyndactyly
cross-eye
cross-gender
crossing over
cross-link
    N-telopeptide cross-links (NTx)
    TSRH c.-l.
cross-linking
Cross-McKusick-Breen syndrome
cross-modal fluency
crossover
    circulatory c.
cross-reaction
cross-sectional
cross-table lateral film
crotamiton
crouch gait
croup
    coryzal c.
    diphtheritic c.
    membranous c.
    C. score
    spasmodic c.
croupette

croupy cough
Crouzon
    C. craniofacial dysostosis
    C. disease
    C. syndrome
crowded teeth
crowding
    dental c.
    fetal c.
    c. theory
Crowe sign
crown-heel length (CHL)
crowning
crown-rump length (CRL)
crow's nest
CRP
    C-reactive protein
CRPF
    chloroquine-resistant *Plasmodium*
      falciparum
CRS
    caudal regression syndrome
    Cell Recovery System
    congenital rubella syndrome
    Conners Rating Scale
CRST
    calcinosis, Raynaud phenomenon,
      sclerodactyly, telangiectasia
    CRST syndrome
cruciferous vegetable
crude risk ratio
cruenta
    lochia c.
Cruex Topical
Cruiser hip abduction brace
cruising
crunch
    mediastinal c.
crura (*pl. of* crus)
cruris (*gen. of* crus)
crus, *gen.* **cruris,** *pl.* **crura**
    paired crura
    tinea cruris
crush injury
crusta lactea
crusted
    c. lesion
    c. scabies
crusting telangiectasia
  keratosis
crutches
    Lofstrand c.
crux
cruzi
    Trypanosoma c.
Cruz trypanosomiasis
cry
    cat's c.
    cephalic c.

    high-pitched c.
    hoarse c.
    uterine c.
    voiceless c.
    weak c.
cryaerophilia
    Campylobacter c.
crying
    c. cat syndrome
    differentiated c.
    c., requires oxygen, increased vital
      signs, expression, sleepless (CRIES)
CRYOcare cryoablation system
cryocauterization
cryocautery
cryoconization
cryofibrinogenemia
cryoglobulin
    polyclonal c.
cryoglobulinemia
Cryogun
CryoHit cryotherapy device
cryoinjury
cryomyolysis
cryoprecipitate transfusion
cryopreservation
    oocyte c.
cryopreserved
    c. embryo (CPE)
    c. embryo from donor oocyte
      (CPEDO)
    c. valved allograft
cryoprotectant
cryosurgery
cryothalamectomy
cryotherapy
Cryovial tube
crypt
    c. abscess
    c. cell
    c. cell mitosis
    c. depth
    c. hyperplasia
    c. hypoplasia
    c. of Lieberkühn
cryptic
    c. hemangioma
    c. hyperandrogenism
    c. tuber
cryptocephalus
cryptococcal
    c. antigen
    c. meningitis
cryptococcosis
    cutaneous c.
    extrapulmonary c.
    pulmonary c.
Cryptococcus neoformans
cryptodidymus

C

cryptogenic
   c. cirrhosis
   c. fibrosing alveolitis
   c. hepatitis
   c. infantile spasm
cryptomenorrhea
cryptomerorachischisis
cryptomicrotia-brachydactyly syndrome
cryptophthalmia (*var. of* cryptophthalmos)
cryptophthalmos, cryptophthalmia
   c. syndrome
cryptophthalmos-syndactyly syndrome
cryptorchidism, cryptorchism
   bilateral c.
   unilateral c.
cryptorchid testis
cryptorchism (*var. of* cryptorchidism)
cryptosporidiosis
Cryptosporidium parvum
cryptotia
cryptozoospermia
crypt-villus architecture
Cryselle tablet
crystal
   calcium c.
   Charcot-Leyden c.
   indinavir c.
   c. methamphetamine
   urate c.
   c. violet
CrystalEyes endoscopic video system
crystallina miliaria
crystalline lens
crystallization
   fern leaf c.
crystalloid
   miliaria c.
   Reinke c.'s
   c. solution
crystalluria
   renal tubular c.
C&S
   culture and sensitivity
CS
   cesarean section
   congenital syphilis
   coronal suture
Cs
   cesium
CSA
   child sexual abuse
   clinically significant arrhythmia
   colony-stimulating activity
CsA
   cyclosporin A
Csaba stain
CSBI
   Child Sexual Behavior Inventory
CS-5 cryosurgical system

CSD
   cat-scratch disease
CSE
   combined spinal-epidural
    CSE anesthesia
C-section
   cesarean section
    LUST C-s.
CSF
   cerebrospinal fluid
   colony-stimulating factor
    bloody CSF
    CSF glycine
    CSF lymphocytic pleocytosis
    CSF otorrhea
    CSF rhinorrhea
    CSF VDRL
    xanthochromic CSF
C-shaped curve
CSI
   chemical shift imaging
CsI
   cesium iodide
Csillag disease
CSOM
   chronic suppurative otitis media
CSPI
   childhood severity of psychiatric illness
CSQI
   continuous subcutaneous infusion
CST
   contraction stress test
    antepartum fetal CST
    fetal CST
CSTR
   complete subtalar release
CSW
   cerebral salt wasting
    CSW syndrome
C3T
   clomiphene citrate challenge test
CT
   Chlamydia trachomatis
   computed tomography
   computerized tomography
    CT guidance
    CT laser mammography
    CT pelvimetry
    CT scan
    CT scanning
CTAF
   conotruncal anomaly face syndrome
CTD
   chronic tic disorder
   clitoral therapy device
CTEI
   communal traumatic experiences inventory

C-telopeptide
　　type I collagen C-t.
C-terminal propeptide of type I collagen
CTG
　　cardiotocography
C-thalassemia
CTL
　　cytotoxic T lymphocyte
　　　　CTL cell
　　　　CTL response
CTLM
　　computed tomography laser
　　mammography
CT1 needle
CTNS gene
CTP
　　carboxyl terminal peptide
CTQ
　　childhood trauma questionnaire
CTS
　　clitoris tourniquet syndrome
CTX
　　cyclophosphamide
CTZ
　　chemoreceptor trigger zone
cube pessary
cubic
　　c. centimeter (cc)
　　c. centimeter per hour (cc/hr)
cubiti (*pl. of* cubitus)
cubitus, *pl.* **cubiti**
　　c. valgus
　　c. valgus deformity
　　c. varus
cuboid, cuboidal
cuboidal (*var. of* cuboid)
CUCS
　　complex unroofed coronary sinus
cued speech
Cue Fertility Monitor
cuff
　　c. cellulitis
　　Ethox c.
　　muscular c.
　　neonatal c.
　　posterior vaginal c.
　　c. test
　　vaginal c.
cuffed
　　c. endotracheal tube
　　c. ET tube
cuffing
　　pericapillary inflammatory c.
Cu-7 intrauterine device
cuirass respirator
culbertsoni
　　Acanthamoeba c.
cul-de-sac
　　c.-d.-s. biopsy

　　Douglas c.-d.-s.
　　c.-d.-s. obliteration
　　c.-d.-s. of Douglas
　　posterior c.-d.-s.
　　rectouterine c.-d.-s.
culdocentesis
　　equivocal c.
　　nondiagnostic c.
culdoplasty
　　Halban c.
　　high McCall c.
　　Marion-Moschcowitz c.
　　Mayo c.
　　McCall c.
　　Moschowitz c.
　　prophylactic c.
　　Torpin-Waters-McCall c.
culdoscope
culdoscopy
culdotomy
Culex
　　C. nigripalpus
　　C. pipiens
　　C. quinquefasciatus
　　C. tarsalis
Culiseta melanura
Cullen sign
cultivable virus
cultural
　　c. artifact
　　c. competence
culture
　　amniotic fluid cell c.
　　c. and sensitivity (C&S)
　　blood c.
　　broth c.
　　cell c.
　　cervical c.
　　colony-forming unit in c.
　　　(CFUC)
　　epiglottic surface c.
　　extended c.
　　c. fertilization
　　fibroblast c.
　　gastric aspirate c.
　　GBS screening c.
　　gonorrhea c. (GC)
　　in vitro human intestinal organ c.
　　nasal swab c.
　　oocyte c.
　　purified chick embryo cell c.
　　　(PCEC)
　　screening c.
　　shell vial c.
　　sputum c.
　　test-of-cure c.
　　tracheal-aspirate c.
　　Ureaplasma c.
　　Uricult c.

C

culture (*continued*)
  urine c. (UC)
  vaginorectal c.
cultured skin fibroblast
culture-negative
  c.-n. cytomegalovirus infection
  c.-n. neutrocytic ascites
culture-specific determinant
culturing
  viral c.
Cumulase
  SynVitro C.
cumulative
  c. conception rate (CCR)
  c. gene
  c. parental dysfunction
cumulus
  c. cell
  c. oophorus
  c. ovaricus
cuneiform bone
cup
  Bird OP c.
  CMI-Mityvac c.
  CMI-O'Neil c.
  cut-away c.
  cut-out c.
  c. ear
  c. feeding
  heel c.
  c. insemination
  Instead feminine protection c.
  Malmstrom c.
  Milex cervical c.
  Mityvac obstetric vacuum
    extractor c.
  Mityvac Super M c.
  M-Style Mushroom vacuum c.
  O'Neil c.
  Tender-Touch vacuum birthing c.
  vacuum c.
  zinc-free plastic specimen c.
Cupid's
  C. bow
  C. bow curve
  C. bow upper lip
cupped metaphysis
cupping
  c. of optic nerve head
  optic nerve c.
Cuprimine
cupriuria
cuprophane hemodialyzer membrane
cuproprotein
Curaderm dressing
Curafil dressing
curage
Curagel Hydrogel dressing
curare

Curasorb calcium alginate dressing
curative
curdy discharge
C-urea
  C-u. breath test
  C-u. serology
curet (*var. of* curette)
curetment
curettage, curettement
  blunt c.
  dilation and c. (D&C)
  endocervical c. (ECC)
  endometrial c. (EMC)
  fractional dilation and c.
  radial c.
  repeat c.
  sharp c.
  suction and c. (S&C)
  suction, dilation, and c.
  vacuum c.
  vaginal interruption of pregnancy
    with dilatation and c. (VIP-DAC)
curette, curet
  banjo c.
  Berkeley suction c.
  Bumm c.
  Duncan c.
  FemSuite endocervical c.
  Green uterine c.
  Heaney c.
  Helix endocervical c.
  Helix uterine biopsy c.
  Kelly-Gray c.
  Kevorkian c.
  Kevorkian-Younge c.
  lighted ear c.
  Meigs c.
  Mi-Mark disposable endocervical c.
  Novak c.
  optic aspirating c. (OAC)
  Pipelle endometrial suction c.
  Pipet C.
  Randall suction c.
  Shapleigh c.
  Sims c.
  St. Clair-Thompson c.
  suction c.
  Thomas c.
  Townsend endocervical biopsy c.
  uterine c.
  Uterine Explora c.
  Vabra suction c.
  Yankauer c.
  Z-Sampler endometrial suction c.
curettement, curetment
curetting
  endocervical c.
curie (Ci)
curly toe

Curosurf
    C. intratracheal suspension
    C. poractant alpha
    C. surfactant
Curran syndrome
currant jelly stool
Currarino triad
currens
    larva c.
current
    diathermy c.
Curretab Oral
Curry-Jones syndrome
Curschmann spiral
curse
    Ondine c.
Curtis syndrome
curtsey sign
curvatura (*var. of* curvature)
curvature, curvatura
    abnormal penile c.
    dorsal penile c.
    excessive penile c.
    lateral c.
    c. of spine
    penile c.
    thoracolumbar kyphotic c.
curve
    Barnes c.
    biologic satiation c.
    Carus c.
    C-shaped c.
    Cupid's bow c.
    flow-volume c.
    Friedman labor c.
    growth c.
    hemoglobin-oxygen dissociation c.
    intrauterine growth c.
    isodose c.
    Kaplan-Meier survival c.
    Liley c.
    lumbar c.
    c. of Spee
    oxygen dissociation c.
    oxygen-hemoglobin dissociation c.
    Risser c.
    saddleback temperature c.
    sexual response c.
    S-shaped c.
    standard c.
curved
    c. finger
    c. hemostat
    c. Mayo scissors
Curvularia lunata
CUSA
    Cavitron ultrasonic surgical aspirator
CUSALap accessory needle
Cusco speculum

Cushing
    C. disease
    C. effect
    C. forceps
    C. syndrome
    C. triad
cushingoid
    c. appearance
    c. body habitus
    c. facies
    c. syndrome
cushion
    birth c.
    c. defect of heart
    endocardial c.
    scintimammography prone breast c.
    sucking c.
cusp
cuspid
custodial care
cut section
cutaneocerebral angioma
cutaneomeningospinal angiomatosis
cutaneous
    c. albinism
    c. angioma
    c. anthrax
    c. atrophy
    c. blanching
    c. candidiasis
    c. cryptococcosis
    c. dimple
    c. diphtheria
    c. ectoderm
    c. fetal blood flow
    c. fibrosis
    c. hemangioma
    c. hepatic porphyria
    c. larva migrans
    c. leishmaniasis
    c. lesion
    c. manifestation
    c. mastocytosis
    c. melanoma
    c. melanosis
    c. mucormycosis
    c. nevus
    c. nodule
    c. pressure pulse
    c. pyelostomy
    c. shunt
    c. sporotrichosis
    c. tag
    c. telangiectasis
    c. tuberculosis
    c. ureterostomy
    c. urticaria
    c. vasculitis

cutaneous (*continued*)
    c. vasoconstriction
    c. vesicostomy
cut-away cup
cutdown
    greater saphenous vein c.
    c. method
cut-down liver
cutis
    aplasia c.
    c. aplasia of scalp
    c. elastica
    c. hyperelastica
    c. laxa
    c. marmorata
    c. marmorata alba
    c. marmorata telangiectatica
    c. marmorata telangiectatica
      congenita
    tuberculosis verrucosa c.
    c. verticis gyrata
    xanthosis c.
Cutivate
    C. cream
    C. lotion
cutoff sign
cut-out cup
cutter
    endoscopic linear c.
    Polaris reusable c.
cutting
    cutting, annoyance, guilt, eye-opener
    (CAGE)
    c. loop
Cuvier
    duct of C.
CVA
    cerebrovascular accident
    costovertebral angle
    CVA tenderness
CVAD
    central venous access device
CVAT
    costovertebral angle tenderness
CVB
    chorionic villus biopsy
CVC
    central venous catheter
CVI
    common variable
      immunodeficiency
    cortical visual impairment
CVID
    common variable immunodeficiency
CVL
    central venous line
      tunneled CVL
CVM
    cardiovascular malformation

CVN
    central venous nutrition
CVP
    central venous pressure
      CVP line
CVS
    cardiovascular system
    chorionic villus sampling
CVVH
    continuous venovenous hemofiltration
CVVHD
    continuous venovenous hemodialysis
CWS
    cotton-wool spot
CWSN
    Children with Special Health Care
      Needs
CXR
    chest x-ray
cyanide toxicity
cyanocobalamin
cyanogen bromide (CNBr)
cyanosis
    acral c.
    cardiac c.
    central c.
    differential c.
    nail bed c.
    neonatal c.
    oral mucosa c.
    perioral c.
    peripheral c.
    pulmonary c.
    slate-gray c.
cyanotic
    c. breath-holding spell
    c. congenital heart disease (CCHD)
    c. congenital heart lesion
    c. flush
    c. heart disease
    c. newborn
cyclacillin
cyclamate
    calcium c.
    sodium c.
cyclandelate
cyclase
    adenyl c.
    adenylate c.
cyclazocine
cycle
    battering c.
    cell c.
    circadian c.
    citric acid c.
    endometrial c.
    estrogen-progestin artificial c.
    female reproductive c.
    fertility c.

fetal sleep c.
futile c.
genesial c.
glutamate c.
initiated c.
intrauterine pressure c.
itch-scratch c.
Krebs c.
c. length
menstrual ovarian c.
micturition c.
c. of violence
ovarian c.
ovulatory menstrual c.
periodic breathing c. (PBC)
c. per second (cps)
reproductive c.
respiratory c.
sexual response c.
S phase of cell c.
spontaneous menstrual c.
stationary c.
urea c.
CycleBeads fertility device
cycle-monitoring detail
cyclencephalus
cycle-nonspecific agent
cycle-specific agent
Cyclessa tablet
cyclic, cyclical
c. adenosine monophosphate (cAMP)
c. adenosine monophosphate test
c. antidepressant poisoning
c. breast pain
c. endoperoxide
c. guanosine monophosphate (cGMP)
c. hormone production
c. mastalgia
c. neutropenia
c. proliferative endometrium
c. sloughing
c. uterine bleeding
c. vomiting
c. vomiting syndrome
c. vulvitis
c. vulvodynia
c. vulvovaginitis
cyclical (*var. of* cyclic)
cyclicity
menstrual c.
postmenarchal c.
cycling
cyclizine lactate
Cyclocort Topical
cyclocryotherapy
cyclodestructive procedure
Cyclofem
cyclofenil citrate
Cyclogyl

cycloheximide
cyclohexylchloroethylnitrosurea (CCNU)
cyclohydrolase
guanosine triphosphate c.
Cyclomen
cyclomethycaine
Cyclomydril
cyclooxygenase (COX)
platelet c.
cyclooxygenase-1 (COX-1)
cyclooxygenase-2 (COX-2)
cyclooxygenase-2-derived prostanoid
cyclopea (*var. of* cyclopia)
cyclopentanoperhydrophenanthrene
cyclopenthiazide
cyclopentolate hydrochloride
cyclophosphamide (CTX)
c., hydroxydaunorubicin,
methotrexate, prednisone (CHOP)
cyclopia, cyclopea
cyclopism
cycloplegic
cyclopropane
Cyclo-Provera
cyclops
c. hypognathus
C. procedure
cycloserine
Cyclospora cayetanensis
cyclosporiasis
cyclosporin
c. A (CsA)
cyclosporine, cyclosporin A
cyclosporine-induced gingival overgrowth
cyclothiazide
cyclothymia
cyclothymic disorder
cycrimine hydrochloride
Cycrin
cyesis
Cyklokapron
Cylert
Cylex
Cylexin
cylinder
c. cast
cesium c.
Delclos c.
muscle c.
cylindrical embryo
cyllosoma
cymbocephaly
Cynapin
CYP11B1 gene
CYP11B2 gene
CYP17 deficiency
CYP21 genotyping
CYP21A gene
CYP21B gene

C

cypionate
    estradiol c.
    hydrocortisone c.
    testosterone c.
Cypress facial neuromusculoskeletal syndrome
cyproheptadine
    c. hydrochloride
    c. receptor blocker
cyproterone acetate
cyst
    acne c.
    adnexal c.
    allantoic c.
    alveolar c.
    aneurysmal bone c.
    apocrine c.
    arachnoid c.
    c. aspiration
    autonomous ovarian follicular c.
    Baker c.
    Bartholin duct c.
    Bartholin gland c.
    benign pineal c.
    bilateral choroid plexus c.
    blue dome c.
    branchial cleft c.
    breast c.
    bronchogenic c.
    calcified outline of c.
    canal of Nuck c.
    chocolate c.
    choledochal c.
    chorionic c.
    choroid plexus c. (CPC)
    colloid c.
    corpus albicans c.
    corpus luteum c.
    Dandy-Walker c.
    dental lamina c.
    dentigerous c.
    dermoid c.
    duplication c.
    dysontogenetic c.
    echinococcal c.
    Echinococcus granulosus hydatid c.
    endometrial c.
    enterogenous c.
    epidermal c.
    epidermal inclusion c. (EIC)
    epidermoid c.
    epithelial inclusion c.
    eruptive vellus hair c.
    esophageal duplication c.
    extraaxial arachnoid c.
    fetal ovarian c.
    follicular c.
    functional ovarian c.

    Gartner duct c.
    gartnerian c.
    germinal inclusion c.
    gingival c.
    glioependymal c.
    hydatid c.
    inclusion c.
    intraabdominal c.
    involution c.
    keratin c.
    keratinized c.
    keratinous c.
    lacteal c.
    leptomeningeal c.
    luteal ovarian c.
    massive ovarian c.
    mesonephric c.
    milk c.
    mucous retention c.
    mucus c.
    müllerian c.
    multilocular c.
    multilocular thymic c. (MTC)
    multiloculated c.
    multiple c.
    Naboth c.
    nabothian c.
    neoplastic c.
    neurenteric c.
    noncommunicating c.
    oil c.
    omental c.
    omphalomesenteric c.
    oophoritic c.
    ovarian c.
    paraovarian c.
    paratubal c.
    paraurethral c.
    parenchymal c.
    pericardial c.
    pilar c.
    pilonidal c.
    pineal c.
    popliteal c.
    porencephalic c.
    posterior fossa arachnoid c.
    pseudoporencephalic c.
    renal cortex c.
    retrocerebellar arachnoidal c.
    Sampson c.
    sebaceous c.
    second branchial cleft c.
    siderophagic c.
    simple c.
    Skene duct c.
    skin c.
    solitary bone c.
    sperm-containing c.
    subcapsular c.

subepidermal keratin c.
suprasellar arachnoid c.
tarry c.
tension c.
theca lutein c.
thyroglossal duct c.
trichilemmal c.
umbilical c.
unicameral bone c.
unilocular ovarian c.
urachal c.
vaginal c.
vaginal dysontogenetic c.
vaginal embryonic c.
vaginal inclusion c.
vestibular c.
vitelline duct c.
vitellointestinal c.
vulvar inclusion c.
wolffian remnant c.

Cystadane
cystadenocarcinoma
mucinous c.
ovarian c.
papillary serous c.
serous c.
cystadenofibroma
cystadenoma
apocrine c.
benign mucinous c.
mucinous c.
ovarian proliferative c.
serous c.
vulvar apocrine c.
Cystagon
cystathionine
c. beta-synthase (CBS)
c. beta-synthase deficiency
c. synthase
c. synthase deficiency
cystathioninemia
cystathioninuria
cystatin C
cysteamine
cystectomy
Bartholin c.
ovarian c.
vulvovaginal c.
cysteine hydrochloride
cystencephalus
cystic
c. adenomatoid malformation (CAM)
c. adenomatoid malformation of lung
c. adenomatous malformation (CAM)
c. adnexal mass
c. brainstem glioma
c. cerebellar neoplasm

c. congenital adenomatoid malformation (CCAM)
c. dilation
c. dilation of intrahepatic bile duct
c. disease of the breast
c. encephalomalacia
c. endometrial hyperplasia
c. fibrosis (CF)
c. fibrosis transmembrane conductance regulator gene
c. fibrosis transmembrane regulator (CFTR)
c. glandular hyperplasia
c. hamartoma
c. hydatid disease
c. hygroma
c. hyperplasia of the breast
c. kidney
c. lesion
c. leukomalacia
c. lymphangioma
c. medial necrosis
c. mole
c. myoma degeneration
c. nephroma
c. ovarian mass
c. periventricular leukomalacia (cPVL)
c. PVL
c. renal disease
c. sac
c. teratoma
c. teratoma of ovary
c. wall
c. Walthard rest
cystica
colpohyperplasia c.
cystitis c.
osteitis fibrosis c.
osteogenesis imperfecta c.
pachyvaginitis c.
spina bifida c.
vaginitis c.
cysticercosis
parenchymatous cerebral c.
Cysticercus cellulosae
cysticum
cranium bifidum c.
epithelioma adenoides c.
lymphangioma c.
cyst-induced pancreatitis
cystine
c. deposition
c. stone
cystinosis
infantile neuropathic c.
neuropathic c.
ocular nonnephropathic c.

cystinuria
  transient neonatal c.
cystitis
  acute c.
  bacterial c.
  c. cystica
  eosinophilic c.
  c. glandularis
  hemorrhagic c.
  honeymoon c.
  Hunner interstitial c.
  interstitial c. (IC)
  irradiation c.
  postoperative c.
  postradiation c.
  radiation c.
cystoblast
Cystocath catheter
cystocele
  paravaginal c.
  c. repair
cystoduodenostomy
cystogastrostomy
cystogram
  sleep c.
cystography
  indirect c.
  radionuclide voiding c. (RVC)
  voiding c.
cystojejunostomy
cystometer
  Lewis recording c.
cystometric capacity
cystometrics
  office c.
cystometrogram (CMG)
  eyeball c.
  multichannel c.
  poor man's c.
cystometrography
cystometry, cystometrography
cystoperitoneal shunt
cystopexy
cystoplasty
  augmentation c.
cystosarcoma phyllodes
cystoscopic transurethral tumor resection
cystoscopy
  rigid c.
  c. table
Cystospaz
Cystospaz-M
cystostomy
  suprapubic c.
cystotomy
  suprapubic c.
cystourethrocele
cystourethrogram
  voiding c. (VCUG)

cystourethrograph
  voiding c. (VCUG)
cystourethrography
  chain c.
  metallic bead-chain c.
  voiding c. (VCU, VCUG)
cystourethropexy
  needle c.
  retropubic c. (RPCV)
  vaginal c.
cystourethroscopy
Cytadren
cytarabine
cytidine
  c. diphosphate-choline
  c. diphosphate-diacylglycerol
  c. monophosphate
cytinosin
cytoarchitectonic
cytoarchitectural development
cytoarchitecture
Cytobrush
  C. cell collector
  C. Plus cell collector
  C. Plus endocervical cell sampler
  C. Plus GT
  C. spatula
  Zelsmyr C.
cytochalasin
cytochrome
  c. *b*
  c. *b* system
  c. *c* oxidase deficiency
  c. *c* oxidative enzyme
  c. oxidase test
  P450 c.
  c. P450scc
CytoGam
cytogenetic
  c. analysis
  c. line
  c. map
  c. study
cytogenetics
  bone marrow c.
cytoid body
cytokine
  c. cascade
  c. granulocyte
  c. modulator
  pleiotropic c.
  proinflammatory c.
cytokinemia
  fetal c.
  maternal c.
cytokine-related dysmotility
cytologic
  c. analysis
  c. atypia

c. screening
c. smear
c. study
c. washing
cytological
c. band
c. map
cytology
aspiration biopsy c. (ABC)
bland c.
c. brush
brush c.
cervical c.
peritoneal c.
scrape c.
sputum c.
urine c.
vaginal c.
cytolysis
cytolytic vaginitis
cytomegalic
c. hypoplasia
c. inclusion disease (CID)
cytomegalovirus (CMV)
congenital c.
c. disease
fetal c.
c. immune globulin intravenous (CMV-IGIV)
c. infection
maternal c.
prenatal c.
c. seropositive
c. total immunoglobulin assay
transfusion-associated c.
cytomegalovirus-specific immunoglobulin
cytomegaly syndrome
Cytomel Oral
cytometer
Epics XL flow c.
cytometry
flow c.
cytopathic effect (CPE)
cytopathogenesis
cytopathologic evaluation
cytopathology
cytopathy
mitochondrial c.
cytopenia
autoimmune c.
intermittent hematologic c.
cytophagocytosis
cytophilic antibody

cytopipette
cytoplasm
bubble gum c.
ground-glass c.
cytoplasmic
c. inheritance
c. lipid droplet (CLD)
c. membrane
c. trait
cytoprotective agent
cytoreduction
cytoreductive surgery
CytoRich process
Cytosar-U
cytosine
c. arabinoside
c. arabinoside, etoposide, methotrexate (CEM)
c. nucleotide
cytosine-adenine-guanine
c.-a.-g. (CAG)
cytosine-guanine-guanine (CGG)
cytoskeleton
cytosol
cytosolic tyrosine transaminase deficiency
Cytospray
cytotechnician
Cytotec induction
cytotoxic
c. agent
c. edema
c. effect
c. factor
c. lymphocyte response
c. memory T cell
c. T lymphocyte (CTL)
cytotoxicity
antibody-dependent cell-mediated c. (ADCC)
cytotoxin
vero c.
cytotrophoblast
malignant c.
Cytovene
Cytoxan
C., Adriamycin, leucovorin, calcium, fluorouracil, ethinyl estradiol (CALF-E)
C., Oncovin, fluorouracil plus Cytoxan, Oncovin, methotrexate (COF/COM)
Czerny anemia

2D

2-dimensional
2D Doppler
2D echocardiogram
2D echocardiography

3D

3-dimensional
3D echocardiography
3D ultrasound

D$_2$

prostaglandin D$_2$

D$_4$

leukotriene D$_4$ (LTD$_4$)

D920

Audio Doppler D920

DA

developmental age
dextroamphetamine
ductus arteriosus

DAA

digital auditory aerobics
double aortic arch

dacarbazine (DTIC)
dacliximab
daclizumab
Dacogen
Dacron

D. fiber
D. fiber-coated coil
D. patch
D. sleeve catheter

dacryoadenitis
dacryocystitis

acute d.

dacryocystorhinostomy
dacryocystostenosis
dacryostenosis
dactinomycin
dactylitis

blistering distal d.
sickle cell d.
tuberculous d.

dactylomegaly
DA-DAPI stain
DAG

diacylglycerol

Dagenan
DAI

diffuse axonal injury

daily

d. activity
d. fetal movement record (DFMR)
d. routine
d. weight measurement

Dakin antibacterial solution

Dalacin C
Dale

D. abdominal binder
D. Foley catheter holder

dalfopristin
Dalkon shield
Dall-Miles cable grip procedure
Dalmane
Dalrymple sign
dam

dental d.

damage

brain d.
corneal d.
hepatocellular d.
macromolecular d.
minimal brain d.
neuronal d.
obstetric d.
obturator nerve d.
parenchymatous d.
pelvic d.
pelvic floor d.
placental d.
tubal d.
tubal inflammatory d. (TID)
vestibular d.
virus-induced epithelial d.
white matter d. (WMD)

d-amino acid
dAMP

deoxyadenylic acid

DAMP

deficits in attention, motor control, perception

D-amphetamine
Damus-Fontan procedure
Damus-Kaye-Stansel

D.-K.-S. anastomosis
D.-K.-S. pulmonary artery to ascending aorta anastomosis procedure
D.-K.-S. pulmonary artery to ascending aorta anastomotic operation

danazol

low-dose d.

dance

hilar d.
D. sign
St. Vitus d.

dancer's ankle
dancing

d. eye
d. eye movement

D

dancing (*continued*)
    d. eyes/dancing feet
    disorder
    d. eye syndrome
    d. feet
dander
    animal d.
    cat d.
Dandy-Walker
    D.-W. cyst
    D.-W. deformity
    D.-W. formation
    D.-W. malformation (DWM)
    D.-W. malformation-basal ganglia
    disease-seizures syndrome
    D.-W. syndrome (DWS)
Dandy-Walker-like syndrome
Dane particle
Danforth sign
danger
    radiation d.
dangerousness
Danlos
    D. disease
    D. syndrome
Danocrine
danthron
D-antigen isoimmunization
Dantrium
dantrolene sodium
Danus-Stanzel repair
DAP
    diastolic arterial pressure
    direct agglutination pregnancy
    DAP test
dapsone
Daranide
Daraprim
Darier
    D. disease
    D. sign
Darier-White disease
darifenacin
darkened reflex
dark-field
    d.-f. examination
    d.-f. microscopy
dark urine
Darrow-Gamble syndrome
darting tongue
Dartos fascia
Darvocet
Darvocet-N 100
Darvon
Darwin
    D. ear
    D. theory of evolution
darwinian
    d. evolution

    d. fitness
    d. reflex
dashboard perineum
DAT
    dementia of Alzheimer type
    direct antiglobulin test
data
    Fibroid Registry for Outcomes Data
    (FIBROID)
    hemodynamic data
    morphologic data
    mortality data
    oximetric data
    sociodemographic data
database
    automatic karyotype system d.
    Cochrane Pregnancy and Childbirth
    D.
    Interstitial Cystitis D.
    National Cancer D.
    POSSUM d.
    Vermont-Oxford Neonatal D.
datalink
    Vaccine Safety D. (VSD)
date
    d. of birth (DOB)
    post d.'s
    d. rape
    small for d.'s
dating
    biopsy d.
    clinical d.
    endometrial d.
    pregnancy d.
daughter
    d. cell
    d. chromosome
    DES d.
daunomycin
daunorubicin
Davidenkow syndrome
David-O'Callaghan syndrome
Davis
    D. bladder catheter
    D. Geck
Davis-Geck Softgut suture
Davydov
    D. vagina construction
    D. vaginoplasty procedure
dawn phenomenon
Dawson
    D. disease
    D. encephalitis
DAX1 gene
day
    Acutrim Late D.
    d. of life (DOL)
daycare
7-day rule

4-day syndrome
Daytrana patch
DAZ
    deleted in azoospermia
        DAZ gene cluster
daze
DAZL1 autosomal homologue
dazzle reflex
dB
    decibel
DBA
    Diamond-Blackfan anemia
DBCP
    dibromochloropropane
d-Biotin
DBP
    double breech presentation
DBS
    diffuse brain swelling
D&C
    dilation and curettage
DCA
    directional coronary atherectomy
DCCT
    diabetes control and complications trial
DCD
    developmental coordination disorder
DCFS
    Department of Children and Family Services
DCIS
    ductal carcinoma in situ
DCL
    diffuse cutaneous leishmaniasis
dCMP
    deoxycytidylic acid
DCS
    Department of Children's Services
DD
    developmental disability
        DD antigen
DDAVP
    desmopressin acetate
        DDAVP nasal spray
ddC
    zalcitabine
DDH
    developmental displacement of hip
    developmental dysplasia of hip
DDI
    decision-to-delivery interval
D-dimer
DDP
    cis-diamminedichloroplatinum
DDS
    Denver Developmental Screening Test
DDSS
    double decidual sac sign

DDST
    Denver Developmental Screening Test
de
    D. Crecchio syndrome
    d. Grouchy syndrome 1, 2
    d. Juan forceps
    d. la Chapelle dysplasia
    d. la Cruz classification
    d. la Cruz classification of congenital aural atresia
    d. Lange syndrome
    d. Lange syndrome 1, 2
    d. Morsier-Gauthier syndrome
    d. Morsier syndrome
    d. novo
    d. novo balanced chromosome rearrangement
    d. novo balanced translocation
    d. novo deletion
    d. Pezzer catheter
    D. Sanctis-Cacchione syndrome
    d. Toni-Fanconi-Debré acute syndrome
    d. Toni-Fanconi syndrome
    D. Vaal disease
    D. Vega tricuspid annuloplasty
D&E
    dilation and evacuation
DE
    diatomaceous earth
dead
    d. fetus syndrome
    full term, born d. (FTBD)
    d. space
    d. space technique
DEAE
    diethylaminoethyl
        DEAE bead
deaf-blindness
deafness
    adventitious d.
    coloboma, heart disease, atresia choanae, retarded growth and development, and/or CNS anomalies, genital hypoplasia, ear anomalies and/or d. (CHARGE)
    congenital nerve d.
    diabetes insipidus and mellitus with optic atrophy and d. (DIDMOAD)
    eighth nerve d.
    goitrous hypothyroidism with d.
    hereditary progressive bulbar paralysis with d.
    d., hypogonadism, hypertrichosis, short stature
    ichthyosiform erythroderma, corneal involvement, d.
    d., imperforate anus, hypoplastic thumbs

deafness (*continued*)
 keratitis, ichthyosis, d. (KID)
 lentigines, electrocardiographic
 abnormalities, ocular hypertelorism,
 pulmonary stenosis, abnormalities
 of genitalia, retardation of growth,
 and d. (LEOPARD)
 maturity onset d.
 neurosensory d.
 pontobulbar palsy with neurosensory
 d.
 prelingual d.
 progressive bulbar palsy with
 perceptive d.
 retardation of growth and d.
 sensorineural d.
deafness-causing allele variant
deafness-craniofacial syndrome
deafness-nephritis syndrome
Deal syndrome
deaminase
 adenosine d. (ADA)
 polyethylene glycol-modified
 adenosine d. (PEG-ADA)
death
 apoptotic cell d.
 brain d.
 d. by calcium
 d. by neurological criteria
 crib d.
 early embryonic d.
 false-negative d.
 fetal brain d.
 infant d.
 injury-related maternal d.
 intrapartum d.
 intrauterine d. (IUD)
 intrauterine fetal d.
 (IUFD)
 maternal d.
 neonatal d. (ND, NND)
 nonmaternal d.
 d. of co-twin
 perinatal d.
 postoperative sudden d.
 d. rattle
 single intrauterine d.
 sudden infant d. (SID)
 sudden intrauterine unexplained d.
 (SIUD)
 sudden unexpected d. (SUD)
Deaver retractor
DEB
 diepoxybutane
DeBakey
 D. aortic clamp
 D. tissue forceps
debrancher enzyme deficiency
debranching enzyme deficiency

Debré-Sémélaigne syndrome
débridement
 broad d.
 thoracoscopic pleural d.
debris
 amniotic d.
 cellular d.
 fetal d.
 keratinous d.
 necrotic cellular d.
 nuclear d.
 stone d.
Debrox Otic
debt
 sleep d.
debulking
 d. of tumor
 optimal d.
 ovarian carcinoma d.
 surgical d.
 tumor d.
debut
 sexual d.
Decadron
 D. Oral
 D. Phosphate Cream
 D. Phosphate Injection
 D. Respihaler
 D. Turbinaire
Decadron-LA Injection
Deca-Durabolin
Decaject Injection
Decaject-LA Injection
decalvans
 keratosis follicularis spinulosa d.
decamethonium bromide
decancellation
 talar d.
decannulate
decanoate
 Haldol D.
 Hybolin D.
decapeptide
decapitate
decapitation
dacarbazaine
 mesna, Adriamycin, Ifosfamide, D.
 (MAID)
decarboxy
decarboxylase
 glutamic acid d. (GAD)
 ornithine d.
 pyruvate d.
decarboxylation
Decavac vaccine
decay
 bottle tooth d.
 tooth d.
decay-accelerating factor

deceleration
    abnormal d.
    early d.
    fetal heart rate d.
    d. injury
    late d.
    nadir of d.
    d. phase
    prolonged variable d.'s
    U-shaped d.
    variable d.
decerebrate
    d. posturing
    d. rigidity
decerebration
decibel (dB)
decidua
    d. basalis
    d. capsularis
    d. compacta
    ectopic d.
    d. menstrualis
    d. parietalis
    d. polyposa
    tuberous subchorial hematoma of d.
    d. vera
decidual
    d. arteriolar atherosis
    d. arteriolopathy
    d. cast
    d. cell
    d. endometritis
    d. fibrinoid necrosis
    d. fibrin thrombosis
    d. floor
    d. lumen
    d. mural thickening
    d. prolactin synthesis
    d. reaction
decidualization
    progestin-induced d.
decidualized endometrium
decidua-macrophage connection
deciduas tuberosa papulosa
deciduate placenta
deciduation
deciduitis
deciduoma
    Loeb d.
deciduous teeth
decision-to-delivery interval (DDI)
decitabine
declining ovarian function
Declomycin
decoding stage
Decofed Syrup
decompensated
    d. cirrhosis
    d. shock

decompensation
decomposition
decompression
    gastric d.
    nasogastric d.
    silo d.
    small intestine d.
    uterine d.
    vaginal d.
decondensation
    sperm chromatin d.
decondensed spermhead injection
decongestant
    Balminil d.
    nasal d.
decontamination
    gastrointestinal d.
decorticate posturing
decortication
    pleural d.
decreased
    d. anal tone
    d. appetite
    d. attending skill
    d. biparietal diameter
    d. breath sound
    d. commissural separation
    d. gastrointestinal motility
    d. libido
    d. mucosal surface
    d. propulsion
    d. red blood cell survival
    d. sphincter tone
    d. talocalcaneal angle
    d. urine output
decrescendo diastolic murmur
decubitus
    d. film
    d. ulcer
decussation
dedicated Doppler probe
deep
    d. cervical node
    d. circumflex iliac artery
    d. dyspareunia
    d. hypothermia and total circulatory arrest (DHCA)
    d. hypothermic circulatory arrest
    d. inferior epigastric perforator (DIEP)
    d. partial-thickness burn
    d. sleep
    d. systemic hypothermia
    d. tendon reflex (DTR)
    d. tendon reflex delayed relaxation phase
    d. transverse arrest
    d. vein thrombophlebitis

D

deep (*continued*)
   d. vein thrombosis (DVT)
   d. venous thrombosis (DVT)
deep-knee bend
deep-set eyes
deer tick
DEET
   diethyltoluamide
   n,n-diethyl-m-toluamide
defasciculation
defecating proctogram
defecation
defecatory dysfunction
defecography
defect
   absence d.
   acyanotic congenital cardiac d.
   alternative pathway d.
   amino acid transport d.
   anatomic support d.
   androgen synthesis d.
   anterior apical vault d.
   anterior neural tube d.
   anterior wall d.
   aorticopulmonary window d.
   arteriovenous canal d.
   atrial septal d. (ASD)
   atrioventricular canal d.
   atrioventricular septal d.
   biochemical d.
   biosynthetic d.
   birth d.
   cardiac septal d.
   central d.
   chromosomal d.
   classical pathway d.
   closed neural tube d.
   coagulation d.
   Coffin-Siris d.
   coloboma, heart defects,
    ichthyosiform dermatosis, mental
    retardation, ear d.'s (CHIME)
   colobomatous d.
   complex heart d.
   conduction d.
   congenital cardiac d.
   congenital ectodermic scalp d.
   congenital heart d. (CHD)
   congenital hemidysplasia with
    ichthyosiform erythroderma and
    limb d.'s (CHILD)
   congenital structural d.
   congenital transport d.
   conotruncal heart d.'s
   coupling d.
   cranial nerve d.
   dehalogenase d.
   dental d.
   diaphragmatic d.

distal sacral d.
early constraint d.
endocardial cushion d. (ECD)
enzyme d.
erythrocyte acquired d.
eustachian tube d.
fetal structural d.
fibrocortical d.
fibrous cortical d.
genetic d.
genetic enzyme d.
genitourinary d.
Gerbode d.
Hartnup d.
heart d.
hydroxylase enzyme d.
intercalary d.
intracardiac d.
intrauterine filling d.
intrauterine positional d.
iodide trap d.
laterality d.
lobulation d.
luteal phase d. (LPD)
metaphysial fibrous d.
microphthalmia with linear skin d.'s
   (MLS)
midline facial d.
mitochondrial respiratory chain d.
müllerian fusion d.
nail d.
neural tube d. (NTD)
nonneural congenital d.
open neural tube d. (ONTD)
opsonin d.
ovulatory d.
paraumbilical d.
paravaginal d.
pelvic support d.
perineal d.
peroxidase d.
Pi type ZZ gene d.
pleiotropic functional d.
posterior wall d.
radial ray d.
recessive disorder d.
red blood cell membrane d.
relative afferent d.
sacral neural tube d.
septal d.
single gene d.
sinus venosus d.
skeletal d.
skin d.
spinal column closure d.
structural brain d.
structural heart d.
subclavian artery d.
supracristal ventricular septal d.

T-cell activation d.
terminal transverse acheiria d.
terminal transverse limb d.
testis migration d.
third-degree d.
thyroid enzyme d.
unbalanced AV canal d.
unrestrictive ventricular septal d.
urea cycle enzyme d.
urinary concentrating d.
uterine lateral fusion d.
ventral wall d.
ventricular septal d. (VSD)
vertebral arch d.
vertebral column d.
visual field d.
X-linked uric aciduria enzyme d.

defectiva
Abiotrophia d.

defective
d. abdominal wall syndrome
d. eye abduction
d. primary platelet aggregation
d. purine metabolism
d. tryptophan absorption

defect-specific repair
defeminization
defense
compromised host d.

defensins
vaginal fluid neutrophil d.

defensiveness
oral tactile d.
tactile d.

defensive obstetrics
deferens
bilateral congenital absence of vas d. (BCAVD)
congenital absence of vas d. (CAVD)
congenital bilateral absence of vas d. (CBAVD)
ductus d.
vas d.

deferiprone
deferoxamine
d. challenge test
d. mesylate

deferred childbearing
defervesced
defervescence
defiant behavior
defibrillation
defibrillator
Lifepak d.

deficiency
abdominal muscle d.
abdominal muscular d.
acid ceramidase d.

acid maltase d. (AMD)
acquired antithrombin III d.
acquired C1 INH d.
acquired growth hormone d.
acquired protein C, S d.
ACTH d.
adenosine deaminase d.
adenylosuccinate d.
adenylosuccinate lyase d. (ASLD)
adrenal cortical d.
adrenocorticotropic hormone d.
AGA d.
aldosterone d.
alpha-antilysin d.
alpha-1 antitrypsin d.
alpha-glucosidase d.
alpha-lipoprotein d.
alpha-N-acetylgalactosaminidase d.
alpha-reductase d.
American Association on Mental D. (AAMD)
Andersen d.
antibody d.
antiplasmin d.
antithrombin III d.
apoenzyme d.
arginase d.
argininosuccinic acid synthetase d.
arylsulfatase-activator d.
ascorbic acid d.
ataxia with isolated vitamin E d.
AT3 d. (types I, II)
B$_6$ d.
beta-galactosidase-1 d.
11-beta-HSD2 d.
11-beta-hydroxysteroid dehydrogenase type 2 d.
biotinidase d.
BLNK d.
brancher d.
branching enzyme d.
calcium d.
carboxylase d.
carnitine acylcarnitine translocase d.
CBS d.
C2–C9 d.
ceruloplasmin d.
C1 esterase inhibitor d.
Chédiak-Higashi d.
cobalamin reductase d.
cofactor d.
cognitive d.
complement d.
congenital growth hormone d.
congenital intrinsic factor d.
congenital lactase d.
congenital lipase/colipase d.
congenital longitudinal d.
congenital TC II d.

D

deficiency (*continued*)
    congenital thyroid d.
    congenital trypsinogen d.
    copper d.
    Cori enzyme d.
    cortisol d.
    CPS d.
    CPT I, II d.
    C1r d.
    creatine d.
    CYP17 d.
    cystathionine beta-synthase d.
    cystathionine synthase d.
    cytochrome *c* oxidase d.
    cytosolic tyrosine transaminase d.
    debrancher enzyme d.
    debranching enzyme d.
    dense body d.
    developmental d.
    dihydropteridine reductase d.
    dihydrotestosterone receptor d.
    (DHTR)
    disaccharidase d.
    EFA d.
    enterokinase d.
    enzyme d.
    epinephrine d.
    erythrocyte enzyme d.
    erythrocyte glutathione peroxidase d.
    erythrocyte phosphoglycerate
    kinase d.
    erythrocyte pyruvate kinase d.
    factor D, H d.
    factor I–XIII d.
    familial APOA-I d.
    familial lecithin:cholesterol
    acyltransferase d.
    femoral d.
    fibrinogen d.
    folate d.
    folic acid d.
    formiminotransferase d.
    fructose galactokinase d.
    FUCA d.
    GABA transaminase d.
    galactokinase d.
    galactosylceramide
    beta-galactosidase d.
    GALC d.
    GALE d.
    GALT d.
    genetic isolated CD59 d.
    GH d.
    glucoamylase d.
    glucocorticoid d.
    glucosamine-6-sulfate d.
    glucuronyl transferase d.
    glutamate formiminotransferase d.
    glutathione synthetase d.

    glycerol kinase d. (GKD)
    glycogen synthetase d.
    GnRH d.
    gonadotropic d.
    granule d.
    growth hormone d. (GHD)
    growth hormone receptor d.
    (GHRD)
    GUSB d.
    HCS d.
    heparin cofactor II d.
    hepatic lipase d.
    hereditary xanthinuria d.
    hexosaminidase A d.
    HGPRT d.
    HMWK d.
    holocarboxylase synthetase d.
    homozygous glucose-6-phosphate
    dehydrogenase d.
    hormone d.
    humoral antibody d.
    11beta-hydroxylase d.
    11-hydroxylase d.
    17-hydroxylase d.
    21-hydroxylase d.
    hyperammonemia due to ornithine
    transcarbamoylase d.
    IDA d.
    idiopathic growth hormone d.
    IDS d.
    IDUA d.
    IgA d.
    IgE d.
    IgG2 d.
    IgG4 d.
    IgM d.
    immune d.
    immunoglobulin G subclass d.
    insulin d.
    interleukin d.
    intrinsic sphincter d. (IDS, ISD)
    iron d.
    isolated gonadotropin d.
    isolated growth hormone d. (IGHD)
    17-ketosteroid reductase d.
    lactase d.
    lactose d.
    late-onset 21-hydroxylase d. (LOHD)
    LCAD d.
    LCAD/MCAD d.
    LCAD/VLCAD d.
    LCHAD d.
    LDH d.
    leukocyte adhesion d. (LAD)
    liver phosphorylase d.
    longitudinal d.
    LPL d.
    luteal phase d.
    magnesium d.

MCAD d.
mental d.
merosin d.
methionine synthase d.
MHC class I antigen d.
micronutrient d.
molybdenum cofactor d. (MCD)
monoamine oxidase A d.
MPO d.
multiple acyl-coenzyme A
  dehydrogenase d. (MADD)
multiple carboxylase d.
multiple pituitary hormone d.
  (MPHD)
multiple sulfatase d. (MSD)
muscle adenosine monophosphate
  deaminase d.
muscle carnitine palmityltransferase
  d.
muscle phosphofructokinase d.
myeloperoxidase d.
myophosphorylase d.
N-acetylgalactosamine-4-sulfatase d.
N-acetylglutamate synthetase d.
neuraminidase d.
neutrophil actin d.
neutrophil chemotactic d.
neutrophil G6PD d.
nonclassic 21-hydroxylase d.
OCT d.
d. of C4-binding protein
d. of C1q
d. of factor B, D
d. of pyruvate carboxylase
ornithine-ketoacid aminotransferase d.
ornithine transcarbamylase d.
  (OTCD)
OTC d.
5-oxoprolinase d.
PAI d.
pancreatic exocrine d.
PDHC d.
PEPCK d.
peroxisomal d.
PFK d.
PGK d.
phosphofructokinase d.
phosphorylase kinase d.
PK d.
placental progesterone d.
placental sulfatase d.
plasminogen activator inhibitor d.
PNP d.
postinfectious secondary lactase d.
prekallikrein d.
primary carnitine d.
primary immune d. (PID)
primary neuraminidase d.
prolactin d.

prolidase d.
properdin d.
propionyl CoA carboxylase d.
prostacyclin d.
protein C d.
protein S d.
proximal femoral focal d.
pseudocholinesterase d.
pyridoxine d.
pyruvate kinase d.
RAG d.
red blood cell enzyme d.
red blood cell phosphoglycerate
  kinase d.
riboflavin d.
SCAD d.
SCOT d.
secondary carnitine d.
selective IgA d.
serotonin d.
skeletal calcium d.
sphincter d.
sphingolipid activator protein d.
steroid sulfatase d.
STS d.
sucrase-isomaltase d.
sulfite oxidase d.
sulfoiduronate sulfatase d. (SIDS)
surfactant protein d.
systemic carnitine d.
systemic fatty acid d.
TBG d.
terminal complement component d.
tetany of vitamin D d.
tetrahydrobiopterin d.
thiamin d.
thymic-dependent d.
thyroid d.
thyroid-binding globulin d.
thyrotropin d.
thyroxine-binding globulin d.
tocopherol d.
TPI d.
TPMT d.
transcobalamin (I, II) d.
transglutaminase d.
trifunctional protein d. (TFP)
triose phosphate isomerase d.
tyrosine aminotransferase d. (TATD)
tyrosine transaminase d.
upper limb d.
urocanase d.
vitamin A d. (VAD)
vitamin B_6 d.
vitamin B_{12} d.
vitamin C d.
vitamin D d.
vitamin E d.
vitamin K d.

D

deficiency (*continued*)
xanthine oxidase d.
X-linked congenital glycerol kinase d.
X-linked monoamine oxidase d.
xylulose dehydrogenase d.
y-cystathionase d.
zinc d.
deficiency-1
leukocyte adhesion d.-1 (LAD-1)
deficiency-2
leukocyte adhesion d.-2 (LAD-2)
deficient
d. enzyme
d. hydroxylation of cholecalciferol
deficit
attention d.
base d.
dichotic listening d.
fluid d.
focal neurologic d.
hemisensory d.
d.'s in attention, motor control, perception (DAMP)
lexical-syntactic d.
naming speed d.
neurodevelopmental d.
posterior column sensory d.
pragmatic and semantic-pragmatic d.'s
sensory d.
spinothalamic sensory d.
d. therapy
definitive
d. surgery
d. therapy
Definity suspension for IV injection
deflection
deflexion abnormality
defloration
defoaming
deformans
cephalhematoma d.
dystonia musculorum d. (DMD)
myodysplasia fetalis d.
myodystrophia fetalis d.
osteochondrodystrophia d.
deformation
plastic d.
shear-strain d.
deformational occipital plagiocephaly
deformity
adduction d.
angular d.
antimongoloid d.
Arnold-Chiari d.
back-knee d.
barrel chest d.

bell-clapper d.
bend d.
bowing d.
bunionette d.
calcaneovalgus d.
cavovarus d.
Chiari d.
cloverleaf skull d.
clubfoot d.
congenital condylar d.
congenital postural d.
coxa vara d.
cubitus valgus d.
Dandy-Walker d.
equinovarus pes d.
equinus d.
fixed flexion d.
flexible positional d.
foot d.
forefoot d.
genu varum d.
gibbous d.
gooseneck d.
gunstock d.
habit tic d.
hindfoot valgus d.
hip d.
hyperextension d.
inversion d.
Jaccoud d.
jaw d.
joint d.
kleeblattschädel d.
limb reduction d. (LRD)
lobster-claw d.
lordotic d.
Madelung d.
Michel d.
mitten hand d.
neurogenic equinus d.
pes cavus d.
ping-pong ball d.
postural d.
protuberant step d.
pseudo-Hurler d.
rachitic bone d.
recurvatum d.
rigid supination d.
round back d.
saber shin d.
saddle-nose d.
shepherd's crook d.
silver fork d.
spinning-top d.
split-foot d.
Sprengel d.
static d.
supratip nasal tip d.
talipes equinovarus d.

thumb in palm d.
torsional d.
Volkmann d.
windswept d.
wryneck d.
defunctionalized bladder
degenerate
d. consensus primer
d. oligonucleotide primer
(DOP)
degenerated fibroadenolipoma
degenerating myoma
degeneration
anterior horn cell d.
axonal d.
carneous d.
cerebellar d.
cerebromacular d.
cochleosaccular d.
congenital macular d.
congenital progressive
oculoacousticocerebral d.
cystic myoma d.
dominant Doyne honeycomb
retinal d.
dying-back axonal d.
familial striatal d.
hepatolenticular d.
hereditary oligophrenic cerebellolental
d.
hyaline myoma d.
hypobetalipoproteinemia,
acanthocytosis, retinitis pigmentosa,
pallidal d. (HARP)
infantile neuronal d.
infantile striatonigral d.
joint d.
Leber congenital tapetoretinal d.
malignant d.
molar d.
mucoid myoma d.
myocardial fiber d.
nuclear d.
oligodendroglial d.
olivopontocerebellar d.
pallidal d.
pulpal d.
red d.
retinal pigmentary d.
sarcomatous myoma d.
spinocerebellar d.
spongy d.
subacute combined d.
tapetoretinal d.
uterine fibroid carneous d.
uterine fibroid red d.
vitelliform d.
wallerian d.
white matter d.

degenerative
d. arthritis
d. osteoarthritis
degloving injury
deglutition
degradable starch microsphere (DSM)
degradation
fibrin d.
ganglioside d.
glycoprotein d.
degranulation
30-degree lens
70-degree lens
degree of kindred
45-degree skin traction
dehalogenase defect
dehiscence
asymptomatic d.
episiotomy d.
uterine scar d.
wound d.
dehydrated
dehydration
d. fever
hemorrhagic d.
hypernatremic d.
hyperosmolar d.
hypertonic d.
hyponatremic d.
hypotonic d.
hypovolemic d.
isonatremic d.
isotonic d.
mild d.
moderate d.
d., poisoning, trauma (DPT)
severe d.
dehydrocholate (DHC)
7-dehydrocholesterol
dehydroepiandrosterone (DHEA)
d. sulfate (DHEAS)
d. sulfate loading test
dehydrogenase
acetyl-CoA d.
17-beta-estradiol d.
3-beta-hydroxysteroid d. (3-betaHSD)
electron transfer flavoprotein d.
(ETF-DH)
glucose-6-phosphate d. (G6PD)
15-hydroxyprostaglandin d.
18-hydroxysteroid d.
isovaleryl-CoA d.
lactate d. (LDH)
lactic acid d. (LDH)
long- and medium-chain acyl-CoA
d. (LCAD/MCAD)
long and very long chain acyl-CoA
d. (LCAD/VLCAD)
long-chain acyl-CoA d. (LCAD)

D

dehydrogenase (*continued*)
    long-chain 3-hydroxyacyl-CoA d.
      (LCHAD)
    long-chain hydroxyacyl-coenzyme A
      d. (LCHAD)
    medium-chain acyl-CoA d. (MCAD)
    pyruvate d.
    short-chain acyl coenzyme A d.
      (SCAD)
    short-chain hydroxyacyl-coenzyme A
      d. (SCHAD)
    succinate d.
    very long chain acyl-CoA d.
      (VLCAD)
dehydrogenation
    pyruvate d.
dehydroisoandrosterone sulfate
dehydroxylase
    phenylalanine d.
Dejerine disease
Dejerine-Klumpke syndrome
Dejerine-Sottas
    D.-S. atrophy
    D.-S. disease
    D.-S. syndrome
Dekasol Injection
Dekasol-L.A. Inject
del
    deletion
    d. 11/aniridia complex
    D. Aqua-10 Gel
    D. Aqua-5 Gel
    d. Castillo syndrome
Delalutin
Delaprem
Delatestryl Injection
delavirdine
Delaxin
delay
    adaptive d.
    atrioventricular conduction d.
    benign maturation d.
    cognitive d.
    constitutional growth d.
    developmental d.
    global developmental d.
    growth d.
    language d.
    neurodevelopmental d.
    physiologic d.
    puberal d.
    radial-femoral d.
    speech d.
    d. syndrome
delayed
    d. bone age
    d. chemotherapy-associated nausea
    d. deep tendon reflex
    d. fertilization

    d. first stage
    d. gastric emptying
    d. hypersensitivity
    d. implantation
    d. menarche
    d. menstruation
    d. motor development
    d. myelopathy
    d. neuropsychological sequela
      (DNS)
    d. orthostatic intolerance
    d. phase computed tomography
    d. primary closure
    d. puberty
    d. relaxation phase
    d. repair
    d. sexual maturation
    d. sleep phase syndrome (DSPS)
    d. thyrotropin elevation
    d. tooth eruption
    d. transfusion reaction
    d. union
delayed-type hypersensitivity (DTH)
**Delbet fracture classification (type
I–IV)**
Delclos
    D. cylinder
    D. ovoid
Delcort Topical
DeLee
    D. forceps
    D. instrumentation
    D. maneuver
    D. suction catheter
    D. suction device
    D. suctioning
    D. Universal retractor
Delestrogen
deleted in azoospermia (DAZ)
deletion (del)
    autosomal d.
    chromosomal d.
    chromosome d.
    de novo d.
    elastin gene d.
    gene d.
    interstitial d.
    d. of chromosome
    d. 1p–22p syndrome
    d. 1q–22q syndrome
    d. 1–22 syndrome
    terminal d.
    Xp d.
    d. Xp21 syndrome
    d. Xp22 syndrome
    d. Xq syndrome
Delfen
delinquency
delinquent

delirium
    d., infection, atrophic urethritis and vaginitis, pharmacologic cause, psychological cause, excessive urine production, restricted mobility, stool impaction (DIAPPERS)
    d., infection, atrophic urethritis/vaginitis, pharmaceuticals, psychological, excess urine
    d., infection, pharmacology, psychology, endocrinopathy, restricted mobility, stool impaction

delivered
    pregnancy, uterine, not d. (PUND)

Deliver formula

delivery
    abdominal d.
    d. area
    arterial oxygen d. (DO_2)
    assisted breech d.
    assisted cephalic d.
    assisted spontaneous vaginal d.
    asynchronous multifetal d.
    breech vaginal d.
    cephalic d.
    cesarean d. (CD)
    controlled vaginal d.
    Duncan mechanism of placental d.
    elective cesarean d.
    en caul d.
    expected date of d. (EDD)
    expeditious d.
    failed forceps d.
    fear-causing d.
    fearless first d.
    fear of d.
    forceps d. (FD)
    high forceps d.
    instrumental d.
    intraventricular opioid d.
    Kiwi ProCup d.
    labor and d. (L&D)
    low forceps d.
    midforceps d. (MFD)
    d. mode
    natural d.
    near-term d.
    normal spontaneous vaginal d. (NSVD)
    normal vaginal d. (NVD)
    operative vaginal d.
    outlet forceps d.
    oxygen d.
    perimortem d.
    postmortem d.
    precipitate labor and d.
    precipitous d.
    premature d.
    preterm d. (PTD)
    previous preterm d.
    d. record
    d. room
    rotational d.
    route of d.
    sequential d.
    soft cup vacuum d.
    spontaneous cephalic d.
    spontaneous preterm d.
    spontaneous vaginal d. (SVD)
    sterile, spontaneous, controlled vaginal d. (SSCVD)
    sterile, spontaneous vaginal d. (SSVD)
    sunny-side up d.
    term d.
    traumatic d.
    twin d.
    underwater d.
    vacuum-assisted d.
    vacuum extraction d.
    vacuum extractor d.
    vaginal breech d.
    vertex d.

Delleman syndrome

Dellepiane hysterectomy

Delorme rectal prolapse repair procedure

del(5p) chromosome

Delsym

delta (Δ)
    d. agent
    d. hepatitis
    d. OD_{450}
    d. phalanx
    D. shunt
    d. sleep
    d. wave

Delta-Cortef Oral

delta-F508 cystic fibrosis

Deltasone

Deltatrac II indirect calorimeter

deltoid
    d. insertion
    d. muscle
    d. paralysis

delusion
    grandiose d.

Demadex
    D. Injection
    D. Oral

demand
    d. effect
    d. feeding

demander
    entitled d.

demarcated

demecarium

D

demeclocycline
dementia
    Heller d.
    d. of Alzheimer type (DAT)
Demerol
demineralization
    acral d.
    bone d.
demise
    fetal d.
    intrapartum d.
    intrauterine fetal d.
    single fetal d.
    single-twin d.
    spontaneous preterm labor with
      intrapartum d.
    twin d.
demodex
    D. brevis
    D. folliculorum
    D. phylloides
demographic
Demons-Meigs syndrome
Demser
Demulen
    D. 1/35
    D. 1/50
demyelinating encephalopathy
demyelination, demyelinization
    inflammatory d.
    symmetric d.
demyelinative
demyelinization (*var. of* demyelination)
demyelinogenic leukodystrophy
denature
denaturing
    d. gradient gel electrophoresis
    d. high-performance liquid
      chromatography
Denavir
dendritic
    d. arborization
    d. cell
    d. cell-related disorder
    d. keratitis
denervation
dengue
    d. fever
    d. hemorrhagic fever
    d. shock syndrome
    d. virus
Denhardt solution
denial stage
denidation
Denis
    D. Browne bar
    D. Browne clubfoot splint
    D. Browne night splint
    D. Browne pouch

Denman spontaneous evolution
Dennen forceps
Dennie
    D. line
    D. line of lower eyelid
Dennie-Marfan syndrome
Dennie-Morgan
    D.-M. fold
    D.-M. line
Dennyson-Fulford extraarticular subtalar
    arthrodesis
Denonvilliers fascia
Denorex
dens
    hypoplastic d.
densa
    sublamina d.
dense
    d. adhesion
    d. band
    d. body
    d. body deficiency
    d. cast
    d. striation
densitometer
    DXA d.
    Expert bone d.
    Hologic 1000 QDR d.
    OsteoAnalyzer d.
    PIXI bone d.
    QDR-1500 bone d.
densitometry
    bone d.
    dynamic spiral CT lung d.
density
    areal bone mineral d. (aBMD)
    arterial linear d.
    bone d.
    bone mineral d. (BMD)
    fat d.
    d. gradient
    hip bone d.
    hypoechoic d.
    increased bone d.
    lamellar body number d.
    optic d.
    radiographic d.
    soft tissue d.
    d. spectral array
    volumetric bone d.
    volumetric bone mineral d. (vBMD)
dental
    d. abscess
    d. avulsion
    d. caries
    d. cementum
    d. crowding
    d. dam
    d. defect

d. enamel hypoplasia
d. extrusion
d. extrusion/lateral luxation
d. intrusion
d. lamina cyst
d. speech appliance
d. trauma
dentate
d. line
d. nucleus
dentatorubral atrophy
dentatorubral-pallidoluysian atrophy (DRPLA)
dentia praecox
denticulate hymen
dentigerous cyst
dentin dysplasia
dentinogenesis imperfecta
dentition
permanent d.
primary d.
dentoalveolar unit
dentoauriculoskeletal
cerebroocular d. (CODAS)
denuded surface
denumerable character
Denver
D. classification
D. Developmental chart
D. Developmental Screening Test (DDS, DDST)
D. Developmental Screening Test II
D. Home Screening Questionnaire
D. hydrocephalus shunt
D. II screening
Denys-Drash syndrome
deodorant artifact
deossification
deoxyadenosine
deoxyadenosylcobalamin
deoxyadenylic acid (dAMP)
deoxycholate
amphotericin B d. (AmBd)
deoxycorticosterone (DOC)
deoxycytidylic acid (dCMP)
deoxy-D-glucose
deoxyguanylic acid (dGMP)
deoxyhemoglobin (MbO2)
deoxynucleotide triphosphate
deoxypyridinoline (Dpd)
deoxyribonuclease (DNAse, DNase)
deoxyribonucleic
d. acid (DNA)
d. acid analysis
d. acid index
deoxyribonucleotide
15-deoxyspergualin
deoxythymidylic acid (dTMP)
Depacon

Depakene
Depakote sprinkle
department
D. of Children and Family Services (DCFS)
D. of Children and Youth Services
D. of Children's Services (DCS)
D. of Public Social Services (DPSS)
pediatric emergency d. (PED)
dependence
coital d.
vitamin D d.
dependency
chemical d.
pyridoxine d.
dependent
d. edema
d. pooling
depersonalization
depigmentation
d. disorder
postinflammatory d.
depigmented nevus
depigmentosus
nevus d.
depilation
depleted
lymphocyte d.
depletion
germ-cell d.
intravascular volume d.
juvenile spermatogonial d.
T-cell d.
Depo-Estradiol Injection
Depogen Injection
depolarization
atrial premature d.
ectopic ventricular d.
ventricular premature d.
Depo-Medrol injection
depo-medroxyprogesterone
depomedroxyprogesterone acetate (DMPA)
depo-MPA
Deponit
Depopred Injection
Depo-Provera Injection
deposit
electron-dense subepithelial d.
granular osmiophilic d.
macrocephaly with feeblemindedness and encephalopathy with peculiar d.'s
deposition
complement d.
copper d.
cystine d.
diffuse perivillous fibrinoid d.

D

deposition (*continued*)
  fat d.
  fibrin d.
  hemosiderin d.
  IgA mesangial d.
  immunoglobulin d.
  neonatal elastin d.
depot
  Androcur D.
  Lupron D.
  Sandostatin LAR D.
Depo-Testadiol
Depo-Testosterone Injection
depot-F
  abarelix d.-F
depot-M
  abarelix d.-M
Depot-Ped
  Lupron D.-P.
depressed
  d. fontanelle
  d. scar
  d. sensorium
  d. skull fracture
depression
  agitated d.
  anaclitic d.
  anxiety d.
  atypical d.
  bipolar d.
  bright white light therapy for
    postpartum d.
  cardiovascular d.
  cortical spreading d.
  double d.
  fetal skull d.
  inbreeding d.
  intimate partner d.
  melancholic d.
  narcotic d.
  neonatal respiratory d.
  paternal postnatal d.
  ping-pong ball d.
  posteromedial articular d.
  postictal d.
  postnatal d. (PND)
  postpartum d. (PPD)
  prepuberal d.
  psychotic d.
  d. rating scale
  respiratory d.
  d. screening
  D. Self-Rating Scale
  d. stage
  treatment-refractory d.
  unipolar d.
depressive
  d. disorder
  d. symptom

depressor
  d. anguli oris
  d. anguli oris muscle
  d. anguli oris muscle hypoplasia
    syndrome
  tongue d.
  torque d.
deprivation
  d. amblyopia
  antagonist-induced
    gonadotropin d.
  estrogen d.
  idiocy by d.
  oxygen d.
  psychosocial d.
  social d.
depth
  crypt d.
  d. dose (E_d)
  Douglas d.
  d. perception
  d. relationship
  vertical pocket d.
derangement
  internal d.
  physiologic d.
Dercum disease
derealization
derecruitment
derepressed gene
derivation
  sexual d.
derivative
  acetoxyprogesterone d.
  17-alpha-acetoxyprogesterone d.
  d. chromosome
  coumarin d.
  19-nortestosterone d.
  purified protein d.
    (PPD)
Dermablend
Dermabond
dermabrasion
Dermacentor
  D. andersoni
  D. variabilis
Dermacort Topical
dermal
  d. erythropoiesis
  d. melanocytosis
  d. melanosis
  d. nevus
  d. sinus
  d. sinus tract
  d. vasculitis
  d. vitiligo
Dermarest Dricort Topical
Derma-Smoothe/FS Topical
Dermasone

dermatan
    d. sulfate
    d. sulfate accumulation
dermatitic
dermatitidis
    Blastomyces d.
dermatitis
    allergic contact d.
    atopic d.
    brawny d.
    burnlike d.
    Candida diaper d.
    candidal diaper d.
    cercarial d.
    chronic bullous d.
    chronic eczematoid d.
    contact d.
    diaper d.
    eczematoid d.
    d. enteropathica
    exfoliative d.
    follicular d.
    friction d.
    d. gangrenosa infantum
    d. herpetiformis (DH)
    d. herpetiformis-associated
      gluten-sensitive enteropathy
    infantile seborrheic d.
    infectious eczematoid d.
    infective d.
    irradiation d.
    irritant contact d.
    irritant diaper d.
    isolated vulvar seborrheic d.
    Jacquet erosive diaper d.
    juvenile plantar d.
      (JPD)
    mask of atopic d.
    monilial diaper d.
    neonatal bullous d.
    neonatal seborrheic d.
    nickel d.
    nummular d.
    occlusion d.
    perianal d.
    periorificial d.
    photosensitive d.
    progesterone d.
    psoriatic d.
    rebound d.
    rhus d.
    scalp seborrheic d.
    scaly d.
    seborrheic d.
    shoe contact d.
    tide mark d.
    d. venenata
    vesiculopustular d.
    vulvar d.

    vulvar seborrheic d.
    weeping d.
dermatofibroma
dermatofibrosarcoma protuberans
dermatofibrosis lenticularis disseminata
dermatoglyphic
    d. abnormality
    d. finding
    d. pattern
dermatoglyphics
dermatoleukodystrophy
dermatology
    neonatal d.
    pediatric d.
dermatomal distribution
dermatomegaly
dermatomyositis (DM)
    amyopathic juvenile d.
    juvenile d. (JDM, JDMS)
    primary idiopathic d.
dermatomyositis/polymyositis
dermatoosteolysis
    Kirghizian d.
Dermatop
dermatophyte
    d. infection
    d. lesion
    d. test medium (DTM)
dermatophytid reaction
dermatophytosis
dermatoses (*pl. of* dermatosis)
dermatosis, *pl.* dermatoses
    acute febrile neurophilic d.
    bullous d.
    dermolytic bullous d.
    ichthyosiform d.
    idiopathic d.
    juvenile plantar d. (JPD)
    lichenoid vulvar d.
    linear IgA d.
    d. of kwashiorkor
    plantar d.
    Siemens-Bloch pigmented d.
    vulvar d.
dermis
    papillary d.
    reticular d.
    thinned d.
dermocyma
dermoepidermal junction
dermographism
    white d.
dermoid
    d. cyst
    d. cyst of ovary
    epibulbar d.
    d. sinus
    d. sinus tract
Dermolate Topical

D

dermolipoma
dermolysis bullosa
dermolytic bullous dermatosis
dermopathy
    nephrogenic fibrosing d.
    restrictive d.
Dermoplast
dermotrichic syndrome
Dermovate
Dermtex HC with Aloe Topical
Derogatis Brief Symptom
 Inventory
Deronil
derotation femoral osteotomy
Derry syndrome
DES
    diethylstilbestrol
    Dissociative Experience Scale
        DES daughter
        DES exposure
25-desacetyl rifapentine
DESAD
    National Collaborative Diethylstilbestrol
    Adenosis Project
desalination
desaturate
desaturation
    red d.
Desbuquois syndrome
Descemet membrane
descending
    d. aorta
    d. aorta anastomosis
    d. colon
    left anterior d. (LAD)
    d. perineum syndrome
    (DPS)
descensus uteri
descent
    aberrant course of testicular d.
    d. during labor
    fetal d.
    identical by d. (IBD)
    perineal d.
    rapid d.
    rotation and d.
    second-degree d.
    spontaneous d.
    testicular d.
    third-degree d.
Deschamps ligature
descriptive embryology
Desenex
    Prescription Strength D.
desensitization
    imaginal d.
    pituitary d.
desert rheumatism
Desferal Mesylate

desferrioxamine
    d. mesylate
    d. therapy
desflurane
desiccate
design
    family-based d.
designated donor blood
designation
    eligibility d.
designed
    Dortmund Nutritional and
      Anthropometrical Longitudinally D.
      (DONALD)
designer
    Pharsight Trial D.
desipramine
desire
    hypoactive sexual d.
    inhibited sexual d. (ISD)
    sexual d.
Desitin
deslanoside
deslorelin
Desmarres
    D. forceps
    D. retractor
desmethylimipramine
desmins
desmiognathus
desmocranium
desmoid tumor
desmolase
    cholesterol 20, 22 d.
Desmons syndrome
desmoplasia
    intratumoral d.
desmoplastic
    d. infantile ganglioglioma (DIG)
    d. medulloblastoma
    d. small round cell tumor
      (DSRCT)
desmopressin
    d. acetate (DDAVP)
    d. acetate nasal spray
    intranasal d.
desmosome
Desocort
Desogen
desogestrel
    d. and ethinyl estradiol
    ethinyl estradiol and d.
desonide
desorption
DesOwen Topical
desoximetasone
desoxycholate amphotericin B
Desoxyn
desquamated epithelial cell

desquamation
    follicular d.
    perineal d.
    periungual d.
desquamative
    d. inflammatory vaginitis
    d. interstitial pneumonia (DIP)
    d. interstitial pneumonitis (DIP)
desquamativum
    erythroderma d.
Desquam-E Gel
Desquam-X Gel
destruction
    hypothalamic-hypophysial d.
    iatrogenic d.
    physial d.
    postirradiation d.
destructive grasping forceps
destruens
    chorioadenoma d.
    molar d.
desultory labor
Desyrel
detach
detachment
    exudative retinal d.
    retinal d.
    rhegmatogenous d.
    serous retinal d.
    tractional retinal d.
    urethral d.
detail
    cycle-monitoring d.
Detect HIV-1 assay
detection
    leucocyte d.
    mammographic d.
    prenatal d.
    d. rate
detector
    Pedi-cap d.
detergens
    liquor carbonis d.
deterioration
    central syndrome of rostrocaudal d.
    fetal d.
determinant
    antigen d.
    culture-specific d.
    d. group
    sialyl Lewis X d.
determination
    blood gas d.
    bone age d.
    cell d.
    emesis pH d.
    fetal sex d.
    gender d.
    hematocrit d.

    hemoglobin A1c d.
    parentage d.
    prenatal sex d.
    scalp pH d.
    selective renal vein renin d.
    sex d.
    sweat chloride d.
    testis d.
    ultrasonographic d.
detorsion
    manual d.
detoxification
Detroit Test of Learning Aptitude 2
detrusor
    d. contraction
    d. hyperactivity with incomplete
      contractility (DHIC)
    d. hyperreflexia
    d. instability
    d. muscle
    d. overactivity
    d. pressure
    d. sphincter dyssynergia
    d. tone
detrusorrhaphy
detumescence
devascularization
development
    abnormal fetal d.
    adaptive d.
    alveolar d.
    alveolar stage of lung d.
    arrested d.
    Assessment in Infancy Ordinal
      Scales of Psychological D.
    axillary hair d.
    Bayley Scales of Infant D. (BSID)
    breast d.
    Brigance Diagnostic Inventory of
      Early D.
    canalicular stage of lung d.
    cardiovascular d.
    cellular and molecular regulation of
      lung d.
    cephalocaudal sequence of d.
    CNS d.
    cytoarchitectural d.
    delayed motor d.
    dissociated motor d.
    early follicular d.
    embryonic d.
    emotional d.
    endometrial d.
    Erikson stages of growth and d.
    excretory system d.
    expressive language d.
    fetal d.
    fetal lung d.
    fetal respiratory d.

D

development (*continued*)
  fine motor d.
  genital d.
  goiter d.
  Griffith Scale of Mental D.
  gross d.
  gross motor d.
  hearing d.
  incomplete alveolar d.
  infant d.
  language d.
  lung growth and d.
  male genital duct d.
  mental d.
  National Institute of Child Health
    and Human D. (NICHD)
  neurologic d. (ND)
  normal fetal d.
  Ordinal Scales of Intellectual D.
  phonological d.
  pseudoglandular stage of lung d.
  psychosocial d.
  pulmonary vascular d.
  receptive language d.
  reproductive system d.
  saccular stage of lung d.
  social d.
  d. specialist
  speech d.
  stromal d.
  Tanner stage of d. (1–5)
  Tanner staging of genital d. (1–5)
  trilineage d.
  visual d.
developmental
  d. age (DA)
  d. area
  d. assessment
  d. assessment score
  D. Behaviour Checklist
  d. cataract
  d. check
  d. coordination disorder (DCD)
  d. crisis
  d. deficiency
  d. delay
  d. delay-multiple strawberry nevi
    syndrome
  d. diapause
  d. disability (DD)
  d. disorder
  d. displacement of hip (DDH)
  d. dissociation
  d. dysfluency
  d. dyslexia
  d. dysphasia
  d. dysplasia of hip (DDH)
  d. flatfoot
  d. genu varum

  d. hip disease
  d. hip dysplasia
  d. issue
  d. language disorder (DLD)
  d. level
  d. milestone
  d. motor quotient (DMQ)
  d. pattern
  d. pattern disorder
  D. Profile-II (DP-II)
  D. Programming for Infants and
    Young Children
  d. quotient (DQ)
  d. screening
  d. stage
  d. surveillance
  D. Test of Visual-Motor Integration
dvelopment-II
  Bayley Scales of Infant D.-II
    (BSID-II)
Deventer pelvis
deviant volitional movement
deviated septum
deviation
  axis d.
  eye d.
  jaw d.
  left axis d.
  right axis d.
  septal d.
  sexual d.
  standard d. (SD)
Devic disease
device
  AcuTrainer d.
  AeroChamber spacer d.
  alternative communication d.
  Amplatzer d.
  antisiphon d.
  aspiration-tulip d.
  Atad Ripener d.
  augmentative communication d.
  AutoPap automated screening d.
  autostapling d.
  barium-impregnated plastic
    intrauterine d.
  BVM d.
  Cameco syringe pistol aspiration d.
  CardioSeal d.
  central venous access d. (CVAD)
  CerviSoft cytology collection d.
  clamshell-type catheter occlusion d.
  clitoral therapy d. (CTD)
  Colpexin sphere intravaginal d.
  Contiform incontinence d.
  contraceptive d.
  Copper T intrauterine d.
  CryoHit cryotherapy d.
  Cu-7 intrauterine d.

CycleBeads fertility d.
DeLee suction d.
Diva laparoscopic morcellator d.
Donnez d.
double-balloon d.
double-umbrella d.
dynamic orthotic cranioplasty d.
EarPopper inflation d.
Eder cord blood collection d.
electric suction d.
Endo Stitch laparoscopic suturing d.
Eros-CTD eroscillator d.
evacuation d.
ExacTech glucose measuring d.
external urethral barrier d.
FemAssist d.
FemCap barrier contraceptive d.
Finapres d.
flutter d.
FNA-21 fine-needle aspiration d.
Gianturco-Grifka vascular
    occlusion d.
GynoSampler endometrial
    sampling d.
handheld flutter d.
HemoCue AB hemoglobin
    measurement d.
Hollister collecting d.
Ilizarov d.
Implanon contraceptive d.
intracavity d.
intrauterine d. (IUD)
intrauterine contraception d.
    (IUCD)
intrauterine contraceptive d. (ICD,
    IUD)
intravaginal support d.
IVS Tunneller d.
Kiwi vacuum-assisted fetal
    delivery d.
knee height measuring d.
left ventricular assist d. (LVAD)
Lippes-type intrauterine d.
Macroplastique implantable d.
Makler insemination d.
McMaster Family Assessment D.
M-cup vacuum extraction d.
Medilog 9000 polysomnography d.
Mirena intrauterine d.
Mucat cervical sampling d.
Multiload Cu-375 intrauterine d.
Multispatula cervical sampling d.
Niplette d.
NovaSure d.
One Step Button gastrostomy d.
OraSure d.
OsteoView d.
Papette d.
ParaGard intrauterine copper d.

Poly CS d.
Progestasert intrauterine d.
progesterone-releasing T-shaped d.
Protocult stool sampling d.
ReliefBand d.
Scopette d.
Seitzinger d.
sequential compression d.
Shug male contraceptive d.
STARFlex d.
STOP nonsurgical permanent
    contraception d.
Tcu-380A intrauterine d.
umbrella d.
vacuum clitoral therapy d.
Venodyne pneumatic compressive d.
ventricular assist d.
Wallach Endocell collection d.
Z sampler endometrial sampling d.

DeWeese axis traction forceps
Dewey obstetrical forceps
deworm
DEXA
    dual-energy x-ray absorptiometry
    DEXA scan
Dexacidin Ophthalmic
Dexacort
    D. Phosphate Respihaler Oral
        Inhaler
    D. Phosphate Turbinaire
    D. Phosphate Turbinaire Intranasal
        Aerosol
Dex-A-Diet
dexamethasone
    methotrexate, bleomycin, doxorubicin,
        cyclophosphamide, Oncovin, d.
        (m-BACOD)
    d., neomycin polymyxin B
    pulse d.
    d. suppression test
    d. suppression testing (DST)
    d. therapy
    vincristine and d.
Dexameth Oral
Dexasone L.A. Injection
Dexasporin Ophthalmic
Dexatrim
dexbrompheniramine
dexchlorpheniramine
Dexedrine Spansule capsule
dexfenfluramine
Dexide
    D. disposable cannula
    D. disposable trocar
dexiocardia (*var. of* dextrocardia)
Dexon
    D. II suture
    D. mesh
    D. Plus suture

D

Dexone
- D. LA
- D. LA Injection
- D. Tablet

dexpanthenol

dexrazoxane

dexter
- cor triatriatum d.

dextran (DX)
- d. 40
- HMW d.
- iron d.
- LMW d.
- low molecular weight d. (LMWD)
- d. sulfate

dextran-70 barrier material

dextrans
- limit d.

dextrin
- d. sulfate
- d. sulfate gel

dextrinosis
- limit d.

dextroamphetamine (DA)
- d. saccharate
- d. sulfate

dextrocardia, dexiocardia
- mirror-image d.

dextrocardia/situs inversus syndrome

dextromethorphan
- guaifenesin and d.

dextroposition
- anomalous right pulmonary vein d.
- d. of heart

dextrose in water

Dextrostix reagent strip

dextrosuria

dextrothyroxine

dextrotransposition (D-transposition)

dextroversion

Dey-Drop Ophthalmic Solution

Dey-Wash skin wound cleanser

DF
- diabetic fetopathy

DFA
- direct fluorescent antibody
- direct fluorescent antigen
- DFA stain
- DFA staining
- DFA test

D-fenfluramine

DFFRY gene

DFMO
- difluoromethyl ornithine

DFMR
- daily fetal movement record

DFNA3
- autosomal dominant nonsyndromic hearing loss

DFNB1
- autosomal-recessive nonsyndromic hearing loss

DFS
- disease-free survival

D-galactose

dGMP
- deoxyguanylic acid

DH
- dermatitis herpetiformis

DHA
- docosahexaenoic acid
- Citracal Prenatal + DHA

DHC
- dehydrocholate

DHCA
- deep hypothermia and total circulatory arrest

DHEA
- dehydroepiandrosterone
- DHEA sulfate

DHEAS
- dehydroepiandrosterone sulfate

DHIC
- detrusor hyperactivity with incomplete contractility

DHT
- dihydrotestosterone

DHTR
- dihydrotestosterone receptor deficiency

DI
- diabetes insipidus
- donor insemination

DIA
- diametric inhibin A
- dot immunobinding assay

DiaBeta

diabetes
- borderline d.
- brittle d.
- bronze d.
- chemical d.
- congenital lipoatrophic d.
- d. control and complications trial (DCCT)
- drug-induced d.
- gestational d. (GD)
- D. in Early Pregnancy Study
- d. insipidus (DI)
- d. insipidus and mellitus with optic atrophy and deafness (DIDMOAD)
- d. insipidus, diabetes mellitus, optic atrophy (DIDMO)
- insulin-dependent d.
- juvenile d.
- juvenile-onset d. (JOD)

ketosis-prone d.
ketosis-resistant d.
latent d.
lipoatrophic d.
maternal d.
maturity-onset d.
d. mellitus, mental retardation, lipodystrophy, dysmorphic traits syndrome
d. mellitus (type 1, 2) (DM)
d. neonatorum
non-insulin-dependent d.
pregestational d.
D. Prevention Trial
streptozocin-induced d.
sugar d.
transient neonatal d. (TND)
diabetes-associated maternal complication
diabetes-deafness syndrome
diabetes-related congenital malformation
diabetic
d. acidosis
d. cardiomyopathy
d. cheiroarthropathy
d. coma
d. embryopathy
d. fetopathy (DF)
insulin-dependent d.
d. ketoacidosis (DKA)
d. mother
d. nephropathy
non-insulin-dependent d.
pregnant d.
d. retinopathy
D. Tussin DM
D. Tussin EX
diabeticorum
necrobiosis lipoidica d. (NLD)
diabetogenic effect of pregnancy
Diabinese
diacetate
diflorasone d.
ethinyl estradiol and ethynodiol d.
ethynodiol d.
propylene glycol d.
diacylglycerol (DAG)
diadochokinesis
diagnosed
acute, critical, unexpected, treatable, easily d. (ACUTE)
diagnosis
antenatal d.
ayurvedic d.
colposcopic d.
computer-aided d. (CAD)
established medical d.
fetal d.
genetic d.
histologic d.

histopathological d.
neonatal d.
preimplantation d.
preimplantation genetic d. (PGD)
prenatal genetic d.
ultrasonographic d.
ultrasound d.
visual d.
diagnostic
d. accuracy
D. and Statistical Manual of Mental Disorders, 4th Edition (DSM-IV)
d. hysteroscope
d. imaging
D. Interview for Genetic Study (DIGS)
D. Interview Schedule for Children (DISC)
D. Interview Schedule for Children-Revised (DISC-R)
d. mammography
d. maneuver
d. overshadowing
d. peritoneal lavage (DPL)
d. procedure
d. radiation
d. ultrasonography
diagnostics
Amplicor PCR d.
DNA d.
Roche D.
diagonal conjugate
diakinesis
d. stage
d. stage of oocyte meiosis
dialectical
dialysate protein loss
dialysis
continuous ambulatory peritoneal d. (CAPD)
continuous cyclic peritoneal d. (CCPD)
kidney d.
peritoneal d. (PD)
dialytic parabiosis
diameter
anteroposterior d. (APD, A-PD)
aortic root d.
AP d.
Baudelocque d.
biischial d.
biparietal d. (BPD)
bitemporal d.
conjugate d. (CD)
decreased biparietal d.
fetal biparietal d.
gestational sac mean d.
increased anteroposterior chest d.
internal d.

D

diameter (*continued*)
 intertuberous d.
 Loehlein d.
 narrow bifrontal d.
 d. obliqua
 oblique d.
 obstetric conjugate d.
 occipitofrontal d. (OFD)
 occipitomental d.
 plane of greatest d.
 plane of least d.
 posterior sagittal d.
 suboccipitobregmatic d.
 trachelobregmatic d.
 d. transversa
 transverse d.
2-diameter pocket technique
diametric inhibin A (DIA)
diaminobenzidine
 3,3′ d.
3,3′ diaminobenzidine
diamniotic
 d. dichorionic placenta
 d. twins
Diamond-Blackfan
 D.-B. anemia (DBA)
 D.-B. congenital hypoplastic
  anemia
 D.-B. juvenile pernicious anemia
 D.-B. syndrome
Diamond medium
diamond-shaped murmur
Diamox Sequels
Diana
 D. complex
 D. Project
Dianabol
Dianeal dialysis solution
Diaparene
diapause
 developmental d.
 embryonic d.
diapedetic leukocyte
diaper
 d. dermatitis
 double d.'s
 d. rash
 d. syndrome
 triple d.'s
 zinc-free plastic-lined d.
diaphanography
diaphoresis
diaphoretic
diaphragm
 arcing spring d.
 coil spring d.
 contraceptive d.
 duodenal d.
 eventration of d.

 everted d.
 flat spring d.
 hinged spring d.
 intrauterine d.
 Ortho All-Flex d.
 d. palsy
 d. paralysis
 pelvic d.
 d. pessary
 plication of d.
 urogenital d.
diaphragmatic
 d. agenesis
 d. atony
 d. defect
 d. eventration
 d. hernia
 d. hiatus
 d. injury
 d. plication
 d. trauma
diaphyseal (*var. of* diaphysial)
diaphysial, diaphyseal
 d. aclasis
 d. dysplasia
 d. fibular osteotomy
 d. fracture
 d. osteomyelitis
diaphysis
Diapid
DIAPPERS
 delirium, infection, atrophic urethritis
 and vaginitis, pharmacologic cause,
 psychological cause, excessive urine
 production, restricted mobility, stool
 impaction
diarrhea
 antibiotic-associated d. (AAD)
 bloody d.
 chloride-losing d.
 chronic nonspecific d.
 Clostridium difficile-associated d.
  (CDAC, CDAD)
 congenital sodium d.
 explosive watery d.
 infantile d.
 nosocomial d.
 osmotic d.
 pediatric viral d.
 protracted d.
 secretory d.
 toddler's d.
 traveler's d. (TD)
 watery d.
diarrhea-associated hemolytic uremic
 syndrome
diarrheal, diarrheic
 d. dehydration illness
 d. shellfish poisoning

diarrhea-malnutrition syndrome
diarrheic (*var. of* diarrheal)
diarthrodial
    d. joint
    d. muscle
diary
    baby's day d.
    bladder d.
    food d.
    headache d.
    retraining d.
    urinary d.
    voiding d.
DiaScreen reagent strip
Diasorb
diastasis
    d. recti
    symphysis pubis d.
diastatic fracture
Diastat rectal delivery system
diastematomyelia
diastole
diastolic
    d. arterial pressure
    (DAP)
    d. blood pressure
    d. component
    d. gradient
    d. murmur
    d. overload
    d. overload pattern
    d. thrill
diastomyelia
diastrophic
    d. dwarf
    d. dwarfism
    d. dysplasia
diathermy
    d. current
    electrocoagulation d.
    excision d.
    laparoscopic ovarian d.
    d. loop excision
diatheses (*pl. of* diathesis)
diathesis, *pl.* diatheses
    bleeding d.
    cognitive-stress d.
    familial d.
    gouty d.
    hemorrhagic d.
diatomaceous earth (DE)
diatrizoate
    meglumine d.
    sodium d.
Diazemuls Injection
diazepam
    D. Intensol
diazo reaction
diazoxide

dibasic
    d. amino acid
    d. aminoaciduria
Dibbell
    D. cleft lip-nasal reconstruction
    D. cleft lip-nasal revision
Dibenzyline
dibromochloropropane (DBCP)
dibromodulcitol (DBD)
dibucaine
DIC
    disseminated intravascular
    coagulation
    disseminated intravascular
    coagulopathy
dicentric chromosome
dicephalus
dicheilia, dichilia
dicheiria, dichiria
dichilia (*var. of* dicheilia)
dichiria (*var. of* dicheiria)
dichloroacetic acid
dichlorphenamide
dichorial, dichorionic
    d. pregnancy
dichorionic (*var. of* dichorial)
    d. diamniotic placenta
    d. placenta
    d. placentation
    d. twins
dichorionic-diamniotic twins
dichotic
    d. listening
    d. listening deficit
dichotomous
dichotomy
Dickinson syndrome
Dick test
diclofenac
    d. potassium
    d. sodium
dicloxacillin sodium
DICOM
    digital imaging and communication in
    medicine
dictyate
    d. stage
    d. stage of oocyte meiosis
dicumarol resistance
dicyclomine hydrochloride
didactic material
didanosine (ddI)
didelphic
didelphys
    uterus d.
DIDMO
    diabetes insipidus, diabetes mellitus,
    optic atrophy
    DIDMO syndrome

D

DIDMOAD
diabetes insipidus and mellitus with
optic atrophy and deafness
DIDMOAD syndrome
Didronel
didymus
Dieckmann intraosseous needle
diembryony
diencephalic
d. syndrome (DS)
d. syndrome of infancy
d. system n
diencephalon
Dienestrol Vaginal
Dientamoeba fragilis
DIEP
deep inferior epigastric perforator
DIEP flap
diepoxybutane (DEB)
diet
ADA d.
ad libitum d.
American Diabetes Association d.
d. and nutrition
Atkins d.
BRAT d.
BRATT d.
elemental d.
elimination d.
fluid d.
galactose-free d.
glutamine-supplemented d.
gluten-free d. (GFD)
glycemic index d.
high-calorie d.
high-fiber d.
high-phosphate d.
K d.
K+2 d.
ketogenic d.
lactose-free d.
Lorenzo's oil d.
low branched chain amino acid d.
low-cholesterol d.
low-fat d.
low-phenylalanine d.
low-protein d.
low-residue d.
low-salt d. (LSD)
low-sodium d. (LSD)
migraine d.
Moro-Heisler d.
non-casein-based d.
polymeric d.
PSMF d.
Pulmocare d.
pureed d.
d. recommendation
semifluid d.

Sippy d.
tea-and-toast d.
traffic-light d.
vegetarian d.
dietary
d. amenorrhea
d. change
d. craving
d. fat
d. fiber
d. habit
d. problem
d. protein enterocolitis
d. supplement
D. Supplement Health and
Education Act (DSHEA)
Dieter forceps
Dieterle stain
diethylamide
lysergic acid d. (LSD)
diethylaminoethyl (DEAE)
diethylcarbamazine
diethyldithiocarbamate
diethylenetriaminepentaacetic acid (DTPA)
diethylpropion
diethylstilbestrol (DES)
diethylstilbestrol-exposed
diethyltoluamide (DEET)
**diet-induced hypochloremic metabolic
alkalosis**
dietitian
Dieulafoy gastric lesion
DIF
direct immunofluorescence
DIF test
DiFerrante syndrome
difference
arteriovenous oxygen d.
gender d.
intrapair birth weight d.
racial d.
differential
d. agglutination test
d. cell count
d. cyanosis
d. detection hypothesis
d. effect
manual d.
d. temperature sensor (DTS)
d. treatment hypothesis
d. vascular resistance
differentiated crying
differentiation
alveolar myofibroblast d.
central nervous system d.
corticomedullary d.
embryonic d.
extraembryonic d.
fetal sexual d.

ganglionic d.
genital d.
gonadal d.
hemopoietic d.
lymphopoietic d.
male sex d.
d. of respiratory tree
schwannian d.
sexual d.
somatic d.
terminal lung d.
testicular d.
Differin gel
difficile
   Clostridium d.
difficulty
attentional d.
feeding d.
d. sleeping
swallowing d.
diffusa
neurospongioblastosis d.
placenta d.
diffuse
d. astrocytoma
d. axonal injury (DAI)
d. brain swelling (DBS)
d. cortical thrombophlebitis
d. cutaneous leishmaniasis (DCL)
d. cutaneous mastocytosis
d. cystic polycystic kidney disease
d. esophageal spasm
d. fasciitis
d. fibrocystic disease
d. globoid body sclerosis
d. globoid cell cerebral sclerosis
d. glomerular sclerosis
d. hyperpigmentation
d. intestinal polyp
d. mesangial sclerosis (DMS)
d. mesangial sclerosis-ocular
abnormalities syndrome
d. mixed lymphocytic plasmacytic
disease
d. morbilliform rash
d. neonatal hemangiomatosis
d. nephroblastomatosis
d. nonmalignant lymphadenopathy
d. periaxial encephalitis
d. perivillous fibrinoid deposition
d. proliferative glomerulonephritis
d. proliferative lupus nephritis
d. small cell cleaved lymphoma
d. tensor brain MRI
diffuse-onset seizure
diffusing
d. capacity
d. capacity of lung for carbon
monoxide (DLCO, DL_{co})

diffusion
diffusion-weighted
d.-w. imaging (DWI)
d.-w. magnetic resonance
imaging
diffusum
angiokeratoma corporis d.
diflorasone diacetate
Diflucan
diflunisal
difluoromethyl ornithine (DFMO)
DIG
desmoplastic infantile ganglioglioma
Digene
D. HPV Assay
D. HPV test
D. Hybrid Capture II HPV Test
DiGeorge
D. anomaly
D. malformation sequence
D. microdeletion syndrome
digestive system
Dighton-Adair syndrome
Digibind
Digilab FTS 40A spectrometer
digit
bambooing of d.
duplicated d.
hypoplastic d.
rudimentary-type d.
sausage d.
D. Span Subtest
supernumerary d.
d. syndactyly
trigger d.
digital
d. auditory aerobics (DAA)
d. clubbing
d. fibroma
d. imaging and communication in
medicine (DICOM)
d. imaging colposcopy
d. mammographic imaging screening
trial (DMIST)
d. mammography
d. mammography system
d. pitting
d. pulp
d. radiography
d. subtraction angiography
d. tuft
d. ulceration
d. ultrasound
digitalis effect
digitalis-induced arrhythmia
digitata
   Laminaria d.
digitorenocerebral syndrome (DRC)
digitotalar dysmorphism

D

digitoxin
Digitrapper portable pH recorder
dignathus
digoxigenin-labeled deoxyuridine triphosphate
digoxin
    d. immune fab
    d. monotherapy
digoxin-like immunoreactive factor (DLIF)
DIGS
    Diagnostic Interview for Genetic Study
digynia (*var. of* digyny)
digyny, digynia
dihybrid cross
dihydoprogesterone
dihydralazine
dihydrate
    azithromycin d.
dihydrochloride
    quinine d.
    triethylene tetramine d.
dihydrocodeine bitartrate
dihydrocodeinone
dihydroergotamine (DHE)
    d. mesylate
dihydrofolate
    d. reductase
    d. reductase inhibitor
dihydromorphinone hydrochloride
dihydropteridine
    d. reductase
    d. reductase deficiency
dihydrotachysterol
5-dihydrotachysterol
dihydrotestosterone (DHT)
    d. cream
    d. receptor deficiency (DHTR)
1,25-dihydroxycholecalciferol
dihydroxyphenylalanine (DOPA, dopa)
dihydroxyprogesterone acetophenide
9-13-dihydroxypropoxymethyl guanine
1,25-dihydroxyvitamin D$_3$
diiodohydroxyquin
diiodohydroxyquinoline
diiodothyronine (T2)
    d. test
diiodotyrosine (DIT)
diisopropyl
    d. fluorophosphate
    d. iminodiacetic acid (DISIDA)
Dilacor XR
Dilantin syndrome
dilatation (*var. of* dilation)
dilatator (*var. of* dilator)
dilated
    d. bowel loop resection
    d. capillary

    d. cardiomyopathy
    d. cisterna magna
    d. collateral vein
    fingertip d.
    d. intestinal loop
    d. optic vessel
    d. posterior urethra
    d. renal pelvis
    d. vein
dilating reflux
dilation, dilatation
    d. and curettage (D&C)
    d. and evacuation (D&E)
    aorta d.
    cervical d.
    congenital choledochal d.
    cystic d.
    esophageal d.
    Frank technique of d.
    fusiform d.
    gastric d.
    lumen d.
    d. of cervix
    d. of ventricle
    persistent ventricular d.
    pneumatic d.
    posthemorrhagic ventricular d. (PHVD)
    premature cervical d.
    saccular d.
    secondary arrest of d.
    urinary tract d.
dilator, dilatator
    bougie d.
    Goodell d.
    Hanks d.
    Hegar d.
    hygroscopic d.
    iris d.
    laminaria cervical d.
    Lucite d.
    mechanical cervical d.
    osmotic d.
    Pharmaseal disposable cervical d.
    Pratt d.
    retained hygroscopic cervical d.
    rocket d.
    Soehendra d.
    vaginal d.
    Walther d.
Dilaudid
    D. injection
    D. Oral
    D. Suppository
Dilaudid-HP injection
dildo, dildoe
dildoe (*var. of* dildo)
dilemma
diltiazem

dilute
    d. Surfaxin
    d. urine
diluted formula
dilutional anemia
dime
    March of D.'s
dimeglumine
    gadopentetate d.
dimelia
dimenhydrinate
dimension
    hyperactive/impulsive d.
    inattention d.
    left ventricular end-diastolic d.
    left ventricular end-systolic d.
    pelvic plane of greatest dimensions
    pelvic plane of least dimensions
2-dimensional (2D)
    2-d. echocardiogram
3-dimensional (3D)
    3-d. ultrasonography
    3-d. ultrasound (3DUS)
    3-d. videoendoscope
dimer
    metalloprotein d.
dimercaprol
dimercaptosuccinic acid (DMSA)
dimeric
    d. inhibin A level
    d. protein
Dimetane Extentabs
Dimetapp ND
dimethindene maleate
dimethothiazine mesylate
dimethyl
    d. phthalate
    d. sulfoxide (DMSO)
dimethyl-triazeno-imidazole carboxamide
dimethylxanthine
dimetria
dimidiata
    placenta d.
dimidiate
diminazene
diminished fremitus
Dimitri disease
dimorphic pathogenic fungus
dimorphism
    sexual d.
dimorphous leprosy
dimple
    acromial d.
    anal d.
    chin d.
    cutaneous d.
    lumbosacral d.
    pilonidal d.
    pretibial skin d.

    sacral d.
    vaginal d.
Dinamap blood pressure monitor
dinitrate
    isosorbide d. (ISDN)
dinitrochlorobenzene (DNCB)
    d. therapy
dinitrofluorobenzene
dinitrophenylhydrazine
dinoprostone cervical gel
dinoprost tromethamine
dinucleotide
    flavin adenine d. (FAD)
Diochloram
Diocto
Diocto-C
diode
    argon d.
    light-emitting d.
Diodoquin
dioecious
Dioeze
Diomycin
dione
    piperazine d.
DIOS
    distal intestinal obstruction syndrome
diosgenin
Diosuccin
Diovan
dioxide
    carbon d. (CO_2)
    end-tidal carbon d. (E_TCO_2)
    fraction in expired gas of carbon d. ($FECO_2$)
    fraction of alveolar carbon d. ($FACO_2$)
    partial pressure of arterial carbon d. ($PaCO_2$)
    partial pressure of carbon d. (PCO_2)
    pressure of carbon d.
    sulfur d.
dioxin
dioxyline
DIP
    desquamative interstitial pneumonia
    desquamative interstitial pneumonitis
dipalmitoyl phosphatidylcholine (DPPC)
Dipentum
diphallia (*var. of* diphallus)
diphallus, diphallia
diphasic
diphemanil methylsulfate
diphenadione
Diphenadryl
Diphenatol
Diphen Cough
diphencyprone

D

Diphenhist
diphenhydramine citrate
diphenoxylate and atropine
diphenylhydantoin
diphenyl tetrazolium bromide
diphenylthiourea
diphosphate
    galactose uridine d.
    menadiol sodium d.
    uridine d. (UDP)
diphosphate-choline
    cytidine d.-c.
diphosphate-diacylglycerol
    cytidine d.-d.
diphosphoglycerate
diphtheria
    d. antitoxin
    cutaneous d.
    laryngeal d.
    nasal d.
    diphtheria, pertussis, tetanus (DPT)
    pharyngeal d.
    diphtheria, tetanus, acellular pertussis vaccine
    tetanus and d. (Td)
    d., tetanus, pertussis immunization
    d., tetanus, pertussis vaccine
    d., tetanus toxoid, acellular pertussis (DTPa)
    d., tetanus toxoid, acellular pertussis vaccine
    tetanus toxoid and d.
    d., tetanus toxoid, pertussis (DTP)
    d., tetanus toxoids, whole-cell pertussis vaccine
    d., tetanus toxoid, whole-cell pertussis (DTPw)
    d. toxin (DT)
    d. toxoids-acellular pertussis
    d. toxoid with pertussis
diphtheriae
    Corynebacterium d.
diphtheritic
    d. croup
    d. membrane
    d. toxic myocarditis
diphtheroid
diphthong
diphyllobothriasis
Diphyllobothrium latum
DIPI
    direct intraperitoneal injection
    direct intraperitoneal insemination
dipivefrin
dipivoxil
    adefovir d.
diplegia
    atonic astatic d.
    congenital facial d.

    facial d.
    faciolingual-masticatory d.
    infantile d.
    spastic d.
diplococcus
    gram-positive d.
    D. pneumoniae
diplogenesis
diploid
    d. distribution
    d. merogony
    d. spermatogonial stem cell
diploid/tetraploid mixoploidy
diploid/triploid mixoploidy
diploidy
diplomyelia
diplopagus
diplopia
    monocular d.
diplosomatia
diplosome
diplotene phase of meiosis
diploteratology
dipodia
dipole
Diprivan Injection
Diprolene
    D. AF Topical
    D. Glycol
dipropionate
    beclomethasone d.
    betamethasone d.
Diprosone Topical
dipstick
    leukocyte esterase d.
    d. test
    urine d.
dipygus parasiticus
dipyridamole
    d. myocardial scintigraphy
    d. stress integrated backscatter
dipyrone
direct
    d. agglutination pregnancy (DAP)
    d. antiglobulin test (DAT)
    d. bilirubin
    d. Coombs test
    d. egg injection
    d. extension
    d. fetal transfusion
    d. fluorescent antibody (DFA)
    d. fluorescent antigen (DFA)
    d. hyperbilirubinemia
    d. immunofluorescence (DIF)
    d. immunofluorescent staining
    d. immunohistochemical staining
    d. insertion technique
    d. intraperitoneal injection (DIPI)
    d. intraperitoneal insemination (DIPI)

d. laryngoscopy
d. microscopy
d. oocyte sperm transfer (DOST)
d. oocyte transfer (DOT)
d. ophthalmoscope
d. orbital floor fracture
d. stimulation
d. stimulation of pancreas
d. suicide risk (DSR)
d. treponemal test
d. vision internal urethrotomy (DVIU)
d. wet mount
directed
d. amplification of minisatellite region DNA
d. biopsy
d. donor
Directigen Flu A
direction
caudal d.
pelvic d.
rostral d.
directional coronary atherectomy (DCA)
directive
advance d.
directly observed therapy (DOT)
direct-reacting bilirubin
dirithromycin
Dirofilaria
D. immitis
D. tenuis
dirty background
disability
cognitive d.
developmental d. (DD)
intellectual d.
language-based learning d.
learning d. (LD)
mobility d.
motor d.
National Joint Committee on Learning Disabilities (NJCLD)
neurodevelopmental d.
neurologic d.
nonverbal learning d. (NVLD)
reading d.
selective reading d.
social-emotional learning d.
specific reading d.
disabled
orthopedically d.
disaccharidase deficiency
disaccharide intolerance
DiSala syndrome
Disalcid
disappearance
fetal d.

disarray
myofiber d.
panlobar d.
disassociation
disaturated
d. lecithin
d. phosphatidylcholine
disc, disk
choked d.
dragged d.
embryonic d.
EMLA anesthetic d.
glandular d.
herniated d.
d. herniation
intervertebral d. (IVD)
juvenile intervertebral d.
Merkel tactile d.
neovascularization of d. (NVD)
optic d.
placental d.
tilted d.
trilaminar embryonic d.
DISC
Diagnostic Interview Schedule for Children
discernment
gustatory d.
discharge
adherent vaginal d.
cheesy d.
cloudy d.
cloudy nipple d.
copious d.
curdy d.
epileptiform d. (ED)
foul-smelling d.
frothy d.
generalized epileptogenic d.
gleety d.
homogeneous vaginal d.
hypersynchronous d.
hypersynchrony of neural discharges
interictal d.
leukorrheal d.
mucous d.
neural d.
newborn rehospitalization after early d.
nipple d.
partial epileptogenic d.
pathologic d.
physiologic d.
polyspike d.
pulsatile d.
purulent nasal d.
sharp-wave d.
urethral d. (UD)
vaginal d.

D

DisCide disinfecting towel
disciform keratitis
discitis, diskitis
    intervertebral d.
discoid
    d. eczema
    d. lateral meniscus
    d. lesion
    d. lupus
    d. rash
discoloration
    heliotropic d.
    prominent skin d.
    skin d.
discomfort
    internal d.
    radiation of d.
    suprapubic d.
discontinuity
    ossicular d.
discontinuous lesion
discoordinated uterine action
discoplacenta
discordance
    atrioventricular d.
    birth weight d.
    twin birth weight d.
discordancy
    growth d.
discordant
    d. artery flow velocity waveform
    d. growth
    d. twin growth
    d. twins
    d. umbilical arteries
DISC-R
    Diagnostic Interview Schedule for Children-Revised
discrepancy
    leg length d. (LLD)
    size-date d.
discrepant
discrete
    d. character
    d. subaortic stenosis (DSS)
discrete-trial learning
discrimination
    auditory d.
    2-point d.
    right-left d.
    tactile d.
discriminatory hCG zone
DISCUS
    Dyskinesia Identification System: Condensed User Scale
discus proligerus
disease
    ABO hemolytic d.
    acid lipase deficiency d.

acid peptic d.
acquired heart d.
acute fulminant d.
acute graft-versus-host d. (AGVHD)
acute neuronopathic Gaucher d.
acute respiratory d. (ARD)
acyanotic congenital heart d.
Addison d.
adhesive d.
adult-onset polycystic kidney d.
adult polycystic d.
adult Refsum d.
advanced-stage d.
Albers-Schönberg d.
Albright d.
Alexander d.
allergic bowel d.
allogenic d.
alloimmune d.
Alpers d.
alpha-1-antitrypsin d.
Alzheimer d.
American Foundation for Urologic D.'s (AFUD)
Andersen d.
Anderson-Fabry d.
anterior horn cell d.
antiglomerular basement membrane antibody d.
Antopol d.
aortic valve d.
Apert d.
Apert-Crouzon d.
Aran-Duchenne d.
arterial occlusive d. (AOD)
arterial vascular d.
atypical Kawasaki d.
autoimmune d.
autosomal dominant medullary cystic kidney d. (ADMCKD)
autosomal dominant polycystic d.
autosomal dominant polycystic kidney d. (ADPKD)
autosomal recessive polycystic kidney d. (ARPKD)
Azorean d.
Baló d.
Barlow d.
Bassen-Kornzweig d.
Batten d.
Batten-Mayou d.
Beck d.
Becker d.
Béguez César d.
Behçet d.
Behr d.
benign breast d. (BBD)
Berger renal d.
Best d.

Bielschowsky-Jansky d.
blistering d.
Bloodgood d.
Blount d.
Bornholm d.
Bourneville d.
Bourneville-Brissaud d.
Bowen d.
Brailsford d.
breast d.
Brill d.
Brill-Zinsser d.
brittle-bone d.
bronze Schilder d.
Brown-Symmers d.
Bruton d.
bubble boy d.
Buhl d.
Byler d.
Caffey d.
Caffey-Kenny d.
Caisson d.
Calvé-Perthes d.
Canavan d.
Canavan-van Bogaert-Bertrand d.
Caroli d.
Castleman d.
cat-scratch d. (CSD)
cavitary lung d.
celiac d. (CD)
central core d.
central nervous system d.
central Recklinghausen d. (type I, II)
cerebrovascular d.
Chagas d.
Charcot d.
Charcot-Marie-Tooth d.
Charlevoix d.
Cheadle d.
cholestatic liver d.
cholesterol ester storage d. (CESD)
Christmas d.
chronic Gaucher d.
chronic granulomatous d. (CGD)
chronic lung d. (CLD)
chronic maternal d.
chronic neuromuscular d. (CNMD)
chronic neuronopathic Gaucher d.
chronic pulmonary d.
chronic sickle cell lung d.
chronic vascular d.
chylomicron retention d.
cicatricial retinal d.
circling d.
classic celiac d.
Coats d.
cold agglutinin d.
cold hemagglutinin d.

collagen vascular d.
colorectal d.
communicable d.
complex congenital heart d.
congenital cardiac d.
congenital heart d. (CHD)
congenital hip d.
congestive heart d. (CHD)
connective tissue d.
Conradi d.
contractural arachnodactyly d.
cooperative study of sickle cell d. (CSSCD)
copper transport d.
Cori d.
Cori-Forbes d.
coronary artery d.
coronary heart d. (CHD)
Cowden d.
cranial sclerosis with striated bone d.
Creutzfeldt-Jakob d. (CJD)
Crigler-Najjar d. (type I, II)
critical illness neuromuscular d.
Crohn d.
Crouzon d.
Csillag d.
Cushing d.
cyanotic congenital heart d. (CCHD)
cyanotic heart d.
cystic hydatid d.
cystic renal d.
cytomegalic inclusion d. (CID)
cytomegalovirus d.
Danlos d.
Darier d.
Darier-White d.
Dawson d.
Dejerine d.
Dejerine-Sottas d.
Dercum d.
De Vaal d.
developmental hip d.
Devic d.
diffuse cystic polycystic kidney d.
diffuse fibrocystic d.
diffuse mixed lymphocytic plasmacytic d.
Dimitri d.
disseminated adenovirus d.
distal tubal d.
diverticular d.
Dorfman-Chanarin d.
duct-dependent heart d.
Dukes d.
Duncan d.
Duroziez d.
early-onset d.
end-stage kidney d.

D

disease (*continued*)
    end-stage liver d.
    Erb-Goldflam d.
    Erdheim d.
    Eulenburg d.
    exanthematous d.
    exertional reactive airway d.
    extraabdominal organ system d.
    extramammary Paget d. (EPD)
    Fabry d.
    Fahr d.
    Fairbank d.
    familial Alzheimer d. (FAD)
    familial cardiovascular d.
    familial Creutzfeldt-Jakob d.
    Farber d.
    Fazio-Londe d.
    Feer d.
    fetal heart d.
    fibrocystic d. (FCD)
    fifth d.
    fifth venereal d.
    FIGO d. (stage I–IV)
    Filatov-Dukes d.
    first d.
    Folling d.
    Fong d.
    Forbes d.
    Fordyce d.
    fourth venereal d.
    Fox-Fordyce d.
    free neuraminic acid storage d.
    free sialic acid storage d.
    Freiberg d.
    Fukuyama d.
    fulminant d.
    functional heart d.
    gallbladder d.
    Gambian d.
    ganglioside storage d.
    gastroesophageal reflux d. (GERD)
    gastrointestinal d.
    Gaucher d. (type 1–3)
    gay bowel d.
    Gee d.
    Gee-Herter d.
    Gee-Herter-Heubner d.
    genetic d.
    genetotrophic d.
    genital ulcer d. (GUD)
    gestational trophoblastic d. (GTD)
    Gianotti d.
    Gierke d.
    Gilbert d.
    gingival d.
    Gitelman d.
    glandular d.
    Glanzmann d.

    Glenárd d.
    glomerular renal d.
    glomerulocystic d.
    glycogen storage d. (type Ia–Id, II–VII)
    Goldstein d.
    graft versus host d. (GVHD)
    granulomatous d.
    Graves d.
    Greenfield d.
    group B streptococcus d.
    Günther d.
    Hailey-Hailey d.
    Hallervorden-Spatz d.
    hand-foot-and-mouth d. (HFMD)
    Hand-Schüller-Christian d.
    Hansen d.
    Hartnup d.
    Hashimoto d.
    HbH d.
    heart d.
    Heller-Döhle d.
    helminthic d.
    hemoglobin C d.
    hemoglobin M d.
    hemoglobin S d.
    hemoglobin SC d.
    hemoglobin SD d.
    hemolytic d.
    hemorrhagic d.
    Henoch d.
    hepatic d.
    hepatic glycogen storage d.
    hepatobiliary d.
    hepatocellular d.
    hereditary d.
    heredodegenerative d.
    Hers d.
    Hirschsprung d.
    Hodgkin d.
    homologous d.
    hookworm d.
    horn cell d.
    Hünermann d.
    Huntington d. (HD)
    Hurler d.
    Hutinel d.
    hyaline membrane d. (HMD)
    hydatid d.
    hydrocephaloid d.
    hypophosphatemic bone d.
    hypothalamic d.
    iatrogenic Creutzfeldt-Jakob d.
    I-cell d.
    idiopathic peptic ulcer d.
    immune complex d.
    immunoproliferative small intestinal d.
    inclusion cell d.

infantile Alexander d.
infantile celiac d.
infantile Gaucher d.
infantile motor neuron d.
infantile polycystic d. (IPCD)
infantile polycystic kidney d.
  (IPKD)
infantile Refsum d.
infectious d.
inflammatory bowel d. (IBD)
International Classification of D.'s
  (ICD)
International Society for the Study
  of Vulvar Diseases (ISSVD)
interstitial lung d. (ILD)
intranuclear hyaline inclusion d.
intraperitoneal endometrial metastatic
  d.
ischemic heart d. (IHD)
isoimmune hemolytic d.
Jaksch d.
Jansky-Bielschowsky d.
Jeune d.
Joseph d.
juvenile Alexander d.
juvenile hereditary motor neuron d.
juvenile neuronopathic Gaucher d.
juvenile-onset inflammatory bowel d.
juvenile-onset multisystem
  inflammatory d.
juvenile Paget d.
juvenile Parkinson d.
juvenile rheumatic d.
Kashin-Bek d.
Kawasaki d. (KD)
Keshan d.
kidney d.
Kienböck d.
Kikuchi d.
Kimmelstiel-Wilson d. (KW)
kinky-hair d. (KHD)
Kirner d.
kissing d.
Köhler bone d.
Kok d.
Kostmann d.
Kozlowski d.
Krabbe d. (KD)
Kramer d.
Krause d.
Kufs d.
Kugelberg-Welander d.
kuru d.
KW d.
kwashiorkor d.
Kyasanur Forest d.
kyphoscoliotic heart d.
Lafora body d.
Langdon Down d.

late hemorrhagic d.
latent celiac d.
Leber d.
Legg-Calvé-Perthes d. (LCPD)
Legg-Perthes d.
Legionnaires d.
Leigh d.
Leiner d.
Lesch-Nyhan d.
Letterer-Siwe d.
Lhermitte-Duclos d.
Libman-Sacks d.
linear IgA d.
lipid storage d.
Little d.
liver d.
Lobstein d.
Lou Gehrig d.
lower airway d.
Luft d.
Lyell d.
Lyme d. (LD)
lymphocyte-depleted Hodgkin d.
lymphocyte-predominant Hodgkin d.
lymphohematogenous d.
lymphoproliferative d.
lymphoproliferative/
  myeloproliferative d.
lysosomal storage d.
Machado-Joseph d.
mad cow d.
Maher d.
maple syrup urine d. (MSUD)
marble bone d.
Marburg d.
Marion d.
Maroteaux-Lamy d.
mast cell d.
maternal cyanotic heart d.
McArdle d.
MEB d.
medullary cystic d.
Melnick-Needles d.
Menetrier d.
Ménière d.
Merzbacher-Pelizaeus d.
metabolic bone d.
metastatic Crohn d. (MCD)
microvillus inclusion d. (MID)
Miege d.
Mikulicz d.
milk precipitin d.
Milroy d.
Minamata d.
minimal-change d.
Minot d.
mitochondrial d.
mitral valve d.
mixed cellularity Hodgkin d.

D

disease (*continued*)

    mixed connective tissue d. (MCTD)
    Moeller-Barlow d.
    Mondor d.
    Morquio d.
    Morquio-Brailsford d.
    Morquio-Ullrich d.
    motor neuron d.
    moyamoya d.
    Mucha-Habermann d.
    mucopolysaccharide storage d.
      (I–VIII)
    multicentric Castleman d.
    multicystic dysplastic kidney d.
      (MCKD)
    multicystic kidney d. (MCKD)
    Münchausen d.
    mycobacterial d.
    N-acetylneuraminic acid storage d.
      (NSD)
    nemaline rod d.
    neonatal chest d.
    neonatal cyanotic congenital heart d.
    neonatal gonococcal d.
    neonatal Graves d.
    neonatal iron-storage d. (NISD)
    neoplastic trophoblastic d.
    neurodevelopmental d.
    neurogenic hip d.
    neurologic demyelinating d.
    neuromuscular d.
    neutral lipid storage d.
    new variant Creutzfeldt-Jakob d.
      (nvCJD)
    Nicolas-Favre d.
    Niemann-Pick d. (type I, II) (NPD)
    nodular sclerosing Hodgkin d.
    nodular thyroid d.
    noncirrhotic ascitic d.
    noncyanotic congenital heart d.
    nonmetastatic gestational
      trophoblastic d. (NMGTD)
    non-Rh D/non-ABO hemolytic d.
    Norrbottnian Gaucher d.
    Norrie d.
    NYHA classification of heart d.
    oasthouse urine d.
    obliterative coronary artery d.
    obstructive lung d.
    obstructive respiratory d.
    occlusive vascular d.
    Oguchi d.
    oligoarticular d.
    Ollier d.
    Oppenheim d.
    optic nerve d.
    oral Crohn d.
    organic brain d.
    organic heart d.

    Osgood-Schlatter d. (OSD)
    Osler-Weber-Rendu d. (OWRD)
    Owren d.
    OXPHOS d.
    oxygen toxicity lung d.
    Paas d.
    Paget d.
    Panner d.
    parathyroid d.
    parenchymal lung d.
    Parkinson d.
    pediatric infectious d. (PID)
    pediatric spectrum of d. (PSD)
    Pelizaeus-Merzbacher d. (PMD)
    pelvic adhesive d. (PAD)
    pelvic Castleman d.
    pelvic inflammatory d. (PID)
    peptic ulcer d. (PUD)
    perianal d.
    periodontal d.
    peripheral arterial d.
    peroxisomal d.
    persistent gestational trophoblastic d.
      (pGTD)
    Perthes d.
    Peyronie d.
    Phocas d.
    phytanic acid storage d.
    ping-pong spread of d.
    pink d.
    Pityrosporum d.
    placental site gestational
      trophoblastic d.
    platelet-type von Willebrand d.
    PNAC liver d.
    polycystic kidney d. (PKD)
    polycystic ovarian d. (PCOD)
    polycystic renal d.
    polyglandular autoimmune d. (type
      I, II)
    Pompe glycogen storage d. (type I,
      II)
    Portuguese d.
    postabortal pelvic inflammatory d.
    postpartum pleuropulmonary and
      cardiac d.
    postrheumatic valve d.
    posttransplant lymphoproliferative d.
      (PTLD)
    Pott d.
    Potter d.
    preinvasive cervical d.
    premalignant d.
    Pringle d.
    prion d.
    pseudo-Crouzon d.
    pseudo-von Willebrand d.
    psychosomatic d.
    puff-of-smoke d.

pulmonary parenchymal d.
pulmonary valve d.
pulmonary venoocclusive d.
pulseless d.
Pyle d.
pyramidal tract d.
radiation-induced heart d. (RIHD)
Ramstedt d.
Raynaud d.
reactive airways d. (RAD)
Recklinghausen d. (type I, II)
Reclus d.
recurrent d.
refractory Crohn d.
Refsum d.
renal cystic d.
Rendu-Osler-Weber d.
restrictive lung d.
restrictive respiratory d.
retroviral d.
Rh D d.
rheumatic heart d.
rheumatic valvular heart d.
Rh hemolytic d.
Rh isoimmune hemolytic d.
Ribbing d.
rickettsial d.
Riga-Fede d.
rippling muscle d.
Ritter d.
Rosai-Dorfman d.
Rotor d.
Roussy-Lévy d.
runt d.
Salla d.
Sandhoff d.
Santavuori d.
Saunders d.
Scheuermann d.
Schilder d.
Schimmelbusch d.
Schindler d.
Scholz d.
Schwartz-Jampel d.
sclerotic skin d.
SD d.
secondary moyamoya d.
secretory d.
Seitelberger d.
Sever d.
sexually transmitted d. (STD)
sialic acid storage d.
sickle cell d. (SCD, SSD)
sickle cell-hemoglobin C, D d.
sickle cell-thalassemia d.
silent celiac d.
silent pelvic inflammatory d.
silo filler's d.
Simmonds d.

sixth d.
skin d.
skin-eye-mouth d.
slapped cheek d.
Sly d.
sphingolipid storage d.
Spielmeyer-Vogt d.
spinocerebellar degenerative d.
sporadic Creutzfeldt-Jakob d. (sCJD)
Stargardt d.
startle d.
Steinert d.
Sticker d.
Still d.
storage d.
stress-related peptic ulcer d.
Strumpell-Lorrain d.
Sturge-Weber d.
subacute neuronopathic Gaucher d.
Swift d.
systemic d.
Takayasu d.
Tangier d.
Tarui d.
Taussig-Bing d.
Tay-Sachs d.
T-cell-mediated d.
Terson d.
Thiemann d.
thin basement membrane d.
 (TBMD)
third d.
Thomsen d.
thromboembolic d. (TED)
thrombohemolytic d.
thyroid d.
Tillaux d.
Tourette d.
transplant coronary artery d.
Trevor d.
triglyceride storage d.
trophoblastic d.
trophoblastic neoplastic d.
tubulointerstitial d.
ulceroglandular d.
Ullrich d.
underlying d.
Underwood d.
Unverricht d.
Unverricht-Lundborg d.
upper motor neuron d.
Urbach-Wiethe d.
urea cycle d.
uveomeningitic d.
valvular heart d.
van Bogaert d.
vascular d.
venereal d. (VD)
venoocclusive d. (VOD)

D

disease (*continued*)
  Vogt-Spielmeyer d.
  Volkmann d.
  Voltolini d.
  von Gierke glycogen storage d.
  von Hippel-Lindau d.
  von Recklinghausen d.
  von Willebrand d. (type IIB, III)
  Vrolik d.
  vulvar Paget d.
  Waldenström d.
  Waldmann d.
  Wegner d.
  Weil d.
  Werdnig-Hoffmann d. (type I–III)
  Werlhof d.
  Wernicke d.
  wet lung d.
  Whipple d.
  Wilkie d.
  Wilkins d.
  Williams d.
  Wilson d.
  Winckel d.
  Wolman d.
  woolly hair d.
  X-linked chronic granulomatous d.
  X-linked dominant d.
  X-linked recessive d.
  Zellweger d.
  Zinsser d.
  Zuska d.
disease-free survival (DFS)
**disease-modifying antirheumatic drug
  (DMARD)**
disengagement
disequilibrium, dysequilibrium
  linkage d.
  d. syndrome
  test of linkage d.
  transmission d.
disfigurement
disfluency (*var. of* dysfluency)
disgerminoma
dish
  d. face
  insemination d.
  Uri-Two petri d.
DISIDA
  diisopropyl iminodiacetic acid
disiens
  Prevotella d.
disinfectant
  Sklar aseptic germicidal d.
disinfection
  vaginal d.
disinhibited
disinhibition
disintegrate

disintegration
disintegrin
Disipal
disjunctum
  ovarium d.
disk (*var. of* disc)
Diskhaler metered-dose inhaler
diskitis (*var. of* discitis)
Diskus
  Advair D.
  D. inhaler
  Serevent D.
dislocated
  d. hip
  d. mandible
  d. patella
  d. testis
dislocating patella
dislocation
  atlantoaxial d.
  atlantooccipital d.
  congenital d.
  congenital hip d. (CHD)
  elbow d.
  facet d.
  femoral head d.
  Galeazzi fracture d.
  habitual shoulder d.
  lens d.
  mandibular d.
  metacarpophalangeal d.
  Monteggia fracture d.
  multiple d.'s
  peroneal d.
  radial head d.
  subluxation d.
  teratologic d.
  testicular d.
dislodged tube
dismissing attachment
dismutase
  extracellular superoxide d.
  recombinant human superoxide d.
    (rhSOD)
dismutase-1
  superoxide d.-1
disodium
  cefotetan d.
  d. cromoglycate
  edetate calcium d.
  etidronate d.
  intermittent cyclical etidronate d.
  moxalactam d.
  ticarcillin d.
disomy
  uniparental d. (UPD)
  uniparental maternal d.
  uniparental paternal d.
disopyramide

disorder

acid-base d.
acquired platelet d.
acute stress d. (ASD)
adjustment d.
affective d.
aggressive conduct d.
alcohol-related neurodevelopmental d.
  (ARND)
alpha-chain d.
amniotic fluid volume d.
androgen excess d.
anterior pituitary d.
antisocial personality d. (ASPD)
anxiety d.
arousal d.
arrest d.
articulation d.
Asperger d.
athetotic movement d.
attachment d.
attention deficit d. (ADD)
attention deficit hyperactivity d.
  (ADHD)
autism spectrum d. (ASD)
autistic d.
autistic spectrum d. (ASD)
autosomal chromosome d.
autosomal dominant genetic d.
autosomal recessive d.
avoidant d.
basal ganglion d.
behavioral, anxiety, mood, and other
  types of d.'s (BAMO)
binge eating d. (BED)
bipolar d. (type 1, 2) (BPD)
body dysmorphic d. (BDD)
borderline personality d.
brain d.
breathing-related sleep d.
cardiac rhythm d.
cardiopulmonary d.
carnitine transferase enzyme d.
central auditory processing d.
  (CAPD)
cerebelloparenchymal d. (I–IV)
Charcot-Marie-Tooth d.
childhood disintegrative d. (CDD)
children and adults with attention
  deficit d. (CHADD)
Children's Interview for Psychiatric
  D.'s (ChIPS)
choreoathetotic movement d.
chromosomal d.
chromosome 9p d.
chronic motor tic d.
chronic tic d. (CTD)
cluster B d.
coagulation d.

collagen vascular d.
communication d.
comorbid anxiety d.
complement deficiency d.
conduct d. (CD)
congenital hip d.
congenital quantitative d.
connective tissue d.
conversion d.
Copeland Symptom Checklist for
  Attention Deficit D.'s
cyclothymic d.
dancing eyes/dancing feet d.
dendritic cell-related d.
depigmentation d.
depressive d.
developmental d.
developmental coordination d.
  (DCD)
developmental language d. (DLD)
developmental pattern d.
disruptive behavior d.
dissociative d.
dominant d.
dysthymic d.
dystonic dyskinetic d.
eating d.
embryogenic induction d.
emotional d.
endocrine d.
epithelial d.
expressive language d.
factitious d.
familial bipolar mood d.
FAO d.
female orgasmic d. (FOD)
female sexual arousal d. (FSAD)
fertility d.
fetal iodine deficiency d. (FIDD)
food avoidance emotion d. (FAED)
fragile X d.
full-syndrome eating d.
functional gastrointestinal d.
gamma-chain d.
gamma-loop d.
gastrointestinal d.
gender identity d. (GID)
generalized anxiety d. (GAD)
genetic d.
glomerular d.
glycogen storage d.
GSH pathway d.
Hartnup d.
hematologic d.
heme metabolism d.
hemopoietic d.
hepatic parenchymal d.
heredodegenerative d.
histiocytic d.

D

disorder (*continued*)

human leukocyte antigen-associated d.
hyperkinetic d.
hypoactive sexual desire d.
hypothalamic-pituitary d.
immunobullous d.
impulse spectrum d.
infantile sialic acid storage d. (ISSD)
inherited bleeding d.
International Classification of Sleep D.'s (ICSD)
intersex d.
intestinal d.
intrinsic renal d.
kifafa seizure d.
lactation d.
language d.
late luteal phase dysphoric d. (LLPDD)
laterality d.
learning d. (LD)
leukorrheal d.
lipid metabolism d.
lipid storage d.
lower respiratory tract d.
lymphoproliferative d.
lysosomal enzyme d.
lysosomal storage d.
major depressive d. (MDD)
manic-depressive d. (MDD)
mendelian genetic d.
metabolic d.
metal metabolism d.
Methods for Epidemiology of Child and Adolescent Mental D.'s (MECA)
migrational d.
minor depressive d.
mitochondrial d.
mixed receptive-expressive language d. (MRELD)
monogenic d.
mood d.
motility d.
multifactorial d.
multigenic d.
multiple complex developmental d. (MCDD)
muscle glycogen storage d.
musculoskeletal d.
myeloproliferative d.
myoneural junction d.
National Organization for Rare D.'s (NORD)
neonatal endocrine d.
neural tube d.
neurocutaneous d.

neurologic d.
neuromuscular d.
neuronal migration d.
neuropsychiatric d.
nonepileptic paroxysmal d.
nonmendelian d.
nonneoplastic epithelial d.
nonspecific esophageal motility d. (NEMD)
nonverbal perceptual-organization-output d.
obsessive-compulsive d. (OCD)
obsessive-compulsive personality d. (OCPD)
oppositional d.
oppositional defiant d. (ODD)
opsoclonus d.
orgasmic d.
ovarian d.
overanxious d. (OAD)
oxidation d.
pain d.
panic d.
paranoid personality d.
parathyroid d.
parkinsonian movement d.
paroxysmal movement d.
partial-syndrome eating d.
periodic movement d.
peripheral auditory d.
peroxisomal congenital d.
peroxisome import d.
personality d. (PD)
pervasive developmental d. (PDD)
petit mal-like seizure d.
phonological d.
phytanic acid oxidation d.
pituitary d.
platelet d.
polygenic d.
polygenic/multifactorial d.
porphyrin metabolism d.
posterior pituitary d.
posttransplant lymphoproliferative d. (PTLD)
posttraumatic stress d. (PTSD)
Practice Parameters for the Assessment and Treatment of Anxiety D.'s
premenstrual dysphoric d. (PMDD)
primary bullous d.
Primary Care Evaluation of Mental Disorders (PRIME-MD)
primary immunodeficiency d.
protraction d.
pulmonary d.

purine metabolism d.
qualitative d.
quantitative d.
recessive d.
recurrent affective d.
REM sleep behavior d.
reproductive d.
Rett d.
rheumatologic d.
rhythmic movement d.
Rome II criteria for functional
  bowel d.
rumination d.
schizoaffective d.
schizoid personality d.
schizophreniform d.
Screen for Child Anxiety-Related
  Emotional D.'s (SCARED)
seasonal affective d. (SAD)
seizure d.
semantic-pragmatic d.
separation anxiety d. (SAD)
sex-linked d.
sexual arousal d.
sexual aversion d.
sexual pain d.
sickling d.
single-gene d.
sleep terror d.
sleep-wake transition d.
sleepwalking d.
social anxiety d.
somatization d.
somatoform d.
speech d.
stereotypical movement d.
storage d.
substance-induced psychotic d.
substance use d. (SUD)
symptomatic primary
  immunodeficiency d.
test of variables of attention
  deficit d.
thought d.
tic d.
Tourette d. (TD)
transient myeloproliferative d.
  (TMD)
transient tic d.
transport d.
triad of head tilt d.
unifactorial d.
urea cycle d.
urinary tract d.
vesicobullous d.
voice d.
vulvovaginal d.
Werdnig-Hoffmann d.
within-the-infant depressive d.

X-linked dominant d.
X-linked recessive d.
year 7 conduct d.
disordered renal acidification
disorganized
  d. behavior
  d. brainstem nuclei
Disotate
dispar
  Entamoeba d.
  Veillonella d.
dispenser
  Baxa oral d.
  Exacta-Med oral d.
DisperDose
dispermia (*var.* of dispermy)
DisperMox oral suspension
dispermy, dispermia
disperse placenta
dispersion
  Taylor d.
displaced
  d. capitellum
  d. pinna
  d. supracondylar fracture
displacement
  d. implantation
  inner canthus d.
  lateral head d. (LHD)
  lateral sperm head d.
  rotatory d.
  uterine d.
display
  M-mode d.
disposable
  d. bottle
  d. butterfly needle
  d. cannula
  d. speculum
  d. wipe
disproportion
  cephalopelvic d. (CPD)
  congenital fiber-type d. (CFTD)
  congenital muscle fiber-type d.
    (CMFTD)
  craniofacial d.
  fetopelvic d. (FPD)
  fiber-type d.
  limb d.
disproportionate dwarfism
disputed maternity
disruption
  anal sphincter d.
  bilateral corticobulbar d.
  inferior vena cava d.
  d. of fetal membranes
  ossicular d.
  perineal sphincter d.
  surgical d.

D

disruption (*continued*)
  synchondrosis d.
  traumatic aortic d.
  tubular d.
disruptive
  d. behavior disorder
  D. Behavior Disorder Scale
  d. proboscis
dissecans
  endometritis d.
  osteochondritis d. (OCD)
dissecting aortic aneurysm
dissection
  aortic d.
  axillary node d. (AND)
  blunt and sharp d.
  carotid artery d.
  gauze d.
  groin d.
  inguinal-femoral node d.
  inverted Y detrusor d.
  partial zona d. (PZD)
  pelvic node d. (PND)
  retroperitoneal d.
  selective inguinal node d.
  sharp d.
  traumatic d.
dissector
  Endo-Assist cutting d.
  Kittner d.
  Maryland d.
  plasma d.
  Polaris reusable d.
  spud d.
disseminata
  dermatofibrosis lenticularis d.
  leiomyomatosis peritonealis d. (LPD)
disseminated
  d. adenovirus disease
  d. candidiasis
  d. CMV
  d. coccidioidomycosis
  d. encephalopathy
  d. gonococcal infection
  d. gonorrhea
  d. granuloma
  d. granulomatous vasculitis
  d. hemangiomatosis
  d. herpes infection
  d. histoplasmosis
  d. intravascular coagulation (DIC)
  d. intravascular coagulation state
  d. intravascular coagulopathy (DIC)
  d. lupus erythematosus
  d. Mycobacterium avium complex (DMAC)
  d. sclerosis
  d. tuberculosis
  d. varicella

dissemination
  iatrogenic d.
  peritoneal d.
disseminatus
  lupus erythematosus d.
dissimilar twins
dissociate
dissociated
  d. motor development
  d. movement
dissociation, disassociation
  albuminocytologic d.
  atrioventricular d.
  d. constant
  craniofacial d.
  developmental d.
  electroclinical d.
  electromechanical d. (EMD)
  hemoglobin-oxygen d.
  immune complex d. (ICD)
dissociative
  d. disorder
  D. Experience Scale (DES)
  d. phenomenon
  d. symptom
dissolution of clot formation
dissymmetry
distal
  d. arthrogryposis (type I, II)
  d. claviclectomy
  d. collecting duct
  d. dilated bowel segment resection
  d. esophageal atresia
  d. esophageal pH monitoring
  d. femoral skeletal traction
  d. humeral physial fracture
  d. ileum
  d. intestinal obstruction
  d. intestinal obstruction syndrome (DIOS)
  d. jejunum
  d. limb deficiency-mental retardation syndrome
  d. occlusion
  d. onycholysis
  d. RTA
  d. sacral defect
  d. shaft hypospadias
  d. splenorenal shunt
  d. symmetric sensorimotor neuropathy
  d. tongue bud
  d. trichorrhexis nodosa
  d. triradius
  d. tubal disease
  d. tubal microsurgery
  d. tubal obstruction
  d. tuft
  d. vagina

distamycin A/4-6-diamidino-2-phenylindole
distance
> genetic d.
> intercapillary d.
> source-to-axis d. (SAD)
> source-to-skin d. (SSD)
> d. vision

distasonis
> *Bacteroides d.*

distemper
> canine d.

distended
> d. abdomen
> d. capillary

distending pressure
distensae
> striae cutis d.

distensible
distension (*var. of* distention)
distention, distension
> abdominal d.
> centrizonal sinusoidal d.
> gaseous d.
> jugular venous d. (JVD)
> lacrimal sac d.
> d. medium

distichiasis
distigmine bromide
distortion
> body-image d.
> lobular d.
> segregation d.
> tubal d.

distractibility
distractible
> hyperactive d.

distraction
distress
> fetal d.
> iatrogenic fetal d.
> intrauterine fetal d. (IUFD)
> neonatal d.
> psychological d.
> pulmonary d.
> respiratory d. (RD)
> transient fetal d.

distribution
> butterfly d.
> Christmas tree d.
> dermatomal d.
> diploid d.
> fluid d.
> gaussian d.
> malar d.
> d. pattern
> tetraploid d.
> trigeminal nerve d.
> watershed d.

distributive shock

disturbance
> architectural d.
> behavioral d.
> cerebral d.
> coagulation d.
> electrolyte d.
> feeding d.
> growth d.
> immunologic d.
> menstrual d.
> mental d.
> neurobehavioral d.
> d. of attachment
> ovulatory d.
> serious emotional d. (SED)
> sleep d.
> thought d.
> visual d.

disturbed
> emotionally d.
> d. equilibrium syndrome

disulfiduria
> mercaptolactate-cysteine d. (MCDU)

disulfiram
disuse
> d. amblyopia
> d. muscular atrophy
> d. syndrome

DIT
> diiodotyrosine

dithiothreitol
Ditropan XL
Diuchlor H
Diurese-R
diuresis
> alkaline d.
> glycosuric d.
> osmotic d.
> solute d.

diuretic
> d. challenge
> loop d.
> mercurial d.
> potassium-sparing d.
> d. renography
> thiazide d.

Diuril
diurnal
> d. enuresis
> d. micturition
> d. rhythm

diurnus
> pavor d.

diva
> D. laparoscopic morcellator
> D. laparoscopic morcellator device

divalproex sodium
divergens
> *Babesia d.*

D

259

divergent
 d. fetal growth
 d. rectus muscle
 d. strabismus
diversion
 bilateral ureteral d.
 biliopancreatic d.
 colonic d.
 colonic conduit d.
 continent supravesical bowel urinary d.
 ileal loop d.
 ileocecal conduit d.
 loop d.
 Mainz pouch d.
 partial external biliary d. (PEBD)
 urinary d.
diversity
 genetic d.
diversus
 Citrobacter d.
diverticula (*pl. of* diverticulum)
diverticular disease
diverticulectomy
 urethral d.
diverticulitis
 suburethral d.
diverticulosis
diverticulum, *pl.* **diverticula**
 bladder d.
 congenital d.
 Hutch d.
 Meckel d.
 Nuck d.
 pharyngeal d.
 porencephalic d.
 tubal d.
 urethral d.
 urinary d.
diverting
 d. colostomy
 d. colostomy with pull-through procedure
 d. enterostomy
dividens
 crista d.
diving reflex
division
 cell d.
 cellular d.
 equatorial d.
 meiotic d.
 miotic d.
 d. of pancreatic ring
 premature centromere d.
 transcervical d.
 urethral plate d.
divisum
 pancreas d.

Dix-Hallpike maneuver
dizygotic twin
dizygous
dizziness
 orthostatic d.
DKA
 diabetic ketoacidosis
DLCO, DLco
 diffusing capacity of lung for carbon monoxide
DLD
 developmental language disorder
DLIF
 digoxin-like immunoreactive factor
DM
 dermatomyositis
 diabetes mellitus (type 1, 2)
  Diabetic Tussin DM
  Fenesin DM
  Genatuss DM
  Guiatuss DM
  Halotussin DM
  Hold DM
  Koffex DM
  Mytussin DM
  Poly-Histine DM
  Robafen DM
  Silphen DM
  Siltussin DM
  Tolu-Sed DM
DMAC
 disseminated *Mycobacterium avium* complex
DMARD
 disease-modifying antirheumatic drug
DMC
 demeclocycline
DMD
 Duchenne de Boulogne muscular dystrophy
 Duchenne muscular dystrophy
 dystonia musculorum deformans
DMD/BMD gene
D-mire test
DMIST
 digital mammographic imaging screening trial
D-mosaic blood type
DMPA
 depomedroxyprogesterone acetate
DMQ
 developmental motor quotient
  fine motor total DMQ
  gross motor total DMQ
DMS
 diffuse mesangial sclerosis
DMSA
 dimercaptosuccinic acid

DMSO
dimethyl sulfoxide
DNA
deoxyribonucleic acid
DNA amplification
DNA amplification fingerprinting
DNA analysis
branched DNA
chloroplast DNA
DNA clone
DNA cloning
complementary DNA (cDNA)
DNA copy
DNA diagnostics
directed amplification of minisatellite region DNA
DNA dual color probe
exogenous DNA
genomic DNA
heterochromatic DNA
heteroduplex DNA
homoduplex DNA
DNA hybridization
DNA hybridization assay
DNA index
kinetoplast DNA
DNA library
DNA ligase
DNA marker
DNA methylation testing
mitochondrial DNA (mtDNA)
DNA nucleotidylexotransferase
DNA nucleotidyltransferase
plasmid DNA
DNA ploidy
DNA polymerase
DNA probe test
randomly amplified polymorphic DNA
recombinant DNA
repetitive DNA
DNA replication
satellite DNA
DNA sequence
synthetic DNA
DNA testing
DNA typing
DNAase
deoxyribonuclease
DNA-based testing
DNA-directed RNA polymerase
DNase, DNAse
deoxyribonuclease
DNase B factor
human recombinant DNase
DNCB
dinitrochlorobenzene
DNCB therapy
d-norgestrel

DNR
do not resuscitate
DNR order
DNS
delayed neuropsychological sequela
DO2
arterial oxygen delivery
Doan's
Extra Strength D.
Original D.
DOB
date of birth
Dobbhoff
D. catheter
D. nasogastric feeding tube
DOBI
dynamic optical breast imaging
DOBI system
Dobrava virus
dobutamine hydrochloride
Dobutrex
DOC
deoxycholate
deoxycorticosterone
docetaxel
docosahexaenoic acid (DHA)
docosapentaenoic acid
doctor
medical d. (MD)
d. of medicine
docusate
d. and casanthranol
d. calcium
sodium d.
d. sodium
Döderlein
D. bacillus
D. hysterectomy technique
D. method of vaginal hysterectomy
D. roll-flap hysterectomy
D. vaginal hysterectomy method
dog
d. bite
d. tick
dogma
central d.
Döhle body
DOL
day of life
Dolacet
dolasetron
dolens
leukophlegmasia d.
phlegmasia d.
phlegmasia alba d.
dolichocephalic, dolichocephalous
dolichocephalism (*var. of* dolichocephaly)
dolichocephalous (*var. of* dolichocephalic)
dolichocephaly, dolichocephalism

D

dolichopellic, dolichopelvic,
dolichopelvic (*var. of* dolichopellic)
dolichostenomelia
doll play
doll's
    d. eye maneuver
    d. eye phenomenon
    d. eye reflex
    d. eye response
    d. eyes
    d. head maneuver
Dolobid
Dolophine
dolphin
    D. hysteroscopic fluid management
    system
    D. instrument
domain
    adaptive d.
    cognitive d.
    communication d.
    fine motor d.
    gross motor d.
    hyperactivity/impulsivity d.
    inattention d.
    language d.
    perceptual d.
    Revised Gesell Language D.
    self-help d.
    shedding d.
    social-emotional d.
Domeboro
    Otic D.
    D. solution
dome cell
domestic
    d. abuse
    d. victimization
    d. violence
    d. violence evaluation
    d. violence treatment
domesticum
    Pyronema d.
domiciliary monitoring
dominance
    eye d.
    incomplete d.
    thromboxane d.
    d. variance
dominant
    d. choroidal sclerosis
    d. disorder
    d. Doyne honeycomb retinal
    degeneration
    d. dystrophic epidermolysis bullosa
    d. follicle
    d. gene
    d. hand
    d. inheritance

    d. lethal trait
    d. recurrent ataxia
    X-linked d. (XLD)
dominantly
    d. hyperactive
    d. hyperactive impulsive type
Dominic-R questionnaire
domino connector
domperidone
Donahue syndrome
DONALD
    Dortmund Nutritional and
    Anthropometrical Longitudinally
    Designed
    DONALD procedure
    DONALD study
Donald-Fothergill uterine suspension
Donath-Landsteiner cold hemolysin
donation
    autologous blood d.
    egg d.
    embryo d.
    oocyte d.
    ovum d.
    sperm d.
Done nomogram
Donnagel
Donnan equilibrium
Donna-Sed
Donnatal
Donnez device
Donohue syndrome
donor
    artificial insemination d. (AID)
    artificial insemination by d.
    (AID)
    cadaveric d.
    directed d.
    egg d.
    d. egg
    embryo d.
    d. human milk
    d. insemination (DI)
    intrafamilial genoidentical d.
    oocyte d.
    d. oocyte
    d. oocyte transfer
    sperm d.
    d. sperm
    d. T cell
    d. twin
    d. venous graft
donor-specific blood
do not resuscitate (DNR)
Donovan body
donovanosis
Doo
    Super Duper Diaper D.
DOOR syndrome

DOP
degenerate oligonucleotide primer
dopa
dihydroxyphenylalanine
DOPA
dihydroxyphenylalanine
Dopamet
dopamine
d. hydrochloride
d. receptor agonist
dopamine-altering drug
dopaminergic
d. agonist
d. system
dopa-responsive dystonia (DRD)
Doppler
Acuson color D.
color-coded duplex D.
color-flow D.
continuous wave D.
2D D.
D. echocardiography
D. effect
D. evaluation
FetalPulse Plus fetal D.
D. flow
D. flow study
D. flow-velocity waveform
Imex Pocket-Dop OB D.
Koven D.
D. myocardial performance index
D. principle
D. probe
pulsed-wave D.
range-gated D. (RGD)
D. scanning
D. shift
D. shift spectra
spectral D.
transcranial D. (TCD)
D. ultrasonography
D. ultrasound
D. umbilical artery velocimetry
D. velocimetry
Doppler-guided ligation
Dopplex
Baby D. 4000
Dopram
Doptone fetal stethoscope
d'orange
peau d.
Dorcol
Dorfman-Chanarin disease
dormant basket cell hypothesis
Dormin Oral
dornase alfa
Dorros infusion and probing catheter
dorsal
d. birthing position

d. bunion
d. chordee
d. extension splint
d. hood
d. kyphosis
d. lithotomy position
d. myeloschisis
d. penile curvature
d. penile nerve block (DPNB)
d. radiculitis
d. rhizotomy
d. supine position
dorsalis
d. pedis
d. pedis pulse
tabes d.
dorsiflexion
dorsogluteal
dorsosuperior lie
dorsum linguae
Dortmund Nutritional and Anthropometrical Longitudinally Designed (DONALD)
DORV
double-outlet right ventricle
Doryx
DOS
dysosteosclerosis
dosage
antepartum d.
dosage-sensitive sex reversal (DSS)
dose
average radiation d.
bolus d.
booster d.
cancericidal d.
central axis depth d.
depth d.
gene d.
maximal permissible d.
minimal effective d. (MED)
minimum lethal d. (MLD)
physiologic replacement d.
priming d.
radiation d.
radiation absorbed d. (rad)
rescue d.
weight-appropriate d.
dosing
extended internal d.
DOST
direct oocyte sperm transfer
Dostinex
dot
black d.
d. ELISA test
glistening d.
d. immunobinding assay (DIA)

D

dot (*continued*)
  Mittendorf d.
  Schüffner d.
DOT
  directly observed therapy
  direct oocyte transfer
dot-blot
  d.-b. HPV hybridization test
  d.-b. hybridization
  d.-b. procedure
  d.-b. technique
dothiepin
double
  d. aortic arch (DAA)
  d. breech presentation (DBP)
  d. cell
  d. collecting system
  d. cortex
  d. cortex syndrome
  d. cortin
  d. decidual sac sign (DDSS)
  d. depression
  d. diapers
  d. diaper treatment
  d. elevator palsy
  d. epiphyses
  d. footling presentation
  d. gloving
  d. helix
  d. hemiplegia
  d. hump sign of an
    enterocele
  d. intussusception
  d. lip
  d. pylorus
  d. ring
  d. setup examination
  d. strength (DS, XX)
  d. thyroid ectopia
  d. ureter
  d. uterus
  d. vacuolization
double-balloon
  d.-b. catheter
  d.-b. device
double-bank
  d.-b. bilirubin lights
  d.-b. phototherapy
double-barrel colostomy
double-blanket phototherapy
double-bleb sign
double-blind
  d.-b. placebo challenge food
    challenge
  d.-b. study
double-bubble
  d.-b. flushing reservoir
  d.-b. gas shadow
  d.-b. isolette

  d.-b. sign
  d.-b. ventriculoperitoneal shunt
double-catheter technique
double-contrast CT scan
Doublecortin
double-focus tube
double-freeze technique
double-inlet
  d.-i. left ventricle
  d.-i. right ventricle
double-insulated incubator
double-J stent
double-lumen
  d.-l. airway
  d.-l. catheter
  d.-l. venovenous ECMO
double-lung transplantation
double-mouthed uterus
double-onlay preputial flap
double-orifice mitral valve
double-outlet
  d.-o. right ventricle (DORV)
  d.-o. ventricle
double-sandwich ELISA
double-setup examination
double-switch procedure
double-tooth tenaculum
double-tract sign
double-umbrella device
double-volume exchange transfusion
double-walled
  d.-w. bubble isolette
  d.-w. incubator
doubling time
douche
  fan d.
  Fritsch d.
  iodine d.
  Massengill d.
  maternal d.
  povidone-iodine d.
  vaginal d.
  yogurt d.
douching
  postcoital d.
  vinegar d.
doughnut pessary
doughnut-shaped mass
doughy
  d. mass
  d. skin
Douglas
  D. abscess
  D. bag
  D. cul-de-sac
  cul-de-sac of D.
  D. depth
  D. mechanism
  D. method

D. pouch
semilunar fold of D.
D. spontaneous evolution
douglascele
doula
dovetail sign
dowager's hump
Dowling-Meara epidermolysis bullosa simplex
down
    bearing d.
    clamped d.
    d. slant
    D. stigmata
    strain d.
    D. syndrome (DS)
    D. syndrome child (DSC)
    D. syndrome growth chart
    talking d.
    testes d.
    tolerance, worried, eye opener, amnesia, kut (cut) d. (TWEAK)
downbeat nystagmus
Downes score
downgaze
    tonic d.
downregulate
downregulation regimen
downslanting
    d. eyes
    d. palpebral fissure
downsloping palpebral fissure
downstream
downturned mouth
downward gaze
doxacurium chloride
doxapram hydrochloride
doxazosin
doxepin
Doxil
doxorubicin hydrochloride
Doxy-100
Doxycin
doxycycline
    d. hyclate
    d. monohydrate
doxylamine
Doxytec
Doyen vaginal hysterectomy
doylei
    Campylobacter jejuni d.
Doyle operation
Dpd
    deoxypyridinoline
D-penicillamine
DPI
    dry powder inhaler
    dynamic pulmonary imaging

DP-II
    Developmental Profile-II
DPL
    diagnostic peritoneal lavage
DPNB
    dorsal penile nerve block
DPPC
    dipalmitoyl phosphatidylcholine
DPSS
    Department of Public Social Services
DPT
    dehydration, poisoning, trauma
    diphtheria, pertussis, tetanus
DQ
    developmental quotient
dracunculiasis, dracunculosis
dracunculosis (*var. of* dracunculiasis)
Dracunculus medinensis
Dräger thermal gel mattress
dragged disc
dragging of retina
dragon
    d. pyelogram
    d. sign
drain
    butterfly d.
    fluted d.
    Freyer suprapubic d.
    Jackson-Pratt d. (JPD)
    Penrose d.
    peritoneal d.
    retroperitoneal d.
    Shirley wound d.
drainage
    anomalous pulmonary venous d.
    chest tube d.
    closed d.
    coffee-ground d.
    felon d.
    hematoma d.
    incision and d. (I&D)
    intercostal d.
    in utero d.
    d., irrigation, fibrinolytic therapy (DRIFT)
    lymphatic d.
    lymph node d.
    mastoid d.
    mediastinal air d.
    nasogastric d.
    open flap d.
    open pericardial d.
    percutaneous catheter d.
    postural d. (PD)
    primary peritoneal d. (PPD)
    d. procedure
    pulmonary venous d.
    suction d.
    surgical d.

D

drainage (*continued*)
    syringopleural d.
    syringosubarachnoid d.
    d. system
    thoracic duct d.
    vaginal d.
    water seal d.
draining otitis media
drain-pipe urethra
Dramamine II
Drapanas mesocaval shunt
drape
    barrier laparoscopy d.
    Ioban d.
    iodophor-impregnated adhesive d.
    Steri-Drape 2 incise d.
Drash syndrome
draught
    Black D.
Draw-a-Person Test
drawing
    human figure d.
    line d.
DRC
    digitorenocerebral syndrome
DRD
    dopa-responsive dystonia
    dystrophia retinae pigmentosa-dysostosis
    DRD syndrome
Drenison
dressing
    alginate wound d.
    AlgiSite d.
    Algosteril d.
    Allevyn d.
    Aquacel d.
    Aquasorb d.
    Biobrane/HF d.
    Biopatch d.
    BlisterFilm d.
    Breakaway wound d.
    Carrasyn Hydrogel d.
    ClearSite hydrogauze d.
    Coban d.
    CollaCote d.
    compressive d.
    Conformant d.
    Coverlet d.
    Curaderm d.
    Curafil d.
    Curagel Hydrogel d.
    Curasorb calcium alginate d.
    Exuderm d.
    d. forceps
    Fuller shield rectal d.
    FyBron calcium alginate d.
    hydrogel d.
    Iodosorb absorptive d.
    Kalginate d.

    Nu Gauze d.
    Nu-Gel d.
    occlusive d.
    PanoPlex d.
    PolyMem d.
    polyurethane d.
    SignaDRESS d.
    Silon wound d.
    StrataSorb d.
    SurePress d.
    SureSite d.
    THINsite d.
    Transorbent d.
    Veingard d.
    Viasorb d.
Drews forceps
Drew-Smythe catheter
dribble
    postmicturition d.
Dri-Dot
    Monosticon D.-D.
drier
    Savant Speed-Vac d.
drift
    genetic d.
    pure random d.
DRIFT
    drainage, irrigation, fibrinolytic therapy
drill
    bladder d.
    bladder retraining d. (BRD)
drilling
    zona d. (ZD)
drink
    Boost nutritional d.
Drinker respirator
drinking
    binge d.
    social d.
drip
    continuous gastric d. (CGD)
    continuous intravenous oxytocin d.
    intravenous d. (IVD)
    postnasal d.
    sterile water gastric d. (SWGD)
dripping
    candle d.
Drisdol
Dristan Sinus caplet
drive
    central respiratory d.
    d. for thinness
    respiratory d.
    ventilatory d.
driver
    Laurus ND-260 needle d.
driving
droloxifene
dromedary hump

dronabinol
drooling
drooping
    d. lily appearance
    d. lily appearance of lower
      collecting system
drop
    d. attack
    Auro ear d.'s
    Ayr saline d.'s
    Coly-Mycin S Otic d.
    E-R-O Ear D.'s
    head d.
    Little Tummys gas relief d.'s
    Mallazine Eye d.
    methylcellulose d.'s
    Murine ear d.'s
    Mylicon d.'s
    parasympathomimetic d.
    Phazyme infant d.'s
    Polytrim eye d.'s
    Robitussin-DM infant d.'s
    Rondec d.'s
    saline nose d.'s
    d. seizure
    silver nitrate d.'s
    sympatholytic d.
    Triaminic Oral Infant D.'s
    vitamin C d.'s
droperidol and fentanyl
droplet
    cytoplasmic lipid d. (CLD)
    d. infection
dropout
    capillary d.
    echo d.
    d. of capillary end loop
dropped beat
dropsy
    iatrogenic preterm birth maternal d.
    d. of fetus
drosophila
    D. melanogaster diaphanous gene
    D. mutation
drospirenone/ethinyl estradiol
Drotic Otic
drowning
    cold water near d.
    dry d.
    near d.
    wet d.
Droxia Hydrea
DRPLA
    dentatorubral-pallidoluysian atrophy
    hereditary DRPLA
DRSP
    drug-resistant *Streptococcus pneumoniae*
drug
    acetylcysteine d.

    d. addiction
    adrenergic d.
    alcohol and other d.'s (AOD)
    alcohol, tobacco, and other d.'s
      (ATOD)
    anthelminthic d.
    antianxiety d.
    antibacterial d.
    antibiotic d.
    anticholinergic d.
    anticonvulsant d.
    antidepressant d.
    antiepileptic d. (AED)
    antifungal d.
    antihistamine d.
    antihypertensive d.
    antimalarial d.
    antineoplastic d.
    antipsychotic d.
    antiretroviral d.
    antispastic d.
    antithyroid d.
    anxiolytic d.
    atypical antipsychotic d.
    d. baby
    bactericidal d.
    bacteriostatic d.
    beta-adrenergic d.
    beta-lactamase-stable d.
    bronchodilator d.
    cell cycle-nonspecific d.
    cell cycle-specific d.
    cholinergic d.
    disease-modifying antirheumatic d.
      (DMARD)
    dopamine-altering d.
    d. fever
    gateway d.
    d. holiday
    illicit d.
    immunosuppressive d.
    d. ingestion
    intramuscular d.
    intranasal d.
    intravenous d.
    musculotropic d.
    narcotic d.
    neuroleptic d.
    nonestrogen d.
    nonsteroidal antiinflammatory d.
      (NSAID)
    orphan d.
    ototoxic d.
    over-the-counter d.
    ovulation-inducing d.
    parasympatholytic d.
    prenatally exposed to d.'s (PED)
    prescription d.
    d. prophylaxis

D

drug (*continued*)
    psychedelic d.
    psychiatric d.
    psychoactive d.
    psychotropic d. (PTD)
    d. reaction pruritus
    d. reaction with eosinophilia and
      systemic signal (DRESS)
    recreational d.
    d. resistant
    social d.
    stimulant d.
    tocolytic d.
    tranquilizer d.
    d. use
drug-depressed infant
drug-induced
    d.-i. acne
    d.-i. diabetes
    d.-i. dystonia
    d.-i. gynecomastia
    d.-i. hematuria
    d.-i. hemolytic anemia
    d.-i. hirsutism
    d.-i. neonatal goiter
    d.-i. neutropenia
    d.-i. pancreatitis
    d.-i. rash
    d.-i. systemic lupus erythematosus
drug-related
    d.-r. anaphylaxis
    d.-r. purpura
drug-resistant
    d.-r. *Streptococcus pneumoniae*
      (DRSP)
    d.-r. tuberculosis
8-drugs-in-1-day treatment series
drusen
dry
    d. birth
    d. chemical burn
    d. drowning
    d. eye
    d. eye syndrome
    d. labor
    d. mucous membranes
    OAB d.
    d. pericarditis
    d. pleurisy
    d. powder inhaler (DPI)
    d. skin
    d. socket
    d. vagina
    d. weight (DW)
dryer
    Sahara DryEar ear d.
dryness
    vaginal d.
Drysol

DS
    diencephalic syndrome
    double strength
    Down syndrome
      Bactrim DS
      Septra DS
      Sulfatrim DS
      Tolectin DS
      WinRho DS
DSC
    Down syndrome child
      Parafon Forte DSC
DSHEA
    Dietary Supplement Health and
      Education Act
DSM
    degradable starch microsphere
DSM-IV
    Diagnostic and Statistical Manual of
      Mental Disorders, 4th Edition
      DSM-IV criteria
1D sodium dodecyl sulfate gel
DSPS
    delayed sleep phase syndrome
DSR
    direct suicide risk
DSRCT
    desmoplastic small round cell tumor
DSS
    discrete subaortic stenosis
    dosage-sensitive sex reversal
DST
    dexamethasone suppression testing
D-stix
    Dextrostix
DT
    diphtheria toxin
D-Tach removal needle
D-TGA
    D-transposition of great arteries
DTH
    delayed-type hypersensitivity
DTIC
    dacarbazine
    dimethyl-triazeno-imidazole
      carboxamide
DTM
    dermatophyte test medium
dTMP
    deoxythymidylic acid
DTP
    diphtheria, tetanus toxoid, pertussis
      DTP vaccine
DTPA
    diethylenetriaminepentaacetic acid
      DTPA radionuclide scan
DTPa
    diphtheria, tetanus toxoid, acellular
      pertussis

DTPw
 diphtheria, tetanus toxoid, whole-cell pertussis
DTR
 deep tendon reflex
D-transposition
 dextrotransposition
  D-transposition of great arteries (D-TGA)
DTS
 differential temperature sensor
Du
 blood group D variant equivalent to Rh-negative
  Du Pen epidural catheter
  Du variant blood type
Duac topical gel
dual-energy
  d.-e. photon absorptiometry
  d.-e. x-ray
  d.-e. x-ray absorptiometry (DEXA, DXA)
  d.-e. x-ray absorptiometry scan
dual nucleoside analog reverse transcriptase inhibitor
Dual-Pak
  Monistat D.-P.
dual-photon absorptiometry
Duane
  D. anomaly
  D. retraction syndrome
Duarte variant galactosemia
DUB
 dysfunctional uterine bleeding
Dubin-Johnson syndrome
dublin
  Salmonella d.
dubliniensis
  Candida d.
Dubois abscess
Dubowitz
  D. evaluation
  D. examination
  neonatal maturity classification of D.
  D. Neurological Assessment
  D. Scale for Infant Maturity
  D. score
  D. syndrome
Dubowitz/Ballard Exam for Gestational Age
Duchenne
  D. de Boulogne muscular dystrophy (DMD)
  D. muscular dystrophy (DMD)
  D. muscular dystrophy/Becker muscular dystrophy
  D. myodystrophy
  D. palsy

D. paralysis
D. syndrome
Duchenne-Griesinger syndrome
Duchenne-type pseudohypertrophic progressive muscular dystrophy
duckbill speculum
Duckett
 D. transverse preputial island flap
 D. tubularized neourethra procedure
duckfoot
Ducrey bacillus
ducreyi
  Haemophilus d.
duct
 allantoic d.
 apocrine d.
 Bartholin d.
 bile d.
 blocked d.
 branchial d.
 cloacal d.
 common hepatic d.
 congenital atresia of bile d.
 congenital obstruction of nasolacrimal d.
 cowperian d.
 cystic dilation of intrahepatic bile d.
 distal collecting d.
 eccrine sweat d.
 d. ectasia
 ejaculatory d.
 focally dilated d.
 follicular d.
 Gartner d.
 gartnerian d.
 genital d.
 gland d.
 greater vestibular gland d.
 imperforate nasolacrimal d.
 inspissated d.
 intrahepatic bile d.
 lacrimal d.
 lactiferous d.
 male genital d.
 mesonephric d.
 metanephric d.
 minor vestibular gland d.
 müllerian d.
 nasolacrimal d. (NLD)
 d. of Cuvier
 omphalomesenteric d.
 paramesonephric d.
 paraurethral d.
 patent omphalomesenteric d.
 paucity of interlobular bile d. (PILBD)
 pilosebaceous d.
 Reichel cloacal d.

D

duct (*continued*)
    sebaceous d.
    Skene d.
    solitary dilated d.
    stenotic nasolacrimal d.
    Stensen d.
    sweat d.
    thyroglossal d.
    vanishing bile d.
    vestibular d.
    vitelline d.
    vitellointestinal d.
    wolffian d.
ductal
    d. adenoma
    d. carcinoma
    d. carcinoma in situ
    (DCIS)
    d. cell
    d. ectasia
    d. epithelium
    d. hyperplasia
    d. inflammation
    d. lavage (DL)
    d. obstruction
    d. papilloma
    d. plate malformation
    d. shunt
    d. shunting
    d. sperm
ductal-dependent
    d.-d. lesion
    d.-d. pulmonary blood
    flow
ductal-independent mixing lesion
duct-dependent
    d.-d. heart disease
    d.-d. pulmonary blood flow
    d.-d. pulmonary circulation
    d.-d. systemic circulation
DuctOcclud coil
ductule
    bile d.
ductuli efferentia
ductus, *pl.* **ductus**
    d. arteriosus (DA)
    bilateral d.
    d. choledochus
    d. closure
    d. deferens
    d. venosus
Duffy
    D. antigen
    D. system
Dufourmentel transpostion flap technique
Duhamel abdominoperineal pullthrough procedure
Dührssen incision

Dukes
    D. classification
    D. disease
Dulbecco
    D. medium
    D. phosphate buffered saline
Dulcolax
Dull-C
dullness, dulness
    absolute cardiac d.
    area of cardiac d. (ACD)
    flank d.
    shifting d.
    span of liver d.
    d. to percussion
dulness (*var. of* dullness)
duloxetine hydrochloride
Duluth model
dumbbell tumor
dummy
    d. source
    d. spacer
Dumontpallier pessary
dumping syndrome (DS)
Duncan
    D. curette
    D. disease
    D. folds
    D. knot
    D. mechanism
    D. mechanism of placental delivery
    D. placenta
    D. position
    D. presentation
    D. slipknot
    D. syndrome
    D. test
Dunedin
    D. birth cohort
    D. longitudinal study
duodenal
    d. atresia
    d. diaphragm
    d. duplication
    d. fluid
    d. ileus
    microcephaly, oculo-digito-esophageal, d. (MODED)
    d. obstruction
    d. resection
    d. stenosis
    d. ulcer
    d. vacuolization
duodenale
    Ancylostoma d.
duodenitis
duodenum
    Z-shaped d.
DuoFilm

Duosol
Duotrate
dup
> duplication
>> dup (10p)/del (10q) syndrome
>> dup (1p)–(22p) syndrome
>> dup (9q)/del(9p) syndrome
>> dup (1q)–(22q) syndrome
>> dup (Xq) syndrome

duplex
> d. kidney
> placenta d.
> d. scanning
> d. ultrasound (DU)
> uterus d.
> d. uterus

duplicated
> d. digit
> d. elastic lamina
> d. ureter
> d. vagina

duplicate uterus
duplication (dup)
> d. anomaly
> bowel d.
> caudal d.
> chromosome 15 inverted d.
> complete vulvar d.
> cranial d.
> d. cyst
> duodenal d.
> enteric d.
> fetal d.
> foregut d.
> gastric d.
> gastrointestinal d.
> gene d.
> intestinal d.
> intrachromosomal d.
> mirror d.
> d. of gallbladder
> d. of ileum
> penile d.
> d. 1p–22p syndrome
> d. 1q–22q syndrome
> renal d.
> ureteral d.
> urethral d.
> d. Xq syndrome

duplication-deficiency syndrome
duplicitas anterior
Du-positive mother
dura
> d. mater
> d. mater allograft

durable power of attorney
Durabolin
Duracillin AS
Duraclon Injection

Dura-Estrin
Duragen
Duragesic Transdermal
dural
> d. arteriovenous malformation
> d. ectasia
> d. sinus thrombosis
> d. spinal angioma
> d. venous thrombosis

Duralon-UV nylon membrane
Duralutin
Duramist Plus
Duramorph injection
DuraNeb portable nebulizer
DuraPrep surgical solution
Duraquin
Durasphere carbon bead
Dura-Tabs
> Quinaglute D.-T.

Duratears
duration
> D. Nasal Solution
> d. of symptoms

Duratuss-G
Duricef
Duroziez disease
3DUS
> 3-dimensional ultrasound

duskiness
dusky skin
dust
> d. mite
> nuclear d.

Dutch
> D. cap
> D. pessary

Duval forceps
Duverney gland
DVIU
> direct vision internal urethrotomy

DVSS
> dysfunctional voiding scoring system

DVT
> deep vein thrombosis
> deep venous thrombosis
>> silent DVT

dwarf
> diastrophic d.
> d. pelvis
> Russell d.
> d. syndrome

dwarfism
> achondroplastic d.
> acromesomelic d.
> alopecia, contracture, d. (ACD)
> Amsterdam d.
> d. and cortical thickening of tubular bones
> asexual d.

D

dwarfism (*continued*)
ateliotic d.
bird-headed d.
Brissaud d.
camptomelic d.
d., cerebral atrophy, keratosis
follicularis
child abuse d.
chondroplastic d.
d., congenital medullary stenosis
syndrome
constitutional d.
d., cortical thickening of tubular
bones, transient hypocalcemia
cretin d.
diastrophic d.
disproportionate d.
d., eczema, peculiar facies
familial bird-headed d.
6-fingered d.
geleophysic d.
genital d.
hypophysial d.
hypothyroid d.
infantile d.
Kniest d.
Langer mesomelic d.
Laron d.
lean spastic d.
Lenz-Majewski hyperostotic d.
lethal neonatal d.
Lorain-Lévi d.
metatropic d.
microcephalic primordial d. 1
micromelic d.
mulibrey d.
nanocephalic d.
d., onychodysplasia syndrome
osteodysplastic primordial d.
osteoglophonic d.
ovarian d.
parastremmatic d.
d., pericarditis syndrome
pituitary d.
d., polydactyly, dysplastic nails
syndrome
polydystrophic d.
primordial d.
psychosocial d.
rhizomelic d.
Robinow d.
Russell-Silver d.
Saldino-Noonan d.
Seckel d.
sexual d.
short-limb d.
short-rib d.
Silver d.
Silver-Russell d.

Smith-McCort d.
thanatophoric d.
Walt Disney d.
DWI
diffusion-weighted imaging
DWM
Dandy-Walker malformation
DWS
Dandy-Walker syndrome
Dwyer
D. correction
D. correction of scoliosis
DX
dextran
Dx
diagnosis
DXA
dual-energy x-ray absorptiometry
DXA densitometer
d-xylose
Dyadic Adjustment Scale
Dyazide
Dyban oocyte fixation technique
Dyclone
dyclonine
dydrogesterone
dye
aniline d.
azo d.
d. decolorization test
d. disappearance test
Evans blue d.
formazan d.
indigo carmine d.
iodinated d.
isosulfan blue d. (IBD)
methylene blue d.
triple d.
Dyggve-Melchior-Clausen syndrome
dying-back axonal degeneration
Dyke-Davidoff syndrome
Dynabac
Dynacin Oral
Dyna-Hex
dynamic
d. exercise testing
d. graciloplasty
d. image on ultrasound
d. mutation
d. optical breast imaging
(DOBI)
d. orthotic cranioplasty device
d. pes varus
d. posturography
d. pulmonary imaging (DPI)
d. spiral CT lung densitometry
d. splint
d. subaortic stenosis (DSAS)
d. testing

dynamics
  androgen d.
  family d.
  flow velocity d.
  toxic d.
Dynamite mattress system
Dynapen
dynein
  left/right d.
dynorphin
dyphylline
Dyrenium
dysacousia, dysacusia, dysacusis
dysacusia (*var. of* dysacousia)
dysacusis (*var. of* dysacousia)
dysadrenalism
dysarthria
dysarthritic speech
dysautonomia
  familial d.
dysbetalipoproteinemia
dyscalculia
dyscephalia
  François d.
  Hallermann-Streiff d.
dyscephaly
  d., congenital cataract, hypotrichosis
    syndrome
  mandibulo-oculofacial d.
  oculomandibular d.
dyschezia
dyschondroplasia
  Voorhoeve d.
dyscinesia (*var. of* dyskinesia)
dyscontrol
  episodic d.
dyscoria
dyscrasia
  blood d.
  sonography blood d.
dysdiadochokinesis
dysembryoma
dysembryoplasia
dysencephalia splanchnocystica
dysenteriae
  Shigella d.
dysentery
  amebic d.
  bacillary d.
  Shigella d.
dysequilibrium (*var. of* disequilibrium)
dyserythropoiesis
dysesthetic vulvodynia
dysfibrinogenemia
dysfibronectinemic Ehlers-Danlos
  syndrome
dysfluency, disfluency
  abnormal d.
  developmental d.

dysfluent speech
dysfunction
  adrenal axis d.
  apomorphine sexual d.
  arm d.
  auditory d.
  autonomic nervous system d.
    (ANSD)
  AV node d.
  B-cell d.
  bilirubin-induced neurologic d.
    (BIND)
  bladder d.
  bone marrow d.
  brain d.
  cardiopulmonary d.
  catheter d.
  cerebellar d.
  cerebral d.
  chromosomal d.
  CNS d.
  cognitive d.
  corpus luteum d.
  corticospinal tract d.
  cumulative parental d.
  defecatory d.
  endocrine pancreatic d.
  endothelial d.
  eustachian tube d.
  exercise-induced hypothalamic d.
  exocrine pancreatic d.
  familial vocal cord d.
  family d.
  female sexual d. (FSD)
  gait d.
  generalized autonomic d.
  global neurologic d.
  gonadal d.
  hepatic d.
  HPA d.
  hypertonic uterine d.
  hypothalamic d.
  hypothalamic-pituitary d.
  hypotonic uterine d.
  left ventricular d. (LVD)
  LV d.
  lymphocyte d.
  metabolic disorder with hepatic d.
  metabolic disorder with
    neurologic d.
  microcirculatory d.
  minimal brain d. (MBD)
  minimal cerebral d.
  minor cerebral d.
  motor perception d.
  neurogenic bladder d.
  neurologic d.
  neuromotor d.
  neutrophil actin d.

D

dysfunction (*continued*)
    oculomotor d.
    oral-motor d.
    ovarian d. (OvDF)
    ovarian axis d.
    palatorespiratory d.
    pancreatic d.
    papillary muscle d.
    placental d.
    postoperative bladder d.
    postoperative voiding d.
    psychosexual d.
    renal d.
    sacroiliac d.
    serotonergic d.
    sexual d. (SDF)
    sinus node d. (SND)
    social-occupational d.
    spinal cord d.
    sudomotor d.
    T-cell d.
    temporomandibular joint d.
    testicular d.
    thyroid d.
    thyroid gland d.
    transient pharyngeal muscle d.
    urinary bladder d.
    uterine d.
    vocal cord d. (VCD)
    voiding d.
dysfunctional
    d. family
    d. labor pattern
    d. uterine bleeding (DUB)
    d. voiding
    d. voiding scoring system (DVSS)
dysgammaglobulinemia
dysgenesia (*var. of* dysgenesis)
dysgenesis, dysgenesia
    autosomal congenital tubular d.
    cerebral d.
    cerebrooccular d. (COD)
    cortical d.
    familial pure gonadal d.
    female gonadal d.
    gonadal d.
    iridocorneal mesodermal d.
    d. mesostromalis anterior
    mixed gonadal d. (MGD)
    müllerian d.
    ovarian d.
    partial gonadal d.
    penile d.
    pure gonadal d. (PGD)
    renal d.
    reticular d.
    seminiferous tubule d.
    d. syndrome
    testicular d.

    tubular d.
    X-linked recessive d.
    XX-type gonadal d.
    XY gonadal d.
dysgenetic
    d. gonad
    d. ovotestis
    d. testis
dysgenic
dysgenitalism
dysgerminoma
    ovarian d.
dysgeusia
dyshidrosis, dysidrosis, dyshydrosis
dyshidrotic eczema
dyshormonogenesis
dyshydrosis (*var. of* dyshidrosis)
dysidrosis (*var. of* dyshidrosis)
dyskaryosis
dyskeratoma
    warty d.
dyskeratosis
    d. congenita
    congenital d.
dyskinesia, dyskinesis, dyscinesia
    ciliary d.
    exertion-induced d.
    D. Identification System: Condensed
      User Scale (DISCUS)
    kinesigenic paroxysmal d.
    nonkinesigenic d.
    orofacial d.
    paroxysmal d.
    primary ciliary d. (PCD)
    sleep-induced d.
    tardive d.
    withdrawal d.
dyskinesis (*var. of* dyskinesia)
dyskinetic cerebral palsy
dyslexia
    developmental d.
dyslexic
dyslipidemia
dysmaturative myopathy
dysmature
    d. infant
    d. neonate
dysmaturity syndrome
dysmegakaryocytopoiesis
dysmenorrhea
    acupuncture for d.
    essential d.
    functional d.
    intrinsic d.
    mechanical d.
    membranous d.
    obstructive d.
    ovarian d.
    primary d.

secondary d.
spasmodic d.
tubal d.
ureteral d.
uterine d.
vaginal d.
dysmenorrheal membrane
dysmetria
ocular motor d.
dysmorphia (*var. of* dysmorphism)
dysmorphic
d. erythrocyte
d. face
d. facial features
d. facies
d. syndrome
dysmorphism, dysmorphia
digitotalar d.
facial d.
major d.
mandibulo-oculofacial d.
minor d.
dysmorphogenesis
otomandibular facial d.
dysmorphologist
dysmorphology
craniofacial d.
d. examination
dysmotile cilia syndrome
dysmotility
ciliary d.
colonic d.
cytokine-related d.
gastric d.
gastrointestinal d.
small bowel d.
d. syndrome
dysmotility-sclerodactyly-telangiectasia
dysmyelinisatus
status d.
dysmyelinogenic
dysmyelopoiesis
dysnomia
dysontogenesis
dysontogenetic cyst
dysosmia
dysosteogenesis
dysosteosclerosis (DOS)
dysostosis
acrocraniofacial d.
acrofacial d. (AFD)
Catania-type acrofacial d.
cleidocranial digital d.
d. cleidocranialis
d. cleidocraniodigitalis
d. cleidocraniopelvina
craniofacial d. (CFD, CFDS)
d. craniofacialis with hypertelorism
craniofrontonasal d. (CFND)

Crouzon craniofacial d.
epiphysial d.
frontofacionasal d.
Genée-Wiedemann acrofacial d.
  (GWAFD)
d. generalisata
hereditary polytopic enchondral d.
hypomandibular faciocranial d.
mandibulofacial d. (MFD)
d. mandibulofacialis
maxillofacial d.
metaphysial d.
d. multiplex
mutational d.
Nager-type acrofacial d.
orodigitofacial d.
otomandibular d.
pelvicocleidocranial d.
preaxial acrofacial d.
preaxial mandibulofacial d.
Rodriguez lethal acrofacial d.
Treacher Collins mandibulofacial d.
unilateral mandibulofacial d.
dyspareunia
deep d.
Friedrich criteria for d.
insertional d.
secondary vestibular d.
vestibular d.
dyspepsia
functional d.
nonulcer d.
dysphagia, dysphagy
motility-related d.
nonneurogenic d.
dysphagy (*var. of* dysphagia)
dysphalangism
brachymorphism, onychodysplasia, d.
  (BOD)
dysphasia
developmental d.
dysphonia
spasmodic d.
spastic d.
dysphoria
premenstrual d.
dysphoric
d. mood
d. reaction
dyspigmentation
dysplasia
acetabular d.
acromelic frontonasal d.
acromesomelic d.
acromicric d.
acropectorovertebral d.
agyria-pachygyria cortical d.
Alagille arteriohepatic d.
alveolar capillary d.

D

dysplasia (*continued*)
anal sphincter d.
angel-shaped phalangoepiphysial d. (ASPED)
anhidrotic ectodermal d.
arrhythmogenic right ventricular d. (ARVD)
arteriohepatic d. (AHD)
asphyxiating thoracic d.
atriodigital d.
azoospermia, renal anomaly, cervicothoracic spine d. (ARCS)
bone d.
bony d.
boomerang d.
BOR d.
bowenoid d.
bronchopulmonary d. (BPD)
3C d.
camptomelic d.
caudal d.
CCC d.
cerebellar d.
cerebellotrigeminal and focal dermal d.
cerebrofaciothoracic syndrome or d.
cervical d.
chondroectodermal d.
cleidocranial d.
d. cleidocranialis
d. cleidofacialis
clubfoot d.
colposcopic grading of cervical d.
congenital alveolar d.
congenital encephalo-ophthalmic d.
congenital glenoid d.
congenital hip d. (CHD)
cortical d. (CD)
costovertebral d.
craniodiaphysial d.
cranioectodermal d. (CED)
craniofrontal d.
craniofrontonasal d. (CFND)
craniometaphysial d.
craniotubular d.
cretinoid d.
de la Chapelle d.
dentin d.
developmental hip d.
diaphysial d.
diastrophic d. (DD)
dyssegmental d.
ectodermal d. (ED)
endocervical glandular d.
d. epiphysealis hemimelica
d. epiphysealis punctata
epiphysial d.
d. epiphysialis hemimelia
facial ectodermal d.

faciocardiomelic d.
faciogenital d.
familial focal facial dermal d.
Fanconi d.
fetal skeletal d.
fibromuscular d.
fibrous d.
focal cortical d.
focal facial dermal d. (type I, II)
focal facial ectodermal d.
frontofacionasal d.
frontometaphysial d.
frontonasal d. (FND)
geleophysic d.
glenoid d.
Goldenhar oculauricular vertebral d.
gonadal d.
gracile bone d.
Grebe d.
hereditary bone d.
hereditary ectodermal d.
hereditary expansile polyostotic osteolytic d.
hereditary retinal d.
hidrotic ectodermal d.
high-grade cervical d.
hip d.
Holt-Oram atriodigital d.
hydrocephalus, agyria, retinal d. (HARD)
hypohidrotic ectodermal d.
immunoosseous d.
intestinal neuronal d.
intraepithelial cervical d.
iridodental d.
ischiopatellar d.
Kniest d.
Kniest-like d.
Kozlowski spondylometaphysial d.
kyphomelic d.
Langer mesomelic d.
lateral facial d. (LFD)
Lenz d.
lethal bone d.
d. linguofacialis
low-grade d. (LGD)
lymphatic d.
mammary d. (MD)
mandibular-acral d.
mandibuloacral d.
Margarita Island type ectodermal d.
d. marginalis posterior
maxillonasal d.
medullary d.
mesectodermal d.
mesomelic d.
metaphoric d.
metaphysial d.
metatropic d.

Mexican cardiomelic d.
microglandular d.
mild acetabular d.
müllerian duct aplasia, renal
 agenesis/ectopia, cervical somite d.
 (MURCS)
multicystic renal d.
multiple epiphysial d.
myxoid d.
necrotic facial d.
neonatal osseous d.
nerve d.
neurogenic hip d.
neuronal d.
oculoauricular d.
oculoauriculovertebral d.
oculodentodigital d.
d. oculodentodigitalis
oculodentoosseous d. (ODOD)
odontoonychodermal d.
OFD with tibial d.
olfactogenital d.
ophthalmomandibulomelic d.
optic nerve d.
osteodental d. (ODD)
osteofibrous d.
osteoglophonic d.
otospondylomegaepliphysial d.
pelvis capsular d.
pelvis-shoulder d.
polycystic fibrous d.
polyostotic fibrous d.
porencephaly cortical d.
posterior urethral valves, unilateral
 reflux, renal d. (VURD)
pseudoachondroplastic d.
pseudodiastrophic d.
ptosis of eyelids, diastasis recti,
 hip d.
pulmonary d.
punctate epiphyseal d.
radial d.
radiation d.
Rapp-Hodgkin ectodermal d.
renal medullary d.
retinal d.
right ventricular d.
Robinow mesomelic d.
Schimke immunoosseous d.
Schmid metaphysial d.
Schneckenbecken d.
septooptic-pituitary d.
Silverman-Handmaker
 dyssegmental d.
skeletal d.
sphenoid d.
sponastrime d.
spondyloepimetaphysial d. (SEMD)
spondyloepiphysial d. (SED)

spondylometaphysial d.
spondyloperipheral d.
spondylothoracic d.
squamous d.
Stickler d.
Streeter d.
d. syndrome
thanatophoric d.
thymic d.
trichorhino-auriculophalangeal
 multiple exostoses d.
trichorhinophalangeal multiple
 exostosis d.
urinary tract d.
ventricular d.
dysplastic
 d. cell
 d. change
 d. cortical architecture
 d. gangliocytoma
 d. gangliocytoma of cerebellum
 d. kidney
 d. nevus
 d. nevus syndrome
dyspnea
 d. of pregnancy
 paroxysmal nocturnal d. (PND)
dyspraxia
dysproteinemia
dysprothrombinemia
dysraphia (*var. of* dysraphism)
 d. of spine
 olfacto-ethmoidohypothalamic d.
 tectocerebellar d.
dysraphism, dysraphia
 occult spinal d.
 spinal d.
dysregulated
 d. behavior
 d. insulin secretion
dysregulation
 autonomic d.
 hypothalamic-pituitary-adrenal axis d.
 immune d.
 temperature d.
dysrhythmia
 cardiac d.
 gastric d.
 ventricular d.
dyssegmental dysplasia
dyssomnia
 circadian rhythm d.
 extrinsic d.
 infant d.
 intrinsic d.
dysspermia
dyssynchrony
dyssynergia, dyssynergy
 detrusor sphincter d.

277

dyssynergy (*var. of* dyssynergia)
dystasia
    hereditary areflexic d.
dystaxia cerebralis infantilis
dysthymia
dysthymic disorder
dysthyroidal infantilism
dystocia
    abdominal d.
    all-fours maneuver for shoulder d.
    cervical d.
    fetal d.
    maternal d.
    placental d.
    shoulder d.
    vaginal soft tissue d.
dystocia-dystrophia syndrome
dystonia
    buccomandibular d.
    craniocervical d.
    dopa-responsive d. (DRD)
    drug-induced d.
    early-onset d.
    focal d.
    generalized d.
    idiopathic torsion d.
    d. musculorum deformans
      (DMD)
    myoclonic d.
    oromandibular d.
    paroxysmal d.
    primary d.
    progressive d.
    secondary d.
    segmental d.
    symptomatic d.
    tardive d.
    torsion d.
    transient d.
dystonia-deafness syndrome
dystonia-parkinsonism
dystonic
    d. cerebral palsy
    d. dyskinetic disorder
    d. hyperextension
    d. posturing
    d. reaction
dystopia canthorum
dystrophia
    d. bullosa hereditaria, typus
      maculosus
    d. retinae-dysacousis syndrome
    d. retinae pigmentosa-dysostosis
      (DRD)
dystrophic
    d. calcification
    d. change
    d. epidermolysis bullosa
    d. myopathy

    d. nail
    d. tooth
dystrophica
    epidermis bullosa d.
dystrophin-associated gene complex
dystrophin gene
dystrophinopathy
dystrophy, dystrophia
    adult pseudohypertrophic muscular d.
    Aran-Duchenne muscular d.
    asphyxiating thoracic d. (ATD)
    autoimmune polyendocrinopathy,
      candidiasis, ectodermal d.
      (APECED)
    autosomal dominant d.
    autosomal recessive muscular d.
    Becker-Kiener muscular d.
    Becker muscular d. (BMD)
    Becker pseudohypertrophic muscular
      d.
    Becker type progressive muscular d.
    benign X-linked recessive muscular
      d.
    cerebroocular dysgenesis-muscular d.
      (COD-MD)
    cerebroocular dysplasia-muscular d.
    cerebroocular muscular d.
    childhood pseudohypertrophic
      muscular d.
    classic X-linked recessive muscular
      d.
    congenital endothelial corneal d.
    congenital muscular d. (CMD)
    congenital myotonic d.
    corneal d.
    craniocarpotarsal d.
    Duchenne de Boulogne muscular d.
      (DMD)
    Duchenne muscular d. (DMD)
    Duchenne muscular dystrophy/Becker
      muscular d.
    Duchenne-type pseudohypertrophic
      progressive muscular d.
    early corneal d.
    Emery-Dreifuss muscular d.
    endothelial d.
    Erb juvenile muscular d.
    fadioscapulohumeral muscular d.
      (FSHD)
    familial osseous d.
    FSH muscular d.
    Fukuyama congenital muscular d.
      (FCMD)
    giant neuroaxonal d.
    gingival fibromatosis-corneal d.
    hereditary bullous d.
    humeroperoneal muscular d.
    hyperplastic d.
    infantile neuroaxonal d.

infantile thoracic d.
Jeune thoracic d.
juvenile epithelial corneal d.
juvenile muscular d.
juvenile myotonic d.
Landouzy d.
Landouzy-Dejerine muscular d.
Leyden-Möbius muscular d.
limb girdle muscular d.
macular d.
Meesmann corneal d.
micropolygyria with muscular d.
mild X-linked recessive muscular d.
muscular d. (MD)
myotonic d. (MD)
myotonic muscular d.
nail d.
neuroaxonal d.
neurovascular d.
ocular muscular d.
oculocerebral d.
oculocerebrorenal d.
oculopharyngeal muscular d.
osteochondromuscular d.
peroneal muscular d.

pseudohypertrophic adult muscular d.
pseudohypertrophic progressive
  muscular d.
reflex sympathetic d. (RSD)
scapulohumeral muscular d.
scapuloperoneal d.
Schnyder crystalline corneal d.
  (SCCD)
scleroatonic muscular d.
secondary nail d.
severe childhood autosomal recessive
  muscular d. (SCARMD)
short-limb d.
spinal muscular d.
Steinert myotonic d.
thoracic asphyxiant d.
thoracic-pelvic-phalangeal d.
twenty-nail d.
vulvar d.
X-linked recessive muscular d.
dysuria, dysury
dysuria-pyuria syndrome
dysuria-sterile pyuria syndrome
dysury (*var. of* dysuria)
dyszoospermia

D

E

E antigen
E autoantibody
E sign

E$_1$

estrone
prostaglandin E$_1$ (PGE$_1$)
synthetic prostaglandin E$_1$

E$_2$

estradiol
eutopic endometrium prostaglandin E$_2$
prostaglandin E$_2$ (PGE$_2$)

E$_3$

unconjugated estriol

E$_4$

leukotriene E$_4$ (LTE$_4$)

EA

early amniocentesis
esophageal atresia

EAA

excitotoxic amino acid

EABT

estrogen add-back therapy

EAC

external auditory canal

EACA

epsilon aminocaproic acid

EAE

experimental allergic encephalomyelitis

Eagle-Barrett syndrome
Eagle test
ear

e. anomaly
Aztec e.
bat e.
e. canal
e. crease/pit
cup e.
Darwin e.
external e.
glue e.
inner e.
laser office ventilation of e.'s (LOVE)
left e.
lop e.
low-set e.'s
malformed e.
middle e.
Morel e.
Mozart e.
Otocalm E.
outer e.
e., patella, short stature (EPS)

prominent e.
satyr e.
scroll e.
e. speculum
swimmer's e.
tugging at e.'s
e. ventilation tube
Wildermuth e.

EAR

early asthmatic response

EarCheck
ear-cough reflex
eardrum

perforated e.
e. perforation

Earle

E. balanced salt solution
E. culture medium

earlobe

bifid e.
e. crease

early

e. adolescence
e. amniocentesis (EA)
e. amnion vascular disruption complex
E. and Periodic Screening, Diagnosis, and Treatment
e. asthmatic reaction
e. asthmatic response (EAR)
e. cardiac motion
e. childhood caries (ECC)
E. Childhood Special Education Program
e. congenital syphilis
e. constraint defect
e. corneal dystrophy
e. deceleration
e. educator
e. embryonic cell
e. embryonic death
e. embryonic loss
e. enteral feeding
e. follicular development
e. infantile autism
e. infantile epileptic encephalopathy (EIEE)
e. intervention
e. interventionist
e. intervention program (EIP)
E. Language Milestone (ELM)
E. Language Milestone scale
e. mature
e. midsystolic closure
e. morning irritability

E

early (*continued*)
    e. neonatal neurobehavioral scale
    e. neonate
    e. onset neonatal pneumonia
    e. pregnancy factor (EPF)
    e. pregnancy loss (EPL)
    e. pregnancy test (EPT)
    e. pregnancy wastage
    e. proliferative phase
    e. satiety
    e. stromal invasion
early-discharge program
early-onset
    e.-o. diabetes mellitus-epiphysial dysplasia syndrome
    e.-o. disease
    e.-o. dystonia
    e.-o. parkinsonism-mental retardation syndrome
    e.-o. preeclampsia
    e.-o. schizophrenia (EOS)
    e.-o. sepsis
EarPopper inflation device
earth
    diatomaceous e. (DE)
EAS
    Emotionality Activity Sociability Scale
    external anal sphincter
ease
    Gebauer's Pain E.
EASI
    extraamniotic saline infusion
    EASI catheter
Easprin
Eastern
    E. blot
    E. blot test
    E. equine encephalitis (EEE)
Eastman-Bixler syndrome
easy
    E. Breathing asthma management program
    e. bruisabilty
    Clearblue E.
    ClearPlan E.
    e. fatigability
eater
    picky e.
eating
    E. Attitudes Test
    binge e.
    e. disorder
    e. disorder not otherwise specified (EDNOS)
    e. disorders examination (EDE)
    E. Disorders Inventory (EDI)
    E. Disorders Inventory Score for Interoceptive Awareness Affect
    e. habit

Eaton-Lambert myasthenic syndrome
EB
    epidermolysis bullosa
EBCT
    electron-beam computed tomography
EBF
    erythroblastosis fetalis
EBLL
    elevation of blood lead level
EBM
    epidermolysis bullosa, macular type
EBNA
    Epstein-Barr nuclear antigen
EBNS
    endoscopic bladder neck suspension
Ebola hemorrhagic fever
Ebstein
    E. anomaly
    E. malformation
EBV
    Epstein-Barr virus
EBV-related B-cell lymphoma
EC
    emergency contraception
E-cadherin protein
ecbolic
ECC
    early childhood caries
    embryonal cell carcinoma
    endocervical curettage
    extracorporeal circulation
eccentric
    e. exercise
    e. gaze
    e. orifice
eccentrochondrodysplasia
eccentrochondroplasia
eccentroosteochondrodysplasia
ecchymosis
    periorbital e.
    postauricular e.
    trocar site e.
ecchymotic Ehlers-Danlos syndrome
ECCL
    encephalocraniocutaneous lipomatosis
Eccocee ultrasound system
eccrine
    e. bromhidrosis
    e. sweat duct
    e. sweat gland
    e. sweating
eccyesis
ECD
    endocardial cushion defect
ECF
    executive cognitive functioning
    extracellular fluid
ECG
    electrocardiogram

echinacea
echinococcal cyst
echinococciasis (*var. of* echinococcosis)
echinococcosis, echinococciasis
    alveolar e.
Echinococcus
    E. granulosus
    E. granulosus hydatid cyst
    E. multilocularis
echinocyte
Echistatin
echo
    e. Doppler gradient
    e. dropout
    e. formation
    scattered e.
    single shot fast spin e.
      (SSFSE)
    specular e.
    ECHO virus
echocardiogram (ECG)
    color e.
    2D e.
    2-dimensional e.
    fetal e.
    M-mode e.
echocardiograph (echo, echoes)
echocardiography
    abdominal fetal e.
    A-mode e.
    2D e.
    3D e.
    Doppler e.
    fetal e.
    M-mode e.
    real-time e.
    transesophageal e. (TEE)
    transpericardial e.
    transthoracic e.
EchoCheck
echodensity
echoencephalogram
echoencephalography
    cranial e.
echo-free zone
echogenic
    e. cardiac focus
    e. fetal bowel
    e. tissue
echogenicity
echogram
    M-mode e.
echo-guided balloon atrial septostomy
echolalia
    compulsive e.
echolucency
    periventricular e. (PVEL)
echolucent area
EchoMark salpingography catheter

echoplanar functional magnetic resonance
  imaging
echopraxia, echopraxis
echopraxis (*var. of* echopraxia)
Echo-Screen
echothiophate iodide
Echotip
    E. Norfolk aspiration needle
    E. percutaneous entry needle
echoviral meningitis
echovirus, ECHO virus
    e. 9 meningitis
Echovist contrast
eclampsia
    e. nutans
    puerperal e.
    superimposed e.
eclamptic
    e. idiocy
    e. retinopathy
    e. seizure
eclamptogenic, eclamptogenous
eclamptogenous (*var. of* eclamptogenic)
ECLS
    extracorporeal life support
ECLT
    euglobulin clot lysis time
ECM
    erythema chronicum migrans
    ECM rash
ECMO
    extracorporeal membrane oxygenation
    double-lumen venovenous ECMO
    venovenous ECMO
ECochG
    electrocochleography
ECoG
    electrocochleography
E-Complex-600
econazole
Econopred Plus Ophthalmic
Ecostatin
Ecotrin
Ecowarm gel warmer
ECP
    emergency contraception pill
    emergency contraceptive pill
    eosinophilic cationic protein
ECR
    endocervical resection
ecstasy
ECT
    electroconvulsive therapy
ectasia, ectasis
    annuloaortic e.
    arterial e.
    duct e.
    ductal e.
    dural e.

E

ectasia (*continued*)
 familial aortic e.
 mammary duct e.
 scoliosis with dural e.
ectasis (*var. of* ectasia)
ecthyma gangrenosum
ectocervical lesion
ectocervix
 friable e.
ectoderm
 cutaneous e.
ectodermal
 e. dysplasia
 e. dysplasia, cleft lip and palate, hand and foot deformity, mental retardation syndrome
 e. dysplasia, cleft lip and palate, mental retardation, syndactyly syndrome (I, II)
 e. dysplasia, mental retardation, syndactyly syndrome
 e. dysplasia of face
 e. ridge
ectolecithal
ectomere
ectomesoblast
ectoneurodermal hamartoma
ectopagus
ectoparasite
ectopia, ectopy
 e. cordis
 crossed fused e.
 double thyroid e.
 infrahyoid e.
 e. lentis
 e. lentis et pupillae
 renal e.
 ureteral e.
ectopic
 e. anus
 e. atrial tachycardia
 e. decidua
 e. endometrial tissue
 e. endometrium
 e. gastric mucosa
 e. implant
 e. implantation
 e. ovarian tissue
 e. pancreatic rest
 e. pinealoma
 e. pregnancy (EP)
 e. testis
 e. thyroid
 e. ureter
 e. ureterocele
 e. ventricular depolarization
ectoplacental cone
ectopy
 cervical e.

Ectosone
ectrodactylia (*var. of* ectrodactyly)
ectrodactylism (*var. of* ectrodactyly)
ectrodactyly, ectrodactylia, ectrodactylism
 e., ectodermal dysplasia and cleft lip/palate syndrome
 e., ectodermal dysplasia, clefting (EEC)
 e., mandibulofacial dysostosis syndrome
ectrodactyly-cleft lip/palate syndrome
ectromelia
ectrometacarpia
ectrometatarsia
ectrophalangia
ectropion, ectropium
 cervical e.
 congenital e.
ectropium (*var. of* ectropion)
ectrosyndactyly
ECV
 external cephalic version
 extracellular volume
eczema
 asteatotic e.
 atopic e.
 discoid e.
 dyshidrotic e.
 e. herpeticum
 infantile e.
 e. marginatum
 e. neonatorum
 nipple e.
 nummular e.
 plaque of nummular e.
 seborrheic e.
 e. vaccinatum
eczematization
eczematoid
 e. dermatitis
 e. lesion
 e. skin rash
eczematous
 e. halo nevus
 e. rash
 e. skin lesion
EDAS
 encephaloduroarteriosynangios
EDC
 estimated date of conception
 estimated date of confinement
 expected date of confinement
EDD
 expected date of delivery
Eddowes syndrome
EDE
 eating disorders examination
Edecrin
 E. Oral
 E. Sodium Injection

edema
    angioneurotic e.
    benign transient optic disc e.
    Berlin e.
    brain e.
    brawny e.
    cardiogenic pulmonary e.
      (CPE)
    cellular e.
    cerebral e.
    corneal e.
    cytotoxic e.
    dependent e.
    focal cerebral e.
    gestational e.
    hereditary e.
    high-altitude cerebral e.
      (HACE)
    high-altitude pulmonary e.
      (HAPE)
    idiopathic scrotal e.
    indurative e.
    intercellular e.
    interstitial e.
    ischemic e.
    labial e.
    laryngeal e.
    leg e.
    lung e.
    malignant brain e.
    menstrual e.
    e. neonatorum
    neurogenic pulmonary e.
    noncardiac pulmonary e.
    optic nerve e.
    periorbital e.
    peritonsillar e.
    pitting e.
    placental e.
    postasphyxial cerebral e.
    postthoracotomy pulmonary e.
    premenstrual e.
    presternal e.
    pulmonary e.
    rebound e.
    retinal e.
    scrotal e.
    segmental e.
    subglottic e.
    suborbital e.
    tonsillar e.
    vasogenic e.
    villous e.
    vulvar e.
edematous papilla
Eden-Lawson hysterectomy
Eder cord blood collection device
edetate calcium disodium
Edex

edge effect
EDH
    epidural hematoma
    extradural hematoma
EDI
    Eating Disorders Inventory
Edinburgh
    E. malformation syndrome
    E. Postnatal Depression Scale
    (EPDS)
Edinger-Westphal nucleus
edition
    Bayley Scales of Infant
      Development-Motor, 2nd E.
    Child Health and Illness Profile,
      Adolescent E. (CHIP-AE)
    Clinical Evaluation of Language
      Fundamentals, 3rd E.
    Diagnostic and Statistical Manual
      of Mental Disorders, 4th E.
      (DSM-IV)
    Receptive-Expressive Emergent
      Language Scale, 2nd E. (REEL-2)
    Stanford-Binet Intelligence Scale,
      4th E.
    Stanford-Binet Memory Scale, 4th
      E.
    Wechsler Adult Intelligence Scale,
      3rd E.
    Wechsler Intelligence Scale, 3rd E.
Edmonston-Zagreb measles vaccine
edrophonium
    e. chloride
    e. test
EDS
    Ehlers-Danlos syndrome
EDTA
    ethylenediaminetetraacetic acid
EDTA-anticoagulated Vacutainer
EDTA-Vacutainer
educable
education
    Bradley childbirth e.
    conductive e. (CE)
    Lamaze childbirth e.
    special e.
educator
    early e.
    infant e.
EDV
    end-diastolic velocity
    end-diastolic volume
    umbilical arterial EDV
Edwards-Gale syndrome
Edwardsiella tarda
Edwards syndrome
EE
    electrosurgical excision
    ethinyl estradiol

E

EEC
    ectrodactyly, ectodermal dysplasia, clefting
      EEC syndrome
EECS
    extraembryonic celomic space
EEG
    electroencephalogram
    electroencephalography
      amplitude-integrated EEG
      interictal EEG
E6-E7 gene
EEG/polygraphic/video monitoring
EELV
    end-expiratory lung volume
eelworm
EENT
    eyes, ears, nose, throat
EEP
    end-expiratory phase
    end-expiratory pressure
EER
    extraesophageal reflux
E.E.S.
    erythromycin ethylsuccinate
    E.E.S. granules
EES
    endometrial stromal sarcoma
    erythromycin ethylsuccinate
    expandable esophageal stent
EFA
    essential fatty acid
      EFA deficiency
EFAS
    embryofetal alcohol syndrome
efavirenz
EFE
    endocardial fibroelastosis
      primary EFE
efface
effacement
    cervical e.
    e. of cervix
effect
    Accutane e.
    adiabatic e.
    adverse maternal e.
    anemic e.
    antiendometriotic e.
    antiestrogen e.
    antiestrogenic e.
    antiinflammatory e.
    Arias-Stella e.
    ball-valve e.
    Bohr e.
    brain-sparing e.
    bystander e.
    cardioprotective e.
    cardiovascular e.
    choroid plexus pulse e.

    chronotropic e.
    Coanda e.
    Compton e.
    Cushing e.
    cytopathic e. (CPE)
    cytotoxic e.
    demand e.
    differential e.
    digitalis e.
    Doppler e.
    edge e.
    Eisenmenger e.
    estrogen e.
    estrogen-agonist uterine e.
    estrogenic e.
    fetal e.
    fetal alcohol e. (FAE)
    first-pass e.
    founder e.
    halo e.
    Hawthorne e.
    hormonal e.
    hypnotic e.
    iatrogenic e.
    inotropic e.
    jet cooling e.
    Mach band e.
    marijuana e.
    mass e.
    maternal e.
    mitogenic e.
    muscarinic e.
    neurologic adverse e.
    perinatal e.
    pituitary gonadotropin e.
    progestational e.
    psychological e.
    returning-soldier e.
    salutary e.
    sedative e.
    side e. (SE)
    siphon e.
    social factor e.
    star e.
    systemic side e.
    teratogenic e.
    waterhammer e.
    white coat e.
    Yom Kippur e.
effective
    e. conjugate
    e. refractory period
effectiveness
    contraceptive e.
effector cell
efferentia
    ductuli e.
efferent limb
Effexor

efficacious
efficacy
    in vitro e.
    oral contraceptive e.
efficiency
    female fertility e.
    sleep e.
effluent
    fetal pulmonary e.
    menstrual e.
effluvium
    anagen e.
    telogen e.
efflux
effort
    respiratory e.
effortless regurgitation
effusion
    bilateral otitis media with e.
        (BOME)
    boggy synovial e.
    chylous pleural e.
    clenched fist and pleural e.
    hemorrhagic pleural e.
    lingular e.
    malignant pleural e.
    middle ear e. (MEE)
    nonchylous pleural e.
    otitis media with e. (OME)
    otitis media without e.
    parapneumonic pleural e.
    pericardial e.
    pleural e.
    subdural e.
    transudative pleural e.
    tuberculous pleural e.
Efidac/24
eflornithine (DMFO)
EFM
    electronic fetal monitoring
    external fetal monitoring
EFNEP
    expanded food nutrition education
        program
EFS
    event-free survival
Efudex Topical
EFW
    estimated fetal weight
EGA
    estimated gestational age
Egan mammography
EG/BUS
    external genitalia/Bartholin, urethral,
        and Skene glands
EGD
    esophagogastroduodenoscopy
EGF
    epidermal growth factor

EGFR
    epidermal growth factor receptor
egg
    e. activation
    e. cell
    e. donation
    e. donor
    donor e.
    frozen e.
    e. membrane
    e. on a string
    e. phospholipid
    e. retrieval
    e. transport
    e. yolk extender
eggbeater running pattern
1-egg twins
2-egg twins
EGNB
    enteric gram-negative bacillary
Egnell
    E. breast pump
    E. vacuum
egodystonic
ego-oriented individual therapy (EOIT)
egophony
egosyntonic
egress
    neutrophil e.
EH
    endometrial hyperplasia
    epidural hematoma
EHEC
    enterohemorrhagic *Escherichia coli*
EHG
    electrohysterography
Ehlers-Danlos syndrome (EDS)
EHM
    embryonic heart motion
Ehrlich catheter
Ehrlichia
    E. chaffeensis
    E. phagocytophila
    E. sennetsu
ehrlichiosis
    granulocytic e.
    human granulocytic e. (HGE)
    human monocytic e. (HME)
EIA
    enzyme immunoassay
    enzyme immunosorbent assay
    exercise-induced asthma
EIB
    erythema induration of Bazin
    exercise-induced bronchospasm
EIC
    epidermal inclusion cyst
    extensive intraductal component
eicosanoid

E

eicosapentaenoic acid
EIEE
 early infantile epileptic encephalopathy
EIFT
 embryo intrafallopian transfer
eighth nerve deafness
Eikenella corrodens
EIM
 extraintestinal manifestation
EI/MV
 endotracheal intubation and mechanical
 ventilation
EIN
 endometrial intraepithelial neoplasia
Einstein
 E. Neonatal Neurobehavioral
 Assessment Scale (ENNAS)
 E. screening test
Einthoven triangle
EIP
 early intervention program
eIPV
 enhanced inactivated polio vaccine
Eisenmenger
 E. complex
 E. effect
 E. physiology
 E. syndrome (Eis)
EITB
 enzyme-linked immunotransfer blot
ejaculate
 sperm-free e.
ejaculation
 e. failure
 premature e.
 retrograde e.
ejaculatory duct
ejection
 e. click
 milk e.
 e. murmur
 e. reflex
EKC
 epidemic keratoconjunctivitis
EKG
 electrocardiogram
 electrocardiography
 pediatric EKG
Eklund
 E. mammography technique
 E. positioning system
ektacytometer
elastance
 respiratory system e. (E_{dyn})
 static e. (E_{st})
elastase
 fecal pancreatic e.
elastic
 e. abdominal retractor

 e. bandaging
 e. canal
 e. lamina
 e. recoil of bronchus
 e. stocking
 e. tissue hyperplasia
elastica
 cutis e.
elasticity
 blood vessel e.
elasticum
 pseudoxanthoma e.
elastin (ELN)
 e. gene deletion
elastogram
elastography
 magnetic resonance e.
 (MRE)
elastolysis
 generalized e.
elastomer catheter
elastosis perforans serpiginosa
Elavil
elbow
 e. dislocation
 e. fracture
 Little League e.
 nursemaid's e.
 pitcher's e.
 prone on e.'s (POE)
 pulled e.
 tennis e.
ELBW
 extremely low birth weight
 ELBW infant
ELBWI
 extremely low birth weight infant
Eldecort Topical
elderly primigravida
EleCare
 E. formula
 E. nutritional supplement
Elecsys 1010 analyzer
elective
 e. abortion
 e. abortion material
 e. cesarean delivery
 e. cesarean section
 e. termination
Electra complex
electric
 e. breast pump
 General E. (GE)
 e. suction device
 e. vacuum aspiration (EVA)
 e. vacuum aspirator
electrical
 e. accustimulation
 e. alternans

e. burn
e. stimulation
electrified scissors
electrocardiogram (ECG, EKG)
    fetal e. (FECG, FEKG)
electrocardiography (ECG, EKG)
    abdominal fetal e.
    fetal e.
electrocautery
    AmpErase e.
    bipolar e.
    Endoclip monopolar e.
    laparoscopic e.
    transurethral e.
    unipolar e.
electroclinical dissociation
electrocoagulation diathermy
electrocochleography (ECochG, ECoG)
    round window e. (RWECochG)
electroconvulsive therapy (ECT)
electrocortical silence
electrode
    Aspen laparoscopy e.
    ball e.
    e. balloon
    bipolar e.
    Bugbee e.
    closed loop system passing e.
    Copeland fetal scalp e.
    endocervical e.
    fetal scalp e. (FSE)
    Kontron e.
    Littmann ECG e.
    LLETZ-LEEP active loop e.
    loop e.
    Medi-Trace e.
    REM PolyHesive II patient return e.
    rollerball e.
    RollerBar e.
    roller-barrel e.
    RollerLoop vaporizing loop e.
    scalp e.
    spiral e.
    St. Mark e.
    unipolar e.
    Valleylab ball e.
    Valleylab loop e.
electrodesiccation
electrodialyzed whey formula
electroejaculation
electroencephalogram (EEG)
    amplitude-integrated e. (aEEG)
electroencephalographic sleep study
electroencephalography (EEG)
    quantitative e. (qEEG)
    video e.
electrogastrography
Electro-Gel conductivity gel
electrographic background abnormality

electrohysterograph
electrohysterography (EHG)
electrolysis
electrolyte
    e. balance
    e. disturbance
    e. imbalance
    e. loss
    e. replacement
    e. therapy
electromagnetic
    e. radiation
    e. spectrum
electromechanical
    e. dissociation (EMD)
    e. morcellation
electromembrane
    therapeutic e. (TEM)
electrometrogram
electromyelogram (EMG)
electromyogram (EMG)
    surface e. (SEMG)
electromyography (EMG)
    anal sphincter e.
    surface e. (SEMG)
    transabdominal uterine e.
electron
    e. microscopy
    e. microscopy of stool
    e. transfer flavoprotein (ETF)
    e. transfer flavoprotein
      dehydrogenase (ETF-DH)
    e. volt (eV)
electron-beam computed tomography (EBCT)
electron-dense subepithelial deposit
electronic
    e. communication aid
    e. fetal heart rate monitoring
    e. fetal monitoring (EFM)
    e. leash
    e. scale
electronystagmography (ENG)
electrooculogram
electrooculography
electrophilic center
electrophoresis
    capillary e.
    denaturing gradient gel e.
    fluorophore-assisted carbohydrate e. (FACE)
    e. gel
    hemoglobin e.
    high-performance capillary e. (HPCE)
    Laurell (rocket) immune e.
    polyacrylamide gel e.
    pulsed field gel e. (PFGE)
    RNA e.
    thermal gel gradient e.

E

electrophoretic mobility shift assay (EMSA)
electrophrenic stimulation
electroporation
electroretinal abnormality
electroretinogram (ERG)
electroretinography (ERG)
Electroscope disposable scissors
Electroshield monitoring system
electroshock
    maximal e. (MES)
    e. therapy
electrospray ionization mass spectrometry (ESIMS)
electrosurgery
electrosurgical
    e. excision (EE)
    e. loop excision
    e. plume
    e. wire
elegance
    sartorial e.
elegans
    Abiotrophia e.
Elejalde syndrome
Elek test
Elema angiocardiogram
element
    estrogen response e. (ERE)
    immature neural e.
    IS e.
    radioactive e.
    transposable e.
elemental
    e. diet
    e. iron
elephant
    E. Ears bottle holder
    e. man
    e. pelvis
elephantiasis
    congenital e.
    genital e.
    e. vulvae
elevate
elevated
    e. bile acid
    e. cardiac output
    e. conjugated bilirubin
    e. enzyme activity
    e. fetal hemoglobin
    e. intracranial pressure
    e. liver enzymes
    e. obstetric risk
    e. renin
    e. sweat chloride concentration
    e. transaminase
elevation
    alpha-fetoprotein e.

    delayed thyrotropin e.
    fetus growth e.
    intraabdominal pressure e.
    e. of blood lead level (EBLL)
    periosteal e.
    posterior pharyngeal wall e.
    rest, ice, compression, e. (RICE)
    ST-segment e.
elevator
    Boyle uterine e.
    lemon-squeezer obstetrical e.
    Somer uterine e.
    U e.
    uterine e.
ELF
    epithelial lining fluid
    pulmonary ELF
elfin facies hypercalcemia syndrome
elfinlike facies
ELIFA
    enzyme-linked immunofiltration assay
eligibility designation
elimination diet
Elimite Cream
ELISA
    enzyme-linked immunosorbent assay
    double-sandwich ELISA
    Lyme ELISA
    ELISA test
ELISpot
    solid-phase enzyme-linked immunospot
    ELISpot assay
    ELISpot test
Elixicon
elixir
    Brofed E.
    Bromaline E.
    Bromanate E.
    Lortab E.
    Tylenol and Codeine E.
Elixophyllin
Elliot forceps
ellipsis
elliptical uterine incision
elliptocyte
elliptocytic anemia
elliptocytosis
    hereditary e. (HE)
    spherocytic hereditary e.
Ellis-Sheldon syndrome
Ellis-van Creveld syndrome
ELM
    Early Language Milestone
    ELM scale
Elmed
    E. BC 50 M/M digital bipolar coagulator
    E. peristaltic irrigation pump
Elmiron

ELN
    elastin
Elocon
elongation
    rete ridge e.
    urethral e.
ELP
    exogenous lipoid pneumonia
ElSahy-Waters syndrome
Elscint ESI-3000 ultrasound
Elspar
ELT
    euglobulin lysis time
Eltor
Eltroxin
elucidation
ELVIS
    enzyme-linked virus-inducible systems
        ELVIS test
EM
    erythema multiforme
EMA
    endomysium antibody
    epithelial membrane antigen
E-Mac
    English MacIntosh
emaciated
E-Mac laryngoscope blade
Emadine
emancipated minor
EMB
    endometrial biopsy
    ethambutol
embarrassment
    respiratory e.
Embden-Meyerhof pathway
embolectomy
    Fogarty arterial e. (FAE)
emboli (*pl. of* embolus)
embolic abscess
embolism
    air e.
    amniotic fluid e. (AFE)
    cerebral e.
    fat e.
    pulmonary e. (PE)
    pulmonary fat e.
embolization
    angiographic e.
    aortopulmonary collateral coil e.
    arterial e.
    catheter e.
    fibroid e.
    patent ductus arteriosis coil e.
    pelvic arterial e.
    selective arterial e.
    e. therapy
    transcatheter coil e.
    transcatheter uterine artery e.

    transvenous coil e.
    uterine artery e. (UAE)
    uterine fibroid e. (UFE)
embolus, *pl.* **emboli**
    air e.
    amniotic fluid e.
    gas e.
    massive pulmonary e.
    occluding spring e.
    pulmonary e.
    septic e.
    trophoblastic e.
Embosphere microsphere
embrace reflex
embryatrics
embryectomy
embryo
    abnormal e.
    e. biopsy
    e. carrier
    2-cell e.
    4-cell e.
    8-cell e.
    cleaved e.
    e. cloning
    cryopreserved e. (CPE)
    cylindrical e.
    e. donation
    e. donor
    e. encapsulation
    endometrial e.
    frozen e.
    gastrulating e.
    e. intrafallopian transfer (EIFT)
    Janosik e.
    multicelled e.
    nodular e.
    preimplantation e. (PIE)
    presomite e.
    previllous e.
    pronuclear e.
    e. reduction
    somite e.
    Spee e.
    e. splitting
    stunted e.
    tetraploid e.
    e. thawing
    e. thawing with transfer
    e. transfer (ET)
    triploid e.
embryoblast
embryocardia
embryocide
embryoctony
embryofetal alcohol syndrome (EFAS)
embryofetoscopy
    transabdominal thin-gauge e. (TGEF)
embryogenesis

E

embryogenic induction disorder
embryography
embryoid
embryologic malformation
embryology
    breast e.
    causal e.
    comparative e.
    descriptive e.
    experimental e.
    genital tract e.
    Leydig cell e.
    reproductive tract e.
embryoma
embryomorphous
Embryon
    E. GIFT catheter
    E. GIFT transfer catheter set
    E. HSG catheter
embryonal
    e. cell carcinoma (ECC)
    e. polyp
    e. rhabdomyosarcoma (ERMS)
    e. RMS
    e. sarcoma
    e. tumor
embryonate
embryonic
    e. anideus
    e. axis
    e. blastoderm
    e. branchial system
    e. cleavage
    e. development
    e. diapause
    e. differentiation
    e. disc
    e. esophagus
    e. genome activation
    e. heart motion (EHM)
    e. hemoglobin
    e. loss
    e. neural retina
    e. neural tube
    e. organ culture study
    e. period
    e. renomedullary interstitial cell
    e. sac
    e. stem cell (ESC)
    e. testicular regression syndrome
    e. tissue
embryoniform
embryonization
embryonum
    smegma e.
embryony
embryopathology
embryopathy
    alcoholic e. (AE)

    diabetic e.
    heparin e.
    isotretinoin e.
    retinoic acid e.
    rubella e.
    thalidomide e.
    trimethadione e.
    valproic acid e.
    warfarin e.
embryoplastic
embryoscope
embryoscopy
embryotome
embryotomy
embryotoxic
embryotoxon
    posterior e.
embryotrophy
EMC
    endometrial curettage
Emcyt
EMD
    electromechanical dissociation
emedastine
emergency
    e. cesarean section
    e. contraception (EC)
    e. contraception pill (ECP)
    e. contraceptive pill (ECP)
    hypertensive e.
    e. medical services for children
      (EMS-C)
    e. medicine
    e. room (ER)
    e. surgery
    surgical e.
emergent injury
Emerson respirator
Emery-Dreifuss
    E.-D. muscular dystrophy
    E.-D. syndrome
emesis
    bile-stained e.
    bilious e.
    coffee-grounds e.
    intractable e.
    e. pH determination
    posttussive e.
    salivation, lacrimation, urination,
      defecation, gastrointestinal distress,
      e. (SLUDGE)
emetic agent
EMG
    electromyelogram
    electromyogram
    electromyography
    exomphalos, macroglossia, gigantism
    MyoTrac EMG
    EMG syndrome

Emgel
eminence
>malar e.
>median e.

emission
>evoked otoacoustic e. (EOAE)
>nasal air e.
>otoacoustic e. (OAE)
>transient evoked otoacoustic e. (TEOAE)

EMIT
>enzyme-multiplication immunoassay technique
>enzyme-multiplied immunoassay technique

Emko
EMLA
>eutectic mixture of local anesthetics
>EMLA anesthetic disc
>EMLA cream
>EMLA disc topical anesthetic adhesive system
>EMLA patch

EMLB
>erythromycin lactobionate

emmenagogic
emmenagogue
emmenia
emmenic
emmeniopathy
emmenology
Emmet operation
emmetropia
Emmett cervical tenaculum
Emo-Cort
emollient cream
emotional
>e. abuse
>e. amenorrhea
>e. development
>e. disorder
>e. lability
>e. milestone
>e. response
>e. state

Emotionality Activity Sociability Scale (EAS)
emotionally
>e. disturbed
>e. impaired

empathy
emphysema
>congenital lobar e. (CLE)
>lobar e.
>perivascular e.
>pulmonary interstitial e. (PIE)
>subcutaneous e.

emphysematosa
>colpohyperplasia e.
>vaginitis e.

empiric
>e. therapy
>e. treatment

empirical
empirically
Empirin
emprosthotonos, emprosthotonus
emprosthotonus (*var. of* emprosthotonos)
empty
>e. scrotum syndrome
>e. sella syndrome

emptying
>abnormal gastric e.
>bladder e.
>delayed gastric e.
>gastric e.

empyema
>encapsulated e.
>epidural e.
>intracranial e.
>e. necessitatis
>subdural e.
>symptomatic chronic e.

EMR
>endomyometrial resection

EMRN
>encephalomyeloradiculoneuropathy

EMS
>encephalomyosynangiosis

EMSA
>electrophoretic mobility shift assay

EMS-C
>emergency medical services for children

EMTAC
>Enhanced Metabolic Testing Activity Chamber

EM/TEN
>erythema multiforme/toxic epidermal necrolysis

emulsion
>fat e.
>Soyacal IV fat e.
>Travamulsion IV fat e.

Emulsoil
en
>e. bloc
>e. bloc resection
>e. caul delivery
>e. face position

EnAbl thermal ablation system
enalapril
enalaprilat
enamel
>e. hypoplasia
>mottled e.

E

enamelogenesis
enanthate
    estradiol e.
    norethindrone e. (NET-EN)
    testosterone e.
enanthem, enanthema
    hemorrhagic e.
    oral e.
enanthema (*var. of* enanthem)
Enbrel
encainide
Encap
    Novo-Rythro E.
encapsulated empyema
encapsulation
    embryo e.
Encare
enceliitis (*var. of* encelitis)
encelitis, enceliitis
encephalitis
    acute chagasic e.
    acute influenza A e.
    allergic e.
    arboviral e.
    brainstem e.
    California e.
    cerebellar e.
    chagasic e.
    chronic focal e.
    chronic granulomatous amebic e.
    chronic mumps e.
    chronic progressive e.
    Dawson e.
    diffuse periaxial e.
    Eastern equine e. (EEE)
    enterovirus e.
    epidemic e.
    equine e.
    focal postviral e.
    giant cell e.
    hemorrhagic e.
    herpes e.
    herpes simplex e. (HSE)
    herpes simplex virus e.
    herpesvirus e.
    influenza A e.
    Japanese e.
    La Crosse e.
    e. lethargica
    Marie-Strümpell e.
    measles inclusion body e.
      (MIBE)
    multinucleated cell e.
    mumps e.
    neonatal HSV-1 e.
    neonatal HSV-2 e.
    periaxial e.
    e. periaxialis concentrica
    postinfectious e.
    postinfluenza vaccination e.
    postmeasles e.
    postviral e.
    Powassan e.
    progressive e.
    Rasmussen e.
    Russian spring-summer e.
    Schilder e.
    septic e.
    St. Louis e. (SLE)
    subacute e.
    tick-borne e. (TBE)
    Toxoplasma e.
    toxoplasmic e.
    varicella e.
    Venezuelan equine e. (VEE)
    viral e.
    Western equine e. (WEE)
encephalitogenic cell
encephalocele
    cranial e.
    frontal e.
    hydrocephalus, agyria, retinal
      dysplasia with or without e.
      (HARD+/-E)
    nasal e.
    parietal e.
    transalar sphenoidal e.
encephaloclastic
encephalocraniocutaneous lipomatosis
  (ECCL)
encephalocraniofacial angiomatosis
encephaloduroarteriosynangios (EDAS)
encephalofacial angiomatosis
encephalofacialis
    angiomatosis e.
encephalomalacia
    cystic e.
    multicystic e.
    periventricular e.
    polycystic e.
encephalomeningocele
encephalomere
encephalomyelitis
    acute disseminated e. (ADEM)
    allergic e.
    experimental allergic e. (EAE)
    fatal e.
    immune-mediated disseminated e.
    inflammatory demyelinating e.
    postinfectious e. (PIE)
    postrabies vaccine e.
    varicella-zoster e.
encephalomyelocele
encephalomyelopathy
    Leigh necrotizing e.
    mitochondrial e.
encephalomyeloradiculoneuropathy
  (EMRN)

encephalomyopathy
mitochondrial e.
e. of Leigh
subacute necrotizing e.
encephalomyosynangiosis (EMS)
encephalopathia (*var. of* encephalopathy)
encephalopathic crisis
encephalopathy, encephalopathia
AIDS e.
anoxic-ischemic e.
bilirubin e.
bovine spongiform e. (BSE)
Brett epileptogenic e.
burn e.
childhood epileptic e.
chronic spongiform e.
demyelinating e.
disseminated e.
early infantile epileptic e.
   (EIEE)
epileptic e.
epileptogenic e.
fatal neonatal hyperammonemic e.
hepatic e. (HE)
human immunodeficiency virus e.
hypertensive e.
hypoxic e.
hypoxic-ischemic e. (HIE)
infantile epileptic e.
infantile subacute necrotizing e.
Kinsbourne e.
late radiation e.
lead e.
Leigh subacute necrotizing e.
metabolic e.
mitochondrial e.
myoclonic e.
necrotizing e.
neonatal e. (NE)
neonatal hypoxic-ischemic e.
nonspecific e.
overt bilirubin e.
phenytoin e.
plateau e.
postasphyxial e.
postvaccinal e.
progressive e.
radiation e.
Reye hepatic e.
Sarnat e.
spongiform e.
static e.
subacute necrotizing e.
transient bilirubin e.
transmissible spongiform e. (TSE)
uremic e.
Wernicke e. (WE)
e. with prolinemia
encephalotomy

encephalotrigeminal
e. angiomatosis
e. syndrome
enchondral ossification
enchondroma, *pl.* **enchondromata**
multiple bone enchondromata
enchondromata (*pl. of* enchondroma)
enchondromatosis
encode
encoding
encopresis
encranius
encu method
encyesis
end
e. bud
e. ileostomy
E. Lice Liquid
endadelphos
Endantadine
endarterectomy
endarteritis, endoarteritis
infective e.
obliterative e.
Endcaps
Glucolet E.
end-diastolic
e.-d. velocity (EDV)
e.-d. volume (EDV)
endemic
e. Burkitt lymphoma
e. cretinism
e. goitrous hypothyroidism
malaria e.
e. syphilis
e. Tyrolean infantile cirrhosis
endemicity
Endermologie LPG system
Enders Edmonston measles strain
end-expiratory
e.-e. lung volume (EELV)
e.-e. phase (EEP)
e.-e. pressure (EEP)
end-inspiratory airway occlusion
Endo
E. GIA 30 suture stapler
E. Stitch laparoscopic suturing
   device
endoanal
e. ultrasonography
e. ultrasound
endoarteritis (*var. of* endarteritis)
Endo-Assist
E.-A. cutting dissector
E.-A. endoscopic forceps
E.-A. endoscopic knot pusher
E.-A. endoscopic ligature carrier
E.-A. endoscopic needle holder
E.-A. retractable blade

E

Endo-Assist (*continued*)
    E.-A. retractable scalpel
    E.-A. sponge aspirator
Endo-Avitene
    E.-A. hemostatic material
    E.-A. microfibrillar collagen
      hemostat
endobronchial tuberculosis
endocardiac (*var. of* endocardial)
endocardial, endocardiac
    e. cushion
    e. cushion defect (ECD)
    e. fibroelastosis (EFE)
    e. fibrosis
    e. sclerosis
    e. thrombus
endocarditis
    acute bacterial e.
    bacterial e.
    enterococcal e.
    fetal e.
    fungal e.
    infectious e. (IE)
    infective e. (IE)
    Libman-Sacks e.
    marantic e.
    nonbacterial thrombotic e.
    e. prophylaxis
    subacute bacterial e. (SBE)
    thrombotic e.
    verrucose e.
endocardium
    mural e.
endocautery
endocavitary radiation therapy
Endocell
    E. endometrial cell collector
    E. endometrial cell sampler
endocervical
    e. aspirator
    e. canal
    e. canal colposcopy
    e. curettage (ECC)
    e. curetting
    e. electrode
    e. glandular dysplasia
    e. mucosa
    e. polyp
    e. resection (ECR)
    e. sample
    e. sampling
    e. sampling brush
    e. sinus tumor
    e. speculum
endocervicitis
endocervix
endochondral ossification
endochondroma
endochorion

Endoclip
    E. cautery
    E. monopolar electrocautery
endocolpitis
endocrine
    e. disorder
    e. factor
    e. gland
    e. manifestation
    e. nonfunctional testis
    e. pancreatic dysfunction
    e. system
endocrinologic sex
endocrinologist
endocrinology
    pediatric e. (PdE)
    reproductive e. (ReEND)
endocrinology-infertility
    reproductive e.-i.
endocrinopathy
endocytosis
    receptor-mediated e.
endoderm
endodermal, endodermic
    e. cell
    e. sinus
    e. sinus tumor (EST)
endodermic (*var. of* endodermal)
endoesophageal pH
endogenic (*var. of* endogenous)
endogenicity/melancholia
endogenous, endogenic
    e. catecholamine
    e. cervicovaginal flora
    e. estrogen
    e. estrogen exposure
    e. estrogenic stimulation
    e. fat
    e. gonadotropin
    e. gonadotropin activity suppression
    e. hormonal production
    e. hormone
    e. opiate
    e. opiate receptor
    e. opioid
    e. opioid peptide
    e. pyrogen
    e. steroid
endoglin
endograsper
Endoloop suture
endoluminal
    e. stent
    e. stenting
endomesenchymal tract
endometria (*pl. of* **endometrium**)
endometrial
    e. ablation
    e. ablator

e. adenoacanthoma
e. adhesion
e. aspirator
e. atrophy
e. biopsy (EMB)
e. breakdown
e. cancer
e. cannula
e. carcinoma
e. cavity
e. clear cell adenocarcinoma
e. curettage (EMC)
e. cycle
e. cycling activity
e. cyst
e. dating
e. development
e. embryo
e. histology
e. hyperplasia (EH)
e. implant
e. intraepithelial neoplasia (EIN)
e. involvement
e. metastasizing leiomyoma
e. milieu
e. morphology
e. neoplasia
e. neoplasm
e. polyp
e. proliferation
e. protein
e. receptor
e. resection
e. resection and ablation (ERA)
e. sampling
e. sarcoma
e. secretory adenocarcinoma
e. shedding
e. spiral artery
e. stimulation
e. stripe
e. stroma
e. stromal sarcoma (EES, ESS)
e. suction
e. thickness
e. tuberculosis
e. tumor
e. vaporization
endometrioid
e. carcinoma
e. epithelial cell tumor
endometrioma
complex adnexal e.
large e.
ovarian e.
ruptured e.
torsion of e.
endometriosis
adhesive e.

AFS Revised Classification of E.
American Fertility Society Revised Classification of E.
E. Association
asymptomatic mild e.
extrapelvic e.
Halban theory of e.
e. interna
internal e.
Meyer theory of e.
nonpigmented e.
e. of scar
ovarian e.
pelvic e.
pulmonary e.
rectosigmoid colon e.
retroperitoneal e.
Sampson theory of e.
small bowel e.
stromal e.
tubal e.
urinary tract e.
vulvar e.
endometriosis-associated infertility
endometriotic
e. focus
e. implant
e. lesion
e. tissue
endometritis
bacteriotoxic e.
decidual e.
e. dissecans
indolent e.
nonpuerperal e.
postpartum e. (PPE)
puerperal e.
endometrium, *pl.* **endometria**
asynchronously shedding e.
atrophic e.
cyclic proliferative e.
decidualized e.
ectopic e.
eutopic e.
hyperechoic e.
hypersecretory e.
inactive e.
menstrual e.
nonpregnant e.
proliferative e.
quiescent e.
secretory e.
shedding e.
Swiss cheese e.
tubal e.
endometropic
endomyocardial
e. biopsy
e. fibrosis

E

endomyometrial resection (EMR)
endomyometritis
    bacterial e.
    postpartum e.
endomyometrium
endomysial staining
endomysium antibody (EMA)
endoneurial fibrosis
endonuclease
    e. analysis
    restriction e.
endoparametritis
Endopath
    E. bladeless trocar
    E. endoscopic articulating stapler
    E. needle tip electrosurgery probe
    E. Optiview optical surgical
    obturator
    E. Tristar trocar
    E. Ultra Veress needle
endopelvic fascia
endopeptidase
endoperoxide
    cyclic e.
endophthalmitis
    nematode e.
endophytic
endoplasm
endoplasmic reticulum (ER)
Endopouch
    E. Pro specimen-retrieval bag
    E. retriever
endorectal
    e. flap
    e. pull-through
endoreduplication
end-organ complication
endorphin, dopamine, prostaglandin
theory
endosalpingiosis
    atypical e.
endosalpingitis
endosalpinx
endoscope
    MicroLap e.
    mother and baby e.
    Olympus GIF-XP10 video e.
    Pentax EG-2430 video e.
    Pentax FG 24-x video e.
    rigid open-tube e.
    Storz e.
endoscopic
    e. bladder neck suspension (EBNS)
    e. cautery
    e. choroid plexus extirpation
    e. correction
    e. elastic band ligation
    e. ethmoidectomy
    fetal e. (FETENDO)

    e. incision
    e. incision with flap
    e. linear cutter
    e. microsurgery
    e. retrograde
    cholangiopancreatography (ERCP)
    e. sclerotherapy
    e. sinus surgery
    e. strip craniectomy
    e. unroofing
    e. variceal ligation (EVL)
    e. variceal sclerotherapy (EVS)
endoscopy
    flexible fiberoptic e.
Endoshears
endosonography
endosperm
Endotek
    E. UDS-1000 monitor
    E. urodynamics system
endothelia (*pl. of* endothelium)
endothelial
    e. cell
    e. cell activation
    e. cell lysate
    e. dysfunction
    e. dystrophy
    e. fibronectin level
    e. nitric oxide synthetase
endothelin
    e. plasma level
    e. receptor-B gene
endothelin-1 (ET-1)
    e.-1 gene
endothelin-2 (ET-2)
    e.-2 gene
endothelin-3 (ET-3)
    e.-3 gene
endotheliochorial placenta
endotheliosis
    glomerular e.
    glomerular capillary e.
endothelium, *pl.* **endothelia**
    fenestrated vascular e.
    vascular e.
endothelium-derived relaxing factor
(EDRF)
endotoxemia
endotoxic shock
endotoxin
    gram-negative e.
    lipopolysaccharide e.
    meningococcal e.
endotracheal (ET)
    e. intubation (ETI)
    e. intubation and mechanical
    ventilation (EI/MV)
    e. suction (ETS)
    e. tube

endotrachelitis
endovaginal
    e. finding
    e. imaging
    multiplane e. (MEVA)
    e. probe
    e. sonography
    e. transducer
    e. ultrasonography
    e. ultrasound (EVUS)
endovascular hemolytic-uremic syndrome
endovasculitis
    hemorrhagic e.
end-point dilution method
Endrate
Endrin
end-stage
    e.-s. cirrhosis
    e.-s. heart failure
    e.-s. kidney disease
    e.-s. liver disease
end-systolic
    e.-s. stress (ESS)
    e.-s. wall stress
end-tidal
    e.-t. breath carbon monoxide
    e.-t. carbon dioxide (E_TCO_2)
    e.-t. CO
    e.-t. CO_2
    e.-t. CO_2 monitoring
    e.-t. CO_2 tension
end-to-side
    e.-t.-s. anastomosis
    e.-t.-s. portocaval shunt
Endtz test
Enduron
enema
    air e.
    air-contrast barium e.
    antegrade continence e. (ACE)
    barium e.
    Cortenema e.
    Fleet Mineral Oil E.
    Gastrografin e.
    hydrogen peroxide e.
    lactulose e.
    oil e.
    phosphate e.
    e. procedure
    rectocolonic saline e.
    retention e.
    Rowasa e.
    soapsuds e.
    water e.
    water-soluble contrast e.
Ener-B
energy
    color Doppler e. (CDE)
    e. expenditure
    e. healing
    e. metabolism
EnfaCare Lipil formula
Enfamil
    E. A.R. Lipil formula
    E. Gentlease Lipil formula
    E. human milk fortifier
    E. human milk fortifier formula
    E. LactoFree Lipil formula
    E. Lipil low iron formula
    E. Lipil with iron formula
    E. Next Step ProSobee Lipil
        formula
    E. Nutramigen Lipil formula
    E. Pregestimil formula
    E. Premature Lipil formula
    E. ProSobee Lipil formula
enflurane
ENG
    electronystagmography
engaged head
engagement in labor
Engerix-B
    E.-B hepatitis B vaccine
    E.-B immunization
engineering
    genetic e.
Englert forceps
English
    E. lock
    E. MacIntosh (E-Mac)
    manual E.
    E. position
    signed E. (SE)
    signed exact E. (SEE)
    E. yew
Engman syndrome
engorged
    e. breast
    e. vessel
engorgement
    breast e.
    clitoral e.
    e. of intussusceptum
    vascular e.
    venous e.
engraftment
    fetal e.
Engstrom respirator
enhanced
    e. inactivated polio vaccine (eIPV)
    E. Metabolic Testing Activity
        Chamber (EMTAC)
    e. urinalysis
enhanced-potency MAb
enhancement
    acoustic e.
    e. factor
    immunologic e.

E

enhancement (*continued*)
    rapid acquisition with resolution e. (RARE)
enhancer
    surfactant-associated protein C e.
enigmatic fever
enjoyment
    sexual e.
Enjuvia
enkephalin
enlarged
    e. cavum septum
    e. cavum septum pellucidum
    e. liver
    e. posterior fossa
enlargement
    abdominal e.
    areolar e.
    bony e.
    breast e.
    clitoris e.
    corneal e.
    left atrial e. (LAE, LAF)
    lymph node e. (LNE)
    muscle e.
    parotid e.
    pelvis e.
    sellar e.
    uterine e.
Enlon
enmeshment
ENNAS
    Einstein Neonatal Neurobehavioral Assessment Scale
enolase
    neuron-specific e. (NSE)
enophthalmia (*var. of* enophthalmos)
enophthalmos, enophthalmia
enoxacin
enoxaparin
Enpresse tablet
Enseals
    potassium iodide E.
ensu method
ensure
    E. Healthy Mom shake
    E. Healthy Mom snack bar
    E. high-protein formula
    E. Plus HN formula
    E. with fiber formula
EN-tabs
    Azulfidine EN-t.
Entamoeba
    E. dispar
    E. gingivalis
    E. histolytica
entanglement
    cord e.
    fetal e.

ENTec coblator plasma system
enteral feeding
enteric
    e. adenovirus
    e. cytopathogenic human orphan (ECHO)
    e. duplication
    e. feeding
    e. fever
    e. gentamicin
    e. gram-negative bacillary (EGNB)
    e. hyperoxaluria
    e. infection
    e. neuropeptide
entericus
    liquor e.
enteritidis
    Salmonella e.
enteritis
    bacterial e.
    Campylobacter e.
    CMV e.
    inflammatory bacterial e.
    regional e.
    rotavirus e.
    tuberculous e.
    viral e.
Enterobacter
    E. cloacae
    E. pneumonia
Enterobacteriaceae
enterobiasis
Enterobius vermicularis
enterocele
    anterior e.
    double hump sign of an e.
    pulsion e.
    e. repair
    traction e.
enterochromaffin
    e. cell
    e. cell stimulation
enterococcal endocarditis
enterococci (*pl. of* enterococcus)
enterococcus
    E. casseliflavus
    E. faecalis
    E. faecium
    glycopeptide-resistant e. (GRE)
    vancomycin-resistant e. (VRE)
    viridans e.
enterocolic fistula
enterocolitica
    Yersinia e.
enterocolitis
    allergic e.
    autistic e.
    dietary protein e.
    Hirschsprung e.

necrotizing e. (NEC)
pseudomembranous e.
e. syndrome
enterocutaneous fistula
enterocyte
enterocytopathogenic human orphan (ECHO)
Enterocytozoon
E. bieneusi
E. intestinalis
enteroenteric fistula
enterogenous cyst
enteroglucagon
enterohemorrhagic *Escherichia coli* **(EHEC)**
enterohepatic
e. recirculation
e. shunt
e. shunting
enterokinase deficiency
enteromammary circulation
enteromenia
enteropathica
acrodermatitis e. (AE)
dermatitis e.
enteropathogenic *Escherichia coli* **(EPEC)**
enteropathy
autoimmune e. (AIE)
dermatitis herpetiformis-associated gluten-sensitive e.
gluten e.
gluten-induced e.
gluten-sensitive e.
protein-losing e.
enteroscopy
small bowel e.
enterostomal therapy
enterostomy
diverting e.
proximal e.
Santulli e.
Entero-Test
enterotoxigenic *Escherichia coli* **(ETEC)**
enterotoxin
e. F
sporulation e.
enterovaginal fistula
enterovesical fistula
enteroviral
e. infection
e. meningitis
e. meningoencephalitis
e. myocarditis
enterovirus
e. 71
e. encephalitis
nonpolio e.
Entex LA
enthesitis

enthesopathy
entitled demander
Entocort
entrapment
head e.
intrapartum head e.
penile zipper e.
saphenous nerve e.
entrapped temporal horn
Entree
E. II trocar and cannula system
E. Plus trocar and cannula system
EntriStar
E. gastrostomy system
E. Skin Level Tube
E. Skin Level Tube for gastrostomy
entropy
enucleation
surgical e.
Enulose
enunciate
enuresis
diurnal e.
head banding e.
nocturnal e.
pad and bell technique for e.
primary nocturnal e.
secondary e.
enuretic episode
envelope
lipid e.
peritoneal e.
envenomation
arachnid e.
snakebite e.
environment
anaerobic e.
Home Observation for the Measurement of the E. (HOME)
hormonal e.
intrauterine e.
least restrictive e. (LRE)
natural e.
thermal neutral e.
environmental
e. risk
e. teratogen
e. tobacco smoke (ETS)
e. toxin
e. trigger
e. variance
Envision endocavity probe
Enzone
enzygotic twins
enzymatic block
enzyme
e. activity
angiotensin-converting e. (ACE)
antioxidant e.

E

enzyme (*continued*)
    e. assay
    cytochrome *c* oxidative e.
    e. defect
    e. deficiency
    deficient e.
    elevated liver e.'s
    exogenous pancreatic e.
    human recombinant antioxidant e.
    e. immunoassay (EIA)
    e. immunosorbent assay (EIA)
    inosinate pyrophosphorylase e.
    major detoxification e.
    peroxidative e.
    proteolytic e.
    rare-cutter e.
    recombinant e.
    e. replacement therapy
    restriction e.
    e. supplement
    *Taq*I e.
    TNF-alpha converting e.
    zinc-dependent e.
enzyme-linked
    e.-l. antiglobulin test
    e.-l. immunofiltration assay (ELIFA)
    e.-l. immunosorbent assay (ELISA)
    e.-l. immunotransfer blot (EITB)
    e.-l. virus-inducible systems (ELVIS)
enzyme-multiplication immunoassay
  technique (EMIT)
enzyme-multiplied immunoassay technique
  (EMIT)
enzymic acid hydrolysis
enzymopathy
EOAE
    evoked otoacoustic emission
EOIT
    ego-oriented individual therapy
EOM
    equal ocular movement
    extraocular movement
    extraocular muscle
EOS
    early-onset schizophrenia
eosin
    hematoxylin and e. (H&E)
    e. stain
eosinopenia
eosinophilia
    nonallergenic rhinitis with e.
    peripheral e.
    pulmonary e.
    pulmonary infiltrate with e. (PIE)
    sputum e.
eosinophilia-myalgia syndrome
eosinophilic
    e. adenoma
    e. allergic colitis

    e. ascites
    e. cationic protein (ECP)
    e. cystitis
    e. esophagitis
    e. fasciitis
    e. gastroenteritis
    e. gastroenteropathy
    e. granuloma
    e. infiltrate
    e. leukemia
    e. meningitis
    e. meningoencephalitis
    e. myocarditis
    e. myositis
    e. nonallergic rhinitis
    e. pleocytosis
    e. pneumonia
    e. pustular folliculitis (EPF)
eosinophilocytic
eosinophil peroxidase
eosin-4 stain
EP
    ectopic pregnancy
    etoposide
EPC
    external pneumatic calf compression
EPD
    extramammary Paget disease
EPDS
    Edinburgh Postnatal Depression
    Scale
EPEC
    enteropathogenic *Escherichia coli*
ependyma
ependymitis
    granular e.
ependymoblastoma
ependymoma
    posterior fossa anaplastic e.
    supratentorial anaplastic e.
eperezolid
EPF
    early pregnancy factor
    eosinophilic pustular folliculitis
ephaptic interaction
ephebiatrics
ephebic
ephebogenesis
ephebogenic
ephebology
ephedra
ephedrine
    racemic e.
    e. sulfate
ephelides (*pl. of* ephelis)
ephelis, *pl.* **ephelides**
    nevi, atrial myxoma, myxoid
    neurofibromas, ephelides
    (NAME)

ephemeral
- e. fever
- e. temperature

Epi
- Epi E-Z Pen
- Epi E-Z Pen-Jr

EPI
- extremely premature infant

epiblast
epiblepharon
epibulbar dermoid
epicanthal fold
epicanthus inversus
epicardial pacing
epicardium
epicomus syndrome
epicondyle
- traction apophysitis of medial e.

epicondylitis
- lateral e.
- medial e.

epicranial aponeurosis
Epics XL flow cytometer
epicutaneous test
epidemic
- e. capillary bronchitis
- e. encephalitis
- e. keratoconjunctivitis (EKC)
- e. keratoconjunctivitis adenovirus
- e. motor polyradiculoneuritis
- e. parotitis
- e. pleurodynia
- e. relapsing fever
- e. vertigo

epidemica
- myalgia cruris e.

epidemiologic, epidemiological
- E. Catchment Program
- e. characteristic
- e. features
- e. genetics
- e. study

epidemiological (*var. of* epidemiologic)
epidemiology
epidermal, epidermatic
- e. covering
- e. cyst
- e. growth factor (EGF)
- e. growth factor receptor (EGFR)
- e. hyperkeratosis
- e. inclusion cyst (EIC)
- e. melanocyte
- e. nevus
- e. nevus syndrome

epidermatic (*var. of* epidermal)
epidermidis
- *Staphylococcus* e.

epidermis bullosa dystrophica

epidermodysplasia verruciformis
epidermoid cyst
epidermolysis
- e. bullosa (EB)
- e. bullosa acquisita
- e. bullosa letalis
- e. bullosa, macular type (EBM)
- e. bullosa simplex
- e. bullosa simplex of feet
- e. bullosa simplex of hands

epidermolytic
- e. hyperkeratosis
- e. toxin

Epidermophyton floccosum
epidermophytosis
epididymal
- e. sperm
- e. sperm aspiration (ESA)
- e. vessel vasculitis

epididymides (*pl. of* epididymis)
epididymis, *pl.* **epididymides**
- appendix e.

epididymitis
- postoperative congestive e.

epididymoorchitis
epididymovasostomy
epidural
- e. abscess
- e. analgesia
- e. anesthesia
- e. empyema
- e. hemangioma
- e. hematoma (EDH, EH)
- e. hemorrhage
- labor e. (LE)
- e. morphine
- e. opioid
- e. PCA

Epifoam
Epifrin
epigastric
- e. artery
- e. hernia
- e. pain
- e. tenderness

epigastrium
epigastrius
epigenesis
epigenetic event
epiglottal blockage
epiglottic surface culture
epiglottiditis (*var. of* epiglottitis)
epiglottis
- omega-shaped e.

epiglottis, epiglottiditis
- acute e.

epignathus
epilepsia (*var. of* epilepsy)
- e. partialis continua

E

303

epilepsy, epilepsia
    abdominal e.
    absence e.
    benign childhood e. (BCE)
    benign focal e.
    benign myoclonic e.
    benign neonatal e.
    benign partial e.
    benign rolandic e. (BRE)
    centralopathic e.
    centrencephalic e.
    centrotemporal e.
    childhood absence e. (CAE)
    complex myoclonic e.
    complex partial e.
    extratemporal e.
    fictitious e.
    focal e.
    E. Foundation
    grand mal e.
    idiopathic e.
    infantile e.
    International League Against E.
      (ILAE)
    jacksonian e.
    juvenile absence e.
    juvenile myoclonic e. (JME)
    e. management
    midtemporal e.
    myoclonic e.
    myoclonus e.
    nocturnal e.
    partial complex e.
    petit mal e.
    photosensitive e.
    posttraumatic e.
    primary generalized e.
    progressive bulbar palsy with e.
    progressive myoclonic e.
    psychomotor e.
    reactive e.
    reflex e.
    rolandic e.
    secondary e.
    e. seizure
    severe myoclonic e.
    startle e.
    sylvian e.
    symptomatic e.
    television e.
    temporal lobe e.
    typical absence e.
    vestibulogenic e.
    video game e.
    visual reflex e.
epileptic
    e. aura
    e. convulsion
    e. encephalopathy

    e. idiocy
    e. myoclonus
    e. seizure
    e. syndrome
epilepticus
    absence status e.
    complex partial status e.
    convulsive status e.
    febrile status e.
    idiopathic status e.
    limbic status e.
    nonconvulsive status e. (NCSE)
    partial status e.
    refractory status e. (RSE)
    status e. (SE)
    symptomatic status e.
epileptiform
    e. activity
    e. discharge
epileptogenesis
epileptogenic, epileptogenous
    e. encephalopathy
    e. lesion
epileptogenicity
epileptogenous (*var. of* epileptogenic)
epileptologist
epileptology
epiloia
epimenorrhagia
epimenorrhea
epimyoepithelial island
Epinal
epinephrine
    aerosolized racemic e.
    e. deficiency
    high-dose therapy with e.
      (HDE)
    lidocaine and e.
    Marcaine with e.
    e. provocation
    racemic e.
    self-injectable e.
    Xylocaine With E.
epineurium
EpiPen
    E. Jr.
    E. Sr.
epipericardial connective tissue
epiphora
epiphyseal (*var. of* epiphysial)
epiphyseolysis (*var. of* epiphysiolysis)
epiphysial, epiphyseal
    e. closure
    e. dysostosis
    e. dysplasia
    e. growth
    e. growth plate
    e. ossification center
    e. plate injury

e. stapling
e. syndrome
epiphysiodesis
epiphysiolysis, epiphyseolysis
epiphysis
    capital femoral e.
    capitellar e.
    congenital stippled e.
    double epiphyses
    femoral e.
    intraarticular e.
    proximal femoral e.
    proximal tibial e.
    radial e.
    slipped e.
    slipped capital femoral e. (SCFE)
    slipped upper femoral e. (SUFE)
    stippled e.
    stippling of epiphyses
    tibial e.
    upper humeral e.
epiplocele
epiploia
epipodophyllotoxin
epipygus
epirubicin
episcleritis, episclerotitis
episclerotitis (*var. of* episcleritis)
episioperineoplasty
episioperineorrhaphy
episioplasty
episiorrhaphy
episiostenosis
episiotomy
    bilateral mediolateral e.'s
    e. dehiscence
    first-degree e.
    fourth-degree e.
    median e.
    mediolateral e.
    midline e.
    prophylactic e.
    e. repair
    ruptured e.
    e. scissors
    second-degree e.
    e. site
    third-degree e.
Episkopi blindness
episode
    enuretic e.
    hyperammonemic e.
    hypomanic e.
    hypotonic-hyporesponsive e.'s
     (HHEs)
    mitochondrial myopathy,
     encephalopathy, lactic acidosis,
     strokelike e.'s (MELAS)
    nonprimary first e.

    present e.
    protracted depressive e.
    Schedule for Affective Disorders
     and Schizophrenia for School-Age
     Children-Present E. (K-SADS-P)
    strokelike e.
    syncopal e.
    vasoocclusive e.
episodic
    e. angioedema
    e. ataxia (1, 2)
    e. blanching
    e. dyscontrol
    e. dyscontrol syndrome
    e. flushing
    e. hypoglycemia
    e. memory
episome
epispadias
    female e.
    simple e.
epispadias-exstrophy complex
epistasis
epistatic
epistaxis
    recurrent e.
    refractory e.
epistemology
episthotonos
epitarsus
epitaxy
17-epitestosterone
epithelia (*pl. of* epithelium)
epithelial
    e. atrophy
    e. autoantibody localization
    e. bud
    e. cell
    e. cell abnormality
    e. cell ovarian carcinoma
    e. cell proliferation
    e. disorder
    e. hyperplasia
    e. inclusion cyst
    e. keratitis
    e. lining fluid (ELF)
    e. liver tumor
    e. membrane antigen (EMA)
    e. ovarian cancer (stage I–IV)
    e. pearl
    e. plate
    e. plug
    e. serous tumor
    e. stromal ovarian neoplasm
    e. stromal tumor
    e. tuft
epithelialization, epithelization
epithelial-mesenchymal interaction
epitheliochorial placenta

E

epithelioid
    e. cell
    e. cell nevus
    e. leiomyosarcoma
epithelioma
    e. adenoides cysticum
    basal cell e.
    calcifying e.
epithelium, *pl.* **epithelia**
    acetowhite e.
    airway e.
    artificial vaginal e.
    atypical e.
    celomic e.
    cervical e.
    ciliated columnar e.
    circumferential eversion of
      urethral e.
    columnar e.
    ductal e.
    germinal e.
    infarction of oral e.
    luminal e.
    native squamous e.
    oral e.
    ovarian germinal e.
    papilla of columnar e.
    respiratory e.
    retinal pigment e. (RPE)
    squamous e.
    stratified squamous e.
    surface e.
    urethral e.
    urogenital e.
    uterine e.
    white e.
epithelization (*var. of* epithelialization)
Epitol
epitope
epitopic
epituberculosis
epitympanic recess
Epivir
Epivir-HBV
EPL
    early pregnancy loss
EPO
    erythropoietin
    evening primrose oil
Epo
    erythropoietin
epoch
    growth e.
    sleep e.
epoetin alfa
Epogen
epoophorectomy
epoophoron
epothilone D

EPP
    erythropoietic protoporphyria
Eppendorfer
    E. biopsy forceps
    E. biopsy punch
Eppy/N
Eprolin
EPS
    ear, patella, short stature
    EPS syndrome
EPSDT
    Early and Periodic Screening,
      Diagnosis, and Treatment
    EPSDT program
epsilon
    e. aminocaproic acid (EACA)
    e. toxin
Epstein-Barr
    E.-B. nuclear antigen (EBNA)
    E.-B. virus (EBV)
Epstein pearls
EPT
    early pregnancy test
epulis
    e. gravidarum
    e. of newborn
    e. of pregnancy
Equagesic
equal
    e. conjoined twins
    e. ocular movement (EOM)
equalization
    pressure e. (PE)
equation
    Hadlock e.
    Harris-Benedict basal energy
      expenditure e.
    Henderson-Hasselbalch e.
    Schofield weight- and height-based
      resting energy expenditure
      prediction e.
    Starling e.
equatorial
    e. division
    e. plane
equi
    Rhodococcus e.
equilibration
equilibrium (eq, EQ)
    acid-base e.
    Donnan e.
    genetic e.
    Hardy-Weinberg e.
    linkage e.
    e. phase
    e. reaction
    Starling e.
equina
    cauda e.

equine
- e. antitoxin
- e. encephalitis
- e. estrogen

equinovalgus
- talipes e.

equinovarus
- fetal talipes e.
- idiopathic talipes e.
- neurogenic talipes e.
- pes e.
- e. pes deformity
- talipes e. (TEV)

equinus
- ankle e.
- e. clubfoot
- e. deformity
- e. gait
- e. position
- talipes e.

equivalent
- genome e. (GE)
- lethal e.
- meconium ileus e.

equivocal culdocentesis
ER
- emergency room
- endoplasmic reticulum
- estrogen receptor
- extended release
- Methylin ER

ERA
- endometrial resection and ablation
- evoked response audiometry
- ERA resectoscope sheath

eradication therapy
Erb
- E. juvenile muscular dystrophy
- E. palsy
- E. syndrome

Erb-Charcot syndrome
Erb-Duchenne
- E.-D. palsy
- E.-D. paralysis

Erbe
- E. electrical coagulation instrument
- E. electrical cutting instrument

Erb-Goldflam
- E.-G. disease
- E.-G. syndrome

Erb-Klumpke palsy
ERCP
- endoscopic retrograde cholangiopancreatography

Erdheim disease
ERE
- estrogen response element

erectile
- e. structure
- e. tissue

erection
- artificial e.
- capillary e.
- penile e.

erethism
ERG
- electroretinogram
- electroretinography

ergocalciferol
ergogenic
ergometer
- bicycle e.

ergonovine maleate
ergosterol
ergot
ergotamine tartrate
Ergotrate
Erhardt
- E. developmental prehension assessment
- E. forceps

erigentes
- nervi e.

Erikson stages of growth and development
Erlacher-Blount syndrome
Erlenmeyer flask appearance
ERM
- extended radical mastectomy

E-R-O Ear Drops
Eronen syndrome
Eros-CTD eroscillator device
E-rosette receptor
erosion
- bony e.
- cervical e.
- mesh e.
- subglottic e.

erosive
- e. adenomatosis of nipple
- e. esophagitis
- e. rhinitis
- e. vulvitis

ERP
- event-related potential

ERPC
- evacuation of retained products of conception

erratic
- e. blood pressure
- e. temperature

erratica
- mamma e.

error
- alpha e.
- beta e.

E

error (*continued*)
- Garrodian inborn e.
- inborn e.
- metabolic e.
- refractive e.

ERT
- estrogen replacement therapy

ertapenem sodium

erucic acid

eructation

eruption
- bullous drug e.
- Christmas tree distribution e.
- creeping e.
- delayed tooth e.
- Kaposi varicelliform e.
- maculopapular e.
- monomorphous papular e.
- morbilliform e.
- papular e.
- papulosquamous e.
- polymorphous light e.
- pruritic vesiculopapular e.
- purpuric light e.
- scarlatiniform e.
- seabather's e.
- vesicobullous e.
- vesiculopapular e.
- violaceous e.

eruptive
- e. fever
- e. hidradenoma
- e. lichen planus
- e. nevus
- e. syringoma
- e. temperature
- e. vellus hair cyst
- e. xanthoma

ERV
- expiratory reserve volume

Er:YAG laser

Erybid

Eryc

Erycette

EryDerm

Erygel

Erymax

EryPed

erysipelas
- e. internum
- necrotizing e.

Erysipelothrix rhusiopathiae

Ery-Tab

erythema
- e. chronicum migrans (ECM)
- fixed e.
- gingival e.
- heliotropic e.
- e. induration of Bazin (EIB)

- e. infectiosum
- Jacquet e.
- linear gingival e.
- e. marginatum
- e. migrans
- e. multiforme (EM)
- e. multiforme exudativum
- e. multiforme/toxic epidermal necrolysis (EM/TEN)
- e. neonatorum toxicum
- e. nodosum
- e. nodosum leprosum
- ocular e.
- orange peel e.
- palmar e.
- periorbital violaceous e.
- periungual e.
- scarlatiniform e.
- toxic e.
- e. toxicum neonatorum
- vasculitic e.
- violaceous e.
- vulvovaginal e.

erythematosus
- disseminated lupus e.
- drug-induced systemic lupus e.
- lupus e. (LE)
- neonatal lupus e. (NLE)
- systemic lupus e. (SLE)

erythematous
- e. blush
- e. confluent plaque
- e. cutaneous plaque
- e. halo
- e. macule
- e. papule
- e. rash
- e. satellite lesion

erythrasma of vulva

erythredema polyneuropathy

erythrityl tetranitrate

Erythro-Base

erythroblastic
- e. anemia
- e. anemia of childhood

erythroblastopenia
- transient e.

erythroblastosis
- ABO e.
- fetal e. (FE)
- e. fetalis (EBF)
- e. neonatorum

Erythrocin

erythrocytapheresis

erythrocyte
- e. acquired defect
- burr-shaped e.
- e. count
- dysmorphic e.

e. enzyme deficiency
e. glutathione peroxidase deficiency
e. membrane
e. mosaicism
neonatal e.
packed e.
e. phosphoglycerate kinase deficiency
e. pyruvate kinase deficiency
e. sedimentation rate (ESR)
e. transfusion
erythrocytopoiesis
erythrocytosis
familial e.
stress e.
erythroderma, erythrodermia
atopic e.
bullous congenital ichthyosiform e.
congenital ichthyosiform e. (CIE)
e. desquamativum
exfoliative e.
generalized e.
ichthyosiform e.
nonbullous congenital ichthyosiform
e. (NBCIE)
erythrodermia (*var. of* erythroderma)
erythrodermic
erythrohepatic
e. porphyria
e. protoporphyria
erythroid
colony-forming unit e. (CFU-E)
e. hyperplasia
e. hypoplasia
mature burst-forming unit e.
(M-BFU-E)
e. progenitor
e. progenitor cell
erythrokeratodermia
symmetric progressive e.
e. variabilis
erythroleukoblastosis
erythromelalgia
Erythromid
erythromycin
e. estolate
e. ethylsuccinate (EES)
e. lactobionate
erythron
erythrophagocytic lymphohistiocytosis
erythroplasia
e. of Queyrat
Queyrat e.
Zoon e.
erythropoiesis
compensatory e.
dermal e.
e. failure
megaloblastic e.
stress e.

erythropoietic
e. heme
e. porphyria
e. porphyria congenita
e. protoporphyria (EPP)
erythropoietin (EPO, Epo)
human e.
recombinant human e. (r-EPO)
serum e.
Erythroxylum coca
Eryzole
ES
Augmentin ES
Pertussin ES
Vicodin ES
ESA
epididymal sperm aspiration
ESA Coulochem multi-electrode
ESC
embryonic stem cell
Escalante syndrome
escape
e. beats
PMS E.
e. rhythm
escharotomy
Escherichia
E. coli
E. coli sepsis
E. coli vaccine
escitalopram
Esclim
E. estradiol transdermal system
E. patch
E. Transdermal
E. transderm system
Escobar syndrome
escutcheon
female e. (FE)
E-selectin
Eserine
Isopto E.
Eskalith
esmolol hydrochloride
esodeviation
esophageal
e. anastomosis
e. atresia (EA)
e. candidiasis
e. carcinoma
e. coin
e. compression
e. dilation
e. duplication cyst
e. foreign body
e. hiatus
e. impedance monitoring
e. manometry
e. obstruction

E

esophageal (*continued*)
 e. perforation
 e. pressur
 e. reflux
 e. replacement
 e. rupture
 e. spasm
 e. sphincter
 e. stenosis
 e. stricture
 e. transection
 e. ulceration
 e. web
esophagectomy
esophagi (*pl. of* esophagus)
esophagitis
 allergic e.
 eosinophilic e.
 erosive e.
 infectious e.
 monilial e.
 peptic e.
 reflux e.
 tetracycline-induced e.
 viral e.
esophago-deglutition response
esophagoduodenostomy
esophagogastroduodenoscopy (EGD)
esophagogram (*var. of* esophagram)
esophagography
 barium e.
esophagomyotomy
 Heller-Nissen thorascopic e.
esophagoscope
 Holinger infant e.
esophagoscopy
esophagostomy
 cervical e.
esophagotracheal primordium
esophagram, esophagogram
 barium e.
 contrast e.
 Gastrografin e.
esophagus, *pl.* **esophagi**
 Barrett e.
 cervical e.
 embryonic e.
 nutcracker e.
 stenosis of e.
EsopHogram software
esophoria
esotropia
 accommodative e.
 congenital e.
 infantile e.
 intermittent e. (E(T))
espundia
ESR
 erythrocyte sedimentation rate

ESS
 endometrial stromal sarcoma
 end-systolic stress
essential
 e. amino acid
 e. benign pentosuria
 e. dysmenorrhea
 e. fatty acid (EFA)
 e. fructosuria
 e. hypertension
 e. menorrhagia
 e. myoclonus
 e. thrombocythemia (ET)
 e. tremor
 e. vulvodynia
Essiac
Essure
 E. micro-insert method
 E. micro-insert method of female
   sterilization
EST
 endodermal sinus tumor
established
 e. medical diagnosis
 e. risk
Estalis
Estar
ester
 cholesterol e.
 L-valine e.
 phorbol e.
 tosylarginine methyl e. (TAME)
esterase
 leucocyte e.
 tosylarginine methyl ester e.
esterified estrogen
Estes
 E. operation
 E. ovarian transfer procedure
estetrol
esthesioneuroblastoma
esthiomene
estimated
 e. date of conception (EDC)
 e. date of confinement (EDC)
 e. fetal weight (EFW)
 e. gestational age (EGA)
estimation
 gestational age e.
 e. of gestational age
estimator
 maximum likelihood e.
Estinyl
estolate
 erythromycin e.
Estrace
 E. Oral
 E. vaginal cream
 E. VR intravaginal ring

Estra-D
Estraderm
E. Transdermal
E. transdermal system
E. TTS
estradiol (E_2)
e. assay
bound e.
e. cypionate
e. cypionate and
medroxyprogesterone acetate
Cytoxan, Adriamycin, leucovorin,
calcium, fluorouracil, ethinyl e.
(CALF-E)
desogestrel and ethinyl e.
drospirenone/ethinyl e.
e. enanthate
ethinyl e. (EE)
ethynodiol diacetate and e.
exogenous e.
free e.
e. level
levonorgestrel and ethinyl e.
micronized 17-beta e.
norethindrone acetate and ethinyl e.
norgestimate and ethinyl e.
pre-hCG e.
e. receptor
e. suppression
e. transdermal system
e. vaginal cream
e. valerate (EV)
estradiol/levonorgestrel
estradiol/norethindrone acetate
estradiol/norgestimate
**estradiol-releasing silicone vaginal
ring**
estramustine phosphate sodium
estrane
Estrasorb
Estratab
Estratest
E. HS
E. Oral
Estren-Dameshek subtype
Estring estradiol vaginal ring
estriol (E_3)
e. level
salivary e.
unconjugated e. (E3, uE3)
EstroGel pump
estrogen
e. add-back therapy (EABT)
e. agonist
e. antagonist
e. breakthrough bleeding
catechol e.
Cenestin synthetic conjugated e.'s
circulating e.

conjugated e. (CE)
conjugated equine e.'s (CEE)
e. deprivation
e. effect
endogenous e.
equine e.
esterified e.
e. excess
fetal e.
health, osteoporosis, progestin, e.
(HOPE)
e. level
e. loss
e. metabolism
oral conjugated e.
orally administered e.
postcoital e.
prevent postmenopausal Alzheimer
with replacement e.'s (PREPARE)
e. receptor (ER)
e. receptor alpha (Er alpha)
e. receptor beta (Er beta)
e. receptor localization
e. replacement
e. replacement therapy (ERT)
e. response element (ERE)
serum e.
e. sulfotransferase
e. surge
e. synthesis
synthetic conjugated e.
transdermal e.
uninterrupted e.
unopposed e.
e. window etiologic hypothesis
e. withdrawal (EW)
e. withdrawal bleeding (EWB)
estrogens with methyltestosterone
women's angiographic vitamins and
e. (WAVE)
estrogen-agonist uterine effect
estrogen-assisted colposcopy
estrogen-dependent
e.-d. endometrial carcinoma
e.-d. neoplasia
estrogenic effect
**estrogen-independent endometrial
carcinoma**
estrogen-induced prolactinoma
estrogenization
introital e.
estrogenized mucosa
estrogen-only HRT
estrogen-progesterone
e.-p. ratio
e.-p. withdrawal bleeding
estrogen-progestin
e.-p. artificial cycle
e.-p. contraceptive

E

estrogen-progestin (*continued*)
    e.-p. replacement therapy
    e.-p. test
estrogen-progestogen combination
estrone (E_1)
    oral e.
    e. sulfate
estropipate
Estrostep
    E. Fe
    E. oral contraceptive
Estroven
estrus
ET
    embryo transfer
    endotracheal
    essential thrombocythemia
    eustachian tube
        K+ Care ET
        ET tube
ET-1
    endothelin-1
ET-2
    endothelin-2
ET-3
    endothelin-3
etanercept
$E_T CO2$
    end-tidal carbon dioxide
ETEC
    enterotoxigenic *Escherichia coli*
E-tegrity test
ETF
    electron transfer flavoprotein
ETF-DH
    electron transfer flavoprotein
      dehydrogenase
ETH
    ethionamide
ethacrynic acid
ethambutol (EMB)
Ethamide
ethane
    exhaled e.
ethanol (EtOH, ETOH)
    blood e.
    e. poisoning
ethchlorvynol
ether
Ethibond polybutilate-coated polyester suture
Ethicon
    E. disposable cannula
    E. disposable trocar
Ethiguard needle
ethinamate
ethinyl
    e. estradiol (EE)
    e. estradiol and desogestrel

    e. estradiol and ethynodiol diacetate
    e. estradiol and levonorgestrel
    e. estradiol and norethindrone
    e. estradiol and norgestimate
    e. estradiol and norgestrel
    e. testosterone
ethiodized oil
Ethiodol
ethionamide (ETH)
ethisterone
ethmocephalus (*var. of* ethmocephaly)
ethmocephaly, ethmocephalus
    e. syndrome
ethmoid
    e. bone
    e. sinus
ethmoidectomy
    endoscopic e.
ethnic heritage
ethnicity
ethoheptazine citrate
ethologic
ethopropazine hydrochloride
ethosuximide
ethotoin
Ethox cuff
ethoxzolamide
Ethrane
ethyl
    e. alcohol (EtOH, ETOH)
    e. biscoumacetate
    e. chloride
ethylenediamine
ethylenediaminetetraacetic acid (EDTA)
ethylene glycol
ethylester
    tryptophan e.
ethylmalonic-adipic aciduria
ethylnorepinephrine
ethylphenylephrine
ethylsuccinate
    erythromycin e. (EES)
ethynodiol
    e. diacetate
    e. diacetate and estradiol
Ethyol
ETI
    endotracheal intubation
etidronate
    e. disodium
    sodium e.
etiocholanolone
etiologic fraction of tubal infertility
etiology
    fever of unknown e. (FUE)
    opsoclonus-myoclonus e.
etiopathogenesis
etiopathogeny
etodolac

ETOH, EtOH
  ethanol
  ethyl alcohol
etomidate
etonogestrel
Etopophos
etoposide (EP)
  e. phosphate
etoricoxib
etretinate
ETS
  endotracheal suction
  environmental tobacco smoke
EUB-405
  EUB-405 ultrasound scanner
  EUB-405 ultrasound system
Eubacterium
eucalcemia
eucapnia
eucaryote (*var. of* eukaryote)
Eucerin Plus Cream
euchromatin
Eudermic surgical glove
eugenics
euglobulin
  e. clot lysis time (ECLT)
  e. lysis time (ELT)
euglycemia
  newborn e.
eugonadal amenorrhea
eugonadism
  constitutional e.
eugonadotropic
  e. amenorrhea
  e. hypogonadism
  e. oligospermia
eukaryote, eucaryote
eukaryotic cell
EULAR
  European League Against Rheumatism
  EULAR classification
Eulenburg disease
Euler and Byrne score
eumelanin
eumenorrheic woman
eunuch
eunuchoid
  e. gigantism
  e. habitus
eunuchoidism
  female e.
  hypergonadotropic e.
  hypogonadotropic e.
euphoria
euphoriant
euploid
  e. abortion
  e. pregnancy
euploidy

eupnea
eupneic
euprolactinemic woman
Eurax Topical
Euro-Med FNA-21 aspiration needle
European League Against Rheumatism (EULAR)
europium
eustachian
  e. tube (ET)
  e. tube defect
  e. tube dysfunction
eutectic mixture of local anesthetics (EMLA)
euthymic
euthyroid sick syndrome
Eutonyl
eutopic
  e. congenital hypothyroidism
  e. endometrium
  e. endometrium prostaglandin E_2
eV
  electron volt
EV
  estradiol valerate
EVA
  electric vacuum aspiration
evacuation
  air e.
  e. device
  dilation and e. (D&E)
  fimbrial e.
  molar e.
  e. of retained products of conception (ERPC)
  e. of uterine contents
  e. proctography
  surgical e.
evacuator
  smoke e.
  uterine e.
evaluation
  Acute Physiology and Chronic Health E.
  audiometric e.
  cervical mucus e.
  Collaborative Home Infant Monitoring E. (CHIME)
  cytopathologic e.
  domestic violence e.
  Doppler e.
  Dubowitz e.
  fluoro-urodynamic e.
  genetic e.
  infertility e.
  intrapartum e.
  longitudinal interval followup e. (LIFE)
  mental status e.

E

evaluation (*continued*)
  midtrimester ultrasonographic e.
  e. of passenger
  physical capacity e. (PCE)
  postpartum e.
  posttreatment e.
  psychomotor e.
  rape crisis e.
  Sexual Assault Nurse E. (SANE)
  sonographic e.
  urologic e.
  uterine e.
  women's ischemia syndrome e.
    (WISE)
evanescent maculopapular rash
Evans
  E. blue dye
  E. calcaneal lengthening
  E. syndrome
Evans-Steptoe procedure
evaporated
  e. milk
  e. milk formula
evaporation
evening primrose oil (EPO)
event
  acute life-threatening e. (ALTE)
  apneic e.
  apparent life-threatening e. (ALTE)
  asphyxial e.
  epigenetic e.
  iatrogenic e.
  idiopathic apparent life-threatening e.
  inciting e.
  intracellular e.
  life e.
  e. monitor
  thromboembolic e. (TE)
  unexplained apparent life-threatening
    e. (UALTE)
  unprotected coital e.
event-free survival (EFS)
eventration
  congenital e.
  diaphragmatic e.
  e. of diaphragm
event-related potential (ERP)
Everard Williams retropubic
  cystourethropexy suspension procedure
Everone
Evershears
  E. bipolar laparoscopic forceps
  E. bipolar laparoscopic scissors
eversion
  cervical e.
  circumferential e.
  e. injury
  vaginal e.
everted diaphragm

Evert-O-Cath drug delivery catheter
evidence
  laparoscopic e.
  e. of anticipation
  rape e.
  sexual assault forensic e. (SAFE)
evisceration
  vaginal e.
Evista
E-Vitamin
EVL
  endoscopic variceal ligation
EVLW
  extravascular lung water
evoked
  e. otoacoustic emission (EOAE)
  e. potential
  e. potential technique
  e. response
  e. response audiometry (ERA)
evolution
  darwinian e.
  Darwin theory of e.
  Denman spontaneous e.
  Douglas spontaneous e.
  spontaneous e.
evolutionarily conserved
Evolution-C kit
Evra
  Ortho E.
EVS
  endoscopic variceal sclerotherapy
EVUS
  endovaginal ultrasound
EW
  estrogen withdrawal
EWB
  estrogen withdrawal bleeding
Ewing
  E. sarcoma (ES, EWS)
  E. sarcoma gene
  E. tumor (ET)
ex
  ex utero intrapartum technique
    (EXIT)
  ex utero intrapartum tracheloplasty
    (EXIT)
  ex utero intrapartum treatment
    (EXIT)
  ex vivo
  ex vivo fertilization
  ex vivo liver-directed gene therapy
EX
  Diabetic Tussin EX
ExAblate fibroid 2000 system
exacerbation
  asthma e.
Exacta-Med oral dispenser
Exact Cream

ExacTech glucose measuring device
Exact-Touch Saccomanno Pap smear
  collection system
exaggerated craniocaudal view
exam (*var. of* examination)
Exami-Gown gown
examination, exam
    abdominal e.
    Allen and Capute neonatal
      neurodevelopmental e.
    audiometric e.
    Ballard e.
    benign breast e.
    bimanual pelvic e.
    buffy coat e.
    cervical e.
    chest e.
    circumferential e.
    clinical breast e. (CBE)
    colposcopic e.
    dark-field e.
    double setup e.
    Dubowitz e.
    dysmorphology e.
    eating disorders e. (EDE)
    eye e.
    manipulative e.
    microscopic e.
    neonate e.
    neurologic e.
    newborn e.
    obstetric ultrasound e.
    pelvic e.
    peripubertal e.
    personality disorder e. (PDE)
    preparticipation sports e. (PSE)
    prepuberal e.
    radiological e.
    rectal e.
    rectoabdominal e.
    rectovaginal e.
    roentgenographic e.
    routine screening cervical e.
    self-breast e. (SBE)
    serial digital e.'s
    serial neurologic e.'s
    speculum e.
    split speculum e.
    sterile speculum e.
    sterile vaginal e. (SVE)
    stool e.
    swab e.
    targeted ultrasonographic e.
    vaginal e.
    VCU e.
    well-woman e.
examnialis
    graviditas e.
exanthem (*var. of* exanthema)

exanthema, exanthem
    bacterial e.
    Boston e.
    laterothoracic e.
    maculopapular e.
    measles e.
    e. multiforme exudativum
    papular e.
    pediatric e.
    polymorphous e.
    rheumatic e.
    scarlet fever e.
    e. subitum
    toxin-induced scarlet fever e.
    unilateral laterothoracic e. (ULE)
    vesicular e.
    viral e.
exanthematous disease
excavator
excavatum
    pectus e.
eXcel-DR Glasser laparoscopic needle
excess
    adrenal e.
    e. androgen
    androgen e.
    apparent mineralocorticoid e.
      (AME)
    base e.
    estrogen e.
    glucocorticoid e.
    hyponatremia of water e.
    iatrogenic androgen e.
    sodium e.
    soluble antigen e.
    TBG e.
excessive
    e. acid secretion
    e. amniotic fluid
    e. blood loss
    e. hoarseness
    e. insulin action
    e. insulin secretion
    e. penile curvature
    e. pulmonary arterial flow
    e. QT prolongation
    e. sleeping
    e. sweating
    e. villous maturation
exchange
    fetal-maternal e.
    maternofetal e.
    e. of body fluids
    perfluorocarbon-assisted gas e.
    plasma e.
    regional gas e. (R_{AW})
    sister chromatid e.
    Starling law of transcapillary e.
    e. transfusion (EXT)

E

excision
- atrial septum e.
- e. diathermy
- diathermy loop e.
- electrosurgical e. (EE)
- electrosurgical loop e.
- laparoscopic cornual e.
- large loop e.
- laser e.
- local e.
- needle e.
- radical e.
- radical local e.
- repeat-loop e.
- surgical e. (SE)
- thyroglossal duct cyst e.
- wide e.

excisional
- e. biopsy
- e. procedure

excitation

excitement
- sexual e.

excitotoxic
- e. amino acid (EAA)
- e. injury
- e. mechanism
- e. necrosis

excitotoxicity

exclamation-mark hair

exclusion
- allelic e.

exclusive breast-feeding

excoriation

excrescence
- internal e.
- ovarian e.

excreta

excrete

excretion
- coproporphyrin e.
- fractional e.
- glucose e.
- sodium e.
- urinary e.
- urobilinogen e.
- water e.

excretory
- e. system development
- e. urogram

excursion
- thoracic wall e.

executive
- e. cognitive functioning (ECF)
- e. function

Exelderm Topical

exemestane

exencephalia
- bifid e.

exencephaly, exencephalia

exenteration
- anterior e.
- anterior pelvic e.
- pelvic e.
- posterior e.
- posterior pelvic e.
- pyelonephritis in e.
- stress reaction in e.
- total pelvic e. (TPE)

exercise
- bladder-stretching e.
- e. bronchial challenge
- eccentric e.
- e. intolerance
- isometric quadriceps e.
- Kegel e.'s
- maternal e.
- pelvic floor muscle e. (PFME)
- pelvic muscle e. (PME)
- pelvic muscle-strengthening e.
- e. physiologist
- e. physiology
- e. recommendation
- visual training e.

exercise-induced
- e.-i. amenorrhea
- e.-i. asthma (EIA)
- e.-i. bronchospasm (EIB)
- e.-i. hematuria
- e.-i. hypothalamic dysfunction
- e.-i. incontinence

exertional reactive airway disease

exertion-induced dyskinesia

exfoliated squamous cell

exfoliation
- e. failure
- lamellar e.

exfoliative
- e. dermatitis
- e. erythroderma

exhaled
- e. ethane
- e. pentane

exhaustion
- maternal e.
- ovarian follicle e.

exhibitionism

exit
- e. plan
- e. plan for abuse

EXIT
- ex utero intrapartum technique
- ex utero intrapartum tracheloplasty
- ex utero intrapartum treatment
- EXIT procedure

Exna

exocelomic
    e. cavity
    e. membrane
exocervical sample
exocervix
exochorialis
    graviditas e.
exocrine
    e. pancreatic dysfunction
    e. pancreatic hypoplasia
    e. pancreatic insufficiency
exocytosis
    cortical granule e.
exodeviation
exogastric lesion
exogenous
    e. DNA
    e. estradiol
    e. estrogen administration
    e. estrogenic stimulation
    e. gonadotropin
    e. gonadotropin stimulation
    e. hormone
    e. insulin
    e. lipoid pneumonia (ELP)
    e. medication
    e. obesity
    e. pancreatic enzyme
    e. steroid
    e. surfactant
    e. surfactant therapy
    e. thyroxine treatment
exomphalos, macroglossia, gigantism (EMG)
exon
exonuclease
Exophiala werneckii
exophoria
exophthalmos, exophthalmus
    apparent e.
    pulsating e.
exophthalmus (*var. of* exophthalmos)
exophytic
    e. lesion
    e. mass
    e. wart
exostoses (*pl. of* **exostosis**)
exostosis, *pl.* **exostoses**
    calcified e.
    multiple cartilaginous exostoses
    pelvic e.
    subungual e.
    trichorhinophalangeal multiple exostoses (TRAMPE)
Exosurf Neonatal
exotoxemia
exotoxin
    e. C
    Pseudomonas e.

exotoxin-A
    streptococcal e.-A (SPEA)
exotropia
    constant e.
    intermittent e.
expandable esophageal stent (EES)
expanded
    e. Ballard score
    e. food nutrition education program (EFNEP)
expander
    AccuSpan tissue e.
    Becker tissue e.
    tissue e.
    volume e.
expander/implant
    Contour Profile Bechert 35 e./i.
expansion
    CAG e.
    CGG e.
    GAA trinucleotide e.
    molecular e.
    e. of chromosome
    palatal e.
    plasma volume e.
    volume e.
Expecta Lipil supplement
expectancy
    life e.
expectant management
expected
    e. date of confinement (EDC)
    e. date of delivery (EDD)
expectorant
    Benylin E.
expectorate
expeditious delivery
expenditure
    energy e.
    nonresting energy e. (NREE)
    resting energy e. (REE)
    total daily energy e. (TDEE)
    total energy e.
experience
    appropriate learning e.
    Calendar of Premenstrual Syndrome E. (COPE)
    Charing Cross e.
    Positive Reinforcement in the Menopausal E. (PRIME)
    separation-reunion e.
experimental
    e. allergic encephalomyelitis (EAE)
    e. embryology
    e. lymphocytic choriomeningitis
    e. obesity
    e. pneumococcal meningitis
Expert bone densitometer
expiration

E

expiratory
  e. apnea
  e. flow volume
  e. grunting
  inspiratory to e. (I/E, I:E, I-E, I:E
    ratio)
  e. noise
  e. reserve volume (ERV)
  e. scan
  e. stridor
expiratory-to-inspiratory ratio (E:I)
expire
explanted
exploration
  oral e.
exploratory celiotomy
explosive watery diarrhea
exponential
exposed
  chemically e.
  e. large venous channel
exposure
  airway, breathing, circulation,
    disability, e. (ABCDE)
  anesthetic gas e.
  DES e.
  endogenous estrogen e.
  fetal androgen e.
  intrauterine e.
  in utero e.
  in utero drug e. (IUDE)
  lead e.
  maternal mercury e.
  methamphetamine e.
  needlestick e.
  prenatal diethylstilbestrol e.
  radiation e.
  teratogen e.
  teratogenic e.
  toxin e.
expressed
  e. milk
  e. sequence tag
expression
  abnormal gene e.
  facial e.
  gender e.
  gene e.
  Human Gene E. (HuGE)
  Human Genome E. (HuGE)
  oncogene e.
expressionless face
expressive
  e. aphasia
  e. language
  e. language development
  e. language disorder
  e. one-word picture vocabulary test
expressivity

expulsion
expulsive
  e. force
  e. pains
exsanguination
  fetal e.
Exsel shampoo
exstrophic
  e. cecum
  e. vagina
exstrophy
  bladder e.
  cloacal e.
  e. of the bladder
EXT
  exchange transfusion
Extencaps
  Micro-K 10 E.
extended
  e. culture
  e. end-to-end anastomosis
  e. family
  e. field irradiation therapy
  e. internal dosing
  e. radical hysterectomy
  e. radical mastectomy (ERM)
  e. release (ER, XL, XR, XT)
  e. rubella syndrome
extended-release methylphenidate
extended-spectrum penicillin
extender
  egg yolk e.
extension
  classical incision e.
  direct e.
  e. in labor
  J e.
  medial hip rotation in e.
  midline vertical uterine e.
  paracervical e.
  parametrial e.
  protective e.
  Score for Neonatal Acute
    Physiology-Perinatal E.
    (SNAP-PE)
  T e.
  vaginal e.
extensive
  e. alveolar exudate
  e. intraductal component (EIC)
  e. support
extensor
  e. fit
  e. hypertonus
  e. leg posture
  e. thrust pattern
Extentabs
  Dimetane E.
  Quinidex E.

exteriorization
  uterine e.
externa
  malignant otitis e.
  otitis e.
  theca e.
external
  e. anal sphincter (EAS)
  e. anal thrombosis
  e. auditory canal (EAC)
  e. auditory meatus
  e. beam irradiation
  e. beam radiation therapy
  e. branchial sinus
  e. cephalic version (ECV)
  e. cephalic version and spontaneous vertex
  e. conjugate
  e. ear
  e. femoral torsion
  e. fetal monitoring (EFM)
  e. genitalia/Bartholin, urethral, and Skene glands (EG/BUS)
  e. hemorrhage
  e. hordeolum
  e. hydrocephalus
  e. iliac artery
  e. jugular vein catheter placement
  e. jugular venipuncture
  e. male genitalia
  e. oblique muscle
  e. ophthalmoplegia
  e. os
  e. otitis
  e. photon beam radiation
  e. pneumatic calf compression (EPC)
  e. radiation therapy
  e. rotation
  e. sphincter muscle
  e. surface
  e. tibial torsion
  e. urethral barrier device
  e. urethral meatus
  e. uterine massage
  e. version
  e. virilization
  e. x-ray therapy
externalizing
  e. behavior
  E. Behavior Scale
  e. score
extinction
extirpation
  Amreich vaginal e.
  endoscopic choroid plexus e.
extirpative surgery
extra
  e. ossification

  e. strength (ES, E.X.)
  E. Strength Doan's
extraabdominal organ system disease
extraamniotic
  e. pregnancy
  e. saline infusion (EASI)
extraaxial
  e. arachnoid cyst
  e. fluid
extracapsular growth
extracardiac
  e. abnormality
  e. anomaly
  e. conduit cavopulmonary anastomosis
  e. malformation
  e. shunt
extracellular
  e. fluid (ECF)
  e. fluid compartment
  e. matrix
  e. matrix component
  e. matrix signal
  e. plasma potassium
  e. superoxide dismutase
  e. volume (ECV)
extrachorales
  placenta e.
extrachorial pregnancy
extrachromosomal inheritance
extracorporeal
  e. circulation (ECC)
  e. CO_2 removal (ECOR)
  e. knot
  e. life support (ECLS)
  e. membrane oxygenation (ECMO)
  e. rewarming
extracortical axial aplasia
extracranial foreign body
extract
  calf lung surfactant e. (CLSE)
  malt soup e.
  modified bovine surfactant e.
  pyrethrum e.
extraction
  breech e.
  cross-brain oxygen e.
  internal podalic version and breech e.
  Marshall-Taylor vacuum e.
  menstrual e.
  microsurgical e.
  partial breech e. (PBE)
  peripheral fractional oxygen e. (PFOE)
  podalic e.
  spontaneous breech e.
  testicular sperm e. (TESE)

E

extraction (*continued*)
    total breech e.
    vacuum e.
extractor
    Bird vacuum e.
    CMI vacuum e.
    comedo e.
    Kobayashi vacuum e.
    Malmstrom vacuum e.
    Mityvac vacuum e.
    M-type e.
    mucus e.
    Murless vacuum e.
    O'Neil vacuum e.
    plastic cup vacuum e.
    silastic cup e.
    soft-cup e.
    Tender-Touch e.
    TRIzol RNA e.
    vacuum e.
extracutaneous
    e. sporotrichosis
    e. vas fixation clamp
extradural
    e. abscess
    e. anesthesia
    e. block
    e. hematoma
extraembryonic
    e. bleed
    e. celomic space (EECS)
    e. differentiation
    e. fetal membrane
    e. location
    e. mesoderm
extraesophageal reflux (EER)
extrafamily offender
extrafascial total abdominal hysterectomy
extraglandular
    e. conversion
    e. testosterone production
extraglomerular
extragonadal
    e. germ cell
    e. germ cell tumor
extrahepatic
    e. bile duct resection
    e. biliary atresia
    e. biliary tract
    e. biliary tree
    e. portal vein obstruction
    e. presinusoidal obstruction
extraintestinal manifestation (EIM)
extralobar sequestration
extra-long artery-pedicled bask fascia skin flap
extraluminal
    e. fluid
    e. gas bubble

extramammary Paget disease (EPD)
extramedullary hemopoiesis
extramembranous pregnancy
extramural upper airway obstruction
extranodal
    e. marginal zone
    e. marginal zone B-cell lymphoma
    e. tumor
extranumerary nipple
extraocular
    e. movement (EOM)
    e. muscle (EOM)
    e. muscle palsy
    e. muscle surgery
extraordinary urinary frequency syndrome
extraosseous Ewing sarcoma
extraovular placement
extrapelvic
    e. endometriosis
    e. malignancy
    e. solid tumor
extraperitoneal
    e. cesarean
    e. insufflation
extraplacental membrane
extrapolate
extrapolation
extrapulmonary
    e. cryptococcosis
    e. extravasation
    e. extravasation of air
    e. tuberculosis
extrapyramidal
    e. cerebral palsy
    e. lesion
    e. manifestation
    e. movement
    e. nervous system
    e. sign
    e. tract
extrapyramidal-pyramidal syndrome
extrarenal
    e. pheochromocytoma
    e. rhabdoid tumor
    e. saline
extra-systole (*var. of* extrasystole)
extrasystole, extra-systole
extratemporal epilepsy
extrathoracic
    e. obstruction
    e. tuberculosis
    e. ventilator
extrauterine
    e. life
    e. pregnancy
extravasation
    blood e.

extrapulmonary e.
   e. injury
extravascular
   e. fluid collection
   e. lung water (EVLW)
extraventricular
extravesical
   e. mass
   e. ureteral reimplantation
extravillous trophoblast
extreme
   e. benign hyperbilirubinemia
   e. leukocytosis
extremely
   e. low birth weight (ELBW)
   e. low birth weight infant (ELBWI)
   e. premature infant (EPI)
extremis
   in e.
extremitas (*var. of* extremity)
extremity, extremitas
   congenital contracture of e.
   flaccid e.
   long thin e.
   lower e. (LE)
   e. lymphedema
   upper e. (UE)
extrinsic
   e. alveolar alveolitis
   e. compression of airway
   e. dyssomnia
   e. extravesical mass
   e. pathway inhibitor
   e. positive end-expiratory pressure
extrophy
   cloacal e.
extrusion
   dental e.
   oocyte e.
   placental e.
   e. reflex
extrusion/lateral luxation
extrusive luxation
extubate
extubation
exuberant callus
exudate
   alveolar fibrinous e.
   cheesy e.
   cotton-ball e.
   extensive alveolar e.
   fibrinopurulent e.
   fibrinous e.
   inflammatory e.
   opaque white e.
   peritoneal e.
   subretinal e.
   tonsillar e.
   tonsillopharyngeal e.

exudative
   e. ascites
   e. conjunctivitis
   e. meningitis
   e. pharyngitis
   e. retinal detachment
   e. tonsillitis
exudativum
   erythema multiforme e.
   exanthema multiforme e.
Exuderm dressing
Eyberg Child Behavior Inventory (ECBI)
eye
   amblyopic e.
   Clear E.'s
   Credé maneuver of e.'s
   dancing e.
   deep-set e.'s
   e. defects-diffuse renal mesangial sclerosis syndrome
   e. deviation
   doll's eyes
   e. dominance
   downslanting e.'s
   dry e.
   e.'s, ears, nose, throat (EENT)
   e. examination
   e. inflammation
   lazy e.
   e. movement
   nonfixing e.
   ox's e.
   e. popping
   raccoon e.'s
   e. retraction with adduction
   e. salvage therapy
   e. slant
   sunset e.'s
   widely spaced e.'s
eyeball cystometrogram
eyebrow
   confluent eyebrows
   ichthyosis, cheek, e. (ICE)
eyeground
eye-hand coordination
eyelash trichomegaly
eyelid
   Dennie line of lower e.
   fusion of eyelids
   heliotrope e.
   e. muscle
   e. squeezing
   e. tumor
eye-of-the-tiger sign
eye-opener
   cutting, annoyance, guilt, e.-o. (CAGE)
Eyesine Ophthalmic

E

EZ-EM
 EZ-EM Bio-Gun automated biopsy
  system
 EZ-EM PercuSet amniocentesis tray

E-Z Heat hot pack
EZ-HSG catheter
Ezide
EZ-On Vest

f

fragile chromosome site F (FRAXF)

F₂ — F_2

prostaglandin F_2

F.A.

Mission Prenatal F.A.

FA

Fanconi anemia
femoral anteversion
fetal age
Nestabs FA
FA screening

FAA

febrile antigen agglutination
FAA gene

Fab

fragment antigen binding
F. classification
digoxin immune f.
F. staging of carcinoma

FABP

finger arterial blood pressure

fabric

Solumbra 30+ SPF f.

Fabricius

bursa of F.

Fabry

F. crisis
F. disease

FAC

fetal abdominal circumference

face

abnormal f.
adenoidal f.
asymmetry of f.
bovine f.
f. chamber
cleft f.
congenital ectodermal dysplasia of f.
dish f.
dysmorphic f.
ectodermal dysplasia of f.
expressionless f.
fetal f.
F. kit
face, legs, activity, cry, consolability (FLACC)
f. mask
f. presentation
round moon f.
f. tent
f. underdevelopment

FACE

fluorophore-assisted carbohydrate electrophoresis

face/chin presentation
face-near-straight-down (FNSD)
face-out, whole-body plethysmograph
FACES

Family Adaptability and Cohesion Evaluation Scale

FACES-III

Family Adaptability and Cohesion Scale-III

face-straight-down (FSD)
facet, facette

f. dislocation
jumped f.
locked f.
medial talocalcaneal f.
subtalar f.
f. syndrome

face-to-pubes fetal position
face-to-side (FTS)
facette (*var. of* facet)
facial

f. affect recognition
f. angioma
f. anomaly
f. asymmetry
f. buttress
f. clefting syndrome, Gypsy type
f. diplegia
f. dysmorphia syndrome
f. dysmorphism
f. dysplasia, hyperextensibility of joints, clinodactyly, growth retardation, mental retardation syndrome
f. ectodermal dysplasia
f. expression
f. expression and sleeplessness
f. nerve
f. nerve injury (FNI)
f. nerve palsy
f. nerve paralysis
f. pain
f. vein insertion

facial-digital-genital syndrome
facialis

herpes f.

faciei

lupus miliaris disseminatus f.

facies

abnormal f.
asymmetric crying f. (ACF)
birdlike f.
f. bovina
bovine f.
Campbell Soup kid f.

F

facies (*continued*)
    cushingoid f.
    dwarfism, eczema, peculiar f.
    dysmorphic f.
    elfinlike f.
    femoral hypoplasia unusual f.
        (FHUF)
    flat f.
    moon f.
    moon-shaped f.
    peculiar f.
    Potter f.
    progeroid f.
    seborrheic-like f.
    soup kid f.
    thalassemia f.
    triangular f.
facilitated communication (F/C)
facility
    intermediate care f. (ICF)
facioauriculovertebral (FAV)
    f. anomalad
    f. malformation complex
    f. spectrum (FAVS)
faciocardiomelic dysplasia
faciocardiorenal syndrome
faciocutaneoskeletal (FCS)
faciodigitogenital syndrome
faciogenital
    f. dysplasia
    f. syndrome
faciolingual-masticatory diplegia
faciooculoacousticorenal (FOAR)
faciopalatoosseous (FPO)
facioscapulohumeral (FSH)
    f. muscular dystrophy (FSHD)
    f. syndrome of Landouzy-Dejerine
faciotelencephalic malformation
Facit polyp forceps
FACO$_2$
    fraction of alveolar carbon dioxide
FACS
    fluorescence-activated cell sorter
fact
    F. Plus
    F. Plus Pro pregnancy test
FACT
    Functional Assessment of Cancer
    Therapy
factitial panniculitis
factitious
    f. disorder
    f. disorder by proxy (FDP)
    f. precocious puberty
factor
    acidic fibroblast growth f.
        (FGFa)
    alloimmune f.
    angiogenic growth f.

antihemophilic f. (AHF)
atrial natriuretic f. (ANF)
autocrine-acting growth f.
autocrine motility f. (AMF)
autocrine/paracrine-acting growth f.
autoimmune f.
azoospermia f. (AZF)
basic fibroblast growth f. (bFGF)
bifidus f.
binding protein-2 insulinlike
    growth f.
binding protein-3 insulinlike
    growth f.
biologic f.
biomedical f.
biotin f.
blocking f.
brain-derived neurotrophic f.
    (BDNF)
cell adhesion f. (CAF)
cervical f.
chemotactic f.
Christmas f.
ciliary neurotrophic f. (CNTF)
citrovorum f.
clotting f. (CF)
coagulation f.
coital f.
colony-stimulating f. (CSF)
complement chemotactic f.
f. concentrate
contact f.
contagion f.
corticotropin-releasing f.
cytotoxic f.
decay-accelerating f.
f. D, H deficiency
digoxin-like immunoreactive f.
    (DLIF)
DNAse B f.
early pregnancy f. (EPF)
endocrine f.
endothelium-derived relaxing f.
    (EDRF)
enhancement f.
epidermal growth f. (EGF)
fecundity f.
fetal f.
fibrin stabilizing f.
fibroblast growth f. (FGF)
fibroblast pneumocyte f.
follicular f.
glass f.
glial cell line derived neurotrophic
    f. (GDNF)
gonadotropin-releasing f. (GnRH,
    GRF)
granulocyte colony-stimulating f.
    (G-CSF)

granulocyte-macrophage
  colony-stimulating f. (GM-CSF)
growth f. (GF)
growth control f.
growth-like f.
Hageman f.
helper f.
hepatocyte growth f. (HGF)
hepatocyte nuclear f. (HNF)
hidden rheumatoid f.
HMWK f.
home f.
hormonal f.
human antihemophilic f.
human sperm cytosolic f.
humoral f.
hyaluronic acid f.
hyaluronidase f.
f. I, II, IIa, III-VIII, X-XIII
immune f.
immunologic f.
infertility f.
insulinlike growth f. (IGF)
intrauterine f.
intrinsic f. (IF)
f. I–XIII deficiency
keratinocyte growth f. (KGF)
kidney-derived growth f.
labile f.
leukemia inhibitory f. (LIG)
lifestyle f.
luteinizing-releasing f. (LRF)
lymphocyte-activating f.
f. M
macrophage-activating f. (MAF)
macrophage colony-stimulating f.
macrophage-inhibition f.
male f.
maternal f.
maturation-promoting f. (MPF)
menarche f.
microbial f.
migration inhibitory f. (MIF)
mitosis-promoting f. (MPF)
mixed lymphocyte reaction blocking
  f.
mortality risk f.
M-phase-promoting f.
M protein f.
müllerian duct inhibitory f.
müllerian inhibiting f. (MIF)
necrotizing f.
nephritic f.
nerve growth f. (NGF)
neurologic f.
obstetric risk f.
ovarian f.
paracrine-acting growth f.
paternal f.

perinatal risk f.
perisphincteric f.
PK f.
placental growth f. (PGF, PlGF)
plasma thromboplastin antecedent f.
platelet-activating f.
platelet-derived growth f.
postnatal f.
precipitating f.
predisposing f.
pregnancy risk f. (PRF)
prenatal risk f.
primary testis-determining f.
prognostic f.
prolactin inhibiting f. (PIF)
prolactin releasing f.
prostacyclin-stimulating f. (PSF)
proteinase f.
psychosocial f.
recombinant antihemophilic f.
Rh f.
rhesus f.
rheumatoid f. (RF)
risk f.
Service Utilization and Risk F.'s
  (SURF)
somatic cell-derived growth f. (SCF)
specific transcription f.
spreading f.
stable f.
streptokinase f.
Stuart f.
Stuart-Prower f.
testis-determining f. (TDF)
tissue f.
transfer f.
transforming growth f. (TGF)
tubal f.
tumor angiogenesis f. (TAF)
tumor-limiting f.
tumor necrosis f. (TNF)
uterine f.
vascular endothelial growth f.
  (VEGF)
vascular permeability f.
f. VIIa (FVIIa)
f. VIII:C
f. VIII hemophilia
f. VII, VIII inhibitor
f. V Leiden (FVL)
f. V Leiden carrier
f. V Leiden mutation
f. V Leiden mutation test
f. V Leiden thrombophilia
f. VIIIa
von Willebrand f. (vWF)
f. V polypeptide
work f.
f. Xa inhibition assay

factor-1
 recombinant human insulin-like
  growth f.-1 (rhIGF-1)
 steroidogenic f.-1 (SF-1)
 thyroid transcription f.-1 (TTF-1)
 transforming growth f. (TGF-1)
Factrel
facultative scotoma
FAD
 familial Alzheimer disease
 flavin adenine dinucleotide
Fadhil syndrome
fading
FADIR
 flexion, adduction, internal rotation
fadir
 flexion, adduction, internal rotation
  fadir sign
FADS
 fetal akinesia deformation sequence
FAE
 fetal alcohol effect
 Fogarty arterial embolectomy
  FAE catheter
  FAE syndrome
faecalis
 Enterococcus f.
faecium
 Enterococcus f.
FAED
 food avoidance emotion disorder
Fagan Test of Infant Intelligence
FAH
 fumarylacetoacetate hydrolase
Fahr disease
failed
 f. breastfeeding
 f. Fontan circuit
 f. forceps delivery
 f. intrauterine pregnancy
 f. physiologic change
 f. reduction
failure
 acute oliguric renal f. (AORF)
 acute renal f. (ARF)
 acute respiratory f. (ARF)
 bilateral gonadal f.
 bone marrow f.
 cardiac f.
 chronic renal f. (CRF)
 congestive heart f. (CHF)
 contraceptive f.
 ejaculation f.
 end-stage heart f.
 erythropoiesis f.
 exfoliation f.
 fertility f.
 fimbrial f.
 fulminant hepatic f. (FHF)

 gonadal f.
 growth f.
 heart f.
 high-output f.
 hypercapnic respiratory f.
 hypothalamic f.
 hypoxic respiratory f.
 impending renal f.
 implantation f.
 kidney f.
 left ventricular f.
 liver f.
 multiorgan system f.
 multiple-organ f.
 multiple-organ system f. (MOSF)
 neurogenic respiratory f.
 ovarian f.
 premature ovarian f. (POF)
 primary ovarian f. (POF)
 primary testicular f.
 progressive central nervous system
  f.
 progressive renal f.
 renal f.
 reproductive f.
 respiratory f.
 right-sided heart f.
 severe growth f.
 testicular f.
 f. to progress
 f. to thrive (FTT)
 treatment f.
 ventilatory f.
faint
 vasovagal f.
Fairbank
 F. disease
 F. skeletal abnormality
Fairbank-Keats syndrome
falces (*pl. of* falx)
falciform
 f. hymen
 f. ligament
falciparum
 chloroquine-resistant *Plasmodium f.*
  (CRPF)
 chloroquine-sensitive *Plasmodium f.*
 f. malaria
 Plasmodium f.
Falk-Shukuris operation
fall-away response
falling
 f. of the womb
 f. sickness
falling-out sensation
fallopian (FALL)
 f. pregnancy
 f. tube
 f. tube carcinoma (FTC)

f. tube mass
f. tube metastasis
f. tube peristalsis
f. tube prolapse
f. tube sperm perfusion (FTSP)
falloposcope
falloposcopy
Fallot
  acyanotic tetralogy of F.
  F. complex
  F. pentalogy
  pentalogy of F.
  pink tetralogy of F.
  F. syndrome
  tetralogy of F. (TET, TF, TOF)
  F. trilogy
  trilogy of F.
Falope
  F. ring
  F. ring applicator
false
  f. acetabulum
  f. conjugate
  f. fontanelle
  f. knot
  f. knot of umbilical cord
  f. labor
  f. localizing sign
  f. mole
  f. pains
  f. pelvis
  f. positive
  f. pregnancy
  f. vocal cord
  f. waters
false-negative death
false-positive
falx, *pl.* **falces**
  cerebral f.
  f. laceration
  f. sign
FAMA
  fluorescent antibody to membrane antigen
  fluorescent antimembrane antibody
  FAMA assay
famciclovir
familial
  f. achalasia
  f. adenomatous polyposis (FAP)
  f. adenomatous polyposis coli
  f. alobar holoprosencephaly
  f. Alzheimer disease (FAD)
  f. aortic ectasia
  f. aortic ectasia syndrome
  f. APOA-I deficiency
  f. ataxia-hypogonadism syndrome
  f. atypical multiple mole melanoma syndrome

f. benign hematuria
f. bipolar mood disorder
f. bird-headed dwarfism
f. cardiac myxoma
f. cardiac myxoma syndrome
f. cardiovascular disease
f. centrolobal sclerosis
f. cholesterolemia
f. chylomicronemia syndrome
f. combined hyperlipidemia (FCHL)
f. congenital fourth cranial nerve palsy
f. congenital superior oblique oculomotor palsy
f. congenital trochlear nerve palsy
f. Creutzfeldt-Jakob disease
f. defective apolipoprotein B-100
f. diathesis
f. dominant thrombocytopenia
f. dysautonomia
f. endocrine-neuroectodermal abnormalities syndrome
f. erythroblastic anemia (FEA)
f. erythrocytosis
f. erythrophagocytic lymphohistiocytosis (FEL)
f. exudative vitreoretinopathy (FEV)
f. focal facial dermal dysplasia
f. glomerulonephritis
f. glycinuria
f. granulomatous arteritis
f. hemiplegic migraine (FHM)
f. hemophagocytic lymphohistiocytosis (FHLH)
f. Hibernian fever
f. hirsutism
f. hypercalcemia
f. hypercalcemia with hypocalciuria (FHH)
f. hypercholesterolemia
f. hyperglycerolemia
f. hyperinsulinemic hypoglycemia
f. hyperinsulinism of infancy
f. hyperlipidemia
f. hyperlysinemia
f. hyperprolinemia
f. hypertriglyceridemia (FHTG)
f. hypoalphalipoproteinemia
f. hypobetalipoproteinemia
f. hypocalciuric hypercalcemia (FHH)
f. hypofibrinogenemia
f. hypokalemic periodic paralysis
f. hypomagnesemia
f. hypophosphatemia
f. hypophosphatemic rickets (FHR)
f. iminoglycinuria
f. infertility

F

familial (*continued*)
   f. insomnia syndrome
   f. intrahepatic cholestasis
   f. inverted choreoathetosis
   f. juvenile gout
   f. juvenile hyperuricemic
    nephropathy
   f. juvenile nephrophthisis (FJN)
   f. lecithin:cholesterol acyltransferase
    deficiency
   f. lipodystrophy
   f. lipoid adrenal hyperplasia
   f. loading
   f. lumbosacral syringomyelia
   f. lymphedema praecox
   f. macrocephaly
   f. macroglossia-omphalocele
    syndrome
   f. male precocious puberty
    (FMPP)
   f. Mediterranean fever (FMF)
   f. multiple endocrine adenomatosis
   f. multiple lipomatosis
   f. muscular atrophy
   f. neonatal seizure
   f. neuroblastoma
   f. neurovisceral lipidosis
   f. olivopontocerebellar atrophy
   f. osseous dystrophy
   f. osteochondrodystrophy
   f. ovarian cancer
   f. panhypopituitarism
   f. polysyndactyly-craniofacial
    anomalies syndrome
   f. protein intolerance
   f. pterygium syndrome
   f. pure gonadal dysgenesis
   f. pyridoxine-dependency
    syndrome
   f. recurrent hematuria
   f. short stature
   f. spastic paraparesis
   f. spastic paraplegia (FSP)
   f. spinal neurofibromatosis
   f. striatal degeneration
   f. tendency
   f. third and fourth pharyngeal
    pouch syndrome
   f. thrombophilia
   f. trait
   f. tremor
   f. Turner syndrome
   f. vasopressin-sensitive diabetes
    insipidus
   f. visceral myopathy
   f. visceral neuropathy
   f. vocal cord dysfunction
familiaris
   osteopathia dysplastica f.

family
   F. Adaptability and Cohesion
    Evaluation Scale (FACES)
   F. Adaptability and Cohesion
    Scale-III (FACES-III)
   f. cancer genetic counseling
   f. cancer history
   CEPH f.
   f. dynamics
   f. dysfunction
   dysfunctional f.
   F. Environment Scale (FES)
   extended f.
   gene f.
   f. history
   f. history research diagnostic criteria
    (FH-RDC)
   F. Inventory of Resources for
    Management (FIRM)
   F. Medical Leave Act (FMLA)
   f. member presence (FMP)
   f. planning
   Poxviridae f.
   f. selection
   f. therapy
family-based
   f.-b. design
   f.-b. test
family-centered
   f.-c. approach
   f.-c. obstetrics
famotidine
Famvir
Fanconi
   F. anemia (FA)
   F. aplastic anemia
   F. dysplasia
   F. pancytopenia
   F. pancytopenia syndrome
Fanconi-Albertini Zellweger syndrome
Fanconi-Bickel syndrome
Fanconi-Prader syndrome
Fanconi-Schlesinger syndrome
fan douche
fanning
fan-shaped hemorrhagic infarction
Fansidar
fantasy, phantasy
   revenge f.
fantasy/make-believe world
FAO
   fatty acid oxidation
   FAO disorder
FAP
   familial adenomatous polyposis
faradism
Farber
   F. disease
   F. lipogranulomatosis

F. syndrome
F. test
farcinica
    Nocardia f.
Fareston
farmeri
    Citrobacter f.
farmer's lung
Farre white line
Farr test
farsightedness
FAS
    fetal alcohol syndrome
    Functional Assessment Scale
fascia, *pl.* **fasciae, fascias**
    f. adherens
    Camper f.
    f. clitoridis
    Colles f.
    Cooper f.
    cremasteric f.
    Dartos f.
    Denonvilliers f.
    endopelvic f.
    Gerota f.
    inferior f.
    f. lata
    f. lata allograft
    f. lata suburethral sling
    obturator f.
    perirectal f.
    plantar f.
    presacral f.
    pubocervical f.
    f. rectovaginalis
    Scarpa f.
    Smead-Jones closure of peritoneum and f.
    subserous f.
    superior f.
    transversalis f.
fasciae (*pl. of* fascia)
fascial
    f. flap
    f. necrosis
    f. reconstruction
    f. replacement
    f. sling procedure
    f. strip
fascias (*pl. of* fascia)
fascicle (fasc)
fasciculata
    zona f.
fasciculation
    muscle f.
    tongue f.
fasciculi (*pl. of* fasciculus)
fasciculus, *pl.* **fasciculi**
    syndrome of median longitudinal f.

fasciitis, fascitis
    cranial f.
    diffuse f.
    eosinophilic f.
    gas gangrene f.
    necrotizing f.
    nodular f.
    plantar f.
Fasciola hepatica
fascioliasis
fascioscapulohumeral
fascitis (*var. of* fasciitis)
fashion
    crescentic f.
    forward roll f.
    Halban f.
    Moschcowitz f.
FASIAR
    follicle aspiration, sperm injection, assisted rupture
Faslodex
fast
    f. channel syndrome
    f. neutron
    protein modified f. (PMF)
    protein-sparing modified f. (PSMF)
FAST
    Focused Assessment by Sonography for Trauma
    FAST blood test
fastener
    ROC XS suture f.
FASTER
    first abarelix depot study for treating endometriosis rapidly
    first and second trimester evaluation of risk
fasting
    f. blood sugar
    f. plasma cholecystokinin
    f. plasma glucose (FPG)
    f. serum insulin
fat
    f. absorption
    f. analysis
    body f.
    f. density
    f. deposition
    dietary f.
    f. distribution pattern
    f. embolism
    f. emulsion
    endogenous f.
    f. flap
    f. flexor hallucis longus tendon
    f. herniation
    f. malabsorption
    f. mass (FM)
    f. metabolism

F

fat (*continued*)
    microscopic f.
    f. necrosis
    percent body f. (PBF)
    f. plane
    preperitoneal f.
    unsaturated f.
    f. wrapping
FAT
    female athlete triad
    feminizing adrenal tumor
fatal
    f. cutaneous aspergillosis
    f. encephalomyelitis
    f. familial insomnia
    f. infantile myopathy
    f. neonatal hyperammonemic encephalopathy
fate mapping
fat-free mass (FFM)
fatigability
    easy f.
    increased f.
fatigue
    f. fracture
    f. syndrome
fat-induced infarction
fatty
    f. acid
    f. acid-coenzyme A
    f. acid content
    f. acid oxidation (FAO)
    f. acid profile
    f. halo
    f. infiltration
    f. liver
    f. liver of pregnancy
    f. milk
faun tail nevus
FAV
    facioauriculovertebral
fava
    f. bean
    f. bean ingestion
favism
favor neoplasia
FAVS
    facioauriculovertebral spectrum
Fazio-Londe
    F.-L. atrophy
    F.-L. disease
FBEP
    Fort Bragg evaluation project
FBM
    fetal bone marrow
    fetal breathing movement
5-FC
    5-flucytosine
    5-fluorocytosine

F&C
    fever and chills
F/C
    facilitated communication
FCHL
    familial combined hyperlipidemia
FCM
    fetal cardiac motion
FCMD
    Fukuyama congenital muscular dystrophy
FCS
    faciocutaneoskeletal
        FCS syndrome
FD
    forceps delivery
FDA
    Food and Drug Administration
FDIU
    fetal death in utero
FDP
    factitious disorder by proxy
    fibrin degradation product
FDS
    fetal distress syndrome
Fe
    iron
        Estrostep Fe
        Loestrin Fe
        Loestrin 24 Fe
        Microgestin Fe 1/29
        Microgestin Fe 1.5/30
        Norlestrin Fe
        Slow Fe
FE
    fetal erythroblastosis
FEA
    familial erythroblastic anemia
fear
    f. food
    f. of delivery
    pregnancy f.
    social-evaluative f.
fear-causing delivery
fearless first delivery
feathery
feature
    coarse facial f.'s
    dysmorphic facial f.'s
    epidemiologic f.'s
    grotesque f.'s
    f. matching
    mongoloid f.'s
    mood-congruent psychotic f.'s
    sharp facial f.'s
febrile
    f. antigen agglutination (FAA)
    f. baby
    f. convulsion

f. morbidity
f. myalgia
f. nonhemolytic transfusion reaction
f. paroxysm
f. seizure
f. status epilepticus
f. UTI

fecal

f. acidity
f. bolus
f. calprotectin
f. diversion colostomy
f. hoarding
f. impaction
f. incontinence (FI)
f. marker
f. microflora
f. occult blood testing (FOBT)
f. pancreatic elastase
f. shedding
f. shedding of virus
f. streptococci
f. water loss

fecalith

appendiceal f.
calcified f.

fecaloma, scatoma
fecal-oral spread
feces
FECO2

fraction in expired gas of carbon
dioxide

fecund
fecundability
fecundate
fecundation
fecundity

f. factor
natural f.
f. selection

fed

bottle f.
nipple f.

feed

bottle f.
full enteral f.
full nipple f.
trophic f.
tube f.

feedback

f. inhibition
tubuloglomerular f.

feeder

Brecht f.
f. layer

feeding

ad lib f.
Alimentum f.
bolus tube f.

f. bradycardia
by-mouth f.
coercive f.
complex enteral f.
continuous tube f.
cup f.
demand f.
f. difficulty
f. disturbance
early enteral f.
enteral f.
enteric f.
finger f.
Finkelstein f.
gastric enteral f.
gastric tube f.
f. gastrostomy
gavage f.
G-tube f.
hydrolyzed f.
f. intolerance
intragastric f.
intravenous f.
liquid f.
nasoduodenal f.
nasogastric drip f.
nasogastric tube f. (NTF)
nipple f.
p.o. f.
poor f.
f. problem
f. regimen
scheduled f.
syringe f.
transpyloric enteral f.
transpyloric tube f.
f. tube (FT)

Feelings About Yourself instrument
Feer disease
feet (*pl. of* foot)
FEF

forced expiratory flow

Feiba VH Immuno
Feilchenfeld forceps
Feingold syndrome
Feinmesser-Zelig syndrome
FEL

familial erythrophagocytic
lymphohistiocytosis

felbamate
Felbatol
Feldene
Feldenkrais method
felis

Afipia f.
Rickettsia f.

Felix-Weil reaction (FWR)
felon drainage
Felty syndrome

F

female
> f. athlete triad (FAT)
> f. circumcision
> f. condom
> f. epispadias
> f. escutcheon
> f. eunuchoidism
> f. factor infertility
> f. fertility efficiency
> f. fertility inefficiency
> f. genital mutilation (FMG)
> f. genital tract mutilation (FGTM)
> f. gonadal dysgenesis
> f. karyotype
> f. orgasmic disorder (FOD)
> phenotypic f.
> f. pseudohermaphroditism (FPH)
> f. pseudo-Turner syndrome
> f. reproductive cycle
> f. reproductive tract
> f. sexual arousal disorder (FSAD)
> F. Sexual Distress Scale (FSDS)
> f. sexual dysfunction (FSD)
> F. Sexual Function Index (FSFI)
> f. sexual response
> f. sterilization
> f. sterilization procedure
> super f.
> triple-X f.
> f. virilization

female-to-male (FTM)
Femara
FemAssist device
FemCap barrier contraceptive device
Femcaps
FemExam kit
femhrt
feminae
> hydrocele f.

feminine
feminization
> complete testicular f.
> male f.
> f. syndrome (FS)
> testicular f. (TF)

feminizing
> f. adrenal tumor (FAT)
> f. surgery
> f. testes syndrome

Feminone
Femiron
Femizol-M
Femogen Forte
Femogex
femora (*pl. of* femur)
femoral
> f. antetorsion
> f. anteversion (FA)
> f. artery catheter
> f. artery catheterization
> f. bulb
> f. circumflex artery
> f. cutaneous nerve
> f. deficiency
> f. epiphysis
> f. head dislocation
> f. hernia
> f. hypoplasia unusual facies (FHUF)
> f. length
> f. lymph node
> f. neck
> f. nerve
> f. nerve, artery, vein, empty space, lymphatics (NAVEL)
> f. neuropathy
> f. osteosarcoma
> f. osteotomy
> f. retroversion
> f. shaft fracture
> f. testis
> f. torsion
> f. triangle

femoral-facial syndrome
femoral-tibial angle
FemPatch
FemSoft continence insert
Femstat 3
FemSuite endocervical curette
FemTest endometrial biopsy pipette
femtomole/milligram
femur, *pl.* **femora**
> biologically plastic femora
> f. length (FL)
> metaphysial lesion of distal f.
> NSA of f.
> rectus femoris

femur-fibula-ulna (FFU)
FEN
> fluids, electrolytes, nutrition

FENa
> fractional excretion of sodium

fencing
> f. position
> f. reflex

Fenesin DM
fenestrata
> placenta f.

fenestrated vascular endothelium
fenestration
> bilateral optic nerve sheath f.
> Fontan f.
> laparoscopic f.
> third ventricle f.

fenfluramine
fenoprofen calcium
fenoterol

fentanyl
 f. citrate
 droperidol and f.
 f. lollipop
 f. patch
 TTS f.
fentendo plug
fentomole/milligram
Fenton vaginoplasty
fenugreek
Fe₃O₄
 magnetite
Feosol
Feostat
FEP
 free erythrocyte protoporphyrin
FER
 frozen embryo replacement
Feratab
ferberizing
Ferber method
Fergon
Ferguson reflex
Fer-In-Sol
 F.-I.-S. supplement
 F.-I.-S. vitamin
Fer-Iron
fermentans
 Mycoplasma f.
fermentum
 Lactobacillus f.
fern
 f. leaf crystallization
 f. leaf pattern
 f. leaf tongue
 f. test
ferning
 f. pattern
 f. technique
 vaginal fluid f.
fern-positive Nitrazine
Ferospace
Ferralyn Lanacaps
ferric
 f. chloride reaction
 f. chloride test
 f. hyaluronate adhesion barrier
 f. sulfate
Ferriman-Gallwey
 F.-G. hirsutism score
 F.-G. hirsutism scoring system
Ferris Smith-Sewall retractor
ferritin
 F. IRMA kit
 f. level test
 serum f.
Ferro-Sequels
ferrous
 f. chloride

 f. fumarate
 f. gluconate
 f. sulfate (FeSO₄)
fertile
 f. period
 f. phase
fertility
 f. agent
 f. control
 f. cycle
 f. disorder
 f. failure
 f. rate
 subsequent f.
fertilizable life span
fertilization
 f. age
 assisted f.
 culture f.
 delayed f.
 ex vivo f.
 in vitro f. (IVF)
 in vivo f. (IVF)
 microassisted f.
 minimal-stimulation in vitro f.
 oocyte f.
fertilized
 f. oocyte
 f. ovum
Fertinex
FES
 Family Environment Scale
 functional bladder stimulation
 functional electrical stimulation
FeSO₄
 ferrous sulfate
fes **protooncogene**
fetal
 f. abdominal circumference (FAC)
 f. Accutane syndrome
 f. acid-base balance
 f. acid-base status
 f. acidemia
 f. acidosis
 f. acoustic stimulation test
 f. activity test
 f. adrenal gland
 f. age (FA)
 f. akinesia deformation sequence (FADS)
 f. akinesia syndrome
 f. alcohol effect (FAE)
 f. alcohol syndrome (FAS)
 f. aminopterin-like syndrome
 f. aminopterin syndrome
 f. anasarca
 f. androgen exposure
 f. anemia
 f. aneuploidy

F

fetal (*continued*)
f. anoxia
f. anticoagulant syndrome
f. aorta
f. aortic blood flow
f. aortic Doppler velocimetry
f. arrhythmia
f. arterial oxygen saturation (FS_pO_2)
f. arterial velocimetry
f. arthrogryposis
f. ascites
f. asphyxia
f. aspiration syndrome
f. assessment technique
f. attitude
f. biometry
f. biophysical profile
f. biparietal diameter
f. birth injury
f. bladder
f. bladder catheterization
f. blood gas
f. blood glucose
f. blood oxygen-carrying capacity
f. blood pH
f. blood study
f. blood value
f. blood volume
f. body movement
f. bone marrow (FBM)
f. BPP
f. bradycardia
f. brain
f. brain death
f. brain disruption sequence
f. brain sparing
f. brainstem auditory evoked potential
f. breathing
f. breathing movement (FBM)
f. capillary branching
f. cardiac activity
f. cardiac control mechanism
f. cardiac function
f. cardiac motion (FCM)
f. cardiac rhabdomyoma
f. cardiomyopathy
f. cardiotocography
f. cardiovascular circulation
f. cartilage
f. cellular growth
f. cerebral oxygenation
f. chromosome abnormality
f. chromosome analysis
f. chromosome complement
f. circulation
f. circulatory centralization
f. cocaine syndrome
f. complications

f. compromise
f. condition
f. congenital hyperplasia
f. cord blood
f. cortisol infusion
f. cotyledon
f. cranial artery
f. crowding
f. CST
f. cystic hygroma
f. cytokinemia
f. cytomegalovirus
f. cytomegalovirus infection
f. death in utero (FDIU)
f. death rate
f. debris
f. demise
f. demise in utero (FDIU)
f. descent
f. deterioration
f. development
f. diabetes insipidus
f. diagnosis
f. Dilantin syndrome
f. disappearance
f. distress
f. distress in labor
f. distress syndrome (FDS)
F. Dopplex monitor
f. dose limit
f. drug therapy
f. ductus arteriosus constriction
f. duplication
f. dysmaturity syndrome
f. dystocia
f. echocardiogram
f. echocardiography
f. effect
f. effects of alcohol
f. electrocardiogram
f. electrocardiography
f. endocarditis
f. endoscopic
f. endoscopic tracheal occlusion
f. engraftment
f. entanglement
f. erythroblastosis (FE)
f. erythroid progenitor
f. estrogen
f. exsanguination
f. face
f. facies syndrome
f. factor
f. fibroblast
f. fibronectin (FFN, fFN)
f. fibronectin assay
f. fibronectin measurement
f. fibronectin test
f. foot length (FFL)

f. fracture
f. gasping
f. gigantism
f. gigantism, renal hamartoma, nephroblastomatosis syndrome
f. goiter
f. goitrous hypothyroidism
f. grasping
f. growth aberration
f. growth measurement
f. growth parameter
f. growth restriction (FGR)
f. growth retardation
f. habitus
f. HC/AC
f. head (FH)
f. head position
f. heart (FH)
f. heart action
f. heart activity
f. heart disease
f. heart frequency (FHF)
f. heart rate (FHR)
f. heart rate deceleration
f. heart rate monitor
f. heart rate monitoring
f. heart rate pattern
f. heart rate reactivity
f. heart rate variability (FHRV)
f. heart sounds
f. hemoglobin (HbF)
f. hemogram
f. hemolysis
f. hemorrhage
f. hiccup
f. histocompatibility antigen
f. hormone
f. hydantoin syndrome (FHS)
f. hydronephrosis
f. hydrops
f. hydrostatic pressure
f. hypercarbia
f. hyperglycemia
f. hyperinsulinism
f. hypotrophy
f. hypoxia
f. imaging
f. inflammatory response
f. inflammatory response syndrome
f. intolerance of labor
f. intracranial anatomy
f. iodine deficiency disorder (FIDD)
f. isotretinoin syndrome
f. jeopardy
f. karyotype
f. kernicterus
f. kick count
f. LDL level
f. leptin concentration

f. lie
f. limb
f. liver
f. lobectomy
f. loss
f. LOU
f. lung development
f. lung fluid
f. lung liquid
f. lung maturation
f. lung maturity (FLM)
f. lung readiness
f. maceration
f. macrosomia
f. magnetocardiography (FMCG)
f. malformation
f. malnutrition
f. malpresentation
f. maturity testing
f. membrane
f. metabolism
f. methotrexate syndrome
f. monitoring strip
f. morbidity
f. mortality
f. movement assessment
f. movement count (FMC)
f. movement counting
f. movement profile
f. neck fold thickness
f. nonimmune hydrops
f. NST
f. nuchal translucency thickness
f. nucleated cell
f. number
f. nutrition
f. nutritional deprivation syndrome
f. oculocerebrorenal syndrome of Lowe
f. organogenesis
f. outcome
f. outline
f. ovarian cyst
f. overgrowth syndrome
f. oximetry monitoring
f. oxygen saturation
f. paramethadione-trimethadione syndrome
f. parathyroid suppression
f. phenytoin syndrome
f. physiologic marker
f. physiologist
f. physiology
f. pole
f. postural abnormality
f. posture
f. prematurity
f. presentation
f. pulmonary circulation

F

fetal (*continued*)
f. pulmonary effluent
f. pulmonary hypoplasia
f. pulmonary maturity
f. pulmonary sequestration
f. pulmonary vascular resistance
f. pulse oximetry (FPO)
f. pyelectasis
f. red blood cell
f. reduction
f. reentrant SVT
f. rejection
f. resorption
f. respiratory acidosis
f. respiratory development
f. retention
f. risk
f. rubella syndrome
f. sac
f. scalp blood pH
f. scalp blood sampling
f. scalp electrode (FSE)
f. scalp monitoring
f. scalp oxygenation
f. scalp platelet sampling
f. scalp stimulation
f. seizure
f. serum
f. sex determination
f. sexual differentiation
f. shoulder extraction force
f. skeletal anomaly
f. skeletal dysplasia
f. skin sampling
f. skull depression
f. sleep cycle
f. small parts
f. somatic activity
f. souffle
f. spine position
f. spleen
f. squame
f. startle response
f. station
f. status
f. stem cell transplantation
f. steroid concentration
f. structural defect
f. structural malformation
f. surgery
f. surgical procedure
f. surveillance
f. surveillance technique
f. surveillance test
f. surveillance testing
f. swallowing
f. tachycardia
f. talipes equinovarus
f. thalidomide

f. thermal regulation
f. thoracic abnormality
f. thrombocytopenia
f. thrombopoietin concentration
f. thrombotic vasculopathy
(FTV)
f. tissue biopsy
f. tissue implant
f. tissue transplant
f. tobacco syndrome (FTS)
f. tone
f. toxoplasmosis
f. tracheal occlusion
f. transfusion
f. transfusion syndrome
f. trauma
f. trimethadione syndrome
f. ultrasound
f. urination
f. urine
f. urine production
f. uropathy
f. valproate syndrome (FVS)
f. varicella syndrome (FVS)
f. vascular anomaly
f. vascular conduit
f. vascular impedance
f. vasculitis
f. ventriculomegaly
f. version in utero
f. viability
f. warfarin syndrome (FWS)
f. wastage
f. weight (FW)
f. well-being
f. zone of adrenal cortex

fetalis
chondromalacia f.
erythroblastosis f. (EBF)
hydrops f.
ichthyosis f.
immune hydrops f.
maternal hydrops f.
maternal parvovirus f.
nonimmune hydrops f. (NIHF)
opisthotonos f.
rachitis f.

fetalism

fetal-maternal
f.-m. communication
f.-m. exchange
f.-m. hemorrhage
f.-m. medicine

fetal-pelvic index

fetal-placental
f.-p. circulation
f.-p. insufficiency
f.-p. steroidogenesis
f.-p. unit

FetalPulse
    F. Plus fetal Doppler
    F. Plus monitor
fetal-to-neonatal transition
fetation
Fetendo
    F. clip
    F. clip procedure
feticide
    selective f.
fetid breath
fetoamniotic shunt
fetofetal
    f. transfusion
    f. transfusion syndrome
fetography
fetology
fetomaternal
    f. alloimmune thrombocytopenia
      (FMAIT)
    f. bleed
    f. hemorrhage (FMH)
    f. transfusion (FMT)
    f. transfusion reaction
fetometry
    ultrasonic f.
    ultrasound f.
fetoneonatal estrogen-binding protein
fetopathy
    diabetic f. (DF)
fetopelvic disproportion (FPD)
fetoplacental
    f. access
    f. anasarca
    f. blood volume
    f. circulation
    f. function
    f. transfusion
fetor
    f. hepaticus
    f. oris
fetoscope
    Hillis-DeLee f.
fetoscopic
    f. laser occlusion
    f. laser occlusion of
      chorioangiopagus vessels (FLOC)
fetoscopy
fetotoxic
fetotoxicity
fetu
    fetus in f. (FIF)
fetus
    acardiac f.
    f. acardius
    amorphous f.
    f. amorphus
    anomalous f.
    asynclitic position of f.

    calcified f.
    Campylobacter f.
    coexistent f.
    f. compressus
    compromised f.
    constitutionally large f.
    dropsy of f.
    f. growth elevation
    growth-restricted f.
    growth-retarded f.
    habitus of f.
    harlequin f. (HF)
    HLA-compatible f.
    ichthyosis f.
    impacted f.
    f. in fetu (FIF)
    just-viable f.
    macerated f.
    mummified f.
    near-viable f.
    nonhydropic f.
    nonstressed f.
    nonvertex f.
    nonviable f.
    nuchal translucency in a f.
    paper-doll f.
    papyraceous f.
    f. papyraceus
    parasitic f.
    postmature f.
    presentation of f.
    previable f.
    retroperitoneal f.
    Rh-sensitized f.
    f. sanguinolentis
    singleton f.
    sireniform f.
    sirenomelic f.
    stressed f.
    stunted f.
    triploid f.
    trisomic f.
    vanishing f.
    viable f.
    Vibrio f.
fetus-to-fetus transplant
Feuerstein-Mims syndrome
Feulgen stain
FEV
    familial exudative vitreoretinopathy
    forced expiratory volume
FEV$_1$
    forced expiratory volume in 1 second
fever
    absorption f.
    acute rheumatic f. (ARF)
    African tick bite f.
    f. and chills (F/C, F&C)
    Argentine hemorrhagic f.

F

fever (*continued*)
arthritis of rheumatic f.
artificial f.
aseptic f.
biphasic f.
blackwater f.
f. blister
Bolivian hemorrhagic f.
boutonneuse f.
cat-scratch f.
childbed f.
Colorado tick f.
Crimean-Congo hemorrhagic f.
dehydration f.
dengue hemorrhagic f.
drug f.
Ebola hemorrhagic f.
enigmatic f.
enteric f.
ephemeral f.
epidemic relapsing f.
eruptive f.
familial Hibernian f.
familial Mediterranean f. (FMF)
Flinders Island spotted f.
glandular f.
Haverhill f.
hay f.
hemorrhagic f.
inanition f.
intermittent f.
intrapartum maternal f.
Katayama f.
Korean hemorrhagic f.
Lassa f.
louse-borne f.
maternal f.
Mediterranean f.
milk f.
f. of undetermined origin (FUO)
f. of unknown etiology (FUE)
f. of unknown origin (FUO)
Omsk hemorrhagic f.
Oriental spotted f.
Oroya f.
paratyphoid f.
parrot f.
parturient f.
PediaCare F.
pediatric f.
Pel-Ebstein f.
periodic f.
pharyngoconjunctival f.
phlebotomus f.
f. phobia
Pontiac f.
postoperative f.
puerperal f.
Q f.

Queensland f.
query f.
quotidian f.
rat-bite f.
recrudescence of f.
relapsing f.
revised Jones criteria for diagnosis of acute rheumatic f.
rheumatic f.
Rift Valley f.
Rocky Mountain spotted f. (RMSF)
saddleback f.
San Joaquin f.
scarlet f.
South African tick f.
spirillary rat-bite f.
spotted f.
staphylococcal scarlet f.
surgical scarlet f.
tactile f.
three-day f.
tick f.
tick-borne relapsing f.
transitory f.
trench f.
tsutsugamushi f.
typhoid f.
typhus f.
undulant f.
unexplained f.
uveoparotid f.
Valley f.
West Nile f.
yellow f.
FeverAll
Fèvre-Languepin syndrome
fexofenadine
FF
flatfoot
FFL
fetal foot length
FFM
fat-free mass
fFN
fetal fibronectin
FFN
fetal fibronectin
FFP
fresh frozen plasma
FFU
femur-fibula-ulna
FFU syndrome
FGF
fibroblast growth factor
FGFa
acidic fibroblast growth factor
FGFR
fibroblast growth factor receptor

FGFR3
  fibroblast growth factor receptor 3
FGR
  fetal growth restriction
fgr protooncogene
FG syndrome
FGTM
  female genital mutilation
  female genital tract mutilation
FH
  fetal head
  fetal heart
  fundal height
FHF
  fetal heart frequency
  fulminant hepatic failure
FHH
  familial hypercalcemia with
    hypocalciuria
  familial hypocalciuric
    hypercalcemia
FHLH
  familial hemophagocytic
    lymphohistiocytosis
FHM
  familial hemiplegic migraine
FHR
  familial hypophosphatemia
  fetal heart rate
    FHR acceleration
    FHR baseline
    nonreassuring FHR
FH-RDC
  family history research diagnostic
    criteria
FHRV
  fetal heart rate variability
FHS
  fetal hydantoin syndrome
FHTG
  familial hypertriglyceridemia
FHUF
  femoral hypoplasia unusual facies
    FHUF syndrome
FI
  fecal incontinence
FIA
  fluorescent immunoassay
fiber, fibra, fibre
  f. bone
  Dacron f.
  dietary f.
  myoclonic epilepsy with ragged red
    f.'s (MERRF)
  myometrial f.
  parasympathetic f.
  Perdiem F.
  postsynaptic f.
  Purkinje fibers

  ragged red f. (RRF)
  Rosenthal f.
Fiberall
  F. Powder
  F. Wafer
FiberCon
fiberglass jacket
fiberoptic
  f. bronchoscopy
  f. headband
  f. phototherapy (FO-PT)
Fibersource HN formula
fiber-type disproportion
fibra (*var. of* fiber)
fibre (*var. of* fiber)
fibril
  anchoring f.
fibrillary
  f. astrocytoma
  f. gliosis
fibrillation
  atrial f.
  f. potential
fibrillatory wave
fibrillin
fibrin
  basal perivillous f.
  f. degradation
  f. degradation product
  f. deposition
  f. sheath
  f. split product (FSP)
  f. stabilizing factor
  f. thrombus
fibrinogen
  f. abnormality
  f. deficiency
  f. degradation product (FDP)
  plasma f.
  radiolabeled f.
  serial maternal serum f.
  f. split product
fibrinogen-fibrin
  f.-f. conversion syndrome
  f.-f. degradation product
fibrinoid
  f. degeneration of astrocytes
  f. leukodystrophy
  f. necrosis
fibrinolysis
  f. inhibitor
  tissue activator-induced f.
fibrinolytic
  f. agent
  f. and clotting system
  f. therapy
fibrinopurulent exudate
fibrinous
  f. coalition

F

fibrinous (*continued*)
f. exudate
f. pericarditis
f. polyp
fibroadenolipoma
degenerated f.
fibroadenoma
giant f.
intracanalicular f.
juvenile f.
pericanalicular f.
fibroareolar tissue
fibroblast
f. culture
cultured skin f.
fetal f.
genital skin f.
f. growth factor (FGF)
f. growth factor-10 null phenotype
f. growth factor receptor (FGFR)
f. growth factor receptor 3
(FGFR3)
human embryo f. (HEF)
f. pneumocyte factor
fibroblastic osteosarcoma
fibroblastoid synoviocyte
fibrochondrogenesis
fibrocortical defect
fibrocystic
f. breast
f. breast change
f. disease
fibrodysplasia ossificans progressiva
(FOP)
fibroelastosis
endocardial f. (EFE)
prenatal f.
fibroepithelial polyp
fibrogenesis
fibroid
calcified uterine f.
f. embolization
intramural f.
lower uterine segment f.
F. Registry for Outcomes Data
(FIBROID)
submucous f.
subserous f.
uterine f.
FIBROID
Fibroid Registry for Outcomes Data
fibroidectomy
fibrolamellar hepatocellular carcinoma
(FL-HCC)
fibroma
benign nasopharyngeal f.
chondromyxoid f.
digital f.
histiocytic f.

infantile digital f.
f. molle gravidarum
nasopharyngeal f.
nonossifying f.
ossifying f.
ovarian f.
periungual f.
sternocleidomastoid f.
subungual f.
vulvar f.
fibromatosis
gingival f.
infantile f.
ovarian f.
pelvic f.
fibromectomy
fibromuscular
f. cervical stroma
f. dysplasia
fibromyalgia
childhood f.
f. syndrome (FMS, FS)
fibromyoma
uterine f.
fibromyxoid stroma
fibronectin
cervicovaginal fetal f.
fetal f. (FFN, fFN)
oncofetal f.
f. receptor
fibroplasia
retrolental f. (RLF)
fibropurulent
fibrosa, *pl.* **fibrosae**
osteitis f.
fibrosae (*pl. of* fibrosa)
fibrosarcoma
congenital f.
fibrosing
f. adenomatosis
f. adenosis
f. colonopathy
f. inflammation
f. mediastinitis
fibrosis
cavernosal f.
cerebellar vermis hypoplasia,
oligophrenia, congenital ataxia,
ocular coloboma, hepatic f.
(COACH)
chronic interstitial f.
coloboma-hepatic f.
congenital hepatic f. (CHF)
cutaneous f.
cystic f. (CF)
delta-F508 cystic f.
endocardial f.
endomyocardial f.
endoneurial f.

focal f.
focal tubulointerstitial f. (FTIF)
gum f.
hepatic f.
horseshoe f.
idiopathic diffuse interstitial f.
interstitial f.
meningeal f.
neoplastic f.
obstructing periuretal f.
peribronchial f.
peritoneal f.
peritubular f.
portal f.
postradiation periureteral f.
pulmonary interstitial f.
reactive f.
retroperitoneal f.
retropubic f.
f. scoring
tubular interstitial f.

fibrosum
corpus f.
molluscum f.
pedunculated molluscum f.

fibrothecoma
fibrotic ophthalmoplegia
fibrous, fibrosa
f. anlage
f. connective tissue
f. cortical defect
f. dysplasia
f. dysplasia of jaw

fibrovascular
f. tissue
f. tumor

fibroxanthoma
fibula
congenital longitudinal deficiency of f.

fibular
f. hemimelia
f. osteotomy
f. shaft fracture

Fick
F. method
F. principle

Ficoll-Hypaque centrifugation
fictitious epilepsy
FIDD
fetal iodine deficiency disorder

fiddle-string adhesion
fidget
fidgety
Fiedler myocarditis
field
f. block
central visual f.
high-power f. (hpf)

involved f. (IF)
low-power f. (lpf)
f. of view
f. of vision
tangential breast f.
visual f.

FIF
fetus in fetu

fifth
f. digit syndrome
f. disease
f. finger clinodactyly
f. phacomatosis
f. venereal disease

fifth-day fit
fight-and-flight response
fighter
Flimm F.

FIGLU
formiminoglutamic acid

FIGLU-uria
formiminoglutamicaciduria

FIGO
International Federation of Gynecology and Obstetrics
FIGO disease (stage I–IV)
FIGO nomenclature
FIGO staging

figure
Gesell f.
Matching Familiar F.'s (MFF)
mitotic f.

figure-of-3 sign
figure-of-4 test
figure-of-8
f.-o.-8 apparatus
f.-o.-8 clavicle strap
f.-o.-8 harness
f.-o.-8 strapping

filament
myosin f.
sarcomeric f.

filamentous hemagglutinin
filariasis
Filatov-Dukes disease
filgrastim
filial generation
filiform
f. adnatum
f. papule
f. plaque
f. wart

Filippi syndrome
Fillauer night splint
filled and spilled
fillet
filling
bladder f.
ventricular f.

F

film
  contraceptive f.
  cross-table lateral f.
  decubitus f.
  scoliosis f.
  spot compression f.
  tear f.
  tibial f.
  upright chest f.
  vaginal contraceptive f. (VCF)
Filmtab
  Rondec F.
filmy adhesion
Filshie
  F. clip
  F. clip applicator
filter
  Greenfield f.
  HEPA f.
  inferior vena cava f. (IVCF)
  leukocyte-depletion f.
  leukocyte-removal f.
  leukodepletion f.
  Millipore f.
  f. paper (FP)
  vena caval f.
filtered specimen trap
filtrate
  glomerular f.
filtration
  f. fraction
  glass-wool f.
  glomerular f.
  rate of fluid f. (Qf)
filum terminale
fimbria, *pl.* **fimbriae**
  flowering-out of f.
  mushrooming of f.
  f. ovarica
fimbriae (*pl. of* fimbria)
fimbrial
  f. adhesion
  f. ectopic pregnancy
  f. evacuation
  f. failure
  f. obstruction
  f. prolapse
fimbriated end of fallopian tube
fimbriectomy
  Uchida f.
fimbriocele
fimbrioplasty
  Bruhat laser f.
Finapres
  F. blood pressure monitor
  F. device
finasteride
find
  Child F.

finding
  clinical f.
  congenital familial lymphedema with
    ocular f.'s
  dermatoglyphic f.
  endovaginal f.
  histopathological f.
  laboratory f.
  pathologic f.
  sonographic f.
  ultrasonic endovaginal f.
Findley folding pessary
fine
  f. inspiratory crackle
  f. lens opacity
  f. Metzenbaum scissors
  f. motor
  f. motor-adaptive skill
  f. motor development
  f. motor domain
  f. motor index
  f. motor milestone
  f. motor total DMQ
Fine-Lubinsky syndrome
fine-needle
  f.-n. aspiration (FNA)
  f.-n. aspiration biopsy (FNAB)
finger
  f. agnosia
  f. arterial blood pressure
    (FABP)
  baseball f.
  bent f.
  boutonnière f.
  coach's f.
  f. cot
  curved f.
  f. feeding
  f. grasp
  index f.
  Madonna f.
  mallet f.
  middle f.
  f. opposition
  overriding f.
  f. plethysmography
  pollicization of index f.
  ring f.
  seal f.'s
  spider f.
  webbed f.'s
fingerbreadth
6-fingered dwarfism
fingernail
finger-nose-finger test
fingerprint
fingerprinting
  DNA amplification f.
  plasmid f.

fingerspelling
fingerstick
finger-tapping test
fingertip
    f. dilated
    f. number writing test
finger-to-nose test
Finkelstein feeding
Finnish
FIO$_2$
    fraction of inspired oxygen
Fioricet With Codeine
fire
    f. ant allergy
    f. setting
    St. Anthony's f.
fire-setting behavior
FIRM
    Family Inventory of Resources for
    Management
firm hepatomegaly
first
    f. abarelix depot study for
    treating endometriosis rapidly
    (FASTER)
    f. and second branchial arch
    syndrome
    f. and second trimester evaluation
    of risk (FASTER)
    f. bicuspid
    f. disease
    f. heart sound
    f. Korotkoff sound
    f. parallel pelvic plane
    f. permanent molar
    f. primary molar
    F. Response ovulation predictor
    f. stage of labor
    f. trimester
    f. trimester screening
    f. trimester termination
first-cycle clinical pregnancy
first-degree
    f.-d. AV block
    f.-d. burn
    f.-d. episiotomy
    f.-d. hypospadias
    f.-d. laceration
    f.-d. prolapse
first-generation
    f.-g. cephalosporin
    f.-g. progesterone
first-line measure
first-morning urine collection
first-order kinetics
first-pass effect
First-Progesterone
    F.-P. VGS 100 vaginal suppository
    F.-P. VGS 50 vaginal suppository

FISCA
    Functional Impairment Scale for
    Children and Adolescents
fish
    f. oil
    f. poisoning
    f. skin
FISH
    fluorescent in situ hybridization
    FISH analysis
Fisher
    F. and Paykel RD1000
    resuscitator
    infantile choreoathetosis of F.
fisherman's knot
Fisher-Race Rh system nomenclature
Fishman syndrome
fishmouth
    f. abnormality
    f. cervix
    f. meatus
    f. vertebra
fish-shaped mouth
fish-tank granuloma
fishy vaginal odor
FISS
    Flint Infant Security Scale
fissure
    abnormal palpebral f.
    Ammon f.
    anal f.
    antimongoloid palpebral f.
    azygos f.
    downslanting palpebral f.
    downsloping palpebral f.
    f. in ano
    mild downslant to palpebral f.
    f. of sternum
    palpebral f.
    rectal f.
    superior vesical f.
    upslanting palpebral f.
fissured
    f. lip
    f. tongue
fissuring
fist
    clenched f.'s
fisting of hands
fistula, *pl.* **fistulae, fistulas**
    anterior rectoperineal f.
    arterioportal f.
    arteriovenous f.
    branchial cleft f.
    bronchobiliary f.
    bronchoesophageal f.
    bronchopleural f.
    bronchopulmonary f.
    (BPF)

F

fistula (*continued*)
    carotid artery-cavernous sinus f.
    carotid-cavernous f.
    cervicovaginal f.
    colovaginal f.
    congenital perilymphatic f.
    coronary arteriovenous f.
    coronary artery f. (CAF)
    coronary-cameral f.
    enterocolic f.
    enterocutaneous f.
    enteroenteric f.
    enterovaginal f.
    enterovesical f.
    gastrointestinal f.
    genitourinary f.
    hepatic arteriovenous f.
    H-type tracheoesophageal f.
    H-type transesophageal f.
    hysterectomy-related f.
    intestinal f.
    intracranial arteriovenous f.
    intrahepatic arterioportal f.
    lacteal f.
    mammary f.
    metroperitoneal f.
    palatal f.
    perianal f.
    perilymphatic f. (PLF)
    perineal f.
    perineovaginal f.
    peripheral arteriovenous f.
    persistent gastrocutaneous f.
    postradiation f.
    rectal fourchette f.
    rectolabial f.
    rectourethral f.
    rectovaginal f.
    rectovestibular f.
    rectovulvar f.
    renal f.
    sinus f.
    spit f.
    systemic arteriovenous f.
    tracheocutaneous f.
    tracheoesophageal f. (TEF, TOF)
    transesophageal f. (TEF)
    tubovaginal f.
    umbilical f.
    urachal f.
    ureter f.
    ureterovaginal f.
    urethrocutaneous f.
    urethrovaginal f.
    urinary f.
    urogenital f.
    uteroperitoneal f.
    vaginorectal f.
    vesicocervicovaginal f.

    vesicocutaneous f.
    vesicouterine f.
    vesicovaginal f.
    vesicovaginorectal f.
    vestibular f.
    vitelline f.
fistulae (*pl. of* fistula)
fistulas (*pl. of* fistula)
fistulogram
fistulotomy
fistulous vascular communication
fit
    arrest/akinetic f.
    extensor f.
    fifth-day f.
    flexor f.
    mixed flexor/extensor f.
    uncinate f.
fitness
    darwinian f.
Fitz-Hugh-Curtis syndrome
Fitzsimmons syndrome
fixation
    buttonpexy f.
    complement f.
    flexible intramedullary f.
    iliococcygeal f.
    intramedullary rod f.
    Nichols sacrospinous f.
    f. nystagmus
    percutaneous pin f.
    sacrospinous ligament f. (SSLF)
fixative
    Carnoy f.
fixator
    Ilizarov external f.
fixed
    f. allele
    f. erythema
    f. flexion deformity
    f. pulmonary hypertension
    f. splitting
    f. stenosis
    f. subvalvular stenosis
fixed-ratio atrioventricular block
FJN
    familial juvenile nephrophthisis
FK binding protein
FLACC
    face, legs, activity, cry, consolability
    FLACC scale
flaccid
    f. contracture
    f. extremity
    f. lesion
    f. paralysis
    f. paraparesis
    f. paraplegia

f. paresis
f. quadriparesis
f. tetraplegia
f. tone
flaccidity
penile f.
flag sign
Flagyl
F. 375
F. Oral
flail
f. chest
f. foot
f. mitral leaflet (FML)
FLAIR
fluid-attenuated inversion recovery
FLAIR sequence
flaking
periungual f.
flame burn
flammeus
nevus f.
flange
tracheostomy tube f.
flank
bluish discoloration of f.
bulging f.
f. dullness
f. mass
f. pain
flanking region
flap
bladder f.
Boari f.
bridging f.
bulbocavernosus fat f.
butterfly f.
Byers hypospadias f.
DIEP f.
double-onlay preputial f.
Duckett transverse preputial
island f.
endorectal f.
endoscopic incision with f.
extra-long artery-pedicled bask fascia
skin f.
fascial f.
fat f.
foreskin f.
gluteal free f.
island f.
lateral transverse thigh f.
latissimus dorsi f.
liver f.
maple leaf f.
Martius bulbocavernosus fat f.
McCraw gracilis myocutaneous f.
Mustardé cheek f.
myocutaneous f.

onlay island f.
Ponten fasciocutaneous f.
preputial f.
Rubens f.
saddlebag f.
f. tracheostomy
TRAM f.
TRAMP f.
vaginal wall f.
vein f.
Warren f.
4-flap Z-plasty
flare
cell and f.
lupus f.
Flarex
flaring
alar f.
f. and grunting
grunting and f.
metaphysial f.
nasal f.
f. of ala nasi
flash
hot f.
f. VEP
flashback
flashlamp-pulsed
f.-p. dye laser
f.-p. laser therapy
Flashtab
flat
f. abdominal radiograph
f. acetabular roof
f. affect
f. back
f. facies
f. fontanelle
f. frontal bone
f. nasal bridge
f. nose
f. pelvis
f. red-black telangiectasia
f. spring diaphragm
f. tire test
f. wart
flatfoot (FF)
calcaneovalgus f.
developmental f.
flexible f.
hypermobile f.
peroneal spastic f.
physiologic f.
flatness to percussion
flattened
f. occiput
f. villus
flatulence
Flatulex

F

flava
　　macula f.
flavimaculatus
　　fundus f.
flavin adenine dinucleotide (FAD)
Flaviviridae
Flavobacterium
flavoprotein
　　electron transfer f. (ETF)
flavoxate
flavus
　　Aspergillus f.
flecainide acetate
Fleet
　　F. Babylax Rectal
　　F. Mineral Oil Enema
　　F. Pain Relief
　　F. Phospho-Soda
fleeting paralysis
Fleming ovoid
Flents breast comfort pack
flesh-colored papule
fleshy mole
Fletcher-Suit applicator
fleur-de-lis breast reconstruction pattern
flexible
　　f. fiberoptic bronchoscopy
　　f. fiberoptic endoscopy
　　f. flatfoot
　　f. hysteroscope
　　f. intramedullary fixation
　　f. kyphosis
　　f. MVA cannula
　　f. pes planovalgus
　　f. positional deformity
　　f. Teflon catheter
flexion
　　flexion, adduction, internal rotation
　　　(FADIR, fadir)
　　f. contracture
　　f. reflex
　　f. spasm
flexion-distraction injury
flexion-extension
Flexi-Seal fecal collector
flexneri
　　Shigella f.
flexor
　　f. fit
　　f. hallucis longus tendon
　　f. tone
flexural
　　f. area
　　f. crease
flexure
　　basicranial f.
　　splenic f.
FL-HCC
　　fibrolamellar hepatocellular carcinoma

flight
　　f. of color
　　f. of ideas
Flimm Fighter
Flinders Island spotted fever
Flint Infant Security Scale (FISS)
Flintstones Complete
FLM
　　fetal lung maturity
　　FLM test
floating
　　f. great toe
　　f. membrane
　　f. thumb
Floating-Harbor syndrome (FHS)
FLOC
　　fetoscopic laser occlusion of
　　chorioangiopagus vessels
floccosum
　　Epidermophyton f.
flocculation
Flonase
flooding
floor
　　decidual f.
　　f. fluoroscopy
　　orbital f.
　　pelvic f.
Flo-Pack
floppy
　　f. infant
　　f. infant syndrome
　　f. larynx
flora
　　commensal f.
　　endogenous cervicovaginal f.
　　microbial f.
　　prepuberal vaginal f.
　　skin f.
　　uterine f.
　　vaginal f.
Florical
florid
　　f. complexion
　　f. pulmonary valvular incompetence
　　f. toxemia
Florida pouch
Florinef Acetate
Florone
flottant
　　pouce f.
flour
　　carob seed f.
Flovent Rotadisk
flow
　　aboral f.
　　f. angulation
　　blood f. (Q)
　　bulk f.

cardiac f.
carotid blood f. (CaBF)
cerebral blood f. (CBF)
coaxial f.
collateral blood f.
cutaneous fetal blood f.
f. cytometric analysis
f. cytometry
Doppler f.
ductal-dependent pulmonary
  blood f.
duct-dependent pulmonary blood f.
excessive pulmonary arterial f.
fetal aortic blood f.
forced expiratory f. (FEF)
gene f.
hyperemic cerebral blood f.
f. karyotyping
menstrual f.
f. murmur
myocardial blood f.
outward menstrual f.
f. pattern
peak expiratory f. (PEF, PEFR)
placental blood f. (PBF)
pulmonary arterial f.
pulmonary blood f. (PBF)
f. rate
renal blood f. (RBF)
renal plasma f.
retrograde axoplasmic f.
retrograde menstrual f.
reversed end-diastolic f.
f. ripening
splanchnic blood f.
systemic f.
to-and-fro f.
torrential pulmonary f.
umbilical blood f.
umbilical venous f.
urine f.
uterine blood f.
uteroplacental blood f.
f. velocity dynamics
f. velocity waveform
venous f.
f. void
volume f.
flowering-out of fimbria
FlowGel barrier material
flowmeter, flow meter
laser-Doppler f.
FlowStat
Flowtron DVT prophylaxis unit
flow-volume
f.-v. curve
f.-v. loop
Floxin Otic
floxuridine in hepatic metastasis

flu
influenza
Fluanxol
flucloxacillin
fluconazole
fluctuance
fluctuant
fluctuating tone
fluctuation
mood f.
flucytosine
5-flucytosine
Fludara
fludarabine
fludrocortisone
fluency
cross-modal f.
verbal f.
flufenamic acid
fluid
amniotic f. (AF)
ascitic f.
BAL f.
Bamberger f.
body f.
f. bolus
bronchoalveolar f.
cerebrospinal f. (CSF)
f. deficit
f. diet
f. distribution
duodenal f.
fluids, electrolytes, nutrition (FEN)
epithelial lining f. (ELF)
excessive amniotic f.
exchange of body f.'s
extraaxial f.
extracellular f. (ECF)
extraluminal f.
fetal lung f.
follicular f.
foul-smelling amniotic f.
hemorrhagic spinal f.
f. homeostasis
human oviduct f. (HOF)
hydrocele f.
hysteroscopy f.
interstitial f.
intracellular f. (ICF)
intravascular f.
intravenous crystallized f.
isotonic f.
maintenance f.
meconium-stained amniotic f.
  (MSAF)
middle ear f. (MEF)
milky f.
negative balance of body f.
nipple aspiration f. (NAF)

F

fluid (*continued*)
f. overload
peripancreatic f.
peritoneal f.
proteinaceous subretinal f.
pseudochylous milky f.
f. replacement
f. replacement therapy
f. restriction
f. resuscitation
retained fetal lung f. (RFLF)
f. retention
seminal f.
serosanguineous f.
f. sift
sperm-counting f.
subretinal f.
synovial f.
third spacing of f.
tracheobronchial aspirate f.
 (TAF)
transcapillary f.
ventricular f.
viscous f.
f. wave
xanthochromic f.
fluid-attenuated inversion recovery (FLAIR)
fluke
lung f.
flulike syndrome
Flumadine Oral
flumazenil
flumecinol
FluMist vaccine
flunisolide
flunitrazepam
fluocinolone acetonide
fluocinonide
Fluoderm
Fluogen
fluorangiography
fluorescein
f. fundus angiography
f. isothiocyanate
f. sodium
f. stain
f. treponema antibody test
fluorescein-conjugated monoclonal antibody test
fluorescein-labeled milk
fluorescence
f. actin staining test
f. depolarization analysis
f. spot test
fluorescence-activated cell sorter (FACS)
fluorescens
 Pseudomonas f.

fluorescent
f. antibody to membrane antigen (FAMA)
f. antimembrane antibody (FAMA)
f. antimembrane antibody test
f. immunoassay (FIA)
f. in situ hybridization (FISH)
f. polarization
f. polarization immunoassay (FPIA)
f. treponemal antibody (FTA)
f. treponemal antibody absorption (FTA-ABS)
f. treponemal antibody absorption test (FTA-ABS)
fluoridation
fluoride
polyvinylidene f. (PVDF)
slow-release sodium f.
sodium f.
Fluorigard
Fluori-Methane
fluorinated corticosteroid
fluorine
Fluorinse
5-fluorocytosine (5-FC)
fluorodeoxyuridine (FUDR)
9-fluorohydrocortisone
fluoroimmunoassay
time-resolved f.
fluorometholone (FML)
fluorophore-assisted carbohydrate electrophoresis (FACE)
fluorophosphate
diisopropyl f.
Fluoroplex Topical
fluoroquinolone
fluoroscope
fluoroscopic guidance
fluoroscopy
airway f.
floor f.
image intensification f.
mini f.
pelvic f.
fluorouracil
5-fluorouracil (5-FU)
intraperitoneal 5-f.
fluoro-urodynamic evaluation
Fluothane
fluoxetine
f. HCl
f. hydrochloride
fluoxymesterone
flupenthixol (*var. of* flupentixol)
flupentixol, flupenthixol
fluphenazine
flurandrenolide
flurazepam
flurbiprofen

flush
    breast f.
    ciliary f.
    cyanotic f.
    heparin-lock f.
    hot f.
    malar f.
    f. method
    orgasmic f.
    vasomotor f.
flushing
    episodic f.
flutamide
fluted drain
fluticasone
    f. propionate
    f. propionate dry powder inhaler
    f. propionate inhalation powder
flutter
    atrial f.
    f. device
    f. isthmus
    ocular f.
    f. wave
flutter-like oscillation
fluvoxamine maleate
flux
    bile acid f.
Fluzone
fly
    Spanish f.
flying squirrel typhus
flying-T pelvis
FM
    fat mass
FMAIT
    fetomaternal alloimmune
      thrombocytopenia
FMC
    fetal movement count
FMCG
    fetal magnetocardiography
FMF
    familial Mediterranean fever
FMG
    female genital mutilation
FMH
    fetal-maternal hemorrhage
    fetomaternal hemorrhage
FML
    flail mitral leaflet
    fluorometholone
      FML Forte
FMLA
    Family Medical Leave Act
FMP
    family member presence
FMPP
    familial male precocious puberty

FMR1
    fragile site mental retardation 1
      FMR1 gene
FMR2
    fragile site mental retardation 2
fMRI
    functional MRI
FMRP
    fragile X mental retardation protein
FMS
    fibromyalgia syndrome
FMT
    fetomaternal transfusion
FNA
    fine-needle aspiration
FNA-21
    FNA-21 fine-needle aspiration device
    FNA-21 needle
FNAB
    fine-needle aspiration biopsy
FND
    frontonasal dysplasia
FNI
    facial nerve injury
FNSD
    face-near-straight-down
FO
    foot orthosis
    foramen ovale
foam
    Because vaginal f.
    f. cell
    contraceptive f.
    intravaginal f.
    f. rubber vaginal form
    Sklar f.
    F. Stability Index (FSI)
    f. stability test (FST)
FoamCare
    F. cleansing system
    F. double scrub brush
FOAR
    faciooculoacousticorenal
    FOAR syndrome
FOBT
    fecal occult blood testing
focal
    f. and segmental glomerular
      sclerosis-hyalinosis
    f. atrophy
    f. axonal swelling
    f. brainstem glioma
    f. cerebral edema
    f. change
    f. clonic seizure
    f. convulsion
    f. cortical dysplasia
    f. dermal hypoplasia
    f. dermal hypoplasia syndrome

F

focal (*continued*)
  f. dystonia
  f. epilepsy
  f. facial dermal dysplasia (type I, II)
  f. facial ectodermal dysplasia
  f. fibrosis
  f. glomerulosclerosis
  f. hemorrhage
  f. heterotopia
  f. lobular carcinoma
  f. lupus nephritis
  f. motor seizure
  f. mucopolysaccharidosis
  f. neurologic deficit
  f. nodular hyperplasia
  f. pontine leukoencephalopathy
  f. postviral encephalitis
  f. scleroderma
  f. segmental glomerular sclerosis
  f. segmental glomerulosclerosis
  f. segmental lupus glomerulonephritis
  f. segmental proliferative glomerulonephritis
  f. spot size
  f. tubulointerstitial fibrosis (FTIF)
  f. villitis
  f. vulvitis
Focalin
  F. tablet
  F. XR
focally dilated duct
focal-onset seizure
foci (*pl. of* focus)
focus, *pl.* foci
  echogenic cardiac f.
  endometriotic f.
  hyperechogenic foci
  occult f.
  Simon f.
focused
  F. Assessment by Sonography for Trauma (FAST)
  f. computed tomography
FOD
  female orgasmic disorder
Foerster sponge-holding forceps
Fogarty
  F. arterial embolectomy (FAE)
  F. arterial embolectomy catheter
  F. atrioseptostomy catheter
fogo selvagem
Foille Medicated First Aid
folacin
folate
  f. antagonist
  f. deficiency
  f. level
  f. supplementation

folate-deficiency anemia
Fol cath
fold
  absent antihelical f.
  antihelical f.
  aryepiglottic f.
  broad ligament f.
  Dennie-Morgan f.
  Duncan folds
  epicanthal f.
  genitocrural f.
  gluteal f.
  head-and-tail f.
  Juvara f.
  lateral umbilical f.
  median umbilical f.
  nuchal f.
  f. of Hoboken
  Pawlik f.
  pleuroperitoneal f.
  rectouterine f.
  rugal f.
  skin f.
  splanchnic f.
  umbilical f.
  urogenital f.
folding frequency
Foley
  F. catheter
  F. tube
folia (*pl. of* folium)
foliaceus
  pemphigus f.
folic
  f. acid
  f. acid antagonist
  f. acid deficiency
folinic acid
folium, *pl.* folia
  cerebellar f.
  folia cerebelli
  folia linguae
  folia of cerebellum
  folia of vermis
folklore-based contraceptive technique
folk medicine
follicle
  antral f.
  f. aspiration, sperm injection, assisted rupture (FASIAR)
  f. aspiration tube
  atretic f.
  dominant f.
  graafian f.
  luteinized unruptured f. (LUF)
  f. maturation stimulation
  Naboth f.

nabothian f.
preantral f.
preovulatory f.
primary f.
primordial f.
f. regulatory protein (FRP)
f. steroidogenesis
follicle-stimulating
f.-s. hormone (FSH)
f.-s. hormone suppression
follicular
f. atrophoderma, basal cell carcinoma syndrome
f. attrition
f. bronchitis
f. conjunctivitis
f. cyst
f. dermatitis
f. desquamation
f. development arrest
f. duct
f. factor
f. fluid
f. function
f. hematoma
f. hyperplasia
f. maturation
f. ostium
f. phase
f. phase gonadotropin secretion
f. plugging
f. scoring
f. tonsillitis
f. urethritis
f. vulvitis
follicularis
dwarfism, cerebral atrophy, keratosis f.
keratosis f.
folliculi
atresia f.
hydrops f.
liquor f.
folliculitis
eosinophilic pustular f. (EPF)
fungal f.
hot tub f.
Staphylococcus epidermidis f.
folliculogenesis
folliculorum
Demodex f.
folliculostatin
Folling disease
follistatin
Follistim/Antagon kit
Follistim Pen drug delivery system
follitropin
f. alpha
f. beta

follow-up (*var. of* followup)
Carnation F.-U.
F.-U. Soy formula
followup, follow-up
f. care
long-term f.
Folvite
folylpolyglutamate
fomepizole
fomite
hand-to-eye f.
Fong disease
Fontaine syndrome
Fontan
F. fenestration
F. operation
F. principle
F. procedure
fontanel (*var. of* fontanelle)
fontanelle, fontanel, fonticulus
anterior f. (AF)
anterolateral f.
bulging f.
Casser f.
casserian f.
depressed f.
false f.
flat f.
Gerdy f.
mastoid f.
posterior f.
posterolateral f.
pulsatile f.
sagittal f.
scaphoid f.
f. sign
sphenoid f.
sunken anterior f.
fonticulus
food
f. allergen
F. and Drug Administration (FDA)
f. avoidance emotion disorder (FAED)
f. challenge test
f. craving
f. diary
fear f.
f. foraging
F. Guide Pyramid
f. impaction
f. insecurity
f. poisoning
f. police
f. seeking
solid f.
thermic effect of f. (TEF)
food-antigen sensitization
foodborne illness

F

food-induced
f.-i. enterocolitis syndrome
f.-i. pulmonary hemosiderosis
foot, *pl.* **feet**
athlete's f.
bilateral club feet
calcaneovalgus f.
cavovarus f.
cavus f.
congenital rocker-bottom f.
dancing feet
f. deformity
epidermolysis bullosa simplex of
feet
flail f.
Friedreich f.
high arch f.
hyperdorsiflexed f.
Madura f.
Morand f.
narrow f.
f. orthosis (FO)
f. presentation
f. presentation
pronated f.
reel f.
rockerbottom f.
spatula f.
Z f.
footballer's migraine
football hold
football-shaped vesicle
footdrop
footling breech presentation
foot-plate (*var. of* footplate)
footplate, foot-plate, foot plate
astrocyte f.
footprinting
foot-progression angle (FPA)
FOP
fibrodysplasia ossificans progressiva
FO-PT
fiberoptic phototherapy
foraging
food f.
foramen, *pl.* **foramina**
bulboventricular f.
Grater sciatic f.
f. magnum
obturator f.
f. of Luschka
f. of Magendie
f. of Monro
f. of Morgagni
f. of Morgagni hernia
outlet foramina
f. ovale (FO)
f. ovale persistence
parietal foramina

pleuroperitoneal f.
f. primum
f. secundum
sternomastoid f.
stylomastoid f.
foramina (*pl. of* foramen)
Forane
Forbes-Albright syndrome
Forbes disease
force
acceleration-deceleration f.
compression f.
expulsive f.
fetal shoulder extraction f.
F. GSU argon-enhanced
electrosurgery system
negative inspiratory f. (NiF, NIF,
NiF n)
oncotic f.
physician-applied f.
shearing f.
Starling f.
United States Preventive Services
Task F. (USPSTF)
U.S. Preventive Services Task F.
(USPSTF)
force
accouchement f.
forced
f. bowel training
f. choice
f. expiratory flow (FEF)
f. expiratory volume (FEV)
f. expiratory volume in 1 second
(FEV$_1$)
f. grasping reflex
f. grasp reflex
f. vital capacity (FVC)
forced-air blanket
forceps
Adson f.
alligator f.
Allis f.
Allis-Abramson breast biopsy f.
Apple Medical bipolar f.
artery f.
ASSI bipolar coagulating f.
atraumatic f.
axis-traction f.
Babcock f.
Backhaus towel f.
Bailey-Williamson f.
Baird f.
Barton f.
bayonet f.
Bellucci alligator f.
BiCOAG f.
Bierer ovum f.
Billroth tumor f.

Bill traction handle f.
biopsy f.
bipolar laparoscopic f.
f. birth trauma
Bishop-Harmon f.
Bozeman uterine dressing f.
Brown-Adson tissue f.
Castroviejo fixation f.
cephalic f.
Chamberlen f.
Clarke ligator scissor f.
coagulation f.
coaptation bipolar f.
cold biopsy f.
Colibri f.
Corey ovum f.
Corson myoma grasping f.
Crile f.
Cushing f.
DeBakey tissue f.
de Juan f.
DeLee f.
f. delivery (FD)
Dennen f.
Desmarres f.
destructive grasping f.
DeWeese axis traction f.
Dewey obstetrical f.
Dieter f.
dressing f.
Drews f.
Duval f.
Elliot f.
Endo-Assist endoscopic f.
Englert f.
Eppendorfer biopsy f.
Erhardt f.
Evershears bipolar laparoscopic f.
Facit polyp f.
Feilchenfeld f.
Foerster sponge-holding f.
Francis f.
Fujinon biopsy f.
Gellhorn f.
Gerald f.
Glassman f.
Greven f.
Haig-Fergusson f.
Halsted mosquito f.
Haugh f.
Hawk-Dennen f.
Heaney-Ballantine f.
Heaney hysterectomy f.
high f.
Hirst placental f.
Hodge f.
hot biopsy f.
Hunt bipolar f.
Iselin f.

Jacobson hemostatic f.
Jaws f.
jeweler's f.
Juers f.
Kelly tissue f.
Kelly vulsellum f.
Kevorkian-Younge biopsy f.
Kjelland f.
Kjelland-Barton f.
Kjelland-Luikart f.
Kleppinger bipolar f.
Lahey f.
Lalonde delicate hook f.
laparoscopic plasma f.
Laufe-Piper f.
Laufe polyp f.
Laurer f.
Leff f.
Levret f.
Livernois-McDonald f.
Llorente dissecting f.
low f.
Luikart f.
Luikart-Simpson f.
f. maneuver
Mazzariello-Caprini f.
McGee f.
McGill f.
McKernan-Adson f.
McKernan-Potts f.
McLane f.
McPherson f.
Nadler f.
Nägele f.
Neville-Barnes f.
nonfenestrated f.
obstetric f.
Ochsner f.
outlet f.
ovum f.
paddle f.
Palmer ovarian biopsy f.
Péan f.
pelvic f.
Pennington f.
Perez-Castro f.
Phaneuf uterine artery f.
Piper f.
Pistofidis cervical biopsy f.
pituitary f.
Polaris reusable f.
Pollock f.
preemie Simpson f.
punch biopsy f.
Quinones uterine-grasping f.
radial jaw biopsy f.
Randall stone f.
Reddick-Saye f.
Reiner-Knight f.

F

forceps (*continued*)
  ring f.
  Rochester-Ochsner f.
  Rochester-Péan f.
  Roger f.
  f. rotation
  Russian tissue f.
  Saenger ovum f.
  Scanzoni f.
  Schroeder tenaculum f.
  Schroeder vulsellum f.
  Schubert uterine biopsy f.
  Seitzinger tripolar cutting f.
  Semken f.
  Shea f.
  Shearer f.
  Simpson f.
  Singley f.
  Sopher ovum f.
  sponge f.
  sponge-holding f.
  spoon f.
  Stolte f.
  suture grasper f.
  Tabb crura tissue f.
  Tarnier axis-traction f.
  tendon f.
  Therma Jaw hot urologic f.
  Thomas-Gaylor biopsy f.
  Tischler cervical biopsy f.
  Tischler-Morgan uterine biopsy f.
  tissue f.
  trial f.
  Tucker-McLane f.
  Tucker-McLane-Luikart f.
  uterine tenaculum f.
  Utrata f.
  Willett f.
  Winter placental f.
  Yeoman f.
  Z-Clamp hysterectomy f.
Forchheimer spot
Fordyce
  F. disease
  F. granule
  F. spot
forebag
forefoot
  f. abduction
  f. adduction
  f. adductus
  f. deformity
  f. valgus
  f. varus
foregut
  f. duplication
  f. malformation
forehead
  broad f.

foreign
  f. body
  f. body aspiration
  f. body salpingitis
forekidney
forelock
  white f.
foremilk
forensic specimen
foreplay
foreskin
  f. flap
  large f.
forest
  conidial f.
forewaters
fork
  replication f.
forking
  aqueductal f.
form
  balsa vaginal f.
  child behavior rating f. (CBRF)
  coccobacillary f.
  connatal f.
  foam rubber vaginal f.
  Lucite f.
  MedWatch f.
  parenchymatous f.
  pelvic pain assessment f.
  phosphorylated drug f.
  racemose f.
  serous f.
  Teacher Rating F. (TRF)
  Teacher Report F. (TRF)
  Vineland Adaptive Behavior Scales, Survey F.
form-35
  Ware Short F.-35
Forma
  F. in vitro incubator
  F. water-jacketed incubator
formaldehyde
formalin
formation
  abscess f.
  alveolar saccule f.
  blood vessel f.
  bone f.
  cataract f.
  chiasma f.
  chylomicron f.
  clot f.
  colostomy f.
  crescent f.
  Dandy-Walker f.
  dissolution of clot f.
  echo f.
  kerion f.

macular star f.
neoaorta f.
onion bulb f.
perivascular pseudorosette f.
pneumatocele f.
popcorn f.
primary lung bud f.
recurrent hernia f.
sequestrum f.
somite f.
subcutaneous catheter tunnel f.
terminal blush f.
uterine window f.
formative yolk
formazan dye
formboard
forme fruste
formic acid
formiminoglutamic acid (FIGLU)
formiminoglutamicaciduria (FIGLU-uria)
formiminotransferase
f. deficiency
f. deficiency syndrome
formula, *pl.* **formulas, formulae**
Accupep HPF enteral f.
Advance f.
Advera f.
AL 110 f.
Alcare f.
Alimentum f.
Alimentum Advance f.
Alitraq f.
Alsoy 1, 2 f.
Bayer Timed-Release Arthritic Pain F.
Bazett f.
BC Cold Powder Non-Drowsy F.
Brozek body fat percentage f.
20-calorie f.
24-calorie f.
Carnation Follow-Up soy f.
Carnation Good Start f.
Carvajal f.
Casec f.
casein hydrolysate f.
Compleat Modified f.
Compleat Pediatric f.
Comtrex Cough F.
Criticare H f.
Deliver f.
diluted f.
EleCare f.
electrodialyzed whey f.
F. EM oral solution
EnfaCare Lipil f.
Enfamil A.R. Lipil f.
Enfamil Gentlease Lipil f.
Enfamil human milk fortifier f.
Enfamil LactoFree Lipil f.

Enfamil Lipil low iron f.
Enfamil Lipil with iron f.
Enfamil Next Step ProSobee Lipil f.
Enfamil Nutramigen Lipil f.
Enfamil Pregestimil f.
Enfamil Premature Lipil f.
Enfamil ProSobee Lipil f.
Ensure high-protein f.
Ensure Plus HN f.
Ensure with fiber f.
evaporated milk f. (EMF)
Fibersource HN f.
Follow-Up Soy f.
fortified f.
full-strength f.
Glucerna f.
glucose f.
goat's milk f.
Good Start f.
Gorlin f.
half-strength f.
Hardy-Weinberg f.
high-caloric density f.
high-calorie f.
high-fructose f.
high-glucose f.
homemade f.
hydrolysate f.
hydrolyzed premature f.
hypercaloric f.
Infalyte f.
Intralipid f.
Isocal HN f.
Isomil DE f.
Isosource 1.5 Cal f.
Isosource HN f.
Isosource Standard f.
I-Soyalac f.
Jevity Plus f.
Kaopectate Advanced F.
Kindercal f.
LactoFree Lipil f.
lactose-containing f.
lactose-free f.
Liposyn f.
Lohman-Brozek body fat percentage f.
Lonalac f.
Lytren f.
Magnacal f.
Mall f.
MCT oil f.
Mead Johnson f.
menstrual f.
Meritene f.
Microlipid f.
milk-based f.
Moducal f.

F

formula (*continued*)
Mollifene Ear Wax Removing F.
Mollison f.
Neocate One+ f.
Newtrition Isofiber f.
Newtrition Isotonic f.
nucleotide-fortified f.
Nutramigen f.
Nutren 1.0, 1,5, 2.0 f.
Nutren 1.0 with Fiber f.
Osmolite HN f.
Oxepa f.
Parent's Choice f.
Parkland f.
Pedialyte f.
PediaSure with Fiber f.
Peptamen Jr. f.
Perative f.
Polycose liquid f.
Polycose powder f.
Portagen f.
powdered milk f.
predigested f.
Pregestimil f.
preterm f.
prethickened f.
Profiber f.
ProMod f.
Promote with Fiber f.
Propac Plus f.
ProSobee f.
protein hydrolysate f.
Pulmocare f.
quarter-strength f.
rapid dissolution f. (RDF)
RCF f.
Rehydralyte f.
Resource Just for Kids with
  Fiber f.
Resource Plus f.
Resource Standard f.
semielemental casein hydrolysate f.
Similac 2 Advance f.
Similac Alimentum Advance f.
Similac human milk fortifier f.
Similac Isomil Advance 2 f.
Similac Isomil DF f.
Similac Lactose Free Advance f.
Similac Natural Care Advance f.
Similac NeoSure Advance f.
Similac PM 60/40 f.
Similac Special Care 20, 24, 40 f.
Similac with iron f.
Siri body fat percentage f.
sodium-free f.
soy-based protein isolate f.
Spearman-Brown prediction f.
sucrose-free f.
Sumacal f.

Suplena f.
Sustacal Plus f.
Sustagen f.
three-quarter strength f.
Tolerex f.
TraumaCal f.
Triaminic AM Decongestant F.
TwoCal HN f.
Ultra Bright Beginnings Lipids f.
vegetable oil fat-based f.
Vicks F. 44
Vital High Nitrogen f.
Vitaneed f.
Vivonex Pediatric f.
Vivonex Plus f.
Vivonex Ten f.
formulae (*pl. of* **formula**)
formula-feeding woman
formulas (*pl. of* **formula**)
fornices (*pl. of* fornix)
fornix, *pl.* **fornices**
posterior f.
posterior vaginal f.
vaginal f.
Forsius-Eriksson type ocular albinism
Forssman
F. antigen
F. titer
Fortaz
Fort Bragg evaluation project (FBEP)
Forte
Biotin F.
Femogen F.
FML F.
Robinul F.
Zone-A F.
Fortel ovulation test
Fortical
fortification spectrum
fortified formula
fortifier
Enfamil human milk f.
human milk f. (HMF)
Similac human milk f. (SHMF)
Fortovase
fortuitum
Mycobacterium f.
Forvade
forward
f. chaining
f. roll fashion
f. roll method
f. tandem gait
forward-bending test
Fosamax
fosamprenavir
foscarnet
Foscavir
fosfomycin tromethamine

fosinopril
fossa, *pl.* **fossae**
    congenital supraspinous f.
    enlarged posterior f.
    iliac f.
    ischiorectal f.
    f. navicularis
    f. of Waldeyer
    olecranon f.
    f. ovalis
    posterior cranial f.
    shallow acetabular fossae
fossae (*pl. of* fossa)
foster care
Fostex
    F. Bar
    F. 10% BPO Gel
Fothergill-Donald operation
Fothergill-Hunter uterine prolapse
  repair
Fothergill operation
Fototar
foul-smelling
    f.-s. amniotic fluid
    f.-s. discharge
foundation
    Children's Digestive Health and
      Nutrition F. (CDHNF)
    Epilepsy F.
    March of Dimes Birth Defects F.
    MedicAlert F.
    National Osteoporosis F.
founder
    f. chromosome
    f. effect
Fountain syndrome
fourchette
    posterior f.
Fourier transform infrared
  microspectroscopy
Fournier tooth
fourth
    Bartholomew rule of f.'s
    f. heart sound
    f. nerve palsy
    f. parallel pelvic plane
    f. phacomatosis
    f. stage of labor
    f. venereal disease
fourth-degree
    f.-d. burn
    f.-d. episiotomy
    f.-d. laceration
foveal hypoplasia
fowleri
    Naegleria f.
Fowler position
Fowler-Stephens orchiopexy
Fox-Fordyce disease

FP
    filter paper
    FP blood lead testing
FPA
    foot-progression angle
FPD
    fetopelvic disproportion
FPG
    fasting plasma glucose
FPH
    female pseudohermaphroditism
FPIA
    fluorescent polarization immunoassay
FPO
    faciopalatoosseous
    fetal pulse oximetry
    FPO syndrome
fra
    fragile
    fragile chromosome site
    fragile gene
FRA
    fragile
    fragile chromosome site
    fragile gene
fraction
    cardiac ejection f.
    filtration f.
    increased globulin f.
    f. in expired gas of carbon dioxide
      ($FECO_2$)
    left ventricular ejection f. (LVEF)
    f. of alveolar carbon dioxide
      ($FACO_2$)
    f. of inspired oxygen (FI_{O2}, FIO_2,
      FIO2)
    plasma f.
    recombination f.
    regurgitant f.
    right ventricular ejection f. (REF,
      RVEF)
    shortening f.
    S phase f.
fractional
    f. dilation and curettage
    f. excretion
    f. excretion of sodium (FENa)
    f. shortening (FS)
fractionated sterotactic radiotherapy
fractionation
fracture
    avulsion f.
    basal skull f.
    basilar skull f.
    bend f.
    birth f.
    blowout f.
    bowing f.
    boxer's f.

F

fracture (*continued*)
  bucket-handle f.
  buckle f.
  bursting f.
  calcaneal f.
  Chance f.
  clavicular f. (CF)
  coccygeal f.
  coexisting f.
  Colles f.
  comminuted f.
  complete f.
  compression f.
  corner f.
  cribriform f.
  depressed skull f.
  diaphysial f.
  diastatic f.
  direct orbital floor f.
  displaced supracondylar f.
  distal humeral physial f.
  elbow f.
  fatigue f.
  femoral shaft f.
  fetal f.
  fibular shaft f.
  Galeazzi f.
  greenstick f.
  growing f.
  growth plate f.
  hangman's f.
  hindfoot f.
  hip f.
  impacted f.
  indirect orbital floor f.
  intertrochanteric f.
  intrauterine f.
  Jefferson f.
  Jones stress f.
  juvenile Tillaux f.
  laryngeal f.
  lateral condylar f.
  Le Fort f. (I, II)
  linear skull f.
  Maisonneuve f.
  Malgaigne f.
  mastoid bone f.
  maternal f.
  medial epicondylar f.
  metacarpal f.
  metaphysial f.
  middle third of clavicle f.
  Monteggia f.
  NOE f.
  nonaccidental spiral tibial f.
  nondisplaced lateral condylar f.
  nonpathologic f.
  oblique f.
  f. of penis

  f. of Tillaux
  olecranon f.
  open f.
  orbital blowout f.
  orbital wall f.
  osteochondral f.
  osteoporotic f.
  patellar f.
  pathologic f.
  f. pattern
  pelvic type A, B, C f.
  physial f.
  ping-pong f.
  plastic deformation f.
  plate f.
  pond f.
  proximal humeral stress f.
  pubic ramus stress f.
  radial head f.
  radial neck f.
  f. reduction
  f. remodeling
  rib f.
  Salter-Harris classification of f.
  Salter-Harris epiphysial f.
  Salter-Harris f. (type I–V)
  scapular f.
  shear f.
  skull f.
  sleeve f.
  spinal compression f.
  spiral tibial f.
  sternal f.
  stress f.
  supracondylar humeral f.
  talar dome f.
  thoracic spine f.
  tibial shaft f.
  tibial stress f.
  Tillaux f.
  toddler's f.
  torus f.
  transverse f.
  triplane f.
  ulnar styloid f.
  vertebral f.
  vertebral compression f.
  zygomaticomaxillary f.
fractured
  f. chromosome
  f. sternum
fragile (fra, FRA)
  f. chromosome site (FRA, fra)
  f. chromosome site E (FRAXE)
  f. chromosome site F (FRAXF)
  f. gene (FRA, fra)
  medically f.
  f. site mental retardation 1 (FMR1)
  f. site mental retardation 2 (FMR2)

f. tissue
f. X analysis
f. X carrier
f. X chromosome
f. X disorder
f. X gene (FRAX)
f. X mental retardation protein (FMRP)
f. X mental retardation syndrome
f. Xq syndrome
f. X syndrome (FRAX, FXS)
f. X type A (FRAXA)
fragilis
    Bacteroides f.
    Dientamoeba f.
fragilitas ossium
fragment
    f. antigen binding (Fab)
    anucleate f.
    Okazaki f.
    placental f.
    restriction f.
    retained placental f.
    urinary beta-core f.
fragmentation
    f. of necrotic bone
    uterine f.
fragmented poikilocyte
Fragmin
frame
    open reading f.
    reading f.
frameshift mutation
Franceschetti-Goldenhar syndrome
Franceschetti-Jadassohn syndrome
Franceschetti-Klein syndrome
Franceschetti syndrome
Franceschetti-Zwahlen-Klein syndrome
Franceschetti-Zwahlen syndrome
Francisella
    F. tularensis
    F. tularensis holarctica
Francis forceps
François
    F. dyscephalia
    F. dyscephalic syndrome
frank
    f. ambiguity
    f. breech
    f. breech presentation
    F. procedure
    F. technique of dilation
    F. vaginal construction
Frankenhäuser
    F. ganglion
    F. plexus
Franklin-Dukes test
Frank-Starling
    F.-S. mechanism

    F.-S. principle
    F.-S. relationship
Frantz tumor
frappage therapy
Fraser-François syndrome
Fraser-like syndrome
Fraser syndrome
FRAST
    Free Running Asthma Test
frataxin
fraternal twins
fra(X)
    fra(X) gene
    fra(X) syndrome
FRAXA
    fragile X type A
FRAXE
    fragile chromosome site E
FRAXE-associated mental retardation
FRAXF
    fragile chromosome site F
FRAXq27 syndrome
Frazier suction tip
FRC
    functional residual capacity
FreAmine
freckling
    axillary f.
    inguinal f.
Fredet-Ramstedt
    F.-R. extramucosal longitudinal myotomy procedure
    F.-R. operation
free
    F. Active
    f. androgen index
    f. beta hCG
    f. bilirubin
    Breathe F.
    f. choline
    f. erythrocyte protoporphyrin (FEP)
    f. estradiol
    f. fatty acid
    f. hydroxyl radical
    f. iron
    f. neuraminic acid storage disease
    f. peritoneal air
    f. radial generation
    f. radical (FR)
    F. Running Asthma Test (FRAST)
    f. sialic acid storage disease
    f. testosterone
    f. testosterone index
    f. thyroxine
    f. thyroxine index
    f. tie
    F. to Be Me body image program
    f. tongue
    f. tracheal autograft

F

free (*continued*)
    f. triiodothyronine
    f. water calculation
freebase cocaine
free-floating loop
free-flow oxygen
freely movable breast mass
Freeman cookie cutter areola marker
Freeman-Sheldon syndrome
freeze-thaw-freeze
freezing process
Freezone Solution
Frei
    F. antibody
    F. test
Freiberg
    F. disease
    F. infraction
Frejka pillow splint
fremitus
    diminished f.
    tactile f.
    vocal f.
frena (*pl. of* frenum)
French
    F. Gesco catheter
    F. hysteroscope
    F. lock
French-American-British (FAB)
24-French Foley balloon
frenectomy
frenoplasty
frenotomy
frenula (*pl. of* frenulum)
frenulum, *pl.* frenula
    f. labiorum pudendi
    f. linguae
    lingual f.
    multiple oral frenula
    f. of clitoris
frenum, *pl.* frena
Frenzel middle ear pressure maneuver
frequency
    allele f.
    f. dysuria syndrome
    fetal heart f. (FHF)
    folding f.
    high f. (HF)
    low f. (LF)
    Nyquist f.
    pulse f.
    recombination f.
    spectral edge f. (SEF)
    urinary f.
fresh frozen plasma (FFP)
fresh-packed RBCs
freshwater near-drowning
freudian
Freud theory

Freund
    F. adjuvant
    F. operation
freundii
    Citrobacter f.
    Clostridium f.
Freyer suprapubic drain
friable
    f. cervix
    f. clot
    f. ectocervix
    f. hair
Fria muscle training device & program
Friberg microsurgical agglutination test
fricative
    glottal f.
friction
    f. dermatitis
    f. diaper rash
    f. rub
frictional trauma
Friedman
    F. labor curve
    F. rabbit test
    F. Splint brace
Friedreich
    F. ataxia
    F. foot
Friedrich criteria for dyspareunia
Fried syndrome
Friend syndrome
frigid
Frigiderm
frigidity
Frin
    Isopto F.
Fritsch
    F. douche
    F. syndrome
Fritsch-Asherman syndrome
Froben-SR
frogleg
    f. lateral radiograph
    f. position
    f. posture
    f. view
frog-legged
Fröhlich syndrome
frondlike
frondosum
    chorion f.
frontal
    f. baldness
    f. bones scalloping
    f. bossing
    f. encephalocele
    f. horn
    f. plagiocephaly

f. pole area
f. suture
frontoanterior
    left f. (LFA)
    f. position
frontodigital syndrome
frontofacionasal
    f. dysostosis
    f. dysplasia
frontometaphysial dysplasia
frontonasal dysplasia (FND)
frontoparietal sensorimotor cortex
frontoposterior position
frontostriatal
frontotemporal cortical atrophy
frontotransverse
    left f. (LFT)
    f. position
front-to-back wiping
frostbite
frothy discharge
frottage
frozen
    f. biopsy
    f. egg
    f. embryo
    f. embryo replacement (FER)
    f. milk
    f. ovum
    f. pelvis
    f. plasma
    f. red blood cell
    f. section (FS)
    f. semen
    f. smile puckered lips
    f. sperm
    f. zygote
frozen-thawed embryo transfer
FRP
    follicle regulatory protein
fructokinase
fructose
    f. galactokinase deficiency
    f. intolerance
    f. intolerance test
fructosemia
fructosuria
    benign f.
    essential f.
fruity breath odor
frusemide
fruste
    forme f.
Frykman-Goldberg resection rectopexy
Fryns-Moerman syndrome
Fryns syndrome (1–3)
Fryns-van den Berghe syndrome
FS
    feminization syndrome

fractional shortening
frozen section
    AmpliTaq DNA polymerase FS
FSAD
    female sexual arousal disorder
FSD
    face-straight-down
    female sexual dysfunction
FSDS
    Female Sexual Distress Scale
FSE
    fetal scalp electrode
FSFI
    Female Sexual Function Index
FSG
    focal segmental glomerulosclerosis
FSGS
    focal segmental glomerulosclerosis
FSH
    facioscapulohumeral
    follicle-stimulating hormone
        FSH antagonist
        FSH binding inhibitor
        highly purified FSH
        FSH inhibition
        FSH level
        FSH MAIAclone immunoradiometric
          assay
        FSH muscular dystrophy
        purified urinary FSH
        FSH secretion
FSHD
    facioscapulohumeral muscular dystrophy
FSI
    Foam Stability Index
FS$_p$O$_2$
    fetal arterial oxygen saturation
FST
    foam stability test
FT
    feeding tube
    full term
FTA
    fluorescent treponemal antibody
        FTA test
FTA-ABS
    fluorescent treponemal antibody
      absorption
FTBD
    full term, born dead
FTC
    fallopian tube carcinoma
FTI
    free thyroxine index
FTIF
    focal tubulointerstitial fibrosis
FTM
    female-to-male
        FTM transition

F

FTNB
  full-term newborn
FTP
  full-term pregnancy
FTS
  face-to-side
  fetal tobacco syndrome
FTSP
  fallopian tube sperm perfusion
FTT
  failure to thrive
    FTT syndrome
Ftube
  feeding tube
FTV
  fetal thrombotic vasculopathy
5-FU
  5-fluorouracil
FUCA
  alpha-L-fucosidase
    FUCA deficiency
Fucidin
fucosidase
fucosidosis
FUDR
  fluorodeoxyuridine
FUE
  fever of unknown etiology
fugax
    amaurosis f.
fugue state
Fuhrmann syndrome
Fuhrman pleural drainage set
Fujinon
  F. biopsy forceps
  F. flexible hysteroscope
Fukuyama
  F. CMD
  F. congenital muscular dystrophy
    (FCMD)
  F. disease
  F. syndrome
FUL
  functional urethral length
fulguration
  direct f.
  indirect f.
  laparoscopic f.
full
  f. breech presentation
  f. enteral feed
  f. inclusion
  f. lepromatous leprosy
  f. mutation
  f. nipple feed
  f. term (FT)
  f. term, born dead (FTBD)
  f. tuberculoid leprosy
  f. venography

Fuller
  F. Albright syndrome 1
  F. shield
  F. shield rectal dressing
fullness
  periorbital f.
full-strength formula
full-syndrome eating disorder
full-term
  f.-t. infant
  f.-t. newborn (FTNB)
  f.-t. pregnancy (FTP)
full-thickness
  f.-t. bowel biopsy
  f.-t. burn
  f.-t. intestinal biopsy
  f.-t. necrosis
  f.-t. skin graft
fulminans
  acne f.
  neonatal purpura f.
  purpura f.
fulminant
  f. disease
  f. early-onset neonatal pneumonia
  f. hepatic failure (FHF)
  f. hepatitis
  f. sepsis
  f. ulcerative colitis
fulminating meningitis
· **fulvestrant**
Fulvicin
  F. P/G
  F. U/F
fumarate
  ferrous f.
  quetiapine f.
fumarylacetoacetate hydrolase (FAH)
fumes
fumigatus
    Aspergillus f.
function
    adrenocortical f.
    atrioventricular node f.
    axon-reflex f.
    binocular f.
    bladder f.
    bowel f.
    brain f.
    brainstem f.
    cardiac f.
    cardiorespiratory f.
    cholinergic sympathetic f.
    ciliary f.
    corpus luteum f.
    declining ovarian f.
    executive f.
    fetal cardiac f.
    fetoplacental f.

follicular f.
global assessment of f. (GAF)
hypothalamic-pituitary f.
impaired cognitive f.
kidney f.
leukocyte f.
luteal f.
mitochondrial f.
mucociliary f.
myocardial f.
oromotor f.
ovarian f.
peroneal nerve f.
pituitary-adrenal f.
pituitary gland f.
pituitary-ovarian f.
placental f.
pulmonary f.
renal tubular f.
reproductive f.
serotonergic f.
sexual f.
sinus node f.
sympathetic adrenergic f.
thyroid f.
urethral f.
ventricular f.

functional
f. abdominal pain
f. age
f. alveolus
f. anemia
f. asplenia
F. Assessment of Cancer Therapy (FACT)
F. Assessment Scale (FAS)
f. behavior
f. bladder stimulation (FES)
f. brain activity
f. brain imaging
f. cloning
f. constipation
f. dysmenorrhea
f. dyspepsia
f. electrical stimulation (FES)
f. gastrointestinal disorder (FGID)
f. heart disease
f. impairment
F. Impairment Scale for Children and Adolescents (FISCA)
f. incontinence
F. Independence Measure for Children (WeeFIM)
f. MRI (fMRI)
f. murmur
f. outlet obstruction
f. ovarian cyst
f. posterior rhizotomy
f. prepuberal castrate syndrome

f. pulmonary atresia
f. residual capacity (FRC)
f. urethral length (FUL)
functionale
stratum f.
functionalis
zona f.
function-enhancing mutation
functioning
executive cognitive f. (ECF)
global level of f. (GLOF)
neurovegetative f.
f. tumor
fundal
f. height (FH)
f. height measurement
f. placentation
f. plication
f. pressure
f. tenderness
fundamentals-preschool
Clinical Evaluation of Language F.-P.
fundectomy
fundi (*pl. of* fundus)
fundic gland polyp
fundoplication
laparoscopic f. (LF)
Nissen f.
Thal f.
fundus, *pl.* **fundi**
f. albipunctatus
f. flavimaculatus
ghost vessel f.
incarcerated f.
optic f.
red f.
salt-and-pepper f.
uterine f.
funduscopic
funduscopy
fundusectomy
fungal
f. ball
f. endocarditis
f. folliculitis
f. id reaction
f. infection
f. meningitis
f. oil
f. sepsis
fungating mass
fungemia
fungi (*pl. of* fungus)
fungiform papilla
Fungizone
fungoid
F. AF Topical Solution
F. Cream

F

fungoides
mycosis f.
fungus, *pl.* **fungi**
f. ball
dimorphic pathogenic f.
lipophilic f.
umbilical f.
funic
f. presentation
f. reduction
f. souffle
funicular souffle
funiculi (*pl. of* funiculus)
funiculus, *pl.* **funiculi**
f. umbilicalis
funipuncture
funis
funisitis
necrotizing f.
funnel
accessory müllerian f.
f. chest
f. length
f. width
funneling
cervical f.
funnel-shaped pelvis
Funston syndrome
FUO
fever of undetermined
origin
fever of unknown
origin
Furadantin
Furalan
furan
furazolidone
furcate insertion of cord
furfur
Malassezia f.
furoate
mometasone f.
furosemide
Furoxone
furrow
furrowing
surface f.
furrowlike umbilicus
furuncle
staphylococcal f.

furunculosis
staphylococcal f.
fusaric acid
Fusarium
fused
f. frontal horn
f. raphe
fusiform
f. aneurysm
f. dilation
f. dilation of urethra
f. nerve thickening
fusion
anterior spinal f.
calcaneonavicular f.
cervical vertebral f.
f. implantation
incomplete müllerian f.
f. inhibitor (FI)
joint f.
labial f.
labioscrotal f.
müllerian duct f.
f. of eyelids
postvaginal f.
robertsonian f.
spinal f.
talocalcaneal f.
thought action f.
Fusobacterium
F. gonidiaformans
F. mortiferum
F. necrophorum
F. nucleatum
fusospirillary gangrenous stomatitis
fusospirochetal gingivitis
futile cycle
FVC
forced vital capacity
FVS
fetal valproate syndrome
fetal varicella syndrome
FW
fetal weight
FWS
fetal warfarin syndrome
FXS
fragile X syndrome
FyBron calcium alginate dressing
fyn protooncogene

G
gravida
G₀
gap₀
G₁
gap₁
primigravida
G₂
gap₂
GA
gestational age
GAA
gossypol acetic acid
GAA trinucleotide expansion
GABA
gamma aminobutyric acid
GABA transaminase deficiency
gabapentin
GABEB
generalized atrophic benign
epidermolysis bullosa
GABHS
group A beta-hemolytic streptococcus
GABHS pharyngitis
Gabitril
GAD
generalized anxiety disorder
glutamic acid decarboxylase
gadolinium
chelated g.
gadopentetate dimeglumine
GAF
global assessment of function
Gaffney joint
GAG
glycosaminoglycan
Gage sign
gag reflex
Gail
G. breast cancer model
G. risk assessment model
Gaillard syndrome
gain
absolute length g.
absolute weight g.
maternal weight g.
poor weight g.
total weight g.
weight g.
gait
antalgic g.
g. apraxia
g. ataxia
ataxic g.
broad-based g.

circumduction g.
crouch g.
g. dysfunction
equinus g.
forward tandem g.
heel-toe g.
g. laboratory
lordotic g.
nonreciprocal g.
outtoe g.
reciprocating g.
shuffling g.
slapping storklike g.
teddy-bear g.
toe-in g.
toe-out g.
Trendelenburg g.
waddling g.
wide-based shuffling g.
galactacrasia
galactagogue
galactic
galactitol
galactobolic
galactocele
galactocerebrosidase (GALC)
galactogram
mammary g.
galactography
galactokinase deficiency
galactokinesis
galactolipid
galactometer
galactopoiesis
galactorrhea
galactorrhea-amenorrhea syndrome
galactosamine
galactose
g. breath test
g. uridine diphosphate
galactose-free diet
galactosemia
African American variant g.
classical g.
Duarte variant g.
hereditary g.
Los Angeles variant g.
transferase deficient g.
galactose-1-phosphate uridyltransferase (GALT)
galactosialidosis
galactosidase
ceramide trihexoside alpha g.
galactosis
galactosuria

G

galactosylceramide beta-galactosidase deficiency
galactosylsphingosine lipidosis
galactotherapy
GALC
  galactocerebrosidase
  GALC deficiency
GALE
  UDP-galactose-4-epimerase
  GALE deficiency
galea
Galeazzi
  G. fracture
  G. fracture dislocation
  G. sign
Galen
  aneurysm of vein of G.
  vein of G.
Galileo rigid hysteroscope
Gallant reflex
gallbladder
  atretic g.
  g. disease
  duplication of g.
  hydropic g.
  g. hydrops
  g. resection
  g. stasis
gallinatum
  pectus g.
gallium
  g. scan
  g. scintography
gallium-67
  g.-6. citrate contrast medium
  g.-6. scan
gallop
  protodiastolic g.
  g. rhythm
  summation g.
Galloway-Mowat syndrome
Galloway syndrome
gallstone
  cholesterol g.
  g. pancreatitis
galoche chin
GALT
  galactose-1-phosphate uridyltransferase
  gastrointestinal-associated lymphoid tissue
  gut-associated lymphoid tissue
  GALT deficiency
galtonian-Fisher genetics
galtonian trait
Galton law of regression
Gambee suture
Gambian
  G. disease
  G. trypanosomiasis

gamble
Gamble-Darrow syndrome
gamekeeper's thumb
gametangium
gamete
  aging g.
  g. intrafallopian transfer (GIFT)
  g. manipulation
  g. micromanipulation
  overmature g.
  unbalanced g.
gametic
  g. chromosome
  g. selection
gametogenesis
  ovarian g.
gametokinetic
Gamimune N
gamma
  g. aminobutyric acid (GABA)
  G. BHC
  g. globulin (GG)
  g. globulin replacement
  g. glutamyl transferase (GGT)
  g. glutamyl transpeptidase
  g. interferon (IFN-G)
  interferon g. (IFN-gamma)
  g. knife surgery
  g. ray
gamma-1b
  interferon g.-1b
gamma-benzene hexachloride
Gammabulin Immuno
gamma-chain disorder
Gammagard S/D
gamma-irradiated cellular products transfusion
gamma-loop disorder
Gammar-IV
Gammar-P IV
Gamper
  G. bowing reflex
  G. method
  G. method of childbirth
gampsodactyly
Gamulin Rh
ganaxolone
ganciclovir
ganglia (*pl. of* ganglion)
gangliocytoma
  dysplastic g.
ganglioglioma
  desmoplastic infantile g. (DIG)
ganglion, *pl.* **ganglia, ganglions**
  basal g.
  g. cell
  Frankenhäuser g.
  gasserian g.
  herpes zoster of geniculate g.

hypoglossal g.
sympathetic g.
g. trigger theory
volar g.
ganglioneuroblastoma
ganglioneuroma
ganglioneuromatosis
mucosal g.
ganglionic
g. blocker
g. differentiation
ganglions (*pl. of* ganglion)
ganglioside
g. degradation
g. storage disease
gangliosidosis
adult generalized g.
cerebral GM1 g.
generalized infantile g.
generalized juvenile g.
GM2 g.
GM3 g.
g. GM1 juvenile type
g. GM1 late onset without bony
involvement
g. GM1 type II
juvenile GM1 g.
juvenile GM2 g.
neuronal GM1 g.
Sandhoff GM2 g. (type I, II)
gangrene
acute streptococcal g.
gas g.
Meleney synergistic g.
pulmonary g.
streptococcal g.
synergistic g.
gangrenosa
varicella g.
gangrenosum
ecthyma g.
pyoderma g.
vulvar pyoderma g.
gangrenous
g. appendicitis
g. stomatitis
ganirelix
g. acetate
g. acetate injection
GANT
gastrointestinal autonomic nerve tumor
gap
anion g.
g. junction
osmotic g.
plasma anion g.
GAP
gonadotropin-releasing
hormone-associated peptide

gap_0 (G_0)
gap_1 (G_1)
gap_2 (G_2)
gape
allergic g.
GAPS
Guidelines for Adolescent Preventive
Services
Garamycin
Garatec
Garcia-Lurie syndrome
Gardasil
Gardner
G. Expressive One-Word Vocabulary
Test-Revised
G. syndrome
Gardnerella
G. vaginalis
G. vaginalis chorioamnionitis
G. vaginitis
Gardner-Silengo-Wachtel syndrome
Gardner-Wells tongs
Gareis-Mason syndrome
gargantuan mastitis
gargoylism
Gariel pessary
garinii
Borrelia g.
Garrodian inborn error
Gartner
G. duct
G. duct cyst
gartnerian
g. cyst
g. duct
gas
g. anesthetic
arterial blood g. (ABG)
g. bloat
blood g.
capillary blood g. (CBG)
carbon dioxide g.
g. chromatography
g. chromatography-mass spectrometry
(GC-MS)
g. chromatography-mass spectroscopy
(GC-MS)
g. collection
cord blood g. (CBG)
g. embolus
fetal blood g.
g. gangrene
g. gangrene fasciitis
inspired g. (I)
intervillous blood g.
intramural g.
Mylanta G.
paucity of g.
sweep g.

G

gas (*continued*)
    g. transfer
    venous blood g. (VBG)
GAS
    group A streptococcus
    GAS infection
GASA
    growth-adjusted sonographic age
gaseous distention
gas-forming bacteria
Gaskin maneuver
gasless laparoscopy
GasPak jar
gasping
    fetal g.
    g. respiration
gasseri
    Lactobacillus g.
gasserian ganglion
Gasser syndrome
GAST
    gonadotropin agonist stimulation test
gastric, gastricus
    g. accommodation
    g. acid hypersecretion
    g. acid hyposecretion
    g. aspirate culture
    g. atony
    g. atrophy
    g. balloon
    g. bubble
    g. bypass
    g. carcinoma
    g. decompression
    g. dilation
    g. duplication
    g. dysmotility
    g. dysrhythmia
    g. emptying
    g. emptying time
    g. enteral feeding
    g. fluid aspiration
    g. inhibitory polypeptide (GIP)
    g. irrigation
    g. lavage
    g. mobilization
    g. mucosa
    g. outlet obstruction (GOO)
    g. perforation
    g. peristaltic wave
    g. pullup
    g. reduction surgery
    g. regurgitation
    g. residual volume (GRV)
    g. residue
    g. stapling
    g. tonometry
    g. tube feeding
    g. tube insertion

    g. visceral hypersensitivity
    g. volvulus
    g. wash
    g. washing
    g. web
gastricus (*var. of* gastric)
gastrinoma
gastritis
    antral g.
    chronic hypertrophic g.
    infectious g.
    lymphocytic g.
    micronodular g.
    nodular g.
    peptic g.
gastroacephalus
gastroamorphus
gastrocnemius
    g. aponeurosis
    g. contracture
    g. muscle
gastrocnemius-semimembranosus bursa
gastrocolic reflex
Gastrocrom
gastrocystoplasty
gastrodidymus
gastroduodenoscopy
gastroenteritis
    allergic eosinophilic g.
    Campylobacter g.
    eosinophilic g.
    parasitic g.
    rotavirus g.
    Salmonella g.
    viral g.
gastroenterologist
gastroenteropathy
    allergic g.
    eosinophilic g.
gastroepiploic
    g. artery (GEA)
    g. artery graft
gastroesophageal (GE)
    g. angle of His
    g. balloon tamponade
    g. incompetence
    g. junction (GEJ)
    g. reflux (GER)
    g. reflux disease (GERD)
    g. reflux-reflex apnea recording
Gastrografin
    G. enema
    G. esophagram
gastrointestinal (GI)
    g. anaphylaxis
    g. anastomosis (GIA)
    g. anomaly
    g. atresia
    g. autonomic nerve tumor (GANT)

g. decontamination
g. disease
g. disorder
g. duplication
g. dysmotility
g. fistula
g. hemorrhage
g. infection
g. loss
g. malignancy
g. manifestation
g. obstruction
g. paraganglioma
g. polyp
g. priming
g. reflux
g. series
g. syndrome
g. tract
g. tract tumor
g. tube
g. tuberculosis
upper g.
gastrointestinal-associated lymphoid tissue (GALT)
gastrojejunostomy
gastromelus
gastropagus
gastroparesis
gastropathy
AIDS g.
congestive g.
hypertrophic g.
gastrophrenic ligament
gastroplasty
gastroschisis
silastic silo reduction of g.
gastrostomy
g. button
EntriStar Skin Level Tube for g.
feeding g.
percutaneous endoscopic g. (PEG)
Stamm g.
g. tube
g. tube placement
gastrothoracopagus
gastrula
gastrulating embryo
Gas-X
gate-control
g.-c. hypothesis
g.-c. theory
gated blood pool scanning
gate-keeper
gateway drug
Gaucher
G. cell
G. disease (type 1–3)
Gaucher-type histiocyte

gauge
strain g.
gaussian distribution
Gauss sign
gauze
Aquaphor g.
Cover-Roll g.
g. dissection
iodoform g.
Oxycel g.
Vaseline-impregnated g.
g. wick
gavage feeding
Gaviscon
Gaw airway conductance
GAX collagen
gay
g. bowel disease
g., lesbian, bisexual (GLB)
g. relationship
gaze
conjugate upward g.
downward g.
eccentric g.
g. palsy
paralysis of conjugate upward g.
upward g.
gaze-evoked nystagmus
gaze-paretic nystagmus
G-banded
G-b. cytogenetic aberration
G-b. karyotype
G-banding
GBM
glomerular basement membrane
GBS
group B streptococcus
Guillain-Barré syndrome
GBS meningitis
GBS screening culture
GBS (type Ia, Ib, Ic, II, III)
GBS vaccine
GBV-C
GB virus C
GC
gonococcus
gonorrhea culture
GCDAS
Gesell Child Development Age Scale
GCI
gestational carbohydrate intolerance
GC-MS
gas chromatography-mass spectrometry
gas chromatography-mass spectroscopy
GCPS
Greig cephalopolysyndactyly syndrome

G

GCS
    Glasgow coma scale
G-CSF
    granulocyte colony-stimulating factor
G-CSF-R
    granulocyte colony-stimulating factor
      receptor
GCU
    gonococcal urethritis
GD
    gestational diabetes
GDH
    gonadotropic hormone
GDM
    gestational diabetes mellitus
GDNF
    glial cell line derived neurotrophic
      factor
GDS
    Gesell Developmental Scale
    Gordon diagnostic system
GE
    gastroesophageal
    General Electric
    genome equivalent
      GE RT 3200 Advantage II
        ultrasound
      GE Senographe 2000D
      GE Senographe 2000D digital
        mammography system
GEA
    gastroepiploic artery
      GEA graft
Gebauer
      G. ethyl chloride
      G. Pain Ease
Geck
      Davis G.
Gee disease
Gee-Herter disease
Gee-Herter-Heubner disease
Gehrung pessary
GEJ
    gastroesophageal junction
gel
      AccuSite injectable g.
      ACTH g.
      Acthar g.
      Adhibit adhesion prevention g.
      Advantage 24 bioadhesive
        contraceptive g.
      amethocaine g.
      Ametop g.
      Aquagel lubricating g.
      Aquasonic 100 ultrasound
        transmission g.
      ATD g.
      Benzac AC G.
      BenzaClin topical g.

      Benzac W G.
      Cerviprost g.
      cidofovir topical g.
      Comfort personal lubricant g.
      Crinone bioadhesive progesterone g.
      Del Aqua-10 G.
      Del Aqua-5 G.
      Desquam-E G.
      Desquam-X G.
      dextrin sulfate g.
      Differin g.
      dinoprostone cervical g.
      1D sodium dodecyl sulfate g.
      Duac topical g.
      Electro-Gel conductivity g.
      electrophoresis g.
      Fostex 10% BPO G.
      H.P. acthar g.
      Itch-X g.
      keratolytic g.
      MetroGel-Vaginal g.
      metronidazole vaginal g.
      miconazole g.
      Monsel g.
      Multidex g.
      Orabase g.
      Panretin topical g.
      Perfectoderm G.
      povidone-iodine g.
      Prepidil Vaginal G.
      PRO 2000 G.
      PRO/Gel ultrasound transmission g.
      prostaglandin E_2 g.
      Protectaid contraceptive sponge with
        F-5 g.
      Rid g.
      Scan ultrasound g.
      SonoMix ultrasound g.
      Spry Infant tooth g.
      Tisit Blue G.
gelastic
    g. convulsion
    g. seizure
gelatin agglutination test
gelatin-encapsulated microbubble
gelatinosa
    substantia g.
gelatinous
    g. skin
    g. varix
geleophysic
    g. dwarfism
    g. dysplasia
Gelfoam
Gel-Kam
Gellhorn
      G. forceps
      G. rigid pessary
gelling

Gelpi perineal retractor
gel-transfer
gemcitabine
Gemella
    G. bergeriae
    G. haemolysans
    G. morbillorum
    G. sanguinis
gemellary pregnancy
gemellipara
gemellology
gemeprost
geminus
gemistocyte
gemmule
    Hoboken g.
Gemonil
Gemzar
Genac
Genahist Oral
Genapap
Genapax
Genaspor
Genatuss DM
Gen-Clobetasol
gender
    g. assignment
    g. determination
    g. difference
    g. dysphoria syndrome
    g. expression
    g. identity disorder (GID)
    g. reassignment
    g. reversal
    g. role
    g. variance
gene
    g. action
    adhalin g.
    AIRE g.
    allelic g.
    g. amplification
    autoimmune regulator g.
    autosomal g.
    BLNK g.
    breast cancer g. 1 (BRCA1)
    breast cancer g. 2 (BRCA2)
    Bruton/B-cell tyrosine kinase g.
    g. carrier
    cell interaction g.
    chimeric g.
    g. chip
    g. cloning
    codominant g.
    COL7A1 g.
    complementary g.
    g. complex
    CTNS g.
    cumulative g.

CYP21A g.
CYP21B g.
CYP11B1 g.
CYP11B2 g.
cystic fibrosis transmembrane
  conductance regulator g.
DAX1 g.
g. deletion
derepressed g.
DFFRY g.
DMD/BMD g.
dominant g.
g. dose
Drosophila melanogaster diaphanous
  g.
g. duplication
dystrophin g.
E6-E7 g.
endothelin-1 g.
endothelin-2 g.
endothelin-3 g.
endothelin receptor-B g.
Ewing sarcoma g.
g. expression
FAA g.
g. family
g. flow
FMR1 g.
fragile g. (FRA, fra)
fragile X g.
GLUT1 g.
GLUT3 g.
GUSB g.
H g.
herpes simplex virus thymidine
  kinase g.
histocompatibility g.
holandric g.
homeobox 2 g.
homeotic g.'s
housekeeping g.
HOX A g.
HPV E7 g.
human jagged-1 g. (JAG1)
ILS17 g.
ILSX g.
immune response g.
immune suppressor g.
immunoglobulin g.
imprinted g.
Ir g.
Is g.
jumping g.
KAL g.
leaky g.
lethal g.
g. library
g. location
g. locus

G

gene (*continued*)
major capsid protein g.
g. map
g. mapping
marker g.
MOMP g.
g. mosaic
MTHFR g.
mutant g.
g. mutation
NF1 g.
nonstructural g.
od g.
operator g.
p53 g.
partner g.
PAX3 g.
penetrant g.
Pi type g.
Pi type 2 g.
Pi type 22 g.
pleiotropic g.
g. pool
pRb tumor suppressor g.
g. probe
g. product
PTEN g.
PTK g.
p53 tumor suppressor g.
RBM g.
recessive g.
reciprocal g.
recombinase activating g.
  (RAG)
regulator g.
repressed g.
repressor g.
RhCE g.
g. sequencing
sex-conditioned g.
sex-influenced g.
sex-limited g.
sex-linked g.
SGLT1 g.
SHOX g.
silent g.
sodium/glucose co-transporter g.
SOX9 g.
g. splicing
structural g.
g. study
sublethal g.
suicide g.
supplementary g.
suppressor g.
syntenic g.
g. targeting
tdy g.
TGF-beta birth defect g.

g. therapy
g. transcription
g. transfer
transmembrane conductance
  regulator g.
tumor suppression g.
tumor suppressor g.
UBE3A g.
vimentin g.
wild-type g.
Wilms tumor suppression g.
X-linked g.
Y-linked g.
GeneAmp PCR test
Genebs
gene-environment interaction
Genée-Wiedemann
G.-W. acrofacial dysostosis
  (GWAFD)
G.-W. syndrome
Genentech
G. biosynthetic human growth
  hormone
G. growth chart
general
G. Electric (GE)
g. endotracheal anesthesia
g. obstetrics
g. practitioner
g. reading backwardness (GRB)
g. triceps contracture
generalisata
dysostosis g.
osteitis condensans g.
generalization
generalized
g. albinism
g. alopecia
g. aminoaciduria
g. anxiety disorder (GAD)
g. atrophic benign epidermolysis
  bullosa (GABEB)
g. autonomic dysfunction
g. bilaterally synchronous
  sharp-wave and slow-wave
  complexes
g. convulsion
g. dystonia
g. elastolysis
g. epileptogenic discharge
g. erythroderma
g. gangliosidosis GM1 adult type
g. gangliosidosis GM1 type I
g. gangliosidosis juvenile type
g. gray matter atrophy
g. infantile gangliosidosis
g. infantile gangliosidosis with bony
  involvement
g. juvenile gangliosidosis

g. linear interactive modeling (GLIM)
g. lipodystrophy
g. obstructive overinflation
g. phlebectasia
g. pustular psoriasis
g. slowing
g. tetanus
g. tonic-clonic seizure
g. vigilance
g. white matter atrophy

generation
filial g.
free radial g.

generational
generator
migraine g.
Valleylab Force IC electrosurgical g.

genesial cycle
genetic
g. aberration
g. abnormality
g. amniocentesis
g. anomaly
g. bit analysis
g. burden
g. code
g. constitution
g. counseling
g. counselor
g. defect
g. diagnosis
g. disease
g. disorder
g. distance
g. diversity
g. drift
g. engineering
g. engineering technology
g. enzyme defect
g. equilibrium
g. evaluation
g. fine structure
g. heterogeneity
g. history
g. inheritance pattern
g. interference
g. isolated CD59 deficiency
g. karyotyping
g. line
g. linkage
g. linkage analysis
g. locus
g. map
g. marker
g. material
g. model
g. mutation
g. myopathy

g. polymorphism
g. predisposition
g. screening
g. sex
g. study
g. susceptibility
g. switch
g. syndrome
g. test
g. testing
g. therapy
g. thrombophilia
g. variance

geneticist
medical g.

genetics
behavioral g.
biochemical g.
cancer g.
classical g.
epidemiologic g.
galtonian-Fisher g.
human g.
medical g.
modern g.
multilocal g.
prenatal g.
reproductive g.

genetotrophic disease
genetous idiocy
Genex
Geneye Ophthalmic
geniculate
g. herpes
lateral g.

geniculostriate
genioglossus muscle
genital
g. actinomycosis
g. ambiguity
g. anomaly-cardiomyopathy syndrome
g. aphthous ulcer
g. cleft
g. cord
g. corpuscle
g. crisis of newborn
g. development
g. differentiation
g. duct
g. dwarfism
g. elephantiasis
g. herpes
g. infection
g. lesion
g. mucosa
g. mutilation
g. mycoplasma
g. outflow tract
g. papule

G

genital (*continued*)
  g. prolapse
  g. prolapse staging
  g. pruritus
  g. ridge
  g. sensation
  g. skin fibroblast
  g. tract embryology
  g. tract infection (GTI)
  g. tract integrity
  g. tract malignancy
  g. tract obstruction
  g. tract trauma
  g. tract tumor
  g. tubercle
  g. tuberculosis
  g. tumor
  g. ulceration
  g. ulcer disease (GUD)
  g. ulcer syndrome
  g. wart
genitalia
  ambiguous external g.
  external male g.
  indifferent g.
  internal g.
  lymphatic drainage of g.
genitalis
  herpes g.
  herpes simplex g. (HSG)
genitalium
  Mycoplasma g.
genitocrural fold
genitofemoral nerve
genitogram with or without IVP
genitopalatocardiac syndrome
genitoplasty
Genitor mini-intrauterine insemination cannula
genitourinary (GU)
  g. abnormality
  g. atrophy
  g. defect
  g. fistula
  g. sphincter (GUS)
  g. tract
Genoa syndrome
genoblast
genocide
genocopy
genodermatosis
genogram
genome
  g. activation
  g. equivalent (GE)
  g. project
genomic
  g. DNA
  g. imprinting

  g. in situ hybridization
  g. library
genomovar
  Burkholderia cepacia g. (III)
  Burkholderia multivorans g. (II)
  g. (I–VI)
Genoptic S.O.P.
Genora
  G. 1/35 contraceptive
  G. 0.5/35 contraceptive
Genotropin Injection
genotype
  AA g.
  ACE g.
genotypic assay
genotyping
  CYP21 g.
  Kell g.
Genpril
Gen-Probe
  G.-P. amplified CT assay
  G.-P. amplified CT test
Gentacidin
Gent-AK
gentamicin
  g. cream
  enteric g.
  prednisolone and g.
  g. sulfate
gentian violet
GentleLASE Plus
Gentran
Gentrasul
genu, *pl.* **genua**
  g. recurvatum
  g. valgum
  g. varum
  g. varum deformity
genua (*pl. of* genu)
genucubital position
genuine stress incontinence (GSI)
genupectoral position
genus-specific monoclonal antibody
Gen-XENE
Geocillin
geographic tongue
geohelminth
geometric
  g. design test
  g. mean titer (GMT)
Geopen
geophagia, geophagism, geophagy
geophagism (*var. of* geophagia)
geophagy (*var. of* geophagia)
georgiae
  Actinomyces g.
geotaxis
GER
  gastroesophageal reflux

Gerald forceps
Gerbode defect
GERD
    gastroesophageal reflux disease
Gerdy fontanelle
Geref
gerencseriae
    Actinomyces g.
Gerhardt syndrome
Gerimed
germ
    g. cell
    g. cell mosaicism
    g. cell neoplasm
    g. cell ovarian neoplasm
    g. cell teratoma
    g. cell testicular tumor
    g. layer
    g. line
    g. line mosaicism
    g. ridge
    g. tube test
German
    G. lock
    G. measles
    G. syndrome
germ-cell depletion
germinal
    g. cell tumor
    g. center
    g. epithelium
    g. epithelium of Waldeyer
    g. inclusion cyst
    g. matrix
    g. matrix hemorrhage (grade 1–4)
    g. membrane
    g. pole
    g. vesicle (GV)
    g. vesicle breakdown (GVBD)
    g. vesicle stage
    g. zone
germinolysis
    subependymal g.
germinoma
    pineal g.
germ-line mutation
germplasm
Gerota fascia
Gerstmann-Sträussler-Scheinker syndrome
Gerstmann syndrome
Gesco
    G. cannula
    G. catheter
Gesell
    G. Adaptive and Personal Behavior Domain, Revised
    G. Child Development Age Scale (GCDAS)
    G. Developmental Model

    G. Developmental Scale (GDS)
    G. Developmental Schedules (GDS)
    G. Developmental Schedules, Revised
    G. figure
    G. Gross Motor Domain, Revised
    G. Infant Scale
    G. Preschool Test
    G. School Readiness Test
    G. test with Knobloch modification
gestagen
gestagenic
Gestalt closure
gestation
    anembryonic g.
    cornual g.
    higher-order g.
    monochorionic g.
    monochorionic-diamniotic g.
    multifetal g.
    multiple g.
    prolonged g.
    stuck twin g.
    term g.
    tubal g.
    twin g.
    unruptured tubal g.
    vascular anastomoses in multifetal g.
gestation-adjusted age
gestational
    g. abnormality
    g. age (GA)
    g. age assessment
    g. age estimation
    g. asthma
    g. carbohydrate intolerance (GCI)
    g. carrier
    g. chickenpox
    g. diabetes (GD)
    g. diabetes mellitus (GDM)
    g. edema
    g. growth
    g. hypertension
    g. lupus
    g. mother
    g. proteinuria
    g. psychosis
    g. ring
    g. sac (GS)
    g. sac mean diameter
    g. sac size (GSS)
    g. surrogacy
    g. surrogate
    g. thrombocytopenia
    g. thyrotoxicosis
    g. trophoblastic disease (GTD)
    g. trophoblastic neoplasia (GTN)
    g. trophoblastic tumor (GTT)

G

gestationis
  herpes g. (HG)
  hydroa g.
  pemphigoid g.
  prurigo g.
gestation-specific nomogram
Gesterol
Gestiva
Gestodene
gestogen
gestosis
  second-trimester acute g.
Gestrinone
gesturing
GF
  growth factor
GFAP
  glial fibrillary acidic protein
GFD
  gluten-free diet
GFR
  glomerular filtration rate
GG
  gamma globulin
  Lactobacillus rhamnosus strain G.
  (L-GG)
GGT
  gamma glutamyl transferase
GH
  growth hormone
    GH deficiency
GHBP
  growth hormone-binding protein
GHD
  growth hormone deficiency
GHI
  growth hormone insensitivity
Ghon
  G. complex
  G. tubercle
ghost
  peroxisomal g.
  g. vessel
  g. vessel fundus
GHR
  growth hormone receptor
GHRD
  growth hormone receptor deficiency
GH-RH
  growth hormone-releasing hormone
GHST
  growth hormone stimulation test
GI
  gastrointestinal
    GI bleeding
    GI cocktail
    GI tract venous malformation
GIA
  gastrointestinal anastomosis

GIA 30
GIA 60 stapler
GIA 80 stapler
Gianotti-Crosti syndrome
Gianotti disease
giant
  g. anorectal condyloma acuminatum
  g. axonal neuropathy
  g. baby
  g. cell
  g. cell arteritis
  g. cell chondrodysplasia
  g. cell encephalitis
  g. cell hepatitis
  g. cell myocarditis
  g. cell pneumonia
  g. chromosome
  g. colon
  g. congenital pigmented nevus
  g. coronary artery aneurysm
  g. fibroadenoma
  g. hemangioma
  g. metamyelocyte
  g. neuroaxonal dystrophy
  g. platelet alpha-granule
  g. platelet granulation
  g. platelet syndrome
giantism (*var. of* gigantism)
Gianturco coil
Gianturco-Grifka vascular occlusion device
Giardia lamblia
giardiasis
gibbous deformity
gibbus
  lumbar g.
  thoracolumbar g.
Gibco BRL sperm preparation medium
Gibson-Coke method
Gibson murmur
GID
  gender identity disorder
giddiness
Giemsa
  G. banding
  G. stain
Gierke disease
GIFT
  gamete intrafallopian transfer
  granulocyte immunofluorescence test
    cervical GIFT
    intrauterine GIFT
    vaginal GIFT
gigantism, giantism
  cerebral g.
  eunuchoid g.
  exomphalos, macroglossia, g. (EMG)
  fetal g.
  hyperpituitary g.

pituitary g.
Sotos cerebral g.
gigantoblast
gigantocellularis
nucleus reticularis g.
gigantomastia
giggle incontinence
Gigli
G. operation
G. saw
Gilbert
G. disease
G. syndrome
Gilbert-Dreyfus syndrome
Gilbert-Lereboullet syndrome
gill
g. arch skeleton
G. respirator
Gilles
G. de la Tourette
G. de la Tourette syndrome
Gillespie-Numerof Burnout Inventory
Gillespie syndrome
Gillette joint
Gilliam
G. operation
G. round ligament
Gilliam-Doleris
G.-D. operation
G.-D. uterine suspension
Gilmore Oral Reading Test (GORT)
Gimbernat reflex ligament
gingiva, *pl.* **gingivae**
gingivae (*pl. of* gingiva)
gingival
g. cyst
g. cyst of newborn
g. disease
g. erythema
g. fibromatosis
g. fibromatosis-corneal dystrophy
g. hyperplasia
g. hypertrophy-corneal dystrophy
syndrome
g. lesion
g. overgrowth
gingivalis
Bacteroides g.
Entamoeba g.
Porphyromanus g.
gingivitis
acute necrotizing ulcerative g.
(ANUG)
fusospirochetal g.
herpetic g.
necrotizing g.
necrotizing ulcerating g. (NUG)
pregnancy-associated g.
Vincent g.

gingivostomatitis
herpetic g.
primary herpetic g.
Ginkgo biloba
ginseng
Giordano suburethral sling operation
GIP
gastric inhibitory polypeptide
girdle
Hitzig g.
limb g. (LG)
g. weakness
girl
premenarchal g.
g.'s, Ritalin LA, and ADHD
(GRACE)
girth
abdominal g.
gitalin
Gitelman
G. disease
G. syndrome
Gittes
G. bladder suspension technique
G. endoscopic bladder neck
suspension
G. endoscopic bladder neck
suspension procedure
G. urethral suspension
GK
glycerol kinase
GKD
glycerol kinase deficiency
glabella
glabellar response
glabrata
Candida g.
Torulopsis g.
gladiatorum
herpes g.
tinea g.
gladioli
Burkholderia g.
gland
accessory sex g.
adrenal g.
apocrine sweat g.
Bartholin g.
Brunner g.
bulbourethral g.
BUS g.'s
Cowper g.
g. duct
g. duct opening
Duverney g.
eccrine sweat g.
endocrine g.
external genitalia/Bartholin, urethral,
and Skene g.'s (EG/BUS)

G

gland (*continued*)
  fetal adrenal g.
  greater vestibular g.
  holocrine sebaceous g.
  hypoplastic parathyroid g.
  g. infection
  Krause lacrimal accessory g.
  lacrimal g.
  late-onset congenital large
   ectopic g.
  Littré g.
  mammary g.
  meibomian g.
  Méry g.
  Moll g.
  Montgomery g.
  Naboth g.
  nabothian g.
  parathyroid g.
  paraurethral g.
  parotid g.
  periurethral g.
  Philip g.
  pilosebaceous g.
  pineal g.
  pituitary g.
  salivary g.
  sebaceous g.
  Skene g.
  sublingual g.
  submaxillary g.
  sweat g.
  thymus g.
  thyroid g.
  urethral g.
  uterine g.
  vestibular g.
  Wolfring lacrimal accessory g.
  Zeis g.
glanders
glandes (*pl. of* glans)
glandular
  g. atypia
  g. atypia lesion
  g. cell
  g. disc
  g. disease
  g. fever
  g. hyperplasia
  g. mastitis
  g. neoplasia
  g. tissue
  g. tularemia
glandularis
  cystitis g.
glans, *pl.* **glandes**
  g. clitoris
  g. penis
  g. proper

glans-cavernosal procedure
glanular
  g. hypospadias
  g. urethral meatus
glanuloplasty
  meatal advancement and g.
  urethral advancement and g.
Glanzmann
  G. disease
  G. syndrome
  G. thrombasthenia
Glanzmann-Riniker syndrome
Glasgow
  G. coma scale (GCS)
  G. Meningococcal Septicemia
   Score
glass factor
Glassman forceps
glass-wool filtration
glassy cell carcinoma
glatiramer acetate
glaucoma
  acute angle closure g.
  congenital g.
  infantile g.
  primary congenital g.
  traumatic g.
Glazer method
Glazunov tumor
GLB
  gay, lesbian, bisexual
  GLB youths
GLB-1
  beta-galactosidase-1
gleet
gleety discharge
Glen Anderson ureteroneocystostomy
Glenárd disease
Glenn
  G. anastomosis
  G. operation
  G. shunt
Glenn-Anderson ureteric reflux repair
  technique
glenohumeral
  g. instability
  g. joint
glenoid dysplasia
glia
gliadin
glial
  g. cell line derived neurotrophic
   factor (GDNF)
  g. fibrillary acidic protein
   (GFAP)
glide consonant
gliding movement
gli family zinc-finger transcriptional
  activators

GLIM
generalized linear interactive modeling
glimepiride
glioblastoma multiforme
glioependymal cyst
glioma
brainstem g.
cervicomedullary brainstem g.
chiasmal g.
chiasmatic-hypothalamic g.
cystic brainstem g.
focal brainstem g.
g. of optic nerve
optic nerve g.
optic pathway g.
pontile g.
spinal cord g.
tectal brainstem g.
gliomatosis peritonei
gliosis
aqueductal g.
astrocytic g.
compensatory g.
fibrillary g.
g. uteri
gliotic
g. reaction
g. tuft
glipizide
Glisson capsule
glistening dot
global
g. aphasia
g. assessment of function
(GAF)
g. brain hypoxia
g. brain swelling
g. developmental delay
g. glomerulosclerosis
g. hypertonia
g. hypoplasia
g. level of functioning (GLOF)
g. neurologic dysfunction
g. seasonality score
G. Severity Index of Brief
Symptom Inventory (GSI-BSI)
globe
g. cell anemia
ruptured g.
globi (*pl. of* globus)
globiformis
Arthrobacter g.
globin chain
globoid
g. body sclerosis
g. cell cerebral sclerosis
g. cell leukodystrophy
globoside
globozoospermia

globule
milk fat g. (MFG)
globulin
antilymphocyte g.
anti-Rh gamma g.
anti-Rho(D) g.
antithymocyte g.
corticosteroid-binding g. (CBG)
cortisol-binding g.
gamma g. (GG)
hepatitis B immune g. (HBIG,
H-BIG)
hyperimmune serum g.
immune g.
immune serum g. (ISG)
intravenous gamma g. (IVGG)
pregnancy-associated g.
purified gamma g.
sex hormone-binding g. (SHBG)
testosterone-estrogen-binding g.
thyroid-binding g. (TBG, TGB)
thyroxine-binding g. (TBG)
varicella-zoster immune g. (VZIG)
zoster immune g. (ZIG)
globus, *pl.* **globi**
g. hystericus
g. pallidus
GLOF
global level of functioning
glomerular, glomerulose
g. basement membrane (GBM)
g. basement membrane antigen
g. capillary endotheliosis
g. change
g. disorder
g. endotheliosis
g. filtrate
g. filtration
g. filtration rate (GFR)
g. insufficiency
g. proteinuria
g. renal disease
g. sclerosis (GS)
g. sialoglycoprotein
g. tuft
glomerulation
glomeruli (*pl. of* glomerulus)
glomerulocystic disease
glomerulonephritides (*pl. of*
glomerulonephritis)
glomerulonephritis, *pl.*
glomerulonephritides
acute g.
acute postinfectious g. (APGN)
acute poststreptococcal g. (APSGN)
acute progressive g.
autoimmune g.
chronic g.
crescentic g.

G

glomerulonephritis (*continued*)
    diffuse proliferative g.
    familial g.
    focal segmental lupus g.
    focal segmental proliferative g.
    hemorrhagic cystitis g.
    hypocomplementemic g.
    idiopathic rapidly progressive g.
    immune complex-mediated g.
    membranoproliferative g. (MPGN)
    membranous g.
    mesangial proliferative g.
    mesangiocapillary g. (type I, II)
     (MPGN)
    necrotizing g.
    pauciimmune g.
    postinfectious g.
    poststreptococcal g.
    proliferative g.
    rapidly progressive g.
glomerulopathy
glomerulosa
    zona g.
glomerulosclerosis
    focal g.
    focal segmental g. (FSG, FSGS)
    global g.
glomerulose (*var. of* glomerular)
glomerulotubular
glomerulus, *pl.* **glomeruli**
glomus tumor
GLORIA
    gold-labeled optical rapid
    immunoassay
glossa
glossitis
    benign migratory g.
    candidal g.
glossodynia
glossopalatine ankylosis syndrome
glossopharyngeal nerve
glossoptosia (*var. of* glossoptosis)
glossoptosis, glossoptosia
glottal
    g. fricative
    g. obstruction
glottic
    g. opening
    g. spasm
glottides (*pl. of* glottis)
glottidospasm (*var. of* laryngospasm)
glottis, *pl.* **glottides**
glove
    g.'s and socks syndrome
    Biogel Reveal g.
    Eudermic surgical g.
    latex g.
    Mylar g.
    Neolon surgical g.

    powder-free g.
    SensiCare surgical g.
    sheepskin g.
gloving
    double g.
glubionate
    calcium g.
glucagon
Glucamide
Glucerna formula
glucoamylase deficiency
glucocerebrosidase
    macrophage-targeted g.
glucocorticoid
    g. deficiency
    g. excess
    g. insufficiency
glucocorticosteroid therapy
glucogenesis
glucoglycinuria
glucokinase
Glucola screen
Glucolet Endcaps
glucometer
    Accu-Chek II g.
    G. Elite diabetes care system
    Glucostat II g.
    G. II
gluconate
    calcium g.
    chlorhexidine g.
    ferrous g.
    potassium g.
    quinidine g.
gluconeogenesis
    hepatic g.
Glucophage
glucosamine
glucosamine-6-sulfate deficiency
glucose
    blood g. (bG)
    casual plasma g.
    g. challenge test
    g. concentration
    g. excretion
    fasting plasma g. (FPG)
    fetal blood g.
    g. formula
    hypertonic g.
    g. intolerance
    g. meter
    g. monitoring
    g. oxidase test tape
    plasma g.
    g. plus insulin
    postprandial g.
    g. production rate (GPR)
    g. reagent stick
    serum g.

g. tolerance
g. tolerance test (GTT)
g. transporter (GLUT)
urinary g.
glucose-dependent insulinotropic peptide
glucose-galactose
    g.-g. intolerance
    g.-g. malabsorption
glucose-intolerant gravida
glucose-6-phosphate dehydrogenase (G6PD)
glucosiduronate
Glucostat II glucometer
Glucostix
glucosuria of pregnancy
Glucotrol
glucuronate pregnanediol
glucuronidation
glucuronide, glucuronoside
    3 alpha-androstanediol g.
    androsterone g.
    isovaleryl g.
    virilizing 3 alpha-androstanediol g.
glucuronoside (*var. of* glucuronide)
glucuronosyltransferase
glucuronyl
    g. transferase
    g. transferase deficiency
    g. transferase inactivity
glue
    airplane g.
    g. ear
glue-sniffing neuropathy
GLUT
    glucose transporter
glutamate
    arginine g.
    g. cycle
    g. formiminotransferase deficiency
glutamic
    g. acid
    g. acid decarboxylase (GAD)
    g. acid decarboxylase antibody
glutamic-oxalacetic
glutamic-pyruvic transaminase
glutamine
glutamine-supplemented diet
glutamyltransferase
glutamyl transpeptidase (GTP)
glutaraldehyde crosslinked collagen injection
glutaric
    g. acidemia (type I, II)
    g. aciduria syndrome (type I, II)
    g. aciduria (type I, II)
glutathione (GSH)
    g. peroxidase
    g. S-transferase

g. S-transferase isoform
g. synthetase deficiency
glutathionemia
gluteal
    g. fold
    g. free flap
    g. lymph node
    g. muscle
    g. trauma
gluten
    g. allergy
    g. challenge
    g. enteropathy
    g. intolerance
    g. sensitivity
gluten-free diet (GFD)
gluten-induced enteropathy
gluten-sensitive enteropathy
glutethimide
gluteus
    g. maximus muscle
    g. medius limp
    g. medius muscle
    g. minimus muscle
GLUT1 gene
GLUT3 gene
glyburide
glycemia
glycemic
    g. control
    g. index
    g. index diet
glycerin
    g., lanolin and peanut oil
    g. suppository
glycerol, glycerin
    iodinated g.
    g. kinase (GK)
    g. kinase deficiency (GKD)
glycerophospholipid
glycerophosphorylcholine
glyceryl
    g. guaiacolate
    g. trinitrate (GTN)
glycine
    blood g.
    CSF g.
    g. distention medium
glycinuria
    familial g.
glycocalyx
glycocorticoid
glycodelin-A
glycogen
    g. accumulation
    g. storage disease (type Ia–Id, II–VII)
    g. storage disorder
    g. synthetase deficiency

G

glycogenesis
  hepatic g.
  g. (type I, II)
glycogenosis
  type 7 g.
  von Gierke g.
glycohemoglobin
glycol
  Diprolene G.
  ethylene g.
  polyethylene g.
  propylene g.
glycol-ADA
  polyethylene g.-ADA
glycolic
  Aqua G.
glycolipid metabolism
glycolysis
  anaerobic g.
**glycopeptide-resistant enterococcus
  (GRE)**
glycophorin C
glycoprotein
  carbohydrate deficient g. (CDG)
  g. degradation
  heterodimeric integral
    membrane g.
  g. hormone
  KL-6 mucinous g.
glycoproteinosis
glycoprotein-producing tumor
Glycopyrrol
glycopyrrolate
glycorrhachia
glycosaminoglycan (GAG)
  g. layer
  urinary g.
glycoside
  cardiac g.
glycosphingolipid
glycosuria
  renal g.
glycosuric diuresis
glycosylated hemoglobin (HgA1c)
glycosylation
Glylorin
Gly-Oxide Oral
Glyset
Glytuss
GM
  grand multiparity
GM-CSF
  granulocyte-macrophage
    colony-stimulating factor
GMDS
  Griffith Mental Developmental
    Scale
GM2 gangliosidosis
GM3 gangliosidosis

GMS
  goniodysgenesis, mental retardation,
    short stature
    GMS syndrome
GMT
  geometric mean titer
gnashing
gnathocephalus
Gnathostoma spinigerum
gnathostomiasis
GNR
  gram-negative rod
GnRH
  gonadotropin-releasing hormone
    GnRH agonist (GNRHa)
    GnRH deficiency
GNRHa
  gonadotropin-releasing hormone agonist
  gonadotropin-releasing hormone analog
GnRH-facilitated
  GnRH-f. FSH release
  GnRH-f. LH release
GnRH-independent sexual precocity
goal
  annual g.
goat's
  g. milk formula
  g. rue
**Goebell-Frangenheim-Stoeckel
  urethrovesical suspension technique**
Goebell procedure
Goebell-Stoeckel-Frangenheim procedure
Go-Evac
Goffe colporrhaphy
goiter
  g. development
  drug-induced neonatal g.
  fetal g.
  simple colloid g.
goiter-deafness syndrome
goitrogen ingestion
goitrous
  g. hypothyroidism
  g. hypothyroidism with deafness
Golabi-Ito-Hall syndrome
Golabi-Rosen syndrome (GRS)
gold (Au)
  radioactive g. (^{198}Au)
  g. salt
  g. seed
  g. sodium thiomalate
  g. therapy
gold-198 (^{198}Au)
Goldberg syndrome
Goldenhar
  G. hemifacial microsomia
  G. microphthalmia syndrome
  G. oculauricular vertebral dysplasia
  G. sequence

Goldenhar-Gorlin syndrome
Golden sign of S
Goldie-Coldman hypothesis
gold-labeled optical rapid immunoassay
  (GLORIA)
Goldmann perimeter visual field test
Goldstein disease
Goldston syndrome
Golgi
  G. apparatus
  G. body
  G. stain
Gollop-Wolfgang complex
Goltz
  G. focal dermal hypoplasia
  G. syndrome
Goltz-Gorlin syndrome
Goltz-Peterson-Gorlin-Ravitz syndrome
GoLYTELY
GOMBO
  growth retardation, ocular
    abnormalities, microcephaly,
    brachydactyly, oligophrenia
    GOMBO syndrome
Gomco
  G. bell
  G. circumcision clamp
  G. circumcision technique
Gomez and López-Hernández syndrome
Gomori
  G. methenamine-silver stain
  G. trichrome reaction
  G. trichrome stain
gompertzian growth
gonad
  dysgenetic g.
  indifferent g.
  maternal g.
  palpable g.
  streak g.
  undifferentiated g.
gonadal
  g. agenesis
  g. agenesis syndrome
  g. aplasia
  g. axis
  g. differentiation
  g. dysfunction
  g. dysgenesis
  g. dysgenesis syndrome
  g. dysplasia
  g. failure
  g. failure, short stature, mitral valve
    prolapse, mental retardation
    syndrome
  g. germ cell neoplasm
  g. hormone treatment
  g. mosaicism
  g. ridge

g. sex
g. steroid
g. steroid suppression
g. streak
g. stroma
g. stromal cell tumor
g. stromal ovarian tumor
gonadarche
gonadectomy
gonadoblastoma
  ovarian g.
gonadocrinin
gonadoliberin
gonadorelin acetate
gonadostat
gonadotoxin
gonadotrope
gonadotropic
  g. deficiency
  g. hormone (GDH, GTH)
gonadotropin
  g. agonist stimulation test (GAST)
  beta-human chorionic g. (beta-hCG,
    beta-HCG)
  chorionic g. (CG, CGT)
  chorionic human recombinant g.
  endogenous g.
  exogenous g.
  human chorionic g. (HCG, hCG)
  human menopausal g. (hMG)
  g. level
  nicked human chorionic g.
  g. ovulation induction
  pituitary g.
  pulsatile human menopausal g.
  g. regimen
  g. regulation
  g. secretion
  g. secretion inhibitor
  g. surge
  urinary chorionic g. (UCG)
  urinary menopausal g.
gonadotropin-dependent precocious
  puberty
gonadotropin-independent precocious
  puberty
gonadotropin-induced ovarian
  hyperstimulation
gonadotropin-releasing
  g.-r. factor (GnRH, GRF)
  g.-r. hormone (GnRH, GRH)
  g.-r. hormone agonist (GnRHa)
  g.-r. hormone analog (GnRHa)
  g.-r. hormone antagonist
  g.-r. hormone-associated peptide (GAP)
  g.-r. hormonelike protein
gonadotropin-resistant
  g.-r. ovary syndrome
  g.-r. testis

G

Gonal-f
gonane
gondii
    Toxoplasma g.
gonidiaformans
    Fusobacterium g.
goniodysgenesis
    g., mental retardation, short stature (GMS)
    g., mental retardation, short stature syndrome
goniometer
goniometry
gonioscopy
gonoblennorrhea
gonococcal (GC)
    g. arthritis
    g. arthritis of newborn
    g. blindness
    g. conjunctivitis
    g. infection
    g. ophthalmia
    g. ophthalmia neonatorum
    g. perihepatitis
    g. septicemia
    g. urethritis (GCU)
gonococcus (GC)
    penicillinase-producing g.
gonorrhea
    g. culture (GC)
    disseminated g.
    Neisseria g.
    pharyngeal g.
gonorrheal
    g. cervicitis
    g. ophthalmia
    g. salpingitis
gonorrhoica
    macula g.
Gonozyme test
Gonzales blood group
Goodell
    G. dilator
    G. sign
Goodenough-Harris Drawing Test
Goodman syndrome
Goodpasture syndrome
Good Start formula
gooseflesh
goose neck
gooseneck, goose neck
    g. deformity
    g. deformity of left ventricular outflow tract
Gordofilm liquid
Gordon
    G. diagnostic system (GDS)
    G. Distractibility Test

    G. reflex
    G. syndrome
Gore-Tex
    G.-T. Soft Tissue Patch
    G.-T. surgical membrane
Gorlin
    G. formula
    G. syndrome (1, 2)
Gorlin-Goltz syndrome
Gorlin-Psaume syndrome
GORT
    Gilmore Oral Reading Test
    Gray Oral Reading Test
GORT-R
    Gray Oral Reading Test-Revised
GOS
    Great Ormond Street
        GOS criteria
goserelin
    g. acetate
    g. acetate implant
gossypiboma
gossypol acetic acid (GAA)
Gott malleable retractor
Gottron
    G. papule
    G. sign
Gougerot-Carteaud syndrome
gout
    familial juvenile g.
gouty
    g. arthritis
    g. diathesis
Gower-1
    hemoglobin G.-1
Gower-2
    hemoglobin G.-2
Gowers
    G. maneuver
    G. sign
gown
    barrier g.
    Exami-Gown g.
gp41
    transmembrane glycoprotein gp41
G6PD
    glucose-6-phosphate dehydrogenase
GPMAL
    gravida, para, multiple births, abortions, live births
GPR
    glucose production rate
G-protein-coupled receptor
graafian
    g. follicle
    g. vesicle
GRACE
    girls, Ritalin LA, and ADHD
gracile bone dysplasia

gracilis
- *Campylobacter* g.
- g. flap neovagina
- g. flap technique
- g. muscle

graciloplasty
- dynamic g.

grade
- placental g.
- Roenigk g.

graded
- g. challenge
- g. compression ultrasonography

Gradenigo syndrome

gradient
- A-a g.
- albumin g.
- alveolar-arterial oxygen g.
- alveolar-arterial pressure g.
- arterial-ascitic fluid pH g.
- blood pressure g.
- density g.
- diastolic g.
- echo Doppler g.
- hepatic venous wedge pressure g.
- peak instantaneous g.
- pressure g.
- g. recalled acquisition in the steady state (GRASS)
- g. refocused acquisition in steady state (GRASS)
- sucrose g.
- transtubular potassium concentration g. (TTKG)
- tympanometric g.

grading
- histopathological g.
- Papile g.
- placental g.
- tumor g.

Graefenberg
- G. ring
- G. spot (G-spot)

Graefe-Usher syndrome

Grafco breast pump

graft
- allogenic fetal g.
- bilateral myocutaneous g.
- bone g.
- buccal mucosa g.
- donor venous g.
- full-thickness skin g.
- gastroepiploic artery g. (GEA graft)
- GEA g.
- heterologous g.
- HLA-identical marrow g.
- isogeneic g.
- Martius labial fat-pad g.
- oral mucous membrane g.
- polytetrafluoroethylene g.
- Prolift g.
- sacrocolpopexy g.
- seromuscular intestinal patch g.
- skin g.
- split-thickness g.
- T-cell-depleted g.
- g. versus host disease (GVHD)
- g. versus leukemia (GVL)
- Xenform g.

Graham
- G. Steell murmur
- G. syndrome

Graham-Rosenblith scale

gram (g)
- G. stain

grammar

gram-negative
- g.-n. acne
- g.-n. bacillus
- g.-n. bacteria
- g.-n. cocci
- g.-n. endotoxic shock
- g.-n. endotoxin
- g.-n. endotoxin-induced shock
- g.-n. organism
- g.-n. pneumonia
- g.-n. rod (GNR)
- g.-n. ventriculitis

gram-positive
- g.-p. bacillus
- g.-p. bacteria
- g.-p. cocci
- g.-p. diplococcus
- g.-p. organism
- g.-p. rod

Gram-Weigert stain

grand
- g. climacteric
- g. mal
- g. mal attack
- g. mal epilepsy
- g. mal seizure
- g. multipara
- g. multiparity (GM)
- g. pregnancy

granddad syndrome

grandiose delusion

grandiosity

grandmother theory

grandmultipara

grandmultiparity

GraNee needle

Granger sign

granisetron

granny knot

G

Grantley
    G. Dick-Read method
    G. Dick-Read method of childbirth
Grant syndrome
Grant-Ward head and neck operation
granular
    g. cell myoblastoma
    g. ependymitis
    g. lung
    g. osmiophilic deposit
    g. urethritis
granulation
    arachnoid g.
    giant platelet g.
    pacchionian g.
    g. tissue
granule
    argyrophilic g.
    Birbeck g.
    Butschli g.
    cortical g.
    g. deficiency
    E.E.S. g's
    Fordyce g.
    Langerhans g.
    large lysosome-like g.
    metachromatic cytoplasmic g.
    Nissl g.
    Reilly g.
    sulfur g.
granulocyte
    g. colony-stimulating factor (G-CSF)
    g. colony-stimulating factor receptor (G-CSF-R)
    g. count
    cytokine g.
    g. immunofluorescence test (GIFT)
    g. transfusion
granulocyte-macrophage colony-stimulating factor (GM-CSF)
granulocytic
    g. ehrlichiosis
    g. leukemia
    g. leukocytosis
    g. sarcoma
granulocytopenia
    congenital g.
granulocytopoiesis
granuloma, *pl.* **granulomata**
    g. annulare
    cholesterol g.
    coccidioidal g.
    disseminated g.
    eosinophilic g.
    fish-tank g.
    g. gluteal infantum
    g. gravidarum
    g. inguinale
    Langhans giant cell g.

    Majocchi g.
    mediastinal g.
    noncaseating sarcoidlike g.
    palisading g.
    progressive g.
    pyogenic g.
    rheumatoid g.
    sperm g.
    swimming pool g.
    telangiectatic g.
    umbilical g.
granulomata (*pl. of* granuloma)
granulomatis
    Calymmatobacterium g.
granulomatosis
    g. infantiseptica
    juvenile systemic g.
    larval g.
    Wegener g. (WG)
granulomatous
    g. amebic meningoencephalitis
    g. angiitis
    g. calcification
    g. colitis
    g. disease
    g. infection
    g. lymphadenitis
    g. mastitis
    g. myocarditis
    g. perivasculitis
    g. salpingitis
    g. vasculitis
granuloplasty
granulopoiesis
    neutrophil g.
granulosa
    g. cell tumor
    g. lutein cell
    membrana g.
    membrane g.
granulosa-stromal cell tumor
granulosa-theca cell tumor
granulosus
    Echinococcus g.
grape mole
graphanesthesia (*var. of* graphesthesia)
graphesthesia, graphanesthesia
grasp
    finger g.
    inferior pincer g.
    neat pincer g.
    palmar g.
    pincer g.
    plantar g.
    radial digital g.
    radial palmar g.
    g. reflex
    toe g.
    ulnar palmar g.

grasper
    Lion's Claw g.
    MetraGrasp ligament g.
    Polaris reusable g.
grasping
    fetal g.
grass
    perennial rye g.
    g. pollen
    timothy g.
GRASS
    gradient recalled acquisition in the steady state
    gradient refocused acquisition in steady state
    GRASS MRI
    GRASS MRI technique
Grater sciatic foramen
grating sound
Graves
    avascular space of G.
    G. bivalve speculum
    G. disease
gravida (G)
    glucose-intolerant g.
    gravida, para, multiple births, abortions, live births (GPMAL)
gravidae
    hydrorrhea g.
gravidarum
    chorea g.
    epulis g.
    fibroma molle g.
    granuloma g.
    hydrops g.
    hydrorrhea g.
    hyperemesis g.
    melasma g.
    molluscum fibrosum g.
    nausea g.
    nephritis g.
    pruritus g.
    striae g.
    tetania g.
gravidic
    g. retinitis
    g. retinopathy
gravidism
graviditas
    g. examnialis
    g. exochorialis
gravidity
gravid uterus
Gravindex test
gravis
    autoimmune myasthenia g.
    congenital myasthenia g.
    icterus g.

    myasthenia g.
    neonatal myasthenia g.
    transient neonatal myasthenia g.
    g. type Ehlers-Danlos syndrome
Gravlee jet washer
Gravol
gray (Gy)
    g. baby
    g. baby syndrome
    g. matter
    g. matter heterotopia
    G. Oral Reading Test (GORT)
    G. Oral Reading Test-Revised (GORT-R)
    g. platelet syndrome
    g. scale
gray-scale
    g.-s. imaging
    g.-s. ultrasonography
gray-white junction
GRB
    general reading backwardness
GRE
    glycopeptide-resistant enterococcus
greasy stool
great
    g. arteries
    G. Ormond Street (GOS)
    G. Smoky Mountains Study of Youth (GSMS)
    g. toe
    g. vessel
    g. vessel of thorax
greater
    g. saphenous vein
    g. saphenous vein cutdown
    g. trochanter
    g. trochanteric bursa
    g. vestibular gland
    g. vestibular gland duct
great-grand multipara
Grebe
    G. chondrodysplasia
    G. dysplasia
green
    g. clay
    G. climacteric scale
    indocyanine g.
    g. light
    G. uterine curette
Greenfield
    G. disease
    G. filter
greenstick
    g. fracture
    g. injury
greeting spasm

G

Greig
> G. cephalopolysyndactyly anomaly
> G. cephalopolysyndactyly syndrome (GCPS)
> G. syndrome

grepafloxacin
Greulich
> G. and Pyle bone age
> G. and Pyle radiographic atlas

Greven forceps
Grey Turner sign
GRF
> gonadotropin-releasing factor

GRH
> gonadotropin-releasing hormone
> GRH antagonist

grid
> Self-Injury G. (SIG)

gridiron incision
grief
> anticipatory g.
> perinatal g.

grieving process
Griffith
> G. General Quotient
> G. Mental Developmental Scale (GMDS)
> G. Scale of Mental Development

Grifulvin V
grimace
grimacing
Grimelius stain
grip, grippe
> milkmaid's g.
> g. myotonia

grippe (*var. of* grip)
grippotyphosa
> *Leptospira* g.

Grisactin
Griscelli syndrome
Grisel syndrome
griseofulvin microcrystalline
griseum
> indusium g.

griseus
> *Streptomyces* g.

Grisolle sign
Grisovin
Gris-PEG
groin
> g. dissection
> g. hernia
> g. ringworm

grommet
groove
> Blessig g.
> Harrison g.
> intercondylar g.

intersphincteric g.
neural g.
primitive g.
g. sign
transverse nail g.
vomerian g.

grooved pegboard
Groshong catheter
gross
> g. development
> g. motor
> g. motor development
> g. motor domain
> g. motor function measure
> g. motor index
> g. motor milestone
> g. motor skill
> g. motor total DMQ

grossly bloody stool
grotesque features
ground-glass
> g.-g. appearance
> g.-g. cytoplasm
> g.-g. osteopenia
> g.-g. pattern

ground itch
group
> g. A beta-hemolytic streptococcal infection
> g. A beta-hemolytic streptococcus (GABHS)
> Adhesion Scoring G. (ASG)
> AIDS Clinical Trials G.
> antepartum support g.
> g. A streptococcal (GAS)
> g. A streptococcal impetigo
> g. A streptococcus
> g. B beta-hemolytic streptococcus
> blood g.
> g. B streptococcal infection
> g. B streptococcal pneumonia
> g. B streptococcal sepsis
> g. B streptococcus (GBS)
> g. B streptococcus disease
> Cartwright blood g.
> g. C autosome
> Children's Cancer G. (CCG)
> Children's Cancer Study G. (CCSG)
> Cochrane Incontinence G.
> Collaborative Antiviral Study G. (CASG)
> g. C pharyngitis
> g. C streptococcus
> determinant g.
> g. D streptococcus
> Gonzales blood g.
> g. G streptococcus
> HACEK g.

Kidd blood g.
Lewis blood g.
linkage g.
Lucarelli bone marrow transplant
  risk g.
Lutheran blood g.
National Wilms Tumor Study G.
  (NWTSG)
Pediatric Oncology G. (POG)
pediatrics AIDS clinical g. (PACTG)
private blood g.
g. problem-solving therapy
Rh blood g.
Scottish Gynecological Cancer Trials
  G. (SCOT-ROC)
spotted fever g.
streptococcal g.
support g.
typhus g.

grouping
blood g.
clinical g.

growing fracture
grows
plug the lung until it g. (PLUG)
growth
g. arrest
bacterial g.
catch-up g.
g. chart
g. control factor
g. curve
g. delay
g. discordancy
discordant g.
discordant twin g.
g. disturbance
divergent fetal g.
epiphysial g.
g. epoch
extracapsular g.
g. factor (GF)
g. failure
g. failure-pericardial constriction
  syndrome
fetal cellular g.
gestational g.
gompertzian g.
g. hormone (GH)
g. hormone-binding protein (GHBP)
g. hormone deficiency (GHD)
g. hormone immunoassay
g. hormone insensitivity (GHI)
g. hormone receptor (GHR)
g. hormone receptor deficiency
  (GHRD)
g. hormone release
g. hormone-releasing hormone
  (GH-RH)

g. hormone-secreting adenoma
g. hormone stimulation test
  (GHST)
g. hormone therapy
g. index
linear g.
longitudinal g.
nonestrogen-regulated g.
g. parameter
g. pattern
placental g.
g. plate
g. plate fracture
g. plate injury
poor linear g.
g. problem
puberal g.
g. rate
g. retardation
g. retardation, ocular abnormalities,
  microcephaly, brachydactyly,
  oligophrenia (GOMBO)
retarded fetal g.
skeletal g.
slow g.
g. spurt
g. stunting
testicular g.
g. velocity (GV)
g. zone
growth-adjusted sonographic age
  (GASA)
growth-discordant twins
growth-like factor
growth-remaining method
growth-restricted fetus
growth-retarded fetus
GRS
Golabi-Rosen syndrome
Grubben syndrome
Gruber syndrome
Grünfelder reflex
grunting
g. and flaring
g. baby syndrome
expiratory g.
flaring and g.
g. respiration
GRV
gastric residual volume
GS
gestational sac
GSD
glycogen storage disorder
GSH
glutathione
GSH pathway disorder
GSI
genuine stress incontinence

G

GSI-BSI
Global Severity Index of Brief
Symptom Inventory
GSMS
Great Smoky Mountains Study of
Youth
G-spot
Graefenberg spot
GSS
gestational sac size
GT
Cytobrush Plus GT
GTD
gestational trophoblastic disease
GTH
gonadotropic hormone
GTN
gestational trophoblastic neoplasia
glyceryl trinitrate
WHO prognostic scoring for GTN
G-to-T transversion mutation
GTP
glutamyl transpeptidase
guanosine triphosphate
guanyltriphosphate
GTT
gestational trophoblastic tumor
glucose tolerance test
G-tube
gastrostomy tube
G-tube feeding
GU
genitourinary
guaiac-negative stool
guaiacolate
glyceryl g.
guaiac-positive stool
guaiac test
guaifenesin
g. and codeine
g. and dextromethorphan
g., phenylpropanolamine,
phenylephrine
Guaifenex DM, LA
guanabenz
guanadrel
guanethidine
guanfacine hydrochloride
guanidine salt
guanidinoacetate
guanine
9-13-dihydroxypropoxymethyl g.
g. nucleotide
guanosine
g. triphosphate (GTP)
g. triphosphate cyclohydrolase
guanyltriphosphate (GTP)
guard
Breast Biopsy G.

high g.
mouth g.
guardian
g. ad litem
G. DNA system
G. vaginal retractor
gubernacular attachment
gubernaculum
GUD
genital ulcer disease
Guerin-Stein syndrome
Guiatuss DM
Guiatussin With Codeine
guidance
concurrent ultrasound g.
CT g.
fluoroscopic g.
hand-over-hand g.
g. officer
pediatric anticipatory g.
pictorial anticipatory g. (PAG)
ultrasonographic g.
ultrasound g.
guide
Pilot suturing g.
trocar g.
winged g.
guideline
Bethesda System g.'s
G.'s for Adolescent Preventive
Services (GAPS)
guidewire
radiopaque g.
Guillain-Barré-Landry syndrome
Guillain-Barré syndrome (GBS)
guilt
survivor g.
guinea worm infection
gulf
Lecat g.
gum
g. arabic rehydration solution
bean g.
g. bleeding
carob g.
g. fibrosis
g. hyperplasia
gumma, *pl.* **gummata, gummas**
pituitary gland g.
tuberculous g.
gummas (*pl. of* gumma)
gummata (*pl. of* gumma)
gum-tooth interface
gun
Bard Biopty g.
coring biopsy g.
Wallach LL100 cryosurgical Cryo
G.
gunstock deformity

Günther disease
gurgling
Gurrieri syndrome
GUS
    genitourinary sphincter
GUSB
    beta-glucuronidase
        GUSB deficiency
        GUSB gene
        GUSB locus
gustatory
    g. discernment
    g. lacrimation
Gustavson syndrome
gut
    g. motility
    g. rest
    g. suture
    g. tonometry
    torsion of g.
    g. vasculitis
gut-associated lymphoid tissue
(GALT)
Guthrie
    bacterial inhibition assay method
      of G.
    G. card
    G. count
    G. muscle
    G. test
guttata
    parapsoriasis g.
    psoriasis g.
guttate
    g. lesion
    g. psoriasis
gutter
    paracolic g.
    pelvic g.
    posterior cul-de-sac g.
GV
    germinal vesicle
    growth velocity
    GV oocyte
GVBD
    germinal vesicle breakdown
GVHD
    graft versus host disease
GVL
    graft versus leukemia
GWAFD
    Genée-Wiedemann acrofacial dysostosis
Gy
    gray
gymnast's wrist
GYN
    gynecologic
    gynecologist
    gynecology

gynandroblastoma
gynandromorph
gynatresia
Gynazole-1 vaginal cream
Gynecare
    G. Thermachoice uterine balloon
      therapy system
    G. TVT obturator system
    G. TVT Secur system
gynecic
gynecogenic
gynecography
gynecoid
    g. fat distribution pattern
    g. obesity
    g. pelvis
gynecologic (GYN), gynecological
    g. cancer
    G. Cancer Foundation - Society of
      Gynecologic Oncologists
    g. cancer patient
    g. carcinoma
    g. history
    g. malignancy
    g. oncology
gynecological (*var. of* gynecologic)
gynecologist (GYN)
    American College of Obstetricians
      and G.'s (ACOG)
gynecology (GYN)
    adolescent g.
    American Board of Obstetrics and
      G.
    obstetrics and g. (O´and´G,
      OB´GYN, OB-GYN, OB/GYN,
      O&G, OG)
    pediatric g.
gynecomastia, gynecomasty
    benign transient g.
    drug-induced g.
    involutional g.
    neonatal g.
    pathologic g.
    physiologic g.
    puberal g.
gynecomasty (*var. of* gynecomastia)
Gynecort Topical
Gyne-Lotrimin Vaginal
Gynemesh
    G. nonabsorbable Prolene mesh
    G. PS polypropylene mesh
    support
Gyne-Sulf
gyniatrics
gyniatry
gynogenetic
Gynol II contraceptive jelly
gynopathy
gynoplastics (*var. of* gynoplasty)

G

gynoplasty, gynoplastics
GynoSampler
    G. endometrial aspirator
    G. endometrial sampling
    device
Gynoscann
gyral
    g. abnormality
    g. anomaly
    g. atrophy
    g. malformation
    g. pattern

gyrata
    cutis verticis g.
gyrate atrophy
gyratum
    ovarium g.
gyri (*pl. of* gyrus)
Gyrocaps
    Slo-Phyllin G.
gyrus, *pl.* **gyri**
    cingulate g. (CG)
    mushroom g.
    orbitofrontal g.

H
    H gene
    H protein
H1
    histamine 1
        H1 receptor
H2
    histamine 2
HA
    hyperalimentation
    hyperandrogenic anovulation
    hypoplastic aorta
Haab stria
HAART
    highly active antiretroviral therapy
    highly active retroviral therapy
Haase rule
Haas intrauterine insemination catheter
HABA
    hydroxybenzoic acid
        HABA binding test
habenula, *pl.* **habenulae**
    Haller h.
    h. urethralis
habenulae (*pl. of* habenula)
habit
    bladder h.
    bowel h.
    h. cough
    dietary h.
    eating h.
    mentalis h.
    sexual h.
    sleeping h.
    h. tic deformity
HabitEX smoking cessation system
habitual
    h. aborter
    h. abortion
    h. shoulder dislocation
    h. shoulder subluxation
    h. snoring (HS)
habituation
habitus
    body h.
    Buddhalike h.
    craniosynostosis-marfanoid h.
    cushingoid body h.
    eunuchoid h.
    fetal h.
    male body h.
    marfanoid h.
    h. of fetus
HAC
    human artificial chromosome

HACE
    high-altitude cerebral edema
HACEK
    Haemophilus aphrophilus,
        Actinobacillus actinomycetemcomitans,
        Cardiobacterium hominis, Eikenella
        corrodens, Kingella kingae
        HACEK coccobacillus
        HACEK group
Hacker hypospadias
Hadlock equation
haematobium
    Schistosoma h.
haemoglobin (*var. of* hemoglobin)
haemolysans
    Gemella h.
haemolyticum
    Arcanobacterium h.
    Corynebacterium h.
Haemophilus
    H. aphrophilus
    H. aphrophilus, Actinobacillus
        actinomycetemcomitans,
        Cardiobacterium hominis, Eikenella
        corrodens, Kingella kingae
        (HACEK)
    H. ducreyi
    H. influenzae
    H. influenzae cellulitis
    H. influenzae meningitis
    H. influenzae type b (Hib)
    H. influenzae type b conjugate
        vaccine
    H. influenzae type b
        immunization
    H. parainfluenzae (HPI)
    H. pertussis vaccine (HPV)
    H. vaginalis
    H. vaginitis
Hagedorn
    neutral protamine H. (NPH)
Hageman factor
Haig-Fergusson forceps
Haight baby retractor
Hailey-Hailey disease
hair
    axillary h.
    bamboo h.
    brittle h.
    h. bud
    h. bulb incubation test
    h. cortex keratin gene type II
    h. cotinine analysis
    exclamation-mark h.
    friable h.

H

hair (*continued*)
    h. groomer's syncope
    h. growth phase
    h. loss
    lumbosacral tuft of h.
    Menkes kinky h.
    moniliform h.
    h. monster
    h. patch
    pubic h.
    h. pulling
    h. sampling
    sexual h.
    sparse h.
    h. spray
    spun glass h.
    terminal h.
    h. tourniquet
    h. tourniquet injury
    tuft of h.
    twisted h.
    vellus h.
    h. whorl
    wispy h.
HAIR-AN
    hirsutism, androgen excess, insulin resistance, acanthosis nigricans
    hyperandrogenism, insulin resistance, acanthosis nigricans
    HAIR-AN syndrome
HAIRAN
    hyperandrogenism, insulin resistance, acanthosis nigricans
hairball
hair-brain syndrome
hairless pseudofemale
hairlike tumor
hairline
    low occipital h.
    pubic h.
hair-on-end appearance
hairpin vessel
hairy
    h. leukoplakia
    h. nevus
    h. patch
    h. tongue
Hajdu-Cheney syndrome
Hakim-Adams syndrome
Hakim syndrome
Halban
    H. culdoplasty
    H. culdoplasty procedure
    H. fashion
    H. syndrome
    H. theory of endometriosis
Halbrecht syndrome
halcinonide
Halcion

Haldol Decanoate
Haley's M-O
half-buried suture
half-desmosome
half-Fourier acquisition single-shot turbo spin-echo (HASTE)
half-kneeling position
half-life
Halfprin
half-strength formula
half-value layer (HVL)
halitosis
Halle
    H. infant nasal speculum
    H. point
Haller
    H. cell
    H. habenula
Hallermann-Streiff
    H.-S. dyscephalia
    H.-S. syndrome
Hallermann-Streiff-François syndrome
Hallermann syndrome
Hallervorden-Spatz
    H.-S. disease
    H.-S. syndrome
Hallopeau-Siemens syndrome
Hall-Pallister syndrome
Hallpike maneuver
Hall-Riggs syndrome
Hall syndrome (1, 2)
halluces (*pl. of* hallucis, hallux)
hallucination
    hypnagogic h.
    olfactory h.
    phobic h.
    tactile h.
    visual phobic h.
hallucinogen
hallucis, *pl.* **halluces**
    spastic abductor h.
hallux
    purple h.
    h. rigidus
    h. valgus
halo
    h. effect
    erythematous h.
    fatty h.
    h. nevus
    osteopenic h.
    h. sign of hydrops
    H. Sleep System
    h. test
    h. traction
halobetasol
halofantrine

Halog-E
halogen
    h. acne
    h. lamp
    h. spotlight phototherapy
halogenated hydrocarbon
haloperidol
haloprogin
Halotestin
Halotex
halothane
Halotussin DM
Halpern syndrome
Halsted
    H. mastectomy
    H. mosquito forceps
    H. operation
halstedian concept of tumor spread
Haltia-Santavuori neural ceroid
  lipofuscinosis
Haltran
HAM
    human T-cell lymphotrophic virus type
    I associated myelopathy
hamartin
hamartoblastoma
    congenital hypothalamic h.
    hypothalamic h.
    renal, anus, lung, polydactyly, h.
    (RALPH)
hamartoma
    cystic h.
    ectoneurodermal h.
    hypothalamic h.
    iris h.
    mesenchymal h.
    neuroectodermal h.
    retinal h.
    smooth muscle h.
hamartomatosis
    hereditary multiple system h.
hamartomatous
    h. malformation
    h. mass
hamartoneoplastic syndrome
hamartopolydactyly syndrome
HAMD
    Hamilton Depression Scale
Hamel syndrome
Ham F10 medium
Hamilton
    H. cardiac output method
    H. Depression Scale (HAMD)
Hamman-Rich syndrome
Hammersmith
    hemoglobin H.
hammer toe, hammertoe
hammertoe (var. of hammer toe)
hammock

    Mersilene gauze h.
    Monarc subfascial h.
    subfascial h.
Hamou
    H. contact microhysteroscope
    H. hysteroscope
    H. hysteroscopic endometrial
    ablation technique
hamster egg penetration assay
hamstring
    lateral h.
    h. lengthening
    lengthening of h.
    medial h.
hand
    h. and head presentation
    ape h.
    choreic h.
    cleft h.
    dominant h.
    epidermolysis bullosa simplex of
    h.'s
    fisting of h.'s
    lobster-claw h.
    mechanic's h.
    milkmaid's h.
    mitten h.
    narrow h.
    h. preference
    vaginal h.
    h. ventilation
    h. wringing
hand-bagging
handbook
    Harriet Lane H.
hand-eye coordination
hand-foot-and-mouth disease (HFMD)
hand-foot-genital syndrome
hand-foot-mouth syndrome
hand-foot syndrome
hand-foot-uterus syndrome
handheld flutter device
handicap
    mental h.
    neurodevelopmental h.
handle
    laryngoscope h.
handling
hand-over-hand guidance
handpiece
    PhotoDerm PL h.
Hand-Schüller-Christian
    H.-S.-C. disease
    H.-S.-C. syndrome
hands-feet position
hand-to-eye fomite
hand-to-mouth movement
handwashing
hand-wringing movement

H

hand-wrist bone age
hanging
    h. panniculus
    h. stirrup
hanging-drop test
hangman's fracture
hangover
Hanhart syndrome
Hank's balanced salt solution (HBSS)
Hanks dilator
Hanoi
    Tower of H. (TOH)
Hansel stain
Hansen disease
Hans Rudolph valve
Hantaan virus
H₂-antagonist
hantavirus
    h. cardiopulmonary syndrome
    (HCPS)
    h. immunoglobulin M antibody
    h. pulmonary syndrome
HAODM
    hypoplasia of anguli oris depressor
    muscle
HAPE
    high-altitude pulmonary edema
haplogroup
haploid
    h. cell
    h. set
    h. sperm
    h. spermatozoon
haploidentical bone marrow
  transplant
haploinsufficiency
haplotype
    maternal HLA h.
    h. relative risk (HRR)
happy
    h. puppet syndrome
    h. wheezer
hapten
hapten-antibody
    hypersensitive h.-a.
haptoglobin
harassing cough
hard hepatomegaly
HARD
    hydrocephalus, agyria, retinal dysplasia
    HARD syndrome
HARD+/-E
    hydrocephalus, agyria, retinal dysplasia
    with or without encephalocele
    HARD+/-E syndrome
Hardikar syndrome
Hardy-Weinberg
    H.-W. equilibrium

    H.-W. formula
    H.-W. law
harelip
harlequin
    h. color change
    h. fetus
    h. ichthyosis
    h. reaction
    h. sign
harmonic
    H. Ace scalpel
    h. tissue imaging
harmony
harness
    figure-of-8 h.
    Kicker Pavlik h.
    Pavlik h.
    Wheaton Pavlik h.
HARP
    hypobetalipoproteinemia, acanthocytosis,
    retinitis pigmentosa, pallidal
    degeneration
    HARP syndrome
Harpenden
    H. calipers
    H. stadiometer
Harriet Lane Handbook
Harrington
    H. retractor
    H. rod
Harris
    H. growth arrest line
    H. uterine injector (HUI)
    H. view
Harris-Benedict basal energy expenditure
  equation
Harris-Kronner uterine
  manipulator-injector (HUMI)
Harrison
    H. atrial end of ventriculoatrial
    shunt method
    H. groove
    H. sulcus
Harrod syndrome
Harry Benjamin International Dysphoria
  Association (HBIGDA)
harsh pansystolic murmur
Hart
    H. line
    H. syndrome
Harter self-esteem questionnaire
Hartmann
    H. sign
    H. solution (HS)
Hartnup
    H. defect
    H. disease
    H. disorder

HAS
 hospitalized attempted suicide
Hashimoto
 H. disease
 H. thyroiditis
hashitoxicosis
Hassall corpuscle
Hasson
 H. cannula
 H. laparoscopy
HASTE
 half-Fourier acquisition single-shot
  turbo spin-echo
 HASTE sequence
HAstV-1
 human astrovirus type 1
hat
 measuring h.
 silver thermal h.
 thermal h.
Hata phenomenon
hatchet face appearance
hatching
 assisted h. (AH)
 assisted zona h. (AZH)
 blastocyst h.
HATT
 hemagglutination treponemal test
Haugh forceps
Haultain inverted uterus operation
HAV
 hepatitis A vaccine
 hepatitis A virus
Haverhill fever
haversian system
Havrix vaccine
Hawaii
 H. agent
 H. Early Learning Profile (HELP)
Hawk-Dennen forceps
Hawkins
 H. breast localization needle
 H. sign
hawkinsinuria
Haw River syndrome
Hawthorne effect
hay fever
Hayflick
 Wistar Institute Susan H. (WISH)
Hay-Wells syndrome
hazard
 Cox proportional h.
haze
 corneal h.
hazy lung
HB
 hepatitis B
 Recombivax HB

Hb
 hemoglobin
HbA
 hemoglobin A
HbA$_2$
 hemoglobin A$_2$
HbA1c
 glycosylated hemoglobin
 hemoglobin A$_{1c}$
HbA$_1$c
 hemoglobin A$_{1c}$
HBAg
 hepatitis B antigen
HBcAb
 hepatitis B core antibody
HbE
 hemoglobin E
HBeAb
 hepatitis B early antibody
HbE beta-thalassemia
HbF
 fetal hemoglobin
 hemoglobin F
HbH
 hemoglobin H
  HbH disease
  HbH disease-mental retardation
   syndrome
  HbH related mental retardation
HBIG
 hepatitis B immune globulin
HBIGDA
 Harry Benjamin International Dysphoria
  Association
HBIR
 Hering-Breuer inflation reflex
HBL
 hepatoblastoma
HBLP
 hyperbetalipoproteinemia
HbOC
 hepatitis B oligosaccharide-CRM197
  vaccine
HbP
 primitive fetal hemoglobin
HBQ
 human health and behavior
  questionnaire
HbS
 hemoglobin S
 sickle cell hemoglobin
HBsAb
 antibody to hepatitis B surface antigen
 hepatitis B surface antibody
HBsAg
 hepatitis B surface antigen
HbSC
 sickle cell hemoglobin C

H

HBSS
  Hank's balanced salt solution
HbS-Thal
  hemoglobin S thalassemia
HBV
  hepatitis B vaccine
  hepatitis B virus
HC
  head circumference
    Bancap HC
    Prevex HC
HC/AC
  head circumference/abdominal
    circumference
    fetal HC/AC
    HC/AC ratio
HCC
  hepatocellular carcinoma
H(c)ELISA
  hemagglutinin enzyme-linked
    immunosorbent assay
HCFA
  Health Care Financing Administration
hCG
  human chorionic gonadotropin
    free beta hCG
    Pro-Step hCG
    Tandem Icon II hCG
    Test Pack hCG
HCII
  heparin cofactor II
  HCII coagulation inhibitor
hck protooncogene
HCl
  hydrochloride
    cefepime HCl
    Cleocin HCl
    fluoxetine HCl
    ondansetron HCl
    oxytetracycline HCl
    phenazopyridine HCl
    ropivacaine HCl
    sertraline HCl
    valacyclovir HCl
    venlafaxine HCl
HCO$_3$
  bicarbonate
HCP
  hereditary coproporphyria
HCPS
  hantavirus cardiopulmonary
    syndrome
HCRM
  home cardiorespiratory monitor
HCS
  holocarboxylase
    HCS deficiency
HCTZ
  hydrochlorothiazide

HCV
  hepatitis C virus
HCW
  healthcare worker
HD
  Huntington disease
HDC
  high-dose chemotherapy
HDC-ABMT
  high-dose chemotherapy with
    autologous bone marrow
    transplantation
HDCV
  human diploid cell rabies
    vaccine
HDE
  high-dose therapy with epinephrine
HDI 3000 ultrasound
HDL
  high-density lipoprotein
HDN
  ABO hemolytic disease of the
    newborn
  hemolytic disease of newborn
  hemorrhagic disease of newborn
HDS
  hematuria-dysuria syndrome
HDV
  hepatitis D virus
H&E
  hematoxylin and eosin
    H&E stain
HE
  hepatic encephalopathy
  hereditary elliptocytosis
  hypophysectomy
    spherocytic HE
head
  after-coming h.
  h. banding enuresis
  h. banging
  h. birth
  h. bobbing
  h. box
  breech h.
  h. circumference
  h. circumference/abdominal
    circumference (HC/AC)
  h. circumference-for-age
    percentile
  h. compression (HC)
  h. control
  cracked-pot h.
  cupping of optic nerve h.
  h. drop
  engaged h.
  h. entrapment
  fetal h. (FH)
  h. growth velocity

hourglass h.
h. lag
h. louse
malformed radial h.
h. mesoderm
molding of h.
h. pole
h. positioner
h. presentation
H. reflex
h. righting
h. size
H. Start
h. tilt
h. titubation
transillumination of h.
h. trauma
h. ultrasound
zygomatic h.

headache
acute h.
analgesic-rebound h.
chronic h.
classic migraine h.
cluster h.
common migraine h.
complicated migraine h.
h. diary
migraine h.
migraine-type h.
migrainous h.
nonmigrainous h.
postdural puncture h.
 (PDPH)
postlumbar puncture h.
preeclampsia h.
primary h.
recurrent h.
secondary h.
sleep-related h.
spinal h.
tension h.
vascular h.

head-and-tail fold
headband
fiberoptic h.
imaging h.
plagiocephaly h.

headlight
Keeler fiberoptic h.
MultArray h.

head-righting
lateral h.-r.

HEADS
home life, education level, activities,
drug use, sexual activity
HEADS question

head-sparing intrauterine growth retardation

HEADSS
home life, education level, activities,
drug use, sexual activity, suicide
ideation/attempts

head-up tilt (HUT)
healing
energy h.

health
H. Care Financing Administration
 (HCFA)
h. maintenance organization
 (HMO)
h. maintenance visit
mental h.
National Institute of Mental H.
 (NIMH)
National Institutes of H. (NIH)
health, osteoporosis, progestin,
estrogen (HOPE)
pediatric public h.
H. Plan Employer Data and
Information Set
H. Scan Assess Plus peak flow
meter
h. status
World Association for Infant
Mental H.

healthcare worker (HCW)
HealthCheck One-Step One Minute pregnancy test
Healthdyne
H. apnea monitor
H. oximeter
H. ventilator

health-related quality of life (HRQOL)
Heaney
H. curette
H. hysterectomy clamp
H. hysterectomy forceps
H. hysterectomy retractor
H. needle holder
H. operation
H. suture
H. vaginal vault closure technique

Heaney-Ballantine
H.-B. forceps
H.-B. hysterectomy clamp

Heaney-Simon retractor
hearing
h. acuity
h. aid
h. development
h. loss
residual h.
h. screening

hearing-loss-nephritis syndrome
heart
air-filled h.

heart (*continued*)
    H. and Estrogen/Progestin
      Replacement Study (HERS)
    h. block
    boot-shaped h.
    crisscross h.
    cushion defect of h.
    h. defect
    h. defect syndrome
    dextroposition of h.
    h. disease
    h. failure
    fetal h. (FH)
    hole in h.
    Holmes h.
    hypoplasia of left h. (HLL)
    hypoplastic left h.
    h. lesion
    h. massage
    midline h.
    h. murmur
    h. rate (HR)
    h. rate monitoring
    h. rate power spectral analysis
      (HRSA)
    h. rate variability (HRV)
    h. shadow
    h. sounds
    h. transplant
    h. transplantation
    upstairs-downstairs h.
    h. valve replacement
heartburn
heart-hand syndrome
heart-shaped
    h.-s. pelvis
    h.-s. uterus
heat
    h. loss
    prickly h.
    h. shock protein
    h. transfer mechanism
heater probe thermal contact
heatstroke, heat stroke
heat-treated
    Profilnine H.-T.
heave
    apical h.
heavy
    h. chain
    h. metal poisoning
heavy-ion
    h.-i. irradiation
    h.-i. mammography
hebephrenia
hebephrenic silliness
hebetic
HEC
    human endothelial cell

Hecht pneumonia
hedgehog
    Sonic H.
heel
    h. capillary sampling
    h. cord
    h. cord lengthening
    h. cup
    h. lance (HL)
    h. pain
    h. strike
    Thomas h.
    h. valgus
heel-cord contracture
heel-stick
    h.-s. hematocrit
    h.-s. procedure
heel-to-ear maneuver
heel-toe gait
heel-to-shin test
Heerfordt syndrome
HEF
    human embryo fibroblast
Hegar
    H. dilator
    H. sign
heidelberg
    Salmonella h.
height
    fundal h. (FH)
    midparental h.
    minimal acceptable h. (MAH)
    sitting h. (SH)
    symphysis-fundus h.
    h. table
    h. velocity (HV)
    h. velocity Z-score
height-for-age (HFA)
heilmannii
    Helicobacter h.
Heimlich maneuver
Heineke-Mikulicz pyloroplasty
Heiner syndrome
Heinz
    H. body
    H. body hemolytic anemia
Hektoen agar
HeLa
    Henrietta Lacks
    HeLa cells
helcomenia
H-7000 electron microscope
helical scan
helices (*pl. of* helix)
Helicobacter
    H. heilmannii
    H. pylori
heliotrope
    h. eyelid

h. pattern
h. rash
heliotropic
h. discoloration
h. erythema
heliox
helium and oxygen
helium and oxygen (heliox)
helix, *pl.* **helices, helixes**
alpha h.
double h.
H. endocervical curette
h. termination peptide
H. uterine biopsy curette
Helixate
helixes (*pl. of* helix)
helix-loop-helix transcription
Hellendall sign
Heller
H. dementia
H. myotomy
H. test
Heller-Belsey esophageal operation
Heller-Döhle disease
Heller-Nissen thorascopic
esophagomyotomy
Hellin law
Hellin-Zeleny law
HELLP
hemolysis, elevated liver enzymes, low
platelet count
HELLP syndrome
helmet
cranial molding h.
plagiocephaly h.
helmet-molding therapy
helminth
helminthic disease
HELP
Hawaii Early Learning Profile
helper
h. factor
h. lymphocyte
T h.
h. T cell
helplessness
Helpline
Bed Rest H.
Hemabate
hemacytometer (*var. of*
hemocytometer)
Hemaflex sheath
hemagglutination
indirect h.
h. inhibition (HI)
h. inhibition antibody (HIA)
h. test
h. treponemal test (HATT)
Treponema pallidum h. (TPHA)

hemagglutinin
h. enzyme-linked immunosorbent
assay (H(c)ELISA)
filamentous h.
hemagogue
hemangiectasia hypertrophica
hemangiectatic hypertrophy
hemangioblastoma
cerebellar h.
hemangioendothelioma
kaposiform h.
hemangioma, *pl.* **hemangiomata**
bone h.
capillary h.
cardiac h.
cavernous h.
cryptic h.
cutaneous h.
epidural h.
giant h.
hepatic h.
infantile hepatic h.
Kaposi-like form of infantile h.
lobular capillary h.
macular h.
port-wine h.
proliferating h.
strawberry h.
vulvar h.
hemangiomata (*pl. of* hemangioma)
hemangioma-thrombocytopenia syndrome
hemangiomatosis
diffuse neonatal h.
disseminated h.
pulmonary h.
hemangiomatous branchial clefts/lip
pseudocleft syndrome
hemangiopericytoma
infantile h.
hemarthrosis
acute h.
hematemesis
coffee-ground h.
Hematest
H. positive
H. test
hemathorax (*var. of* hemothorax)
hematobilia
hematocele
pelvic h.
pudendal h.
hematocephalus
hematochezia
hematocolpometra
hematocolpos
hematocrit (hct)
automated h.
h. determination
heel-stick h.

H

hematocrit (*continued*)
mean menstrual cycle h.
posttransfusion h.
spun h.
hematogenous
h. infection
h. metastasis
h. osteomyelitis
h. primary tuberculosis
h. seeding
h. septic arthritis
h. spread
hematogenously
hematologic
h. crisis
h. disorder
h. neoplasia
h. toxicity
hematological change
hematology
American Society of H.
British Society of H.
hematoma
acute subdural h.
adrenal h.
auricular h.
axillary h.
central hepatic h.
cerebellar h.
cerebral h.
h. drainage
epidural h. (EDH, EH)
extradural h.
follicular h.
hepatic h.
infected cuff h.
interhemispheric subdural h.
interstitial and loculated h.
intracerebral h.
intracranial h.
intraparenchymal h.
intrauterine h.
puerperal h.
rectus h.
retroperitoneal h.
retroplacental h.
secondary h.
subcapsular hepatic h.
subchorionic h.
subdural h. (SDH)
subgaleal h. (SGH)
sublingual h.
submental h.
testicular h.
traumatic h.
umbilical cord h.
uterine h.
vaginal h.
vulvar h.

hematometra, hemometra
hematometrocolpos
hematometry
hematomphalocele
hematophagocytic syndrome
hematopoiesis (*var. of* hemopoiesis)
hematopoietic (*var. of* hemopoietic)
h. system
hematosalpinx, hemosalpinx
hematotrachelos
hematotympanum (*var. of* hemotympanum)
hematoxylin and eosin (H&E)
hematuria
benign familial h. (BFH)
benign recurrent h.
congenital hereditary h.
drug-induced h.
exercise-induced h.
familial benign h.
familial recurrent h.
macroscopic h.
hematuria, nephropathy, deafness syndrome
painless h.
recurrent gross h. (RGH)
sickle cell associated h.
transient h.
hematuria-dysuria syndrome (HDS)
heme
h. arginate
erythropoietic h.
h. iron
h. metabolism disorder
nonerythropoietic h.
h. oxygenase
h. oxygenase inhibitor
hemelytrometra
heme-negative stool
heme-positive stool
Hemet Rectal
hemiacardius
hemiacephalus
hemianencephaly
hemianopia, hemianopsia, hemiopia
bitemporal h.
homonymous h.
transient h.
hemianopsia (*var. of* hemianopia)
hemiatrophy
progressive facial h.
hemiatrophy-hemihypertrophy
hemiblock
left anterior h.
hemibody irradiation
hemicardia
hemicephalia
hemicervix
hemichorea

hemicolectomy
hemicord
hemicortectomy
hemicrania
    migraine sine h.
hemidesmosome
hemidystonia
hemiepiphysiodesis
hemifacial
    h. microsomia (HM)
    h. spasm
hemi-Fontan procedure
hemifusion
hemignathia and microtia
  syndrome
hemihyperplasia
hemihypertrophy
hemihypoplasia
hemihysterectomy
hemimegalencephaly
    unilateral h.
hemimelia
    congenital fibular h.
    congenital tibial h.
    dysplasia epiphysialis h.
    fibular h.
    paraxial fibular h.
    paraxial tibial h.
    tibial h.
    transverse h.
hemimelica
    dysplasia epiphysealis h.
hemimelus
hemin
heminasal
    h. aplasia
    h. hypoplasia
hemineural plate
hemiopia (var. of hemianopia)
hemipagus
hemiparesis
    congenital h.
    postconvulsive h.
    spastic h.
hemiparetic
    h. cerebral palsy
    h. posture
hemiplegia
    acute infantile h.
    alternating h.
    congenital h.
    double h.
    infantile h.
    postmigrainous stroke h.
    spastic h.
    syndrome of acute h.
hemiplegic
    h. cerebral palsy
    h. migraine

hemisection
    h. of cord
    h. uterine morcellation technique
hemisensory deficit
hemisphere
    cerebral h.
hemispherectomy
    total h.
hemispheric tumor
hemisyndrome
    left h.
hemiuterus
hemivagina
hemivertebra
hemivulvectomy
hemizona assay (HZA)
hemizygosity
hemizygous
hemobilia, hematobilia
    traumatic h.
hemoblastic leukemia
Hemoccult II test
hemochorial placenta
hemochromatosis
    hereditary h.
    neonatal h. (NH)
hemoconcentration
HemoCue
    H. AB hemoglobin measurement
    device
    H. blood glucose analyzer
    H. blood glucose system
    H. blood hemoglobin analyzer
    H. blood hemoglobin system
    H. glucose test
    H. hemoglobin photometer
    H. hemoglobin test
    H. microcurette
hemocystinuria
Hemocyte
hemocytometer, hemacytometer
    Neubauer h.
hemodiafiltration
hemodialysis
    continuous venovenous h. (CVVHD)
hemodilution
hemodynamic
    h. abnormality
    h. data
    h. instability
    h. monitoring
    h. parameter
    h. performance
    h. response
hemodynamics
    maternal central h.
    uterine h.
Hemofil M
hemofilter

H

hemofiltration
  continuous arteriovenous h.
    (CAVH)
  continuous venovenous h. (CVVH)
hemoglobin (Hb, hgb), haemoglobin
  h. A
  h. A_2 (HbA$_2$)
  h. A_{1c} HbA$_1$c)
  h. A_{1c} determination
  h. Bart
  h. Bart hydrops fetalis syndrome
  h. C
  h. CC
  h. C disease
  h. Chesapeake
  h. concentration
  cord blood h.
  h. E (HbE)
  h. electrophoresis
  elevated fetal h.
  embryonic h.
  h. F (HbF)
  fetal h. (HbF)
  glycosylated h. (HgA1c)
  h. Gower-1
  h. Gower-2
  h. H (HbH)
  h. Hammersmith
  hereditary persistence of fetal h.
    (HPFH)
  high-affinity h.
  h. Kempsey
  h. Lepore
  h. level
  h. M disease
  mean cell h. (MCH)
  mean corpuscular h. (MCH)
  h. M Hyde Park
  h. M Saskatoon
  h. Portland
  primitive fetal h. (HbP)
  reduced h.
  h. S (HbS)
  h. SC
  h. SC disease
  h. SC phenotype
  h. SD
  h. SD disease
  h. S disease
  serum free h.
  sickle cell h. (HbS)
  h. SS (HbSS)
  h. S solubility test
  h. SS phenotype
  h. S thalassemia (HbS-Thal)
  h. S-Thal phenotype
  h. subtype method
  unstable h.
  variant h.

hemoglobinemia
hemoglobinopathy
  sickle cell h.
hemoglobin-oxygen
  h.-o. dissociation
  h.-o. dissociation curve
hemoglobinuria
  march h.
  paroxysmal nocturnal h.
    (PNH)
hemoglobulinopathy
hemogram
  fetal h.
hemolymphatic stage
hemolysin
  Donath-Landsteiner cold h.
hemolysis
  antibody-mediated h.
  chronic intravascular h.
  h., elevated liver enzymes, low
    platelet count (HELLP)
  fetal h.
  immune h.
  massive intravascular h.
  mechanical h.
  microangiopathic h.
  nonimmune h.
hemolysis-derived black pigment stone
hemolytic
  h. anemia
  h. complement (CH$_{50}$)
  h. crisis
  h. disease
  h. disease of newborn (HDN)
  h. uremia syndrome associated with
    pregnancy
  h. uremic syndrome (HUS)
hemolyzed specimen
hemometra (*var. of* hematometra)
hemomonochorial
Hemonyne
Hemopad
hemopathy
  maternal h.
hemopericardium
hemoperitoneum
  ovulation-associated h.
hemophagocytic
  h. lymphohistiocytosis
  h. syndrome
hemophilia
  h. A, B, C
  acquired h.
  factor VIII h.
hemophiliac
hemophilic arthropathy
hemopneumothorax
hemopoiesis, hematopoiesis
  extramedullary h.

hemopoietic, hematopoietic
    h. differentiation
    h. disorder
    h. stem cell (HSC)
    h. stem cell transplantation (HCT, HSCT)
    h. syndrome
    h. system stimulator
hemoptysis
    catamenial h.
HemoQuant assay
hemorrhage
    accidental h.
    adrenal h.
    antepartum h. (APH)
    catastrophic h.
    cerebellar h.
    cervical h.
    CNS h.
    concealed h.
    cortical h.
    epidural h.
    external h.
    fetal h.
    fetal-maternal h. (FMH)
    fetomaternal h. (FMH)
    focal h.
    gastrointestinal h.
    germinal matrix h. (grade 1–4)
    idiopathic pulmonary h. (IPH)
    iliopsoas h.
    interhemispheric subarachnoid h.
    intracerebellar h.
    intracranial h. (ICH)
    intraoperative h.
    intraparenchymal h.
    intrapartum h.
    intraretinal h. (IH)
    intraventricular h. (grade 1–4) (IVH)
    last postpartum h.
    maternal-fetal h.
    h. of newborn (HN)
    orbital h.
    perinatal cerebral h.
    periventricular h. (grade 1–4) (PVH)
    periventricular-intraventricular h. (PIVH)
    petechial h.
    pinpoint h.
    placental h.
    postcesarean h.
    posterior fossa h.
    postpartum h. (PPH)
    primary postpartum h. (PPH)
    pulmonary h.
    retinal h.
    retroplacental h.

    scleral h.
    secondary postpartum h.
    splinter h.
    sternocleidomastoid h.
    subarachnoid h.
    subcapsular hepatic h.
    subchorionic h.
    subconjunctival h.
    subdural h.
    subependymal h. (SEH)
    subependymal germinal matrix h.
    subgaleal h.
    subhyaloid h.
    transplacental h. (TPH)
    trauma-related acute pelvic h.
    unavoidable h.
    uterine h.
hemorrhagic
    h. colitis
    h. cystitis
    h. cystitis glomerulonephritis
    h. dehydration
    h. diathesis
    h. disease
    h. disease of newborn (HDN)
    h. edema of infancy
    h. enanthem
    h. encephalitis
    h. endovasculitis
    h. *Escherichia coli*
    h. familial nephritis
    h. fever
    h. fever with renal syndrome (HFRS)
    h. hereditary nephritis
    h. pleural effusion
    h. scurvy
    h. shock
    h. shock and encephalopathy syndrome (HSES)
    h. shock syndrome
    h. spinal fluid
    h. telangiectasia
hemorrhagica
    metropathia h.
    purpura h.
hemorrhagicum
    corpus h.
hemorrhoid
hemorrhoidal
    h. artery
    h. nerve
    h. preparation
hemosalpinx (*var. of* hematosalpinx)
hemosiderin
    h. deposition
    h. laden macrophage
hemosiderinuria

H

hemosiderosis
food-induced pulmonary h.
primary pulmonary h.
pulmonary h.
transfusion-induced h.
hemospermia
hemostasia (*var. of* hemostasis)
hemostasis, hemostasia
intrapartum h.
surgical h.
hemostat
Crile h.
curved h.
Endo-Avitene microfibrillar collagen h.
hemostatic staple line
Hemotene
hemothorax, hemathorax
hemotympanum, hematotympanum
HEMPAS
hereditary erythroblastic multinuclearity with positive acidified serum
HEMPAS test
Hem-Prep
Hemril-HC Uniserts
Henderson-Hasselbalch equation
Henle
loop of H.
Hennebert sign
Hennekam lymphangiectasia-lymphedema syndrome
Henoch disease
Henoch-Schönlein purpura (HSP)
Henrietta Lacks (HeLa)
Henschke colpostat
henselae
Bartonella h.
Rochalimaea h.
Hensen node
HEP
hepatoerythropoietic porphyria
HEPA
high-efficiency particulate air
HEPA filter
hepadnavirus
Hepalean
heparan
h. sulfate
h. sulfate accumulation
h. sulfate urine test
heparin
calcium h.
h. challenge test
h. cofactor II (HCII)
h. cofactor II deficiency
h. cofactor II inhibitor
h. embryopathy
intravenous h.
h. lock (hep lock)

low-dose h.
low molecular weight h. (LMWH)
minidose h.
prophylactic h.
h. sodium
unfractionated h.
heparin-binding site mutation
heparin-induced thrombocytopenia (HIT)
heparinization
therapeutic h.
heparinized
h. lactated Ringer
h. saline
heparin-lock flush
HepatAmine
hepatectomy
left h.
partial h.
right h.
total h.
hepatic
h. amebiasis
h. arteriovenous fistula
h. capillariasis
h. capsular calcification
h. cirrhosis
h. coma
h. copper
h. copper overload syndrome
h. crisis
h. disease
h. ductular hypoplasia
h. ductular hypoplasia-multiple malformations syndrome
h. dysfunction
h. encephalopathy (HE)
h. fibrosis
h. focal nodular hyperplasia
h. gluconeogenesis
h. glycogenesis
h. glycogen storage disease
h. hemangioma
h. hematoma
h. infantilism
h. iron concentration (HIC)
h. lipase deficiency
h. lobe
h. metastasis
h. necrosis
h. neoplasm
h. parenchymal disorder
h. porphyria
h. pregnancy
h. rupture
h. sinusoid
h. transaminase
h. transplantation
h. venous wedge pressure gradient
h. wedged venography

hepatica
    Fasciola h.
hepaticojejunostomy, hepatojejunostomy
hepaticus
    fetor h.
hepatis
    bacillary peliosis h.
    peliosis h.
    porta h.
hepatitides (*pl. of* hepatitis)
hepatitis, *pl.* **hepatitides**
    h. A
    acute h.
    h. A immunization
    anicteric h.
    autoimmune chronic acute h.
    h. A vaccine (HAV)
    h. A virus (HAV)
    h. B (HB)
    h. B antigen (HBAg)
    h. B arthritis-dermatitis syndrome
    h. B core antibody (HBcAb)
    h. B early antibody (HBeAb)
    biliary neonatal h.
    h. B immune globulin (HBIG, H-BIG)
    h. B immunization
    h. B oligosaccharide-CRM197 vaccine (HbOC)
    h. B surface antibody (HBsAb)
    h. B surface antigen (HbsAg)
    h. B vaccine (HBV)
    h. B virus (HBV)
    h. C
    chronic h.
    chronic active h.
    chronic cryptogenic h. (CCH)
    chronic non-A-E h.
    h. C immunization
    cryptogenic h.
    h. C virus (HCV, HVC)
    h. D
    delta h.
    h. D virus (HDV)
    h. E
    h. E virus (HEV)
    fulminant h.
    h. F virus (HFV)
    h. G
    giant cell h.
    h. G virus (HGV)
    herpes h.
    hyperalimentation h.
    icteric h.
    idiopathic neonatal giant-cell h.
    h. immunoglobulin
    infectious h.
    maternal h.
    neonatal cholestatic h.

    non-A h.
    non-ABCDE h.
    non-A, non-B h. (NANBH)
    non-B h.
    h. screening
    serum h.
    toxic h.
    viral h.
hepatobiliary
    h. disease
    h. scintigraphy
    h. ultrasonography
hepatoblastoma (HBL)
hepatocellular
    h. carcinoma (HCC)
    h. damage
    h. disease
    h. injury
    h. lysome
hepatoclavicular (Hep/Clav)
hepatocyte
    h. growth factor (HGF)
    h. nuclear factor (HNF)
    pleomorphism of h.
hepatoerythropoietic porphyria (HEP)
hepatofacioneurocardiovertebral syndrome
hepatojejunostomy (*var. of* hepaticojejunostomy)
hepatolenticular degeneration
hepatoma
hepatomegalia (*var. of* hepatomegaly)
hepatomegaly, hepatomegalia
    firm h.
    hard h.
hepatonephoric syndrome
hepatonephric (*var. of* hepatorenal)
hepatopathy
    sickle h.
hepatoportoenterostomy
hepatopulmonary syndrome (HPS)
hepatorenal, hepatonephric
    h. syndrome
    h. tyrosinemia
hepatosplenic candidiasis
hepatosplenomegaly
hepatotoxicity
    nutritional h.
hepatotoxic syndrome
hepatotoxin
hepatotropic virus
heptavalent
Heptavax-B
Heptest Xa assay
HER
    HIV Epidemiology Research
herald
    h. bleed
    h. patch

H

herb
    moxa h.
herbal
    h. medicine
    h. tea
herbarum
    Cladosporium h.
herbicide
Herbst registry
Herceptin
Hercules
    infant H.
hereditaria
    adynamia episodica h.
    alopecia h.
    atrophia bulborum h.
    keratitis fugax h.
    porphyria cutanea tarda h.
hereditary
    h. abductor vocal cord paralysis
    h. agenesis of corpus callosum
    h. angioedema (type I)
    h. areflexic dystasia
    h. autonomic neuropathy
    h. benign chorea
    h. benign intraepithelial dyskeratosis syndrome
    h. bone dysplasia
    h. bullous dystrophy
    h. bullous skin dystrophy, macular type
    h. chin trembling
    h. chondrodysplasia
    h. clubbing
    h. coagulopathy
    h. coproporphyria (HCP)
    h. cutaneomandibular polyoncosis
    h. deforming chondrodystrophy
    h. disease
    h. DRPLA
    h. dysplastic nevus syndrome
    h. ectodermal dysplasia
    h. ectodermal polydysplasia
    h. edema
    h. elliptocytosis (HE)
    h. erythroblastic multinuclearity
    h. erythroblastic multinuclearity with positive acidified serum (HEMPAS)
    h. expansile polyostotic osteolytic dysplasia
    h. familial congenital nephritis
    h. fructose intolerance
    h. galactosemia
    h. hematuria syndrome
    h. hemochromatosis
    h. hemolytic anemia
    h. hemorrhagic telangiectasia (HHT)
    h. interstitial pyelonephritis
    h. lymphedema

    h. macular epidermolysis bullosa
    h. methemoglobinemia
    h. motor-sensory neuropathy (type IA, II–VII) (HMSN)
    h. multiple system hamartomatosis
    h. nephritis, deafness, abnormal thrombogenesis syndrome
    h. neuropathy with liability to pressure palsy (HNPP)
    h. nonpolyposis cancer
    h. nonpolyposis colon cancer (HNPCC)
    h. nonpolyposis colorectal cancer (HNPCC)
    h. nonpolyposis colorectal cancer syndrome
    h. nonspherocytic anemia
    h. oligophrenic cerebellolental degeneration
    h. optic neuron atrophy
    h. orotic aciduria
    h. osteoarthrophthalmopathy
    h. osteochondrodysplasia
    h. osteodysplasia with acroosteolysis
    h. ovarian cancer
    h. pancreatitis
    h. paroxysmal ataxia
    h. persistence of fetal hemoglobin (HPFH)
    h. polytopic enchondral dysostosis
    h. progressive arthroophthalmopathy
    h. progressive bulbar paralysis with deafness
    h. pyropoikilocytosis (HPP)
    h. renal adysplasia
    h. renal agenesis
    h. retinal aplasia
    h. retinal dysplasia
    h. retinoblastoma
    h. retinoschisis
    h. sensory autonomic neuropathy
    h. sensory radicular neuropathy
    h. spastic paraplegia
    h. spherocytosis
    h. spinal muscular atrophy
    h. stomatocytosis
    h. thrombophilia
    h. trait
    h. tremor
    h. trichodysplasia
    h. tyrosinemia
    h. urogenital adysplasia
    h. xanthinuria deficiency
heredity
    autosomal h.
    sex-linked h.
    X-linked h.
heredoataxia
heredodegeneration

heredodegenerative
- h. disease
- h. disorder

heredodiathesis
heredofamilial
heredoimmunity
heredopathia
- h. atactica
- h. atactica polyneuritiformis

heredoretinopathia congenitalis
Hering-Breuer inflation reflex (HBIR)
heritability
heritable coagulopathy
heritage
- Ashkenazi Jewish h.
- ethnic h.
- H. Panel genetic screening test

Herlitz epidermolysis bullosa letalis
Hermansky-Pudlak syndrome
hermaphrodism (*var. of* hermaphroditism)
hermaphrodite
hermaphroditism, hermaphrodism
- true h.
- XX h.

Hernandez syndrome
hernia, *pl.* **hernias, herniae**
- abdominal h.
- Bochdalek h.
- broad ligament h.
- complete h.
- congenital diaphragmatic h. (CDH)
- contralateral h.
- diaphragmatic h.
- epigastric h.
- femoral h.
- foramen of Morgagni h.
- groin h.
- hiatal h.
- immunotherapy h.
- incarcerated inguinal h.
- incisional h.
- incomplete h.
- indirect inguinal h.
- inguinal h.
- h. inguinale
- internal h.
- labial h.
- linea alba h.
- lung h.
- Morgagni h.
- ovary in inguinal h.
- paraduodenal h.
- paraesophageal hiatal h.
- peritoneal h.
- Petit h.
- pleuroperitoneal h.
- port site h.
- reducible h.
- retrocecal h.

- retrosternal h.
- Richter h.
- h. sac
- sliding hiatal h.
- spigelian h.
- strangulated h.
- transmesenteric h.
- trocar h.
- umbilical h.
- uncomplicated h.
- h. uteri inguinale
- ventral h.

herniae (*pl. of* hernia)
hernias (*pl. of* hernia)
herniated
- h. disc
- h. stomach
- h. viscera

herniation
- brain h.
- brainstem h.
- cerebral h.
- chronic tonsillar h.
- disc h.
- fat h.
- midbrain h.
- muscle h.
- syndrome of uncal h.
- transtentorial h.
- uncal h.

herniorrhaphy
herniotomy
- Petit h.

herpangina
Herp-Check test
herpes
- acute neonatal h.
- h. aseptic meningitis
- cervical h.
- congenital h.
- h. encephalitis
- h. facialis
- geniculate h.
- genital h.
- h. genitalis
- h. gestationis (HG)
- h. gladiatorum
- h. hepatitis
- intrauterine h.
- h. keratitis
- neonatal h.
- h. neonatorum
- ophthalmic h.
- orolabial h.
- perinatal h.
- h. simplex (HS)
- h. simplex encephalitis (HSE)
- h. simplex genitalis (HSG)
- h. simplex labialis

H

herpes (*continued*)
  h. simplex pneumonia
  h. simplex viral conjunctivitis
  h. simplex virus (HSV)
  h. simplex virus 1 (HSV-1, HSV1)
  h. simplex virus 2 (HSV-2, HSV2)
  h. simplex virus encephalitis
  h. simplex virus thymidine kinase
    gene
  h. stomatitis
  h. virus
  h. virus entry mediator (HVEM)
  h. vulvitis
  h. whitlow infection
  h. zoster
  h. zoster meningitis
  h. zoster of geniculate ganglion
  h. zoster ophthalmicus (HZO)
  h. zoster oticus
  h. zoster virus (HZV)
HerpeSelect-1
  H.-1 ELISA IgG assay
  H.-1 Immunoblot IgG assay
HerpeSelect-2
  H.-2 ELISA IgG assay
  H.-2 Immunoblot IgG assay
Herpesviridae
herpesvirus (HV), herpes virus
  h. encephalitis
  h. hominis
  human h. 1–8 (HHV1–8)
  Kaposi sarcoma-associated h.
  suid h.
herpetic
  h. corneal infection
  h. gingivitis
  h. gingivostomatitis
  h. keratitis
  h. keratopathy
  h. stomatitis
  h. whitlow
herpeticum
  eczema h.
herpetiform
  h. aphthous ulcer
  h. corneal ulcer
herpetiformis
  dermatitis h. (DH)
  h. epidermolysis bullosa simplex
  impetigo h.
Herplex Liquifilm
Herrick anemia
herringbone pattern
HERS
  Heart and Estrogen/Progestin
    Replacement Study
Hers disease
Herson-Todd score
Herter infantilism

Hertig-Rock ovum
Hertoghe sign
hertz (Hz)
hesitancy
Hespan
Hesselbach triangle
hetacillin
hetastarch solution
heteradelphus
heteralius
heterocephalus
heterochromatic DNA
heterochromatin
heterochromia
  congenital h.
  h. iridis
  h. of inner canthus
  h. of iris
heterochromosome
heterocyclic antidepressant
heterodimer
heterodimeric integral membrane
  glycoprotein
heterodisomy
  maternal uniparental h.
heteroduplex
  h. analysis
  h. DNA
heterodymus
heterogamete
heterogeneic (*var. of* heterogenic)
heterogeneity, heterogenicity
  allelic h.
  genetic h.
  locus h.
  loss of h. (LOH)
heterogeneous
heterogenic, heterogeneic
heterogenicity (*var. of*
  heterogeneity)
heterograft
heteroinoculation
heterokaryon
heterologous
  h. graft
  h. insemination
  h. surfactant
  h. uterine sarcoma
heteromorphous
heteropagus
heterophil, heterophile
  h. antibody
  h. antigen
  h. test
heterophile (*var. of* heterophil)
heterophilic
heteroplasmy
heteroploid
heteroprosopus

heterosexism
heterosexual
    h. high-risk behavior
    h. precocious puberty
    h. relationship
heterosomal aberration
heterosome
heterotaxia syndrome
heterotaxy
    abdominal h.
    h. syndrome
    visceral h.
heterotopia, heterotopy
    band h.
    bilateral periventricular
      nodular h.
    focal h.
    gray matter h.
    leptomeningeal h.
    mesodermal h.
    neuroglial h.
    neuronal h.
    periventricular nodular gray
      matter h.
    subcortical band h.
    subcortical laminar h.
    subependymal h.
heterotopic
    h. gray matter
    h. liver transplantation
    h. pregnancy
heterotopy (*var. of* heterotopia)
heterotropic
    h. chromosome
    h. pregnancies
heterotypic
heterotypical chromosome
heterozygosis (*var. of* heterozygosity)
heterozygosity, heterozygosis
heterozygote
    compound h.
    obligate h.
heterozygous
    h. carrier
    h. familial hypercholesterolemia
Heuser membrane
HEV
    hepatitis E virus
hew mutation
Hexa-Betalin
hexacetonide
    triamcinolone h.
hexachloride
    gamma-benzene h.
hexachlorocyclohexane
hexachlorophene)
    h. bath
    h. wash
hexadactylism (*var. of* hexadactyly)

hexadactyly, hexadactylism
    postaxial h.
    preaxial h.
Hexadrol
    H. Phosphate Injection
    H. Tablet
Hexalen
Hexalite cast
hexamethonium chloride
hexamethyldislazane (HMDS)
hexamethylmelamine
**hexamethyl propylene amine oxime
  (HMPAO)**
hexamine
hexaploidy
Hexastat
hexestrol
Hexit
hexocyclium methylsulfate
hexoprenaline sulfate
hexosamine
hexosaminidase
    h. A
    h. A deficiency
    h. B
hexose
hexylresorcinol
Heyer-Schulte valve
Heyman capsule
Heyman-Herndon clubfoot procedure
**Heyns abdominal decompression
  apparatus**
HF
    high frequency
HFA
    height-for-age
    high-functioning autism
      Proventil HFA
      Xopenex HFA
HFEA
    Human Fertilization and Embryology
    Authority
HFFI
    high-frequency flow interruption
HFJ
    high-frequency jet
      HFJ ventilation
      HFJ ventilator
HFJV
    high-frequency jet ventilation
HFMD
    hand-foot-and-mouth disease
HFO
    high-frequency oscillation
      HFO ventilation
      HFO ventilator
HFOV
    high-frequency oscillatory
    ventilation

H

411

HFPP
  high-frequency positive-pressure
    HFPP ventilation
    HFPP ventilator
HFPPV
  high-frequency positive-pressure
  ventilation
HFRS
  hemorrhagic fever with renal
  syndrome
hFSH
  human follicle-stimulating hormone
HFV
  hepatitis F virus
  high-frequency ventilation
HG
  herpes gestationis
HgA1c
  glycosylated hemoglobin
HGE
  human granulocytic ehrlichiosis
HGF
  hepatocyte growth factor
hGH
  human growth hormone
HGH
  human growth hormone
HGPRT
  hypoxanthine-phosphoribosyltransferase
    HGPRT deficiency
HGSIL
  high-grade squamous intraepithelial
  lesion
HGV
  hepatitis G virus
HHA
  hereditary hemolytic anemia
  hyposmia-hypogonadotropic
  hypogonadism
HHEs
  hypotonic-hyporesponsive episodes
HHH
  hyperornithemia, hyperammonemia,
  homocitrulinemia
    HHH syndrome
HHHO
  hypotonia, hypopigmentia,
  hypogonadism, obesity
    HHHO syndrome
HHS
  Hoyeraal-Hreidarsson syndrome
HHT
  hereditary hemorrhagic telangiectasia
HHV1–8
  human herpesvirus 1–8
HI
  hemagglutination inhibition
    HI antibody
    HI titer

5-HIAA
  5-hydroxyindoleacetic acid
21-HIAA
  21-hydroxyindoleacetic acid
hiatal hernia, hiatus hernia
hiatus, *pl.* **hiatus**
  diaphragmatic h.
  esophageal h.
  h. hernia, microcephaly, nephrosis
  syndrome
  h. leukemicus
  urogenital h.
HIB
  hypoxia, intussusception, brain
  mass
Hib
  Haemophilus influenzae type b
    HiB conjugate vaccine
    HiB polysaccharide vaccine
Hibiclens
Hibistat
HibTITER vaccine
HIC
  hepatic iron concentration
hiccough (*var. of* hiccup)
hiccup, hiccough
  fetal h.
hickey
Hickman catheter
Hicks version
Hi-Cor-1.0 Topical
Hi-Cor-2.5 Topical
hidden
  h. penis
  h. rheumatoid factor
  h. testis
hidradenitis suppurativa
hidradenoma, hydradenoma
  clear cell h.
  eruptive h.
  papillary h.
hidrotic ectodermal dysplasia
HIE
  hypoxic-ischemic encephalopathy
HIFT
  high-frequency ventilation trial
high
  h. airway obstruction syndrome
  h. anular testis
  h. arch foot
  h. bladder pressure
  h. fetal order
  h. forceps
  h. forceps delivery
  h. frequency (HF)
  h. frontal bone
  h. gastrin level
  h. guard
  h. hymenal opening

h. imperforate anus
h. intrauterine insemination
h. McCall culdoplasty
h. molecular weight (HMW)
h. molecular weight kininogen (HMWK)
h. myopia
h. output
h. oxygen percentage (HOPE)
h. oxygen percentage in retinopathy of prematurity (HOPE-ROP)
h. pain threshold
h. risk
h. scrotal testis
h. sensory threshold
h. stirrups
h. tone
h. urogenital sinus
h. uterosacral ligament suspension
high-affinity hemoglobin
high-altitude
h.-a. cerebral edema (HACE)
h.-a. perinatal mortality
h.-a. pulmonary edema (HAPE)
high-arched palate
high-caloric density formula
high-calorie
h.-c. diet
h.-c. formula
high-contrast Bucky imaging
high-density lipoprotein (HDL)
high-dose
h.-d. chemotherapy (HDC)
h.-d. chemotherapy with autologous bone marrow transplantation (HDC-ABMT)
h.-d. therapy
h.-d. therapy with epinephrine (HDE)
high-efficiency particulate air (HEPA)
higher-order
h.-o. birth
h.-o. gestation
high-fiber diet
high-flow
h.-f. nasal cannula
h.-f. nonrebreather
high-frequency
h.-f. flow interruption (HFFI)
h.-f. hearing loss
h.-f. jet (HFJ)
h.-f. jet ventilation (HFJV)
h.-f. oscillation (HFO)
h.-f. oscillator
h.-f. oscillatory ventilation (HFOV)
h.-f. positive-pressure (HFPP)
h.-f. positive-pressure ventilation (HFPPV)
h.-f. ventilation (HFV)

h.-f. ventilation trial (HIFT)
h.-f. ventilator
high-fructose formula
high-functioning autism (HFA)
high-glucose formula
high-grade
h.-g. cervical dysplasia
h.-g. squamous intraepithelial lesion (ASC-H, HGSIL, HSIL)
high-intensity click stimulus
highly
h. active antiretroviral therapy (HAART)
h. active retroviral therapy
h. purified factor IX
h. purified FSH
high-oscillation ventilator
high-output failure
high-performance
h.-p. capillary electrophoresis (HPCE)
h.-p. liquid chromatography (HPLC)
high-phosphate diet
high-pitched
h.-p. bowel sounds
h.-p. cry
h.-p. voice
h.-p. wheeze
high-power
h.-p. field
h.-p. liquid chromatography (HPLC)
high-pressure liquid chromatography (HPLC)
high-resolution
h.-r. banding
h.-r. chest computed tomography
h.-r. computed tomography (HRCT)
h.-r. ultrasonography
h.-r. ultrasound
high-risk (HR)
h.-r. consort
h.-r. infant
h.-r. mother
h.-r. obstetrician
h.-r. partner
h.-r. patient
h.-r. pregnancy (HRP)
h.-r. pregnancy assessment
h.-r. register (HRR)
h.-r. sex
high-tone hearing loss
high-voltage slow activity (HVSA)
Higoumenakis sign
hilar
h. cell hyperplasia
h. cell pathology
h. cell tumor
h. dance

hilar (*continued*)
    h. lymphadenopathy
    h. region
Hilgenreiner line
Hillis-DeLee fetoscope
Hillis-Müller maneuver
hilus cell tumor
hindbrain
hindfoot
    h. fracture
    h. valgus
    h. valgus deformity
hindgut
hind milk
hindwaters
hinge
    knee h.
hinged spring diaphragm
Hinman syndrome
Hinton test
hip
    h. adduction release
    h. bone density
    h. click
    h. clunk
    congenital dislocated h. (CDH)
    congenital dislocation of h. (CDH)
    h. deformity
    developmental displacement of h. (DDH)
    developmental dysplasia of h. (DDH)
    dislocated h.
    h. dysplasia
    h. fracture
    incongruent h.
    irritable h.
    neurogenic dysplasia of h. (NDH)
    nonspherical congruent h.'s
    observation h.
    h. pointer
    h. rotation
    h. rotation test
    snapping h.
    spherical congruent h.'s
    h. spica cast
    subluxed h.
    transient marrow edema syndrome of h. (TMES)
hip-knee-ankle angle
hip-knee-ankle-foot orthosis (HKAFO)
hippocampal
    h. neuron
    h. pathologic injury
    h. sclerosis (HS)
hippocampus
hippocratic nail
hippurate
    methenamine h.

hippus
    respiratory h.
Hiprex
Hirschberg
    H. corneal reflex test
    H. light reflex test
hirschfeldii
    Salmonella h.
Hirschsprung
    H. colitis
    H. disease
    H. enterocolitis
Hirst placental forceps
hirsute woman
hirsuties (*var. of* hirsutism)
hirsutism, hirsuties
    h., androgen excess, insulin resistance, acanthosis nigricans (HAIR-AN)
    constitutional h.
    drug-induced h.
    familial h.
    hormonal h.
    idiopathic h.
    male-pattern h.
    moderate h.
    postmenopausal h.
    h., skeletal dysplasia, mental retardation syndrome
hirudin
his
    angle of H.
    bundle of H.
    gastroesophageal angle of H.
    H. rule
Hispanic
His-Purkinje system
Histadyl
Histalet Forte Tablet
histaminase
histamine (H)
    h. 1 (H_1)
    h. 2 (H_2)
    h. 1 antihistamine
    h. fish poisoning
    h. interleukin
Histantil
Histatan
histidase
histidine
histidinemia
histidinuria
histiocyte, histocyte
    Gaucher-type h.
    sea-blue h.
histiocytic
    h. disorder
    h. fibroma
    h. lymphoma

histiocytoid cardiomyopathy
histiocytoma
 malignant fibrous h. (MFH)
histiocytosis, histocytosis
 acute disseminated h.
 Langerhans cell h. (LCH)
 malignant h.
 sinus h.
 h. X
histochemical
histocompatibility
 h. gene
 h. locus antigen
 maternal-fetal h.
histocyte (*var. of* histiocyte)
histocytic necrotizing lymphadenitis
histocytosis (*var. of* histiocytosis)
Histofreezer portable cryosurgical
 system
histogenesis
histoimmunological origin
histoincompatibility
 maternal-fetal h.
histologic, histological
 h. abnormality
 h. architecture
 h. chorioamnionitis
 h. classification
 h. diagnosis
 h. placental inflammation
 h. sampling
 h. subtype
histological (*var. of* histologic)
histology
 endometrial h.
 proliferative h.
 Shimada h.
 Shimada-Chatten h.
histolytica
 Entamoeba h.
histomorphometry
histone
 h. antigen
 h. H1 kinase
histopathological
 h. diagnosis
 h. finding
 h. grading
 h. study
histopathologic subtype
histopathology
Histoplasma capsulatum
histoplasmosis
 chronic pulmonary h.
 disseminated h. (DH)
 infantile disseminated h.
 pulmonary h.
history
 climacteric h.

 contraceptive h.
 family h.
 family cancer h.
 genetic h.
 gynecologic h.
 maternal h.
 menstrual h. (MH)
 obstetric h.
 occupational h.
 h. of present illness (HPI)
 paternal h.
 personal hygiene h.
 prenatal h.
 reproductive h.
 sexual h.
 sudden infant death unexplained by
  h.
 urologic h.
histrelin acetate
HIT
 heparin-induced thrombocytopenia
Hitachi
 H. EUB 420 digital ultrasound
 H. EUB 405 imaging system
 H. UB 420 digital ultrasound
  system
hitchhiker's thumb
2-hit hypothesis
HITS
 hurt, insult, threat, scream
 HITS scale
Hitzig girdle
HIV
 human immunodeficiency virus
 HIV classification
 HIV Classification for Children (P0,
  P1, P2)
 HIV Epidemiology Research
  (HER)
 HIV immunization
 HIV infected
 HIV infection
 HIV microangiopathy
 HIV test
HIV-1
 human immunodeficiency virus-1
 HIV-1 p24 antigen
 HIV-1 RNA PCR assay
HIVAGEN test
HIVAN
 HIV-associated nephropathy
HIV-associated nephropathy
 (HIVAN)
Hi-Vegi-Lip
hives
Hivid
HIVIG, HIVIg
 human immunodeficiency virus
  immunoglobulin

H

hiving
HIV-seropositive
HKAFO
    hip-knee-ankle-foot orthosis
        Rochester HKAFO
HL
    heel lance
    humerus length
HLA
    human leukocyte antigen
        HLA typing
HLA-A3
HLA-A10
HLA-B
HLA-B27 antigen
HLA-B5/B51
HLA-B27-positive
HLA-compatible fetus
HLA-DR
HLA-DR7
HLA-DRw11
HLA-DRw53
HLA-identical
        HLA-i. haploidentical bone marrow
          stem cell
        HLA-i. marrow graft
HLA-matched platelet transfusion
HLA-mismatch
HLHS
    hypoplastic left heart syndrome
HLI
    human leukocyte interferon
HLL
    hypoplasia of left heart
HLP
    hyperlipoproteinemia
HM
    hemifacial microsomia
    human milk
HMB
    hydroxy beta methylbutyrate
HMC
    hypertelorism, microtia, clefting
        HMC syndrome
HMD
    hyaline membrane disease
        neonatal HMD
HMDS
    hexamethyldislazane
HME
    human monocytic ehrlichiosis
HMF
    human milk fortifier
hMG
    human menopausal gonadotropin
HMG-CoA reductase inhibitor
hMG/IUI
HMO
    health maintenance organization

HMPAO
    hexamethyl propylene amine oxime
        HMPAO leukocyte scintigraphy
HMS Liquifilm
HMSN
    hereditary motor-sensory neuropathy
        (type IA, II–VII)
HMW
    high molecular weight
        HMW dextran
HMWK
    high molecular weight kininogen
        HMWK deficiency
        HMWK factor
HN
    hemorrhage of newborn
HNF
    hepatocyte nuclear factor
HNPCC
    hereditary nonpolyposis colon
        cancer
    hereditary nonpolyposis colorectal
        cancer
HNPP
    hereditary neuropathy with liability to
        pressure palsy
HNU
    human *neu* unit
H_2O
    water
        H_2O syndrome
HOA
    hypertrophic osteoarthropathy
hoarding
    fecal h.
hoarse
    h. cry
    h. voice
hoarseness
    excessive h.
hobnail cell
Hoboken
    fold of H.
    H. gemmule
    H. nodule
HOBT
    hyperbaric oxygen therapy
hockey stick incision
Hodge
    H. forceps
    H. maneuver
    H. with knob pessary
Hodgkin
    H. disease
    H. lymphoma
Hoehne sign
HOF
    human oviduct fluid
Hofbauer cell

Hoffer procedure
Hoffmann
   H. clamp
   H. reflex
Hogben test
Hogness box
Hohn catheter
holandric
   h. gene
   h. inheritance
holarctica
   Francisella tularensis h.
hold
   h. clot
   h. clot order
   H. DM
   football h.
   Madonna h.
   h. technique
   type and h. (T&H)
holder
   Cameco syringe h.
   Crile-Wood needle h.
   Dale Foley catheter h.
   Elephant Ears bottle h.
   Endo-Assist endoscopic
    needle h.
   Heaney needle h.
   Mayo-Hegar needle h.
   needle h.
   Wangensteen needle h.
   Wolf-Castroviejo needle h.
holding
   breath h.
   h. chamber
hole
   h. in heart
   Murphy h.
holiday
   drug h.
   weekend drug h.
Holinger
   H. infant bougie
   H. infant bronchoscope
   H. infant esophageal speculum
   H. infant esophagoscope
   H. infant laryngoscope
Holliday-Segar method
Hollingshead 5-factor index
Hollister collecting device
hollow
   h. of sacrum
   h. viscera
Holmes heart
holmium:yttrium-aluminum-garnet
  (Ho:YAG)
holoacardius
holoacranial
holoblastic ovum

holocarboxylase (HCS)
   h. synthetase
   h. synthetase deficiency
holocrine sebaceous gland
hologastroschisis
Hologic
   H. 1000 QDR densitometer
   H. 1000 QDR dual-energy
    absorptiometer
hologynic inheritance
holoprosencephalic proboscis
holoprosencephaly (HPE)
   alobar h.
   h. anomalad
   familial alobar h.
   lobar h.
   semilobar h.
holorachischisis
holosphere
   cerebral h.
holosystolic murmur
holovisceral
Holtain height stadiometer
Holter monitor
Holt-Oram
   H.-O. atriodigital dysplasia
   H.-O. syndrome
Holzgreve syndrome
Homans sign
homatropine
HOME
   Home Observation for the
   Measurement of the Environment
   HOME scale
home
   h. antibiotic infusion therapy
   h. birth
   h. blood glucose monitoring
   h. cardiorespiratory monitor
   (HCRM)
   h. care service
   h. cognitive score
   h. conservative management
   h. factor
   h. life, education level, activities,
   drug use, sexual activity
   (HEADS)
   h. life, education level, activities,
   drug use, sexual activity, suicide
   ideation/attempts (HEADSS)
   h. management
   H. Observation for the Measurement
   of the Environment (HOME)
   h. oxygen
   h. parenteral nutrition (HPN)
   h. pregnancy test
   h. uterine activity monitor (HUAM)
   h. uterine activity monitoring
   (HUAM)

H

417

home (*continued*)
    h. uterine monitoring (HUM)
homemade formula
homeobox (HOX)
    h. 2 gene
    short stature h. (SHOX)
homeopathy
homeostasis
    bacterial h.
    body h.
    carbohydrate h.
    cardiorespiratory h.
    copper h.
    fluid h.
    thermal h.
homeostatic lag
homeothermy
    servocontrolled h.
homeotic genes
Homer Wright rosette
homicide
    intimate partner h.
hominis
    Blastocystis h.
    Cardiobacterium h.
    herpesvirus h. (HVH)
    Mycoplasma h.
    Poliovirus h.
homochronous inheritance
homocitrulinemia
    hyperornithemia, hyperammonemia,
    h. (HHH)
homocitrullinemia
homocitrullinuria
    hyperammonemia, hyperornithinemia,
    h.
homocysteine loading test
homocystine
homocystinemia
homocystinuria
homoduplex DNA
homogamete
homogeneity
    tissue h.
homogeneous vaginal discharge
homogenize
homogenous
homograft conduit
homokaryon
homolateral weakness
homolog (*var. of* homologue)
HomoloGene
homologous
    h. chromosome
    h. disease
    h. insemination
    h. recombination
    h. surfactant
    h. uterine sarcoma

homologue, homolog
    DAZL1 autosomal h.
homology
homonymous hemianopia
homophilic
homoplasmy
    mutant h.
homosexuality
homothermic
homotropic inheritance
homotypic, homotypical
homotypical (*var. of* homotypic)
homovanillic acid (HVA)
homozygote
homozygous
    h. achondroplasia
    h. familial hypercholesterolemia
    h. glucose-6-phosphate dehydrogenase
    deficiency
    h. hemoglobin E
    h. hyperlipidemia (type I, II)
    h. sickle cell anemia
    h. thalassemia
honei
    Rickettsia h.
honeybee allergy
honeycombed appearance
honeycomb lung
honey-crusted plaque
honeymoon cystitis
Honvol
hood
    clitoral h.
    dorsal h.
    h. mist
    h. O_2
    h. oxygen
    oxygen h.
    Oxyhood oxygen h.
    H. procedure
    Rock-Mulligan h.
    vaginal h.
hook
    Mayo h.
    tenaculum h.
    h. traction technique
hooking maneuver
hookworm
    h. disease
    h. infection
Hootnick-Holmes syndrome
HOP
    hypothalamic-pituitary-ovarian
    hypothyroxinemia of prematurity
HOPE
    health, osteoporosis, progestin,
    estrogen
    high oxygen percentage
hopelessness

Hope resuscitation bag
HOPE-ROP
    high oxygen percentage in retinopathy
    of prematurity
      HOPE-ROP study
Hopkins
    H. Lupus Pregnancy Center
    H. symptom checklist
    H. syndrome
hopping
    bunny h.
5-hop test
hora somni
hordeolum
    external h.
    internal h.
horizon
    H. 2000
    Streeter h.
horizontal
    h. nystagmus
    h. saccadic gaze paresis
    h. supranuclear gaze palsy
    h. suspension
    h. suspension in newborn
    h. transmission
    h. transmission of virus
hormonal
    h. abnormality
    h. antineoplastic therapy
    h. balance change
    h. contraceptive
    h. effect
    h. emergency contraception
    h. environment
    h. factor
    h. hirsutism
    h. implant
    h. level
    h. manipulation
    h. pregnancy test tablet
    h. treatment
hormonally responsive tumor
hormone
    adrenal androgen-stimulating h.
      (AASH)
    adrenocortical h.
    adrenocorticotropic h. (ACTH)
    alpha-melanocyte-stimulating h.
      (alpha-MSH)
    antenatal thyrotropin releasing h.
    anterior pituitary-like h.
    antidiuretic h. (ADH)
    antimüllerian h. (AMH)
    h. assay
    atrial natriuretic h. (ANH)
    bioactive h.
    bioidentical h.
    calciotropic h.

cancer and steroid h. (CASH)
h. chemoprevention
chorionic gonadotropic h. (CGH)
chorionic growth h.
circulating h.
h. complex receptor
cortical androgen-stimulating h.
    (CASH)
corticotropin-releasing h. (CRH)
h. deficiency
endogenous h.
exogenous h.
fetal h.
follicle-stimulating h. (FSH)
Genentech biosynthetic human
    growth h.
glycoprotein h.
gonadotropic h. (GDH, GTH)
gonadotropin-releasing h. (GnRH,
    GRH)
growth h. (GH)
growth hormone-releasing h.
    (GH-RH)
human chorionic adrenocorticotropic
    h.
human follicle-stimulating h.
    (hFSH)
human growth h. (hGH, HGH)
human urinary follicle-stimulating h.
    (hu-FSH)
Humatrope growth h.
hypothalamic luteinizing
    hormone-releasing h.
inappropriate antidiuretic h. (IADH)
LATS h.
luteinizing h. (LH)
luteinizing hormone-releasing h.
    (LH-RH)
lutein-stimulating h. (LSH)
luteotropic h.
melanocortin-stimulating h. (MSH)
melanocyte-stimulating h.
müllerian inhibiting h. (MIH)
ovarian h.
parathyroid h. (PTH)
peptide h.
pituitary h.
placental h.
placental growth h. (PGH)
pregnancy h.
purified h.
recombinant follicle stimulating h.
    (rFSH)
recombinant human growth h.
    (rhGH)
h. replacement therapy (HRT)
serum parathyroid h.
sex h. (SH)
Somatrem growth h.

H

hormone (*continued*)
Somatropin growth h.
steroid h.
syndrome of inappropriate secretion
of antidiuretic h. (SIADH)
h. therapy
thyroid h.
thyroid-stimulating h. (TSH)
thyrotropic h.
thyrotropin releasing h. (TRH)
tropic h.
urinary-derived human
follicle-stimulating h. (u-hFSH)
urinary luteinizing h. (uLH)
hormone-producing neoplasm
hormone-receptor complex
internalization
hormone-secreting tumor
hormone-stimulated endometrial
change
hormonogenesis
hormonotherapy
horn
h. cell disease
entrapped temporal h.
frontal h.
fused frontal h.
iliac h.
noncommunicating uterine h.
h. of uterus
rudimentary uterine h.
uterine h.
1-horned uterus
Horner syndrome
hornet sting
horse-riding stance
horseshoe
h. fibrosis
h. kidney
h. placenta
HOS
hypoosmotic swelling
hospice care
hospital
H. for Sick Children (HSC)
H. Recliner seat
h. stabilization
St. Jude Research H.
tertiary referral h.
Texas Scottish Rite H. (TSRH)
hospitalization
antepartum h.
prolonged delivery h.
hospitalized
h. attempted suicide (HAS)
h. bed rest
host
h. defense mechanism
h. response mechanism

hot
h. biopsy
h. biopsy forceps
h. cross bun skull
h. flash
h. flush
h. knife conization
h. nodule
h. potato voice
h. tub folliculitis
hotline center
Hottentot apron
hour
cubic centimeter per h. (cc/hr)
h. of sleep
Sudafed 12 H.
1-hour
1-h. glucose challenge
1-h. glucose challenge test
1-h. glucose tolerance test
1-h. PG
1-h. prostaglandin
24-hour
Claritin-D 24-H.
24-h. urinary free cortisol
24-h. urine collection
hourglass
h. configuration
h. head
h. uterus
5-hour glucose tolerance test
8-hour polysomnography
4-hour rule
hour-specific total serum bilirubin
72-hour stool collection
house dust mite
household
housekeeping gene
housemaid's knee
Howell biopsy aspiration needle
Howell-Jolly body
HOX
homeobox
HOX A gene
Hoxa5 null mutant
Ho:YAG
holmium:yttrium-aluminum-garnet
Ho:YAG laser
Hoyeraal-Hreidarsson syndrome (HHS)
H.P.
H.P. acthar gel
Mission Prenatal H.P.
HP
Ku-Zyme HP
Profasi HP
HPA
human pancreatic amylase
human platelet antigen
hypothalamic-pituitary-adrenal

hypothalamic-pituitary axis
  HPA axis
  HPA dysfunction
HPCE
  high-performance capillary
  electrophoresis
HPE
  holoprosencephaly
hpf
  high-power field
HPFH
  hereditary persistence of fetal
  hemoglobin
HPH
  hypoxia-induced pulmonary
  hypertension
HPI
  history of present illness
hPL
  human placental lactogen
HPL
  human placental lactogen
HPLC
  high-performance liquid chromatography
  high-power liquid chromatography
  high-pressure liquid chromatography
HPN
  home parenteral nutrition
HPO
  hypothalamic-pituitary-ovarian
    HPO axis
HPOA
  hypothalamic-pituitary-ovarian axis
HPP
  hereditary pyropoikilocytosis
HPS
  hepatopulmonary syndrome
  hypertrophic pyloric stenosis
HPV
  Haemophilus pertussis vaccine
  human papillomavirus
  human parvovirus
    HPV B19
    HPV E7 gene
    HPV screen
    HPV type 16 capsid antibody
    HPV vaccine
HPV-associated lesion
HR
  heart rate
H-*ras*
    H-*ras* oncogene
    H-*ras* p21 protein
HRCT
  high-resolution computed tomography
HRIG
  human rabies immunoglobulin
HRP
  high-risk pregnancy

HRQOL
  health-related quality of life
    HRQOL assessment
    HRQOL questionnaire
HRR
  haplotype relative risk
  high-risk register
HRSA
  heart rate power spectral analysis
HRT
  hormone replacement therapy
    estrogen-only HRT
HRV
  heart rate variability
h.s.
  hora somni
HS
  habitual snoring
  herpes simplex
  hysterosalpingography
    Estratest HS
HSC
  hemopoietic stem cell
  Hospital for Sick Children
    HSC Scale
HSD2
  hydroxysteroid dehydrogenase
    type 2
HSDD
  hypoactive sexual desire disorder
HSE
  herpes simplex encephalitis
H/S Elliptosphere catheter set
HSES
  hemorrhagic shock and encephalopathy
  syndrome
HSG
  herpes simplex genitalis
  hysterosalpingogram
  hysterosalpingography
    HSG tray
HSI
  human seminal inhibitor
HSIL
  high-grade squamous intraepithelial
  lesion
HSP
  Henoch-Schönlein purpura
HS-tk gene therapy
HSV
  herpes simplex virus
HSV-1, HSV1
  herpes simplex virus 1
HSV-2, HSV2
  herpes simplex virus 2
    HSV2 proctitis
HTA
  hydrothermablation
  Hydro ThermAblator

H

HTLV
    human T-cell leukemia virus
HTLV-I
    human T-cell lymphotropic virus
      type I
      HTLV-I associated
        myelopathy/tropical spastic
        paraparesis
HTLV-II
    human T-cell lymphotropic virus
      type II
HTP
    hypothalamic, pituitary, thyroid
5-HTT
    serotonin transporter 5-H.
H-type
    H-t. tracheoesophageal fistula
    H-t. transesophageal fistula
HUAM
    home uterine activity monitor
    home uterine activity monitoring
huang
    ma h.
HuCNS-SC stem cell
HuCV
    human calicivirus
Hudson
    H. prongs
    H. T Up-Draft II disposable nebulizer
hue
    blue scleral h.
    purple h.
    violaceous h.
    white scleral h.
huffing
Huffman
    H. adolescent speculum
    H. vaginal speculum
    H. vaginoscope
hu-FSH
    human urinary follicle-stimulating
    hormone
HuGE
    Human Gene Expression
    Human Genome Expression
    HuGE index
HuGENet
    Human Genome Epidemiology
    Network
Hughes syndrome
Huguier circle
Huhner-Sims test
Huhner test
HUI
    Harris uterine injector
    HUI Mini-Flex
Hulka
    H. clip
    H. tenaculum

Hulka-Clemens clip
hum
    benign venous h.
    cervical venous h.
    venous h.
Humalog
    H. insulin lispro injection
    H. Pen
human
    h. antihemophilic factor
    h. artificial chromosome
    (HAC)
    h. astrovirus type 1 (HAstV-1)
    h. bite
    h. calicivirus (HuCV)
    h. chorionic adrenocorticotropic
    hormone
    h. chorionic gonadotropin (HCG,
    hCG)
    h. chorionic gonadotropin level
    h. diploid cell rabies vaccine
    (HDCV)
    h. diploid cell vaccine
    h. embryo fibroblast (HEF)
    h. endothelial cell (HEC)
    h. epidermal growth factor-2
    oncogene
    h. EP1 receptor
    h. erythropoietin
    h. factor IX complex
    H. Fertilization and Embryology
    Authority (HFEA)
    h. figure drawing
    H. Figure Drawing Test
    h. follicle-stimulating hormone
    (hFSH)
    H. Gene Expression (HuGE)
    h. gene therapy
    h. genetics
    H. Genome Epidemiology Network
    (HuGENET, HuGENet)
    H. Genome Expression (HuGE)
    H. Genome Project
    h. granulocytic ehrlichiosis
    (HGE)
    h. growth hormone (hGH, HGH)
    h. health and behavior questionnaire
    (HBQ)
    h. herpesvirus 1–8 (HHV1–8)
    h. immunodeficiency virus (HIV)
    h. immunodeficiency virus-1
    (HIV-1)
    h. immunodeficiency virus
    encephalopathy
    h. immunodeficiency virus
    immunoglobulin (HIVIg,
    HIVIG)
    h. immunodeficiency virus infected
    children

h. immunoglobulin
Insulatard NPH h.
h. insulin
h. insulin-induced lipoatrophy
h. jagged-1 gene (JAG1)
h. leukocyte antigen (HLA)
h. leukocyte antigen-associated
disorder
h. leukocyte interferon (HLI)
h. lymphocyte antigen-locus DR
h. menopausal gonadotropin (hMG)
h. metapneumovirus
h. milk (HM)
H. Milk Banking Association of
North America
h. milk-fed
h. milk fortifier (HMF)
h. monocytic ehrlichiosis (HME)
Nabi-HB hepatitis B immune
globulin h.
h. neutrophil collagenase
h. *neu* unit (HNU)
h. oviduct fluid (HOF)
h. ovum fertilization test
h. pancreatic amylase (HPA)
h. papillomavirus (HPV)
h. papovavirus BK
h. parvovirus (HPV)
h. parvovirus arthropathy
h. placental lactogen (hPL)
h. platelet antigen (HPA)
h. rabies immunoglobulin (HRIG)
h. recombinant antioxidant
enzyme
h. recombinant DNase
h. scabies
h. seminal inhibitor (HSI)
h. sperm cytosolic factor
H. Surf surfactant
h. T-cell leukemia virus (HTLV)
h. T-cell leukemia virus type I, II,
III
h. T-cell lymphotrophic virus type I
associated myelopathy (HAM)
h. T-cell lymphotropic virus 1
tropic meloneuropathy
h. T-cell lymphotropic virus type I
(HTLV-I)
h. T-cell lymphotropic virus type II
(HTLV-II)
h. umbilical vein endothelial cell
(HUVEC)
h. urinary follicle-stimulating
hormone (hu-FSH)
Velosulin H.
humanus
Pediculus h.
Humate-P
Humatin

Humatrope
H. growth hormone
H. Injection
HumatroPen
Humegon
humeroperoneal muscular dystrophy
humeroradial synostosis
humerus length (HL)
HUMI
Harris-Kronner uterine
manipulator-injector
HUMI catheter
Humibid L.A.
humidification
h. therapy
h. ventilator
humidified
h. air
h. isolette
humidifier
bubbler h.
cool-mist h.
Ohio h.
humid stertor
humor
aqueous h.
vitreous h.
humoral
h. antibody
h. antibody deficiency
h. factor
h. immune system
h. immunity
h. immunodeficiency
hump
buffalo h.
dowager's h.
dromedary h.
rib h.
Humulin
H. 50/50
H. 70/30
H. L
H. N
H. Pen
H. R
H. U
Hünermann disease
Hünermann-Happle syndrome
hunger
air h.
unusual h.
Hunner
H. interstitial cystitis
H. ulcer
Hunt bipolar forceps
hunter
H. canal
H. syndrome

H

Hunter-Fraser syndrome
Hunter-Hurler phenotype
hunterian chancre
Hunter-MacMurray syndrome
Hunter-McAlpine craniosynostosis
syndrome
Huntington
    H. chorea
    H. disease (HD)
    polyglutamine-expanded H.
Hunt-Reich cannula
Hurler
    H. disease
    H. syndrome
    H. variant
Hurler-like
    H.-l. facial appearance
    H.-l. syndrome
Hurler-Pfaundler syndrome
Hurler-Scheie syndrome
hurry
    intestinal h.
Hurst syndrome
Hürthle cell
hurt, insult, threat, scream (HITS)
Hurwitz catheter
HUS
    hemolytic uremic syndrome
husband
    artificial insemination by h. (AIH)
    therapeutic insemination, h. (TIH)
HUT
    head-up tilt
Hutch diverticulum
Hutchinson
    H. incisor
    H. sign
    H. syndrome
    H. teeth
    H. triad
Hutchinson-Gilford progeria
syndrome
hutchinsonian molar
Hutinel disease
Hutterite cerebroosteonephrodysplasia
HUVEC
    human umbilical vein endothelial
    cell
HUVS
    hypocomplementemic urticarial
    vasculitis syndrome
Huxley respirator
HV
    height velocity
    herpesvirus
HVA
    homovanillic acid
HVC
    hepatitis C virus

HVEM
    herpes virus entry mediator
HVL
    half-value layer
HVSA
    high-voltage slow activity
hyaline, hyaloid
    h. body
    h. cast
    h. eosinophilic inclusion
    h. membrane
    h. membrane disease (HMD)
    h. membrane syndrome
    h. myoma degeneration
hyalinosis
    h. cutis et mucosae
    infantile system h.
hyaloid (var. of hyaline)
hyaluronic acid factor
hyaluronidase factor
H-Y antigen
Hyate:C
Hybolin
    H. Decanoate
    H. Improved
hybrid
    H. Capture DNA Assay
    somatic h.
hybridization
    allele-specific oligonucleotide h.
    colorimetric reverse dot blot h.
    comparative genomic h.
    (CGH)
    DNA h.
    dot-blot h.
    fluorescent in situ h. (FISH)
    genomic in situ h.
    in situ nucleic acid h.
    multispectral fluorescent in situ h.
    (M-FISH)
    nucleic acid h.
    papillomavirus h.
    polar body in situ h.
    prenatal interphase fluorescence in
    situ h.
    reverse dot blot h.
hybridoma technique
Hybritech
Hycamtin
hyclate
    doxycycline h.
Hycodan
Hycort Topical
hydantoin syndrome
hydatid
    h. cyst
    h. cyst of Morgagni
    h. disease
    h. mole

h. polyp
h. pregnancy
hydatidiform
h. change
h. mole
hydatidosis
alveolar h.
Hyde-Förster syndrome
Hyderm
hydermia
hydradenoma (*var. of* hidradenoma)
hydralazine
hydramnion (*var. of* hydramnios)
hydramnios, hydramnion
idiopathic h.
hydranencephaly
hydrate
chloral h.
hydration
intravenous h.
maternal h.
hydraulic UF
hydrazide
isonicotinic acid h. (INH)
hydrazine sulfate
Hydrea
Droxia H.
hydrencephalocele, hydrocephalocele,
hydroencephalocele
hydrencephalomeningocele
hydriodic acid
hydroa
h. aestivale
h. gestationis
h. puerorum
h. vacciniforme
hydroalcoholic
hydrocarbon
aliphatic h.
halogenated h.
h. pneumonia
hydrocele
abdominoscrotal h.
h. feminae
h. fluid
Maunoir h.
h. muliebris
Nuck h.
owl's eye view of h.
transitory h.
hydrocelectomy
hydrocephalic
h. brain swelling
h. idiocy
h. lissencephaly
hydrocephalocele
hydrocephaloid disease
hydrocephalus, hydrocephaly
acquired h.

acute h.
h., agyria, retinal dysplasia (HARD)
h., agyria, retinal dysplasia with or
without encephalocele (HARD+/-E)
arrested h.
benign external h.
chronic h.
communicating h.
compensated h.
corpus callosum hypoplasia,
retardation, adducted thumbs,
spastic paraparesis, h. (CRASH)
external h.
h. ex vacuo
h. internus
LICAM gene for X-linked h.
new-onset h.
noncommunicating h.
normal pressure h. (NPH)
obstructive h.
otitic h.
permanent posthemorrhagic h.
posthemorrhagic h. (PHH)
shunt-dependent h.
shunted h.
h., skeletal anomalies, mental
disturbances syndrome
symptomatic progressive h.
uncompensated h.
h. with features of VATER
X-linked h.
hydrocephalus-cerebellar agenesis
syndrome
hydrocephaly (*var. of* hydrocephalus)
Hydrocet
Hydro-chlor
hydrochloride (HCl)
arginine h.
Aventyl H.
betaine h.
bupropion h.
buspirone h.
butriptyline h.
cetirizine h.
chlorcyclizine h.
ciprofloxacin h.
clomipramine h.
clonidine h.
cyclopentolate h.
cycrimine h.
cyproheptadine h.
cysteine h.
dicyclomine h.
dihydromorphinone h.
dobutamine h.
dopamine h.
doxapram h.
doxorubicin h.
duloxetine h.

H

hydrochloride (*continued*)
    esmolol h.
    ethopropazine h.
    fluoxetine h.
    guanfacine h.
    imipramine h.
    isoprenaline h.
    levalbuterol h.
    liposomal doxorubicin h.
    loperamide h.
    mechlorethamine h.
    meclizine h.
    mefloquine h.
    meperidine h.
    mepivacaine h.
    methacycline h.
    methadone h.
    methamphetamine h.
    methdilazine h.
    methixene h.
    methoxamine h.
    methylphenidate h.
    metoclopramide h.
    mitoxantrone h.
    Mustargen H.
    naftifine h.
    naloxone h.
    nortriptyline h.
    nylidrin h.
    olopatadine h.
    opipramol h.
    OROS methylphenidate h.
    paroxetine h.
    phenazopyridine h.
    piperidolate h.
    proguanil h.
    promethazine h.
    propranolol h.
    pseudoephedrine h.
    quinacrine h.
    ranitidine h.
    ritodrine h.
    ropivacaine h.
    sertraline h.
    sulfamethoxazole/phenazopyridine h.
    sulfisoxazole/phenazopyridine h.
    tetracycline h.
    thioridazine h.
    thiphenamil h.
    tolazoline h.
    topotecan h.
    trifluoperazine h.
    triflupromazine h.
    trimethobenzamide h.
    tripelennamine h.
    triprolidine h.
    valacyclovir h.
    vancomycin h.
    venlafaxine h.

hydrochloroquine
hydrochlorothiazide (HCTZ)
    h. and spironolactone
Hydrocil
hydrocodone and acetaminophen
hydrocolloid
hydrocolpocele, hydrocolpos
hydrocolpos (*var. of* hydrocolpocele)
hydrocortisone
    Bactine H.
    h. base
    h. butyrate
    h. cypionate
    neomycin, polymyxin B, h.
    h. sodium succinate
    h. valerate
Hydrocortone
    H. Acetate Injection
    H. Oral
    H. Phosphate Injection
Hydrocort Topical
hydrocystoma
    apocrine h.
    vulvar apocrine h.
hydrodensitometry
hydrodissection
hydrodistention
HydroDIURIL
hydroencephalocele (*var. of* hydrencephalocele)
hydroflotation
hydroflumethiazide
Hydrofluoroaklane (HFA)
hydrogel dressing
hydrogen
    h. bond
    h. breath test
    h. ion concentration (pH)
    h. peroxide
    h. peroxide enema
    h. peroxide-producing *Lactobacillus*
    h. pump inhibitor
Hydrogesic
hydrolase
    fumarylacetoacetate h. (FAH)
hydrolethalus syndrome
hydrolysate
    casein h.
    h. formula
    milk protein h. (MPH)
    protein h.
hydrolysis
    enzymic acid h.
    steroid conjugate h.
hydrolysis-resistant
hydrolyzed
    h. cow's milk
    h. feeding

h. premature formula
h. protein
h. whey
hydroma (*var. of* hygroma)
hydromeningocele
hydrometra
hydrometrocolpos
hydromicrocephaly
hydromorphone
hydromphalus
hydromucocolpos
hydromyelia
hydromyelocele
hydromyelomeningocele
**hydronephrocolpos-postaxial
  polydactyly-congenital heart disease
  syndrome**
hydronephrosis
congenital h.
fetal h.
intermittent h.
neonatal h.
perinatal h.
prenatal h.
progressive h.
unilateral neonatal h.
hydronephrotic kidney
hydroparasalpinx
hydroperoxide
total h. (TH)
hydropertubation
hydrophila
Aeromonas h.
hydrophilic ointment
hydrophobia
hydrophobic
**hydrophthalmia, hydrophthalmos,
  hydrophthalmus**
hydrophthalmos (*var. of* hydrophthalmia)
hydrophthalmus (*var. of* hydrophthalmia)
hydropic
h. chorionic villus
h. gallbladder
h. infant
h. placental villus
hydrops
fetal h.
h. fetalis
fetal nonimmune h.
h. folliculi
gallbladder h.
h. gravidarum
halo sign of h.
immune fetal h.
intrauterine h.
Kell h.
maternal h.
nonimmune fetal h.
h. ovarii

placental h.
h. tubae profluens
hydrops-like cholecystitis
hydroquinone
hydrorrhea
h. gravidae
h. gravidarum
hydrosalpinx
intermittent h.
hydrostatic
h. pressure
h. reduction
hydrosyringomyelia
Hydro-Tex Topical
hydrotherapy
hydrothermablation
hydrothorax
tension h.
hydrotubation
hydroureter
hydroureteronephrosis
hydrovarium
hydroxide
aluminum h.
magnesium h.
potassium h. (KOH)
sodium h.
hydroxocobalamin
11-hydroxyandrosterone
hydroxybenzoic acid (HABA)
hydroxy beta methylbutyrate (HMB)
hydroxybutyrate
hydroxychloroquine sulfate
25-hydroxycholecalciferol
17-hydroxycorticosteroid
hydroxyeicosatetraenoic acid
11-hydroxyetiocholanolone
5-hydroxyindoleacetic
5-h. acid (5-HIAA)
5-h. assay
21-hydroxyindoleacetic acid (21-HIAA)
hydroxyindole-*o*-methyltransferase
hydroxylase
h. enzyme defect
phenylalanine h. (PAH)
17-hydroxylase
17-h. deficiency
17-h. deficiency syndrome
21-hydroxylase
21-h. deficiency
21-h. deficiency syndrome
11-hydroxylase deficiency
hydroxylation
kynurenine h.
hydroxyl radical (OH)
hydroxylysine
3-hydroxy-3-methylglutaric aciduria
3-hydroxy-3-methylglutaryl coenzyme A
hydroxyphenyluria

H

17-hydroxypregnenolone
hydroxyprogesterone
    h. and estradiol valerate
    h. caproate
17-hydroxyprogesterone (17-OHP)
    1.-h. caproate
hydroxyproline
    proline h.
hydroxyprolinemia
15-hydroxyprostaglandin
  dehydrogenase
18-hydroxysteroid dehydrogenase
hydroxysteroid dehydrogenase type 2
  (HSD2)
hydroxytryptophan
    L-5 h.
hydroxyurea
1,25-hydroxyvitamin D
25-hydroxyvitamin-D3
hydroxyzine
hyfrecation
hyfrecator
Hy-Gestrone
hygiene
    perineal h.
    poor dental h.
    sleep h.
hygroma, hydroma
    cystic h.
    fetal cystic h.
    nuchal cystic h.
hygroscopic
    h. dilator
    h. rod
Hylorel
Hylutin
hymen
    h. bifenestratus
    h. biforis
    cribriform h.
    denticulate h.
    falciform h.
    imperforate h.
    infundibuliform h.
    microperforate h.
    redundant h.
    h. sculptatus
    septate h.
    stenotic h.
    h. subseptus
    vertical h.
    virginal h.
hymenal
    h. band
    h. injury
    h. membrane
    h. opening
    h. ring
    h. tag

hymenalis
    caruncula h.
hymenectomy
hymenitis
Hymenoptera
    H. sign
    H. venom
hymenorrhaphy
hymenotomy
hyobranchial cleft
hyoid
    h. bar
    h. bone
hyointestinalis
    Campylobacter h.
hyoscine
    Isopto H.
    h. methylbromide
hyoscyamine sulfate
Hyosophen
hypamnion, hypamnios
hypamnios (*var. of* hypamnion)
Hypaque Meglumine
Hyperab
hyperabduction
    thumb h.
hyperacidity
hyperactive
    h. bowel sounds
    h. distractible
    dominantly h.
    h. impulsivity
hyperactive/impulsive dimension
hyperactivity
    bronchial h.
    central serotonergic h.
    motor h.
hyperactivity/impulsivity domain
hyperacusia (*var. of* hyperacusis)
hyperacusis, hyperacusia
hyperacute
    h. infarction
    h. rejection
hyperadrenalism
hyperaeration
hyperaesthesia (*var. of* hyperesthesia)
hyperalaninemia
hyperaldosteronism
hyperalimentation (HA)
    central h.
    h. hepatitis
    Intralipid h.
    intravenous h. (IVH)
    parenteral h.
    Pedtrace-4 h.
    peripheral h.
    TrophAmine h.
hyperalimentation-associated cholestasis
hyperalphalipoproteinemia

hyperammonemia, hyperammoniemia
  cerebroatrophic h.
  h. due to ornithine
    transcarbamoylase deficiency
  h., hyperornithinemia,
    homocitrullinuria
  transient h.
  h. variant
hyperammonemic
  h. episode
  h. hepatic coma
  h. state
  h. syndrome
hyperammoniemia (var. of
  hyperammonemia)
hyperamylasemia
hyperandrogenemia
hyperandrogenemic chronic anovulation
  syndrome
hyperandrogenic
  h. anovulation (HA)
  h. chronic anovulation
hyperandrogenism
  adrenal h.
  cryptic h.
  h., insulin resistance, acanthosis
    nigricans (HAIRAN, HAIR-AN)
  ovarian h.
  h. reversal
hyperargininemia
hyperarousal
hyperbaric
  h. chamber
  h. oxygen
  h. oxygen therapy (HOBT)
  h. oxygen treatment
hyperbetalipoproteinemia (HBLP)
hyperbilirubinemia
  congenital nonhemolytic
    unconjugated h.
  conjugated h.
  direct h.
  extreme benign h.
  idiopathic h.
  indirect h.
  neonatal h.
  prolonged indirect h.
  prolonged unconjugated h.
  transient familial neonatal h.
  unconjugated h.
hyperbilirubinemic
hypercalcemia
  h. elfin-facies syndrome
  familial h.
  familial hypocalciuric h. (FHH)
  hypocalciuric h.
  idiopathic infantile h.
  infantile h.
  maternal h.

hypercalcemia/Williams-Beuren
  syndrome
hypercalcemic crisis
hypercalcinuria (var. of hypercalciuria)
hypercalciuria, hypercalcinuria,
  hypercalcuria
  absorptive h.
  autosomal recessive renal proximal
    tubulopathy and h. (ARPTH)
  renal h.
hypercalcuria (var. of hypercalciuria)
hypercaloric formula
hypercapnia, hypercarbia
  permissive h.
hypercapnic respiratory failure
hypercarbia
  fetal h.
hypercarotenemia
hypercellularity
  mesangial h.
  segmental mesangial h.
hyperchloremia
hyperchloremic
  h. metabolic acidosis
  h. renal acidosis
hypercholesteremia (var. of
  hypercholesterolemia)
hypercholesterinemia (var. of
  hypercholesterolemia)
hypercholesterolemia, hypercholesteremia,
  hypercholesterinemia
  familial h.
  heterozygous familial h.
  homozygous familial h.
hyperchromic acidosis
hypercinesia (var. of hyperkinesis)
hypercinesis (var. of hyperkinesis)
hypercoagulability
hypercoagulable state
hypercoagulation
hypercortisolism
hypercyanotic spell
hypercyesia (var. of hypercyesis)
hypercyesis, hypercyesia
hyperdactyly
hyperdibasicaminoaciduria
hyperdiploid
hyperdorsiflexed foot
hyperdynamia uteri
hyperdynamic
  h. precordium
  h. ventricle
  h. ventricle with high
    output
hyperechogenic
  h. foci
  h. material
hyperechogenicity
  renal h.

H

hyperechoic
  h. bowel
  h. endometrium
  h. mass
hyperekplexia
hyperelastica
  cutis h.
hyperemesis
  h. gravidarum
  h. lactentium
hyperemia
  conjunctival h.
  mucosal h.
  optic disc h.
  postprandial h.
  posttraumatic h.
hyperemic cerebral blood flow
hyperencephalus
hypereosinophilic
  h. mucoid cast
  h. syndrome
hyperesthesia, hyperaesthesia
hyperestrogenism
hyperexcitability
hyperexpansion
hyperexplexia
hyperextensibility
  knee joint h.
hyperextensible joint
hyperextensile skin
hyperextension
  h. deformity
  dystonic h.
hyperferritinemia
hyperfiltration
hyperfolliculoidism
hyperfractionated
  h. radiation therapy
  h. radiotherapy
hyperfunction
  adrenal cortical h.
hypergalactosis
hypergammaglobulinemia
  polyclonal h.
hypergastrinemia
  infant h.
hypergenitalism
hyperglycemia
  fetal h.
  ketotic h.
  nonketotic h. (NKHG)
  rebound h.
hyperglycemic clamp technique
hyperglycerolemia
  familial h.
hypergonadal hypogonadism
hypergonadism
hypergonadotrophic (*var. of* hypergonadotropic)

hypergonadotropic, hypergonadotrophic
  h. amenorrhea
  h. eunuchoidism
  h. hypogonadism
hypergynecosmia
hyperhaploidy
hyperhemolysis
HyperHep
hyperhidrosis, hyperidrosis
  volar h.
hyperhomocysteinemia
hyperhydroxyprolinemia
hyperidrosis (*var. of* hyperhidrosis)
hyper-IgD syndrome
hyper-IgE
  hyperimmunoglobulin E
  hyper-IgE syndrome
hyper-IgM syndrome
hyperimmune
  h. Ig
  h. serum globulin
hyperimmunoglobulin
  h. E (hyper-IgE)
  h. E syndrome
hyperimmunoglobulinemia A
hyperinflation
hyperinsulinemia, hyperinsulinism
  compensatory h.
hyperinsulinemic
  h. hypoglycemia
  h. infant
hyperinsulinemic-euglycemic clamp technique
hyperinsulinism, hyperinsulinemia
  fetal h.
  h. hyperammonemia syndrome
  h. with hyperammonemia variant
hyperintensity
hyperinvolution
hyperirritable stage
hyperirritant spot
hyperkalemia, hyperkaliemia
hyperkalemic
  h. periodic paralysis
  h. RTA
hyperkaliemia (*var. of* hyperkalemia)
hyperkeratosis
  epidermal h.
  epidermolytic h.
  palmar and plantar punctate h.
  punctate h.
  striate h.
hyperkeratotic
  h. dry skin
  h. ridge
hyperketonemia
hyperkinesia (*var. of* hyperkinesis)
hyperkinesis, hyperkinesia, hypercinesis, hypercinesia

hyperkinetic
  h. behavior pattern
  h. child syndrome
  h. disorder
  h. pulmonary hypertension
hyperkyphosis
hyperlactation
hyperlacticacidemia
hyperlaxity
  joint h.
  skin h.
hyperleukocytosis
hyperlexia
hyperlinearity
  palmar h.
hyperlipemia (*var. of* hyperlipidemia)
hyperlipidemia, hyperlipemia
  familial h.
  familial combined h. (FCHL)
  homozygous h. (type I, II)
  mixed h.
  triglyceride h.
hyperlipoproteinemia (HLP)
hyperlordosis
hyperlucency
hyperlucent
  h. lung
  h. lung syndrome
hyperluteinization
hyperlysinemia
  familial h.
hypermagnesemia
  iatrogenic acute h.
hypermastia
hypermenorrhea
hypermetabolism
hypermethioninemia
hypermetropia
hypermobile
  h. Ehlers-Danlos syndrome
  h. flatfoot
  h. joint
  h. pes planus
hypermobility
  joint h.
  posterior occipitoatlantal h. (POAH)
  h. syndrome
  urethral h.
hypermyelination
hypernasality
hypernasal speech
hypernatremia
hypernatremic
  h. dehydration
  h. state
hypernitrosopnea
hyperolfaction
hyperopia, hypermetropia
  asymmetric h.

hyperornithemia, hyperammonemia, homocitrulinemia (HHH)
hyperornithinemia
hyperosmolality
hyperosmolar
  h. dehydration
  h. nonketotic coma
  h. state
hyperosmotic agent
hyperostosis
  calvarial h.
  cortical h.
  h. generalisata with striation
  infantile cortical h. (ICH)
hyperovarianism
hyperoxaluria
  enteric h.
  primary h.
  secondary h.
hyperoxia test
hyperoxygenation
hyperparasitemia
hyperparathyroidism
  maternal h.
  neonatal h.
hyperperfusion
  ictal h.
hyperphagia
hyperphagic
hyperphenylalaninemia (MHP)
  benign h.
  malignant h.
hyperphosphatemia
hyperphosphaturic syndrome
hyperpigmentation
  brawny h.
  diffuse h.
  periorbital h.
  reticulated h.
  whorled macular h.
hyperpigmented
  h. lesion
  h. lichenified plaque
hyperpipecolic acidemia
hyperpituitary gigantism
hyperplasia
  adenomatous h. (AH)
  adenomatous endometrial h.
  adrenal h.
  adrenocortical h.
  adult onset adrenal h. (AOAH)
  adult-onset congenital adrenal h.
  angiofollicular lymph node h.
  atypical h.
  atypical adenomatous h.
  atypical ductal h. (ADH)
  atypical lobular h.
  basal cell h.
  benign lymphoid h.

H

hyperplasia (*continued*)
    cellular h.
    complex h.
    congenital adrenal h. (CAH)
    congenital adrenal lipoid h.
    crypt h.
    cystic endometrial h.
    cystic glandular h.
    ductal h.
    elastic tissue h.
    endometrial h. (EH)
    epithelial h.
    erythroid h.
    familial lipoid adrenal h.
    fetal congenital h.
    focal nodular h.
    follicular h.
    gingival h.
    glandular h.
    gum h.
    hepatic focal nodular h.
    hilar cell h.
    intimal h.
    Kupffer cell h.
    late-onset h.
    late-onset adrenal h.
    Leydig cell h.
    lipoid adrenal h.
    lymphoid h.
    lymphonodular h.
    microglandular cervical h.
    neonatal breast h.
    nodular adrenal h.
    nodular lymphoid h.
    nonclassic adrenal h. (NCAH)
    nonclassic congenital adrenal h.
      (NC-CAH)
    h. of beta cell
    21-OH nonclassical adrenal h.
    parietal cell h.
    pigmented nodular adrenal h.
    polypoid h.
    pseudoepitheliomatous h.
    pulmonary lymphoid h. (PLH)
    salt-wasting congenital adrenal h.
      (SW-CAH)
    sebaceous gland h.
    simple h.
    simple virilizing congenital adrenal
      h. (SV-CAH)
    squamous cell h.
    stromal h.
    Swiss cheese h.
    thymus h.
    vulvar squamous h.
hyperplastic
    h. dystrophy
    h. joint
    h. lymphoid tissue

    h. polyp (HP)
    h. right heart syndrome
hyperploidy
hyperpnea
hyperpolarization
hyperprogesteronemia
hyperprolactinemia
    nontumoral h.
    tumorous h.
**hyperprolactinemia-associated luteal
phase**
hyperprolactinemic amenorrhea
hyperprolinemia
    familial h.
hyperpronate
hyperpronation
hyperprostaglandin E$_2$ syndrome
hyperprostaglandinuric tubular syndrome
hyperpyrexia
    malignant h.
hyperreactio luteinalis
hyperreactivity
hyperreflexia
    detrusor h.
hyperreflexic apnea
hyperreninemia
    chronic h.
hyperreninemic hypertension
hyperresonance to percussion
hyperresonant calvarial percussion note
hyperresponsive
hypersecretion
    gastric acid h.
hypersecretory endometrium
hypersegmentation
hypersegmented neutrophil
hypersensitive hapten-antibody
hypersensitivity
    h. angiitis
    delayed h.
    delayed-type h. (DTH)
    gastric visceral h.
    h. pneumonitis
    h. reaction
    h. vasculitis
    visceral h.
hypersensitization
hypersensitize
hypersexual behavior
hypersexuality
hypersomnia
    menstrual-associated periodic h.
    primary h.
hypersomnolence
hypersplenism
Hyperstat I.V.
hyperstimulation
    controlled ovarian h. (COH)
    gonadotropin-induced ovarian h.

ovarian h.
spontaneous h.
uterine h.
hypersynchronization
hypersynchronous discharge
hypersynchrony of neural discharges
hypertelorism
Bixler h.
dysostosis craniofacialis with h.
h., microtia, clefting (HMC)
h., microtia, clefting syndrome
ocular h.
hypertelorism-hypospadias syndrome
hypertension
accelerated h.
benign intracranial h. (BIH)
borderline h.
chronic h.
essential h.
fixed pulmonary h.
gestational h.
hyperkinetic pulmonary h.
hyperreninemic h.
hypoxia-induced pulmonary h.
(HPH)
iatrogenic h.
idiopathic intracranial h. (IIH)
infantile h.
intracranial h.
malignant h.
maternal h.
nonproteinuric h.
pediatric h.
persistent pulmonary h. (PPH)
portal h.
postoperative h.
postpartum h.
pregnancy-associated h.
pregnancy-induced h. (PIH)
presinusoidal h.
primary pulmonary h. (PPH)
pulmonary h.
rebound h.
renal h.
renovascular h.
transient h.
white coat h.
hypertension-preeclampsia
hypertensive
h. crisis
h. emergency
h. encephalopathy
h. xiphoid syndrome
hyperthecosis
ovarian stromal h.
h. ovarii
stromal h.
hyperthermia
h. in newborn

malignant h. (MH)
neonatal h.
hyperthermic rhabdomyolysis
hyperthyroid
hyperthyroidism
pulmonary h.
hyperthyrotropinemia
transient h.
hypertonia, hypertonicity
axial h.
global h.
hypertonic
h. dehydration
h. glucose
h. saline (HS, HTS)
h. saline solution
h. uterine dysfunction
hypertonicity
hypertonus
extensor h.
uterine h.
hypertransaminasemia
hypertransfusion regimen
hypertrichosis
h., coarse face, brachydactyly,
obesity, mental retardation
syndrome
h. lanuginosa
h. universalis congenita
vellus h.
hypertrichotic osteochondrodysplasia
hypertriglyceridemia
familial h. (FHTG)
hypertrophia (*var. of* hypertrophy)
hypertrophic
h. bundle
h. bundle of smooth muscle
h. cardiomyopathy
h. cirrhosis
h. gastropathy
h. growth zone
h. interstitial neuropathy of infancy
h. nail
h. osteoarthropathy (HOA)
h. pyloric stenosis (HPS)
h. scar
h. stenosis
h. vulvitis
h. zone (HZ)
hypertrophica
hemangiectasia h.
hypertrophied tissue
hypertrophy, hypertrophia
adenoidal h.
adenotonsillar h.
atrial h.
biventricular h.
cellular h.
cerebellar h.

H

hypertrophy (*continued*)
    clitoral h.
    congenital thyroid deficiency with muscular h.
    contralateral h.
    hemangiectatic h.
    infantile myxedema-muscular h.
    juxtaglomerular apparatus h.
    labial h.
    left atrial h.
    left ventricular h. (LVH)
    massive breast h.
    myocardial h.
    myocytic h.
    h. of labium
    ovarian h.
    pontile h.
    right atrial h.
    right ventricular h. (RVH)
    septal h.
    synovial h.
    testicular h.
    trigonal h.
    ventricular h.
    virginal breast h.
hypertropia
    ipsilateral h.
hypertrypsinemia
hypertryptophanemia
hypertyrosinemia II
hyperuricemia
    X-linked primary h.
hyperuricosuria
hypervalinemia
hyperventilation
    central neurogenic h.
    h. provocative test
    h. syndrome
hypervigilance manifestation
hyperviscosity syndrome
hypervitaminosis A
hypervolemia
hypesthesia, hypoesthesia
    bilateral stocking h.
hyphae
hyphema
    8-ball h.
    traumatic h.
hyphemia (*var. of* hypovolemia)
hypnagogic hallucination
hypnotherapeutic
hypnotherapy
hypnotic effect
hypoactive
    h. bowel sounds
    h. sexual desire
    h. sexual desire disorder (HSDD)
hypoactivity

hypoadrenalism neural ceroid lipofuscinosis
hypoalbuminemia
hypoalbuminemic
hypoaldosteronism
    congenital h.
hypoallergenic
hypoalphalipoproteinemia
    familial h.
    primary h.
hypoandrogenism
hypoarousal
    sustained autonomic h.
hypobetalipoproteinemia
    h., acanthocytosis, retinitis pigmentosa, pallidal degeneration (HARP)
    familial h.
hypocalcemia
    h. and microdeletion 22q11 syndrome
    cardiac abnormality, abnormal facies, thymic hypoplasia, cleft palate, h. (CATCH, CATCH 22)
    dwarfism, cortical thickening of tubular bones, transient h.
    h., dwarfism, cortical thickening syndrome
    late h.
    late neonatal h.
    neonatal h. (NHC)
hypocalcemic
    h. seizure
    h. tetany
hypocalcification
    linear h.
hypocalciuria
    familial hypercalcemia with h. (FHH)
hypocalciuric hypercalcemia
hypocalvaria
hypocapnia, hypocarbia
hypocarbia (*var. of* hypocapnia)
hypocarnitinemia
hypocellularity
hypochloremia
hypochloremic metabolic alkalosis
hypochlorhydria
hypochlorous acid
hypochondriasis
    primary h.
    secondary h.
hypochondrogenesis
hypochondroplasia syndrome
hypochromic microcytic anemia
hypocitraturia
hypocoagulability
hypocomplementemia
    intermittent h.

hypocomplementemic
  h. glomerulonephritis
  h. urticarial vasculitis syndrome
  (HUVS)
hypocycloidal tomography
hypodactylia (*var. of* hypodactyly)
hypodactylism (*var. of* hypodactyly)
hypodactyly, hypodactylia, hypodactylism
hypodense
hypodermoclysis
hypodiploid
hypodontia
hypodysplasia
  renal h.
hypoechogenic area
hypoechoic
  h. density
  h. structure
hypoesthesia
  corneal h.
hypoesthesic skin lesion
hypoestrogenemia
hypoestrogenic woman
hypoestrogenism
hypoferremia
hypofertility
hypofibrinogenemia
  congenital h.
  familial h.
hypofluorescent
hypofunction
  adrenal h.
hypogalactia
hypogalactous
hypogammaglobinemia (*var. of*
  hypogammaglobulinemia)
hypogammaglobulinemia,
  hypogammaglobinemia
  acquired h.
  adult-onset h.
  common variable h.
  congenital h.
  late-onset h.
  physiologic h.
  transient h.
  X-linked h.
hypoganglionic segment of Aldrich
hypoganglionosis
hypogastric
  h. artery
  h. artery ligation
  h. lymph node
  h. pain
  h. plexus
  h. vein
hypogastropagus
hypogastroschisis
hypogenesis
  cerebellar vermis h.

hypogenital dystrophy with diabetic
  tendency syndrome
hypogenitalism
hypoglossal, hypoglossus
  h. ganglion
  h. nerve
hypoglossia-hypodactyly syndrome
hypoglossus (*var. of* hypoglossal)
hypoglycemia
  episodic h.
  familial hyperinsulinemic h.
  hyperinsulinemic h.
  hypoketotic h.
  insulin-induced h.
  ketotic h.
  neonatal h.
  nonfamilial hyperinsulinemic h.
  nonhyperinsulinemic h.
  nonketotic h.
  refractory h.
  severe refractory h.
  transient h.
hypoglycemic
  oral h.
  h. seizure
hypoglycin
hypoglycorrhachia
hypoglycosylation
hypognathus
  cyclops h.
hypogonadal woman
hypogonadism
  alopecia, anosmia, deafness, h.
  (AADH)
  congenital hypogonadotropic h.
  eugonadotropic h.
  hypergonadal h.
  hypergonadotropic h.
  hypogonadotropic h.
  hyposmia-hypogonadotropic h.
  (HHA)
  idiopathic hypothalamic h.
  (IHH)
  isolated hypogonadotropic h.
  (IHH)
  primary h.
hypogonadism-anosmia syndrome
hypogonadotrophic (*var. of*
  hypogonadotropic)
hypogonadotropic, hypogonadotrophic
  h. amenorrhea
  h. eunuchoidism
  h. hypogonadism
hypogonadotropism
hypohaploidy
hypohidrotic
  h. ectodermal dysplasia
  h. sweating
hypokalemia, hypopotassemia

H

435

hypokalemic
    h. acidosis
    h. alkalosis
    h. periodic paralysis
    h. salt-losing tubulopathy
hypoketotic hypoglycemia
hypokinesia
hypokinetic
hypokyphosis
hypolactasia
    adult-type h.
hypoleptinemia
hypolordosis
hypomagnesemia
    congenital h.
    familial h.
    ionized h.
    neonatal h.
    primary h.
hypomagnesemic tetany
hypomandibular faciocranial dysostosis
hypomania
    pharmacologically induced h.
hypomanic episode
hypomastia, hypomazia
hypomaturation-hypoplasia
hypomazia (*var. of* hypomastia)
hypomelanosis
    Ito h.
    h. of Ito
hypomelanotic
hypomenorrhea
hypomenorrheic woman
hypomentia
hypometabolic
hypometabolism
    caudate h.
hypomyelination, hypomyelinogenesis
    congenital h.
hypomyelinogenesis (*var. of* hypomyelination)
hyponasality
hyponasal speech
hyponatremia of water excess
hyponatremic
    h. dehydration
    h. seizure
    h. state
hypoosmotic swelling (HOS)
hypoovarianism
hypoparathyroidism
    idiopathic h. (IHP)
    physiologic transient h.
hypoperfusion
    cerebral h.
    interictal h.
    splanchnic h.
hypoperistalsis

hypopharyngeal-glottal obstruction
hypopharynx
hypophosphatasia
    congenital lethal h.
    h. tarda
hypophosphatemia
    familial h. (FHR)
    X-linked h.
hypophosphatemic
    h. bone disease
    h. rickets
hypophyseal (*var. of* hypophysial)
hypophysectomy
hypophysial, hypophyseal
    h. amenorrhea
    h. dwarfism
    h. infantilism
    h. portal circulation
hypophysis
hypophysitis
    lymphocytic h.
hypopigmentation
    perianal h.
    vulvar h.
hypopigmented
    h. lesion
    h. macule
    h. mycosis
hypopituitarism
    congenital h.
hypopituitary syndrome
hypoplasia
    adrenal h.
    bilateral lung h.
    bilateral optic nerve h.
    biliary h.
    bone marrow h.
    cartilage-hair h. (CHH)
    cerebellar vermis h.
    congenital adrenal h.
    congenital megakaryocytic h.
    congenital universal muscular h.
    crypt h.
    cytomegalic h.
    dental enamel h.
    enamel h.
    erythroid h.
    exocrine pancreatic h.
    fetal pulmonary h.
    focal dermal h.
    foveal h.
    global h.
    Goltz focal dermal h.
    heminasal h.
    hepatic ductular h.
    ipsilateral lung h.
    iris h.
    laryngeal h.
    Leydig cell h.

linear h.
lipoid adrenal gland h.
malar h.
mandibular h.
maxillary h.
midface h.
miniature h.
müllerian h.
odontoid process h.
h. of anguli oris depressor muscle (HAODM)
h. of left heart (HLL)
h. of lung
h. of vermis
optic nerve h. (ONH)
orbital bone h.
oromandibular limb h.
pancreatic h.
pontocerebellar h.
pulmonary h.
right lung h.
right ventricular h.
secondary adrenal h.
segmental h.
spondylohumerofemoral h.
thymic h.
transient erythroid h.
transverse arch h.
tubular h.
velofacial h.
vermis h.
hypoplasia/hydrocephalus
X-linked cerebral h./h.
hypoplastic
h. anemia
h. aorta (HA)
h. congenital anemia syndrome
h. dens
h. digit
h. kidney
h. labium
h. left heart
h. left heart syndrome (HLHS)
h. left ventricle
h. lung
h. mandible
h. nail
h. parathyroid gland
h. patella
h. penis
h. philtrum
h. pulmonary vascular bed
h. radius
h. right heart syndrome (HRHS)
h. sacrum
h. superior cerebral vermis
h. teeth
h. thumb
h. tongue

h. uterus
h. zygomatic arch
hypopnea
hypopotassemia
hypoproliferative anemia
hypoproteinemia
idiopathic h.
hypoprothrombinemia
hypopyon
hyporeflexia
hyposecretion
gastric acid h.
hyposegmentation
hyposensitization
hyposmia
hyposmia-hypogonadotropic hypogonadism (HHA)
hyposomatotropism
obesity-related h.
hypospadias
anterior h.
balanic h.
distal shaft h.
first-degree h.
glanular h.
Hacker h.
middle h.
midshaft h.
penoscrotal h.
perineal h.
perineoscrotal h.
posterior h.
proximal shaft h.
pseudovaginal perineoscrotal h. (PPSH)
h. repair
scrotal h.
second-degree h.
subcoronal h.
third-degree h.
hypospadias-dysphagia syndrome
hypospadias-mental retardation syndrome
hyposplenia
hyposplenism
hypostatic pneumonia
hyposthenuria
hyposulfite
sodium h.
hypotelorism
ocular h.
orbital h.
hypotension
hypovolemic h.
instantaneous orthostatic h. (INOH)
maternal h.
neurally mediated h.
orthostatic h.
hypotensive anesthesia

H

hypothalamic
    h. amenorrhea
    h. disease
    h. dysfunction
    h. failure
    h. GnRH secretion
    h. hamartoblastoma
    h. hamartoblastoma syndrome
    h. hamartoma
    h. hypothyroidism
    h. lesion
    h. luteinizing hormone-releasing
    hormone
    h., pituitary, thyroid
    h. set point
    h. thermoregulating center
    h. thermoregulation
    h. tumor
hypothalamic-hypophysial
    h.-h. destruction
    h.-h. portal circulation
hypothalamic-hypophysial-ovarian-
  endometrial
  axis
hypothalamic-hypopituitary
  hypothyroidism
hypothalamic-pituitary
    h.-p. amenorrhea
    h.-p. axis (HPA)
    h.-p. disorder
    h.-p. dysfunction
    h.-p. function
    h.-p. system
hypothalamic-pituitary-adrenal (HPA)
    h.-p.-a. axis dysregulation
hypothalamic-pituitary-gonadal axis
hypothalamic-pituitary-ovarian (HOP,
  HPO)
    h.-p.-o. axis (HPOA)
hypothenar
hypothermia
    cerebral h.
    chronic scrotal h.
    cranial h.
    deep systemic h.
hypotheses (*pl. of* hypothesis)
hypothesis, *pl.* **hypotheses**
    alternative h.
    Barker low birth weight h.
    bayesian h.
    critical weight h.
    differential detection h.
    differential treatment h.
    dormant basket cell h.
    estrogen window etiologic h.
    gate-control h.
    Goldie-Coldman h.
    2-hit h.
    Knudson 2-hit tumorigenesis h.

    Korenman estrogen window h.
    Lyon h.
    school failure h.
    serotonin h.
    susceptibility h.
hypothesize
hypothyroid
    h. dwarfism
    h. myopathy
hypothyroidism
    acquired h.
    athyrotic h.
    central h.
    congenital h. (CH, CHT)
    congenital goitrous h.
    endemic goitrous h.
    eutopic congenital h.
    fetal goitrous h.
    goitrous h.
    hypothalamic h.
    hypothalamic-hypopituitary h.
    maternal thyrotropin receptor
      blocking antibody-induced
      congenital h.
    mixed h.
    neonatal nongoitrous h.
    primary h.
    secondary h.
    subclinical h.
    h. syndrome
    tertiary h.
    transient congenital h.
hypothyroid-large muscle syndrome
hypothyroxinemia
    h. of prematurity (HOP)
    transient h.
hypotonia, hypotonus, hypotony
    benign congenital h.
    benign infantile h.
    bladder h.
    congenital h.
    h., hypopigmentia, hypogonadism,
      obesity (HHHO)
    infantile muscular h.
    muscle h.
    muscular h.
    nonparalytic h.
    Oppenheim congenital h.
    paralytic h.
    transient h.
    uterine h.
hypotonic
    h. bladder
    h. cerebral palsy
    h. dehydration
    h. myometrium
    h. saline
    h. uterine dysfunction
    h. weakness

hypotonic-hyporesponsive episodes (HHEs)
hypotonicity
hypotonus (*var. of* hypotonia)
hypotony
    ocular h.
hypotransferrinemia
hypotrichosis
    Marie-Unna h.
hypotrophy
    fetal h.
hypotropia
hypouricemia
hypovarianism
hypoventilation
    central alveolar h.
    congenital central h.
    h. syndrome
hypovitaminemia
    thiamin h.
hypovitaminosis
hypovolemia, hyphemia
hypovolemic
    h. dehydration
    h. hypotension
    h. shock
hypoxanthine-phosphoribosyltransferase (HGPRT)
hypoxemia
    acute-on-chronic tissue h.
    perinatal h.
hypoxia
    alveolar h.
    cellular h.
    centrizonal h.
    fetal h.
    global brain h.
    intestinal h.
    intrauterine h.
    h., intussusception, brain mass (HIB)
    in utero h.
    maternal h.
    perinatal h.
    subacute fetal h.
hypoxia-induced pulmonary hypertension (HPH)
hypoxia-ischemia
hypoxic
    h. cell sensitizer
    h. encephalopathy
    h. respiratory failure
    h. spell
    h. vasoconstriction
hypoxic-ischemic
    h.-i. brain injury
    h.-i. cerebral injury
    h.-i. encephalopathy (HIE)
Hyprogest
hypsarrhythmia

hypsarrhythmic pattern
hypsicephaly, hypsocephaly
hypsocephaly (*var. of* hypsicephaly)
Hyrexin
Hyrexin-50 Injection
Hyskon
hysteralgia
hysteratresia
hysterectomized
hysterectomy
    abdominal h. (AH)
    abdominovaginal h.
    Bell-Buettner h.
    Bonney abdominal h.
    cesarean h.
    h. clamp
    classic abdominal Semm h. (CASH)
    Dellepiane h.
    Döderlein method of vaginal h.
    Döderlein roll-flap h.
    Doyen vaginal h.
    Eden-Lawson h.
    H. Educational Resources and Services
    extended radical h.
    extrafascial total abdominal h.
    laparoscopically assisted radical vaginal h.
    laparoscopic-assisted abdominal h. (LAAH)
    laparoscopic-assisted vaginal h. (LAVH)
    laparoscopic Döderlein h.
    laparoscopic supracervical h. (LSH)
    Mayo h.
    Meigs-Werthein h.
    modified radical h.
    Munro and Parker classification for laparoscopic h.
    obstetric h.
    paravaginal h.
    partial exenteration operation class V h.
    Pelosi vaginal h.
    pelviscopic intrafascial h.
    Porro h.
    radical abdominal h.
    Reis-Wertheim vaginal h.
    Rutledge classification of extended h.
    h. scissors
    Semm h.
    subtotal h. (STH)
    supracervical h. (SCH)
    total abdominal h. (TAH)
    transvaginal h.
    vaginal h. (VH)

H

hysterectomy (*continued*)
    Ward-Mayo vaginal h.
    Wertheim h.
hysterectomy-related fistula
hysteresis
hysteria
hysteric, hysterical
    h. amnesia
    h. convulsion
    h. glottic closure
    h. mother
    h. paralysis
    h. seizure
    h. syncope
    h. visual loss
hystericus
    globus h.
hysterocele
hysterocleisis
hysterocolposcope
hysterocystopexy
hysterodynia
hysterofiberscope
    Olympus flexible h.
hysterogram
hysterograph
hysterography
hysteroid convulsion
hysterolith
hysterolysis
hysterometer
hysteromyoma
hysteromyomectomy
hysteromyotomy
hystero-oophorectomy
hysteropathy
hysteropexy
    abdominal h.
    Alexander-Adams h.
hysterophore
hysteroplasty
hysterorrhaphy
hysterorrhexis
hysterosalpingectomy
hysterosalpingogram (HSG)
hysterosalpingography (HS, HSG)
    h. catheter
hysterosalpingo-oophorectomy
hysterosalpingosonography
hysterosalpingostomy
hysteroscope
    Baggish h.
    Circon-ACMI h.
    diagnostic h.

    flexible h.
    French h.
    Fujinon flexible h.
    Galileo rigid h.
    Hamou h.
    Karl Storz flexible h.
    Liesegang LM-Flex 7 flexible h.
    Olympus h.
    OPERA Star SL h.
hysteroscopic
    h. approach
    h. endometrial ablation
    h. insufflator
    h. metroplasty
    h. myomectomy
    h. removal
    h. septum resection
    h. surgery
    h. tubal ligation
hysteroscopy
    h. fluid
    laparoscopic-assisted vaginal h. (LAVH)
    office h.
hysterosonography
hysterospasm
hysterothermometry
hysterotomy
    abdominal h.
    low transverse h.
    Pelosi h.
    vaginal h.
hysterotrachelectomy
hysterotracheloplasty
hysterotrachelorrhaphy
hysterotrachelotomy
hysterotubography
hystersonography
hystrix
    ichthyosis h.
Hytakerol
Hytone Topical
Hytuss
Hytuss-2X
Hyzine-50 Injection
HZ
    hypertrophic zone
Hz
    hertz
HZA
    hemizona assay
HZO
    herpes zoster ophthalmicus
HZV
    herpes zoster virus

I

inspired gas
I antigen score
I IFG-binding protein

123I

iodine-123

125I

iodine-125

127I

iodine-127

131I

iodine-131

132I

iodine-132

IA

infantile autism

IAA

ileoanal anastomosis
intraabdominal abscess

IAB

incomplete abortion
induced abortion

IAC

indwelling arterial catheter
interatrial communication

IADH

inappropriate antidiuretic hormone
IADH syndrome

IAHS

infection-associated hemophagocytic
syndrome

IAI

intraabdominal infection
intraamniotic infection

IALT

intestine-associated lymphoid tissue

IAP

intrapartum antibiotic prophylaxis

IAS

internal anal sphincter

IASA

idiopathic acquired sideroblastic anemia

iatrogenic

i. acute hypermagnesemia
i. airway injury
i. androgen excess
i. anemia
i. bladder
i. CJD
i. complete heart block
i. Creutzfeldt-Jakob disease
i. destruction
i. dissemination
i. effect
i. event

i. fetal distress
i. hypertension
i. infertility
i. menopause
i. multiple pregnancy (IMP)
i. pneumothorax
i. precocious puberty
i. preterm birth maternal dropsy
i. pyopneumothorax
i. ureteral injury
i. urethral obstruction

IB

ibuprofen
infantile botulism
Midol IB

ibandronate sodium

IBC

inflammatory breast cancer
iron-binding capacity

IBD

identical by descent
inflammatory bowel disease

IBDQ

Inflammatory Bowel Disease
Questionnaire

IBIDS

ichthyosis, brittle hair, impaired
intelligence, decreased fertility, short
stature
IBIDS syndrome

IBR

Infant Behavior Record

IBS

irritable bowel syndrome

IBSN

infantile bilateral striatal necrosis

IBT

immunobead test

ibuprofen (IB)

Ibuprohm

Ibu-Tab Junior Strength Motrin

ibutilide

IBW

ideal body weight

%IBW

percent of ideal body weight

IC

immune complex
inspiratory capacity
interstitial cystitis
invasive cancer

ICA

islet cell antibody

iCa

ionized calcium

ICAM1
  intercellular adhesion molecule 1
iC3b receptor
ICC
  Indian childhood cirrhosis
  Interagency Coordinating Council
  invasive cervical cancer
ICCR
  International Committee for
    Contraceptive Research
ICD
  immune complex dissociation
  International Classification of Diseases
  intrauterine contraceptive device
ICD-p24 test
ICE
  ichthyosis, cheek, eyebrow
    ICE syndrome
iced
    i. saline
    i. saline submersion
I-cell
  inclusion cell
    I-cell disease
ICF
  immunodeficiency, centromeric
    instability, facial anomalies
  intermediate care facility
  intracellular fluid
    ICF syndrome
ICFM
  isolated congenital folate
    malabsorption
ICH
  infantile cortical hyperostosis
  intracranial hemorrhage
ichthyosiform
    congenital i.
    i. dermatosis
    i. erythroderma
    i. erythroderma, corneal involvement,
      deafness
    i. erythroderma, hair abnormality,
      mental and growth retardation
ichthyosis
    i., brittle hair, impaired intelligence,
      decreased fertility, short stature
      (IBIDS)
    i., cheek, eyebrow (ICE)
    i. congenita
    congenital i.
    i. fetalis
    i. fetus
    i., follicularis, atrichia, photophobia
      (IFAP)
    harlequin i.
    i. hystrix
    lamellar i.
    i. linearis circumflexa

    i. spinosa
    i. uteri
    i. vulgaris
    i. with keratitis and deafness
      syndrome
    X-linked i.
ichthyotic idiocy
ICI
  intracranial injury
ICN
  intensive care nursery
icon
    I. serum pregnancy test
    I. strep B test
    I. urine pregnancy test
ICON1
  International Collaborative Ovarian
    Neoplasm Trial 1
ICP
  incubation period
  intracranial pressure
  intrahepatic cholestasis of pregnancy
    ICP monitoring
ICPS
  intrauterine contraceptive progesterone
    system
ICR
  intercostal retraction
ICS
  International Continence Society
    ICS bladder prolapse
      (stage I–III)
ICSD
  International Classification of Sleep
    Disorders
    ICSD criteria
ICSHI
  intracytoplasmic sperm head
    injection
ICSI
  intracytoplasmic sperm injection
    ICSI Massachusetts clamp
ictal hyperperfusion
icteric
    i. hepatitis
    i. leptospirosis
    i. phase
icterogenic breast milk
icterometer
    Ingram i.
icterus
    i. gravis
    i. gravis neonatorum
    i. neonatorum
    physiologic i.
    i. praecox
    scleral i.
I&D
  incision and drainage

IDA
    alpha-L-iduronidase
    iron deficiency anemia
        IDA deficiency
Idaho syndrome
Idamycin PFS
idarubicin
IDC
    infiltrating ductal carcinoma
    intervertebral disc calcification
IDDM
    insulin-dependent diabetes mellitus
IDEA
    Individuals with Disabilities Education
        Act
idea
    flight of i.'s (FOI)
ideal body weight (IBW)
ideation
    paranoid i.
    suicidal i.
ideation/attempts
    home life, education level, activities,
        drug use, sexual activity, suicide
        i./a.
identical
    i. by descent (IBD)
    i. twins
identification
    cord vessel i.
identity matrix
ideogram
IDI
    intractable diarrhea of infancy
idiocy
    amaurotic familial i. (AFI)
    Aztec i.
    Batten-Bielschowsky type of late
      infantile and juvenile amaurotic i.
    i. by deprivation
    cretinism i.
    eclamptic i.
    epileptic i.
    genetous i.
    hydrocephalic i.
    ichthyotic i.
    inflammatory i.
    juvenile amaurotic i. (JAI)
    Kalmuk i.
    late infantile amaurotic i.
    microcephalic i.
    paralytic i.
    Spielmeyer-Vogt type of late
      infantile and juvenile
      amaurotic i.
    traumatic i.
    xerodermic i.
idioglossia
idiolalia

idiopathic
    i. abortion
    i. acquired sideroblastic anemia
      (IASA)
    i. apnea
    i. apnea of prematurity
    i. apparent life-threatening event
    i. cavernous sinusitis
    i. cholestasis of pregnancy
    i. chronic arthritis
    i. clubfoot
    i. constipation
    i. copper toxicosis
    i. dermatosis
    i. detrusor overactivity
    i. diffuse interstitial fibrosis
    i. diffuse interstitial fibrosis of lung
    i. dilated cardiomyopathy (IDC,
      IDCM)
    i. epilepsy
    i. facial paralysis
    i. growth hormone deficiency
    i. heel-cord tightness
    i. hemolytic uremia syndrome
    i. hirsutism
    i. hydramnios
    i. hyperbilirubinemia
    i. hypercalcemia-supravalvular aortic
      stenosis syndrome
    i. hypertrophic subaortic stenosis
      (IHSS)
    i. hypoparathyroidism (IHP)
    i. hypoproteinemia
    i. hypothalamic hypogonadism (IHH)
    i. infantile hypercalcemia
    i. infantile hypercalcemia syndrome
    i. infertility
    i. intracranial hypertension (IIH)
    i. intussusception
    i. isosexual precocious puberty
    i. juvenile avascular necrosis
    i. long QT syndrome
    i. low molecular weight proteinuria
    i. megalencephaly
    i. minimal lesion nephrotic
      syndrome (IMLNS)
    i. neonatal giant-cell hepatitis
    i. nephrotic syndrome (INS)
    i. neutropenia
    i. pancreatitis
    i. peptic ulcer disease
    i. polyserositis
    i. premature adrenarche
    i. premature thelarche
    i. primary renal hematuric
      proteinuric syndrome
    i. pulmonary hemorrhage (IPH)
    i. rapidly progressive
      glomerulonephritis

idiopathic (*continued*)
    i. recurrent jaundice of pregnancy
    i. respiratory distress syndrome
    (IRDS)
    i. scoliosis
    i. scrotal edema
    i. seizure
    i. short stature (ISS)
    i. status epilepticus
    i. steatorrhea
    i. steroid-resistant
    proteinuria/nephrotic syndrome
    i. talipes equinovarus
    i. thrombocytopenic purpura (ITP)
    i. tibia vara
    i. toe walking (ITW)
    i. torsion dystonia
    i. torticollis
    i. ulcer
    i. urticaria
    i. venous thromboembolism
    i. vulvodynia
idiosome
idiosyncratic marrow aplasia
idiot
    mongolian i.
IDI-Strep B test
IDM
    infant of diabetic mother
    intensive diabetes management
IDMS
    isolated diffuse mesangial
    sclerosis
idoxifene
idoxuridine
id reaction
IDS
    iduronate sulfatase
    intrinsic sphincter deficiency
    IDS deficiency
IDU
    intravenous drug use
    5-iodo-2'-deoxyuridine
IDUA
    alpha-L-iduronidase
    IDUA deficiency
iduronate sulfatase (IDS)
iduronic acid
I/E
    inspiratory to expiratory
IE
    infectious endocarditis
    infective endocarditis
IEM
    inborn error of metabolism
IEP
    Individualized Education Program
IES
    Impact of Events Scale

IF
    intrinsic factor
    involved field
    IF radiation
IFA
    immunofluorescent antibody
    immunofluorescent assay
    indirect fluorescent antibody
    IFA test
IFAP
    ichthyosis, follicularis, atrichia,
    photophobia
    IFAP syndrome
IFDC
    infiltrating ductal carcinoma
ifenprodil
IFI
    intrafollicular insemination
**iFind handheld device for breast cancer
  screening**
ifosfamide
IFSP
    Individualized Family Service Plan
Ig
    immunoglobulin
IgA
    IgA A
    IgA AGA test
    IgA antiendomysial
    IgA antiendomysium antibody
    IgA antigliadin
    IgA antireticulin antibody
    IgA deficiency
    IgA HIV antibody test
    IgA mesangial deposition
    secretory IgA (sIgA)
IgA1
    immunoglobulin A subclass 1
IgA2
    immunoglobulin A subclass 2
IgD
    immunoglobulin D
    IgD antibody
IgE
    immunoglobulin E
    IgE antibody
    antistaphylococcal IgE
    IgE deficiency
    IgE syndrome
IGF
    insulinlike growth factor
IgF
    immunoglobulin F
IGFBP
    insulinlike growth factor-binding
    protein
IGFBP-3
    insulinlike growth factor-binding
    protein-3

IgG
immunoglobulin G
IgG antibody
IgG antibody titer
IgG anti-HAV
serovar-specific IgG
IgG2
immunoglobulin G2
IgG2 deficiency
IgG4
immunoglobulin G4
IgG4 deficiency
IgG-IFA test
IGHD
isolated growth hormone deficiency
IGIV
immunoglobulin, intravenous
IgM
Immmunoglobulin M
IgM antibody
IgM antibody titer
IgM deficiency
IgM indirect fluorescent antibody
test
serovar-specific IgM
X-linked immunodeficiency with
hyper IgM
IgM-IFA test
ignoring
active i.
IGT
impaired glucose tolerance
IH
intraretinal hemorrhage
IHA
indirect hemagglutination antibody
IHA test
IHD
ischemic heart disease
IHH
idiopathic hypothalamic hypogonadism
isolated hypogonadotropic
hypogonadism
IHP
idiopathic hypoparathyroidism
IHPS
infantile hypertrophic pyloric stenosis
IHSS
idiopathic hypertrophic subaortic
stenosis
IIF
indirect immunofluorescence
IIF assay
IIH
idiopathic intracranial hypertension
iInjection
Key-Pred-SP i.
IIQ
Incontinence Impact Questionnaire

IIQ-R
Incontinence Impact
Questionnaire-Revised
IL
interleukin
ILAE
International League Against Epilepsy
ILAR
International League of Associations
for Rheumatology
ILAR peripheral arthritis
classification
ILC
infiltrating lobular carcinoma
ILD
interstitial lung disease
ileal
i. atresia
i. conduit
i. interposition
i. intussusception
i. limb
i. loop
i. loop diversion
i. perforation
i. pouch-anal anastomosis (IPAA)
i. reservoir
i. stoma
i. ureter
ileitis
backwash i.
nonspecific i.
regional i.
terminal i.
ileoanal
i. anastomosis (IAA)
i. pull-through
ileocecal
i. conduit diversion
i. intussusception
ileocolic, ileocolonic
i. artery
i. intussusception
ileocolitis
ileocolonic (*var. of* ileocolic)
ileocystoplasty
Camey i.
ileoentectropy
ileoileal
i. anastomosis
i. intussusception
ileoileocolic intussusception
ileostomy
Bishop-Koop i.
continent i.
end i.
ileovesicostomy
Yang-Monti i.
Iletin

ileum
    distal i.
    duplication of i.
    native i.
ileus
    adynamic i.
    complicated meconium i.
    duodenal i.
    meconium i. (MI)
    paralytic i.
    postinfectious i.
    postoperative i.
    simple meconium i.
    i. subparta
ilia (*pl. of* ilium)
iliac
    i. apophysis maturation index
    i. artery
    i. crest
    i. crest apophysitis
    i. crest contusion
    i. fossa
    i. horn
    i. node
    i. spine
    i. vein
iliococcygeal
    i. fixation
    i. muscle
iliococcygeus
    i. fascia suspension
    i. muscle
iliofemoral artery
ilioneoureterocystotomy
iliopagus
iliopectineal
    i. bursa
    i. line
iliopsoas
    i. hemorrhage
    i. sign
iliothoracopagus
iliotibial
    i. band
    i. band friction syndrome
ilioxiphopagus
ilium, *pl.* **ilia**
Ilizarov
    I. device
    I. external fixator
    I. limb-lengthening procedure
ill-defined mass
illegal substance
illegitimacy
illegitimate
illicit
    i. drug
    i. drug use
    i. sex

Illinois Test of Psycholinguistic Abilities (ITPA)
illness
    acute i.
    childhood severity of psychiatric i. (CSPI)
    chronic i.
    communicable i.
    diarrheal dehydration i.
    foodborne i.
    history of present i. (HPI)
    Integrated Management of Childhood I. (IMCI)
    leptospiral i.
    lower respiratory i. (LRI)
    manic-depressive i. (MDI)
    maternal i.
    mental i.
    nonthyroidal i. (NTI)
    present i. (PI)
    prodromal i.
    psychiatric i.
    roseolalike i.
    seroconversion i.
    systemic i.
    upper respiratory i.
    viral lower respiratory i. (VLRI)
illocutionary stage
illuminated vaginal speculum
illumination
    chemiluminescent i.
illuminator
    LightMat surgical i.
Illum syndrome
iLook 15 handheld ultrasound system
iloprost
Ilotycin
ILS17 gene
ILSX gene
IM
    infectious mononucleosis
    intestinal malrotation
    intramuscular
image
    body i.
    i. intensification fluoroscopy
    i. intensifier
    i. recording system
image-degradation amblyopia
image-guided breast biopsy
imager
    peripheral instantaneous X-ray i. (PIXI)
imagery
    traumatic i.
imaginal desensitization
imaging
    chemical shift i. (CSI)
    color Doppler flow i. (CDFI)

Color Power Angio i.
continuous-wave ultrasound i.
diagnostic i.
diffusion-weighted i. (DWI)
diffusion-weighted magnetic
   resonance i.
dynamic optical breast i.
dynamic pulmonary i. (DPI)
echoplanar functional magnetic
   resonance i.
endovaginal i.
fetal i.
functional brain i.
gray-scale i.
harmonic tissue i.
i. headband
high-contrast Bucky i.
magnetic resonance i. (MRI)
magnetic source i. (MSI)
mediastinal i.
medical optimal i. (MOI)
MIGB i.
M-mode i.
neuraxis tumor i.
OB-View i.
OPS i.
phosphorus-31 magnetic resonance i.
   (^{31}P MRI)
plantar i.
prenatal magnetic resonance i.
radionuclide i.
rhod-2 i.
SieScape i.
thallium i.
tissue Doppler i. (TDI)
tissue specific i.
ultrafast magnetic resonance i.

IMB
intermenstrual bleeding
imbalance
asymmetric muscle i.
electrolyte i.
neuromuscular i.
neurotransmitter i.
ventilation/perfusion i.
IMC
immunohistochemical
IMCI
Integrated Management of Childhood
   Illness
Imelab vascular diagnostic system
Imerslünd-Grasbeck syndrome
Imerslünd syndrome
Imex
I. antepartum monitor
I. Pocket-Dop OB Doppler
Imexlab vascular diagnostic system
imidazole
topical i.

imidazopyridine
imiglucerase
iminoglycinuria
familial i.
imipemide
imipenem and cilastatin
imipenem-cilastatin sodium
imipramine hydrochloride
imiquimod cream
imitative play
Imitrex Injection
Imlach ring
IMLNS
idiopathic minimal lesion nephrotic
   syndrome
immature
i. infant
i. lung
i. malignant teratoma
i. neural element
i. ovarian teratoma
i. placenta
i. social behavior
i. teratoma (grade 0–3)
immaturity
parathyroid gland i.
pulmonary i.
immediate
i. extrauterine adaptation
i. hypersensitivity reaction
immersion
i. burn
i. oil
static i.
imminent abortion
immitis
Coccidioides i.
Dirofilaria i.
immobilization
cervical spine i.
Treponema pallidum i. (TPI)
immobilizer
straight-leg i.
immotile
i. cilia
i. cilia syndrome
Immulite
immune
i. clearance
i. complex (IC)
i. complex disease
i. complex dissociation (ICD)
i. complex-mediated
   glomerulonephritis
i. complex-mediated pericarditis
i. complex-mediated vasculitis
i. complex vasculitis
i. deficiency
i. dysregulation

immune (*continued*)
    i. factor
    i. fetal hydrops
    i. globulin
    i. hemolysis
    i. hydrops fetalis
    i. modulator
    i. monitoring technique
    i. neutropenia
    i. phase
    i. process
    i. response
    i. response gene
    rubella i.
    i. separation technique
    i. serum globulin (ISG)
    i. suppressor gene
    i. surveillance
    i. system
    i. system anatomy
    i. thrombocytopenia
    i. thrombocytopenic purpura (ITP)
immune-competent child
immune-mediated
    i.-m. abnormality
    i.-m. disseminated encephalomyelitis
    i.-m. neutropenia
    i.-m. thrombocytopenia
immunity
    adaptive i.
    Burnet acquired i.
    cell-mediated i. (CMI)
    cellular i.
    humoral i.
    passive i.
    previous maternal i.
immunization
    active i.
    antipregnancy i.
    blood group i.
    diphtheria, tetanus, pertussis i.
    Engerix-B i.
    *Haemophilus influenzae type
      b* i.
    hepatitis A i.
    hepatitis B i.
    hepatitis C i.
    HIV i.
    influenza i.
    invasive pneumococcal disease i.
    MMR i.
    I. Monitoring Program, Active
      (IMPACT)
    passive i.
    pneumococcal i.
    poliomyelitis i.
    preconception i.
    prophylactic i.
    Recombivax HB i.

    Rh i.
    rubella i.
    rubeola i.
    tetanus-diphtheria i.
    varicella i.
immunizing unit (IU)
Immuno
    Feiba VH I.
    Gammabulin I.
immunoassay
    alpha-fetoprotein enzyme i.
      (AFP-EIA)
    BioStar Flu optical i.
    chemiluminescent i. (CIA)
    Chlamydiazyme i.
    enzyme i. (EIA)
    fluorescent i. (FIA)
    fluorescent polarization i. (FPIA)
    gold-labeled optical rapid i.
      (GLORIA)
    growth hormone i.
    microparticle enzyme i.
    nonradioactive i.
    nonreactive i.
    optic i. (OIA)
    PhiCal fecal calprotectin i.
    Quantikine human IL-6 I.
    radioactive i.
    SalEst i.
    solid-phase enzyme i.
immunobead test (IBT)
immunobiologic
immunoblastic
    i. lymphoma
    i. sarcoma
immunoblot, immunoblotting
    i. assay
    Western i.
immunoblotting (*var. of* immunoblot)
immunobullous disorder
ImmunoCap specific IgE blood test
immunochemiluminometric insulin assay
immunochemistry
immunochemotherapy
immunocompetence
    maternal i.
immunocompetent cell
immunocompromised child
immunocytochemical
immunocytochemistry
immunodeficiency
    acquired i.
    cell-mediated i.
    cellular i.
    i. centromeric heterochromatin
      instability, facial anomalies
      syndrome
    i., centromeric instability, facial
      anomalies (ICF)

combined i. (CID)
common variable i. (CVI, CVID)
humoral i.
primary i. (PID)
severe combined i. (SCID)
X-linked severe combined i.
 (X-SCID)
immunodeficient
immunodiagnosis
immunoelectrophoresis
immunofluorescence
3-color i.
direct i. (DIF)
indirect i. (IIF)
i. study
immunofluorescent
i. antibody (IFA)
i. assay (IFA)
i. *Chlamydia* test
immunofunctional assay
immunogen
immunogenetics
immunogenic
immunogenicity
immunoglobulin (Ig)
i. A (IgA)
i. A nephropathy
antenatal anti-D i.
i. antibody
anti-D i. (anti-D)
anti-D i.
i. A subclass 1 (IgA1)
i. A subclass 2 (IgA2)
botulinum i.
cytomegalovirus-specific i.
i. D (IgD)
i. deposition
i. E (IgE)
i. E level
i. F (IgF)
i. G (IgG)
i. G2 (IgG2)
i. G4 (IgG4)
i. gene
i. G subclass deficiency
hepatitis i.
human i.
human immunodeficiency virus i.
 (HIVIg)
human rabies i. (HRIG)
intravenous i. (IVIG)
immunoglobulin, intravenous (IGIV)
intravenous i. (IVIG, IVIg)
intravenous anti-D i.
lymphocyte i. (LIG)
i. M (IgM)
i. M fluorescent treponemal
 antibody
quantitative i.

rabies i. (RABig, RIG)
regular i.
respiratory syncytial virus i.
 (RSV-IG, RSVIG)
Rh i.
Rh i. (RhIg)
RhD i.
Rho(D) i. (RhoGAM)
specific i.
surface i.
tetanus i. (TIg, TIG)
thyroid-stimulating i.
Venilon human i.
immunohistochemical
i. change
i. stromal leukocyte
 characterization
immunologic, immunological
i. assay
i. change
i. disturbance
i. enhancement
i. factor
i. maladaptation
i. paralysis
i. pregnancy test
i. reaction
i. screening
i. study
i. suppression
i. surveillance
i. tolerance
i. unresponsiveness
immunological (*var. of* immunologic)
i. infertility
immunology
maternal i.
nutritional i.
placental i.
transplantation i.
tumor i.
immunomodulation
immunomodulator
immunomodulatory treatment
immunoosseous dysplasia
immunoperoxidase
i. stain
i. technique
immunoproliferative small intestinal
 disease
immunoprophylaxis
immunoprotein
immunoradiometric assay (IRMA)
immunoreaction
immunoreactive trypsinogen (IRT)
immunoreactivity
immunoresistance
immunosorbent agglutination assay
 (ISAGA)

immunospot
>solid-phase enzyme-linked i.
>(ELISpot)

immunosuppression
>pharmacologic i.

immunosuppressive
>i. agent
>i. drug
>i. therapy

immunotherapy
>active specific i. (ASI)
>adoptive i.
>allergen i.
>i. hernia
>nonspecific i.
>Pacis BCG i.
>rush i.
>specific i.
>systemic-active nonspecific i.
>tumor i.

Imodium
>I. A-D
>I. Advanced

Imogam

Imovax

IMP
>iatrogenic multiple pregnancy

IMPACT
>Immunization Monitoring Program,
>Active

impacted
>i. bowel
>i. fetus
>i. fracture
>i. twin
>i. uterus

impaction
>delirium, infection, atrophic urethritis
>and vaginitis, pharmacologic cause,
>psychological cause, excessive
>urine production, restricted
>mobility, stool i. (DIAPPERS)
>delirium, infection, pharmacology,
>psychology, endocrinopathy,
>restricted mobility, stool i.
>fecal i.
>food i.
>stool i.

Impact of Events Scale (IES)

impaired
>i. cognitive function
>emotionally i.
>i. glucose tolerance (IGT)
>i. rectal sensation
>i. secretion
>i. taste
>i. vision

impairment
>auditory i.

bilateral hearing i.
cognitive i.
conductive hearing i.
cortical visual i. (CVI)
functional i.
inherited androgen uptake i.
intrauterine growth i.
mixed hearing i.
neurocognitive i.
neurologic i.
neurosensory i. (NSI)
opioidergic control i.
renal i.
sensorineural hearing i.
sensory i.
somatosensory i.
unilateral hearing i.

impedance
>acoustic i.
>i. audiometry
>bioelectrical i. (BEI)
>i. cardiogram
>fetal vascular i.
>i. plethysmography
>i. pneumography
>transcephalic i.
>i. tympanometry

impending renal failure

imperfecta
>amelogenesis i.
>dentinogenesis i.
>osteogenesis i. (type I–IV) (OI)
>perinatal lethal osteogenesis i.
>progressive deforming
>osteogenesis i.
>Sillence classification of osteogenesis
>i. (type I, IA, IB, II, III, IV,
>IVA, IVB)

imperforate
>i. anus
>i. anus, hand, and foot anomalies
>i. anus repair
>i. hymen
>i. nasolacrimal duct
>i. urethra
>i. vagina

impervious
>i. sheet
>i. stockinette

impetigo
>Bockhart i.
>bullous i.
>i. contagiosa
>group A streptococcal i.
>i. herpetiformis
>i. neonatorum
>nonbullous i.
>staphylococcal i.
>i. strain

impingement
    i. syndrome
    i. test
Implanon contraceptive device
implant
    benign i.
    Biocell RTV saline-filled breast i.
    breast i.
    cesium i.
    Clarion hearing i.
    cochlear i.
    collapsed subpectoral i.
    Contigen Bard collagen i.
    Contigen glutaraldehyde cross-linked
      collagen i.
    contraceptive i.
    ectopic i.
    endometrial i.
    endometriotic i.
    fetal tissue i.
    goserelin acetate i.
    hormonal i.
    Inamed silicone-filled breast i.
    interstitial i.
    iridium i.
    Jadelle i.
    levonorgestrel i.
    Macroplastique urinary sphincter i.
    McGhan i.
    Mentor MemoryGel silicone
      gel-filled breast i.
    metastatic i.
    Norplant i.
    NovaSaline prefilled breast i.
    Organon percutaneous E2 i.
    peritoneal i.
    progestin-only i.
    radioactive i.
    radium i. (rad imp)
    saline i.
    silicone i.
    single rod i.
    subdermal i.
    subdermal levonorgestrel i.
      (SLI)
    subpectoral i.
    Supprelin-LA 12-month i.
    Tegress urethral i.
    transperineal i.
    transvaginal i.
    Zoladex I.
implantable hormonal contraceptive
implantation
    artificial sphincter i.
    bilateral PC-IOL i.
    blastocyst i.
    i. bleeding
    cortical i.
    delayed i.

    displacement i.
    ectopic i.
    i. failure
    fusion i.
    intrusive i.
    i. phase
    placental i.
    prosthetic graft i.
    i. protein
    radioactive seed i.
    i. theory
    tubouterine i.
impotence, impotency
    psychogenic i.
impotency (*var. of* impotence)
impotent
impregnate
impregnated vaginal packing
impressio (*var. of* impression)
impression, impressio
    basilar i.
    Clinical Global I.'s (CGI)
Impress Softpatch
imprint
    touch i.
imprinted gene
imprinting
    genomic i.
improper formula preparation
improved
    Clearblue I.
    Hybolin I.
impulse
    apical i.
    point of maximal i. (PMI)
    point of maximum i. (PMI)
    i. spectrum disorder
impulsive
impulsivity
    hyperactive i.
IMR
    infant mortality rate
Imuran
Imuthiol
IMV
    intermittent mandatory ventilation
    intermittent mechanical ventilation
IMx Estradiol Assay
in
    i. extremis
    rooming i.
    i. situ
    i. situ nucleic acid hybridization
    i. situ pinning
    i. situ tubularization
    toeing i.
    i. toto
    i. utero (IU)
    i. utero drainage

I

in (*continued*)
  i. utero drainage of fetal bladder
  i. utero drug exposure (IUDE)
  i. utero exposure
  i. utero hypoxia
  i. utero percutaneous umbilical cord ligation
  i. utero reduction
  i. utero reduction of herniated viscera
  i. utero resection
  i. utero sensitization
  i. utero stem cell therapy
  i. utero transplantation
  i. vitro (IV)
  i. vitro antibody production (IVAP)
  i. vitro efficacy
  i. vitro fertilization
  i. vitro fertilization-embryo transfer (IVF-ET)
  i. vitro human intestinal organ culture
  i. vitro maturation
  i. vitro resistance
  i. vivo (IV)
  i. vivo fertilization (IVF)
  i. vivo gene therapy

¹¹¹In
  indium-111
In-111
  indium-111
inactivated
  i. poliomyelitis vaccine
  i. polio vaccine
  i. poliovirus
  i. poliovirus vaccine (IPV)
  i. virus vaccine
  i. X chromosome
inactivation
  i. pattern
  random X i.
  X i.
inactive endometrium
inactivity
  alert i.
  glucuronyl transferase i.
inadequacy
  luteal phase i.
inadequate
  i. body awareness
  i. luteal phase
  i. maternal nutrition
Inamed silicone-filled breast implant
inanition fever
inapparent poliomyelitis
inappropriate
  i. antidiuretic hormone (IADH)
  i. antidiuretic hormone secretion
  i. lactation

Inapsine
inattention
  i. dimension
  i. domain
inattention-overactivity with aggression (IOWA)
inattentive
inborn
  i. error
  i. error of bile acid biosynthesis
  i. error of bile acid synthesis
  i. error of metabolism (IEM)
inbreeding
  i. coefficient
  coefficient of i.
  i. depression
INCA
  infant nasal cannula assembly
incadronate
incapacitating pain
incarcerated
  i. fundus
  i. gravid uterus
  i. inguinal hernia
  i. placenta
incarceration
  uterine i.
incentive spirometry
incessant ovulation
incest
incestuous
incidence
incidentaloma
incidental thrombocytopenia
incipient
  i. abortion
  i. coagulopathy
incision
  abdominal i.
  i. and drainage
  Bevan i.
  bikini cut i.
  bilateral subcostal i.'s
  boutonnière i.
  buttonhole i.
  cervical i.
  Cherney i.
  classic i.
  classical transverse i.
  classical uterine i.
  i. closure
  colpotomy i.
  counter stab wound i.
  Dührssen i.
  elliptical uterine i.
  endoscopic i.
  gridiron i.
  hockey stick i.
  infraumbilical i.

inverted T uterine i.
Joel-Cohen i.
Kehr i.
Lanz i.
laparoscopic i.
laparotomy i.
lazy S i.
longitudinal i.
low-segment transverse i.
low transverse uterine i. (LTUI)
low vertical uterine i.
Maylard i.
McBurney i.
midline longitudinal i.
paramedian i.
periumbilical i.
Pfannenstiel i.
prior low transverse uterine i.
prior low vertical uterine i.
Rockey-Davis i.
rooftop i.
saber cut i.
Sanger i.
Schuchardt i.
Sellheim i.
smiling i.
subcostal i.
supraumbilical i.
transverse i.
transverse skin i.
uterine i.
vertical i.
Y i.
incisional
    i. cellulitis
    i. cellulitis
    i. hernia
    i. neuroma
incision-to-clamp time
incision-to-delivery time
incisor
    barrel-shaped upper central i.
    central i.
    Hutchinson i.
    intruded i.
    lateral i.
    peg-shaped upper central i.
    prominent maxillary i.
    single central maxillary i. (SCMI)
incisura, incisure, *pl.* **incisurae**
incisurae (*pl. of* incisura)
incisure (*var. of* incisura)
    Schmidt-Lantermann i.
inciting event
inclination
    pelvic i.
incline
inclusion
    i. body

i. body of chlamydial conjunctivitis
i. cell (I-cell)
i. cell disease
i. cyst
full i.
hyaline eosinophilic i.
intracytoplasmic i.
lipid i.
Paneth cell i.
paracrystalline i.
incognito
    tinea i.
incoherence
income
    Supplemental Security I. (SSI)
incomitant strabismus
incompatibility
    ABO i.
    blood group i.
    minor group antigen i.
    platelet-antigen i.
    Rh i.
incompatible blood group antigen
incompetence, incompetency
    cervical i. (CI)
    congenital palatopharyngeal i. (CPI)
    florid pulmonary valvular i.
    gastroesophageal i.
    organic tricuspid i.
    palatopharyngeal i.
    pelvic vein i.
    pharyngeal i.
    sphincteric i.
    velopharyngeal i. (VPI)
incompetency (*var. of* incompetence)
incompetent
    i. cervix
    i. lower esophageal sphincter
incomplete
    i. abortion (IAB)
    i. alveolar development
    i. androgen insensitivity
    i. bowel obstruction
    i. breech presentation
    i. cleft
    i. conjoined twins
    i. dominance
    i. foot presentation
    i. hernia
    i. knee presentation
    i. müllerian fusion
    i. precocious puberty
    i. rectal prolapse
    i. syndactyly
    i. uterine inversion
incompletus
    coitus i.

incongruent hip
inconsequential occurrence
inconspicuous penis
incontinence, incontinentia
    anal i.
    anorectal i.
    Blaivas classification of urinary i.
    i. dish pessary
    exercise-induced i.
    fecal i. (FI)
    functional i.
    genuine stress i. (GSI)
    giggle i.
    I. Impact Questionnaire (IIQ)
    I. Impact Questionnaire-Revised
      (IIQ-R)
    key-in-lock i.
    mixed i.
    Miyazaki-Bonney test for stress i.
    i. of milk
    overflow i.
    paradoxical i.
    passive i.
    postpartum i.
    I. quality of life (I-QOL)
    quality of life in persons with
      urinary i. (I-QOL)
    reflex i.
    I. Severity Index
    stress i.
    I. Stress Questionnaire (ISQ)
    stress urinary i. (SUI)
    true i.
    unconscious i.
    urge i.
    urinary exertional i.
    urinary stress i. (USI)
    urodynamic stress i.
incontinentia
    i. pigmenti achromians
    i. pigmenti syndrome
    i. pigmenti (type I, II)
incorporation
    meatal advancement and
      glanduloplasty i. (MAGPI)
    meatal advancement and glansplasty
      i. (MAGPI)
increase
    plasma prorenin i.
increased
    i. anteroposterior chest diameter
    i. bone density
    i. fatigability
    i. femoral anteversion
    i. globulin fraction
    i. intracranial pressure
    i. renin release
    i. resting oxygen requirement
    i. vascular resistance

increta
    placenta i.
incubate
incubation period (ICP)
incubator
    Air Shields i.
    convection-warmed i.
    double-insulated i.
    double-walled i.
    Forma in vitro i.
    Forma water-jacketed i.
    Ohmeda Care-Plus i.
    single-walled i.
incudes (*pl. of* incus)
incudiformis
    uterus i.
incudiform uterus
incus, *pl.* **incudes**
indapamide
independence
    causal i.
independent
Inderal LA
indeterminate
    i. leprosy
    i. sleep
indeterminus
    situs i.
    situs inversus i.
index (I, ind), *pl.* **indices**
    acetabular i. (AI)
    age i.
    amniotic fluid i. (AFI)
    anal i. (AI)
    anxiety sensitivity i. (ASI)
    axial acetabular i. (AAI)
    Bailey Physical Development I.
    Bayley Mental Developmental I.
    Bayley Psychomotor
      Developmental I.
    blood cell indices
    body mass i. (BMI)
    borderline amniotic fluid i.
    Broders i.
    cardiac i. (CI)
    i. case
    Charlson comorbidity i.
    Clinical Colitis Activity I. (CCAI)
    clinical global i. (CGI)
    Colour I. (CI, C.I.)
    Conners Hyperactivity indices
    deoxyribonucleic acid i.
    DNA i.
    Doppler myocardial performance i.
    Female Sexual Function I. (FSFI)
    fetal-pelvic i.
    fine motor i.
    i. finger
    Foam Stability I. (FSI)

free androgen i.
free testosterone i.
free thyroxine i.
glycemic i.
gross motor i.
growth i.
Hollingshead 5-factor i.
HuGE i.
iliac apophysis maturation i.
Incontinence Severity I.
Karnofsky Performance Scale I.
karyopyknotic i.
Kessner I.
Kruger i.
Kupperman i.
left ventricular stroke work i.
  (LVSWI)
Lloyd-Still i.
McGoon i.
Mengert i.
mental development i. (MDI)
Mentzer i.
migration i. (MI)
mixed obstructive apnea/hypopnea i.
  (MOAHI)
neural i.
nonverbal developmental i.
oxygenation i. (OI)
Parental Stress I. (PSI)
Pearl i.
Pediatric Crohn Disease Activity I.
  (PCDAI)
pelvic i.
pelvic support i. (PSI)
Penetrating Abdominal Trauma I.
  (PATI)
PGWB i.
Physiologic Stability I. (PSI)
placental maturity i.
ponderal i. (PI)
Pourcelot i.
Prehospital I. (PHI)
prepregnancy body mass i.
Psychological General Well-Being i.
psychomotor development i. (PDI)
pulmonary vascular restrictive i.
  (PVRI)
pulsatility i. (PI)
quantitative insulin sensitivity check
  i. (QUICKI)
Quetelet body mass i.
radiographic bone strength i. (RBSI)
rapid shallow breathing i. (RSBI)
resistance i. (RI)
right ventricular stroke work i.
  (RVSWI)
Rohrer i.
sexual maturation i.
short-increment sensitivity i. (SISI)

Silverman-Anderson i.
stroke volume i. (SVI)
Stuart i.
sun protection behavior i.
  (SBPI)
testosterone i.
thyroid i.
Tobin i.
total testosterone i.
umbilical coiling i. (UCI)
urinary diagnostic i. (UDI)
weight/height i.
W/H i.
Wintrobe i.
Index-I
  State-Trait Anxiety I.-I
India
  I. ink stain
  I. ink test
  I. rubber skin
Indiana pouch
Indian childhood cirrhosis (ICC)
indican
indicanuria
indications
  maternal i.
indicator
  Bioself fertility i.
  prognostic i.
indices (*pl. of* index)
Indiclor test
indifferent
  i. genitalia
  i. gonad
  i. gonadal stage
indigenous neoplasm
indigo
  i. carmine
  i. carmine dye
indigotin
indinavir
  i. calculi
  i. crystal
indirect
  i. bilirubin
  i. calorimetry
  i. Coombs test
  i. cystography
  i. fluorescent antibody (IFA)
  i. hemagglutination
  i. hemagglutination antibody (IHA)
  i. hyperbilirubinemia
  i. immunofluorescence (IIF)
  i. inguinal hernia
  i. laryngoscopy
  i. laser ophthalmoscope
  i. ophthalmoscope
  i. ophthalmoscopy
  i. orbital floor fracture

indirect (*continued*)
    i. placentography
    i. visualization
indium-111 (^{111}In, In-111)
indium-labeled leukocyte scan
individualized
    I. Education Program (IEP)
    I. Family Service Plan (IFSP)
Individuals with Disabilities Education Act (IDEA)
Indocin
    I. I.V.
    I. I.V. Injection
    I. SR
    I. SR Oral
indocyanine green
indolamine
indolent
    i. carditis
    i. endometritis
    i. granular CMV retinitis
indomethacin
indrawing
    intercostal i.
    supraclavicular i.
induced
    i. abortion (IAB)
    i. labor
    i. remission
    i. sputum analysis (ISA)
inducing
    syncytium i.
induction
    i. chemotherapy
    Cytotec i.
    gonadotropin ovulation i.
    labor augmentation i.
    menstrual cycle i.
    ovulation i.
    Pitocin i.
    prostaglandin gel i.
    rapid sequence i.
    Spemann i.
    superovulation i.
    i. therapy
induction-to-delivery interval
induration
    nonpitting i.
indurative edema
indusium griseum
indwelling
    i. arterial catheter (IAC)
    i. cannula
    i. catheter
    i. optode
    i. thumb
    i. venous catheter (IVC)
    i. venous line (IVL)
ineffective myelopoiesis

inefficiency
    female fertility i.
inequality
    limb length i.
inertia
    primary uterine i.
    secondary uterine i.
    true uterine i.
    uterine i.
inertially induced injury
inevitable abortion
Infalyte formula
infancy
    acropustulosis of i.
    acute hemorrhagic edema of i. (AHEI)
    anaclitic depression of i.
    apnea of i. (AOI)
    autoimmune neutropenia of i. (ANI)
    benign myoclonus of i.
    benign paroxysmal torticollis of i.
    chronic nonspecific diarrhea of i.
    chronic pneumonitis of i. (CPI)
    cricopharyngeal incoordination of i.
    diencephalic syndrome of i.
    familial hyperinsulinism of i.
    hemorrhagic edema of i.
    hypertrophic interstitial neuropathy of i.
    intractable diarrhea of i. (IDI)
    nonfamilial hyperinsulinism of i.
    normal gastroesophageal reflux of i.
    persistent hyperinsulinemic hypoglycemia of i. (PHHI)
    physiologic anemia of i.
    protracted diarrhea of i.
    severe myoclonic epilepsy in i. (SMEI)
    spongy degeneration of i.
    transient hypogammaglobulinemia of i. (THI)
infancy-onset diabetes mellitus, multiple epiphysial dysplasia syndrome
Infanrix vaccine
infant
    acid-loaded i.
    aneuploidy i.
    asphyctic i.
    at-risk i.
    I. Behavior Record (IBR)
    i. bronchoscope
    i. death
    i. development
    i. development program
    i. development specialist
    i. dietary supplement
    drug-depressed i.
    dysmature i.

i. dyssomnia
i. educator
ELBW i.
extremely low birth weight i.
  (ELBWI)
extremely premature i. (EPI)
i. face scale
floppy i.
I. Flow nCPAP system
full-term i.
i. Hercules
high-risk i.
hydropic i.
i. hypergastrinemia
hyperinsulinemic i.
immature i.
jittery i.
large-for-dates i.
LBW i.
LGA i.
liveborn i.
low birth weight i. (LBWI)
macrosomic i.
MAS-ECMO i.
mature i.
i. morbidity
i. mortality
i. mortality rate (IMR)
i. nasal cannula assembly (INCA)
near-term i.
Neurodevelopmental Assessment of
  Preterm Infants (NAPI)
i. of diabetic mother
i. of substance-abusing mother
periodic breathing in i.'s
postmature i.
postterm i.
premature i. (PI, preemie)
preterm i.
i. respiratory distress syndrome
  (IRDS)
Rh-positive i.
i. safety
SGA i.
singleton i.
i. size (IS)
sleepy i.
small premature i.
i. Star high-frequency ventilator
I. Star 8000 oscillator
stillborn i.
i. stimulation program
i. subdural tap
i. suffocation
i. teacher
term i.
very low birth weight i.
viable i.
vigorous i.

VLBW i.
well-oxygenated i.
infanticide
infantile
  i. achalasia
  i. acquired aphasia
  i. acropustulosis
  i. agranulocytosis
  i. Alexander disease
  i. anorexia
  i. arteriosclerosis
  i. asthma
  i. autism (IA)
  i. beriberi
  i. bilateral striatal necrosis syndrome
    (IBSN)
  i. botulism (IB)
  i. breath-holding response
  i. cataract
  i. celiac disease
  i. cerebellooptic atrophy
  i. cerebral sphingolipidosis
  i. choreoathetosis of Fisher
  i. colic
  i. corneal clouding
  i. cortical hyperostosis (ICH)
  i. diarrhea
  i. diarrhea rotavirus
  i. digital fibroma
  i. diplegia
  i. disseminated histoplasmosis
  i. dwarfism
  i. eczema
  i. embryonal carcinoma
  i. epilepsy
  i. epileptic encephalopathy
  i. esotropia
  i. fibromatosis
  i. Gaucher disease
  i. glaucoma
  i. hemangiopericytoma
  i. hemiplegia
  i. hepatic hemangioma
  i. hypercalcemia
  i. hypertension
  i. hypertrophic pyloric stenosis
    (IHPS)
  i. idiopathic scoliosis
  i. masturbation
  i. monoclonic seizure
  i. motor neuron disease
  i. muscular hypotonia
  i. muscular torticollis
  i. myoclonic jerk
  i. myoclonic seizure
  i. myofibrillar myopathy
  i. myofibromatosis
  i. myxedema
  i. myxedema-muscular hypertrophy

infantile (*continued*)
   i. NCL
   i. neuroaxonal dystrophy
   i. neuronal degeneration
   i. neuropathic cystinosis
   i. obstructive cholangiopathy
   i. onset
   i. optic atrophy-ataxia syndrome
   i. osteopetrosis
   i. paralysis
   i. periarteritis nodosa (IPN)
   i. PKD
   i. poikiloderma
   i. polyarteritis nodosa (IPAN, IPN)
   i. polycystic disease (IPCD)
   i. polycystic kidney
   i. polycystic kidney disease
     (IPKD)
   i. polyneuritis
   i. progressive spinal muscular
     atrophy (type I–III)
   i. purulent conjunctivitis
   i. pustulosis
   i. pyknocytosis
   i. Refsum disease
   i. Refsum disease continuum
   i. respiratory distress syndrome
   i. salaam
   i. scurvy
   i. seborrhea
   i. seborrheic dermatitis
   i. sialic acid storage disorder
     (ISSD)
   i. sleep apnea
   i. spasm (IS)
   i. spasms, hypsarrhythmia, mental
     retardation syndrome
   i. spasms with mental retardation
   i. spastic paraplegia
   i. spinal muscular atrophy (ISMA)
   i. striatonigral degeneration
   i. subacute necrotizing
     encephalopathy
   i. syncope
   i. system hyalinosis
   i. tetany
   i. thoracic dystrophy
   i. tibia vara
   i. tremor syndrome
infantile-onset spinocerebellar ataxia
infantilis
   dystaxia cerebralis i.
   poliodystrophia cerebri
     progressiva i.
infantilism
   Brissaud i.
   cachectic i.
   celiac i.
   dysthyroidal i.

   hepatic i.
   Herter i.
   hypophysial i.
   Lorain-Lévi i.
   muscular i.
   myxedematous i.
   pseudonuchal i.
   regressive i.
   sexual i.
infantis
   Bifidobacterium i.
infantiseptica
   granulomatosis i.
InfantSEE vision program
infantum
   anemia pseudoleukemica i.
   cholera i.
   dermatitis gangrenosa i.
   granuloma gluteal i.
   Leishmania i.
   lichen i.
   roseola i.
   tabes i.
infarct
infarction
   acute myocardial i. (AMI)
   bilirubin i.
   bowel i.
   cavernosal i.
   cerebral i.
   chorionic villus i.
   CNS i.
   fan-shaped hemorrhagic i.
   fat-induced i.
   hyperacute i.
   limb i.
   maternal floor i.
   multiple villous i.
   myocardial i. (MI)
   i. of herniated stomach
   i. of oral epithelium
   i. of skinfold
   parasagittal cortical i.
   periventricular i.
   placental i.
   pulmonary i.
   renal i.
   uric acid i.
   white i.
In-Fast bone screw system
Infasurf
   I. intratracheal suspension
   I. surfactant
Infatab
infected
   i. abortion
   i. cuff hematoma
   HIV i.
   vertically i.

infection

acute lower respiratory i. (ALRI)
acute lower respiratory tract i. (ALRTI)
acute respiratory i. (ARI)
adenovirus i.
adnexal i.
amniotic fluid i.
ascending intrauterine i.
astrovirus i.
asymptomatic i.
asymptomatic urinary tract i. (AUTI)
bacterial i.
Bartonella henselae i.
benign papillomavirus i.
bloodstream i. (BSI)
bone i.
Calicivirus i.
Campylobacter i.
Candida i.
cervical i.
cervicovaginal i.
chlamydial i.
chorioamnion i.
chorioamnionic i.
chronic conjunctival i.
chronic parvoviral i.
chronic pelvic i.
chronic urinary tract i.
congenital i.
congenital intrauterine i.
congenital rubella i. (CRI)
congenital STORCH i.
congenital syphilitic i.
conjunctival i.
Coxsackievirus A16 i.
Coxsackievirus B enterovirus i.
culture-negative cytomegalovirus i.
cytomegalovirus i.
dermatophyte i.
disseminated gonococcal i.
disseminated herpes i.
droplet i.
enteric i.
enteroviral i.
fetal cytomegalovirus i.
fungal i.
GAS i.
gastrointestinal i.
genital i.
genital tract i.
gland i.
gonococcal i.
granulomatous i.
group A beta-hemolytic streptococcal i.
group B streptococcal i.
guinea worm i.

hematogenous i.
herpes whitlow i.
herpetic corneal i.
HIV i.
hookworm i.
intraabdominal i. (IAI)
intraamniotic i. (IAI)
intraarticular i.
intractable viral i.
intrauterine i. (IUI)
intrauterine parvovirus B19 i.
invasive bacterial i.
IUD-related i.
latent herpes simplex virus i.
lower genital tract i.
lower respiratory i. (LRI)
lower respiratory tract i. (LRTI)
lower urinary tract i.
lytic i.
MAI i.
i. marker
maternal i.
middle ear i.
multiple opportunistic pathogen i.
multiplicity of i. (MOI)
mycotic i.
nail-fold i.
neisserial i.
neonatal herpes simplex virus i.
nonprimary i.
nontuberculous mycobacterial i.
nosocomial i.
nosocomial bacterial i. (NBI)
opportunistic i.
overwhelming i.
papillomavirus i.
parameningeal i.
parasitic i.
paronychial i.
parvoviral i.
pediatric gonococcal i.
pelvic i.
perinatally acquired HIV i.
pharyngeal gonococcal i.
i. point
polymicrobial pelvic i.
posthysterectomy i.
postoperative i.
postpartum i.
prenatal i.
primary i.
puerperal i.
pyogenic i.
recurrent staphylococcal i.
respiratory i.
respiratory tract i. (RTI)
retroperitoneal i.
rhinocerebral i.
rickettsial i.

I

primary i.
secondary i.
i. treatment
tubal factor i.
tuboperitoneal i.
unexplained i.
infestation
louse i.
mite i.
pinworm i.
threadworm i.
infibulation
infiltrate
cellular i.
eosinophilic i.
inflammatory i.
interstitial i.
leukemia i.
liver i.
lung i.
miliary i.
patchy i.
perihilar i.
perivascular eosinophilic i.
perivascular inflammatory i.
perivascular polymorphonuclear
    i.
plasma cell i.
pleomorphic cellular i.
polymorphonuclear i.
pulmonary i.
retinal i.
streaky i.
white retinal i.
xanthogranulomatous i.
yellow retinal i.
infiltrating
i. ductal carcinoma (IDC)
i. lobular carcinoma (ILC)
i. small cell lobular
    carcinoma
infiltration
bone marrow i.
fatty i.
leukocyte i.
lidocaine i.
lymphohistiocytic i.
lymphomatous i.
lymphoplasmacytic i.
nodular i.
patchy i.
peribronchial i.
peribronchiolar i.
perineal i.
Inflamase
I. Forte Ophthalmic
I. Mild Ophthalmic
inflammation
acute renal parenchymal i.

chronic synovial i.
ductal i.
eye i.
fibrosing i.
histologic placental i.
intraamniotic i.
lymphoplasmacytic i.
maternal intravascular i.
orbital i.
pelvic i.
portal i.
transmural i.
vulvovaginal i.
inflammatory
i. arteritis
i. bacterial enteritis
i. bowel disease (IBD)
I. Bowel Disease Questionnaire
    (IBDQ)
i. bowel malignancy
i. breast cancer (IBC)
i. Brown syndrome
i. carcinoma
i. cascade
i. colitis
i. demyelinating encephalomyelitis
i. demyelination
i. exudate
i. idiocy
i. infiltrate
i. molecule
i. myopathy
i. myositis
i. osteochondrosis
i. polyp
i. process
i. pseudotumor (IPT)
i. response
inflatable ball pessary
inflection, inflexion
voice i.
inflexion (*var. of* inflection)
infliximab
influence
neurobiologic i.
influenza (flu)
i. A
i. A encephalitis
i. B
i. C
Haemophilus influenzae
i. immunization
i. vaccine
i. virus
influenza-like syndrome
influenzal meningitis
informatics
information
integrate sensory i.

information (*continued*)
    pediatric dosing i.
    sensory i.
informed
    i. consent
    i. consent disclosure rules
informosome
infraclavicular
    i. area
    i. node
infraction
    Freiberg i.
infrahyoid ectopia
inframammary
infraorbital nerve
infrapubic ramus
infrared
    i. photocoagulation (IRC)
    i. spectroscopy
    i. thermographic calorimetry (ITC)
infratentorial
    i. tuberculoma
    i. tumor
infraumbilical incision
infravesical obstruction
infundibula (*pl. of* infundibulum)
infundibular
    i. chamber
    i. pulmonic stenosis
    i. stalk
infundibuliform hymen
infundibulopelvic (IP)
    i. ligament
    i. vessel
infundibulum, *pl.* **infundibula**
    i. of fallopian tube
    right ventricular i.
infusate
Infuse-A-Port catheter
infusion
    alkali i.
    apotransferrin i.
    bicarbonate i.
    colloid i.
    continuous glucose i.
    continuous milk i.
    continuous subcutaneous i. (CSQI)
    continuous subcutaneous insulin i.
    extraamniotic saline i. (EASI)
    fetal cortisol i.
    insulin i.
    intraarterial i.
    intralymphatic i.
    intraosseous i. (IOI)
    intravenous i.
    IO i.
    laminaria i.
    i. pump
    vasopressin i.

Ingelman-Sundberg gracilis muscle vesicovaginal fistula repair procedure
ingestion
    accidental caustic i.
    alcohol i.
    caustic i.
    coin i.
    copper sulfate i.
    drug i.
    fava bean i.
    goitrogen i.
    intentional i.
    iron i.
    lead i.
    organophosphate i.
    paraquat i.
    toxic i.
Ingram
    I. bicycle seat
    I. icterometer
ingrown toenail
inguinal
    i. adenitis
    i. adenopathy
    i. area
    i. canal
    i. freckling
    i. hernia
    i. ligament
    i. lymphadenectomy
    i. lymphadenitis
    i. lymph node
    i. lymph node metastasis
    i. triangle
inguinale
    granuloma i.
    hernia i.
    hernia uteri i.
    lymphogranuloma i.
inguinal-femoral node dissection
inguinofemoral lymph node
INH
    isoniazid
    isonicotinic acid hydrazide
inhalation
    i. anesthesia
    Atrovent Aerosol I.
    i. bronchial challenge testing
    i. injury
    INOmax for i.
    intrapulmonary i.
    NebuPent I.
    nitrogen dioxide i.
    i. of nitrous oxide
    smoke i.
    i. suspension
    tobramycin solution for i. (TOBI)
inhaled
    i. beta-2 agonist

i. bronchodilator
i. corticosteroid (ICS)
i. nitric oxide (iNO, INO)
i. nitric oxide therapy
i. steroid

inhaler
AeroBid-M Oral aerosol i.
AeroBid Oral aerosol i.
Azmacort Oral I.
Beconase AQ Nasal I.
Dexacort Phosphate Respihaler Oral
I.
Diskhaler metered-dose i.
Diskus i.
dry powder i. (DPI)
fluticasone propionate dry
powder i.
metered-dose i. (MDI)
Nasalide Nasal I.
steroid i.
Vancenase Nasal I.
Vanceril Oral I.

inheritance
amphigonous i.
autosomal dominant i.
autosomal recessive i.
biparental i.
codominant i.
complemental i.
cytoplasmic i.
dominant i.
extrachromosomal i.
holandric i.
hologynic i.
homochronous i.
homotropic i.
maternal i.
matroclinous i.
mendelian i.
mitochondrial i.
monofactorial i.
multifactorial i.
oligogenic i.
polygenic i.
quantitative i.
quasicontinuous i.
recessive i.
sex-linked i.
unit i.
X-linked dominant i.
X-linked recessive i.
Y-linked i.

inherited
i. androgen uptake impairment
i. bleeding disorder
i. coagulopathy
i. hemolytic uremia syndrome
i. infertility
i. thrombophilia in pregnancy

inhibin
i. A
i. A subunit
i. B
i. concentration
i. subunit
i. test

inhibited sexual desire

inhibition
agglutination i.
behavioral i.
callosal i.
feedback i.
FSH i.
hemagglutination i. (HI)
labor i.
luteinization i.
pituitary gonadotropin i.
premature uterine contraction i.
prostaglandin synthesis i.
response i.
steroid secretion i.
vagal i.

inhibitive casting

inhibitor
ACE i.
alpha-2 antiplasmin coagulation i.
alpha-2 antitrypsin i.
alpha-2AP coagulation i.
alpha-2AT coagulation i.
alpha-glucosidase i.
alpha-2 macroglobulin coagulation i.
alpha-2M coagulation i.
alpha-1 protease i.
alpha-1 proteinase i. (A1PI)
angiotensin-converting enzyme i.
antithrombin III coagulation i.
aromatase i.
AT3 coagulation i.
calcineurin i.
CAMP-specific phosphodiesterase i.
carbonic anhydrase i.
cell growth i.
C1 esterase i.
cholinesterase i.
C1INH coagulation i.
corticotropin-releasing i.
COX-2 i.
dihydrofolate reductase i.
dual nucleoside analog reverse
transcriptase i.
extrinsic pathway i.
factor VII, VIII i.
fibrinolysis i.
FSH binding i.
fusion i.
gonadotropin secretion i.
HCII coagulation i.
heme oxygenase i.

inhibitor (*continued*)
    heparin cofactor II i.
    HMG-CoA reductase i.
    human seminal i. (HSI)
    hydrogen pump i.
    leukotriene i.
    lupus i.
    luteinization i.
    luteinizing hormone receptor-binding
      i.
    M2 i.
    mitogen activated protein kinase i.
    monoamine oxidase i. (MAOI)
    myocardial phosphodiesterase i.
    neuraminidase i.
    nonnucleoside reverse transcriptase i.
      (NNRTI)
    norepinephrine reuptake i.
    nucleoside reverse transcriptase i.
      (NRTI)
    oocyte maturation i. (OMI)
    ovum-capture i.
    phosphodiesterase i. (PDI)
    plasminogen activator i. (PAI)
    prostaglandin synthetase i.
      (PGSI)
    protease i. (PI)
    protein C coagulation i.
    protein S coagulation i.
    proton pump i. (PPI)
    reverse transcriptase i. (RTI)
    secretory leukocyte protease i.
    selective serotonin reuptake i.
      (SSRI)
    serine protease i. (SERPIN)
    serotonin reuptake i. (SRI)
    serum protease i.
    specific phosphodiesterase i.
    tissue factor pathway i. (TFPI)
    topoisomerase-1 i.
    urinary trypsin i.
inhibitory reflex
in-hospital postpartum care
iniencephaly
iniopagus
iniops
initial apnea
initiated cycle
initiation
    labor i.
    lactation i.
    puberty i.
    sexual i.
initiative
    Women's Health I. (WHI)
inject
    Dekasol-L.A. I.
injectable
    i. bromocriptine

    Cardizem I.
    i. hormonal contraceptive
injection
    adrenaline i.
    Adrucil I.
    A-hydroCort I.
    A-methaPred I.
    Antispas I.
    Apresoline I.
    AquaMEPHYTON I.
    Arfonad I.
    Aristocort Forte I.
    Aristocort intralesional i.
    Aristospan intraarticular i.
    Aristospan intralesional i.
    Astramorph PF i.
    Baci-IM I.
    Benadryl i.
    Bentyl Hydrochloride I.
    bulbar conjunctival i.
    Celestone Phosphate i.
    Cel-U-Jec I.
    Cetrorelix for i.
    Chloromycetin I.
    Chlor-Trimeton I.
    choriogonadotropin alfa for i.
    Cipro I.
    combined estrogen and progesterone
      i.
    conjunctival i.
    continuous subcutaneous insulin i.
    Decadron-LA I.
    Decadron Phosphate I.
    Decaject I.
    Decaject-LA I.
    decondensed spermhead i.
    Definity suspension for IV i.
    Dekasol I.
    Delatestryl I.
    Demadex I.
    Depo-Estradiol I.
    Depogen I.
    Depo-Medrol i.
    Depopred I.
    Depo-Provera I.
    Depo-Testosterone I.
    Dexasone L.A. I.
    Dexone LA I.
    Diazemuls I.
    Dilaudid i.
    Dilaudid-HP i.
    Diprivan I.
    direct egg i.
    direct intraperitoneal i. (DIPI)
    Duraclon I.
    Duramorph i.
    Edecrin Sodium I.
    ganirelix acetate i.
    Genotropin I.

glutaraldehyde crosslinked collagen i.
Hexadrol Phosphate I.
Humalog insulin lispro i.
Humatrope I.
Hydrocortone Acetate I.
Hydrocortone Phosphate I.
Hyrexin-50 I.
Hyzine-50 I.
Imitrex I.
Indocin I.V. I.
intracardiac i.
intracytoplasmic sperm i. (ICSI)
intracytoplasmic sperm head i.
  (ICSHI)
intraurethral bulk i.
Isuprel I.
Kefurox I.
Kenalog I.
Key-Pred I.
Kytril I.
Lasix I.
Levothroid I.
local methotrexate i.
medroxyprogesterone i.
menotropins for i.
Minocin IV i.
myofascial i.
Nebcin i.
Neut I.
nonexudative conjunctival i.
Norditropin I.
Nuromax I.
Nutropin AQ I.
Nydrazid I.
Octocaine I.
Osmitrol I.
paracervical i.
Pentam-300 I.
periurethral bulk i.'s
periurethral collagen i.
pessary i.
Phenergan i.
Prednisol TBA i.
Prorex i.
Protropin I.
pudendal i.
Regonol I.
retrograde ureteral dye i.
Romazicon I.
round spermatid nuclei i. (ROSNI)
Saizen I.
i. sclerotherapy
Serostim I.
silicone i.
Solu-Cortef I.
Solu-Medrol i.
Solurex LA I.
Sublimaze i.
subtrigonal i.

subureteric Teflon i.
subzonal i. (SUZI)
Sufenta i.
Synthroid I.
Tac-3 I.
Teflon periurethral i.
Terramycin IM i.
Ticon I.
Tigan I.
Toposar I.
Toradol i.
transurethral collagen i.
Triam-A i.
Triam Forte i.
Triostat I.
urofollitropin for i.
Valium I.
Vancocin i.
Vancoled i.
Vistaril I.
Zinacef i.

injector

Harris uterine i. (HUI)
MadaJet XL needle-free i.
Mini-Flex flexible Harris uterine i.

injury

AAST organ injury scaling of
  vulva, vagina, bladder, urethral,
  rectal i. (grade I–V)
acceleration i.
accidental fetal i.
acute i.
airbag i.
anoxic-ischemic i.
asphyxial birth i.
asphyxial brain i.
avulsion i.
axonal i.
birth i.
bladder i.
blowout i.
blunt cardiac i. (BCI)
bowel i.
brachial plexus i. (BPI)
brain i.
capillary leak i.
cardiovascular i.
catastrophic i.
caustic i.
cerebral i.
cervical spinal cord i.
cervical spine i.
clavicular i.
clenched fist i.
closed fist i.
closed head i. (CHI)
compression i.
congenital i.
contrecoup i.

injury (*continued*)
coup i.
crush i.
deceleration i.
degloving i.
diaphragmatic i.
diffuse axonal i. (DAI)
emergent i.
epiphysial plate i.
eversion i.
excitotoxic i.
extravasation i.
facial nerve i. (FNI)
fetal birth i.
flexion-distraction i.
greenstick i.
growth plate i.
hair tourniquet i.
hepatocellular i.
hippocampal pathologic i.
hymenal i.
hypoxic-ischemic brain i.
hypoxic-ischemic cerebral i.
iatrogenic airway i.
iatrogenic ureteral i.
inertially induced i.
inhalation i.
intracranial i. (ICI)
intraoperative gastrointestinal i.
intrapleural i.
irradiation i.
ischemic brain i.
Kehr sign for splenic i.
large bowel i.
Lauge-Hansen mechanism of i.
life-threatening i.
ligamentous i. (grade I–III)
lumbosacral plexus i.
mechanical birth i.
meniscal i.
mitochondrial i.
muscular i.
musculoskeletal i.
neonatal brain i.
neonatal cold i.
nerve i.
neurologic i.
neuromuscular i.
obstetric traction i.
overuse i.
oxidative brain i.
parasagittal cerebral i.
pelvic nerve i.
penetrating brain i.
peripheral nerve i.
physial i.
popsicle i.
i. prevention
pulmonary i.

radiation-induced physial i.
rectal i.
reperfusion i.
Salter-Harris classification of
epiphysial plate i.
scalding i.
i. severity score (ISS)
small bowel i.
spinal cord i.
splenic i.
sports-related i.
straddle i.
stress i.
submersion i.
thermal i.
tracheobronchial tree i.
traction i.
transfusion-associated lung i.
(TRALI)
traumatic birth i.
traumatic brain i. (TBI)
ureteral i.
urologic i.
vaginal i.
vascular i.
ventilator-induced lung i.
(VILI)
ventilatory-associated lung i.
(VALI)
vessel i.
whiplash i.
injury-related maternal death
inlet
anteroposterior diameter of the
pelvic i.
conjugate diameter of
pelvic i.
conjugate of i.
pelvic plane of i.
in-line probe
innate
inner
i. amnion
i. canthus
i. canthus displacement
i. cell mass
i. ear
innervated
innervation
autonomic i.
somatic sensory i.
sympathetic i.
innocent murmur
innocuous
innominate
i. artery
i. bone
i. osteotomy
i. vein

Innova
> I. electrotherapy system
> I. feminine incontinence treatment system
> I. pelvic floor stimulator

Innovar

iNO
> inhaled nitric oxide

inoculate

inoculation

inoculum
> intranasal i.

INOH
> instantaneous orthostatic hypotension

INOmax for inhalation

inorganic mercury salt

inosinate pyrophosphorylase enzyme

inosiplex

inositide
> polyphosphol i.

inositol trisphosphate

inotropic
> i. agent
> i. effect
> i. support
> i. therapy

inotropy

Inoue-Melnick virus

INOvent delivery system

inpatient
> i. management
> i. monitoring

InPouch TV subculture kit

input
> abnormal cortical visual i.
> labyrinthine afferent i.
> proprioceptive i.
> unequal visual i.
> vestibular i.

INR
> international normalized ratio

INS
> idiopathic nephrotic syndrome

insect
> i. bite
> i. repellent
> i. sting reaction

insecticide
> organophosphate i.

insecurity
> food i.

insemination
> artificial i. (AI)
> artificial intravaginal i.
> cervical i.
> cup i.
> direct intraperitoneal i. (DIPI)
> i. dish

> donor i. (DI)
> heterologous i.
> high intrauterine i.
> homologous i.
> intrafollicular i. (IFI)
> intraperitoneal i. (IPI)
> intratubal i. (ITI)
> intrauterine i. (IUI)
> intravaginal i. (IVI)
> Makler i.
> subzonal i. (SUZI)
> i. swim-up technique
> therapeutic i.
> therapeutic donor i. (TDI)
> washed intrauterine i.

insensible
> i. fluid loss
> i. water loss (IWL)

insensitive ovary syndrome

insensitivity
> androgen i.
> congenital i.
> growth hormone i. (GHI)
> incomplete androgen i.
> partial androgen i. (PAI)

insert
> Cervidil vaginal i.
> Cookie I.
> FemSoft continence i.
> miconazole 7 vaginal i.
> Monistat 1 combination pack vaginal i.
> urethral occlusion i.

inserter
> IUD i.

insertion
> Achilles tendon i.
> catheter i.
> cord i. (CI)
> deltoid i.
> facial vein i.
> gastric tube i.
> interchromosomal i.
> laminaria tent i.
> marginal cord i.
> i. of chromosome
> i. potential
> saphenous vein catheter i.
> i. sequence
> i. site selection
> subzonal i. (SUZI)
> transpyloric tube i.
> umbilical cord i.
> velamentous cord i.

insertional
> i. dyspareunia
> i. mutagenesis

insipidus
> diabetes i. (DI)

insipidus (*continued*)
    familial vasopressin-sensitive
      diabetes i.
    fetal diabetes i.
    nephrogenic diabetes i.
    neurogenic diabetes i.
    X-linked recessive-type diabetes i.
InSite HER2/neu monoclonal antibody
insomnia
    fatal familial i.
    primary i.
    i. syndrome
insonation
inspiration time (I-time)
inspiratory
    i. capacity (IC)
    i. pressure
    i. reserve volume (IRV)
    i. stridor
    i. time (IT)
    i. to expiratory
    i. whoop
inspire
inspired
    i. gas (I)
    i. oxygen
inspissated
    i. bile
    i. bile syndrome
    i. duct
    i. milk syndrome
    i. mucus
inspissation
    amorphous i.
    mucous i.
    i. of breast secretion
INSS
    International Neuroblastoma Staging
    System
instability
    atlantoaxial i.
    bladder i.
    detrusor i.
    glenohumeral i.
    hemodynamic i.
    neurogenic detrusor i.
    occipitoatlantal i.
    vasomotor i.
instantaneous orthostatic hypotension
(INOH)
Instead feminine protection cup
instillation of hypertonic saline
institute
    National Cancer I. (NCI)
    I. of Medical Safety Review
      Committee
    I. of Personality and Ability Testing
      (IPAT)
institutionalize

instruction
    adult-directed i.
    child-directed i.
instrument
    Acute Surgical and Scientific
      Instruments
    Dolphin i.
    Erbe electrical coagulation i.
    Erbe electrical cutting i.
    Feelings About Yourself i.
    I-QOL i.
    Kevorkian-Younge cervical biopsy i.
    Keyes biopsy i.
    Kocher i.'s
    LDS i.
    Lusk i.
    myoma fixation i.
    narrow-band i.
    Newport medical i.
    PlasmaKinetic i.
    Polaris reusable i.
    RigiScan i.
    Welch Allyn AudioPath Platform
      hearing acuity i.
instrumental
    i. delivery
    i. vertex
instrumentation
    anterior spinal i.
    bladder i.
    Cotrel-Dubousset i. (CDI)
    DeLee i.
    Miami Moss i.
    posterior segmental fixation i.
    segmental spinal i.
    TSRH i.
insufficiency
    ACTH i.
    adrenal i.
    adrenocortical i.
    adrenocorticotropic hormone i.
    alacrima, achalasia, adrenal i.
    aortic valve i.
    caloric i.
    chronic adrenal i.
    chronic mitral i.
    chronic pulmonary i.
    chronic renal i.
    corpus luteum i.
    exocrine pancreatic i.
    fetal-placental i.
    glomerular i.
    glucocorticoid i.
    intrapartum uteroplacental i.
    mitral valve i.
    pancreatic exocrine i.
    placental i.
    prerenal i.
    primary adrenal i.

primary ovarian i.
pulmonary i.
renal i.
respiratory i.
secondary adrenal cortical i.
tricuspid i.
uterine i.
uteroplacental i. (UPI)
valvular i.
insufficient milk production
insufflation
continuous tracheal gas i.
extraperitoneal i.
i. needle
peritoneal i.
tubal i.
insufflator
hysteroscopic i.
Kidde tubal i.
laparoscopic i.
Insulatard NPH human
insulin
beef i.
i. deficiency
exogenous i.
fasting serum i.
glucose plus i.
human i.
i. infusion
I. Lente L
i. lipoatrophy
i. lispro
maternal i.
neutral protamine Hagedorn i.
Novolin i.
NPH i.
i. pen
pork i.
i. pump
regular purified pork i.
i. resistance
i. response
I. RIA 100
i. secretion
i. sensitivity
i. sensitivity test
i. shock
i. tolerance test
insulinase
insulin-dependent
i.-d. diabetes
i.-d. diabetes mellitus (IDDM)
i.-d. diabetic
insulinemia
insulin-induced hypoglycemia
insulinlike
i. growth factor (IGF)
i. growth factor-binding protein (IGFBP)

i. growth factor-binding protein-3 (IGFBP-3)
insulinoma
insulinopenia
insulinotropic peptide
insulin-secreting pancreatic tumor
insulitis
insult
perinatal i.
insurance
Social Security Disability I. (SSDI)
InSure
InSync miniform pad
intact membrane
intake
i. and output (I&O, I/O)
caloric i.
maximal oxygen i. (MOI)
oral i.
periconceptual i.
poor caloric i.
poor oral i.
Intal
Integra
integrate
i. sensation
i. sensory information
integrated
I. Management of Childhood Illness (IMCI)
i. visual and auditory (IVA)
integration
Developmental Test of Visual-Motor I.
sensorimotor i.
sensory i.
structural i.
visual-motor i. (VMI)
integrin
beta-1 i.
beta-2 i.
integrin-binding
integrity
genital tract i.
perineal body i.
intellectual disability
intelligence
borderline i.
Fagan Test of Infant I.
normal i.
i. quotient (IQ)
subaverage i.
i. test
Wechsler preschool and primary scale of i. (WPPSI)
intelligence-revised
Wechsler Preschool and Primary Scale of I.-R. (WPPSI-R)

intense emotional state
intensifier
    image i.
intensity
intensity-duration ratio
intensity-time ratio
intensive
    i. care nursery (ICN)
    i. diabetes management (IDM)
    i. phototherapy
    i. special care nursery (ISCN)
    i. special care unit (ISCU)
intensivist
Intensol
    Diazepam I.
intention
    i. myoclonus
    secondary i.
    i. tremor
intentional
    i. ingestion
    i. poisoning
interaction
    actin-myosin i.
    androgen i.
    caregiver-child i.
    ephaptic i.
    epithelial-mesenchymal i.
    gene-environment i.
    Interview Schedule for Social I.
    mother-child i.
    parent-child i.
    poor feeding i.
    sperm-cervical mucus i.
    sperm-oocyte i.
    stromal-epithelial i.
interactive play therapy
Interagency Coordinating Council (ICC)
interarticularis
    pars i.
interarytenoid notch
interassay
interatrial communication (IAC)
interbody ankylosis
intercalary
    i. defect
    i. defect of pollical ray
intercalatum
    Schistosoma i.
intercapillary distance
Interceed
    I. barrier material
    I. TC7 absorbable adhesion barrier
intercellular
    i. adhesion molecule 1 (ICAM1)
    i. edema
interchange

interchromosomal insertion
intercondylar, intercondylic, intercondyloid
    i. groove
    i. notch
    i. radiograph
intercondylic (*var. of* intercondylar)
intercondyloid (*var. of* intercondylar)
intercostal
    i. drainage
    i. indrawing
    i. perforating artery
    i. retraction (ICR)
    i. space
intercourse
    anal i.
    interfemoral i.
    sexual i.
    timed i.
    vulvar i.
intercross
interdigital
    i. candidasis
    i. web
interdigitation
interdisciplinary team
interest
    atypical i.
interface
    gum-tooth i.
    maternal-fetal i.
    placental i.
    tendon-bone i.
interfemoral intercourse
interference
    acoustical i.
    centromere i.
    chiasma i.
    genetic i.
    negative i.
    positive i.
interferon (IFN)
    alfa i.
    i. alfa-2a
    i. alfa-2b
    i. alfa-N1
    i. alfa-N2
    i. alfa-N3
    i. alfa-NL
    i. alpha
    i. alpha-2a
    i. alpha-2b
    alpha-recombinant i.
    i. beta
    beta i.
    i. beta-1a
    i. beta-1b
    i. beta-recombinant
    gamma i.

i. gamma (IFN-gamma)
i. gamma-1b
human leukocyte i. (HLI)
leukocyte i.
lymphoblastoid i.
pegylated i.
i. therapy
interfetal membrane
Intergel irrigating solution
intergluteal cleft
interhemispheric
i. subarachnoid hemorrhage
i. subdural hematoma
interictal
i. discharge
i. EEG
i. hypoperfusion
i. myokymia
i. spike
interior
i. epigastric artery
i. hemorrhoidal nerve
interkinesis
interleukin (IL)
i. (1–30)
i. deficiency
histamine i.
recombinant i. 2
interleukin-1
interleukin-1B
interlobar
intermaxillary narrowness
InterMed Bear
intermedia
thalassemia i.
intermediate
i. care facility (ICF)
i. dystonic stage
i. trophoblast (IT)
intermedius
Staphylococcus i.
intermenstrual
i. bleeding (IMB)
i. pain
intermittent
i. cyclical etidronate disodium
i. esotropia
i. exotropia
i. fever
i. hematologic cytopenia
i. hydronephrosis
i. hydrosalpinx
i. hypocomplementemia
i. mandatory ventilation
(IMV)
i. mechanical ventilation
(IMV)
i. pneumatic compression
i. porphyria

i. positive pressure breathing (IPPB)
i. positive-pressure ventilation
(IPPV)
i. self-catheterization
i. sterilization
i. strabismus
i. support
i. urinary leakage
intermuscular abscess
intern, interne
interna
endometriosis i.
theca i.
internal
i. anal sphincter (IAS)
i. branchial sinus
i. conjugate
i. derangement
i. diameter
i. discomfort
i. endometriosis
i. excrescence
i. femoral torsion
i. generative organ
i. genitalia
i. hernia
i. hordeolum
i. iliac artery
i. jugular vein
i. jugular vein catheter placement
i. mammary artery
i. monitoring
i. oblique muscle
i. ophthalmoplegia
i. os
i. podalic version
i. podalic version and breech
extraction
i. pudendal artery
i. radiation therapy
i. representation
i. respiration
i. rotation
i. septation
i. tibial torsion
internalization
hormone-receptor complex i.
receptor i.
internalize
internalizing
I. Behavior Scale
i. problem
i. score
international
i. classification of cancer of cervix
I. Classification of Diseases (ICD)
I. Classification of Sleep Disorders
I. Collaborative Ovarian Neoplasm
Trial 1 (ICON1)

international (*continued*)
I. Committee for Contraceptive Research (ICCR)
I. Continence Society (ICS)
I. Federation of Gynecology and Obstetrics (FIGO)
I. League Against Epilepsy (ILAE)
I. League Against Rheumatism
I. League of Associations for Rheumatology (ILAR)
I. Neuroblastoma Staging System
i. normalized ratio (INR)
I. Reference Preparation (IRP)
I. Society for Gynecologic Pathology
I. Society for Heart Transplantation (ISHT)
I. Society for the Study of Vulvar Diseases (ISSVD)
I. Society of Gynecologic Pathologists (ISGYP)
I. Staging System (INSS)
I. Study of Kidney Disease in Children
I. Union Against Cancer (UICC)
I. Unit (IU)
interne (*var. of* intern)
interneuron
aspiny i.
internist
internuclear ophthalmoplegia
internum
erysipelas i.
internus
hydrocephalus i.
obturator i.
interpeak latency
interpectoral node
Interpersonal Support Evaluation List
interphase
interplant
interposition
antiperistaltic intestinal i.
cartilage i.
colonic i.
costal cartilage i.
ileal i.
intestinal i.
isoperistaltic intestinal i.
interpretation
mirror image i.
i. variability
interrogans
Leptospira i.
interrogation
continuous wave Doppler i.
interrupted
i. aortic arch (type A, B)

i. bites
i. suture
interrupted-bite technique
interruption
high-frequency flow i. (HFFI)
tubal i.
vena caval i.
interruptus
coitus i.
intersex
i. abnormality
i. condition
i. disorder
i. problem
intersexuality
intersphincteric
i. abscess
i. groove
i. space
InterStim therapy
interstitial
i. and loculated hematoma
i. brachytherapy
i. cell
i. cystitis (IC)
I. Cystitis Database
i. deletion
i. edema
i. fibrosis
i. fluid
i. implant
i. infiltrate
i. irradiation
i. keratitis
i. lung disease (ILD)
i. mastitis
i. myocarditis
i. nephritis
i. plasma cell pneumonia
i. pneumonitis
i. positive-pressure interferon alpha
i. pregnancy
i. space
i. therapy
interstitium
renal i.
interthreshold zone
intertriginous
i. area
i. candidiasis
i. candidosis
intertrigo
chronic i.
intertrochanteric fracture
intertuberous diameter
interval (int)
atlantodens i. (ADI)
decision-to-delivery i. (DDI)
induction-to-delivery i.

PR i.
prolonged QT i.
pulse i.
QT i.
short PR i.
intervention
antiinflammatory i.
behavioral i.
court-ordered obstetrical i.
crisis i.
early i.
legal i.
mind-body i.
pharmacologic i.
postmenopausal estrogen and
progestin i. (PEPI)
prenatal smoking i.
psychopharmacological i.
pulsed i.
salvage i.
school-based i.
interventional procedure
interventionist
early i.
interventricular septum
intervertebral
i. disc (IVD)
i. disc calcification (IDC)
i. discitis
interview
Autism Diagnostic I. (ADI)
Brown and Harris i.
LEDS i.
life events and difficulties schedule
i.
prenatal i.
psychiatric diagnostic i. (PDI)
I. Schedule for Children and
Adolescents (ISCA)
I. Schedule for Social Interaction
interview-revised
Autism Diagnostic I.-R.
(ADI-R)
intervillositis
massive chronic i. (MCI)
placental i.
intervillous
i. blood
i. blood gas
i. space
i. thrombus (IVT)
interweaving pattern
intestinal
i. aganglionosis
i. atresia
i. bag
i. bladder augmentation
i. bypass procedure
i. conduit

i. disorder
i. duplication
i. fistula
i. hurry
i. hypoxia
i. interposition
i. ischemia
i. lesion
i. malrotation (IM)
i. mesentery
i. metaplasia
i. motility
i. mucosa
i. neuronal dysplasia
i. obstruction
i. ostomy
i. parasite
i. peristalsis
i. permeability (IP)
i. polyp
i. polyposis
i. pseudoobstruction
i. telangiectasia
i. tract
i. transit time
i. transplantation
i. villous atrophy
i. volvulus
intestinalis
Campylobacter fetus i.
Enterocytozoon i.
pneumatosis i.
pneumatosis cystoides i.
Septata i.
intestine
barber pole small i.
large i.
small i.
whirlwind small i.
intestine-associated lymphoid tissue
(IALT)
intima
intimacy
physical i.
intimal
i. hyperplasia
i. thickening
intimate
i. partner
i. partner depression
i. partner homicide
i. partner violence
intoeing
intolerance
carbohydrate i.
cold i.
cow's milk i.
delayed orthostatic i.
disaccharide i.

intolerance (*continued*)
    exercise i.
    familial protein i.
    feeding i.
    fructose i.
    gestational carbohydrate i.
     (GCI)
    glucose i.
    glucose-galactose i.
    gluten i.
    hereditary fructose i.
    lactose i.
    lysinuric protein i.
    milk protein i.
    orthostatic i.
    primary lactose i.
    protein i.
    soy protein i.
    transient protein i.
intoxicate
intoxication
    acute scombroid i.
    aluminum i.
    anticonvulsant i.
    barbiturate i.
    botulinus i.
    chronic vitamin A i.
    ciguatera i.
    intrarenal androgenic i.
    lead i.
    manganese i.
    mepivacaine i.
    metal i.
    methylmercury i.
    phenothiazine i.
    salicylate i.
    scombroid i.
    sugar i.
    thallium i.
    vitamin A, D i.
    water i.
intraabdominal
    i. abscess (IAA)
    i. cyst
    i. infection (IAI)
    i. pressure
    i. pressure elevation
    i. streak
    i. surgery
    i. testis
intraamniotic
    i. infection (IAI)
    i. inflammation
intraaortic balloon
  counterpulsation
intraarterial
    i. chemotherapy
    i. infusion
    i. sensor

intraarticular
    i. epiphysis
    i. infection
intraassay
intraatrial
    i. redirection
    i. repair
intrabronchial obstruction
intrabronchiolar obstruction
intracanalicular fibroadenoma
intracardiac
    i. defect
    i. injection
    i. shunt
    i. tunnel
intracavitary
    i. brachytherapy
    i. irradiation
    i. lesion
    i. myoma
    i. radium
intracavity device
intracellular
    i. calcium
    i. event
    i. fluid (ICF)
    i. hydrogen ion concentration (pHi)
    i. mediator
    i. myometrial protein
    i. pH (pHi)
    i. progesterone receptor
intracerebellar hemorrhage
intracerebral
    i. aneurysm
    i. hematoma
    i. seeding of bacteria
intracervical
    i. adhesion
    i. placement
    i. purified porcine relaxin
    i. tent
intrachromosomal duplication
intracisternal therapy
intraclass correlation coefficient
intracoronary ultrasound
intracorporeal
intracranial
    i. anatomy
    i. arterial aneurysm
    i. arteriovenous fistula
    i. bleeding
    i. calcification
    i. cystic space
    i. dural vascular anomaly
    i. empyema
    i. foreign body
    i. hematoma
    i. hemorrhage (ICH)
    i. hypertension

i. injury (ICI)
i. malformation
i. neoplasm
i. pathology
i. pressure (ICP)
i. pressure monitoring
i. suppuration
i. tumor
i. venous sinus thrombosis
i. volume
intractable
  i. diarrhea of infancy (IDI)
  i. emesis
  i. pain
  i. uterine bleeding
  i. viral infection
intracystic papillary carcinoma
intracytoplasmic
  i. inclusion
  i. sperm head injection (ICSHI)
  i. sperm injection (ICSI)
intradermal, intradermic
  i. nevus
  i. test
intradermic (*var. of* intradermal)
IntraDop probe
intraductal
  i. cancer
  i. papillary carcinoma (IPC)
  i. papilloma
intradural spinal angioma
intraepidermal
  i. blister
  i. spongiosis
  i. vesiculation
intraepithelial
  i. cervical dysplasia
  i. disease progression
  i. dyskeratosis syndrome
  i. endometrial cancer
  i. lesion
  i. neoplasia
intrafallopian transfer
intrafamilial genoidentical donor
intrafamily offender
intrafollicular insemination (IFI)
intragastric
  i. feeding
  i. pH
intrahepatic
  i. arterioportal fistula
  i. bile duct
  i. bile duct paucity
  i. biliary atresia
  i. cholestasis
  i. cholestasis of pregnancy (ICP)
  i. cholestatic syndrome
  i. vasoocclusive crisis
intralesional steroid therapy

intraligamentary ectopic pregnancy
intraligamentous myoma
Intralipid
  I. formula
  I. hyperalimentation
intralobar
  i. pulmonary sequestration
  i. rest
intralobular connective tissue
intraluminal
  i. agent
  i. clot
  i. electrical impedance technique
  i. nutrient
  i. plug
  i. pressure
  i. upper airway obstruction
  i. web
intralymphatic infusion
intramammary lymph node
intramedullary
  i. rod
  i. rod fixation
  i. spinal abscess
intramural
  i. fibroid
  i. gas
  i. leiomyoma
  i. myoma
  i. pregnancy
  i. thrombus
  i. upper airway obstruction
intramuscular (IM)
  i. block
  i. drug
intramyometrial
  i. coring
  i. mass
intranasal (IN)
  i. desmopressin
  i. drug
  i. inoculum
  i. live influenza vaccine
  i. spray
intranatal
intranuclear
  i. hyaline inclusion disease
  i. inclusion body
  i. virion
intraocular
  i. lymphoma
  i. malignancy
  i. optic neuritis
  i. pressure (IOP)
  i. tumor
intraoperative
  i. complication
  i. gastrointestinal injury
  i. hemorrhage

intraoperative (*continued*)
i. lymphatic mapping
i. radiation
i. ureteral catheterization
intraosseous (IO)
i. infusion (IOI)
i. line placement
i. needle
intrapair birth weight difference
intraparenchymal
i. bleed
i. hematoma
i. hemorrhage
intrapartum
i. antibiotic prophylaxis (IAP)
i. asphyxia
i. asphyxiation
i. cardiotocography
i. chemoprophylaxis
i. complication
i. cord prolapse
i. death
i. demise
i. evaluation
i. fetal heart rate abnormality
i. fetal monitoring
i. fetoplacental transfusion
i. glucose control
i. head entrapment
i. hemorrhage
i. hemostasis
i. management
i. maternal fever
i. monitor
i. period
i. treatment
i. uteroplacental insufficiency
intrapelvic
intraperitoneal
i. blood transfusion
i. chemotherapy
i. cisplatin
i. endometrial metastatic disease
i. fetal transfusion
i. 5-fluorouracil
i. insemination (IPI)
i. involvement
i. pregnancy
i. radiation therapy
intrapleural injury
intrapsychic phenomenon
intrapulmonary
i. inhalation
i. shunt
i. shunting
i. shunt ratio (Qs/Qt)
i. tumor
intrarenal
i. anastomosis

i. androgenic intoxication
i. reflux
i. venous radical
intraretinal hemorrhage (IH)
intraspinous vascular anomaly
intratesticularly
intrathecal
i. anti-HIV antibody
i. medication
i. methotrexate
i. narcotic
i. neurolysis
intrathoracic
i. airway obstruction
i. tracheomalacia
i. tuberculosis
intratonsillar
intratracheal
i. magnesium (ITMg)
i. pulmonary ventilation (ITPV)
i. suspension
intratubal insemination (ITI)
intratumoral desmoplasia
intraurethral bulk injection
intrauterine (IU)
i. acquisition
i. adhesion
i. amputation
i. asphyxia
i. balloon-type cannula
i. blood transfusion
i. cavity
i. circulation
i. cirsoid aneurysm
i. compression
i. contraception device (IUCD)
i. contraceptive device (ICD, IUCD)
i. contraceptive progesterone system (ICPS)
i. death (IUD)
i. device (IUD)
i. diaphragm
i. environment
i. exposure
i. facial necrosis
i. factor
i. fetal death (IUFD)
i. fetal demise (IUFD)
i. fetal distress (IUFD)
i. fetal monitoring
i. filling defect
i. fracture
i. GIFT
i. growth curve
i. growth impairment
i. growth restriction (IUGR)
i. growth retardation (IUGR)

i. growth retardation, microcephaly,
mental retardation syndrome
i. hematoma
i. herpes
i. hydrops
i. hypoxia
i. infection (IUI)
i. insemination (IUI)
i. insemination cannula
i. insemination cannula with
mandrel
i. intraperitoneal fetal transfusion
i. intussusception
i. involvement
i. laser ablation of vascular
anastomoses
i. lymphedema
i. maternofetal transfusion
i. parabiotic syndrome
i. parvovirus B19 infection
i. pneumonia
i. position
i. positional defect
i. positioning
i. pregnancy (IUP)
i. pressure catheter (IUPC)
i. pressure cycle
i. pressure measurement
i. radiation
i. resuscitation
i. sac
i. synechia
i. system (IUS)
i. ureteral obstruction
i. viral myositis
i. volume

intravaginal
i. agent
i. condom
i. contraceptive
i. cream
i. foam
i. foreign body use
i. insemination (IVI)
i. physical therapy
i. pouch
i. prostaglandin
i. radiation
i. sponge
i. support device
i. suppository
i. testicular torsion

intravasation
intravascular
i. fluid
i. oncotic pressure
i. sickling
i. transfusion
i. ultrasonography

i. ultrasound (IVUS)
i. volume
i. volume depletion

intravenous (IV, I.V.)
i. alimentation
i. antibiotic
i. anti-D immunoglobulin
i. crystallized fluid
cytomegalovirus immune globulin i.
(CMV-IGIV)
i. drip (IVD)
i. drug
i. drug use (IDU)
i. excretory urography
i. feeding
i. fluid therapy
i. gamma globulin (IVGG)
i. glucose challenge
i. heparin
i. hydration
i. hyperalimentation (IVH)
i. immunoglobulin (IVIG)
immunoglobulin, i.
i. immunoglobulin (IVIg)
i. infusion
i. leiomyomatosis
i. line
i. line placement
i. medication
i. oxytocin
peripheral i. (PIV)
i. pyelogram (IVP)
i. pyelography (IVP)
respiratory syncytial virus
immunoglobulin i. (RSV-IGIV)
scalp i.
i. urogram (IVU)
i. urography (IVU)

intraventricular (IVT)
i. bleed
i. fibrinolytic therapy
i. hemorrhage (grade 1–4)
(IVH)
i. neurocysticercosis
i. opioid delivery
i. ribavirin

intravesical pressure
intrinsic
i. asthma
i. dysmenorrhea
i. dyssomnia
i. factor (IF)
i. flow resistance (R_{int})
i. PEEP
i. positive and end-expiratory
pressure
i. pulsatility
i. renal disorder
i. sphincter deficiency (IDS, ISD)

intrinsic (*continued*)
    i. tumor
    i. weakness
introducer
    P.D. Access with Peel-Away
      needle i.
introital estrogenization
introitus
    marital i.
    parous i.
    vaginal i.
    virginal i.
Introl bladder neck support prosthesis
intromission
Intron A
intruded incisor
intrusion
    dental i.
    i. symptom
intrusive
    i. implantation
    i. luxation
    i. stress reaction
intubated
intubation
    controlled i.
    endotracheal i. (ETI)
    nasal tube i.
    nasotracheal i. (NTI)
    neonatal i.
    oral tube i.
    orotracheal i.
    rapid sequence i. (RSI)
    silastic tube i.
    stenosis post i.
    tracheal i.
intussusception
    apex of i.
    appendiceal i.
    cecocolic i.
    colic i.
    colocolic i.
    double i.
    idiopathic i.
    ileal i.
    ileocecal i.
    ileocolic i.
    ileoileal i.
    ileoileocolic i.
    intrauterine i.
    jejunogastric i.
    prolapsing apex of i.
    retrograde i.
intussusceptum
    engorgement of i.
invaginata
    trichorrhexis i.
invaginated bowel

invagination
    basilar i.
Invanz
invasion
    early stromal i.
    lymphovascular space i. (LVSI)
    myometrial i.
    trophoblastic i.
invasive
    i. bacterial infection
    i. cancer (IC)
    i. candidiasis
    i. cervical cancer (ICC)
    i. duct carcinoma
    i. hemodynamic monitoring
    i. hydatidiform mole
    i. management
    i. mole
    i. neoplasia
    i. pneumococcal disease immunization
    i. sinusitis
    i. squamous cell carcinoma (ISCC)
    i. testing
invecta
    Solenopsis i.
inventory
    Battelle Developmental I. (BDI)
    Beck Depression I. (BDI)
    Behavior Problem I. (BPI)
    Children's Depression I. (CDI)
    Child Sexual Behavior I. (CSBI)
    colorectal-anal distress i. (CRADI)
    communal traumatic experiences i. (CTEI)
    communicative development i. (CDI)
    Derogatis Brief Symptom I.
    Eating Disorders I. (DI, EDI)
    Eyberg Child Behavior I. (ECBI)
    Gillespie-Numerof Burnout I.
    Global Severity Index of Brief Symptom I. (GSI-BSI)
    infertility perceptions i. (IPI)
    18-item Birleson Depression I.
    Leyton Obsessional I.
    Marital Dyadic I.
    Maslach Burnout I.
    Minnesota Multiphasic Personality I. (MMPI)
    Neonatal Perception I. (NPI)
    Neonatal Withdrawal I. (NWI)
    Pediatric Evaluation of Disability I. (PEDI)
    peer conformity i.
    pelvic floor distress i. (PFDI)
    Spielberger State Anxiety I.

standardized reading i.
State-Trait Anxiety I. (STAI)
Urinary Distress I. (UDI)
Urogenital Distress I. (UDI)
Weinberger Adjustment I. (WAI)
West Haven-Yale Multidimensional
Pain I.
inventory-adolescent
Minnesota Multiphasic Personality
I.-A. (MMPI-A)
inverse
i. cerebellum
i. polymerase chain reaction
i. ratio ventilation (IRV)
i. square law
Inversine
inversion
acute uterine i.
appendiceal i.
chromosomal i.
i. deformity
i. duplication (15) chromosome
syndrome
i. duplication (8p) syndrome
incomplete uterine i.
nipple i.
i. of chromosomes
i. of the uterus
i. of viscera
paracentric i.
parental i.
pericentric i.
puerperal i.
i. stress tilt test
i. 9 syndrome
T-wave i.
uterine i.
ventricular i.
inversion-ligation appendectomy
inversus
blepharophimosis, ptosis, epicanthus
i. (BPEI)
epicanthus i.
situs i.
visceroatrial situs i.
inverted
i. appendiceal stump
i. duplication of chromosome
15
i. nipple
i. pelvis
i. repeat
i. subcuticular suture
i. T uterine incision
i. V mouth
i. X chromosome
i. Y detrusor dissection
inverting baseball stitch
invertogram

Investa suture
investigation
infertility i.
Invirase
involucre (*var. of* involucrum)
involucrum, involucre
involuntary
i. movement
i. sterilization
involute
involuting nevus
involution
aberration of normal development
and i. (ANDI)
i. cyst
i. of uterus
spontaneous thymic i.
uterine i.
involutional
i. gynecomastia
i. melancholia
i. psychosis
involved field (IF)
involved-field radiation
involvement
adnexal i.
congenital muscular dystrophy with
central nervous system i.
endometrial i.
gangliosidosis GM1 late onset
without bony i.
generalized infantile gangliosidosis
with bony i.
intraperitoneal i.
intrauterine i.
lymph node i.
lymphovascular space i.
metastatic axillary i.
multisite lower genital tract i.
neurologic i.
nodal i.
ocular i.
pelvic i.
pleuropulmonary i.
postponing sexual i. (PSI)
Tay-Sachs disease with visceral i.
Invos 3100 cerebral oximeter
I&O
intake and output
I/O
intake and output
IO
intraosseous
IO infusion
Ioban
I. 2 cesarean sheet
I. drape
iocetamic acid
iodamide

iodide
  cesium i. (CsI)
  echothiophate i.
  isopropamide i.
  potassium i.
  propidium i.
  saturated solution of potassium i. (SSKI)
  sodium i.
  i. therapy
  i. trap defect
iodide-containing medication
iodinated
  i. dye
  i. glycerol
iodine
  i. douche
  i. 125-labeled fibrinogen scan
  i. povidone solution
  i. stain
  i. supply
  tincture of i.
  urinary i.
iodine-123 (^{123}I)
iodine-125 (^{125}I)
iodine-127 (^{127}I)
iodine-131 (^{131}I)
iodine-132 (^{132}I)
iodipamide
5-iodo-2′-deoxyuridine (IDU)
iodoform
  i. gauze
  i. gauze packing
iodomethyl-norcholesterol scanning
Iodopen
iodophor
iodophor-impregnated adhesive drape
iodoquinol
Iodosorb absorptive dressing
iodothyronine level
Iofed PD
iohexol
IOI
  intraosseous infusion
ion
  calcium i.
  quarternary ammonium i.
  i. trapping
Ionamin
Ionasescu syndrome
ionic contrast medium
Ionil-T shampoo
ionization
ionized
  i. calcium (iCa)
  i. hypomagnesemia
  i. magnesium
ionizing radiation
ionKids monitoring system

ionophore challenge
Iontocaine
iontophoresis
  pilocarpine i.
  sweat chloride i.
IOP
  intraocular pressure
iopanoic acid
iothalamate sodium
IOWA
  inattention-overactivity with aggression
Iowa
  I. bone development study
  I. trumpet
  I. Women's Health Study
IP
  infundibulopelvic
  intestinal permeability
  IP ligament
IPA
  incontinentia pigmenti achromians
  isopropyl alcohol
IPAA
  ileal pouch-anal anastomosis
IPAN
  infantile polyarteritis nodosa
IPAT
  Institute of Personality and Ability Testing
  IPAT Depression Scale
IPC
  intraductal papillary carcinoma
IPCD
  infantile polycystic disease
ipecac
  i. cardiomyopathy
  i. syrup
  syrup of i.
IPH
  idiopathic pulmonary hemorrhage
IPI
  infertility perceptions inventory
  intraperitoneal insemination
IPKD
  infantile polycystic kidney disease
IPN
  infantile periarteritis nodosa
  infantile polyarteritis nodosa
ipodate sodium
Ipol poliovirus vaccine
IPPB
  intermittent positive pressure breathing
IPPV
  intermittent positive-pressure ventilation
ipratropium
  i. bromide
  i. bromide nasal spray
  i. nebulization

ipriflavone
iprindole
iproniazid
ipsilateral
    i. anhidrosis
    i. anisocoria
    i. hypertropia
    i. lateral rectus muscle
    i. lung hypoplasia
    i. miosis
ipsilon zone
IPT
    inflammatory pseudotumor
IPV
    inactivated poliovirus vaccine
    intimate partner violence
        Salk IPV
        IPVvaccine
IQ
    intelligence quotient
        Raven IQ
I-QOL
    Incontinence quality of life
    quality of life in persons with urinary
      incontinence
        I-QOL instrument
¹⁹²Ir
    iridium-192
IRC
    infrared photocoagulation
Ircon
IRDS
    idiopathic respiratory distress
      syndrome
    infant respiratory distress syndrome
Ir gene
iridectomy
irides (*pl. of* iris)
iridis
    heterochromia i.
iridium (Ir)
    i. implant
    i. wire
iridium-192 (¹⁹²Ir)
iridocorneal mesodermal dysgenesis
iridocyclitis
    acute i.
    chronic i.
    relapsing i.
iridodental dysplasia
iridodonesis
iridogoniodysgenesis with somatic anomalies
irinotecan
iris, *pl.* **irides**
    i., coloboma, ptosis, hypertelorism,
      mental retardation syndrome
    i. dilator
    i. hamartoma

    heterochromia of i.
    i. hypoplasia
    i. lesion
    i. Lisch nodule
    speckled irides
    stellate i.
    i. vessel
iritis
    i. catamenialis
    photophobic i.
IRMA
    immunoradiometric assay
Iromin-G
iron
    carbonyl i.
    i. chelation
    i. chelation therapy
    i. chelator
    i. deficiency
    i. deficiency anemia (IDA)
    i. dextran
    i. dextran complex
    elemental i.
    free i.
    heme i.
    i. ingestion
    I. Intern retractor
    nonheme i.
    i. overload
    Pedicran with I.
    plasma-free i.
    i. poisoning
    i. requirement
    serum i.
    i. supplement
    total body i.
    i. toxicity
    i. turnover
    unbound i.
iron-binding
    i.-b. capacity (IBC)
    i.-b. protein
iron-catalyzed pseudoperoxidation
Irospan
IRP
    International Reference Preparation
irradiated
irradiation
    abdominal i.
    abdominopelvic i.
    axillary i.
    cesium i.
    i. cystitis
    i. dermatitis
    external beam i.
    heavy-ion i.
    hemibody i.
    i. injury
    interstitial i.

irradiation (*continued*)
- intracavitary i.
- local i.
- low-dose involved field i.
- low-dose splenic i.
- ovarian-sparing i.
- paraaortic node i.
- pelvic i.
- surface i.
- total body i. (TBI)
- whole abdomen i.
- whole body i.
- whole pelvis i.

irrational

irregular
- i. cortex
- i. menses
- i. rhythm
- i. stereotyped movement
- i. stereotyped vocalization
- i. tooth placement

irregularity
- menstrual i.

irrigant
- Neosporin GU i.

irrigation
- antibiotic i.
- bowel i.
- copious antibiotic i.
- gastric i.
- i. solution
- i. survey
- whole bowel i. (WBI)

irritability
- early morning i.
- reflex i.

irritable
- i. bowel syndrome
- i. breast
- i. colon of childhood
- i. hip

irritant
- i. contact dermatitis
- i. diaper dermatitis
- i. receptor

irritation
- i. diaper rash
- meningeal i.
- perineal i.

irritative vulvovaginitis

IRT
- immunoreactive trypsinogen

IRV
- inspiratory reserve volume
- inverse ratio ventilation

Irving
- I. method
- I. tubal ligation

IS
- infantile spasm
- infant size
- IS element

ISA
- induced sputum analysis

Isaac-Merton syndrome

Isaac syndrome

ISAGA
- immunosorbent agglutination assay

ISAM
- infant of substance-abusing mother

ISCA
- Interview Schedule for Children and Adolescents

ISCC
- invasive squamous cell carcinoma

ischemia
- cerebral i.
- chorionic villus i.
- clitoral i.
- intestinal i.
- myocardial i.
- penile i.

ischemic
- i. brain injury
- i. decidual necrosis
- i. edema
- i. exercise test
- i. heart disease (IHD)

ischiadelphus

ischial spine

ischiocavernosus muscle

ischiocavernous

ischiodidymus

ischiomelus

ischiopagus
- i. tripus separation
- i. tripus twins

ischiopatellar dysplasia

ischiopubica
- osteochondritis i.

ischiopubic ramus

ischiorectal
- i. abscess
- i. fossa

ischiothoracopagus

ischium

ISCN
- intensive special care nursery

ISCU
- intensive special care unit

ISD
- inhibited sexual desire
- intrinsic sphincter deficiency

ISDN
- isosorbide dinitrate

Iselin forceps

isethionate
    pentamidine i.
ISG
    immune serum globulin
ISGYP
    International Society of Gynecologic
    Pathologists
Ishihara
ISHT
    International Society for Heart
    Transplantation
island
    epimyoepithelial i.
    i. flap
    Langerhans islands
    Pander i.
islander
    Pacific I.
islet
    i. cell adenoma
    i. cell adenomatosis
    i. cell antibody
    (ICA, ICAb)
    i. cell tumor
    islets of Langerhans
ISMA
    infantile spinal muscular atrophy
Ismelin
isoametropic amblyopia
isoamylase
isoantibody
isoantigen
Iso-Bid
isobutyric acid
Isocal HN formula
isocarboxazid
isochromatic
isochromosome
    i. 10p syndrome
    i. 12p syndrome
    i. Xq
isodense lesion
isodisomy
    paternal uniparenteral i.
isodose curve
isoechoic
isoenzyme, isozyme
    MB i.
    myocardial muscle creatine kinase i.
    (CK-MB)
isoetharine
isoflavone
    Novasoy soy i.
isofluorphate
isoflurane
isoform
    glutathione S-transferase i.
isogeneic graft
isograft

isohemagglutinin
    anti-A i.
    anti-B i.
isoimmune
    i. anemia
    i. fetal thrombocytopenia
    i. hemolytic disease
isoimmunization
    antepartum Rh i.
    blood group i.
    D i.
    D-antigen i.
    i. in pregnancy
    Kell i.
    Rh i.
    rhesus i.
isointense
Isoject
    Permapen I.
Isojima test
isolate
    chloramphenicol-resistant i.
isolated
    i. autosomal dominant syndrome
    i. cleft palate
    i. congenital folate malabsorption
    (ICFM)
    i. diffuse mesangial sclerosis
    (IDMS)
    i. double outlet right ventricle
    i. gonadotropin deficiency
    i. growth hormone deficiency
    (IGHD)
    i. hypogonadotropic hypogonadism
    (IHH)
    i. premature menarche
    i. TGA
    i. vulvar seborrheic dermatitis
isolating
isolation
    social i.
isolette
    Airshields i.
    bubble i.
    double-bubble i.
    double-walled bubble i.
    humidified i.
    temperature-controlled i.
isoleucine
isologous neoplasm
isomer
isomerase
    i. reductase
    triose phosphate i. (TPI)
isomerism
isometric quadriceps exercise
Isomil DE formula
isomorphic presentation
isonatremia

isonatremic dehydration
isoniazid (INH)
    prophylactic i.
isonicotinic acid hydrazide (INH)
Isopaque
isoperistaltic intestinal interposition
isoprenaline hydrochloride
Isoprinosine
isopropamide iodide
isopropanol
isopropyl alcohol
isoproterenol
Isoptin SR
Isopto
    I. Atropine Ophthalmic
    I. Carbachol
    I. Carpine
    I. Carpine Ophthalmic
    I. Cetamide
    I. Eserine
    I. Frin
    I. Hyoscine
Isordil
isosexual
    i. idiopathic precocious puberty
    i. precocity
    i. sexual characteristic
isosorbide dinitrate (ISDN)
Isosource
    I. 1.5 Cal formula
    I. HN formula
    I. Standard formula
Isospora belli
isosporiasis
isosthenuria
isosulfan blue dye
Isotamine
isothiocyanate
    fluorescein i.
isotonic
    i. bolus
    i. dehydration
    i. electrolyte solution
    i. fluid
    i. PBS
    i. saline
    i. sodium chloride
isotope
    i. cisternography
    radioactive i.
    i. scanning
Isotrate
isotretinoin
    i. dysmorphic syndrome
    i. embryopathy
    i. teratogenic syndrome
Isotrex
isovaleric
    i. acid

    i. acidemia
    i. aciduria
isovaleryl-CoA dehydrogenase
isovaleryl glucuronide
isovolumic
    i. relaxation (IVR)
    i. relaxation time (IVR, IVRT)
iso-X chromosome
isoxsuprine
I-Soyalac formula
isozyme (*var. of* isoenzyme)
ISQ
    Incontinence Stress Questionnaire
isradipine
israelii
    Actinomyces i.
ISS
    idiopathic short stature
    injury severity score
ISSD
    infantile sialic acid storage
    disorder
issue
    developmental i.
    legal i.
    quality of life i.
    sexual i.
    social i.
    socioeconomic i.
    spiritual i.
ISSVD
    International Society for the Study of
    Vulvar Diseases
isthmi (*pl. of* isthmus)
isthmic
    i. occlusion
    i. pregnancy
isthmica nodosa
isthmorrhaphy
isthmus, *pl.* **isthmi, isthmuses**
    cervical i.
    flutter i.
isthmuses (*pl. of* isthmus)
I-Stop midurethral sling
I-Sulfacet
Isuprel Injection
IT
    inspiratory time
    intermediate trophoblast
ITC
    infrared thermographic calorimetry
itch
    ground i.
    i. mite
    swimmer's i.
itchiness
itching
    perineal i.
    vulvovaginal i.

itch-scratch cycle
Itch-X
    I.-X gel
    I.-X spray
18-item Birleson Depression
 Inventory
itersonii
    Aquaspirillum i.
ITI
   intratubal insemination
I-time
   inspiration time
ITMg
   intratracheal magnesium
Ito
   I. cell
   I. hypomelanosis
   hypomelanosis of I. (HI, HMI)
   I. method
   I. nevus
   nevus of I.
   I. syndrome
I-to-E ratio
ITP
   idiopathic thrombocytopenic purpura
   immune thrombocytopenic purpura
   acute childhood ITP
   chronic ITP
   recurrent ITP
ITPA
   Illinois Test of Psycholinguistic
   Abilities
ITPV
   intratracheal pulmonary ventilation
itraconazole
ITW
   idiopathic toe walking
IU
   immunizing unit
   International Unit
   intrauterine
   in utero
IUCD
   intrauterine contraceptive device
IUD
   intrauterine death
   intrauterine device
   copper-releasing I.
   copper T-380A IUD
   Copper T-380 nonhormonal
    IUD
   IUD inserter
   Mirena I.
   ParaGard T380 copper IUD
   progestin-releasing IUD
   Saf-T-Coil IUD
IUDE
   in utero drug exposure
IUD-related infection

IUGR
   intrauterine growth restriction
   intrauterine growth retardation
   asymmetric IUGR
   symmetric IUGR
IUI
   intrauterine infection
   intrauterine insemination
   IUI disposable cannula
IUP
   intrauterine pregnancy
IUPC
   intrauterine pressure catheter
IUS
   intrauterine system
I.V.
   intravenous
   Hyperstat I.V.
   Indocin I.V.
   Metro I.V.
   Monistat I.V.
   Vasotec I.V.
IV
   intravenous
   in vitro
   in vivo
   IV anti-D therapy
   brachymetatarsus IV
   Gammar-P IV
   Merrem IV
   scalp IV
IVA
   integrated visual and auditory
   IVA visual consistency test
IVAP
   in vitro antibody production
   IVAP assay
IVD
   intervertebral disc
   intravenous drip
   Quantikine IVD
Iveegam
Ivemark syndrome
ivermectin
IVF
   in vitro fertilization
IVF-ET
   in vitro fertilization-embryo transfer
IVF-induced abdominal pregnancy
IVGG
   intravenous gamma globulin
IVH
   intravenous hyperalimentation
   intraventricular hemorrhage (grade
   1–4)
IVI
   intravaginal insemination
IVIG, IVIg
   intravenous immunoglobulin

IVL
indwelling venous line
ivory bones
IVP
intravenous pyelogram
intravenous pyelography
IVR
isovolumic relaxation
isovolumic relaxation time
IVRT
isovolumic relaxation time
IVS Tunneller device
IVT
intervillous thrombus
intraventricular

IVU
intravenous urogram
intravenous urography
IVUS
intravascular ultrasound
ivy
I. bleeding time
i. leaf
IWL
insensible water loss
Ixodes
I. pacificus
I. persulcatus
I. ricinus
I. scapularis

J

joule
> J extension
> J needle
> J pulmonary receptor
> J tracking

JA

juvenile arthritis
jabbering
Jaboulay amputation
Jabs syndrome
Jaccoud deformity
jacket
> body j.
> fiberglass j.
> Orthoplast j.
> yellow j.

jackknife
> j. position
> j. seizure
> j. spasm

Jackson
> J. axiom
> J. membrane
> J. right-angle retractor

jacksonian
> j. epilepsy
> j. march
> j. seizure

Jackson-Pratt drain (JPD)
Jackson-Weiss syndrome (JWS)
Jacobs
> J. cannula
> J. tenaculum

Jacobsen syndrome
Jacobson hemostatic forceps
Jacob syndrome
Jacquemier sign
Jacquet
> J. erosive diaper dermatitis
> J. erythema

Jadassohn
> nevus of J.
> J. nevus phakomatosis (JNP)
> nevus sebaceus of J. (SNJ)
> J. test

Jadassohn-Lewandowski syndrome
Jadassohn-Tièche nevus
Jadelle implant
Jaeken syndrome
Jaffe-Campanacci syndrome
Jaffe-Lichtenstein syndrome
JAG1
> human jagged-1 gene

Jahnke syndrome

JAI
> juvenile amaurotic idiocy

Jakob-Creutzfeldt (JC)
> J.-C. syndrome

Jaksch
> J. anemia
> J. disease
> J. syndrome

Jamaican vomiting sickness
James syndrome
Jancar syndrome
Janeway lesion
janiceps
> j. asymmetrus
> j. parasiticus

Janosik embryo
Jansen
> J. metaphysial chondrodysplasia
> J. syndrome

Jansky-Bielschowsky
> J.-B. disease
> J.-B. neural ceroid lipofuscinosis
> J.-B. syndrome

Jansky classification
Janus
> J. report
> J. syndrome

Janz syndrome
Japanese
> J. B encephalitis virus
> J. encephalitis

japonica
> *Laminaria j.*
> *Rickettsia j.*

japonicum
> *Schistosoma j.*

jar
> GasPak j.

Jarcho-Levin syndrome
Jarisch-Herxheimer (J-H)
> J.-H. reaction

Jarit
> J. disposable cannula
> J. disposable trocar

JAS
> juvenile ankylosing spondylitis

Jatene
> J. arterial switch procedure
> J. operation
> J. valve

jaundice
> benign j.
> black j.
> breast-feeding j.
> breast milk j. (BMJ)

jaundice (*continued*)
    catarrhal j.
    central j.
    cholestatic j.
    congenital hemolytic j.
    congenital nonhemolytic j.
    congenital obliterative j.
    neonatal j. (NNJ)
    neonatal cholestatic j.
    nuclear j.
    obstructive j.
    j. of newborn
    peripheral j.
    physiologic j.
    prolonged j.
    Schmorl j.
    unexplained j.
javanica
    Rhus j.
jaw
    bird-beak j.
    cleft j.
    j. deformity
    j. deviation
    fibrous dysplasia of j.
    Jaws forceps
    j. jerk
    lumpy j.
    j. myoclonus
    parrot j.
    small j.
    j. thrust
    j. thrust-spine stabilization
      maneuver
JC
    Jakob-Creutzfeldt
    joint contracture
    polyomavirus JC
    JC syndrome
    JC virus
JCA
    juvenile chronic arthritis
JDM
    juvenile dermatomyositis
    juvenile diabetes mellitus
    juvenile-onset diabetes mellitus
    amyopathic JDM
    new-onset JDM
JDMS
    juvenile dermatomyositis
Jefferson fracture
Jehovah's Witness
jejunal
    j. atresia
    j. biopsy
    j. ulcer
jejuni
    Campylobacter j.
    Campylobacter fetus j.

jejunitis
    necrotizing j.
jejunogastric intussusception
jejunoileal
    j. atresia
    j. bypass
jejunojejunal anastomosis
jejunostomy
jejunum
    distal j.
    proximal j.
    villous atrophy of j.
jelly
    Aci-Jel vaginal j.
    j. bean
    contraceptive j.
    Gynol II contraceptive j.
    K-Y lubricating j.
    petroleum j.
    Wharton j.
    Xylocaine j.
Jenamicin
Jenest-28
Jensen syndrome
jeopardy
    fetal j.
jerk
    infantile myoclonic j.
    jaw j.
    myoclonic j.
    j. nystagmus
Jervell and Lange-Nielsen long QT syndrome
Jeryl Lynn mumps strain
Jessner-Cole syndrome
JET
    junctional ectopic
      tachycardia
jet
    j. cooling effect
    high-frequency j. (HFJ)
    j. nebulizer
    Plus J.
    pulsatile air j.
    ureteral j.
    j. ventilation
    j. ventilator
Jeune
    J. disease
    J. syndrome
    J. thoracic dystrophy
Jevity Plus formula
Jew
    Ashkenazi J.
    Sephardic J.
jeweler's forceps
Jewett classification
JGCT
    juvenile granulosa cell tumor

J

juxtaglomerular cell tumor
    JGCT of ovary
J-H
    Jarisch-Herxheimer
JIA
    juvenile idiopathic arthritis
Jirasek gestation stage
jiroveci
        Pneumocystis j.
JIS
    juvenile idiopathic scoliosis
jitteriness
jitters
jittery
    j. baby
    j. infant
JME
    juvenile myoclonic epilepsy
JMML
    juvenile myelomonocytic leukemia
JMS
    Juberg-Marsidi syndrome
JNA
    juvenile nasopharyngeal
      angiofibroma
JNB
    jaundice of newborn
JNP
    Jadassohn nevus phakomatosis
Jo-1 antibody
Job syndrome
Jocasta complex
JOD
    juvenile-onset diabetes
JODM
    juvenile-onset diabetes mellitus
Joel-Cohen incision
jogger's
    j. amenorrhea
    j. ankle
Johanson-Blizzard syndrome
Johnson
    J. maneuver
    Mead J.
    J. method
    J. neuroectodermal syndrome
    J. score 1–10
    J. transtracheal oxygen catheter
Johnson-McMillin syndrome
Johnson's Head-to-Toe Baby Wash
joint
    j. attention
    j. bleed
    j. capsule
    Charcot j.
    Clutton j.'s
    j. compression
    j. contracture (JC)
    cricoarytenoid j.

j. deformity
j. degeneration
diarthrodial j.
j. fusion
Gaffney j.
Gillette j.
glenohumeral j.
hyperextensible j.
j. hyperlaxity
hypermobile j.
j. hypermobility
hyperplastic j.
lax j.
j. laxity
j. line tenderness
metacarpophalangeal j.
metatarsophalangeal j. (MPJ)
naviculocuneiform j.
neural arch j.
Oklahoma ankle j.
painful j.
pelvic j.
j. probability
sacroiliac j.
Select j.
septic j.
j. stability
j. suppuration
swollen j.
synovial j.
temporomandibular j. (TMJ)
JOMID
    juvenile-onset multisystem inflammatory
    disease
Jones
    J. and Jones wedge technique
    J. procedure
    J. rheumatic fever diagnostic
      criteria
    J. stress fracture
    J. wedge metroplasty
Jorgenson scissors
Joseph
    J. disease
    J. syndrome
Josephs-Diamond-Blackfan syndrome
Joshi criteria
Joubert syndrome
joule (J)
JPD
    juvenile plantar dermatitis
    juvenile plantar dermatosis
J-pouch
JR
    junctional rhythm
    Aerolate JR
Jr.
    EpiPen Jr.
    Peptamen Jr.

JRA

juvenile rheumatoid arthritis (type I,
II)
pauciarticular JRA
pauciarticular-onset JRA
polyarticular JRA
systemic-onset JRA

J-shaped sella
JSMA

juvenile spinal muscular
atrophy

Juberg-Hayward syndrome
Juberg-Marsidi syndrome (JMS)
Judkins catheter
Juers forceps
jug handle view
jugular

j. bulb catheter
j. bulb catheterization
j. bulb monitoring
j. occlusion plethysmography
j. shunt
j. vein
j. vein thrombosis
j. venous A wave
j. venous cannulation
j. venous distention (JVD)
j. venous pressure (JVP)
j. venous pulse

juice

j. baby
white grape j.

jumped facet
jumper's knee
jumping

chromosome j.
j. Frenchmen of Maine syndrome
j. gene
j. translocation

junction

cardioesophageal j.
cervicomedullary j.
cervicovaginal j.
corticomedullary j.
costochondral j.
craniocervical j.
dermoepidermal j.
gap j.
gastroesophageal j. (GEJ)
gray-white j.
lumbosacral j.
mesencephalic-diencephalic j.
mucocutaneous j.
neuromuscular j. (NMJ)
pontomedullary j.
squamocolumnar j. (SCJ)
sternochondral j.
striatothalamic j.
ureteropelvic j. (UPJ)

ureterovesical j. (UVJ)
uterotubal j. (UTJ)

junctional

j. ectopic tachycardia (JET)
j. epidermolysis bullosa
j. nevus
j. rhythm (JR)
j. tachycardia

Junin virus
Junior Strength Motrin
Junius-Kuhnt syndrome
junky lung
justifiable abortion
just-viable fetus
JustVision diagnostic ultrasound system
Juvara fold
juvenile

j. absence epilepsy
j. aldosteronism
j. Alexander disease
j. amaurotic idiocy (JAI)
j. amyotrophic lateral sclerosis
j. ankylosing spondylitis (JAS)
j. arthritis (JA)
j. avascular necrosis
j. carcinoma
j. cataract
j. cataract, cerebellar atrophy,
mental retardation, myopathy
syndrome
j. chronic arthritis (JCA)
j. colonic polyp
j. dermatomyositis (JDM, JDMS)
j. diabetes
j. diabetes mellitus (JDM)
j. dystonic lipidosis
j. epithelial corneal dystrophy
j. fibroadenoma
j. GM1 gangliosidosis
j. GM2 gangliosidosis
j. granulosa cell tumor (JGCT)
j. hereditary motor neuron disease
j. hyperuricemia syndrome
j. idiopathic arthritis (JIA)
j. idiopathic polyarticular arthritis
j. idiopathic scoliosis (JIS)
j. intervertebral disc
j. kyphosis
j. melanoma
j. MLD
j. muscular dystrophy
j. muscular torticollis
j. myasthenia
j. myelomonocytic leukemia (JMML)
j. myoclonic epilepsy (JME)
j. myotonic dystrophy
j. nasopharyngeal angiofibroma
(JNA)
j. NCL

j. nephronophthisis
j. neuronopathic Gaucher disease
j. onset
j. osteomalacia
j. osteoporosis
j. Paget disease
j. papillomatosis
j. Parkinson disease
j. pelvis
j. periodontitis
j. pernicious anemia
j. pilocytic astrocytoma
j. plantar dermatitis (JPD)
j. plantar dermatosis (JPD)
j. polyarthritis
j. polymyositis
j. psoriatic arthritis
j. rheumatic disease
j. rheumatoid arthritis (JRA)
j. rheumatoid arthritis (type I, II) (JRA)
j. spermatogonial depletion
j. spinal muscular atrophy (JSMA)
j. spondyloarthropathy
j. sulfatidosis
j. systemic granulomatosis
j. tabes
j. tibia vara
j. Tillaux fracture
J. Wellness and Health Survey (JWHS)
j. xanthogranuloma (JXG)
j. X-linked retinoschisis (JXRS)
juvenile-onset
j.-o. diabetes (JOD)
j.-o. diabetes mellitus (JDM, JODM)
j.-o. inflammatory bowel disease
j.-o. multisystem inflammatory disease (JOMID)
juvenilis
arcus j.
kyphoscoliosis dorsalis j.
kyphosis dorsalis j.
osteochondritis deformans j.
osteodystrophia j.
juxtaarticular osteopenia
juxtacardiac
juxtaductal aortic coarctation
juxtaglomerular
j. apparatus hypertrophy
j. cell tumor (JGCT)
j. hyperplasia syndrome
juxtamedullary
juxtapleural inflammatory lesion
juxtapose
juxtaposition
Juzo-Hostess 2-way stretch compression stocking
JVD
jugular venous distention
JVP
jugular venous pressure
JWHS
Juvenile Wellness and Health Survey
J-wire placement
JWS
Jackson-Weiss syndrome
JXG
juvenile xanthogranuloma
JXRS
juvenile X-linked retinoschisis

K

potassium
K cell
K diet

k

constant
lysine

K+

K+ 8
K+ 10
K+ Care ET

KABC

Kaufman Assessment Battery for Children

Kabuki

K. makeup syndrome (KMS)
K. syndrome (KS)

Kadian sustained-release morphine capsule

KAFO

knee-ankle-foot orthosis

Kagan staging system

Kahn

K. approach
K. cannula
K. test

Kajava supernumerary breast tissue classification

KAL

KAL gene
KAL protein

kala azar

Kaletra

Kalginate dressing

Kalicinski ureteral folding technique procedure

Kalischer syndrome

kaliuresis

kallikrein

kallikrein-kinin system

Kallmann-de Morsier syndrome

Kallmann syndrome

Kalmuk idiocy

Kaltostat packing

kaluresis

kanamycin

Kanana Banana

kangaroo

k. care
k. contact
K. enteral feeding pump
K. infusion pump
k. pouch

kangarooing

Kanner syndrome

kansasii

Mycobacterium k.

Kantor sign

Kantrex

Kaochlor

Kao Lectrolyte

kaolin

k. and pectin
k. clotting time

Kaon

S-F K.

Kaopectate

K. Advanced Formula
K. II
K. Maximum Strength

Kao-Spen

Kapectolin

Kapeller-Adler test

Kaplan

K. model
K. syndrome

Kaplan-Meier

K.-M. method
K.-M. survival curve

Kaposi

K. sarcoma (KS)
K. sarcoma-associated herpesvirus
K. varicelliform eruption
K. varicelliform sarcoma

kaposiform hemangioendothelioma

Kaposi-like form of infantile hemangioma

kappa (κ)

k. chain
k. coefficient

Kapur-Toriello syndrome

karaya

Kariva

Karl

K. Storz flexible hysteroscope
K. Storz flexible ureteropyeloscope
K. Storz rigid TTTS fetoscopy instrument set

Karman cannula

Karnofsky

K. Performance Scale Index
K. performance status

Karo syrup

Kartagener syndrome

karyogenesis

karyokinesis

karyopyknosis

karyopyknotic index

karyorrhexis

karyosome

K

karyotheca
karyotype
    abnormal k.
    k. analysis
    atypical k.
    chromosomal k.
    female k.
    fetal k.
    G-banded k.
    male k.
    maternal k.
    parental k.
    paternal k.
    spectral k.
    Turner phenotype with
      normal k.
    45,X k.
    XO k.
    XX k.
    46,XX k.
    47,XX k.
    XXX k.
    XXY k.
    47,XXY k.
    XY k.
    46,XY k.
    47,XY k.
karyotyping
    flow k.
    genetic k.
    spectral k. (SKY)
Kasabach-Merritt
    K.-M. phenomenon
    K.-M. syndrome
Kasai
    K. operation
    K. peritoneal venous shunt
    K. portoenterostomy
    K. portoenterostomy
    procedure
Kashin-Bek disease
Kass criteria
katadidymus
Katayama fever
Katz-Wachtel phenomenon
Kaufman
    K. Assessment Battery for Children
    (KABC)
    K. Factor Score
    K. oculocerebrofacial syndrome
    K. pneumonia
    K. Survey of Early Academic and
    Language Skills (K-SEALS)
    K. Test of Educational Achievement
    (K-TEA)
Kaufman-McKusick syndrome
kava kava
Kaveggia syndrome
Kawasaki

    K. disease (KD)
    K. syndrome (KS)
Kay Ciel
Kayexalate
Kayser-Fleischer ring
Kaznelson syndrome
KBG syndrome
kb
    kilobase
kcal
    kilocalorie
K-cell
KCl
    potassium chloride
KD
    Kawasaki disease
    Krabbe disease
KDC-Healthdyne nonfluorescent spotlight
91kD cytochrome b peptide
K+2 diet
kDNA
    kinetoplast deoxyribonucleic acid
K-Dur
Kearns-Sayre syndrome (KSS)
KEDS
    Kids Eating Disorder Survey
keel chest
keeled breast
Keeler
    K. fiberoptic headlight
    K. loupe
keep vein open (KVO)
Keflex
Keftab
Kefurox Injection
Kefzol
Kegel exercises
Kehr
    K. incision
    K. sign for splenic injury
Keipert syndrome
Keith-Wagener retinopathy
Kell
    K. alloimmunization
    K. antibody
    K. antigen
    K. autoantibody
    K. genotyping
    K. hydrops
    K. isoimmunization
    K. sensitization
    K. series
    K. test
Keller syndrome
Kelley-Seegmiller syndrome
Kelly
    K. clamp
    K. operation
    K. plication

K

K. retractor
K. suture
K. syndrome
K. tissue forceps
K. urethrovesical plication procedure
K. vulsellum forceps
Kelly-Gray curette
Kelly-Kennedy
K.-K. plication
K.-K. procedure
Kelnor
keloid
Kemadrin
Kempsey
hemoglobin K.
Kenalog
K. Injection
K. in Orabase
K. Topical
Kendall
K. double-lumen catheter
K. McGaw Intelligent pump
**Kennedy-Pacey urinary stress
incontinence operation**
Kennedy procedure
Kenny-Caffey syndrome
Kenny-Linarelli-Caffey syndrome
Kenny-Linarelli syndrome
Kenny syndrome
Kent Infant Development Scale (KIDS)
Keofeed tube
keratan
k. sulfate
k. sulfaturia
keratin cyst
keratinization
keratinized
k. cyst
k. papule
keratinizing nasopharyngeal carcinoma
keratinocyte
k. growth factor (KGF)
k. growth factor receptor (KGFR)
keratinous
k. cyst
k. debris
k. plug
keratitis
Acanthamoeba k.
bacterial k.
dendritic k.
disciform k.
epithelial k.
k. fugax hereditaria
herpes k.
herpetic k.
keratitis, ichthyosis, deafness
(KID)
interstitial k.

neurotrophic k.
palmar and plantar keratosis and k.
punctate epithelial k.
k. sicca
syphilitic k.
transient k.
keratoacanthoma
keratoconjunctivitis
epidemic k. (EKC)
microsporidial k.
k. sicca
tuberculous k.
keratoconus
keratocyst
odontogenic k.
keratocyte
keratoderma
k. blennorrhagicum
mutilating k.
palmoplantar k.
k. palmoplantaris transgrediens
keratolysis
k. neonatorum
pitted k.
keratolytic gel
keratoma hereditarium mutilans
keratomalacia
keratopathy
band k.
herpetic k.
keratoses (*pl. of* keratosis)
keratosis, *pl.* **keratoses**
crusting telangiectasia k.
k. follicularis
k. follicularis spinulosa decalvans
k. palmaris
k. palmaris et plantaris
k. palmaris et plantaris-corneal
dystrophy syndrome
k. palmoplantaris
k. palmoplantaris-corneal dystrophy
syndrome
k. pilaris
seborrheic k.
keratotic
k. papule
k. scaling
Kergaradec sign
kerion formation
Kerley B lines
Kerlix gauze bandage
kernicterus
fetal k.
Kernig sign
Kernohan sign
Kerr cesarean
Keshan disease
Kessner Index
Kestrone

Ketalar
ketamine sedation
ketanserin
ketoacid
    k. accumulation
    branched chain k.
    serum k.
    urine k.
ketoacidosis
    diabetic k. (DKA)
    severe k.
    starvation k.
ketoaciduria
    ADR syndrome with k.
    ataxia-deafness-retardation syndrome
      with k.
    branched chain k.
ketoaciduria-mental deficiency syndrome
ketoconazole
3-ketodesogestrel
11-ketoetiocholanolone
ketogenic diet
17-ketogenic steroid
ketone
    k. body
    k. production
ketonemia
ketonuria
    branched chain k.
ketoprofen (KT)
ketorolac tromethamine
ketosis
    starvation k.
ketosis-prone diabetes
ketosis-resistant diabetes
17-ketosteroid (17-KS)
    l.-k. reductase deficiency
17-ketosteroids (17-KS)
ketotic
    k. hyperglycemia
    k. hypoglycemia
ketotifen
Kety-Schmidt cerebral blood flow
  measurement technique
Keutel syndrome (1, 2)
keV
    kilo-electronvolt
Kevorkian
    K. curette
    K. punch biopsy
Kevorkian-Younge
    K.-Y. biopsy forceps
    K.-Y. cervical biopsy instrument
    K.-Y. curette
Keyes
    K. biopsy instrument
    K. dermatologic punch
    K. punch biopsy
    K. vulvar punch

keyhole pupil
key-in-lock
    k.-i.-l. incontinence
    k.-i.-l. maneuver
Key-Pred Injection
Key-Pred-SP iInjection
kg
    kilogram
KGF
    keratinocyte growth factor
KGFR
    keratinocyte growth factor receptor
KHD
    kinky-hair disease
kHz
    kilohertz
Ki67 antibody
Kibrick
    K. method
    K. test
kick count
Kicker Pavlik harness
KID
    keratitis, ichthyosis, deafness
kid
    Caladryl for K.'s
    K.'s Eating Disorder Survey (KEDS)
    K. syndrome
Kidd blood group
Kidde
    K. cannula hysterosalpingogram
    technique
    K. tubal insufflator
KidKart
kidney
    Ask-Upmark k.
    k. biopsy
    cystic k.
    k. dialysis
    k. disease
    duplex k.
    dysplastic k.
    k. failure
    k. function
    horseshoe k.
    hydronephrotic k.
    hypoplastic k.
    infantile polycystic k.
    k. internal splint/stent (KISS)
    medullary sponge k.
    mesonephric k.
    k. morphology
    multicystic k.
    multicystic dysplastic k. (MDK)
    palpable k.
    palpably enlarged k.
    pelvic k.
    k. pole
    polycystic k.

single k.
solitary k.
k. stone
supernumerary k.
k. transplantation
k.'s, ureters, bladder
kidney-derived growth factor
KidO's aerosol and oxygen therapy bear
KIDS
Kent Infant Development Scale
Kienböck disease
Kiesselbach
K. area
K. plexus
K. triangle
kifafa seizure disorder
Kikuchi disease
Kilian pelvis
kill
cell k.
killed virus vaccine
killer
k. cell
natural k. (NK)
Killian syndrome
kilobase (kb)
kilocalorie (kcal)
kilocycle (kc)
kilo-electronvolt (keV)
kilogram (kg)
kilohertz (kHz)
kilohm
kilovolt (kV)
kilowatt (kW)
Kimmelstiel-Wilson
K.-W. disease (KW)
K.-W. syndrome
Kimura procedure
kinase
creatine k. (CK)
glycerol k. (GK)
histone H1 k.
myosin light-chain k.
phosphoglycerate k. (PGK)
pyruvate k. (PK)
serine-threonine k.
tyrosine k.
viral thymidine k.
Kindercal formula
kindergarten
kindred
degree of k.
Kinesed
kinesigenic paroxysmal dyskinesia
kinesiologic
kinesthesia, kinesthesis
kinesthesis (*var. of* kinesthesia)
kinesthetic learner
kinetic

kinetics
cell k.
first-order k.
kinetochore
kinetoplast
k. deoxyribonucleic acid (kDNA)
k. DNA
king
K. arytenoidopexy
K. classification
kingae
Haemophilus aphrophilus,
Actinobacillus
actinomycetemcomitans,
Cardiobacterium hominis, Eikenella
corrodens, Kingella k. (HACEK)
King's Health Questionnaire
kinin
kininogen
high molecular weight k. (HMWK)
kinked
k. cord
k. midbrain
kinky
kinky-hair, kinky hair
k.-h. disease (KHD)
k.-h. syndrome
Kinsbourne
K. encephalopathy
K. syndrome
Kinyoun
K. acid-fast stain
K. acid-fast staining test
K. carbol fuchsin stain
Kionex
Kirby-Bauer method
Kirghizian dermatoosteolysis
Kirner disease
Kirschner wire (K-wire)
Kish urethral illuminating catheter
KISS
kidney internal splint/stent
kiss
angel's k.
kissing
k. disease
k. lesions
k. patellae
k. ulcer
kit
ABI Prism dye terminator cycle
sequencing ready reaction k.
Acceava Trichomonas test k.
Amplicor HIV-1 test k.
Amplicor PCR k.
Amplicor typing k.
ApopTag Plus k.
AutoDELFIA PRL molecule k.
AutoDELFIA unconjugated E3 k.

K

kit (*continued*)
  biokit HSV-2 rapid test k.
  Centocor CA 125
    radioimmunoassay k.
  cervical block k.
  Coat-A-Count neonatal 17
    hydroxyprogesterone k.
  Confide HIV test k.
  Evolution-C k.
  FACE k.
  FemExam k.
  Ferritin IRMA k.
  Follistim/Antagon k.
  InPouch TV subculture k.
  Male FactorPak seminal fluid
    collection k.
  Metra PS procedure k.
  newborn screening k.
  Ortho diaphragm k.
  Otovent autoinflation k.
  OvuDate fertility test k.
  OvuGen test k.
  OvuKit self-test k.
  ovulation detection k.
  OvuQuick self-test k.
  OvuQuick 1-step ovulation k.
  Perkin Elmer rhodamine dye
    terminator k.
  PICC k.
  Pneumotest k.
  Preven emergency
    contraception k.
  Progesterone Radioimmunoassay K.
  QIAamp Tissue k.
  qualitative detection k.
  rape evidence k.
  SAFE k.
  ScheBo pancreatic elastase k.
  SureCell chlamydia test k.
  Tago diagnostic k.
  TCI OcuLook saliva ovulation
    tester k.
  urinary ovulation detection k.
  urinary ovulation predictor k.
  Uri-Three urine culture k.
  UroVysion bladder cancer k.
  Vesica sling k.
  Vidas estradiol II assay k.
Kitano knot
Kitchen postpartum gauze packer
Kittner dissector
Kitzinger method of childbirth
Kiuchi histocytic necrotizing
  lymphadenitis
Kiwi
  K. OmniCup
  K. PalmPump
  K. ProCup
  K. ProCup delivery

  K. ProCup vacuum delivery
    system
  K. vacuum
  K. vacuum-assisted fetal delivery
    device
Kjelland
  K. forceps
  K. rotation
Kjelland-Barton forceps
Kjelland-Luikart forceps
Kjer-type dominant optic atrophy
KlaasKids Foundation for Children
Klavikordal
Klebsiella
  K. oxytoca
  K. ozaenae
  K. pneumoniae
***Klebsiella-Enterobacter* species**
kleeblattschädel
  k. deformity
  k. syndrome
Kleihauer
  K. fetomaternal hemorrhage
    estimation technique
  K. stain
  K. test
Kleihauer-Betke
  K.-B. stain
  K.-B. test
Kleine-Levin syndrome
Klein-Waardenburg syndrome
Kleppinger
  K. bipolar forceps
  K. envelope sign
kleptomania
Klinefelter
  K. syndrom
  K. variant
Klinefelter-Reifenstein-Albright
  syndrome
Klinefelter-Reifenstein syndrome
Kling bandage
Klippel-Feil
  K.-F. anomaly
  K.-F. syndrome
Klippel-Trenaunay-Parkes-Weber
  syndrome
Klippel-Trenaunay syndrome
Klippel-Trenaunay-Weber syndrome
KL-6 mucinous glycoprotein
Kloepfer syndrome
Klonopin
K-Lor
Klor-Con
Klor-Con/25
Klorvess
Klotrix
Klotz syndrome
Kluge method

Klumpke
  K. brachial palsy
  K. paralysis
Klumpke-Dejerine paralysis
Klüver-Bucy syndrome
KM-1 breast pump
K-Medic
KMS
  Kabuki makeup syndrome
knee
  k. angle
  anterior translation of k.
  breaststroker's k.
  k. height measuring device
  k. hinge
  housemaid's k.
  k. jerk reflex
  k. joint hyperextensibility
  jumper's k.
  k. presentation
knee-ankle-foot orthosis
  (KAFO)
knee-chest position
knee-elbow position
kneel-stand position
knemometry
Kniest
  K. dwarfism
  K. dysplasia
  K. syndrome
Kniest-like dysplasia
knife, *pl.* **knives**
  X-acto k.
knives (*pl. of* knife)
knob
  aortic k.
  chromosome k.
knock
  pericardial k.
knock-knees
  physiologic k.-k.
knot
  Aberdeen k.
  clinch k.
  Duncan k.
  extracorporeal k.
  false k.
  fisherman's k.
  granny k.
  Kitano k.
  laparoscopic slip k.
  modified Roeder k.
  primitive k.
  k. pusher
  Roeder k.
  square k.
  surgeon's k.
  syncytial k.
  Weston k.

known, not treatable
knuckle of tube
Knudson
  K. 2-hit genetic model
  K. 2-hit tumorigenesis hypothesis
Koala intrauterine pressure catheter
Koate-DVI
Kobayashi vacuum extractor
Kobberling-Dunnigan syndrome
Köbner
  K. epidermolysis bullosa simplex
  K. phenomenon
  K. reaction
  K. response
Koby syndrome
Kocher
  K. clamp
  K. instruments
Kocher-Debré-Sémélaigne syndrome
Kock pouch
Kodak
  K. hCG serum test
  K. SureCell Chlamydia Test
  K. SureCell hCG-Urine Test
  K. SureCell Herpes Test
  K. SureCell LCH in-office
    pregnancy test
  K. SureCell Strep A test
Koenen tumor
Koeppe iris nodule
Koerber-Salus-Elschnig syndrome
Koffex DM
Kogan endocervical speculum
Kogenate
KOH
  potassium hydroxide
    KOH colpotomizer system
    KOH preparation
    KOH stain
    KOH test
    KOH whiff test
Köhler bone disease
Kohn canal
koilocyte
koilocytic atypia
koilocytosis
koilocytotic
  k. atypia
  k. cell
koilonychia
Kok disease
Kolmer test
Kolobow membrane lung
Kondremul
Konsyl
Konsyl-D
Kontron electrode
Konyne 80
konzo

K

Koplik spot
Korean hemorrhagic fever
Korenman estrogen window hypothesis
Koromex
Korotkoff
 K. phase
 K. sound
 K. test
koseri
 Citrobacter k.
Kostmann
 K. disease
 K. infantile agranulocytosis
 K. neutropenia
 K. syndrome
Kovalevsky canal
Koven Doppler
Kowarski syndrome
Koyanagi procedure
Kozlowski
 K. disease
 K. spondylometaphysial dysplasia
K-Phos
 K-P. M.F.
 K-P. Neutral
 K-P. Original
Krabbe
 K. disease (KD)
 K. leukodystrophy
 K. syndrome
Kramer
 K. disease
 K. syndrome
Kraske position
K-*ras* oncogene
kraurosis vulvae
Krause
 K. disease
 K. lacrimal accessory gland
 K. syndrome
Krause-Kivlin syndrome
Krause-van Schooneveld-Kivlin syndrome
Krebs cycle
Kreiselman infant warmer
Kremer penetration test
Kristalose
Kristeller
 K. maneuver
 K. method
Kroener tubal ligation, Kronner
Kronner
 K. Manipujector
 K. Manipujector uterine
  manipulator-injector
 K. manipulator
Kruger index
Krukenberg tumor
krusei
 Candida k.

KS
 Kabuki syndrome
 Kaposi sarcoma
 Kawasaki syndrome
17-KS
 17-ketosteroids
K-SADS
 Schedule for Affective Disorders and
  Schizophrenia for School-Age
  Children
K-SADS-E
 Schedule for Affective Disorders and
  Schizophrenia for School-Age
  Children-Epidemiologic Version
K-SADS-P
 Schedule for Affective Disorders and
  Schizophrenia for School-Age
  Children-Present Episode
K-SEALS
 Kaufman Survey of Early Academic
  and Language Skills
KSS
 Kearns-Sayre syndrome
KT
 ketoprofen
 Orudis KT
K-Tab
K-TEA
 Kaufman Test of Educational
  Achievement
KTP
 potassium titanyl phosphate
KUB
 kidneys, ureters, bladder
Kufs disease
Kugel artery
Kugelberg-Welander (KW)
 K.-W. disease
Küntscher rod
Kupffer
 K. cell (KC)
 K. cell hyperplasia
Kupperman
 K. index
 K. menopausal distress
  test
kuru disease
Kurzrok-Miller test
Kurzrok-Ratner test
Kussmaul
 K. respiration
 K. sign
Küstner sign
Ku-Zyme HP
kV
 kilovolt
Kveim
 K. antibody
 K. test

KVO
  keep vein open
KW
  Kimmelstiel-Wilson disease
  Kugelberg-Welander
    KW disease
    KW test
kW
  kilowatt
kwashiorkor
  dermatosis of k.
  k. disease
Kwellada
K-wire
  Kirschner wire
Kyasanur Forest disease
K-Y lubricating jelly
kynocephalus
kynurenine hydroxylation
Kyotest

kyphomelic dysplasia
kyphoscoliosis
  cataract, microcephaly, failure to
    thrive, k. (CAMFAK)
  k. dorsalis juvenilis
kyphoscoliotic heart disease
kyphosis
  cataract, microcephaly, arthrogryposis,
    k. (CAMAK)
  congenital k.
  dorsal k.
  k. dorsalis juvenilis
  flexible k.
  juvenile k.
  Scheuermann juvenile k.
    (SJK)
  thoracic k.
  thoracolumbar k.
kyphotic pelvis
Kytril Injection

K

L
    liter
L1
    neural cell adhesion molecule L1
    (LICAM)
L-A
    long-acting
    Bicillin L-A
L.A.
    long-acting
    Humibid L.A.
LA
    long-acting
    Comhist LA
    LA Crosse (LAC)
    LA Crosse
     encephalitis
    Dexone LA
    Entex LA
    Guaifenex DM, LA
    Inderal LA
    LA Leche League
    LA (SS-B) autoantigen
    Zephrex LA
LAAH
    laparoscopic-assisted abdominal
    hysterectomy
lab (*see also* **laboratory**)
    Breathmobile mobile asthma
     testing l.
Laband syndrome
Labcath catheter
labeling
    primed in situ l. (PRINS)
    terminal deoxyribonucleotidyl
     transferase-mediated biotin-16-dUTP
     nick-end l. (TUNEL)
labetalol
labia (*pl. of* labium)
labial
    l. adhesion
    l. agglutination
    l. commissure
    l. edema
    l. fusion
    l. hernia
    l. hypertrophy
    l. reflex
    l. traction technique
labialis
    herpes simplex l.
    micropapillomatosis l.
labile
    l. asthma
    l. factor

lability
    emotional l.
    mood l.
labiodental speech sound
labioscrotal
    l. fusion
    l. swelling
    l. Y-V plasty
labium, *pl.* **labia**
    caruncle of l.
    hypertrophy of l.
    hypoplastic l.
    l. majus
    l. majus pudendi
    l. minus
    l. minus pudendi
labor, stages of labor
    abnormal l.
    accelerated painless l. (APL)
    acceleration phase of l.
    active phase of l.
    l. analgesia
    l. and delivery (L&D)
    arrest of l.
    l. augmentation
    l. augmentation induction
    cardinal movements of l.
    l., delivery, and recovery (LDR)
    descent during l.
    desultory l.
    dry l.
    engagement in l.
    l. epidural (LE)
    extension in l.
    false l.
    fetal distress in l.
    fetal intolerance of l.
    first stage of l.
    fourth stage of l.
    induced l.
    l. induction abortion
    l. inhibition
    l. initiation
    latent phase of l.
    mechanism of l.
    mimetic l.
    missed l.
    obstructed l.
    oxytocin stimulation of l.
    l. pains
    phase of maximum slope of l.
    placental stage of l.
    postmature l.
    postponed l.
    precipitate l.

L

labor (*continued*)
 precipitous l.
 premature l. (PML)
 preterm l. (PTL)
 primary dysfunctional l. (PDL)
 prodromal l.
 prolonged l.
 second stage of l.
 spontaneous l.
 stages of l.
 third stage of l.
 l. trial
 trial of l. (TOL)
 true l.
 vaginal birth after cesarean trial of l. (VBAC-TOL)
laboratory (*see also* **lab**)
 l. finding
 gait l.
 l. test
 Venereal Disease Research L. (VDRL)
Labotect catheter
labra (*pl. of* labrum)
labrum, *pl.* **labra**
 acetabular l.
labyrinth
labyrinthine
 l. afferent input
 l. concussion
 l. placenta
 l. reflex
 l. stimulation
labyrinthitis
 acute l.
 bacterial l.
 progressive l.
 suppurative l.
 traumatic l.
LAC
 La Crosse
 lupus anticoagulant
laceration
 anal sphincter l.
 aortic l.
 birth canal l.
 bladder l.
 cerebral l.
 cervical l.
 falx l.
 first-degree l.
 fourth-degree l.
 perineal l.
 posterior pharyngeal l.
 scalp l.
 second-degree l.
 stellate l.
 suture penile l.
 tentorial l.

 third-degree l.
 vaginal l.
Lachman test
lachrymal (*var. of* lacrimal)
Lac-Hydrin
lack of natural killer cells
Lacks
 Henrietta L. (HeLa)
lacmoid staining solution
Lacri-Lube SOP lubricant eye ointment
lacrimal, lachrymal
 l. bone
 l. duct
 l. duct obstruction
 l. duct stenosis
 l. gland
 l. sac distention
 l. sac massage
lacrimation
 gustatory l.
lacrimoauriculodentodigital syndrome
lactacidemia
lactacidosis
Lactaid
 L. fat-free milk
 L. reduced fat milk
 L. Ultra lactase enzyme supplement
Lact-Aid nursing trainer system
lactalbumin
 alpha l. (ALA)
lactamase
 beta l.
lactase
 congenital absence of l.
 l. deficiency
lactate
 ammonium l.
 amrinone l.
 arterial l.
 blood l.
 cyclizine l.
 l. dehydrogenase (LDH)
 plasma l.
 Ringer l.
lactated
 l. Ringer
 l. Ringer solution (LRS)
lactating
 l. adenoma
 l. breast
 l. woman
lactation
 l. amenorrhea
 l. consultant (LC)
 l. disorder
 inappropriate l.
 l. initiation
 l. letdown response

lactational
l. amenorrhea method (LAM)
l. amenorrhea method of contraception
l. mastitis
lactea
crusta l.
lacteal
l. calculus
l. cyst
l. fistula
lactentium
hyperemesis l.
lactic
l. acid
l. acid dehydrogenase (LDH)
l. acidemia
l. acidosis
lacticacidemia
LactiCare
LactiCare-HC Topical
lactiferous duct
lactifugal
lactifuge
lactigenous
Lactina Select breast pump
Lactinex
lactobacilli (*pl. of* Lactobacillus, lactobacillus)
Lactobacillus
L. acidophilus
L. bifidus
L. bulgaricus
L. fermentum
L. gasseri
hydrogen peroxide-producing *L.*
L. plantarum
L. rhamnosus
L. rhamnosus strain *GG* (L-GG)
lactobezoar
lactobionate
erythromycin l.
lactocele
lactoferrin
plasma l.
lactoflavin
LactoFree Lipil formula
lactogen
human placental l. (hPL)
placental l.
lactogenesis
lactogenic
lactoovovegetarian
lactorrhea
lactose
l. breath hydrogen test
l. deficiency
l. intolerance

l. malabsorption
l. monohydrate
l. tolerance test
lactose-containing formula
lactose-free
l.-f. diet
l.-f. formula
Lactosorb
lactosuria
lactotropin
lactovegetarian
lactulose enema
lacuna, *pl.* **lacunae**
lacunae (*pl. of* lacuna)
lacunar
l. sinusoid
l. skull
LAD
left anterior descending
leukocyte adhesion deficiency
LAD-1
leukocyte adhesion deficiency-1
LAD-2
leukocyte adhesion deficiency-2
Ladd
L. band
L. mobilization of intestine procedure
L. monitor
L. operation
L. syndrome
Ladin sign
LAE
left atrial enlargement
Laerdal
L. mask
L. resuscitator
laetrile
laeve
chorion l.
Lafora
L. body
L. body disease
Laforin
lag
anaphase l.
head l.
homeostatic l.
lid l.
lagophthalmia, lagophthalmos, lagophthalmus
lagophthalmos (*var. of* lagophthalmia)
lagophthalmus (*var. of* lagophthalmia)
Lahey
L. clamp
L. forceps
LA-HFOV
liquid-assisted high-frequency oscillatory ventilation

L

LAIT
    latex agglutination inhibition test
lait
    café au l. (CAL)
LAIV
    live attenuated influenza vaccine
LAK
    lymphokine-activated killer cell
LAKC
    lymphokine-activated killer cell
lake
    subchorial l.
    venous l.
lallation
Lalonde delicate hook forceps
LALT
    larynx-associated lymphoid tissue
LAM
    lactational amenorrhea method
    laser-assisted myringotomy
    LAM contraceptive method
Lamarck theory
Lamaze
    L. childbirth education
    L. method
LAMB
    lentigines, atrial myxomas, cutaneous
    papular myxomas, blue nevi
    LAMB syndrome
lambda
    l. sign
    l. suture line
lambdoid synostosis
Lambert-Eaton syndrome
Lambert syndrome
lamblia
    Giardia l.
Lambotte syndrome
lamellar
    l. body (LB)
    l. body count (LBC)
    l. body number density
    l. bone
    l. desquamation of newborn
    l. exfoliation
    l. ichthyosis
    l. inclusion body
lamellated appearance
Lamictal
lamina, *pl.* **laminae**
    basal l.
    l. cribrosa
    duplicated elastic l.
    elastic l.
    l. lucida
    l. propria
    l. terminalis
laminae (*pl. of* lamina)
laminar airflow

laminaria
    l. cervical dilator
    L. digitata
    l. infusion
    L. japonica
    l. tent
    l. tent insertion
lamination
laminin
l-amino acid
Lamisil Cream
lamivudine
lamotrigine
lamp
    halogen l.
    Nightingale examining l.
    Sunnex Tri-Star l.
    Wood ultraviolet l.
lamp-brush chromosome
lampbrush chromosome, lamp-brush chromosome
Lamprene
Lanacaps
    Ferralyn L.
Lanacort Topical
lance
    heel l. (HL)
Lancefield streptococcal typing system
lancet
    Quikheel l.
Landau
    L. reflex
    L. response
    L. test
Landau-Kleffner
    L.-K. syndrome (LKS)
    L.-K. syndrome variant
Landing syndrome
Landmark catheter
Landouzy-Dejerine
    facioscapulohumeral syndrome of
    L.-D.
    L.-D. muscular dystrophy
Landouzy dystrophy
Landry
    L. palsy
    L. type of paralysis
Landry-Guillain-Barré syndrome
landscape
    adaptive l.
Langdon Down disease
Lange
    Brachmann-Cornelia de L. (BCDL)
    Cornelia de L. (CDL)
    L. test
Lange-Nielsen syndrome
Langer
    L. line
    L. mesomelic dwarfism

L. mesomelic dysplasia
L. syndrome
Langer-Giedion syndrome
Langerhans
L. cell
L. cell histiocytosis (LCH)
L. granule
L. islands
islets of L.
Langer-Saldino syndrome
Langhans
L. giant cell
L. giant cell granuloma
L. layer
L. stria
language
American Sign L. (ASL)
body l.
l. delay
l. development
l. disorder
l. domain
expressive l.
l. milestone
receptive l.
sign l.
l. skill
language-based learning disability
lanolin
Lanophyllin
Lanoxicaps
Lanoxin
lansoprazole
Lanterman cleft
lanuginosa
hypertrichosis l.
lanuginous
lanugo
Lanvis
Lanz incision
LAO
left anterior oblique
lap
laparotomy
l. count
L. Sac
l. tape
laparoelytrotomy
laparohysterectomy
laparohystero-oophorectomy
laparohysteropexy
laparohysterosalpingo-oophorectomy
laparohysterotomy
Laparolift system
laparomyomectomy
LaparoSAC single-use obturator and cannula
laparosalpingectomy
laparosalpingo-oophorectomy

laparosalpingotomy
laparoscope
Lent l.
MiniSite l.
Storz l.
Surgiview l.
Weerda l.
Wolf l.
laparoscopic
l. cautery
l. cholecystectomy (LC)
l. cornual excision
l. Döderlein hysterectomy
l. electrocautery
l. evidence
l. fenestration
l. fulguration
l. full-thickness intestinal biopsy
l. fundoplication (LF)
l. incision
l. insufflator
l. laser-assisted autoaugmentation
l. leash
l. lymphadenectomy
l. management
l. microsurgery
l. multiple-punch resection
l. myomectomy
l. oophorectomy
l. oophoropexy
l. ovarian diathermy
l. plasma forceps
l. retropubic colposuspension
l. sacrocolpopexy
l. salpingectomy
l. scissors
l. slip knot
l. sonography
l. supracervical hysterectomy (LSH)
l. suspension
l. treatment
l. trocar
l. tubal ligation (LTL)
l. unipolar coagulation procedure
l. ureterosacral ligament resection (LUSLR)
l. uterine nerve ablation (LUNA)
l. uterosacral nerve ablation
l. uterosacral plication
l. vault suspension
laparoscopically
l. assisted anorectoplasty
l. assisted radical vaginal hysterectomy
laparoscopic-assisted
l.-a. abdominal hysterectomy (LAAH)
l.-a. vaginal hysterectomy (LAVH)
l.-a. vaginal hysteroscopy (LAVH)

L

laparoscopist
American Association of
Gynecologic Laparoscopists
laparoscopy
gasless l.
Hasson l.
laser l.
pelvic l.
l. port
second-look l.
**LaparoSonic coagulating shears
(LCS)**
laparotomy (lap)
l. incision
l. pad
salvage l.
second-look l.
laparotrachelotomy
laparouterotomy
lapatinib
**Lap-Band adjustable gastric banding
system**
lap-belt
l.-b. complex
l.-b. trauma
Lapides vesicourethropexy technique
Laplace law
LAR
laryngeal adductor reflex
late asthmatic response
Largactil
large
l. B-cell lymphoma
l. bowel injury
l. bowel stasis
l. cell anaplastic Ki-1 lymphoma
l. cell immunoblastic lymphoma
l. cisterna magna
l. endometrioma
l. foreskin
l. for gestational age (LGA)
l. intestine
l. intestine neoplasm
l. loop excision
l. loop excision of transformation
zone (LLETZ)
l. lysosome-like granule
l. single copy
l. tongue
large-bore catheter
large-for-dates
l.-f.-d. infant
l.-f.-d. uterus
large-volume
l.-v. blood study
l.-v. nonobstruction
L-arginine
lari
Campylobacter l.

Laron
L. dwarfism
L. syndrome
Larsen syndrome
larva
l. currens
l. migrans
larval granulomatosis
larvicide
laryngeal
l. abductor paralysis
l. adductor paralysis
l. adductor reflex (LAR)
l. atresia
l. atresia syndrome
l. chemoreflex
l. cleft
l. closure
l. diphtheria
l. edema
l. fracture
l. hypoplasia
l. mask airway (LMA)
l. nerve
l. nerve paralysis
l. papilloma
l. papillomatosis
l. paresis
l. spasm
l. stenosis
l. stridor
l. vagal reflex
l. wart
l. web
larynges (*pl. of* larynx)
laryngitis
acute spasmodic l.
viral l.
laryngocele
laryngologist
laryngomalacia
laryngopharyngeal
l. sensory stimulation
(LPSS)
l. sensory stimulation
testing
laryngopharynx
laryngoscope
Andrews infant l.
l. blade
l. handle
Holinger infant l.
pencil-handled l.
Pentax l.
laryngoscopy
direct l.
indirect l.
mirror l.
laryngospasm, glottidospasm

laryngotracheal
    l. reconstruction
    l. stenosis (LTS)
laryngotracheitis
laryngotracheobronchitis
    bacterial l.
    membranous l.
    viral l.
laryngotracheoesophageal cleft
larynx, *pl.* **larynges**
    atresia of l.
    floppy l.
larynx-associated lymphoid tissue (LALT)
Larzel anemia
laser
    l. ablation
    alexandrite l.
    ArF excimer l.
    argon l.
    l. blanching
    Candela l.
    carbon dioxide l.
    l. cervical conization
    CO_2 l.
    Er:YAG l.
    l. excision
    l. excisional conization
    flashlamp-pulsed dye l.
    Ho:YAG l.
    l. laparoscopy
    Merrimack 1040 CO_2 l.
    l. method
    l. myringotomy
    Nd:YAG l.
    l. office ventilation of ears (LOVE)
    l. office ventilation of ears with insertion of tubes (LOVE IT)
    Opmilas CO_2 l.
    l. photocoagulation
    l. photocoagulation of the communicating vessels (LPCV)
    l. photovaporization
    l. plume
    l. reaction
    SPTL vascular lesion l.
    l. surgery
    Surgicenter 40 CO_2 l.
    Surgilase 55W l.
    l. therapy
    l. treatment
    l. uterosacral nerve ablation (LUNA)
    l. vaporization
    Xanar 20 Ambulase CO_2 l.
    YAG l.
    yttrium-aluminum-garnet l.
laser-assisted myringotomy (LAM)
laser-Doppler flowmeter

lasered
lash
    L. laparoscopic supracervical hysterectomy procedure
    L. operation
Lasix
    L. Injection
    L. Oral
L-asparaginase
Lassa
    L. fever
    L. virus
La/SSB antigen
last
    l. menstrual period (LMP)
    l. normal menstrual period (LNMP)
    l. postpartum hemorrhage
LAT
    lateral atrial tunnel
    lidocaine, adrenaline, tetracaine
    LAT cavopulmonary anastomosis
latae
    tensor fasciae l. (TFL)
LATCH
    Lower Anchorages and Tethers for children
    LATCH system
latching on
latching-on process
late
    l. adolescence
    l. apnea
    l. arrhythmia
    l. asthmatic reaction
    l. asthmatic response (LAR)
    l. complication
    l. complication of transfusion
    l. congenital syphilis
    l. deceleration
    l. embryonic testicular regression syndrome
    l. hemorrhagic disease
    l. hypocalcemia
    l. infantile amaurotic idiocy
    l. infantile MLD
    l. infantile NCL
    l. infantile neural ceroid lipofuscinosis (LINCL)
    l. infantile systemic lipidosis
    l. luteal phase dysphoric disorder (LLPDD)
    l. luteal phase syndrome
    l. mature
    l. neonatal hypocalcemia
    l. phase
    l. pregnancy
    l. radiation encephalopathy
    l. replicating chromosome
    l. uterine wedge resection

L

latency
  interpeak l.
  l. period
  pudendal nerve terminal motor l.
    (PNTML)
  REM l.
  response l.
  sleep l.
  terminal motor l.
latent
  l. carrier
  l. celiac disease
  l. class analysis (LCA)
  l. diabetes
  l. herpes simplex virus infection
  l. nystagmus
  l. phase
  l. phase of labor
  l. syphilis
latent-stage syphilis
late-onset
  l.-o. adrenal hyperplasia
  l.-o. congenital large ectopic gland
  l.-o. 21-hydroxylase deficiency
    (LOHD)
  l.-o. hyperplasia
  l.-o. hypogammaglobulinemia
  l.-o. local junctional epidermolysis
    bullosa-mental retardation syndrome
  l.-o. SED
  l.-o. sepsis
latera (*pl. of* latus)
lateral
  l. atrial tunnel (LAT)
  l. collateral ligament complex
  l. compartment
  l. condylar fracture
  l. condyle
  l. curvature
  l. curvature of spine
  l. displacement of inner canthus
  l. epicondylitis
  l. facial dysplasia (LFD)
  l. femoral torsion (LFT)
  l. geniculate
  l. geniculate body
  l. hamstring
  l. head displacement (LHD)
  l. head-righting
  l. head tilt
  l. hip rotation
  l. incisor
  l. lemniscus
  l. luxation
  l. malleolus
  l. nasal proboscis
  l. oblique view
  l. ovarian transposition
  l. pelvic wall

  l. plate mesoderm
  l. position
  l. radiograph
  l. rectus muscle
  l. rectus palsy
  l. recumbent position
  l. resolution
  l. rotation (LR)
  l. shoulder sway
  l. sinus thrombosis
  l. sperm head displacement
  l. thoracic artery
  l. tibial bowing
  l. tibial torsion (LTT)
  l. transverse thigh flap
  l. umbilical fold
  l. wall retractor
lateralis
  proboscis l.
  vastus l.
laterality
  l. defect
  l. disorder
  l. sequence
lateralization process
lateralizing sign
laterally extended endopelvic resection
lateromedial oblique view
laterothoracic exanthema
lateroversion
latex
  l. agglutination (LA)
  l. agglutination assay
  l. agglutination inhibition test
    (LAIT)
  l. allergy
  l. fixation test
  l. glove
  l. particle agglutination (LPA)
  l. particle agglutination test
  l. sensitization
  l. test for *pneumococcus*
lathyrism
latissimus dorsi flap
lato
  Borrelia burgdorferi sensu l.
latrodectism
LATS
  long-acting thyroid stimulator
  LATS hormone
  LATS protector
latum
  condyloma l.
  Diphyllobothrium l.
  fascia lata
latus, *pl.* **latera**
  nevus unius lateris
Latzko
  L. cesarean

L. colpocleisis
L. operation
L. procedure
laudanum
Lauenstein
L. lateral radiograph
L. pelvic x-ray
Laufe-Piper forceps
Laufe polyp forceps
Lauge-Hansen mechanism of injury
Laugier-Hunziker syndrome
Launois-Cléret syndrome
Launois syndrome
Laurell (rocket) immune electrophoresis
Laurence-Moon-Biedl (LMB)
L.-M.-B. syndrome
Laurence-Moon-Biedl-Bardet (LMBB)
L.-M.-B.-B. syndrome (LMBBS)
Laurence-Moon syndrome
Laurer forceps
Laurus ND-260 needle driver
LAV
lymphadenopathy-associated virus
lavage
alveolar l.
antral l.
bronchoalveolar l. (BAL)
bronchopulmonary l.
diagnostic peritoneal l. (DPL)
ductal l.
gastric l.
nasal l.
nonbronchoscopic bronchoalveolar l.
oral colonic l. (OCL)
peritoneal l.
pulmonary l.
saline l.
surfactant l.
therapeutic pulmonary l.
tracheal l.
LAVH
laparoscopic-assisted vaginal hysterectomy
laparoscopic-assisted vaginal hysteroscopy
law
Collins l.
Hardy-Weinberg l.
Hellin l.
Hellin-Zeleny l.
inverse square l.
Laplace l.
Leopold l.
Mendel first l.
Mendel second l.
l. of mass action
Pflüger l.
Lawford syndrome
Lawrence-Seip syndrome

Lawrence syndrome
lax
l. joint
l. ligament
laxa
acquired cutis l.
cutis l.
laxative
bulk-forming l.
osmotic l.
stimulant l.
laxity
anteroposterior l.
joint l.
ligamentous l.
pelvic floor l.
suspensory ligament l.
layer
Bowman l.
buffy coat l.
feeder l.
germ l.
glycosaminoglycan l.
half-value l. (HVL)
Langhans l.
musculoaponeurotic l.
myofascial l.
Nitabuch l.
l. of Brun
Rauber l.
skeletal muscle l.
subcutaneous l.
Waldeyer l.
lazaroid
Lazarus-Nelson closed peritoneal lavage technique
LazerSporin-C Otic
lazy
l. bladder syndrome
l. colon syndrome
l. eye
l. leukocyte syndrome
l. S incision
LB
lamellar body
LBC
lamellar body count
LBGT
lesbian, bisexual, gay, transsexual
LBM
lean body mass
LBW
low birth weight
LBW infant
LBWC
limb-body wall complex
LBWI
low birth weight infant

L

511

LBW-MES
low birth weight-maternal employment study
LC
lactation consultant
laparoscopic cholecystectomy
living children
LCA
latent class analysis
Leber congenital amaurosis
LCAD
long-chain acyl-CoA dehydrogenase
LCAD deficiency
LCAD/MCAD
long- and medium-chain acyl-CoA dehydrogenase
LCAD/MCAD deficiency
LCAD/VLCAD
long and very long chain acyl-CoA dehydrogenase
LCAD/VLCAD deficiency
L-Caine
L-carnitine
L-Cath peripherally inserted neonatal catheter
LCH
Langerhans cell histiocytosis
LCHAD
long-chain 3-hydroxyacyl-CoA dehydrogenase
long-chain hydroxyacyl-coenzyme A dehydrogenase
LCHAD deficiency
LCIS
lobular carcinoma in situ
lck protooncogene
LCL
localized cutaneous leishmaniasis
LCMV
lymphocytic choriomeningitis virus
LCMV syndrome
LCP
Legg-Calvé-Perthes
LCPD
Legg-Calvé-Perthes disease
LCPUFA
long-chain polyunsaturated fatty acid
LCR
ligase chain reaction
LCR assay
LCS
LaparoSonic coagulating shears
LCx Probe System test
L&D
labor and delivery
LD
learning disability
learning disorder
Lyme disease

LDH
lactate dehydrogenase
lactic acid dehydrogenase
LDH deficiency
LDL
low-density lipoprotein
LDL apheresis
LDL cholesterol
L-DOPA
levodopa
l-dopa
levodopa
LDR
labor, delivery, and recovery
LDR room
LDS
ligate, divide, staple
LDS clip applier
LDS instrument
LE
labor epidural
lower extremity
lupus erythematosus
Le
Lewis
Le cell preparation
Le Fort craniofacial dysjunction operation
Le Fort fracture (I, II)
Le Fort fracture pattern
Le Fort partial colpocleisis
LEA
local education agency
lumbar epidural anesthesia
lead
l. agency
l. block
blood l.
l. bra
l. encephalopathy
l. exposure
l. ingestion
l. intoxication
limb l.
l. line
organic l.
l. pipe stiffness
l. pipe urethra
l. point
l. poisoning
tetraethyl l.
l. tracing
l. triphosphate
l. wire
Leadbetter-Politano
L.-P. ureteroneocystostomy procedure
L.-P. ureterovesicoplasty
LeadCare handheld blood lead analyzer
leading ancestor

leaf, *pl.* **leaves**
  cabbage leaves
  ivy l.
  l. of broad ligament
4-leaf clover pattern
leaflet
  flail mitral l. (FML)
league
  La Leche L.
leak
  air l.
  capillary l.
  cerebrospinal fluid l.
  phosphate l.
  staple line l.
leakage
  intermittent urinary l.
  placental l.
  silicone implant l.
  urine l.
leak-point
  l.-p. pressure (LPP)
  l.-p. pressure test
leaky gene
lean
  l. body mass (LBM)
  l. spastic dwarfism
  l. tissue mass (LTM)
Lear complex
learner
  active l.
  auditory l.
  kinesthetic l.
  visual l.
learning
  l. disability (LD)
  discrete-trial l.
  l. disorder (LD)
  Mullen Scales of Early L. (MSEL)
  situated l.
  slow rate of l.
  l. style
  wide range assessment of memory
    and l. (WRAML)
leash
  electronic l.
  laparoscopic l.
Lea's Shield female barrier contraceptive
least restrictive environment (LRE)
leather-bottle stomach
leaves (*pl. of* leaf)
Leber
  L. abiotrophy
  L. congenital amaurosis (LCA)
  L. congenital retinal amaurosis
  L. congenital tapetoretinal
    degeneration
  L. disease
  L. hereditary atrophy

  L. hereditary optic neuropathy
    (LHON)
  L. optic neuropathy
Leboyer
  L. episiotomy technique
  L. method
LEC
  life events checklist
lecanopagus
Lecat gulf
lecithin
  disaturated l.
lecithin/sphingomyelin (L/S, l/s)
  l. ratio
Lecompte arterial switch maneuver
lectin
Lectrolyte
  Kao L.
Leder stain
LEDS
  life events and difficulties schedule
    LEDS interview
LEEP
  loop electrosurgical excision procedure
    LEEP Redi-kit
LeeSpec disposable vaginal speculum
Lee-White clotting time
Leff forceps
left
  l. anterior descending (LAD)
  l. anterior hemiblock
  l. anterior oblique (LAO)
  l. arterial pressure
  l. atrial enlargement (LAE)
  l. atrial hypertrophy
  l. atrium
  l. axis deviation
  l. bundle branch block
  l. common carotid
  l. ear
  l. frontoanterior (LFA)
  l. frontoanterior position
  l. frontoposterior position (LFP)
  l. frontotransverse (LFT)
  l. frontotransverse position
  l. hemisyndrome
  l. hepatectomy
  l. lateral decubitus position
    (LLDP)
  l. lateral position
  l. lower quadrant (LLQ)
  l. main coronary artery
  l. mentoanterior (LMA)
  l. mentoanterior position
  l. mentoposterior (LMP)
  l. mentoposterior position (LMP)
  l. mentotransverse (LMT)
  l. mentotransverse position
  l. occipitoanterior (LOA)

L

left (*continued*)
    l. occipitoanterior position
    l. occipitoposterior position (LOP)
    l. occipitotransverse (LOT)
    l. occipitotransverse position
    l. renal vei
    l. sacroanterior (LSA)
    l. sacroanterior position
    l. sacroposterior position (LSP)
    l. sacrotransverse (LST)
    l. sacrotransverse position
    l. scapuloanterior (LScA)
    l. scapuloanterior position
    l. scapuloposterior position (LScP)
    l. to right
    l. upper quadrant (LUQ)
    l. ventricle (LV)
    l. ventricular (LV)
    l. ventricular apical aneurysm
    l. ventricular assist device
      (LVAD)
    l. ventricular dysfunction (LVD)
    l. ventricular ejection fraction
      (LVEF)
    l. ventricular end-diastolic dimension
    l. ventricular end-systolic dimension
    l. ventricular failure
    l. ventricular hypertrophy (LVH)
    l. ventricular outflow tract (LVOT)
    l. ventricular outflow tract
      obstruction (LVOTO)
    l. ventricular outlet obstruction
    l. ventricular paced beat
    l. ventricular stroke work index
      (LVSWI)
    l. vertical vein
left-angle suture
left/right
    l./r. asymmetry
    l./r. dynein
left-sided lesion
left-sidedness
    bilateral l.-s.
left-to-right
    l.-t.-r. shunt
    l.-t.-r. shunting
    l.-t.-r. shunt lesion
Lefty-1
Lefty-2
leg
    l. atrophy
    baker's l.
    bayonet l.
    l. cramp
    l. edema
    l. length discrepancy (LLD)
    milk l.
    white l.
    W position of l.'s

legal
    l. abortion
    l. intervention
    l. issue
legally blind
Legat point
Legatrin
leg-compression stocking
Legg-Calvé-Perthes (LCP)
    L.-C.-P. disease (LCPD)
Legg-Perthes disease
Legionella **(L)**
    L. micdadei
    L. pneumophila
legionellosis
Legionnaires disease
Leiden
    factor V L.
    L. mutation
Leigh
    L. disease
    encephalomyopathy of L.
    L. necrotizing encephalomyelopathy
    L. subacute necrotizing
      encephalopathy
    L. syndrome
Leiner
    L. disease
    L. syndrome
leiomyoblastoma
leiomyoma, *pl.* **leiomyomas, leiomyomata**
    cellular l.
    cervical l.
    endometrial metastasizing l.
    intramural l.
    metastasizing l.
    ovarian l.
    parasitic l.
    pedunculated l.
    submucosal l.
    submucous l.
    l. uteri
    uterine leiomyomata
    vascular l.
leiomyomas (*pl. of* leiomyoma)
leiomyomata (*pl. of* leiomyoma)
leiomyomatosis
    intravenous l.
    l. peritonealis disseminata (LPD)
leiomyosarcoma (LMS)
    epithelioid l.
Leisegang colposcope
Leishmania
    L. braziliensis
    L. infantum
    L. major
    L. mexicana
    L. panamensis
    L. tropica

leishmaniasis, leishmaniosis
    cutaneous l.
    diffuse cutaneous l. (DCL)
    localized cutaneous l. (LCL)
    mucocutaneous l.
    mucosal l.
    post-kala azar dermal l. (PKDL)
    visceral l.
leishmaniosis (*var. of* leishmaniasis)
Leiter International Performance
  Scale
Lejeune syndrome
Lejour-type modified breast
  reduction
Lembert stitch
Lemierre syndrome
Lemli-Opitz syndrome
lemniscus
    lateral l.
lemon
    l. balm
    l. sign
lemon-squeezer obstetrical elevator
length
    birth l.
    cervical l.
    clitoral l.
    crown-heel l. (CHL)
    crown-rump l. (CRL)
    cycle l.
    femoral l.
    femur l. (FL)
    fetal foot l. (FFL)
    functional urethral l. (FUL)
    funnel l.
    humerus l. (HL)
    long bone l.
    penile l.
    sinus cycle l.
    stretched penile l.
    stretched phallic l.
    subischial leg l. (SILL)
    supine l.
lengthening
    Achilles tendon l. (ATL)
    Evans calcaneal l.
    hamstring l.
    heel cord l.
    muscle l.
    l. of hamstring
    l. osteotomy
    tendo Achillis l. (TAL)
    tendon l.
length-for-age percentile
Lennox syndrome
Lennox-Gastaut syndrome, Lennox
  syndrome
lens
    Barkan infant l.

crystalline l.
L. culinaris agglutinin
30-degree l.
70-degree l.
l. dislocation
Morgan therapeutic l.
l. opacity
posterior chamber intraocular l.
  (PCIOL, PC-IOL)
Sauflon PW contact l.
Silsoft extended wear
  contact l.
Lente Iletin II
lenticonus
    anterior l.
    posterior l.
lenticular
    l. cataract
    l. opacity
lentiform nucleus, lenticular nucleus,
  lenticular nucleus
lentigines (*pl. of* lentigo)
lentiginosis profusa
lentiginous nevus
lentigo, *pl.* **lentigines**
    agminated l.
    lentigines, atrial myxomas, cutaneous
      papular myxomas, blue nevi
      (LAMB)
    lentigines, electrocardiographic
      abnormalities, ocular hypertelorism,
      pulmonary stenosis, abnormalities
      of genitalia, retardation of growth,
      and deafness (LEOPARD)
    l. simplex
lentis
    ectopia l.
    simple ectopia l.
lentivirus
Lent laparoscope
Lenz
    L. dysmorphogenic syndrome
    L. dysplasia
    L. microphthalmia syndrome
Lenz-Majewski
    L.-M. hyperostotic dwarfism
    L.-M. syndrome
Leonard catheter
LEOPARD
    lentigines, electrocardiographic
      abnormalities, ocular hypertelorism,
      pulmonary stenosis, abnormalities of
      genitalia, retardation of growth, and
      deafness
      LEOPARD syndrome
Leopold
    L. law
    L. maneuver
Lepiota cristata

L

Lepore
  hemoglobin L. (Hb$_{Lepore}$)
  L. thalassemia
lepori
  Brugia l.
leprae
  Mycobacterium l.
leprechaunism
lepromatous leprosy
leprosum
  erythema nodosum l. (ENL)
leprosy
  borderline lepromatous l.
  borderline tuberculoid l.
  dimorphous l.
  full lepromatous l.
  full tuberculoid l.
  indeterminate l.
  lepromatous l.
  tuberculoid l.
leprous salpingitis
leptin
  cord plasma l.
  maternal plasma l.
  l. receptor
  serum l.
  umbilical cord l.
leptomeningeal
  l. angioma
  l. angiomatosis
  l. cyst
  l. heterotopia
leptomeningitis
  acute syphilitic l.
  mumps l.
leptometacarpy
Leptospira
  L. canicola
  L. grippotyphosa
  L. interrogans
  L. pomona
leptospiral
  l. illness
  l. meningitis
leptospire
leptospirosis
  anicteric l.
  icteric l.
leptotene
  l. phase of meiosis
  l. stage
leptotrichosis
Leri
  L. pleonosteosis
  L. syndrome
Leri-Weill syndrome
Leroy
  L. syndrome
  L. ventricular catheter

LES
  lower esophageal sphincter
lesbian
  l., bisexual, gay, transsexual (LBGT)
  l. relationship
lesbianism
Leschke syndrome
Lesch-Nyhan
  L.-N. disease
  L.-N. syndrome (LNS)
lesion
  acetowhite l.
  acquired hypothalamic l.
  acral skin l.
  acyanotic l.
  anal squamous intraepithelial l.
    (ASIL)
  anesthetic skin l.
  anular l.
  arciform l.
  atypical squamous cells-cannot
    exclude high-grade l. (ASC-H)
  axillary skin l.
  Bankart l.
  barrel-shaped l.
  benign l.
  blanching wheal and flare l.
  blueberry muffin skin l.
  brain l.
  brainstem l.
  brown skin l.
  cannonball l.
  cardiac l.
  cavitary white-matter l.
  central cord l.
  cervical l.
  cicatricial l.
  clastic l.
  coin l.
  collapse-consolidation l.
  confetti l.
  congenital l.
  coronary artery l. (CAL)
  correctable l.
  crescentic l.
  crusted l.
  cutaneous l.
  cyanotic congenital heart l.
  cystic l.
  dermatophyte l.
  Dieulafoy gastric l.
  discoid l.
  discontinuous l.
  ductal-dependent l.
  ductal-independent mixing l.
  ectocervical l.
  eczematoid l.
  eczematous skin l.
  endometriotic l.

epileptogenic l.
erythematous satellite l.
exogastric l.
exophytic l.
extrapyramidal l.
flaccid l.
genital l.
gingival l.
glandular atypia l.
guttate l.
heart l.
high-grade squamous intraepithelial l. (ASC-H, HGSIL, HSIL, H-SIL)
HPV-associated l.
hyperpigmented l.
hypoesthesic skin l.
hypopigmented l.
hypothalamic l.
intestinal l.
intracavitary l.
intraepithelial l.
iris l.
isodense l.
Janeway l.
juxtapleural inflammatory l.
kissing l.'s
left-sided l.
left-to-right shunt l.
linear l.
local l.
low-grade squamous intraepithelial l. (LGSIL, LSIL)
lumbosacral plexus l.
lumbosacral root l.
Lynch and Crues type 2 l.
lytic l.
macular-papular-vesicular l.
maculopapular l.
mass l.
metaphysial l.
metastatic l.
microvascular l.
mixing l.
morphogenetic l.
mucosal l.
multifocal white matter inflammatory l.
multiple ring-enhancing mass l.
nipplelike l.
nodulocystic l.
Noonan-like giant cell l.
oculocutaneous l.
organic brain l.
osseous BA l.
osteochondrotic l.
palmar l.
papular l.
papulonodular l.
papulovesicular l.

parenchymal brain l.
pebbly skin l.
pedunculated l.
perineal l.
photodistributed l.
pigmented l.
plexus l.
plucked chicken skin l.
powder-burn endometrial l.
precancerous l.
precursor l.
preinvasive l.
premalignant l.
proliferative l.
pseudoencapsulated l.
psoriasiform l.
punched-out lytic l.
pyramidal l.
radial sclerosing l.
raised l.
right-sided l.
satellite l.
sclerosing l.
seborrheic-looking skin l.
SIL/ASCUS l.
Sinding-Larsen l.
single ring-enhancing mass l.
skin l.
skip l.
solitary bone l.
space-occupying l.
spiculated l.
squamous intraepithelial l. (SIL)
target l.
targetoid l.
total mixing l.
tubulointerstitial l.
umbilication of l.
upper GI l.
urticarial raised l.
vascular proliferative l.
vasculitic skin l.
vermiform l.
vesicobullous skin l.
vesicopustular l.
vesicular palmar l.
vesicular skin l.
vesiculoulcerative l.
violaceous l.
vulvar pigmented l.
vulvovaginal l.
watershed l.
weeping l.
zosteriform l.

Lessina
lesson
speech l.
LET
lidocaine, epinephrine, tetracaine

letalis
    epidermolysis bullosa l.
    Herlitz epidermolysis bullosa l.
letdown
    milk l.
    l. reflex
lethal
    l. bone dysplasia
    l. catatonia
    l. equivalent
    l. gene
    l. multiple pterygium syndrome
    l. neonatal dwarfism
lethargic
lethargica
    encephalitis l.
lethargy
    postictal l.
letrozole
letter chart
Letterer-Siwe disease
Letter-R intelligence test
LETZ
    loop excision of transformation zone
    LETZ procedure
leucine
    l. aminopeptidase
    l. tolerance test
leucocoria
leucocyte
    l. detection
    l. detection strip
    l. esterase
Leuconostoc
leucovorin
leukapheresis
leukemia
    acute lymphatic l.
    acute lymphoblastic l. (ALL)
    acute lymphocytic l. (ALL)
    acute megakaryoblastic l.
    acute myeloblastic l. (AML)
    acute myelogenous l.
    acute myeloid l. (AML)
    acute nonlymphoblastic l.
     (ANLL)
    acute nonlymphocytic l.
    amyeloid l.
    aplastic l.
    basophilic l.
    chronic lymphocytic l. (CLL)
    chronic myelocytic l.
    chronic myelogenous l. (CML)
    CNS l.
    congenital l.
    eosinophilic l.
    graft versus l. (GVL)
    granulocytic l.
    hemoblastic l.

    l. infiltrate
    l. inhibitory factor (LIG)
    juvenile myelomonocytic l. (JMML)
    leukopenic l.
    lymphatic l.
    lymphoblastic l.
    lymphocytic l.
    lymphosarcoma cell l.
    mast cell l.
    megakaryoblastic l.
    megakaryocytic l.
    micromyeloblastic l.
    myeloblastic l.
    myelocytic l.
    myelogenous l.
    myeloid l.
    myelomonocytic l.
    nonlymphoblastic l.
    nonlymphocytic l.
    promyelocytic l.
    testicular l.
leukemia/lymphoma
    adult T-cell l./l. (ATLL)
leukemic
    l. blast
    l. cell
leukemicus
    hiatus l.
leukemogenesis
leukemoid reaction
Leukeran
Leukine
leukoclastic angiitis
leukocoria, leukokoria
leukocyte
    l. adhesion deficiency (LAD)
    l. adhesion deficiency-1 (LAD-1)
    l. adhesion deficiency-2 (LAD-2)
    l. count
    diapedetic l.
    l. esterase dipstick
    l. function
    l. hexosaminidase A
    l. histamine release test
    l. infiltration
    l. integrin lymphocyte
     function-associated antigen 1
    l. interferon
    polymorphonuclear l.
    l. transfusion
leukocyte-depletion filter
leukocyte-removal filter
leukocytoclastic
    l. angiitis
    l. vasculitis
leukocytosis
    extreme l.
    granulocytic l.
    mild l.

neutrophilic l.
synovial l.
leukocytospermia
leukocyturia
leukodepletion filter
leukoderma
l. acquisitum centrifugum
l. of vulva
leukodystrophy
adrenal l.
cerebral l.
demyelinogenic l.
fibrinoid l.
globoid cell l.
Krabbe l.
melanodermic l.
metachromatic l. (MLD)
sudanophilic l.
leukoencephalopathy
focal pontine l.
multifocal l.
perinatal telencephalic l.
progressive multifocal l. (PML)
l. syndrome
leukoerythroblastic syndrome
leukokeratosis
oral l.
leukokoria (*var. of* leukocoria)
leukokraurosis
leukoma
corneal l.
leukomalacia
cerebral l.
cystic l.
cystic periventricular l. (cPVL)
periventricular l. (PVL)
leukopenia
leukopenic leukemia
leukophlegmasia dolens
leukoplakia
hairy l.
oral hairy l.
l. vulvae
leukoplakic vulvitis
leukorrhagia
leukorrhea
menstrual l.
physiologic l.
leukorrheal
l. discharge
l. disorder
leukospermia
leukostasis
pulmonary l.
Leukotrap red cell collector
leukotriene
l. C_4 (LTC$_4$)
l. D_4 (LTD$_4$)
l. E_4 (LTE$_4$)

l. inhibitor
l. modifier
l. receptor antagonist (LTRA)
leukovorin
calcium l.
leuprolide acetate
leuprorelin acetate
Leustatin
levalbuterol hydrochloride
levallorphan tartrate
levamisole
Levaquin
levarterenol
Levate
levator
l. ani
l. ani muscle
l. ani spasm
l. ani syndrome
l. palpebrae muscle
l. plate
l. sling
Levbid
LeVeen shunt
level
ACD l.
air-fluid l.
alpha-2 antiplasmin l.
alpha antitrypsin l.
amniotic fluid l.
arachidonic acid l.
arousal l.
bile chenodeoxycholic acid l.
biparietal diameter l.
blood alcohol l. (BAL)
blood ammonia l.
blood lead l. (BLL)
CA126 l.
CD4+ l.
ceruloplasmin l.
complement C3 l.
cord blood erythropoietin l.
cord IgG l.
cord serum l.
cortisol l.
cotinine l.
C-peptide l.
^{137}Cs l.
developmental l.
dimeric inhibin A l.
elevation of blood lead l. (EBLL)
endothelial fibronectin l.
endothelin plasma l.
estradiol l.
estriol l.
estrogen l.
fetal LDL l.
folate l.
FSH l.

L

level (*continued*)
    gonadotropin l.
    hemoglobin l.
    high gastrin l.
    hormonal l.
    human chorionic gonadotropin l.
    l. III ultrasonography
    immunoglobulin E l.
    iodothyronine l.
    magnesium l.
    maternal estriol l.
    maternal serum marker l.
    methemoglobin l.
    midluteal phase progesterone l.
    l. 1–3 nursery
    l. of consciousness (LOC)
    operant l.
    peak and trough l.'s
    peripheral hormone l.
    phosphatidylglycerol l.
    plasma estrogen l.
    plasma ornithine l.
    plasminogen l.
    platelet calmodulin l.
    postmenopausal l.
    prepregnancy l.
    progesterone l.
    progesterone myometrial l.
    prolactin l.
    quantitative beta hCG l.
    RBC adenosine deaminase l.
    relaxin serum l.
    serum acetaminophen l.
    serum amylase l.
    serum anticonvulsant l.
    serum bile salt l.
    serum carotene l.
    serum copper l.
    serum cortisol l.
    serum digoxin l.
    serum histamine l.
    serum lead l.
    serum leptin l.
    sodium serum l.
    somatomedin l.
    sweat chloride l.
    theophylline l.
    therapeutic blood l.
    troponin I l.
    trough tacrolimus l.
    unconjugated estriol l.
    uterine lysosome l.
    vitamin B_{12} l.
levetiracetam
Levin syndrome
Levlen contraceptive pill
Levlite tablet
levoamphetamine
levobunolol

levocardia
levocarnitine
levodopa (LD, L-DOPA)
Levo-Dromoran
levofloxacin
levonorgestrel
    l. and ethinyl estradiol
    ethinyl estradiol and l.
    l. implant
Levophed
levoposition
Levoprome
Levora
levorotatory alkaloid
levorphanol tartrate
levoscoliosis
Levo-T
Levothroid
    L. Injection
    L. Oral
levothyroxine test
levotransposition (L-transposition)
levoversion
levre de tapir
Levret
    L. breech delivery maneuver
    L. forceps
Levsin
Levsinex
Levsin/SL
Levy-Hollister syndrome
Lewandowsky
    nevus elasticus of L.
Lewis
    L. antigen
    L. blood group
    L. recording cystometer
Lexapro
lexical cohesion
lexical-syntactic
    l.-s. deficit
    l.-s. syndrome (LSS)
lexicon
Lexiva
Leyden-Möbius muscular dystrophy
Leydig
    L. cell
    L. cell aplasia
    L. cell atrophy
    L. cell embryology
    L. cell hyperplasia
    L. cell hypoplasia
    L. cell tumor
Leyton Obsessional Inventory
LF
    laparoscopic fundoplication
    low frequency
LFA
    left frontoanterior

LFD
　lateral facial dysplasia
LFS
　Li-Fraumeni syndrome
LFT
　lateral femoral torsion
　left frontotransverse
LG
　limb girdle
LGA
　large for gestational age
　　LGA infant
　　postterm LGA
　　term LGA
LGD
　low-grade dysplasia
L-GG
　*Lactobacillus rhamnosus*strain GG
LGS
　limb girdle syndrome
LGSIL
　low-grade squamous intraepithelial
　lesion
LGV
　lymphogranuloma venereum
LH
　luteinizing hormone
　　LH color test
　　LH surge
LHD
　lateral head displacement
Lhermitte-Duclos
　　L.-D. disease
　　L.-D. syndrome
Lhermitte sign
LHON
　Leber hereditary optic neuropathy
　　LHON syndrome
LHR
　lung-to-head ratio
LH-RH
　luteinizing hormone-releasing hormone
　　LH-RH agonist therapy
　　LH-RH analog
LHRH
　luteinizing hormone-releasing hormone
L-5 hydroxytryptophan
liability to pressure palsy
liberty
　reproductive l.
libidinal change
libido
　decreased l.
Libman-Sacks
　　L.-S. disease
　　L.-S. endocarditis
library
　arrayed l.
　cDNA l.

DNA l.
gene l.
genomic l.
l. ligation
Librax
Librium
LICAM
　neural cell adhesion molecule L1
　　LICAM gene for X-linked
　　hydrocephalus
Licentiate in Midwifery (LM)
lichen
　l. infantum
　l. nitidus
　l. planus
　l. ruber planus (LRP)
　l. sclerosis of vulva
　l. sclerosus
　l. sclerosus et atrophicus (LS)
　l. scrofulosorum
　l. simplex
　l. simplex chronicus (LSC)
　l. spinulosus
　l. striatus
lichenification
lichenified plaque
lichenoid
　l. papule
　l. vulvar dermatosis
lichenoides
　pityriasis l.
Lich-Gregoire technique
Lich vesicoureteral reflux repair technique
Liddle
　　L. syndrome
　　L. test
Lidemol
Lidex-E
lid lag
lidocaine (L, LCN)
　lidocaine, adrenaline, tetracaine (LAT)
　l. and epinephrine
　l. and prilocaine
　buffered l. (BL)
　lidocaine, epinephrine, tetracaine (LET)
　l. infiltration
　l. toxicity
lidocaine-prilocaine cream
lidofilcon B
lie
　abnormal l.
　anterior l.
　back-up transverse l.
　breech transverse l.
　dorsosuperior l.
　fetal l.

L

lie (*continued*)
>> longitudinal l.
>> oblique l.
>> posterior l.
>> transverse fetal l.
>> unstable l.
>> vertical l.

Lieberkühn
>> crypt of L.

lienorenal ligament
Liesegang LM-Flex 7 flexible hysteroscope
LIFE
>> longitudinal interval followup evaluation

life
>> change of l.
>> day of l. (DOL)
>> l. event
>> l. events and difficulties schedule (LEDS)
>> l. events and difficulties schedule interview
>> l. events checklist (LEC)
>> l. expectancy
>> extrauterine l.
>> health-related quality of l. (HRQOL)
>> incontinence quality of l. (I-QOL)
>> quality of l. (QOL)
>> l. stress
>> l. support
>> l. table method
>> l. table survival
>> wrongful birth and l.

Lifepak
>> L. AEDS
>> L. defibrillator
>> L. nutritional supplement

LifeScan blood glucose meter
lifestyle factor
life-support machine
life-threatening injury
Li-Fraumeni
>> L.-F. cancer syndrome
>> L.-F. syndrome (LFS)

lift
>> chin l.
>> parasternal l.

LIG
>> leukemia inhibitory factor

Ligaclip
ligament
>> acromioclavicular l.
>> Adams advancement of round l.'s
>> anterior cruciate l. (ACL)
>> anterior talofibular l. (ATFL)
>> broad l.
>> calcaneocuboid l. (CCL)

>> calcaneofibular l. (CFL)
>> Carcassonne l.
>> cardinal l.
>> cardinal-uterosacral l.
>> congenital laxity of l.
>> coracoclavicular l.
>> falciform l.
>> gastrophrenic l.
>> Gilliam round l.
>> Gimbernat reflex l.
>> infundibulopelvic l.
>> inguinal l.
>> IP l.
>> lax l.
>> leaf of broad l.
>> lienorenal l.
>> Mackenrodt l.
>> medial collateral l. (MCL)
>> median umbilical l.
>> l. of Marshall
>> l. of Treitz
>> ovarian l.
>> patellar l.
>> Petit l.
>> phrenoesophageal l.
>> posterior talofibular l. (PTFL)
>> posterior uterosacral l.
>> Poupart l.
>> pubocervical l.
>> pubovesical l.
>> reflex l.
>> round l.
>> sacrospinous l.
>> sacrotuberous l.
>> subcutaneous suspensory l.
>> transverse cervical l.
>> triangular l.
>> ulnar collateral l.
>> umbilical l.
>> uteroovarian l.
>> uterosacral l.
>> Waldeyer preurethral l.

ligamenta (*pl. of* ligamentum)
ligamentopexis, ligamentopexy
ligamentopexy (*var. of* ligamentopexis)
ligamentous
>> l. ectopic pregnancy
>> l. injury (grade I–III)
>> l. laxity

ligamentum, *pl.* **ligamenta**
>> l. pubovesicam
>> l. teres
>> l. venosum

ligand
>> l. binding
>> l. receptor

ligase
>> l. chain reaction (LCR)
>> l. chain reaction assay

l. chain reaction testing
DNA l.

LigaSure
L. vessel sealing system
L. V sealer/divider

ligated
suture l.

ligate, divide, staple (LDS)
ligation
Aldridge tubal l.
arterial l.
bilateral tubal l. (BTL)
bilateral uterine artery l.
bleeding site l.
Cook tubal l.
Doppler-guided l.
endoscopic elastic band l.
endoscopic variceal l. (EVL)
hypogastric artery l.
hysteroscopic tubal l.
in utero percutaneous umbilical
cord l.
Irving tubal l.
Kroener tubal l.
laparoscopic tubal l. (LTL)
library l.
liver lobe l.
Madlener tubal l.
modified Irving-type tubal l.
l. of appendix
Parkland tubal l.
Pomeroy tubal l.
reversal of tubal l.
suture l.
thoracic duct l.
tubal l. (TL)
Uchida tubal l.
uterine artery l.
uterosacral nerve l.

ligature
absorbable l.
chromic gut pelviscopic
loop l.
Deschamps l.
suture l.

light
ambient l.
bilirubin l.
broad-spectrum white l.
l. chain
double-bank bilirubin l.'s
green l.
l. microscopy
narrow-spectrum blue l.
l. perception (LP)
Phillips phototherapy l.
Questran L.
l. response
Right Light examination l.

Sabre FreeHand high-intensity
medical pocket l.
Solar Beam medical examination l.
Speculite chemiluminescent l.
super blue l.
l. therapy
ultraviolet l.
Wood l.

lighted ear curette
light-emitting diode
lightening
LightMat surgical illuminator
lightning
l. attack
l. pain
l. seizure

LighTouch Neonate thermometer
Lightwood-Albright syndrome
Lignac syndrome
lignocaine
Likert scale
Liley
L. curve
L. 3-zone chart

Lilliput neonatal oxygenator
limb
l. abnormality syndrome
l. actigraphy
l. bud
circumferential ringed crease
of l.
circumferential skin crease of l.
l. disproportion
efferent l.
fetal l.
l. girdle (LG)
l. girdle muscular dystrophy
l. girdle muscular weakness and
atrophy
l. girdle syndrome (LGS)
ileal l.
l. infarction
l. lead
l. length inequality
l. motion
multiple benign circumferential skin
creases on l.
l. pain of childhood
phantom l.
l. reduction
l. reduction deformity (LRD)
l. salvage
short l.
tripus l.

limb-body wall complex (LBWC)
Limberg flap technique
limbic
l. band
l. GABAergic system

limbic (*continued*)
    l. status epilepticus
    l. structure
limbus
liminal
limit
    l. dextrans
    l. dextrinosis
    fetal dose l.
    radiation dose l.
limited
    l. neck motion
    l. support
    l. systemic scleroderma
    l. venography
limited-exposure intravenous pyelogram
limp
    antalgic l.
    gluteus medius l.
    l. infant syndrome
    psychogenic l.
    Trendelenburg l.
limulus
    l. amebocyte lysate assay
    l. lysate test
LINCL
    late infantile neural ceroid
      lipofuscinosis
Lincocin
lincomycin
lindane shampoo
line
    arcuate l.
    Beau l.
    black l.
    Blaschko l.
    breeding l.
    Burton gum lead l.
    canthomeatal l.
    central venous l. (CVL)
    Chamberlain l.
    coronal suture l.
    CVP l.
    cytogenetic l.
    Dennie l.
    Dennie-Morgan l.
    dentate l.
    l. drawing
    Farre white l.
    genetic l.
    germ l.
    Harris growth arrest l.
    Hart l.
    hemostatic staple l.
    Hilgenreiner l.
    iliopectineal l.
    indwelling venous l. (IVL)
    intravenous l.
    Kerley B l.'s

    lambda suture l.
    Langer l.
    lead l.
    long l.
    midaxillary l.
    midclavicular l.
    milk l.
    multiple resistant cell l.'s
    murine myeloid leukemia cell l.
    neonatal l.
    Pastia l.
    pectinate l.
    percutaneous l.
    peripheral arterial l.
    Perkin l.
    PICC l.
    l. placement
    radial arterial l.
    radiolucent l.
    railroad track l.
    recombinant substitution l.
    sagittal suture l.
    Shenton l.
    simian l.
    suture l.
    Sydney l.
    tympanomastoid suture l.
    tympanosquamous suture l.
    umbilical l.
    umbilical artery l. (UAL)
    umbilical venous l. (UVL)
    V l.
    venous l.
linea, *pl.* **lineae**
    l. alba
    l. alba hernia
    lineae albicantes
    lineae atrophicae
    l. nigra
    l. semicircularis
    l. terminalis
lineae (*pl. of* linea)
lineage
    B-cell l.
    neural crest-derived cell l.
linear
    l. accelerator
    l. atelectasis
    l. atrophy
    l. branching pattern
    l. energy transfer
    l. gingival erythema
    l. growth
    l. growth retardation
    l. growth velocity
    l. hyperkeratotic plaque
    l. hypocalcification
    l. hypoplasia
    l. IgA dermatosis

l. IgA disease
l. IgM disease of pregnancy
l. in-line ligature carrier
l. Koebner reaction
l. lesion
l. nevus sebaceus syndrome
l. probe
l. salpingostomy
l. scleroderma
l. sebaceous nevus syndrome
l. skull fracture
l. verrucous epidermal nevus
l. visual analog scale
linearis
nevus sebaceus l.
linezolid
Lin-Gettig syndrome
lingua, *pl.* **linguae**
apex linguae
dorsum linguae
folia linguae
frenulum linguae
l. nigra
l. plicata
short frenulum linguae
linguae (*pl. of* lingua)
lingual
l. appliance
l. frenulum
l. surface
linguistic
lingula, *pl.* **lingulae**
lingulae (*pl. of* lingula)
lingular effusion
linguofacialis
dysplasia l.
linitis plastica
linkage
l. analysis
complete l.
l. disequilibrium
l. equilibrium
genetic l.
l. group
l. map
partial l.
Y l.
link antibody
linogram
linoleic acid
linolenic acid
Linton tube
Lion's Claw grasper
Lioresal
liothyronine
liotrix
LIP
lipoid interstitial pneumonitis
lymphocytic interstitial pneumonitis

lymphoid interstitial pneumonitis
lip
cleft l. (CL)
l. closure
Cupid's bow upper l.
double l.
fissured l.
frozen smile puckered l.'s
nodular blueberry l.
l. phenomenon
l. pit
l. pseudocleft-hemangiomatous branchial cyst syndrome
l. reflex
l. scar revision
vermilion border of l.
lipase
bile salt-stimulated l. (BSSL)
lipoprotein l. (LPL)
l. unit
lipemia
lipid
l. accumulation
l. cell
l. cell neoplasm
l. cell ovarian tumor
l. envelope
l. inclusion
l. metabolism
l. metabolism disorder
myelin l.
l. myopathy
l. peroxidation
l. peroxide
l. profile assessment
l. storage disease
l. storage disorder
lipid-associated sialic acid
lipid-laden macrophage
lipidosis
cerebroside l.
familial neurovisceral l.
galactosylsphingosine l.
juvenile dystonic l.
late infantile systemic l.
neurovisceral l.
psychosine l.
Lipidox
lipiduria
Lipiodol
Lipisorb
lipoatrophic diabetes
lipoatrophy
human insulin-induced l.
insulin l.
localized l.
lipoblastoma
primitive l.

lipochondrodystrophy
lipodystrophy
 congenital generalized l.
 familial l.
 generalized l.
 partial l.
 protease inhibitor-induced l.
lipodystrophy-acromegaloid gigantism
 syndrome
lipofuscin material
lipofuscinosis
 ceroid l.
 Haltia-Santavuori neural ceroid l.
 hypoadrenalism neural ceroid l.
 Jansky-Bielschowsky neural
  ceroid l.
 late infantile neural ceroid l.
  (LINCL)
 neural ceroid l.
 neuronal ceroid l. (CLN, NCL)
 Spielmeyer-Vogt neural ceroid l.
lipoglycan antigen
lipogranulomatosis
 Farber l.
 l. subcutanea
lipohypertrophy
lipoic acid
lipoid
 l. adrenal gland hypoplasia
 l. adrenal hyperplasia
 l. interstitial pneumonitis (LIP)
 l. ovarian neoplasm
 l. ovarian tumor
 l. pneumonia
 l. proteinosis
lipoidica
 necrobiosis l.
lipolysis
lipoma, *pl.* **lipomata**
 cord l.
 lumbosacral l.
 vulvar l.
lipomata (*pl. of* lipoma)
lipomatosis
 encephalocraniocutaneous l. (ECCL)
 familial multiple l.
lipomeningocele
Lipomul
lipomyelomeningocele
 skin-covered l.
liponecrosis microcystica calcificans
lipooligosaccharide (LOS)
lipophilic fungus
lipoplasty
 suction-assisted l. (SAL)
lipopolysaccharide (LPS)
 l. coat
 l. endotoxin
 Shiga l.

lipoprotein
 l. concentration
 high-density l. (HDL)
 l. lipase (LPL)
 low-density l. (LDL)
 l. metabolism
 l. receptor-related protein (LRP)
 very low density l. (VLDL)
lipoprotein(a) (Lp(a))
lipoprotein-cholesterol metabolism
liposarcoma
 myxoid l.
liposomal
 l. amphotericin B
 l. doxorubicin hydrochloride
Liposyn
 L. formula
 L. II
lipotropin
5-lipoxygenase
lipoxygenase
lip-palate syndrome
Lippes loop
Lippes-type intrauterine device
lipreading
Lipschütz ulcer
liquefaction
 semen l.
liquefactive necrosis
Liquibid
Liqui-Char
liquid
 chylous l.
 End Lice L.
 l. feeding
 fetal lung l.
 Gordofilm l.
 Lotrimin AF spray l.
 l. nitrogen
 Occlusal-HP l.
 perfluorochemical l.
 l. petrolatum
 Pyrinyl II L.
 Rid l.
 Ryna L.
 Sklar Kleen l.
 Tisit L.
 Titralac Plus L.
 Triple X L.
 l. ventilation (LV)
 X-Prep L.
liquid-assisted high-frequency oscillatory
 ventilation (LA-HFOV)
liquified powder cocaine
Liquifilm
 Herplex L.
 HMS L.
 Poly-Pred L.
 P.V. Carpine L.

Liqui-Gel
Liquiprin
LiquiVent
liquor
l. amnii
amniotic fluid l.
l. carbonis detergens
l. carbonis detergens ointment
l. cerebrospinalis
l. cotunii
l. entericus
l. folliculi
meconium staining of l.
Lisch nodule
LIS1 gene for lissencephaly
lisinopril
Lison syndrome
lisp
lispro
insulin l.
Lissauer tract
lissencephalia (*var. of* lissencephaly)
lissencephaly, lissencephalia
classical l.
hydrocephalic l.
LIS1 gene for l.
l. (type I, II)
list
Amsterdam Depression L. (ADL)
Interpersonal Support Evaluation L.
national recipient waiting l.
listening
dichotic l.
Listeria
L. meningitis
L. monocytogenes
L. monocytogenes sepsis
listeriosis
congenital l.
neonatal l.
Lister scissors
listlessness
litem
guardian ad l.
liter (L, l)
l.'s per minute (L/min, L/M)
milliequivalent per l. (mEq/L)
lithiasis
biliary l.
uric acid l.
lithium
l. carbonate
l. citrate
l. resistance
Lithobid
lithokelyphopedion, lithokelyphopedium
lithokelyphopedium (*var. of* lithokelyphopedion)
lithopedion, lithopedium

lithopedium (*var. of* lithopedion)
lithotomy
marian l.
l. position
vaginal l.
little
L. area
L. disease
L. League elbow
L. League shoulder
L. Tummys gas relief drops
Littmann ECG electrode
Littré gland
Litzmann obliquity
Livaditis circular myotomy
live
l. attenuated
l. attenuated influenza vaccine (LAIV)
BCG l.
l. birth
l. poliovirus vaccine
live-attenuated
l.-a. virus
l.-a. virus vaccine
livebirth, live birth
liveborn infant
livedo reticularis
liver
acute fatty l.
l. biopsy
l. bud
l. cirrhosis
cirrhosis of l.
cut-down l.
l. disease
enlarged l.
l. failure
fatty l.
fetal l.
l. flap
l. function tests
l. infiltrate
l. lobe ligation
l. lobe resection
l. metastasis
l. parenchyma
l. phosphorylase deficiency
shock l.
l. span
l. steatosis
l. transplant
l. transplantation
l. tumor
Livernois-McDonald forceps
live-virus vaccine
Livial
livida
asphyxia l.

L

527

lividity
  postmortem l.
living
  activities of daily l. (ADL)
  l. children (LC)
  l. will
Livostin
LJP
  localized juvenile periodontitis
LKS
  Landau-Kleffner syndrome
LLD
  leg length discrepancy
LLDP
  left lateral decubitus position
LLETZ
  large loop excision of transformation
  zone
LLETZ-LEEP active loop
  electrode
l-loop
Llorente dissecting forceps
Lloyd-Davies stirrup
Lloyd-Still index
LLPDD
  late luteal phase dysphoric
  disorder
LLQ
  left lower quadrant
L/M
  liters per minute
LM
  lactose malabsorption
  lateral malleolus
  leptomeningeal
  Licentiate in Midwifery
  light microscopy
  lincomycin
  Listeria monocytogenes
  longitudinal muscle
LMA
  lactose malabsorption
  laryngeal mask airway
  left mentoanterior
LMB
  Laurence-Moon-Biedl
  leiomyoblastoma
  LMB syndrome
LMBB
  Laurence-Moon-Biedl-Bardet
LMBBS
  Laurence-Moon-Biedl-Bardet
  syndrome
L/min
  liters per minute
LMP
  last menstrual period
  left mentoposterior
  left mentoposterior position

low malignant potential
lumbar puncture
LMS
  leiomyosarcoma
LMT
  left mentotransverse
LMW
  low molecular weight
  LMW dextran
  LMW proteinuria
LMWD
  low molecular weight dextran
LMWH
  low molecular weight heparin
LNE
  lymph node enlargement
LNM
  lymph node metastasis
LNMP
  last normal menstrual period
LNS
  Lesch-Nyhan syndrome
LOA
  left occipitoanterior
load
  axial l.
  plasma viral l.
  potential renal solute l. (PRSL)
  pressure l.
  renal solute l. (RSL)
  task l.
  viral l.
  volume l.
loading
  familial l.
lobar
  l. consolidation
  l. emphysema
  l. holoprosencephaly
  l. panniculitis
  l. pneumonia
  l. sclerosis
lobatum
  ovarium l.
lobe
  hepatic l.
  mesial temporal l.
  quadrate hepatic l.
  Riedel l.
  sequestered l.
  temporal l.
lobectomy
  fetal l.
Lobstein
  L. disease
  L. syndrome
lobster-claw
  l.-c. deformity
  l.-c. hand

l.-c. with ectodermal defects syndrome

lobster seat

lobular

l. architecture
l. capillary hemangioma
l. carcinoma
l. carcinoma in situ (LCIS)
l. distortion
l. neoplasia

lobulation defect

lobulation-polydactyly syndrome

lobule

placental l.
sebaceous gland l.
tense l.

LOC

level of consciousness
local
loss of consciousness

local

l. anesthesia
l. anesthetic
l. block
l. education agency (LEA)
l. excision
l. inflammatory response
l. irradiation
l. lesion
l. methotrexate injection
l. ovarian condition
l. seizure
l. treatment

localization

epithelial autoantibody l.
estrogen receptor l.
needle l.
placental l.

localization-related epilepsy seizure

localize

localized

l. albinism
l. cutaneous leishmaniasis (LCL)
l. intravascular coagulation
l. juvenile periodontitis (LJP)
l. lipoatrophy
l. pachygyria
l. peritonitis
l. scleroderma
l. vulvar pemphigoid of childhood (LVPC)

localizing sign

location

breech l.
extraembryonic l.
gene l.
placental l.

locator

Wherify GPS l.

lochia

l. alba
l. cruenta
l. purulenta
l. rubra
l. sanguinolenta
l. serosa

lochial

lochiometra

lochiometritis

lochioperitonitis

lochiorrhagia

lochiorrhea, lochiorrhagia

loci (*pl. of* locus)

lock

English l.
French l.
German l.
heparin l. (hep lock)
pivot l.
sliding l.

locked

l. facet
l. twins

Locke solution

Locke-Wallace Marital Adjustment test

Locoid Topical

locomotion

locomotor

locoregional node

loculate

locus, *pl.* **loci**

l. caeruleus
gene l.
genetic l.
GUSB l.
l. heterogeneity
L. of Control Scale
operator l.
quantitative trait l. (QTL)

locus-specific probe

locutionary stage

lodoxamide tromethamine

Loeb deciduoma

Loehlein diameter

Loestrin

L. 1.5/30
L. 21 1/20
L. Fe
L. 24 Fe

Löffler syndrome

Löfgren syndrome

Lofstrand crutches

Log-a-Rhythm Signal Acquisition unit

logarithm of odds (lod, LOD)

logroll maneuver

LOH

loop of Henle
loss of heterogeneity

L

LOHD
late-onset 21-hydroxylase deficiency
Lohman-Brozek body fat percentage formula
lollipop
fentanyl l.
Oralet l.
lomefloxacin
Lomotil
lomustine
Lonalac formula
lone
L. Star retractor system
L. Star tick
loneliness
long
l. and very long chain acyl-CoA dehydrogenase (LCAD/VLCAD)
l. arm of chromosome (q)
l. arm of chromosome X (Xq)
l. arm of Y chromosome
l. atraumatic retractor
l. axis
l. bone
l. bone length
l. course
l. leg cast
l. leg sitting
l. line
l. Q-T syndrome (LQTS)
l. thin extremity
l. weighted speculum
long-acting (L-A)
l.-a. contraception
l.-a. contraceptive
l.-a. contraceptive steroid
Sinex L.-A.
l.-a. thyroid stimulator (LATS)
long- and medium-chain acyl-CoA dehydrogenase (LCAD/MCAD)
long-axis view
long-chain
l.-c. acyl-CoA dehydrogenase (LCAD)
l.-c. fatty acid (LCFA)
l.-c. 3-hydroxyacyl-CoA dehydrogenase (LCHAD)
l.-c. hydroxyacyl-coenzyme A dehydrogenase (LCHAD)
l.-c. polyunsaturated fatty acid (LCPUFA)
longitudinal
l. deficiency
l. dense striation
l. growth
l. incision
l. interval followup evaluation (LIFE)
l. lie

l. muscle
l. oval pelvis
l. presentation
l. proton MR spectroscopy
l. scan
l. study
long-segment
l.-s. aganglionosis
l.-s. congenital tracheal stenosis (LSCTS)
long-term
l.-t. followup
l.-t. sequelae
l.-t. survival
long-tract sign
longum
Bifidobacterium l.
Loniten Oral
Lonox
loop
bipolar cutting l.
bipolar urological l.
capillary end l.
cine l.
cutting l.
l. diathermy cervical conization
dilated intestinal l.
l. diuretic
l. diversion
dropout of capillary end l.
l. electrode
l. electrosurgical excision procedure (LEEP)
l. excision of transformation zone (LETZ)
flow-volume l.
free-floating l.
ileal l.
Lippes l.
low-voltage diathermy l.
obstructed bowel l.
l. of Henle (LH, LOH)
physiologic endometrial ablation/resection l. (PEARL)
polysomnogram with flow-volume l.
Schroeder tenaculum l.
sentinel l.
somatic nervous system feedback l.
tenaculum hook l.
vaginal speculum l.
looping
cardiac l.
loose body
Loosett maneuver
Lo/Ovral contraceptive pill
LOP
left occipitoposterior position
lop ear
loperamide hydrochloride

lophosphamide
lopinavir
Lopressor
Loprox
Lorabid
loracarbef
Lorain-Lévi
    L.-L. dwarfism
    L.-L. infantilism
    L.-L. syndrome
loratadine
lorazepam
Lorber criteria
Lorcet
    L. 10/650
    L. Plus
Lorcet-HD
lordosis
    lumbar l.
lordotic
    l. deformity
    l. gait
Lorenz night splint
Lorenzo's
    L. oil
    L. oil diet
Loroxide
Lortab
    L. 2.5/500
    L. 5/500
    L. 10/500
    L. Elixir
LOS
    lipooligosaccharide
    low cardiac output syndrome
Los Angeles variant galactosemia
Losec
losoxantrone
loss
    acute interpersonal l.
    autosomal dominant nonsyndromic hearing l. (DFNA3)
    autosomal-recessive nonsyndromic hearing l. (DFNB1)
    average blood l.
    blood l.
    bone l.
    conductive hearing l.
    congenital hearing l.
    consecutive l.
    covert l.
    dialysate protein l.
    early embryonic l.
    early pregnancy l. (EPL)
    electrolyte l.
    embryonic l.
    estrogen l.
    excessive blood l.
    fecal water l.

    fetal l.
    gastrointestinal l.
    hair l.
    hearing l.
    heat l.
    high-frequency hearing l.
    high-tone hearing l.
    hysteric visual l.
    insensible fluid l.
    insensible water l. (IWL)
    menstrual blood l. (MBL)
    mixed hearing l.
    nephron l.
    normal blood l.
    l. of consciousness (LOC)
    l. of correction
    l. of heterogeneity (LOH)
    overt l.
    perioral tissue l.
    permanent hearing l. (PHL)
    postmenopausal bone l.
    pregnancy l.
    protein l.
    range l.
    rapid bone l.
    recurrent early pregnancy l. (REPL)
    recurrent pregnancy l. (RPL)
    renal l.
    repeated pregnancy l. (RPL)
    repetitive pregnancy l.
    RP with progressive sensorineural hearing l.
    sensorineural hearing l. (SNHL)
    sensory l.
    spinal bone l.
    status l.
    stocking-glove sensory l.
    stool l.
    surgical weight l.
    third space l.
    tissue l.
    tooth l.
    transepidermal water l. (TEWL)
    vertebral bone l.
    visual l.
    water l.
    weight l.
Lossen rule
loss-of-resistance technique
Lostorfer body
lost surgical specimen
LOT
    left occipitotransverse
lotion
    calamine l.
    Cutivate l.
    Ovide l.
    Polysonic ultrasound l.
    Sarna l.

L

lotion (*continued*)
    thiosulfate l.
    Total Eclipse moisturizing skin l.
Lotrimin
    L. AF spray liquid
    L. AF spray powder
    L. Topical
Lotronex
LOU
    lower obstructive uropathy
    fetal LOU
    Lou Gehrig disease
loudness
Louis-Bar syndrome
loupe
    Keeler l.
    l. magnification
louse
    body l.
    crab l.
    head l.
    l. infestation
    pubic lice
louse-borne
    l.-b. fever
    l.-b. typhus
Lovaas
    L. method
    L. program
    L. training
lovastatin
Lovaxin C cancer vaccine
LOVE
    laser office ventilation of ears
LOVE IT
    laser office ventilation of ears with
    insertion of tubes
Lovenox
Lovset maneuver
low
    l. back pain
    l. birth weight (LBW)
    l. birth weight infant (LBWI)
    l. birth weight-maternal employment
    study (LBW-MES)
    l. blood sugar
    l. branched chain amino acid diet
    l. cardiac output syndrome
    l. cervical cesarean
    l. forceps
    l. forceps delivery
    l. frequency (lf, LF)
    l. imperforate anus
    l. malignant potential (LMP)
    l. molecular weight (LMW)
    l. molecular weight dextran
    (LMWD)
    l. molecular weight heparin (LMWH)
    l. muscle tone

    l. nasal bridge
    l. occipital hairline
    l. output
    l. pain threshold
    l. pressure bladder
    l. rectal resection
    l. sensory threshold
    l. steroid content combined oral
    contraceptive
    l. transverse cesarean (LTC)
    l. transverse hysterotomy
    l. transverse uterine incision
    (LTUI)
    l. T3 syndrome
    l. vertical uterine incision
    l. vision aid
low-cholesterol diet
low-density lipoprotein (LDL)
low-dose
    l.-d. danazol
    l.-d. heparin (LDH)
    l.-d. involved field irradiation
    l.-d. oral contraceptive
    l.-d. splenic irradiation
    l.-d. steroid
Lowe
    fetal oculocerebrorenal syndrome of
    L.
    oculocerebrorenal disease of L.
    L. oculocerebrorenal syndrome
    oculocerebrorenal syndrome of L.
    L. syndrome (LS)
low-energy sound wave
Löwenstein-Jensen medium
lower
    l. abdominal pain
    l. abdominal tenderness
    l. airway disease
    L. Anchorages and Tethers for
    children (LATCH)
    l. collecting system
    l. esophageal sphincter (LES)
    l. esophageal transection
    l. extremity (LE)
    l. genital tract
    l. genital tract infection
    l. limb ossification center
    l. lip paralysis
    l. motor neuron palsy
    l. obstructive uropathy (LOU)
    l. respiratory illness (LRI)
    l. respiratory infection (LRI)
    l. respiratory tract
    l. respiratory tract disorder
    l. respiratory tract infection (LRTI)
    l. segment cesarean (LSCS)
    l. segment scar
    l. segment transverse cesarean
    section (LSTCS)

l. segment vertical cesarean section (LSVCS)
l. triceps skinfold Z score
l. urinary tract infection
l. uterine segment (LUS)
l. uterine segment fibroid
l. uterine segment transverse (LUST)
lower-angle suture
Lowe-Terry-MacLachlan syndrome
low-fat diet (LFD)
low-flow
  l.-f. cardiopulmonary bypass
  l.-f. oxygen system
  l.-f. sidestream capnography
low-grade
  l.-g. B-cell lymphoma
  l.-g. diffuse astrocytoma
  l.-g. dysplasia (LGD)
  l.-g. fibrillary astrocytoma
  l.-g. mosaicism
  l.-g. positive smear
  l.-g. squamous intraepithelial lesion (LGSIL, LSIL)
Lowila soap
low-lying placenta previa
Lown-Ganong-Levine syndrome
Low-Ogestrel-21, -28
low-phenylalanine diet
low-power field
low-pressure
  l.-p. breast pump
  l.-p. urethra
low-protein diet
Low-Quel
low-residue diet
low-resolution banding
Lowry-MacLean syndrome
Lowry syndrome
Lowry-Wood syndrome (LWS)
low-salt diet (LSD)
low-segment transverse incision
low-set ears
low-sodium
  l.-s. diet (LSD)
  l.-s. syndrome
low-voltage
  l.-v. diathermy loop
  l.-v. electrocortical activity (LVECoG, LV ECoG)
  l.-v. fast activity (LVFA)
loxapine
Loxitane
lozenge
  benzocaine l.
  Cough-X l.
  Suppress l.

Lozol
LPA
  latex particle agglutination
Lp(a)
  lipoprotein(a)
L-PAM
  l-phenylalanine mustard
LPAM
  l-phenylalanine mustard
l-PAM
  l-phenylalanine mustard
LPCV
  laser photocoagulation of the communicating vessels
LPD
  leiomyomatosis peritonealis disseminata
  luteal phase defect
lpf
  low-power field
l-phenylalanine mustard (L-PAM, l-PAM, LPAM)
LPL
  lipoprotein lipase
    LPL deficiency
LPP
  leak-point pressure
LPS
  lipopolysaccharide
LPSS
  laryngopharyngeal sensory stimulation
    LPSS testing
LQTS
  long Q-T syndrome
L-R
  left to right
LRD
  limb reduction deformity
LRE
  least restrictive environment
LRF
  luteinizing-releasing factor
LRI
  lower respiratory illness
  lower respiratory infection
LRP
  lichen ruber planus
  lipoprotein receptor-related protein
LRS
  lactated Ringer solution
LRTI
  lower respiratory tract infection
L/S
  lecithin/sphingomyelin
  lumbosacral
    L/S ratio
LS
  lichen sclerosus et atrophicus
  Lowe syndrome
  lumbosacral

L

LSA
    left sacroanterior
LSC
    lichen simplex chronicus
LScA
    left scapuloanterior
LScP
    left scapuloposterior position
LSCS
    lower segment cesarean
LSCTS
    long-segment congenital tracheal
      stenosis
LSD
    low-salt diet
    low-sodium diet
    lysergic acid diethylamide
LSD-25
    lysergic acid diethylamide
LSH
    laparoscopic supracervical hysterectomy
    lutein-stimulating hormone
L-shaped cautery
LSIL
    low-grade squamous intraepithelial
      lesion
        LSIL Pap smear
LSO
    lumbosacral orthosis
LSP
    left sacroposterior position
LSS
    lexical-syntactic syndrome
LST
    left sacrotransverse
LSTCS
    lower segment transverse cesarean
      section
LSVCS
    lower segment vertical cesarean
      section
LTC
    low transverse cesarean
LTC_4
    leukotriene C_4
LTD_4
    leukotriene D_4
LTE
    laryngotracheoesophageal
LTE4
    leukotriene E_4
L-TGA
    L-transposition of great arteries
LTL
    laparoscopic tubal ligation
LTM
    lean tissue mass
LTRA
    leukotriene receptor antagonist

L-transposition
    levotransposition
    L-transposition of great arteries
      (L-TGA)
LTS
    laryngotracheal stenosis
LTT
    lateral tibial torsion
LTUI
    low transverse uterine incision
Lubchenco nomogram
lube
    Sklar l.
Lübke uterine vacuum cannula
lubricant
    Astroglide personal l.
    Maxilube personal l.
    ocular l.
    personal l.
    Replens l.
    vaginal l.
lubrication
    vaginal l.
Lubri-Flex ureteral stent
Lub syndrome
Lucarelli bone marrow transplant risk
 group
lucency
    white matter l.
lucent band
Lucey-Driscoll syndrome
lucida
    lamina l.
luciferase assay
lucinactant
Lucite
    L. dilator
    L. form
Lückenschadel
Ludiomil
Ludorum
Ludwig angina
Luekens trap
Luer
    L. lock site
    L. Lok syringe
    L. retractor
lues ascites
luetic
LUF
    luteinized unruptured follicle
LUFS
    luteinized unruptured follicle syndrome
Luft disease
Lugol
    L. iodine solution
    L. iodine stain
Luikart forceps
Luikart-Simpson forceps

Lujan-Fryns syndrome
luliberin
Lumadex-FSI test
lumbar
    l. artery
    l. curve
    l. epidural anesthesia (LEA)
    l. extensor muscle
    l. gibbus
    l. lordosis
    l. meningocele
    l. puncture
    l. puncture manometry
    l. theca
lumboperitoneal shunt
lumbosacral (LS, L/S)
    l. agenesis
    l. dimple
    l. junction
    l. lipoma
    l. meningomyelocele
    l. neurofibroma
    l. orthosis (LSO)
    l. plexus injury
    l. plexus lesion
    l. root lesion
    l. sinus
    l. skin pigment change
    l. tuft of hair
lumbricoides
    Ascaris l.
lumen, *pl.* **lumina, lumens**
    appendiceal l.
    decidual l.
    l. dilation
    urethral l.
lumens (*pl. of* lumen)
Lumex PT fiberoptic cystometry system
lumina (*pl. of* lumen)
luminal epithelium
Lumopaque
lumpectomy
lumpy
    l. breast
    l. jaw
LUNA
    laparoscopic uterine nerve ablation
    laser uterosacral nerve ablation
Luna-Parker acid fuscin stain
Lunar DPX dual-energy absorptiometer
lunata
    Curvularia l.
Lund and Browder chart for burn
  assessment
Lundh test
Lunelle
lung
    l. abscess
    l. aeration

    agenesis of l.
    azygos lobe of l.
    azygos lobe of right l.
    bubbly l.'s
    l. cancer
    l. capacity (CL)
    l. carcinoma
    compliance of l. (CL)
    l. consolidation
    cystic adenomatoid malformation
      of l.
    l. edema
    farmer's l.
    l. fluke
    granular l.
    l. growth and development
    hazy l.
    l. hernia
    honeycomb l.
    hyperlucent l.
    hypoplasia of l.
    hypoplastic l.
    idiopathic diffuse interstitial fibrosis
      of l.
    immature l.
    l. infiltrate
    junky l.
    Kolobow membrane l.
    lymphangiomyomatosis of l.
    malt worker's l.
    l. morphogenesis
    l. overdistention
    paraquat l.
    premature l.
    l. profile
    l. recruitment
    sequestered l.
    shock l.
    SP-A of l.
    SP-B of l.
    SP-C of l.
    l. strip
    surfactant-deficient l.
    l. surgery
    l. tap
    l. transplantation
    unilateral hyperlucent l.
    l. volume
lung-to-head ratio
Lupron
    L. add-back therapy
    L. Depot
    L. Depot-Ped
lupus
    ANA-negative l.
    l. angiitis
    l. anticoagulant (LAC)
    l. anticoagulant activity
    l. anticoagulant antibody

L

lupus (*continued*)
  l. anticoagulant syndrome
  l. cerebritis
  l. crisis
  discoid l.
  l. erythematosus (LE)
  l. erythematosus disseminatus
  l. erythematosus profundus
  l. flare
  gestational l.
  l. inhibitor
  l. miliaris disseminatus faciei
  neonatal l.
  l. nephritis
  l. obstetric syndrome
  l. pernio
  l. vulgaris
lupus-like syndrome
LUQ
  left upper quadrant
lurch
  abductor l.
Luride
Lurline PMS
LUS
  lower uterine segment
Luschka
  foramen of L.
Lusk instrument
LUSLR
  laparoscopic ureterosacral ligament resection
LUST
  lower uterine segment transverse
  LUST cesarean section
  LUST C-section
lutea
  corpora l.
  macula l.
luteal
  l. cell
  l. function
  l. ovarian cyst
  l. phase
  l. phase defect (LPD)
  l. phase deficiency
  l. phase inadequacy
  l. phase support
luteectomy
lutein cell
luteinalis
  hyperreactio l.
luteinization
  l. inhibition
  l. inhibitor
  l. stimulator
luteinized
  l. thecoma
  l. unruptured follicle (LUF)

  l. unruptured follicle syndrome (LUFS)
luteinizing
  l. hormone (LH)
  l. hormone receptor-binding inhibitor
  l. hormone-releasing hormone (LH-RH, LHRH)
  l. hormone-releasing hormone analog
  l. hormone secretion
luteinizing-releasing factor (LRF)
luteinoma
lutein-stimulating hormone (LSH)
Lutembacher syndrome
luteolysis
luteolytic action
luteoma
  l. of pregnancy
  pregnancy l.
  stromal l.
luteoplacental shift
luteotropic hormone
luteum
  corpus l. (CL)
  prolapse of corpus l.
  ruptured corpus l.
Lutheran blood group
Lutrepulse
Lutz-Jeanselme nodule
Lutz-Splendore-Almeida blastomycosis
luxation
  dental extrusion/lateral l.
  extrusion/lateral l.
  extrusive l.
  intrusive l.
  lateral l.
  rotary atlantoaxial l.
luxury perfusion
LV
  LV afterload
  LV contractility
  LV dysfunction
  LV preload
LVAD
  left ventricular assist device
L-valine ester
LVD
  left ventricular dysfunction
LVECoG
  low-voltage electrocortical activity
LVEF
  left ventricular ejection fraction
LVFA
  low-voltage fast activity
LVH
  left ventricular hypertrophy
LVOT
  left ventricular outflow tract

LVOTO
  left ventricular outflow tract
  obstruction
LVPC
  localized vulvar pemphigoid of
  childhood
LVSI
  lymphovascular space invasion
LVSWI
  left ventricular stroke work index
lwoffii
  Achromobacter l.
  Acinetobacter l.
LWS
  Lowry-Wood syndrome
lyase
Lyderm
Lyell
  L. disease
  L. syndrome
lyer
  side l.
Lyme
  L. arthritis
  L. disease (LD)
  L. disease vaccine
  L. ELISA
  L. meningitis
  L. neuroborreliosis
  L. radiculoneuritis
**Lyme-associated peripheral facial nerve
  palsy**
lymph
  l. node
  l. node biopsy
  l. node drainage
  l. node endometriotic
    adenoacanthoma
  l. node enlargement (LNE)
  l. node involvement
  l. node metastasis (LNM, LN-met)
  l. node positivity
lymphadenectomy
  inguinal l.
  laparoscopic l.
  Meigs pelvic l.
  paraaortic l.
  pelvic l.
  retroperitoneal l.
lymphadenitis
  cervical l.
  chronic pyogenic l.
  granulomatous l.
  histocytic necrotizing l.
  inguinal l.
  Kiuchi histocytic necrotizing l.
  mediastinal l.
  mesenteric l.
  necrotizing granulomatous l.

  periauricular l.
  pyogenic l.
  recurrent pyogenic l.
  regional l.
  submental l.
  suppurative l.
  tuberculous cervical l.
lymphadenopathy
  acute suppurative cervical l.
  axillary l.
  cervical l.
  diffuse nonmalignant l.
  hilar l.
  mediastinal l.
  shotty cervical l.
  submental l.
  Toxoplasma l.
lymphadenopathy-associated virus (LAV)
lymphangiectasia
  congenital pulmonary l.
  pulmonary l.
lymphangiography
  bipedal l.
lymphangioma
  alveolar l.
  cavernous l.
  l. circumscriptum
  cystic l.
  l. cysticum
lymphangiomatosis
lymphangiomyomatosis of lung
lymphangiosarcoma
lymphangitis
lymphatic
  l. drainage
  l. drainage of genitalia
  l. dysplasia
  femoral nerve, artery, vein, empty
    space, lymphatics (NAVEL)
  l. leukemia
  l. obstruction
  paracervical lymphatics
  l. spread
  l. system
lymphaticus
  status l.
Lymphazurin
lymphedema
  congenital extremity l.
  extremity l.
  hereditary l.
  intrauterine l.
  l. praecox
  primary l.
  secondary l.
  l. tarda
lymphoblastic
  l. leukemia
  l. lymphoma

L

lymphoblastoid
    l. cell
    l. interferon
lymphocyst
    l. omentum
    pelvic l.
lymphocytapheresis
lymphocyte
    l. activator
    B l.
    cytotoxic T l. (CTL)
    l. depleted
    l. dysfunction
    l. function-associated antigen 1
    helper l.
    l. immunoglobulin
    natural killer l.
    peripheral blood l. (PBL)
    polymorphonuclear l.
    l. predominant
    T l.
    T1–T10 l.
lymphocyte-activating factor
lymphocyte-depleted Hodgkin disease
lymphocyte-predominant Hodgkin disease
lymphocytic
    l. adenohypophysitis
    l. choriomeningitis
    l. choriomeningitis virus (LCMV)
    l. gastritis
    l. hypophysitis
    l. interstitial pneumonitis (LIP)
    l. leukemia
    l. meningitis
    l. meningoradiculoneuritis
    l. myocarditis
    l. pleocytosis
    l. thyroiditis
    l. vasculitis
lymphocytosis
    infectious l.
lymphogranuloma
    l. inguinale
    venereal l.
    l. venereum (LGV)
lymphography
lymphohematogenous disease
lymphohistiocytic infiltration
lymphohistiocytosis
    erythrophagocytic l.
    familial erythrophagocytic l. (FEL)
    familial hemophagocytic l. (FHLH)
    hemophagocytic l.
lymphoid
    l. cell
    l. hyperplasia
    l. interstitial pneumonitis (LIP)
    l. tissue
lymphokine

lymphokine-activated killer cell (LAK, LAKC)
lymphoma
    African Burkitt l.
    AIDS-related l.
    American Burkitt l.
    anaplastic large cell l.
    B-cell l.
    Burkitt l. (BL)
    central nervous system l.
    colonic B-cell l.
    diffuse small cell cleaved l.
    EBV-related B-cell l.
    endemic Burkitt l.
    extranodal marginal zone B-cell l.
    histiocytic l.
    Hodgkin l.
    immunoblastic l.
    intraocular l.
    large B-cell l.
    large cell anaplastic Ki-1 l.
    large cell immunoblastic l.
    low-grade B-cell l.
    lymphoblastic l.
    malignant l.
    Mediterranean l.
    metastatic l.
    non-Hodgkin l. (NHL)
    ovarian l.
    primary central nervous system l. (PCNSL)
    recurrent l.
    retroorbital l.
    small cell cleaved l.
    small noncleaved cell l. (SNCCL)
    sporadic Burkitt l.
    T-cell l.
    true histiocytic l. (THL)
lymphomatous infiltration
lymphonodular
    l. hyperplasia
    l. pharyngitis
lymphopenia
lymphoplasmacytic
    l. colitis
    l. infiltration
    l. inflammation
lymphopoietic differentiation
lymphoproliferative
    l. disease
    l. disorder
    l. process
    l. syndrome
lymphoproliferative/myeloproliferative disease
lymphoreticular
    l. malignancy
    l. neoplasia
    l. system

lymphoreticulosis
lymphorrhage
lymphosarcoma
lymphoscintigram
lymphotoxin antitumor activity
lymphovascular
    l. space
    l. space invasion (LVSI)
    l. space involvement
lynch
    L. and Crues type 2 lesion
    L. family syndrome II
    l. suture
    L. syndrome
    L. 2 syndrome
lynestrenol
lyn protooncogene
Lynx midurethral sling
Lyodura sling procedure
Lyon hypothesis
lyonization
lyophilize
lyosomal
Lyphocin
lypressin
lysate
    cell l.
    endothelial cell l.

lysergic
    l. acid
    l. acid diethylamide (LSD)
lysine
    l. malabsorption syndrome
    l. 6-oxidase
lysinuric protein intolerance
lysis
    l. of adhesions
    l. test
Lysodren
lysome
    hepatocellular l.
lysoPC diagnostic ovarian cancer test
lysosomal
    l. enzyme disorder
    l. hydrolase enzyme assay
    l. metabolite
    l. storage disease
    l. storage disorder
lysosome
lysozyme
lysyl bradykinin
lytic
    l. cocktail
    l. infection
    l. lesion
Lytren formula

L

M

M antigen
M protein factor

MA

maternal age
menstrual age
mental age
metatarsus adductus

mA

milliampere

MAA

microphthalmia or anophthalmos with
associated anomalies

Maalox Anti-Gas

MAAP

multiple arbitrary amplicon profiling

MAB

monoclonal antibody

MAb

monoclonal antibody
enhanced-potency MAb
OvaRex MAb

mAb

monoclonal antibody

MABP

mean arterial blood pressure

MAC

midarm circumference
monitored anesthesia care
Mycobacterium avium *complex*
Mycobacterium avium-intracellulare
complex

MacArthur

M. Longitudinal Twin Study
M. Story Stem Battery (MSSB)

MacCallum patch

MacConkey II agar

MacDermot-Winter syndrome

MACDP

Metropolitan Atlanta Congenital
Defects Program

macerated fetus

maceration

fetal m.

Macewen sign

Machado-Joseph

M.-J. ataxia
M.-J. disease
M.-J. syndrome

Mach band effect

Macherey-Nagel strep test

machine

Acuson 128XP ultrasound m.
Berkeley suction m.
BiPAP m.

cobalt megavoltage m.
CPAP m.
life-support m.
Mayo-Gibbon heart-lung m.
megavoltage m.

machinery

m. murmur
m. murmur in patent ductus
arteriosus

Machupo virus

MacIntosh

English M. (E-Mac)

Mackenrodt ligament

MacLean

Macleod syndrome

macrencephalia (*var. of* macrencephaly)

macrencephaly, macrencephalia

macroadenoma

prolactin-secreting m.

macrobead

methyltestosterone m.

Macrobid

macroblepharon

macrocalcification

breast m.

macrocardius

macrocarpon

Vaccinium m.

macrocephalia (*var. of* macrocephaly)

macrocephaly, macrocephalia

benign familial m. (BFM)
familial m.
m. with feeblemindedness and
encephalopathy with peculiar
deposits

macrocephaly-hamartomas syndrome

macrocirculatory

macrocrania

macrocrystal

monohydrate m.
nitrofurantoin monohydrate m.

macrocytic

m. anemia of pregnancy
m. megaloblastic anemia

macrocytosis

macrodactyly

primary m.
secondary m.

Macrodantin

Macrodex

**macrodontia, macrodontism,
megadontism, megalodontia**

macrodontism (*var. of* macrodontia)

Macroduct coil system

macroevolution

M

macrogamete
macrogenitosomia praecox
macroglobinemia
    Waldenström m.
macroglobulin
    alpha-2 m.
macroglobulinemia
macroglossia, megaloglossia
    relative m.
    true m.
macroglossia-omphalocele syndrome
macroglossia-omphalocele-visceromegaly
  syndrome
macrognathia, megagnathia
macrogyria
macrolecithal
macrolide therapy
macromastia, macromazia
macromazia (*var. of* macromastia)
macromelus
macromineral
macromolecular damage
macronodular cirrhosis
macronutrient balance
macroorchidism-marker X
  (MOMX)
macrophage
    m. activation syndrome
      (MAS)
    m. colony-stimulating factor
    hemosiderin laden m.
    m. inflammatory protein (MIP)
    m. inflammatory protein-1 alpha
      (MIP-1 alpha)
    lipid-laden m.
    peritoneal m.
    m. tropic
macrophage-activating factor (MAF)
macrophage-inhibition factor
macrophage-targeted glucocerebrosidase
macrophage-tropic strain
macrophallus
Macroplastique
    M. implantable device
    M. urinary sphincter implant
macroprolactinoma
macrorestriction map
macroscopic hematuria
macrosomia
    m. adiposa congenita
    fetal m.
    neonatal m.
    m., obesity, macrocephaly, ocular
      (MOMO)
macrosomia-mental retardation
  syndrome
macrosomic infant
macrostomia
macrothrombocytopenia

macrovascular
MacroView otoscope
MACS
    magnetically activated cell sorter
    Multicenter AIDS Cohort Study
macula, *pl.* maculae
    m. cerulea
    m. communis
    m. cribrosa
    m. flava
    m. gonorrhoica
    m. lutea
    m. of retina
    m. pellucida
    m. retinae
maculae (*pl. of* macula)
macular, maculate
    m. atrophy
    m. cherry-red spot
    m. dystrophy
    m. hemangioma
    m. light reflex
    m. pseudocoloboma
    m. rash
    m. stain
    m. star formation
macular-papular-vesicular lesion
maculate (*var. of* macular)
macule
    ash-leaf m.
    blanching m.
    bluish-black m.
    café au lait m. (CALMs)
    cherry-red m.
    crop of m.'s
    erythematous m.
    hypopigmented m.
maculopapular
    m. eruption
    m. exanthema
    m. lesion
    m. nodosa
    m. rash
maculosus
    dystrophia bullosa hereditaria,
      typus m.
MACV
    Machupo virus
MadaJet XL needle-free injector
madarosis
mad cow disease
MADD
    multiple acyl-coenzyme A
      dehydrogenase deficiency
Maddacrawler walker
Madelung deformity
Madlener
    M. operation
    M. tubal ligation

Madonna
    M. finger
    M. hold
madurae
    Actinomadura m.
Madura foot
Maestre de San Juan-Kallmann-de Morsier syndrome
MAF
    macrophage-activating factor
mafenide
Mafucci syndrome
Mag-200
magaldrate
Magan
Mag-Carb
MAG-3 diuretic renogram
Magendie
    atresia of foramina of Luschka and M.
    foramen of M.
Maggi disposable biopsy needle guide for ultrasound
magic mouthwash
magma reticulare
magna
    chorea m.
    cisterna m.
    coxa m.
    dilated cisterna m.
    large cisterna m.
    mega cisterna m.
Magnacal formula
magnesia
    milk of m. (MOM)
    Phillips' Milk of M.
magnesium (mag)
    m. chloride
    m. citrate (mag cit)
    m. deficiency
    m. hydroxide
    intratracheal m. (ITMg)
    ionized m.
    m. level
    m. oxide
    m. pemoline
    m. salicylate
    m. sulfate (mag sulf, $MgSO_4$)
    m. supplement
    total m.
magnesium-containing cathartic
magnetic
    m. resonance angiography (MRA)
    m. resonance cholangiography (MRC)
    m. resonance cholangiopancreatography (MRCP)
    m. resonance elastography (MRE)

    m. resonance imaging (MRI)
    m. resonance mammography (MRM)
    m. resonance spectroscopy (MRS)
    m. resonance urography (MRU)
    m. source imaging (MSI)
magnetically
    m. activated cell sorter (MACS)
    m. responsive microsphere
magnetite (Fe_3O_4)
magnetocardiography
    fetal m. (FMCG)
magnetoencephalography (MEG)
magnification
    area of interest m. (AIM)
    loupe m.
    m. mammography
    spot m.
magnum
    asymmetric small foramen m.
    foramen m.
Magnus and de Kleijn tonic neck reflex
Magonate
Mag-Ox 400
MAGPI
    meatal advancement and glanduloplasty incorporation
    meatal advancement and glansplasty incorporation
    MAGPI operation
    MAGPI procedure
Magsal
Mag-Tab SR
Magtrate
MAH
    minimal acceptable height
Maher disease
ma huang
MAI
    Mycobacterium avium-intracellulare
    MAI infection
MAIC
    Mycobacterium avium-intracellulare
MAID
    mesna, Adriamycin, Ifosfamide, Dacarbazine
maidenhead
Maigret-50
main
    m. bronchus
    m. duct of Wirsung
    m. renal vein
Mainstay urologic soft tissue anchor
mainstreaming
maintenance
    m. fluid
    m. medication
    m. therapy

M

Mainz
- M. pouch
- M. pouch diversion
- M. pouch urinary reservoir

Maisonneuve fracture

Majewski
- M. short rib polydactyly
- M. syndrome

Majocchi granuloma

major
- m. aortopulmonary collateral artery (MAPCA)
- m. basic protein (MBP)
- m. capsid protein gene
- m. depressive disorder (MDD)
- m. detoxification enzyme
- m. dysmorphism
- m. histocompatibility antigen
- m. histocompatibility complex (MHC, MHC molecule)
- *Leishmania m.*
- m. motor seizure
- pelvis m.
- pelvis justo m.
- thalassemia m.

majus
- labium m.

Makler
- M. insemination
- M. insemination device
- M. reusable semen analysis chamber

mal
- m. de Meleda
- grand m. (GM)
- myoclonic petit m.
- petit m.

malabsorption
- bile acid m.
- carbohydrate m.
- congenital carbohydrate m.
- congenital folate m.
- fat m.
- glucose-galactose m.
- isolated congenital folate m. (ICFM)
- lactose m.
- methionine m.
- primary bile acid m.
- starch m.
- m. syndrome
- tryptophan m.
- m. workup

malacia

malacoplakia, malakoplakia

maladaptation, maladaption
- immunologic m.

maladaption (*var. of* maladaptation)

maladaptive coping strategy

maladie
- m. de Roger
- m. des tics

malaise

malakoplakia (*var. of* malacoplakia)

malalignment
- patellofemoral m.
- rotational m.
- m. syndrome

malar
- m. distribution
- m. eminence
- m. fat pad
- m. flush
- m. hypoplasia
- m. rash

malaria
- cerebral m.
- chloroquine-resistant m.
- m. endemic
- falciparum m.

malariae
- *Plasmodium m.*

Malassezia
- M. furfur
- M. furfur pustulosis
- M. pachydermatitis

malate

malathion

male
- m. body habitus
- m. condom
- m. factor
- m. factor infertility
- M. FactorPak seminal fluid collection kit
- m. feminization
- m. genital duct
- m. genital duct development
- m. karyotype
- m. pseudohermaphroditism (MPH)
- m. reproductive system
- m. sex differentiation
- m. sterilization
- m. Turner syndrome
- 46,XX m.
- XXY m.
- XYY m.
- ZZ m.

maleate
- carbinoxamine m.
- carphenazine m.
- dimethindene m.
- ergonovine m.
- fluvoxamine m.
- methylergometrine m.
- methylergonovine m.
- methysergide m.

pyrilamine m.
timolol m.
Malecot
M. catheter
M. tube
male-pattern hirsutism
male-to-female (MTF)
malformation
adenomatoid m.
airway m.
aortic arch m.
Arnold-Chiari m.
arteriovenous m. (AVM)
arteriovenous fistula m. (AVFM)
AV m.
body stalk m.
bronchopulmonary m.
cardiac m.
cardiovascular m. (CVM)
cerebral arteriovenous m. (CAVM)
Chiari m. (type I–IV)
cloacal m.
clomiphene fetal m.
congenital bronchopulmonary m.
congenital cardiovascular m.
(CCVM)
congenital cystic adenomatoid m.
(CCAM)
congenital lung m.
congenital obstructive mullerian m.
congenital upper airway m.
conotruncal cardiac m.
cystic adenomatoid m. (CAM)
cystic adenomatous m. (CAM)
cystic congenital adenomatoid m.
(CCAM)
Dandy-Walker m. (DWM)
diabetes-related congenital m.
ductal plate m.
dural arteriovenous m.
Ebstein m.
embryologic m.
extracardiac m.
faciotelencephalic m.
fetal m.
fetal structural m.
foregut m.
GI tract venous m.
gyral m.
hamartomatous m.
intracranial m.
obstructive m.
ocular m.
pelvic arteriovenous m.
pictures of syndromes and
undiagnosed m.'s (POSSUM)
prenatal embryologic m.
pulmonary arteriovenous m.
(PAVM)

Rieger m.
m. sequence
split cord m. (SCM)
split spinal cord m. (SSCM)
submucosal arterial m.
m. syndrome
teratogen-induced m.
thoracic m.
thyroid gland m.
urinary tract m. (UTM)
uterine arteriovenous m.
vascular m.
vein of Galen m.
venous m. (VM)
Walker-Warburg m.
malformed
m. ear
m. pinna
m. radial head
malfunction
congenital cystic adenomatoid m.
shunt m.
Malgaigne fracture
malignancy
borderline m. (BLM)
breast m.
CNS m.
extrapelvic m.
gastrointestinal m.
genital tract m.
gynecologic m.
inflammatory bowel m.
intraocular m.
lymphoreticular m.
metastatic m.
ovarian m.
vulvar m.
malignant
m. arrhythmia
m. brain edema
m. brain tumor
m. calcification
m. cytotrophoblast
m. degeneration
m. epithelial tumor
m. extrarenal rhabdoid tumor
m. fibrous histiocytoma (MFH)
m. germ cell tumor
m. histiocytosis
m. hyperphenylalaninemia
m. hyperpyrexia
m. hypertension
m. hyperthermia (MH)
m. hyperthermic rhabdomyolysis
m. infantile osteopetrosis
m. lymphoma
m. melanoma
m. mesenchymal stroma
m. mesodermal tumor

M

malignant (*continued*)
   m. mesothelioma (MM)
   m. mixed müllerian tumor (MMMT)
   m. nephrosclerosis
   m. nerve sheath tumor
   m. neurilemoma
   m. osteoid
   m. otitis externa
   m. ovarian germ cell tumor
   m. ovarian neoplasm
   m. ovarian teratoma
   m. phenylalaninemia
   m. pilocytic astrocytoma
   m. pleural effusion
   m. schwannoma
   m. syncytiotrophoblast
   m. transformation
   m. tumor of cervix
malignum
   adenoma m.
malingering
Malis CMC-II bipolar coagulator
Mallamint
Mallazine Eye drop
malleable
   m. retractor
   m. splint
mallei (*pl. of* malleus)
malleolar ossification center
malleoli (*pl. of* malleolus)
malleolus, *pl.* **malleoli**
   lateral m.
   medial m.
Mallergan-VC With Codeine
mallet
   m. finger
   m. toe
malleus, *pl.* **mallei**
   Burkholderia mallei
   short process of m.
Mall formula
Mallory-Weiss
   M.-W. syndrome
   M.-W. tear (MWT)
malmoense
   Mycobacterium m.
Malmstrom
   M. cup
   M. vacuum extractor
malnourished
malnutrition
   fetal m.
   protein-calorie m.
   protein-energy m.
malocclusion
malodorous
   m. breath
   m. urine

malondialdehyde (MDA)
Malouf syndrome
malplacement
malposition
   cardiac m.
   uterine m.
malpositioned catheter
malpresentation
   fetal m.
Malpuech facial clefting syndrome
malrotation
   intestinal m. (IM)
   m. of bowel
   renal m.
   volvulus m.
   m. with midgut volvulus
MALT
   mucosa-associated lymphoid tissue
   MALT type
malt
   barley m.
   m. soup extract
   m. worker's lung
maltase
   acid m.
maltophilia
   Stenotrophomonas m.
   Xanthomonas m.
maltreatment
Maltsupex
malunion
   pancreaticobiliary m.
MAMC
   mean arm muscle circumference
   midarm muscle circumference
mamma, *pl.* **mammae**
   m. accessoria
   m. erratica
   supernumerary m.
mammae (*pl. of* mamma)
mammaglobin B breast cancer marker
mammalgia
mammalian transgenesis
mammaplasty, mammoplasty, mastoplasty
   augmentation m.
   postreduction m.
   reconstructive m.
   reduction m.
mammary
   m. calculus
   m. duct ectasia
   m. dysplasia (MD)
   m. fistula
   m. galactogram
   m. gland
   m. neuralgia
   m. sclerosing adenosis
   m. souffle
mammectomy

**Mammex TR computer-aided
  mammography diagnosis system**
mammillaplasty
mammillitis
mammitis
mammogram
  cephalocaudal film-screen m.
  x-ray m. (XMG)
mammographic
  m. abnormality
  m. detection
  m. screening
mammography
  computed tomography laser m.
   (CTLM)
  contoured tilting compression m.
  Corometrics Model 900SC in-office
   m.
  CT laser m.
  diagnostic m.
  digital m.
  Egan m.
  heavy-ion m.
  magnetic resonance m. (MRM)
  magnification m.
  preaspiration m.
  screening m.
  x-ray m.
Mammomat C3 mammography system
mammoplasty (*var. of* mammaplasty)
**MammoReader computer-aided detection
  system**
MammoScan digital imaging system
mammose
Mammotest breast biopsy system
Mammotome breast biopsy system
mammotomy
mammotrophic (*var. of* mammotropic)
mammotropic, mammotrophic
man
  azoospermic m.
  elephant m.
  Mendelian Inheritance in M. (MIM)
managed care organization (MCO)
management
  active third-stage m.
  aggressive m.
  airway m.
  antenatal m.
  antepartum m.
  anxiety m.
  behavioral m.
  brace m.
  burn m.
  conservative m.
  epilepsy m.
  expectant m.
  Family Inventory of Resources for
   M. (FIRM)

home m.
home conservative m.
infertility m.
inpatient m.
intensive diabetes m. (IDM)
intrapartum m.
invasive m.
laparoscopic m.
metabolic m.
MTF medical m.
noninvasive m.
operative m.
pharmacologic m.
physiologic third-stage m.
postevacuation m.
postnatal m.
pregnancy m.
m. protocol
risk m.
routine wound m.
surgical m.
total quality m. (TQM)
manager
  case m.
Manchester
  M. operation
  M. ovoid
Manchester-Fothergill uterine suspension
Mancini plate
mandated reporter
Mandelamine
mandelate
  methenamine m.
mandelic acid
mandible
  acroosteolysis with osteoporosis and
   changes in skull and m.
  dislocated m.
  hypoplastic m.
  prominent m.
  underdeveloped m.
mandibular
  m. advancement
  m. dislocation
  m. hypoplasia
  m. prognathism
mandibular-acral dysplasia
mandibuloacral dysplasia
mandibulofacial dysostosis (MFD)
mandibulofacialis
  dysostosis m.
mandibulo-oculofacial
  m.-o. dyscephaly
  m.-o. dysmorphism
mandibulo-oculofacialis
Mandol
mandrel, mandril
  intrauterine insemination cannula
   with m.

mandril (*var. of* mandrel)
mandrillaris
    Balamuthia m.
maneuver
    all-fours m.
    Barlow m.
    Bill m.
    Bracht m.
    Brandt-Andrews m.
    corkscrew m.
    Credé placental removal m.
    DeLee m.
    diagnostic m.
    Dix-Hallpike m.
    doll's eye m.
    doll's head m.
    forceps m.
    Frenzel middle ear pressure m.
    Gaskin m.
    Gowers m.
    Hallpike m.
    heel-to-ear m.
    Heimlich m.
    Hillis-Müller m.
    Hodge m.
    hooking m.
    jaw thrust-spine stabilization m.
    Johnson m.
    key-in-lock m.
    Kristeller m.
    Lecompte arterial switch m.
    Leopold m.
    Levret breech delivery m.
    logroll m.
    Loosett m.
    Lovset m.
    Massini m.
    Mauriceau m.
    Mauriceau-Levret m.
    Mauriceau-Smellie-Veit m.
    McDonald m.
    McRoberts m.
    midforceps m.
    modified Ritgen fetal head delivery m.
    modified Zavanelli m.
    Müller-Hillis 2nd stage labor m.
    Munro-Kerr m.
    Nylen m.
    Ortolani m.
    ostrich m.
    Pajot m.
    physical m.
    Pinard m.
    Prague m.
    reverse form McRoberts m.
    Ritgen m.
    Rubin shoulder dystocia m.
    Saxtorph forceps delivery m.
    Scanzoni m.
    Scanzoni-Smellie forceps delivery m.
    scarf m.
    Schatz fetal position m.
    Sellick m.
    vagal m.
    vagotonic m.
    Valsalva m.
    Wigand m.
    Woods corkscrew m.
    Zavanelli m.
manganese intoxication
mange
    sarcoptic m.
mania
    prepuberal m.
manic
manic-depressive
    m.-d. disorder (MDD)
    m.-d. illness (MDI)
manifestation
    cardiovascular m.
    congenital m.
    cutaneous m.
    endocrine m.
    extraintestinal m. (EIM)
    extrapyramidal m.
    gastrointestinal m.
    hypervigilance m.
    metabolic m.
    ocular m.
    renal m.
    systemic m.
manifold
Manipujector
    Kronner M.
manipulation
    gamete m.
    hormonal m.
    preorthognathic surgery m.
manipulative examination
manipulator
    ClearView uterine m.
    Kronner m.
    uterine m.
    Valtchev uterine m.
    Vcare uterine m.
manipulator-injector
    Harris-Kronner uterine m.-i. (HUMI)
    Kronner Manipujector uterine m.-i.
    Rowden uterine m.-i. (RUMI)
    Zinnanti uterine m.-i. (ZUMI)
Manning score of fetal activity
Mann isthmic cerclage
mannitol
mannose-type sugar
mannosidase
mannosidosis
manometer

manometric
manometry
    anal m.
    anorectal perfusion m.
    esophageal m.
    lumbar puncture m.
    rectal balloon m.
mansoni
    Schistosoma m.
Mantel-Haenszel procedure
mantle
    acid m.
    cortical m.
    m. sclerosis
    visible cortical m.
Mantoux
    M. method
    M. tuberculin skin test
manual
    m. alphabet
    m. breast pump
    m. cleavage
    m. detorsion
    m. differential
    m. English
    m. healing method
    m. muscle testing
    m. pelvimetry
    m. reduction
    m. rotation
    m. splinting of thoracic cage
    m. thrust
    m. vacuum aspiration (MVA)
    m. vacuum aspirator
    m. ventilation bag (MVB)
manubria (*pl. of* manubrium)
manubrium, *pl.* **manubria**
manuum
    tinea m.
MAO
    monoamine
    monoamine oxidase
MAO-A
    monoamine oxidase type A
MAOA
    monoamine oxidase type A
MAOI
    monoamine oxidase inhibitor
MAP
    mean airway pressure
    mean arterial pressure
map
    brain electrical activity m. (BEAM)
    chromosome m.
    contig m.
    cytogenetic m.
    cytological m.
    gene m.
    genetic m.

    linkage m.
    macrorestriction m.
    physical m.
    recombination m.
    restriction m.
Mapap
MAPCA
    major aortopulmonary collateral artery
maple
    m. leaf flap
    m. syrup urine
    m. syrup urine disease (MSUD)
maplike skull
MapMarkers fluorescent DNA sizing standard
mapping
    brain m.
    brain electrical activity m. (BEAM)
    chromosome m.
    comparative m.
    conscious pain m.
    fate m.
    gene m.
    intraoperative lymphatic m.
    pressure m.
maprotiline
MAR
    mixed agglutination reaction
    MAR test
Marañón syndrome
Maranox
marantic (*var. of* marasmic)
    m. endocarditis
marasmic, marantic
marasmus
Marbaxin
marble
    m. bone disease
    m. bones
marbled hypopigmented streak
Marburg
    M. disease
    M. variant multiple sclerosis
    M. virus
Marcaine with epinephrine
marcescens
    Serratia m.
march
    m. hemoglobinuria
    jacksonian m.
    M. of Dimes
    M. of Dimes Birth Defects Foundation
Marchand
    M. adrenals
    M. rest
Marchetti test
Marcillin
Marckwald cervical os repair

M

Marcus
    M. Gunn jaw-winking ptosis
    M. Gunn phenomenon
    M. Gunn pupil
    M. Gunn sign
Marden-Walker syndrome
Marezine
Marfan
    M. sign
    M. syndrome
marfanoid
    m. craniosynostosis syndrome
    m. habitus
Margarita Island type ectodermal dysplasia
Margesic
    M. A-C
    M. H
margin
    anal m.
    blurring of left psoas m.
    costal m.
    placental m.
    psoas m.
    tentorial m.
marginal
    m. alopecia
    m. cord insertion
    obtuse m.
    m. previa
    m. sinus
    m. sinus rupture
    m. zone
marginalis
    placenta previa m.
marginata
    placenta m.
marginatum
    eczema m.
    erythema m.
marian lithotomy
Marie-Sainton syndrome
Marie-Strümpell encephalitis
Marie syndrome
Marie-Unna hypotrichosis
marihuana (*var. of* marijuana)
marijuana, marihuana
    m. effect
Marinesco-Garland syndrome
Marinesco-Sjögren-Garland syndrome
Marinesco-Sjögren-like syndrome
Marinesco-Sjögren syndrome
Marinol
marinum
    Mycobacterium m.
Marion disease
Marion-Moschcowitz culdoplasty
marital
    M. Dyadic Inventory

    m. introitus
    m. rape
    m. therapy
mark
    belt m.
    Caitlin m.
    choke m.
    port-wine m.
    stork's beak m.
    strawberry m.
    stretch m.
    Unna m.
marked asynchrony
markedly decreased reflex
marker
    adrenal hyperandrogenism m.
    assay m.
    biallelic m.
    CA 15-3 breast cancer m.
    CA 125 endometrial cancer m.
    CA 549 tumor m.
    CD4 m.
    chromosomal m.
    chromosome 22 supernumerary m. (SMG22)
    DNA m.
    fecal m.
    fetal physiologic m.
    Freeman cookie cutter areola m.
    m. gene
    genetic m.
    infection m.
    mammaglobin B breast cancer m.
    maspin breast cancer m.
    maternal serum m.
    neonatal m.
    pericentromeric m.
    peripheral androgen activity m.
    protein m.
    radiopaque m.
    serologic m.
    sigma tumor m.
    tumor m.
    m. X (marX)
    m. X chromosome
    m. X syndrome
marking
    pulmonary vascular m.
    m. time pattern
Marlex
Marlow
    M. disposable cannula
    M. disposable trocar
Marmine Oral
marmorata
    cutis m.
marmoratus
    status m.

marneffei
    Penicillium m.
Maroteaux-Lamy
    M.-L. disease
    M.-L. syndrome (MLS)
Maroteaux-Malamut syndrome
Marplan
marrow
    adult bone m. (ABM)
    bone m. (BM)
    fetal bone m. (FBM)
    m. transplantation
marrow-ablative chemotherapy
MARS
    mixed antiinflammatory syndrome
    molecular adsorbent recirculating
      system
    motion artifact rejection system
Marshall
    ligament of M.
    M. syndrome
    M. test
Marshall-Marchetti-Krantz
(MMK)
    M.-M.-K. operation
    M.-M.-K. retropubic
      cystourethrography suspension
      procedure
Marshall-Marchetti procedure
Marshall-Smith syndrome (MSS)
Marshall-Tanner
    M.-T. pubertal stage (1–5)
    M.-T. pubertal staging (1–5)
Marshall-Taylor vacuum extraction
Mars pulse oximetry
marsupial
    M. belt
    M. pouch
marsupialization
    Spence and Duckett m.
    m. technique
    transurethral m.
Marthritic
Martin-Bell-Renpenning syndrome
Martin-Bell syndrome (MBS)
Martin modification
Martius
    M. bulbocavernosus fat flap
    M. flap and fascial sling
    M. labial fat flap urinary fistula
      repair procedure
    M. labial fat-pad graft
Martsolf syndrome
Mary Jane breast pump
Maryland dissector
MAS
    macrophage activation syndrome
    Maternal Attitude Scale
    meconium aspiration syndrome

MASA
    mental retardation, aphasia, shuffling
      gait, adducted thumb
    MASA syndrome
masculine pelvis
masculinization
masculinovoblastoma
MAS-ECMO
    meconium aspiration syndrome
    extracorporeal membrane oxygenation
    MAS-ECMO infant
Masimo
    M. SET home monitor
    M. SET signal extraction pulse
      oximetry
mask
    m. and bag ventilation
    bag and m.
    bag, valve, m. (BVM)
    face m.
    m. inhalation anesthesia
    Laerdal m.
    Neutrogena Acne M.
    Nic the Dragon pediatric aerosol
      m.
    nonrebreather face m.
    N95 particulate respirator surgical
      m.
    m. of atopic dermatitis
    m. of pregnancy
    oxygen m.
    ventilation by m.
    Venturi m.
Maslach Burnout Inventory
maspin breast cancer marker
masquerade syndrome
MASS
    mitral valve, aorta, skeleton, skin
mass
    abdominal m.
    m. accretion
    adnexal m.
    benign m.
    benign breast m.
    bilateral flank m.'s
    bone m.
    bone mineral m. (BMM)
    calcified m.
    cervical m.
    circumscribed m.
    complex m.
    cortical m.
    cystic adnexal m.
    cystic ovarian m.
    doughnut-shaped m.
    doughy m.
    m. effect
    exophytic m.
    extravesical m.

M

mass (*continued*)
    extrinsic extravesical m.
    fallopian tube m.
    fat m. (FM)
    fat-free m. (FFM)
    flank m.
    freely movable breast m.
    fungating m.
    hamartomatous m.
    hyperechoic m.
    hypoxia, intussusception, brain m.
    (HIB)
    ill-defined m.
    inner cell m.
    intramyometrial m.
    lean body m. (LBM)
    lean tissue m. (LTM)
    m. lesion
    maternal pelvic m.
    mediastinal m.
    mixed-density m.
    neonatal abdominal m.
    noncalcified nodular m.
    ovarian m.
    paraspinal m.
    pelvic m.
    persistent ovarian m.
    M. phenotype
    poorly marginated m.
    postmenopausal body m.
    potato-like m.
    pyloric m.
    scrotal m.
    m. spectrometer
    m. spectrometry (MS)
    spongy m.
    stellate m.
    submucosal m.
    suprapubic m.
    total fat m. (TFM)
    tubal m.
    tumor m.
    umbilical cord m.
    unilateral flank m.
    unilocular cystic ovarian m.
    uterine m.
    vertebral bone m.
    (VBM)
    virilizing ovarian m.
    well-defined m.
massage
    bimanual m.
    cardiac m.
    closed chest m.
    external uterine m.
    heart m.
    lacrimal sac m.
    perineal m.
    Shiatsu therapeutic m.

    m. therapy
    uterine m.
Masse Breast Cream
Massengill douche
masseter muscle
Massini maneuver
massive
    m. ascites
    m. atelectasis
    m. breast hypertrophy
    m. chronic intervillositis (MCI)
    m. genital prolapse
    m. intravascular hemolysis
    m. ovarian cyst
    m. pulmonary embolus
    m. transfusion
Masson-Fontana stain
MAST
    military antishock trousers
    MAST suit
mast
    m. cell (MC)
    m. cell disease
    m. cell leukemia
    m. cell stabilizer
mastadenitis
mastadenoma
mastalgia
    cyclic m.
mastatrophia (*var. of* mastatrophy)
mastatrophy, mastatrophia
mastectomy
    Auchincloss modified radical m.
    extended radical m. (ERM)
    Halsted m.
    McWhirter m.
    modified radical m.
    prophylactic m.
    radical m.
    simple m.
    skin-sparing m.
    subcutaneous m.
    total m.
    Willy Meyer m.
MasterFlex fetal perfusion pump
Masters-Allen syndrome
Masterson clamp
mastitis
    bacterial m.
    chronic cystic m. (CCM)
    gargantuan m.
    glandular m.
    granulomatous m.
    interstitial m.
    lactational m.
    m. neonatorum
    nonpuerperal m.
    parenchymatous m.
    phlegmonous m.

plasma cell m.
postpartum m.
puerperal m.
retromammary m.
stagnation m.
submammary m.
suppurative m.
mastocytoma
mastocytosis
bullous m.
cutaneous m.
diffuse cutaneous m.
nasal m.
primary nasal m.
systemic m.
mastodynia
mastoid
m. air cell
m. bone fracture
m. cortex
m. drainage
m. fontanelle
m. osteitis
m. process
mastoidectomy
mastoiditis
acute coalescent m.
acute surgical m.
chronic m.
coalescent m.
pneumococcal m.
surgical m.
mastology
mastoncus
mastopathy
mastopexy
Benelli m.
mastoplasia, mazoplasia
mastoplasty (*var. of* mammaplasty)
mastoptosis
mastorrhagia
mastoscirrhus
mastotomy
masturbation
infantile m.
MAT
microscopic agglutination test
matching
M. Familiar Figures (MFF)
feature m.
İ V/İ Q m.
mater
dura m.
pia m.
material
absorbent gelling m. (AGM)
Avitene hemostatic m.
coffee-grounds m.
dextran-70 barrier m.

didactic m.
elective abortion m.
Endo-Avitene hemostatic m.
FlowGel barrier m.
genetic m.
hyperechogenic m.
Interceed barrier m.
lipofuscin m.
metal suture m.
mobile hyperechogenic m.
nonionic contrast m.
nylon suture m.
other potentially infectious m.
 (OPIM)
Poloxamer 407 barrier m.
polyester suture m.
polyethylene suture m.
polypropylene suture m.
radiocontrast m.
spontaneous abortion m.
suture m.
synthetic suture m.
white pseudomembranous m.
Materna
M. prenatal vitamin
M. Tablet
maternal
m. abdominal pressure
m. activity restriction
m. age
m. age-related risk
m. age screening
m. alcohol consumption
m. alcoholism
m. anesthesia
m. antibodies
m. antiplatelet antibody
m. antithyroid antibody
m. assessment
m. assessment of fetal movement
m. asthma
M. Attitude Scale (MAS)
m. B-cell
m. Bernard-Soulier syndrome
m. birthing position
m. blood clot patch therapy
m. breast milk
m. care
m. central hemodynamics
m. cholestasis
m. coagulopathy
m. cocaine use
m. complications
m. cortical vein
m. cortical vein thrombosis
m. cotyledon
m. cyanotic heart disease
m. cytokinemia
m. cytomegalovirus

M

maternal (*continued*)
- m. death
- m. death rate
- m. deprivation syndrome
- m. diabetes
- m. douche
- m. drug abuse
- m. dystocia
- m. effect
- m. estriol level
- m. estrogen withdrawal
- m. exercise
- m. exhaustion
- m. factor
- m. febrile morbidity
- m. fever
- m. floor infarction
- m. fracture
- m. gonad
- m. hemodynamics
- m. hemopathy
- m. hepatitis
- m. history
- m. HLA haplotype
- m. hydration
- m. hydrops
- m. hydrops fetalis
- m. hydrops syndrome
- m. hypercalcemia
- m. hyperparathyroidism
- m. hypertension
- m. hypotension
- m. hypoxia
- m. idiopathic thrombocytopenic purpura (MITP)
- m. IgG antibody
- m. illness
- m. immune response
- m. immunocompetence
- m. immunology
- m. indications
- m. infection
- m. inflammatory response
- m. inheritance
- m. insulin
- M. Interview of Substance Use (MISU)
- m. intravascular inflammation
- m. karyotype
- m. meiosis I (MMI)
- m. meiosis II (MMII)
- m. mercury exposure
- m. mortality
- m. mortality rate (MMR)
- m. nutrition
- m. ocular adaptation
- m. outcome
- m. parvovirus fetalis
- m. pelvic mass
- m. peripheral blood
- m. phenylketonuria
- m. physiology
- m. plasma leptin
- m. plasma volume
- m. position
- m. pulse
- m. pyrexia
- m. respiratory alkalosis
- m. rubella
- m. rubella syndrome
- m. serum
- m. serum alpha-fetoprotein (MSAFP)
- m. serum marker
- m. serum marker level
- m. serum screening
- m. serum triple screen
- m. size
- m. smoking
- m. sperm antibody
- m. stature
- m. steroid concentration
- m. stress
- m. substance abuse
- m. surveillance
- m. systemic condition
- m. tachycardia
- m. T-cell
- m. thrombocytopenia
- m. thyrotropin receptor blocking antibody-induced congenital hypothyroidism
- m. tissue
- m. titer
- m. trauma
- m. undernourishment
- m. uniparental heterodisomy
- m. vascular response
- m. weight
- m. weight gain
- m. well-being

maternal-child bonding

maternal-fetal
- m.-f. hemorrhage
- m.-f. histocompatibility
- m.-f. histoincompatibility
- m.-f. HLA compatibility
- m.-f. interface
- m.-f. medicine
- m.-f. medicine unit (MFMU)
- m.-f. microtransfusion
- m.-f. physiology
- m.-f. transmission
- m.-f. transmission of antibody

maternal-infant
- m.-i. attachment
- m.-i. bonding

maternally inherited myopathy and cardiomyopathy (MIMyCA)

maternal-placental-fetal unit
maternal-placental unit
maternity
    m. blues
    disputed m.
maternofetal
    m. exchange
    m. transfusion
mating
    assortative m.
    backcross m.
    consanguineous m.
    nonrandom m.
    random m.
    m. type
matrices (*pl. of* matrix)
matrilineal
matrilysin
Matritech NMP22 bladder cancer
  test
matrix, *pl.* **matrices**
    bone m.
    calcified m.
    collagen m.
    extracellular m.
    germinal m.
    identity m.
    m. metalloproteinase (MMP)
    myxoid m.
    nail m.
    Raven Progressive Matrices (RPM)
    square m.
    telencephalic subependymal
      germinal m.
    uncalcified bone m.
matroclinous inheritance
matted
    m. omentum
    m. peritoneum
matter
    gray m.
    heterotopic gray m.
    particulate m.
    spongy degeneration of white m.
    supratentorial white m.
    white m.
mattress
    apnea alarm m.
    Dräger thermal gel m.
    NightForm infant sleep m.
Matulane
maturation
    adrenal m.
    delayed sexual m.
    excessive villous m.
    fetal lung m.
    follicular m.
    in vitro m.
    m. of cell

    ovum m.
    premature accelerated lung m.
      (PALM)
    pulmonary m.
    secondary sexual m.
    sexual m.
    skeletal m.
    terminal m.
    vaginal cellular m.
    m. value
maturation-promoting factor (MPF)
mature
    m. burst-forming unit erythroid
      (M-BFU-E)
    m. cystic ovarian teratoma
    m. cystic teratoma
    early m.
    m. infant
    late m.
    m. neutrophil
    m. teratoma
maturity
    chronic lung disease of m.
    Dubowitz Scale for Infant M.
    fetal lung m. (FLM)
    fetal pulmonary m.
    neurologic m.
    neuromuscular m.
    m. onset deafness
    physical m.
    social m.
maturity-onset
    m.-o. diabetes
    m.-o. diabetes of young
      (MODY)
    m.-o. diabetes of youth (MODY)
Maturna bra system
Maunoir hydrocele
Mauriac syndrome
Mauriceau-Levret maneuver
Mauriceau maneuver
Mauriceau-Smellie-Veit maneuver
Maxafil
Maxalt
Maxaquin
Maxeran
Maxidex Ophthalmic
Maxiflor
maxilla, *pl.* **maxillae**
    short m.
maxillae (*pl. of* maxilla)
maxillary
    m. advancement
    m. bone
    m. hypoplasia
    m. sinus
    m. sinus aspiration
    m. sinus mucosal specimen
maxillofacial dysostosis

M

maxillonasal dysplasia
Maxilube personal lubricant
maximal
- m. cardiac width
- m. chest width
- m. electroshock (MES)
- m. oxygen intake (MOI)
- m. permissible dose

maximum
- m. breathing capacity
- m. inspiratory pressure
- m. likelihood estimator
- m. oxygen uptake (VO_2 max, VO_2max)
- m. temperature (T_{max}, T-max, T-MAX)
- m. urethral closure pressure (MUCP)

maximum-intensive phototherapy
Maxipime
Maxitrol Ophthalmic
Maxivate Topical
Maxon delayed absorbable suture
Mayaro virus
Mayer
- M. pessary
- M. sign
- M. wave

Mayer-Rokitansky-Küster-Hauser syndrome
May-Hegglin anomaly
Maylard incision
Mayo
- M. culdoplasty
- M. hook
- M. hysterectomy
- M. scissors

Mayo-Fueth inversion procedure
Mayo-Gibbon heart-lung machine
Mayo-Hegar needle holder
MAYV
- Mayaro virus

mazindol
mazolysis
mazoplasia (*var. of* mastoplasia)
Mazzariello-Caprini forceps
Mazzini test
MB
- myocardial band
  - creatine kinase MB
  - MB isoenzyme

m-BACOD
- methotrexate, bleomycin, doxorubicin, cyclophosphamide, Oncovin, dexamethasone

MBC
- minimal bacterial concentration

MBD
- minimal brain dysfunction

M-BFU-E
- mature burst-forming unit erythroid

MBL
- menstrual blood loss

MBM
- mother's breast milk

MBP
- major basic protein
- modified Bagshawe protocol

MBPP
- modified biophysical profile

MBS
- Martin-Bell syndrome
- modified barium swallow

MCA
- middle cerebral artery

MCAD
- medium-chain acyl-CoA dehydrogenase
  - MCAD deficiency

McAllister grading system
MCAO
- middle cerebral artery occlusion

McArdle disease
McBurney
- M. incision
- M. point

McCall
- M. culdoplasty
- M. stitch

McCall-Schumann enterocele procedure
McCaman-Robins test
McCarthy
- M. Memory Scale
- M. reflex
- M. Scales of Children's Abilities

McCraw gracilis myocutaneous flap
McCune-Albright syndrome (MAS)
MCD
- metastatic Crohn disease
- molybdenum cofactor deficiency

MCDD
- multiple complex developmental disorder

McDonald
- M. cervical cerclage
- M. maneuver
- M. measurement
- M. operation
- M. procedure
- M. rule

McDonough syndrome
MCDU
- mercaptolactate-cysteine disulfiduria

MCFA
- medium-chain fatty acid

MCF-7 breast cancer cell
mcg
- microgram

McGee forceps
McGhan implant
McGill forceps
mcg/kg min
McGoon index
McGovern nipple
McGrath scale
MCH
    mean cell hemoglobin
    mean corpuscular hemoglobin
MCHC
    mean cell hemoglobin concentration
    mean corpuscular hemoglobin
      concentration
MCI
    massive chronic intervillositis
MCi
    megacurie
McIndoe
    M. operation
    M. vaginal construction procedure
McIndoe-Hayes procedure
MCKD
    multicystic dysplastic kidney disease
McKernan-Adson forceps
McKernan-Potts forceps
McKissock method
McKusick-Kaufman syndrome
MCL
    medial collateral ligament
McLane forceps
McLeod syndrome
MCLS
    mucocutaneous lymph node
      syndrome
McMaster Family Assessment Device
McMurray
    M. sign
    M. test
McNemar test
MCNS
    minimal change nephrotic
      syndrome
MCO
    managed care organization
MCP
    medical control physician
    metacarpophalangeal
McPherson forceps
MCR
    metabolic clearance rate
m-cresyl acetate
McRoberts maneuver
MCS
    Miles-Carpenter syndrome
MCT
    medium-chain triglyceride
      MCT oil
      MCT oil formula

MCTD
    mixed connective tissue disease
M-cup vacuum extraction device
MCV
    mean corpuscular volume
    methotrexate, cisplatin,
      vinblastine
    molluscum contagiosum virus
McWhirter mastectomy
MD
    mammary dysplasia
    medical doctor
    muscular dystrophy
    myotonic dystrophy
MDA
    malondialdehyde
    multichannel discrete analyzer
MDAC
    multidose activated charcoal
MDD
    major depressive disorder
    manic-depressive disorder
MDI
    manic-depressive illness
    mental development index
    metered-dose inhaler
MDK
    multicystic dysplastic kidney
MDLS
    Miller-Dieker lissencephaly
      syndrome
MDMA
    methylenedioxymethamphetamine
MDR
    minimum daily requirement
    multidrug resistance
MDR-TB
    multidrug-resistant tuberculosis
MDS
    maternal deprivation syndrome
    myelodysplastic syndrome
MDT
    multidrug therapy
M/E
    myeloid-to-erythroid
MEA
    mercaptoethylamine
    microwave endometrial ablation
    multiple endocrine abnormalities
    multiple endocrine adenomatosis
MEAC
    minimal effective analgesic
      concentration
Mead
    M. Johnson
    M. Johnson bottle
    M. Johnson formula
Meadows syndrome
meal-time skill

M

mean

m. age
m. airway pressure (MAP)
m. aortic pressure
m. arm muscle circumference (MAMC)
m. arterial blood pressure (MABP, MBP)
m. arterial pressure (MAP)
m. birth weight
m. cell hemoglobin (MCH)
m. cell hemoglobin concentration (MCHC)
m. corpuscular hemoglobin (MCH)
m. corpuscular hemoglobin concentration (MCHC)
m. corpuscular volume (MCV)
m. developmental quotient
m. hemoglobin concentration
m. intercriterion correlation (MIC)
m. left atrial pressure
m. length of utterance (MLU)
m. length of utterance in morphemes (MLUm)
m. menstrual cycle hematocrit
m. plasma iron concentration
m. platelet volume (MPV)
m. pulmonary artery pressure
m. right atrial pressure
means-end problem solving (MEPS)
measles

atypical m.
black m.
m. exanthema
German m.
m. inclusion body encephalitis (MIBE)
modified m.
measles, mumps, rubella (MMR)
m. pneumonia
m. strain
three-day m.
typical m.
uncomplicated m.
m. vaccine
m. virus (MV)
m. virus enzyme-linked immunosorbent assay (MV(c)ELISA)
measure

anthropometric m.
first-line m.
gross motor function m.
Prematurity Risk Evaluation M. (PREM)
process-oriented m.
second-line m.
third-line m.

measurement

acid-base m.
anthropometric m.
anthropomorphic m.
blood pressure m.
body proportion m.
bone density m.
bone mineral m.
bone strength m.
daily weight m.
fetal fibronectin m.
fetal growth m.
fundal height m.
intrauterine pressure m.
McDonald m.
midluteal progesterone m.
noninvasive blood pressure m. (NIBPM)
nuchal translucency m.
optic density m.
peak flow m.
POWSBP m.
sequential peak flow m.
somatic growth m.
third-trimester m.
transcutaneous m.
measuring hat
meatal

m. advancement and glanduloplasty incorporation
m. advancement and glansplasty incorporation (MAGPI)
m. advancement and glanuloplasty (MAGPI)
m. stenosis
meatus, *pl.* **meatus**

auditory m.
bilateral atresia of external auditory m.
external auditory m.
external urethral m.
fishmouth m.
glanular urethral m.
penile urethral m.
penopubic urethral m.
urethral m.
MEB

muscle-eye-brain
MEB disease
mebanazine
Mebaral
mebendazole
MEBS

muscle-eye-brain syndrome
MECA

Methods for Epidemiology of Child and Adolescent Mental Disorders
MECA study
MECA T score

mecamylamine
mechanical
    m. birth injury
    m. buttress
    m. cervical dilator
    m. compression
    m. dead space
    m. dysmenorrhea
    m. hemolysis
    m. obstruction
    m. respirator
    m. suffocation
    m. tubal occlusion
    m. ventilation (MV)
mechanic's hand
mechanism
    alloimmune m.
    autoimmune m.
    bypass continence m.
    2-cell m.
    cellular cytotoxic m.
    cerebroprotective m.
    Douglas m.
    Duncan m.
    excitotoxic m.
    fetal cardiac control m.
    Frank-Starling m.
    heat transfer m.
    host defense m.
    host response m.
    neural m.
    normal flap-valve m.
    m. of labor
    ovum pickup m.
    pathophysiologic m.
    peptide growth factor
      signaling m.
    Schultze m.
    Starling m.
mechanobullous
mechanosensitive reflex
mechlorethamine
    m. hydrochloride
Meckel
    M. cave
    M. diverticulum
    M. scan
    M. syndrome
Meckel-Gruber syndrome
meclizine, meclozine
    m. hydrochloride
meclofenamate
meclozine (*var. of* meclizine)
mecometer
meconial colic
meconiorrhea
meconium
    m. aspiration
    m. aspiration syndrome (MAS)

    m. aspiration syndrome
      extracorporeal membrane
      oxygenation (MAS-ECMO)
    m. blockage syndrome
    m. corpuscle
    m. ileus (MI)
    m. ileus appearance
    m. ileus equivalent
    m. obstruction
    m. passage
    passage of m.
    m. peritonitis
    m. plug
    m. plug syndrome
    m. stain
    m. stained
    m. staining
    m. staining of liquor
meconium-stained
    m.-s. amniotic fluid (MSAF)
    m.-s. skin
MeCP2
    methyl-CpG-binding protein 2
MED
    minimal effective dose
Meda-Cap
MedaSonics first beat ultrasound
  stethoscope
Meda Tab
Medela
    M. Dominant vacuum delivery
      pump
    M. manual breast pump
    M. membrane regulator
Mederma
Medex
Medfusion 1001 syringe infusion
  pump
media (*pl. of* medium)
    acute otitis m. (AOM)
    acute suppurative otitis m.
    chronic otitis m. (COM)
    chronic suppurative otitis m.
      (CSOM)
    clostridial otitis m.
    draining otitis m.
    mucoid otitis m. (MOM)
    otitis m. (OM)
    recurrent otitis m.
    secretory otitis m. (SOM)
    serous otitis m. (SOM)
    suppurative otitis m. (SOM)
medial
    m. collateral ligament (MCL)
    m. collateral ligament syndrome
    m. compartment
    m. condyle
    m. epicondylar fracture
    m. epicondylitis

M

medial (*continued*)
   m. femoral torsion (MFT)
   m. hamstring
   m. hip rotation
   m. hip rotation in extension
   m. longitudinal arch
   m. longitudinal arch support
   m. malleolus
   m. metaphysial beak
   m. necrosis
   m. oblique view
   m. rotation (MR)
   m. rotation clubfoot
   m. snapping hip syndrome
   m. talocalcaneal facet
   m. tibial torsion (MTT)
medialis
   vastus m.
median
   m. alveolar notch
   m. eminence
   m. episiotomy
   m. facial cleft syndrome
   m. fecal calprotectin
   multiples of m. (MoM)
   m. plane
   m. raphe
   m. umbilical fold
   m. umbilical ligament
mediastinal
   m. air drainage
   m. collagenosis
   m. crunch
   m. granuloma
   m. imaging
   m. lymphadenitis
   m. lymphadenopathy
   m. mass
   m. teratoma
   m. tumor
   m. widening
mediastinitis
   fibrosing m.
   pyogenic m.
   suppurative m.
mediastinum
   narrow m.
mediating action
mediator
   herpes virus entry m. (HVEM)
   intracellular m.
medibottle
   Rx m.
Medicaid
medical
   m. abortion
   m. control physician (MCP)
   m. doctor (MD)
   m. geneticist

   m. genetics
   M. Manager software
   m. noncompliance
   m. oophorectomy
   m. optical spectroscopy (MOS)
   m. optimal imaging (MOI)
   m. record (MR)
   m. termination
   m. worry beads
MedicAlert
   M. bracelet
   M. Foundation
medicalization
medically fragile
medicamentosa
   rhinitis m.
Medicare
medicated
   Zilactin-B M.
medication
   adjuvant m.
   aerosolized m.
   anticholinesterase m.
   antiemetic m.
   antipruritic m.
   antiretroviral m.
   antispastic m.
   antitussive m.
   anxiolytic m.
   base m.
   exogenous m.
   intrathecal m.
   intravenous m.
   iodide-containing m.
   maintenance m.
   medications, monitors, suction,
      oxygen, airway equipment,
      personnel (MSOAP)
   neuroleptic m.
   opioid m.
   organ-specific m.
   over-the-counter m.
   parenteral m.
   postcoital contraceptive m.
   pressor m.
   prophylactic m.
   psychostimulant m.
   quick-relief m.
   rescue m.
   sustained-release m.
   teratogenic m.
medication-induced stuttering
medicine
   adolescent m.
   Alka-Seltzer Plus Children's Cold M.
   American Institute of Ultrasound in
      M. (AIUM)
   American Society for Reproductive
      M.

Chinese m.
community m.
complementary and alternative m.
(CAM)
digital imaging and communication
in m. (DICOM)
doctor of m.
emergency m.
fetal-maternal m.
folk m.
herbal m.
maternal-fetal m.
neonatal m.
osteopathic m.
pediatric emergency m. (PEM)
pediatric pulmonary m.
perinatal m.
pulmonary m.
Reese's Pinworm M.
medicolegal
Medicone
Rectal M.
MED-IDDM
multiple epiphysial dysplasia-early
onset diabetes mellitus
**Medilog 9000 polysomnography
device**
medinensis
Dracunculus m.
mediolateral
m. episiotomy
m. view
Mediplast Plaster
Medipore H soft cloth surgical tape
MediPort catheter
Medi-Quick Topical Ointment
meditation
Transcendental M. (TM)
Mediterranean
M. anemia
M. fever
M. lymphoma
M. myoclonus
Medi-Trace electrode
medium, *pl.* **media**
acute otitis media (AOM)
acute suppurative otitis media
Biggers m.
Bordet-Gengoi m.
charcoal-blood m.
chronic otitis media (COM)
chronic suppurative otitis media
(CSOM)
clostridial otitis media
CPS ID chromogenic m.
dermatophyte test m. (DTM)
Diamond m.
distention m.
draining otitis media

Dulbecco m.
Earle culture m.
gallium-67 citrate contrast m.
Gibco BRL sperm preparation m.
glycine distention m.
Ham F10 m.
ionic contrast m.
Löwenstein-Jensen m.
mucoid otitis media (MOM)
Nickerson m.
nonionic contrast m.
OncoScint CR/OV contrast m.
otitis media (OM)
recurrent otitis media
Regan-Lowe m.
Sabouraud m.
secretory otitis media
selective broth m. (SBM)
serous otitis media
sperm capacitation m.
suppurative otitis media
Thayer-Martin m.
thioglycollate broth m.
transfer m.
transmission m.
transport m.
Whitten m.
Whittingham m.
medium-chain
m.-c. acyl-CoA dehydrogenase
(MCAD)
m.-c. fatty acid (MCFA)
m.-c. triglyceride (MCT)
medius
saccus m.
Med-Neb respirator
Medrol Oral
medroxyprogesterone
m. acetate (MPA)
m. injection
medrysone
MEDS
microsurgical extraction of ductal
sperm
medulla, *pl.* **medullae**
adrenal m.
m. oblongata
rostral ventromedial m.
medullae (*pl. of* medulla)
medullaris
tethered conus m.
medullary
m. canal
m. cord
m. cystic disease
m. dysplasia
m. necrosis
m. parenchyma
m. recycling

M

medullary (*continued*)
   m. sponge kidney
   m. thyroid carcinoma
medulloblastoma
   classic m.
   desmoplastic m.
   melanotic m.
   primitive neuroectodermal tumor m.
    (PNET/MB)
medullomyoblastoma
medusae
   caput m.
MedWatch form
MEE
   middle ear effusion
Meesmann corneal dystrophy
MEF
   middle ear fluid
mefenamic acid
mefloquine hydrochloride
Mefoxin
MEG
   magnetoencephalography
megabase
megabladder
megacalycosis
megacardia
megacaryocyte (*var. of*
  megakaryocyte)
Megace
megacephaly, megalocephalia
mega cisterna magna
megacolon
     aganglionic m.
     congenital aganglionic m.
     toxic m.
megacurie (MCi)
megacystis (MMIH), microcolon,
  intestinal hypoperistalsis
  m.
megacystis-megaureter syndrome
megadontism (*var. of*
  macrodontia)
megadosing
megaelectron volt (MeV)
megaesophagus
megagnathia (*var. of* macrognathia)
megahertz (MHz)
megakaryoblastic leukemia
megakaryocyte, megacaryocyte
megakaryocytic
   m. leukemia
   m. thrombocytopenia
megakaryocytopoiesis
megakaryopoiesis
megalencephaly, megaloencephaly
   benign familial m.
   idiopathic m.
   primary m.

   unilateral m.
   m. with hyaline panneuropathy
megaloblastic
   m. anemia
   m. crisis
   m. erythropoiesis
megaloblastoid
megaloblastosis
megalocardia
megalocephalia
megalocephaly, megalocephalia
megaloclitoris
megalocornea (MMMM)
megalocornea-mental retardation
  syndrome (MMR)
megalodactyly
megalodontia (*var. of* macrodontia)
megaloencephaly
megaloglossia (*var. of* macroglossia)
megalomelia
Megalone
megalopenis
megalophthalmos
megalosyndactylia (*var. of*
  megalosyndactyly)
megalosyndactyly, megalosyndactylia
megaloureter, megaureter
   obstructive m.
megalourethra
meganeurite
megarectum
megaterium
   Bacillus m.
megaureter, megaloureter
megavitamin therapy
megavolt (MV)
megavoltage machine
megestrol acetate
meglumine
   m. diatrizoate
   Hypaque M.
meibomian gland
meibomianitis, meibomitis
meibomitis (*var. of* meibomianitis)
Meier-Gorlin syndrome
Meigs
   M. pelvic lymphadenectomy
   M. syndrome
Meigs-Kass syndrome
Meigs-Okabayashi radical hysterectomy
  procedure
Meigs-Werthein hysterectomy
meiosis
   diakinesis stage of oocyte m.
   dictyate stage of oocyte m.
   diplotene phase of m.
   m. I (MI)
   m. II (MII)
   leptotene phase of m.

oocyte m.
pachytene phase of m.
zygotene phase of m.
meiotic division
Meissner
M. corpuscle
M. plexus
mekongi
Schistosoma m.
melancholia
involutional m.
melancholic depression
Melanex topical solution
melanin-like pigment
melaninogenicus
Bacteroides m.
melanization
melanoblastoma
Bloch-Sulzberger m.
melanocortin-stimulating hormone (MSH)
melanocyte
epidermal m.
pigmented m.
melanocyte-stimulating hormone
melanocytic nevus
melanocytosis
congenital dermal m.
dermal m.
meningeal m.
melanoderma
melanodermic leukodystrophy
melanoma
benign juvenile m.
Clark classification of vulvar m.
cutaneous m.
juvenile m.
malignant m.
metastatic m.
nodular m.
m. specific antigen
superficial spreading m.
vulvar m.
melanosarcoma
melanosis
Becker m.
cutaneous m.
dermal m.
neonatal pustular m.
m. oculi
pustular m.
transient neonatal pustular m.
m. vaginae
m. vulvae
melanotic medulloblastoma
melanura
Culiseta m.

MELAS
mitochondrial myopathy, encephalopathy, lactic acidosis, strokelike episodes
MELAS syndrome
melasma gravidarum
melatonin
m. secretion
urinary excreted m.
Meleda
mal de M.
melena
m. neonatorum
m. spuria
Meleney synergistic gangrene
Melfiat
melioidosis
melitensis
Brucella m.
Melkersson-Rosenthal syndrome
Melkersson syndrome
Mellaril
mellituria
mellitus
A2 diabetes m.
A1 diabetes m.
adult-onset diabetes m. (AODM)
diabetes m. (type 1, 2) (DM)
gestational diabetes m. (GDM)
insulin-dependent diabetes m. (IDDM)
juvenile diabetes m. (JDM)
juvenile-onset diabetes m. (JDM, JODM)
multiple epiphysial dysplasia-early onset diabetes m. (MED-IDDM)
neonatal diabetes m.
new-onset diabetes m.
non-insulin-dependent diabetes m. (NIDDM)
overt insulin-dependent diabetes m.
pregestational diabetes m. (PDM)
transient neonatal diabetes m. (TNDM)
type 1 diabetes m.
type 2 diabetes m.
Melnick-Fraser syndrome
Melnick-Needles
M.-N. disease
M.-N. syndrome
meloneuropathy
human T-cell lymphotropic virus 1 tropic m.
melorheostosis
melphalan
membranacea
placenta m.
membrana granulosa

M

563

membrane
allograft m.
amniotic m.
artificial rupture of m.'s (AROM)
m. attack complex
basal m. (BM)
basement m.
m. bridge
chorioallantoic m. (CAM)
cloacal m.
cracked mucous m.
cricothyroid m.
cuprophane hemodialyzer m.
cytoplasmic m.
Descemet m.
diphtheritic m.
disruption of fetal m.'s
dry mucous membranes
Duralon-UV nylon m.
dysmenorrheal m.
egg m.
erythrocyte m.
exocelomic m.
extraembryonic fetal m.
extraplacental m.
fetal m.
floating m.
germinal m.
glomerular basement m. (GBM)
Gore-Tex surgical m.
m. granulosa
Heuser m.
hyaline m.
hymenal m.
intact m.
interfetal m.
Jackson m.
milk fat globule m. (MFGM)
mucous m.
otitis media with perforated
    tympanic m.
parched mucous m.
perforated tympanic m.
perineal m.
persistent pupillary m.
placental m.
plasma m.
platelet m.
Preclude peritoneal m.
prelabor rupture of m.'s (PROM)
premature rupture of m.'s (PROM)
preterm premature rupture of m.'s
    (PPROM)
preterm rupture of m.'s (PROM)
preterm spontaneous rupture of m.'s
    (PSROM)
prolonged premature rupture of m.'s
    (PPROM)
prolonged rupture of m.'s (PROM)

m. protein
pupillary m.
red blood cell m.
Reissner m.
retained m.
m. rupture
rupture of chorioamniotic m.
Seprafilm bioresorbable m.
Slavianski m.
spontaneous rupture of m.'s (SROM)
m. stripping
subaortic m.
tympanic m.
ultrafiltration m.
vernix m.
Viresolve ultrafiltration m.
vitelline m.
Wachendorf m.
yolk m.

**membranoproliferative glomerulonephritis
(MPGN)**
membranous
m. conjunctivitis
m. croup
m. dysmenorrhea
m. glomerulonephritis
m. laryngotracheobronchitis
m. lupus nephritis
m. nephropathy
m. septum
memory
autobiographical m.
m. cell
episodic m.
m. phenomenon
recovered m.
rote m.
semantic m.
sequential m.
spatial m.
visual sequential m.
visual spatial m.
MEMR
multiple exostosis-mental retardation
    MEMR syndrome
**MEMS 6 TrackCap Monitor medication
monitoring system**
MEN
multiple endocrine neoplasia (type I,
    II, III)
menacme
Menactra
menadiol sodium diphosphate
menadione
Menadol
menarche
delayed m.
m. factor
isolated premature m.

precocious m.
premature m.
menarcheal, menarchial
menarchial (*var. of* menarcheal)
MenCon vaccine
Mendel
    M. first law
    M. second law
mendelian
    m. genetic disorder
    m. inheritance
    M. Inheritance in Man (MIM)
    m. syndrome
    m. trait
mendelizing
Mendelson syndrome
Mendenhall syndrome
Menest
Menetrier disease
Menge pessary
Mengert
    M. index
    M. shock syndrome
Meni-D
Ménière
    M. disease
    M. syndrome
    M. vertigo
meningeal
    m. capillary angiomatosis
    m. carcinomatosis
    m. fibrosis
    m. irritation
    m. melanocytosis
    m. sign
meninges (*pl. of* meninx)
meningioma
    acoustic m.
    optic nerve sheath m.
    perioptic m.
    suprasellar m.
meningism
meningismus
meningitides (*pl. of* meningitis)
meningitidis
    Neisseria m.
meningitis, *pl.* **meningitides**
    aseptic m.
    bacillary m.
    bacterial m.
    basilar m.
    Candida m.
    chronic lymphocytic m.
    chronic syphilitic m.
    coccidioidomycosis m.
    cryptococcal m.
    echoviral m.
    echovirus 9 m.
    enteroviral m.

eosinophilic m.
experimental pneumococcal m.
exudative m.
fulminating m.
fungal m.
GBS m.
Haemophilus influenzae m.
herpes aseptic m.
herpes zoster m.
influenzal m.
leptospiral m.
*Listeria*m.
Lyme m.
lymphocytic m.
meningococcal m.
Mollaret m.
neonatal m.
nosocomial bacterial m.
pneumococcal m.
postnatal bacterial m.
purulent m.
pyogenic m.
recurrent bacterial m.
recurrent fungal m.
recurrent purulent m.
*Salmonella*m.
septic m.
serous form of tuberculous m.
streptococcal m.
syphilitic m.
tuberculous m.
viral m.
meningocele
    cranial m.
    lumbar m.
    spinal m.
meningococcal
    m. conjugate
    m. conjugate vaccine
    m. endotoxin
    m. meningitis
    m. multifocal osteomyelitis
    m. polysaccharide
    m. polysaccharide vaccine (MENps)
    m. septicemia
meningococcemia
    chronic m.
meningococcus
    serogroup B m.
meningoencephalitic stage
meningoencephalitis
    amebic m.
    aseptic m.
    bacterial m.
    Balamuthia m.
    enteroviral m.
    eosinophilic m.
    granulomatous amebic m.
    mumps m.

M

meningoencephalitis (*continued*)
    primary amebic m. (PAM, PAME)
    m. syndrome
    viral m.
meningoencephalocele
meningoencephalomyelitis
meningomyelocele
    lumbosacral m.
    sacral m.
meningooculofacial angiomatosis
meningoradiculomyelitis
    chronic m.
meningoradiculoneuritis
    lymphocytic m.
meningoulofacialis
    angiomatosis m.
meningovascular syndrome
meningoventriculitis
meninx, *pl.* **meninges**
meniscal injury
menisci (*pl. of* meniscus)
meniscoplasty
meniscus, *pl.* **menisci**
    discoid lateral m.
    m. tear
Menkes
    M. kinky hair
    M. kinky-hair syndrome (MKHS)
    M. syndrome
Menkes-Kaplan syndrome
menocelis
menometrorrhagia
menopausal
    m. estrogen replacement
      therapy
    m. syndrome
menopause
    iatrogenic m.
    premature m.
menophania
Menopur
menorrhagia
    essential m.
menorrhalgia
menoschesis
menostasia (*var. of* menostasis)
menostasis, menostasia, menostaxis
menostaxis (*var. of* menostasis)
menotropin
menotropins for injection
menouria
menoxenia
MENps
    meningococcal polysaccharide vaccine
    MENps vaccine
menses
    absent m.
    irregular m.
    m. phase

menstrual
    m. age
    m. aspiration
    m. blood
    m. blood loss (MBL)
    m. colic
    m. cramp
    m. cycle hemodynamic response
    m. cycle induction
    m. cycle regulation
    m. cycle resumption
    m. cyclicity
    m. disturbance
    m. edema
    m. effluent
    m. endometrium
    m. extraction
    m. extraction abortion
    m. flow
    m. formula
    m. history (MH)
    m. irregularity
    m. leukorrhea
    m. migraine
    m. molimina
    m. ovarian cycle
    m. pain
    m. pattern
    m. period (MP)
    m. phase
    m. prodrome
    m. reflux
    m. sclerosis
    m. state
menstrual-associated periodic
  hypersomnia
menstrualis
    decidua m.
menstrual-like cramp
menstruant
menstruate
menstruation
    abnormal m.
    anovular m.
    delayed m.
    painful m.
    Premenstrual Record of Impact and
      Severity of M.
    retained m.
    retrograde m.
    supplementary m.
    suppressed m.
    vicarious m.
mentagrophytes
    Trichophyton m.
mental
    m. age
    m. and growth retardation-amblyopia
      syndrome

m. arithmetic test
m. clouding
m. deficiency
m. development
m. development index (MDI)
m. disturbance
m. handicap
m. health
m. illness
m. retardation
m. retardation-adducted thumbs syndrome
m. retardation, aphasia, shuffling gait, adducted thumb (MASA)
m. retardation-clasped thumb syndrome
m. retardation-distal arthrogryposis syndrome
m. retardation, macroorchidism syndrome
m. retardation-overgrowth sequence
m. retardation-overgrowth syndrome
m. retardation-psoriasis syndrome
m. retardation-sparse hair syndrome
m. scale
m. status evaluation
m. subnormality
mentalis habit
mentoanterior
left m. (LMA)
m. presentation
mentoposterior
left m. (LMP)
m. presentation
mentor
M. catheter
M. female self-catheter
M. MemoryGel silicone gel-filled breast implant
mentotransverse
left m. (LMT)
mentum
m. anterior fetal position
m. posterior fetal position
m. transverse fetal position
Mentzer index
MEP
motor evoked potential
mepenzolate bromide
meperidine hydrochloride
mephentermine
mephenytoin
mephobarbital
Mephyton Oral
mepivacaine
m. hydrochloride
m. intoxication
meprobamate
conjugated estrogen and m.

Mepron
MEPS
means-end problem solving
mepyramine
mEq
milliequivalent
mEq/L
milliequivalent per liter
MER
methanol extraction residue
meralgia paresthetica
mercaptoacetyl triglycine
2-mercaptoethane sulfonate (MESNA, mesna)
mercaptoethylamine (MEA)
mercaptolactate-cysteine disulfiduria (MCDU)
mercaptopurine
mercaptotriglycine
Merchant view
Mercier bar
Merck respirator
mercurial diuretic
mercuric chloride
mercury-free vaccine
mercury vapor poisoning
Meritene formula
Merkel
M. cell
M. cell carcinoma
M. tactile disc
meroacrania
meroanencephaly
merocyte
merogastrula
merogenesis
merogony
diploid m.
meromelia
meromicrosomia
meropenem
merorachischisis, merorrhachischisis
merorrhachischisis (*var. of* merorachischisis)
merosin deficiency
merozygote
Merrem IV
MERRF
myoclonic epilepsy with ragged red fibers
MERRF syndrome
Merrill program
Merrimack 1040 CO_2 laser
Mersilene
M. fascial strip
M. gauze hammock
M. mesh
M. mesh sling
M. suture

M

Merthiolate spray
Meruvax II
merycism
Méry gland
Merzbacher-Pelizaeus disease
MES
    maximal electroshock
MESA
    microsurgical epididymal sperm
    aspiration
mesalamine
mesangial
    m. cell proliferation
    m. hypercellularity
    m. lupus nephritis
    m. proliferative glomerulonephritis
    m. sclerosis
mesangiocapillary glomerulonephritis
(type I, II) (MPGN)
mesangium
mesaraic (*var. of* mesenteric)
mesaraica (*var. of* mesenterica)
mesareic (*var. of* mesenteric)
mesatipellic pelvis
mesectodermal dysplasia
mesencephalic-diencephalic junction
mesencephalic tectum
mesencephalon
mesenchyma (*var. of* mesenchyme)
mesenchymal
    m. cell
    m. hamartoma
    m. neoplasm
mesenchyme, mesenchyma
    nonspecific m.
    portal m.
mesenchymoma
mesenteric, mesaraic, mesareic
    m. adenitis
    m. artery
    m. lymphadenitis
    m. root
    m. stalk
    m. vein
mesenterica, mesaraica
    tabes m.
mesenteroaxial volvulus
mesentery
    intestinal m.
    ventral m.
mesh
    Advantage m.
    Apogee m.
    Brennen biosynthetic surgical m.
    Dexon m.
    m. erosion
    Gynemesh nonabsorbable
     Prolene m.
    Mersilene m.

mesial
    m. temporal lobe
    m. temporal sclerosis (MTS)
mesiodens-cataracts syndrome
mesna, MESNA
    2-mercaptoethane sulfonate
    mesna, Adriamycin, Ifosfamide,
     Dacarbazine (MAID)
Mesnex
mesoappendix
mesoaxial hexadactyly-cardiac
 malformation syndrome
mesoblast
mesoblastic nephroma
mesoblastoma ovarii
mesocardia
mesocaval shunt
mesocephalic
mesoderm
    extraembryonic m.
    head m.
    lateral plate m.
    paraxial m.
mesodermal
    m. dysgenesis of anterior segment
    m. heterotopia
    m. sarcoma
    m. tumor
mesogaster
mesogastrium
mesolimbic dopamine tract
mesomelic
    m. dwarfism-small genitalia
    syndrome
    m. dysplasia
    m. shortening
mesometanephric carcinoma
mesometric pregnancy
mesometritis
mesonephric
    m. adenocarcinoma
    m. carcinoma
    m. cyst
    m. duct
    m. kidney
    m. rest
    m. ridge
    m. tubule
mesonephroi (*pl. of* mesonephros)
mesonephroid
    m. clear cell carcinoma
    m. tumor
mesonephroma
mesonephros, *pl.* **mesonephroi**
mesoporphyrin
    tin m. (SnMP)
mesorchium
mesoridazine besylate
mesosalpingeal

mesosalpinx
mesoteres
mesothelioma
    malignant m. (MM)
mesothelium
    peritoneal m.
mesovarium
MesPGN
    mesangial proliferative
    glomerulonephritis
messenger
    m. ribonucleic acid (mRNA)
    m. RNA
    second m.
Mestatin
Mestinon Oral
mestranol
    m. and norethindrone
    m. and norethynodrel
mesylate
    benztropine m.
    bromocriptine m.
    deferoxamine m.
    Desferal M.
    desferrioxamine m.
    dihydroergotamine m.
    dimethothiazine m.
meta-analysis, metaanalysis
metaanalysis (var. of meta-analysis)
metabolic
    m. abnormality
    m. acidemia
    m. acidosis
    m. acidosis syndrome
    m. alkalosis
    m. bone disease
    m. clearance rate (MCR)
    m. disease in newborn
    m. disorder
    m. disorder with hepatic dysfunction
    m. disorder with neurologic
    dysfunction
    m. encephalopathy
    m. error
    m. management
    m. manifestation
    m. myopathy
    m. response
    m. syndrome X
    m. test
metabolism
    aberrant vitamin D m.
    aerobic m.
    alteration of lipoprotein m.
    amino acid m.
    ammonia m.
    androgen m.
    bone mineral m.
    brain m.

    carbohydrate m.
    cerebral glucose m.
    copper m.
    defective purine m.
    energy m.
    estrogen m.
    fat m.
    fetal m.
    glycolipid m.
    inborn error of m. (IEM)
    m. in intraperitoneal chemotherapy
    lipid m.
    lipoprotein m.
    lipoprotein-cholesterol m.
    methionine m.
    mineral m.
    neonatal m.
    organic acid m.
    partition of energy m.
    phosphorus m.
    placental m.
    progesterone m.
    prostaglandin m.
    purine m.
    steroid m.
    vitamin m.
    water m.
metabolite
    arachidonic acid m.
    lysosomal m.
    steroid m.
metacarpal
    m. fracture
    m. shortening
metacarpophalangeal (MCP)
    m. dislocation
    m. joint
metacentric
    m. chromosome
    m. metaphase
metachromatic
    m. cytoplasmic granule
    m. leukodystrophy (MLD)
metachromosome
metacognition
metacognitive
metacyesis
Metadate
    M. CD
    M. ER tablet
metafemale
metaiodobenzylguanidine (MIBG, MIGB)
metal
    m. coil
    m. intoxication
    m. metabolism disorder
    m. poisoning
    m. suture material
    trace m.

M

metallic
    m. bead-chain cystourethrography
    m. skin staple
metalloenzyme
metalloproteinase
    matrix m. (MMP)
    tissue inhibitors of m.
metalloprotein dimer
metamorphopsia
Metamucil Instant Mix
metamyelocyte
    m. cell
    giant m.
Metandren
metanephric
    m. blastema
    m. bud
    m. duct
metanephros
metaphase
    m. chromosome
    metacentric m.
metaphoric dysplasia
metaphyseal (*var. of* metaphysial)
metaphyses (*pl. of* metaphysis)
metaphysial, metaphyseal
    m. anadysplasia
    m. aspiration
    m. cortex
    m. dysostosis
    m. dysplasia
    m. fibrous defect
    m. flaring
    m. fracture
    m. lesion
    m. lesion of distal femur
    m. sclerosis
metaphysial-diaphysial angle
metaphysis, *pl.* **metaphyses**
    m. angulation
    cupped m.
    popcorn m.
    rachitic m.
    tibial m.
    widened m.
metaplasia
    agnogenic myeloid m. (AMM)
    apocrine m.
    celomic m.
    ciliated m.
    intestinal m.
    squamous m.
    tubal m.
    vaginal squamous m.
metaplastic carcinoma
metapneumovirus
    human m.
metaproterenol sulfate
metaraminol bitartrate

metastases (*pl. of* metastasis)
metastasis, *pl.* **metastases**
    adnexal m.
    aortic node m.
    blood-borne m.
    bone m.
    bony m.
    brain m.
    cerebral m.
    fallopian tube m.
    floxuridine in hepatic m.
    hematogenous m.
    hepatic m.
    inguinal lymph node m.
    liver m.
    lymph node m. (LNM, LN-met)
    ovarian cancer m.
    placental m.
    pulmonary m.
    spinal m.
    stomach cancer m.
    trocar implantation m.
    tumor, node, metastases (TNM)
    uterine sarcoma m.
    vaginal m.
    vascular m.
metastasizing leiomyoma
metastatic
    m. adenocarcinoma
    m. axillary involvement
    m. carcinoma
    m. Crohn disease (MCD)
    m. gynecologic tumor
    m. implant
    m. lesion
    m. lymphoma
    m. malignancy
    m. melanoma
    m. neuroblastoma
    m. tuberculous abscess
Metastron
metatarsal
    m. head osteochondritis
    m. shortening
metatarsophalangeal joint (MPJ)
metatarsus
    m. adductus (MA)
    m. primus varus
    rigid m.
    m. varus
metatropic
    m. dwarfism
    m. dysplasia
metencephalon
Metenier sign
metenkephalin
meter
    Airshields jaundice m.
    Astech Peak Flow M.

glucose m.
Health Scan Assess Plus peak flow
m.
LifeScan blood glucose m.
Mini-Wright Peak Flow M.
Parkinson-Cowan dry gas m.
peak flow m. (PFM)
Pocketpeak peak flow m.
transcutaneous jaundice m.
US 1005 uroflow m.
Wright peak flow m.
metered-dose inhaler (MDI)
metergoline
metformin
methacholine
m. challenge
m. provocation testing
methacycline hydrochloride
methadone hydrochloride
methamphetamine
crystal m.
m. exposure
m. hydrochloride
methandrostenolone
methanol
m. extraction residue (MER)
m., uremia, diabetes, paraldehyde,
isoniazid, infection, lactic acidosis,
ethylene glycol, salicylate
(MUDPILES)
methantheline bromide
methapyrilene
methaqualone
metharbital
methazolamide
methdilazine hydrochloride
methemoglobin
m. level
m. reduction test
methemoglobinemia
hereditary m.
methemoglobinuria
methenamine
m. hippurate
m. mandelate
m. silver stain
Methergine
methergoline
methicillin-resistant Staphylococcus aureus
(MRSA)
methicillin sodium
methimazole
methionine
m. malabsorption
m. malabsorption syndrome
m. metabolism
m. synthase
m. synthase deficiency
methioninemia

Methitest tablet
methixene hydrochloride
methocarbamol
method
amniotomy plus oxytocin m.
arithmetic m.
Astrand 30-beat stopwatch m.
Attwood staining m.
barrier m.
Bayley and Pinneau height-predicting
m.
Billings m.
bone-age determination m.
Bonnaire femoral neck screw
fixation m.
Bradley m.
breath-by-breath m.
brine flotation m.
bromelin m.
Buist intraabdominal pressure
measurement m.
caloric m.
cluster-stratified sampling m.
Cobb m.
cold knife m.
contraceptive m.
Corning m.
CorrTest m.
cotton swab m.
cutdown m.
Döderlein vaginal hysterectomy m.
Douglas m.
encu m.
end-point dilution m.
ensu m.
Essure micro-insert m.
Feldenkrais m.
Ferber m.
Fick m.
flush m.
M.'s for Epidemiology of Child and
Adolescent Mental Disorders
(MECA)
M.'s for the Epidemiology of Child
and Adolescent Disorders score
forward roll m.
Gamper m.
Gibson-Coke m.
Glazer m.
Grantley Dick-Read m.
growth-remaining m.
Hamilton cardiac output m.
Harrison atrial end of
ventriculoatrial shunt m.
hemoglobin subtype m.
Holliday-Segar m.
Irving m.
Ito m.
Johnson m.

M

method (*continued*)
  Kaplan-Meier m.
  Kibrick m.
  Kirby-Bauer m.
  Kluge m.
  Kristeller m.
  lactational amenorrhea m. (LAM)
  Lamaze m.
  LAM contraceptive m.
  laser m.
  Leboyer m.
  life table m.
  Lovaas m.
  Mantoux m.
  manual healing m.
  McKissock m.
  Mosteller m.
  Narula sinoatrial conduction time m.
  m. of Politzer
  oscillometric m.
  per square meter m.
  pilocarpine iontophoresis m.
  Plastibell circumcision m.
  Pomeroy m.
  Prochownik neonatal resuscitation m.
  Puzo endoscopic cancer findings m.
  reverse dot blot sequence-specific oligonucleotide m.
  rhythm m.
  Rodeck m.
  saline drop m.
  shotgun m.
  simplistic m.
  Smellie m.
  Smellie-Veit m.
  sperm washing insemination m. (SWIM)
  Spiegel m.
  Strauss m.
  Stroganoff m.
  symptothermal m.
  symptothermic contraceptive m.
  Tanner-Whitehouse II bone/age determination m.
  Tarkowski m.
  terminal heating m.
  thermodilution m.
  Towako transvaginal-transmyometrial embryo transfer m.
  twin m.
  Uchida m.
  Vecchietti neovagina construction m.
  Victor Gomel microsurgical reconstruction m.
  Video Overlay M.
  Volpe m.
  Wardill 4-flap m.
  Wardill-Kilner advancement flap m.
  Watson scapholunate treatment m.
  Yuzpe contraceptive m.
methodology study
methohexital
methotrexate (MTX)
  Adriamycin, fluorouracil, m. (AFM)
  m., bleomycin, doxorubicin, cyclophosphamide, Oncovin, dexamethasone (m-BACOD)
  m., cisplatin, vinblastine (MCV)
  cytosine arabinoside, etoposide, m. (CEM)
  Cytoxan, Oncovin, fluorouracil plus Cytoxan, Oncovin, m. (COF/COM)
  intrathecal m.
methotrimeprazine
methoxamine hydrochloride
methoxyflurane
methscopolamine
methsuximide
methyclothiazide
methyl
methylation
methylbenzethonium chloride
methylbromide
  hyoscine m.
  scopolamine m.
methylbutyrate
  hydroxy beta m. (HMB)
methyl-CCNU
methylcellulose drops
methylcobalamin
methyl-CpG-binding protein 2 (MeCP2)
methyldopa
methylene
  m. blue
  m. blue dye
  m. tetrahydrofolate reductase (MTHFR)
methylenedioxymethamphetamine (MDMA)
5,10-methylenetetrahydrofolate
methylergometrine maleate
methylergonovine maleate
3-methylglutaconic aciduria
Methylin
  M. C
  M. ER
methylmalonic
  m. acid
  m. acidemia
  m. aciduria (MMA)
methylmercury
  m. intoxication
  m. neurotoxicity
  m. toxicity
methylphenidate (MPH)
  extended-release m.
  m. hydrochloride

methylprednisolone
- m. acetate
- m. base
- pulse m.

15-methyl prostaglandin

15-methylprostaglandin $F^{2\alpha}$

methylsuccinic acid

methylsulfate
- diphemanil m.
- hexocyclium m.

methyltestosterone
- estrogens with m.
- m. macrobead

methyltransferase
- thiopurine m. (TPMT)

methylxanthine

methysergide maleate

Meticorten

metoclopramide hydrochloride

metolazone

metopagus

metopic
- m. craniosynostosis
- m. ridging

Metopirone test

metoprolol tartrate

MetraGrasp ligament grasper

MetraPass suture passer

Metra PS procedure kit

MetraTie knot pusher

metratonia

metratrophia (var. of metratrophy)

metratrophy, metratrophia

metrectomy

Metreton Ophthalmic

metria

metritis
- postpartum m.

metrizamide

metrizoate sodium

Metrodin

metrodynamometer

metrodynia

MetroGel Topical

MetroGel-Vaginal gel

metrography

Metro I.V.

metrolymphangitis

metromalacia

metromalacoma, metromalacosis

metromalacosis (var. of metromalacoma)

metromenorrhagia

metronidazole vaginal gel

metroparalysis

metropathia hemorrhagica

metropathic

metropathy

metroperitoneal fistula

metroperitonitis

metrophlebitis

metroplasty
- abdominal m.
- hysteroscopic m.
- Jones wedge m.
- Strassman m.
- Tompkins m.

Metropolitan Atlanta Congenital Defects Program (MACDP)

metrorrhagia myopathica

metrorrhea

metrorrhexis

metrosalpingitis

metrosalpingography

metroscope

metrostaxis

metrostenosis

metrotomy

metyrapone test

metyrosine

Metzenbaum scissors

MeV
- megaelectron volt

MEVA
- multiplane endovaginal
  - MEVA probe
  - MEVA Probe for endovaginal scanning

mevalonic
- m. acidemia
- m. aciduria

mexicana
- Leishmania m.

Mexican cardiomelic dysplasia

mexiletine

Mexitil

meyeri
- Actinomyces m.

Meyer-Schwickerath and Weyers syndrome

Meyerson nevus

Meyer theory of endometriosis

Mezlin

mezlocillin sodium

MF
- K-Phos MF

MFD
- mandibulofacial dysostosis
- midforceps delivery

MFF
- Matching Familiar Figures

MFG
- milk fat globule

MFGM
- milk fat globule membrane

MFH
- malignant fibrous histiocytoma

M

M-FISH
    multispectral fluorescent in situ
    hybridization
      M-FISH cytogenetic technique
MFMU
    maternal-fetal medicine unit
MFNS
    mometasone furoate aqueous nasal
    spray
MFPR
    multifetal pregnancy reduction
MFR
    monthly fecundity rate
MFT
    medial femoral torsion
mg
    milligram
mg%
    milligram percent
MGD
    mixed gonadal dysgenesis
MgSO$_4$
    magnesium sulfate
MH
    malignant hyperthermia
    menstrual history
MHA
    microhemagglutination assay
MHC
    major histocompatibility complex
      MHC antigen
      MHC class I antigen
      deficiency
      MHC molecule
MHP
    hyperphenylalaninemia
MHz
    megahertz
MI
    meconium ileus
    meiosis I
    migration index
    myocardial infarction
Miacalcin Nasal Spray
Miami Moss instrumentation
MIBE
    measles inclusion body
    encephalitis
Mibelli
    M. angiokeratoma
    angiokeratoma of M.
    porokeratosis of M.
MIBG
    metaiodobenzylguanidine
      MIBG scan
MIC
    mean intercriterion correlation
    minimal inhibitory concentration
    minimum inhibitory concentration

MICA
    microinvasive carcinoma
    microinvasive cervical cancer
Micardis
Micatin Topical
micdadei
    Legionella m.
micellar nanoparticle testosterone
micelle
Michaelis-Menten dissociation constant
Michel
    M. anomaly
    M. aplasia
    M. deformity
Michelin-tire baby syndrome
Michels syndrome
Michigan
    M. Alcoholism Screening Test
    M. 4-wall sacrospinous suspension
miconazole
    m. gel
    m. nitrate
    m. nitrate vaginal cream
    m. 7 vaginal insert
Micral
    M. Chemstrip
    M. urine dipstick test
micrencephalia (*var. of* micrencephaly)
micrencephaly, micrencephalia,
  microencephaly
MICRhoGAM
microabscess
    Munro m.
microadenoma
microaerophilic
microalbuminuria
microangiopathic
    m. hemolysis
    m. hemolytic anemia
    m. hemolytic uremic syndrome
    m. process
microangiopathy
    HIV m.
    mineralizing m.
    thrombotic m. (TMA)
microarousal
microaspiration
microassisted fertilization
microatelectasis
microbe
microbial
    m. factor
    m. flora
    m. sensitivity
microbiology
microbrachia
microbrachycephaly
microbubble
    gelatin-encapsulated m.

microcalcification
microcephalia (*var. of* microcephaly)
microcephalic
    m. idiocy
    m. primordial dwarfism 1
    m. primordial dwarfism-cataracts syndrome
microcephalus, imperforate anus, syndactyly, hamartoblastoma, abnormal lung lobulation, polydactyly (MISHAP)
microcephaly, microcephalia
    microcephaly, microphthalmia, ectrodactyly, prognathism (MMEP)
    microcephaly, oculo-digito-esophageal, duodenal (MODED)
    primary m.
    secondary m.
microcephaly-cardiomyopathy syndrome
microcephaly-cervical spine fusion anomalies
microcephaly-chorioretinopathy syndrome
microcephaly-deafness syndrome
microcephaly-digital anomalies syndrome
microcephaly-spastic diplegia syndrome
microcirculation
microcirculatory
    m. compromise
    m. dysfunction
microcolon
microcolpohysteroscope
microcolpohysteroscopy
microcomedone
microcoria
microcornea
microcrania
microcrystalline
    griseofulvin m.
microcurettage
microcurette
    HemoCue m.
microcyst
    milk of calcium m.
microcystica
microcytic anemia
microcytosis
microdactylia (*var. of* microdactyly)
microdactyly, microdactylia
microdeletion
    chromosome m.
    m. of chromosome 22q11
    m. syndrome
microdialysis
microdysgenesis
microembolization
microencephaly
microendoscopic optical catheter
microendoscopy
microenvironment

microfibrillar collagen
microfilament
microflora
    fecal m.
    neonate gut m.
    vaginal m.
microfracture
    vertebral m.
microgastria
microgenitalism
Microgestin
    M. Fe 1/29
    M. Fe 1.5/30
microglandular
    m. adenosis
    m. cervical hyperplasia
    m. dysplasia
microglia
microglobulin
    beta-2 m.
microglossia
micrognathia
    severe m.
micrognathia-glossoptosis syndrome
microgram (mcg)
    m. per kilogram per minute (mcg/kg min)
microgyria
microhamartoma
    biliary m.
microhemagglutination
    m. assay (MHA)
    m. test
microhyphema
Microhysteroflator
microhysteroscope
    Hamou contact m.
microimmunofluorescence (MIF)
    m. test
microimplant
    silicone m.
microinfarct
microinjection
microinvasion
    stromal m.
microinvasive
    m. adenocarcinoma
    m. carcinoma (MICA)
    m. carcinoma classification
    m. cervical cancer (MICA)
Micro-K 10 Extencaps
MicroLap
    M. endoscope
    M. Gold system
microlaparoscopic sterilization
microlaparoscopy
Microline Re-New II 5-mm modular laparoscopic scissors
Microlipid formula

M

microlithiasis
    biliary m.
    pulmonary alveolar m. (PAM)
micromanipulation
    gamete m.
micromanipulator
micromazia
micromelia
micromelic dwarfism
Micro-Mist disposable nebulizer
micromyeloblastic leukemia
Micronase
microneedle
micronized
    m. 17-beta estradiol
    m. progesterone
    m. testosterone
micronodular
    m. gastritis
    m. liver cirrhosis
Micronor
micronutrient deficiency
microorchidism
microorganism
micropapillomatosis labialis
microparticle enzyme immunoassay
micropenis
microperforate hymen
microphallus
microphthalmia, microphthalmus, microphthalmos
    anterior m.
    m., dermal aplasia, sclerocornea (MIDAS)
    m. or anophthalmos with associated anomalies (MAA)
    m. with linear skin defects (MLS)
microphthalmia-arhinia
microphthalmia-mental deficiency syndrome
microphthalmos (*var. of* microphthalmia)
microphthalmus (*var. of* microphthalmia)
micropinocytosis
micropodia
micropolygyria with muscular dystrophy
micropreemie
microprosopus
microretrognathia
microsatellite
    sequence tagged m.
microscope
    H-7000 electron m.
    Zoomscope portable m.
microscopic, microscopical
    m. agglutination test (MAT)
    m. confirmation
    m. examination
    m. fat
    m. polyarteritis

microscopical (*var. of* microscopic)
microscopy
    dark-field m.
    direct m.
    electron m.
    light m.
    phase-contrast m.
    saline m.
    scanning electron m. (SEM)
    transmission electron m. (TEM)
microsomia
    Goldenhar hemifacial m.
    hemifacial m. (HM)
    unilateral facial m.
MicroSpan
    M. microhysteroscopy system
    M. sheath
microspectroscopy
    Fourier transform infrared m.
microsphere
    degradable starch m. (DSM)
    Embosphere m.
    magnetically responsive m.
    perflutren m.
    radioactive m.
microspherocyte
microspherophakia
microsporidial keratoconjunctivitis
Microsporum
    M. audouinii
    M. canis
microstomia
Microstream capnograph
Microsulfon
microsurgery
    distal tubal m.
    endoscopic m.
    laparoscopic m.
    transanal endoscopic m. (TEM)
    tubal m.
    tubocornual m.
microsurgical
    m. epididymal sperm aspiration (MESA)
    m. extraction
    m. extraction of ductal sperm (MEDS)
    m. tubal reanastomosis (MTR)
    m. tubocornual anastomosis
microthelia
microthrombocytopenia
microthromboembolism
microti
    Babesia m.
microtia
    m., absent patellae, micrognathia syndrome
    aural atresia and m.
    unilateral m.

Microtip catheter
MicroTrak test
Micro-Transducer catheter
microtransfusion
    maternal-fetal m.
microtrauma
microvascular
    m. complication
    m. lesion
microvasculopathy
microvesicular steatosis
microvessel
microvilli (*pl. of* microvillus)
microvillus, *pl.* microvilli
    m. atrophy (MVA)
    m. inclusion disease (MID)
microviscometry
microwave endometrial ablation (MEA)
Microzide
micturition
    m. cycle
    diurnal m.
    nocturnal m.
    m. syncope
Midamor
midarm
    m. circumference (MAC)
    m. muscle circumference
      (MAMC)
MIDAS
    microphthalmia, dermal aplasia,
    sclerocornea
    MIDAS syndrome
midaxillary line
midazolam
    m. nasal spray
    transmucosal m.
midbrain
    m. abnormality
    m. herniation
    kinked m.
midclavicular line
midcycle
    m. cervical mucus
    m. spotting
    m. surge
middiastolic
    m. murmur
    m. rumble
middle
    m. adolescence
    m. cerebellar peduncle
    m. cerebral artery (MCA, mCA)
    m. cerebral artery occlusion
      (MCAO)
    m. ear
    m. ear effusion (MEE)
    m. ear fluid (MEF)
    m. ear infection

    m. finger
    m. hypospadias
    m. meatus nasal antral window
    m. sacral artery
    m. third of clavicle fracture
    m. third of face underdevelopment
midface hypoplasia
midfetal testicular regression syndrome
midfoot breech
midforceps
    m. delivery (MFD)
    m. maneuver
midgestational
midgut volvulus
midline
    m. cleft palate
    m. cleft syndrome
    m. craniofacial tumor
    m. episiotomy
    m. facial defect
    m. heart
    m. longitudinal incision
    m. shift
    m. vertical uterine extension
midluteal
    m. phase progesterone level
    m. progesterone measurement
midmenstrual
midodrine
Midol IB
midpain
midparental height
midpelvis
    plane of m.
midplane arrest
midposition uterus
midsecretory
midshaft hypospadias
midstream
    m. catch
    m. urine sample
    m. urine specimen
midsystolic click
midtemporal epilepsy
midtrimester ultrasonographic
  evaluation
midureteral stricture
midurethra
midurethral sling
midvaginal transverse septum
midwife
    American College of Nurse
    Midwives
midwifery
    Licentiate in M. (LM)
Miege disease
Miescher syndrome
Mietens syndrome
Mietens-Weber syndrome

M

MIF
   microimmunofluorescence
   microimmunofluorescence test
   migration inhibitory factor
   müllerian inhibiting factor
   MIF test
Mifeprex
mifepristone
mifepristone-misoprostol
MIGB
   metaiodobenzylguanidine
   MIGB imaging
miglitol
migraine
   abdominal m.
   acute confusional m.
   basilar artery m.
   classic m.
   classical m.
   common m.
   complicated m.
   confusional m.
   m. diet
   familial hemiplegic m. (FHM=)
   footballer's m.
   m. generator
   m. headache
   hemiplegic m.
   menstrual m.
   ophthalmoplegic m.
   m. sine hemicrania
   m. syndrome
   m. variant
   m. with aphasia
   m. with aura
   m. without aura
migraine-type headache
migrainous
   m. attack
   m. headache
migrans
   cutaneous larva m.
   erythema m.
   erythema chronicum m. (ECM)
   larva m.
   ocular larva m.
   visceral larva m.
migration
   cellular m.
   m. index (MI)
   m. inhibitory factor (MIF)
   placental m.
migrational disorder
migratory
   m. path
   m. peripheral arthritis
   m. polyarthritis
MIH
   müllerian inhibiting hormone

MII
   meiosis II
Mikity-Wilson syndrome
Mikulicz
   M. disease
   M. procedure
   M. syndrome
Milch fracture classification
mild
   m. acetabular dysplasia
   m. anemia
   m. anorexia nervosa
   m. dehydration
   m. downslant to palpebral fissure
   m. leukocytosis
   m. mental retardation (MMR)
   m. pulmonic stenosis
   m. scoliosis
   m. spastic diplegic cerebral palsy
   m. ulcerative colitis
   m. X-linked recessive muscular
     dystrophy
mild-to-moderate obesity
Miles
   M. Nervine caplet
   M. syndrome
Miles-Carpenter syndrome (MCS)
milestone
   anticipated behavioral m.
   anticipated developmental m.
   behavioral m.
   cognitive developmental m.
   developmental m.
   Early Language M. (ELM)
   emotional m.
   fine motor m.
   gross motor m.
   language m.
   motor m.
   puberal m.
   social m.
   social-adaptive m.
Milex
   M. cervical cup
   M. incontinence ring
   M. spatula
   M. syringe sampler
milia (*pl. of* milium)
miliaria
   apocrine m.
   crystallina m.
   m. crystalloid
   m. profunda
   m. pustulosa
   m. rubra
   sebaceous m.
   sudoral m.
miliary
   m. calcified necrosis

m. infiltrate
m. sudamina
m. tuberculosis

milieu
endometrial m.
m. therapy

military
m. antishock trousers (MAST)
m. presentation

milium, *pl.* **milia**
milia neonatorum

milk
m. abscess
m. allergy
atomic m.
m. bank
banked breast m. (BBM)
m. bolus obstruction
breast m.
m. composition
m. cyst
donor human m.
m. ejection
m. ejection reflex
evaporated m.
expressed m.
m. fat globule (MFG)
m. fat globule membrane (MFGM)
fatty m.
m. fever
fluorescein-labeled m.
frozen m.
hind m.
human m. (HM)
hydrolyzed cow's m.
icterogenic breast m.
incontinence of m.
Lactaid fat-free m.
Lactaid reduced fat m.
m. leg
m. letdown
m. line
m. lines of abdomen
m. lines of thorax
maternal breast m.
mother's breast m. (MBM)
nonfat m.
nuclear m.
m. of calcium bile
m. of calcium microcyst
m. of magnesia (MOM)
m. precipitin disease
preterm m.
m. production
m. protein hydrolysate (MPH)
m. protein intolerance
m. scan
soy m.
m. stool

m. supply
term m.
m. thistle
m. tooth
m. triglyceride
unfortified human m.
uterine m.
volume percent of cream in m.
witch's m.

milk-alkali syndrome
milk-based formula
milk-bottle teeth caries
milk-fed
human m.-f.
milking
m. of umbilical cord
m. of urethra
milkmaid's
m. grip
m. hand
m. sign
milk-plasma ratio
milk-protein allergy
milk/soy-protein allergy
milky fluid
Millar microtransducer urethral catheter
Millen-Read modification
Miller
M. Assessment for Preschoolers
M. blade (#0, #1)
M. ovum
M. syndrome
Miller-Abbott tube
Miller-Dieker
M.-D. lissencephaly syndrome
(MDLS)
M.-D. syndrome
Miller-Fisher variant of Guillain-Barré syndrome
milleri
Streptococcus m.
milliampere (mA)
milliequivalent (mEq, meq)
m. per liter (mEq/L)
milligram (mg)
m. percent (mg%)
millijoule (mJ)
milliliter (ml, mL)
million
parts per m. (ppm, PPM)
Millipore filter
millirad (mrad)
milliroentgen (mR)
millivolt (mV)
mill wheel murmur
milrinone
Milroy disease
MILTA
mucosal intact laser tonsillar ablation

M

Miltex disposable biopsy punch
Miltown
Milwaukee brace
MIM
    Mendelian Inheritance in
    Man
Mima polymorpha
Mi-Mark
    M.-M. disposable endocervical
      curette
    M.-M. endocervical curette set
    M.-M. endometrial curette set
mimetic labor
mimicry
    antigenic m.
    molecular m.
Mims
MIMyCA
    maternally inherited myopathy and
      cardiomyopathy
    MIMyCA syndrome
MimyX cream
Minamata disease
mind
    theory of m.
mind-body
    m.-b. intervention
    m.-b. therapy
mineral
    m. balance study
    bone m.
    m. metabolism
    m. oil (M-O)
    m. requirement
mineralization
    bone tissue m.
    skeletal m.
mineralizing microangiopathy
mineralocorticoid
mineralocorticoid-deficiency RTA
mineralocorticosteroid
Minesse
M2 inhibitor
mini
    m. fluoroscopy
    m. Vidas automated immunoassay
      system
MiniArc single incision sling system
miniature hypoplasia
minicore myopathy
minidose heparin
Mini-Flex
    M.-F. flexible Harris uterine
      injector
    HUI M.-F.
miniform
miniguard
    M. CO$_2$ sensor
    M. Patch

minilaparoscope
    Aslan 2-mm m.
    Pixie m.
minilaparotomy
minimal
    m. acceptable height (MAH)
    m. bacterial concentration (MBC)
    m. brain damage
    m. brain dysfunction (MBD)
    m. cerebral dysfunction
    m. change nephrotic syndrome
      (MCNS)
    m. deviation adenocarcinoma
    m. effective analgesic concentration
      (MEAC)
    m. effective dose (MED)
    m. inhibitory concentration (MIC)
    m. lesion nephrotic syndrome
      (MLNS)
minimal-change disease (MCD)
minimal-incision pubovaginal suspension
minimally invasive surgical technique
(MIST)
minimal-stimulation in vitro fertilization
MiniMed continuous glucose monitoring
system
Mini-Med tubing
minimum
    m. daily requirement (MDR)
    m. inhibitory concentration (MIC)
    m. lethal dose (MLD)
MiniOX I, II, III, 100-IV oxygen
monitor
mini-Pena procedure
minipill
Minipress
minisatellite
MiniSite laparoscope
Minitran Patch
Mini-Wright Peak Flow Meter
Minizide
Minkowski-Chauffard syndrome
Minnesota
    M. Multiphasic Personality Inventory
      (MMPI)
    M. Multiphasic Personality
      Inventory-Adolescent (MMPI-A)
Minocin IV injection
minocycline
minor
    m. cerebral dysfunction
    chorea m.
    m. depressive disorder
    m. dysmorphism
    emancipated m.
    m. group antigen incompatibility
    m. motor seizure
    pelvis m.
    pelvis justo m.

thalassemia m.
m. vestibular gland duct
Minot disease
Minot-von Willebrand syndrome
minoxidil
Mintezol
minus
labium m.
Spirillum m.
minute
beats per m. (BPM, bpm)
breaths per m. (BPM, bpm)
liters per m. (L/M, L/min)
microgram per kilogram per m.
(mcg/kg min)
oxygen consumption per m. (VO_2,
Vo_2, VO_2max)
m. oxygen uptake
m. ventilatory volume
minutissimum
Corynebacterium m.
Miocarpine
Miochol-E
miodidymus, miodymus
miodymus (*var. of* miodidymus)
miopus
miosis
congenital m.
ipsilateral m.
Miostat
miotic division
MIP
macrophage inflammatory protein
MIP-1a
macrophage inflammatory protein-1
alpha
mirabilis
Proteus m.
Miradon
MiraLax
Miraluma test
Mircette tablet
Mirena
M. intrauterine device
M. IUD
Mirhosseini-Holmes-Walton syndrome
mirror
m. duplication
m. image breast biopsy
m. image interpretation
m. laryngoscopy
pharyngeal m.
m. syndrome
mirror-image dextrocardia
misarticulation
misbehavior
miscarriage
missed m.
recurrent m. (REMIS)

spontaneous m.
threatened m.
unexplained recurrent m.
miscarry
MISHAP
microcephalus, imperforate anus,
syndactyly, hamartoblastoma, abnormal
lung lobulation, polydactyly
MISHAP syndrome
mismatch
ventilation/perfusion m.
Ì V/Ì Q m.
misonidazole
misoprostol
oral m.
vaginal m.
mispairing
MISS
Modified Injury Severity Score
missed
m. abortion
m. labor
m. miscarriage
m. period
missense mutation
missing teeth
Mission
M. Prenatal F.A.
M. Prenatal H.P.
M. Prenatal Rx
missionary position
MIST
minimally invasive surgical technique
mist
Ayr saline nasal m.
child-adult m. (CAM)
hood m.
Ocean Nasal M.
Primatene M.
m. tent
m. therapy
MISU
Maternal Interview of Substance Use
mite
dust m.
house dust m.
m. infestation
itch m.
scabies m.
Mitex GII mini anchor
Mithracin
mithramycin
mitis
Streptococcus m.
m. type Ehlers-Danlos syndrome
mitochondria (*pl. of* mitochondrion)
mitochondrial
m. chromosome
m. cytopathy

M

mitochondrial (*continued*)
  m. deoxyribonucleic acid (mtDNA)
  m. disease
  m. disorder
  m. DNA (mtDNA)
  m. encephalomyelopathy
  m. encephalomyopathy
  m. encephalopathy
  m. encephalopathy, lactic acidosis, stroke
  m. function
  m. glycine cleavage system
  m. inheritance
  m. injury
  m. myopathy
  m. myopathy and sideroblastic anemia (MLASA)
  m. myopathy, encephalopathy, lactic acidosis, strokelike episodes (MELAS)
  m. oxidative phosphorylation
  m. respiratory chain defect
mitochondrion, *pl.* **mitochondria**
  abnormal m.
mitogen
  m. activated protein kinase inhibitor
  pokeweed m. (PWM)
mitogenic
  m. activity
  m. effect
  m. peptide
mitomycin C
mitoplasm
mitoses (*pl. of* mitosis)
mitosis, *pl.* **mitoses**
  crypt cell m.
  m. phase
mitosis-promoting factor (MPF)
mitotane
mitotic
  m. chromosome
  m. figure
mitoxantrone (DHAD, M, MITOX, MTZ)
  m. hydrochloride
MITP
  maternal idiopathic thrombocytopenic purpura
mitral
  m. arcade
  m. commissurotomy
  m. regurgitation
  m. stenosis
  m. valve
  m. valve, aorta, skeleton, skin (MASS)
  m. valve atresia
  m. valve disease

  m. valve insufficiency
  m. valve prolapse (MVP)
Mitrofanoff
  M. appendicovesicostomy
  M. continent urinary diversion technique
  M. principle
Mitsuda reaction
mittelschmerz
mitten
  m. hand
  m. hand deformity
Mittendorf dot
Mittendorf-Williams rule
Mityvac
  M. obstetric vacuum extractor cup
  M. reusable vacuum pump
  M. Super M cup
  M. vacuum delivery system
  M. vacuum extractor
Mivacron
mivacurium
mix
  CeraLyte drink m.
  Metamucil Instant M.
mixed
  m. agglutination reaction (MAR)
  m. antiinflammatory syndrome (MARS)
  m. cellularity Hodgkin disease
  m. cerebral palsy
  m. connective tissue disease (MCTD)
  m. cystic/solid architecture
  m. flexor/extensor fit
  m. germ cell tumor
  m. gonadal dysgenesis (MGD)
  m. hearing impairment
  m. hearing loss
  m. hyperlipidemia
  m. hypothyroidism
  m. incontinence
  m. infantile spasm
  m. iron and folate deficiency anemia
  m. lymphocyte reaction blocking factor
  m. mesodermal sarcoma (MMS)
  m. mesodermal tumor
  m. müllerian mesodermal tumor (MMMT)
  m. müllerian sarcoma
  m. müllerian tumor (MMT)
  m. obstructive apnea/hypopnea index (MOAHI)
  m. ovarian mesodermal sarcoma
  m. pattern
  m. porphyria

m. receptive-expressive language
disorder (MRELD)
m. sensory polyneuritis
m. sleep apnea
m. TAPVR
m. umbilical arterial acidemia
m. uterine tumor
m. venous oxygen content
mixed-density mass
mixed-type cerebral palsy
mixing lesion
mixoploid
mixoploidy
diploid/tetraploid m.
diploid/triploid m.
Mixtard
Miya hook ligature carrier
Miyazaki-Bonney
M.-B. test
M.-B. test for stress incontinence
Miyazaki technique
mizoribine
mJ
millijoule
MKHS
Menkes kinky-hair syndrome
ML
mucolipidosis
mL
milliliter
MLASA
mitochondrial myopathy and
sideroblastic anemia
MLASA syndrome
MLD
metachromatic leukodystrophy
minimum lethal dose
juvenile MLD
late infantile MLD
ML-II
mucolipidosis II
ML-III
mucolipidosis III
MLNS
minimal lesion nephrotic syndrome
mucocutaneous lymph node
syndrome
MLS
microphthalmia with linear skin
defects
MLU
mean length of utterance
MLUm
mean length of utterance in
morphemes
MM
malignant mesothelioma
MMA
methylmalonic aciduria

MMEP
microcephaly, microphthalmia,
ectrodactyly, prognathism
MMEP syndrome
MMIH
megacystis
MMIH syndrome
MMII
maternal meiosis II
MMK
Marshall-Marchetti-Krantz
MMK colposuspension
MMK retropubic cystourethropexy
suspension procedure
MMMM
megalocornea
MMMT
malignant mixed müllerian tumor
mixed müllerian mesodermal
tumor
M-mode
M-m. analysis
M-m. display
M-m. echocardiogram
M-m. echocardiography
M-m. echogram
M-m. imaging
M-m. ultrasound
MMPI
Minnesota Multiphasic Personality
Inventory
MMPI-A
Minnesota Multiphasic Personality
Inventory-Adolescent
MMR
maternal mortality rate
measles, mumps, rubella
megalocornea-mental retardation
syndrome
mild mental retardation
mouth-to-mouth resuscitation
MMR II vaccine
MMR immunization
MMR vaccine
MMS
mixed mesodermal sarcoma
MMT
mixed müllerian tumor
MMT syndrome
MNBCC
multiple nevoid-basal cell carcinoma
MNBCC syndrome
M-O
mineral oil
Haley's M-O
MOAHI
mixed obstructive apnea/hypopnea
index
Moban

M

Mobenol
Mobidin
mobile hyperechogenic material
mobility
m. aid
bladder neck m.
m. disability
Q-tip test for determining
urethral m.
m. specialist
mobilization
gastric m.
tarsometatarsal m.
Mobitz (I, II) block
Mobius retractor
Möbius
M. anomaly
M. sequence
M. syndrome
modafinil acetamide
modality
Modane Bulk
mode
delivery m.
multiplanar display m.
polygenic m.
pressure support m.
transparency m.
Modecate
MODED
microcephaly, oculo-digito-esophageal,
duodenal
model
APLS m.
cognitive-diathesis m.
Cox proportional hazard m.
Duluth m.
Gail breast cancer m.
Gail risk assessment m.
genetic m.
Gesell Developmental M.
Kaplan m.
Knudson 2-hit genetic m.
pathologic m.
random regression m.
Rossavik growth m.
statistical m.
modeling
generalized linear interactive m.
(GLIM)
moderate
m. dehydration
m. hirsutism
m. mental retardation
m. ulcerative colitis
modern genetics
Modicon
modification
behavior m.

Burch m.
Gesell test with Knobloch m.
Martin m.
Millen-Read m.
posttranslational m.
modified
m. Bagshawe protocol (MBP)
m. barium swallow (MBS)
m. barium swallow with
videofluoroscopy
m. Beighton criteria
m. biophysical profile (MBPP)
m. Blalock-Taussig shunt
m. bovine surfactant extract
m. BPP
m. Burch colpourethropexy
m. Dieterle stain
m. Fontan operation
m. Fontan procedure
m. Gomori trichrome reaction
m. Ham F-10 solution
M. Injury Severity Score
(MISS)
m. Irving-type tubal ligation
m. Kinyoun acid-fast stain
m. measles
m. Pomeroy tubal ligation
technique
m. radical hysterectomy
m. radical mastectomy
m. Ritgen fetal head delivery
maneuver
m. Roeder
m. Roeder knot
m. Shirodkar cerclage
m. sling
m. trichrome stain
m. Zavanelli maneuver
modifier
biologic response m. (BRM)
leukotriene m.
Moditen
MODM
maturity-onset diabetes
MODS
multiorgan dysfunction syndrome
multiple organ dysfunction syndrome
Moducal formula
modulation
antigenic m.
cardiac autonomic m.
sex steroid m.
modulator
benzothiophene-derived selective
estrogen receptor m.
cytokine m.
immune m.
selective estrogen receptor m.
(SERM)

triphenylethylene selective estrogen receptor m.

MODY
maturity-onset diabetes of young
maturity-onset diabetes of youth
Moeller-Barlow disease
mofetil
mycophenolate m.
Mogen
M. circumcision
M. clamp
Mohr-Claussen syndrome
Mohr syndrome
Mohr-Tranebjaerg syndrome (MTS)
MOI
maximal oxygen intake
medical optimal imaging
multiplicity of infection
moiety
moist
Nasal M.
moisture
vaginal m.
moisturizer
Vagisil intimate m.
molar
m. degeneration
m. destruens
m. evacuation
first permanent m.
first primary m.
hutchinsonian m.
Moon m.'s
mulberry m.
permanent m.
m. pregnancy
primary m.
second permanent m.
second primary m.
third permanent m.
mold
Counsellor vaginal m.
m. spore
molding of head
mole
amniography in hydatidiform m.
blood m.
Breus m.
carneous m.
complete hydatidiform m.
cystic m.
false m.
fleshy m.
grape m.
hydatid m.
hydatidiform m.
invasive m.
invasive hydatidiform m.

partial hydatidiform m.
penetrating m.
prior complete m.
prior partial m.
repeated complete m.
tuberous m.
vesicular m.
molecular
m. adsorbent recirculating system (MARS)
m. clone
m. expansion
m. genetic analysis
m. genetic study
m. genetic technique
m. mimicry
m. regulation
molecule
adhesion m.
cell adhesion m. (CAM)
inflammatory m.
intercellular adhesion m. 1 (ICAM1)
soluble intercellular adhesion m. 1
vascular cell adhesion m. (VCAM)
molestation
sexual m.
molimina
menstrual m.
molindone
Mol-Iron
Moll
apocrine gland of M.
M. gland
Mollaret meningitis
Mollica-Pavone-Anterer syndrome
Mollica syndrome
Mollifene Ear Wax Removing Formula
Mollison formula
molluscum
m. contagiosum
m. contagiosum of vulva
m. contagiosum virus (MCV)
m. fibrosum
m. fibrosum gravidarum
m. fibrosum pendulum
Staphylococcus aureus m.
molybdenum
m. cofactor
m. cofactor deficiency (MCD)
m. rotating anode x-ray tube
Molypen
MOM
milk of magnesia
mucoid otitis media
MoM
multiples of median

M

mometasone
    m. furoate
    m. furoate aqueous nasal spray
      (MFNS)
MOMO
    macrosomia, obesity, macrocephaly,
    ocular
    MOMO abnormality
    MOMO syndrome
MOMP gene
MOMX
    macroorchidism-marker X
    MOMX syndrome
Monafed
Monaghan respirator
monamine (*var. of* monoamine)
Monarc subfascial hammock
monarticular arthritis
Monday morning colic
Mondini
    M. anomaly
    M. aplasia
Mondor disease
money spot
mongolian
    m. idiot
    m. spot
mongolism
mongoloid
    m. features
    m. slant
monilia
monilial
    m. diaper dermatitis
    m. diaper rash
    m. esophagitis
    m. vaginitis
moniliasis
    oral m.
moniliform hair
moniliformis
    Streptobacillus m.
Monistat
    M. 1 combination pack vaginal
    insert
    M. 1 1-day vaginal ointment
    M. Dual-Pak
    M. I.V.
    M. Vaginal
    M. 3 vaginal cream
    M. 3 vaginal cream combination
    pack
    M. 3 vaginal suppository
Monistat-Derm Topical
monitor
    Accu-Chek Easy glucose m.
    Accu-Chek II Freedom blood
    glucose m.
    Aequitron 9200 apnea m.

antepartum m. (APM)
apnea m.
Arvee Medical model 2400 infant
  apnea m.
Baby Dopplex 3000 antepartum
  fetal m.
Baby Sense m.
BASC m.
Behavior Assessment System for
  Children m.
blood pressure m.
CA m.
Camino m.
cardiac-apnea m.
cardiac event m.
cardiorespiratory m.
cerebral function m. (CFM)
ClearPlan Easy fertility m.
Corometrics fetal m.
Corometrics 118 maternal/fetal m.
Cue Fertility M.
Dinamap blood pressure m.
Endotek UDS-1000 m.
event m.
Fetal Dopplex m.
fetal heart rate m.
FetalPulse Plus m.
Finapres blood pressure m.
Healthdyne apnea m.
Holter m.
home cardiorespiratory m. (HCRM)
home uterine activity m. (HUAM)
Imex antepartum m.
intrapartum m.
Ladd m.
Masimo SET home m.
MiniOX I, II, III, 100-IV oxygen
  m.
Nellcor N-499 fetal oxygen
  saturation m.
Nellcor N-200 home m.
Nellcor N-3000 home m.
Nellcor Puritan Bennett home m.
Nellcor Puritan Bennett oxygen
  saturation m.
neonatal m.
Neotrend premature infant blood
  gas/temperature m.
NOxBOX+ m.
NOxBOXmobile m.
Omron m.
peak flow meter m.
Pocket-Dop 3 m.
Press-Mate model 8800T blood
  pressure m.
ProDynamic m.
Propaq Encore vital signs m.
QuietTrak m.
Quik Connect fetal m.

Tokos m.
transcutaneous blood gas m.
uterine activity m.
VersaLab APM2 portable antepartum m.
Viasys Doppler and antepartum m.
virtual labor m. (VLM)
VitaGuard m.
monitored anesthesia care (MAC)
monitoring
ambulatory m.
ambulatory blood pressure m. (ABPM)
ambulatory urodynamic m. (AUM)
beat-to-beat continuous blood pressure m.
blood sugar m.
cardiac m.
central m.
continuous blood gas m.
continuous fetal heart m.
continuous long-term m. (CLTM)
contraction m.
critical care m.
distal esophageal pH m.
domiciliary m.
EEG/polygraphic/video m.
electronic fetal m. (EFM)
electronic fetal heart rate m.
end-tidal CO_2 m.
esophageal impedance m.
external fetal m. (EFM)
fetal heart rate m.
fetal oximetry m.
fetal scalp m.
glucose m.
heart rate m.
hemodynamic m.
home blood glucose m.
home uterine m. (HUM)
home uterine activity m. (HUAM)
ICP m.
inpatient m.
internal m.
intracranial pressure m.
intrapartum fetal m.
intrauterine fetal m.
invasive hemodynamic m.
jugular bulb m.
prolonged EEG m.
pulmonary artery pressure m.
tactile sensory m.
tissue pH m.
transcutaneous blood gas m.
transcutaneous oxygen tension m.
transtelephonic m. (TTM)
video m.
monitrice
monkeybars

monkey polyoma virus
monk's pepper
mono
monocyte
mononucleosis
monoamine (MAO), monamine
m. oxidase (MAO)
m. oxidase A deficiency
m. oxidase inhibitor (MAOI)
m. oxidase type A (MAO-A, MAOA)
monoaminergic
monoamnionicity
monoamniotic
m. sac
m. twins
monoarticular synovitis
monobactam
monobrachius
monocaprin
monocephalus
monochorial twins
monochorionic
m. diamniotic placenta
m. gestation
m. monoamniotic placenta
m. placentation
m. twin pregnancy
m. twins
monochorionic-diamniotic
m.-d. gestation
m.-d. twins
monochromatism
blue cone m.
pi cone m.
Monoclate-P
monoclonal
m. antibody (MAB, MAb)
m. antibody coagglutination test
m. antibody therapy
m. antiendotoxin antibody
m. anti-IgE antibody
monoclonic seizure
monocranius
Monocryl suture
monocular
m. diplopia
m. nystagmus
monocyte
monocytogenes
Listeria m.
monocytopenia
monocytosis
monodactylism (*var. of* monodactyly)
monodactyly, monodactylism
monodermal tumor
Monodox
monoecious
monofactorial inheritance
monofluorophosphate

M

monogamous
monogamy
monogenic disorder
Mono-Gesic
monoglutamate
monohybrid cross
monohydrate
    cefadroxil m.
    doxycycline m.
    lactose m.
    m. macrocrystal
    nitrofurantoin m.
monokine
monolaurin
monomelic
monomorphous papular eruption
mononeuritis
    m. multiplex
    m. with paralysis
mononeuropathies
    multiple m.
mononeuropathy
    peripheral m.
Mononine
mononuclear
    m. phagocyte
    m. pleocytosis
mononucleosis (mono)
    infectious m. (IM)
mononucleosis-type syndrome
4-monooxygenase
    phenylalanine 4-m.
monophasic
    m. oral contraceptive
    m. regimen
monophonic wheeze
monophosphate
    adenosine m. (AMP)
    cyclic adenosine m. (cAMP)
    cyclic guanosine m. (cGMP)
    cytidine m.
monoplegia
    spastic m.
monoploid
monopodia
monopolar cautery
MonoPrep Pap test
monops
monopus
monorchid (*var. of* monorchidic)
monorchidic, monorchid
monosialoganglioside
monosodium glutamate poisoning
monosome
monosomy
    m. 1–22
    autosomal m.
    chromosome 1p–22p m.
    chromosome 1q–22q m.

chromosome Xp21 m.
chromosome Xq m.
    m. G
    m. G syndrome
    m. 1p–22p
    m. 1p36 syndrome
    m. 11q23
    m. 22q13,3 deletion syndrome
    m. 7 syndrome
    m. X
    m. Xp21
    m. Xp22
    m. Xq
Monospot
    M. screen
    M. test
Monosticon
    M. Dri-Dot
    M. Dri-Dot test
monostotic
Mono-Sure
monosymptomatic delusional pseudocyesis
Mono-Test
monotherapy
    digoxin m.
    zidovudine m.
monotonically
Mono-Vacc Test (O.T.)
monovular twins
monoxide
    carbon m. (CO)
    diffusing capacity of lung for carbon m. (DLCO, DL_{co})
    end-tidal breath carbon m.
monozygosity
monozygotic twins
monozygous
Monro
    foramen of M.
Monro-Kellie doctrine of intracranial pressure
mons
    m. pubis
    m. veneris
Monsel
    M. gel
    M. paste
    M. solution
monsplasty
monster
    m. cell
    hair m.
monstrosity
Montefiore syndrome
Monteggia
    M. fracture
    M. fracture dislocation
montelukast

Montenegro skin test
Montevideo unit
Montgomery
    M. County virus
    M. gland
    M. strap
    M. tubercle
monthly fecundity rate (MFR)
Monurol
mood
    m. disorder
    dysphoric m.
    m. fluctuation
    m. lability
    m. state
mood-congruent psychotic
  features
moodiness
moon
    m. facies
    M. molars
    M. teeth
moon-shaped facies
Moore-Federman syndrome
Morand foot
Moraxella catarrhalis
morbidity
    m. and mortality
    antenatal m.
    asthma m.
    childbirth-related m.
    febrile m.
    fetal m.
    infant m.
    maternal febrile m.
    neonatal m.
    perinatal m.
    postpartum febrile m.
    m. predictor
    puerperal febrile m.
morbilliform
    m. eruption
    m. skin rash
Morbillivirus
morbillorum
    Gemella m.
morcellation, morcellement
    electromechanical m.
    m. operation
    uterine m.
    vaginal m.
morcellator
    Diva laparoscopic m.
    motorized m.
    OPERA Star m.
    Steiner electromechanical m.
morcellement (*var. of* morcellation)
morcellize, morselize
Morch respirator

More-Dophilus acidophilus powder
Morel ear
Morgagni
    anterior retrosternal hernia of M.
    foramen of M.
    M. hernia
    hydatid cyst of M.
    M. tubercle
Morgagni-Adams-Stokes syndrome
morgagnian
Morgagni-Turner-Albright syndrome
Morgagni-Turner syndrome
Morganella morganii
morganii
    Morganella m.
    Proteus m.
Morgan therapeutic lens
moribund
moricizine
Morison pouch
morning
    m. glory disc anomaly
    m. glory syndrome
    m. osmolality
    m. sickness
morning-after
    m.-a. contraception
    m.-a. pill
Moro
    M. reflex
    M. response
Moro-Heisler diet
morphea
morpheme
    mean length of utterance in m.'s
    (MLUm)
morphine
    epidural m.
    m. sulfate
morphogen
morphogenesis
    branching m.
    lung m.
    parenchymal lung m.
morphogenetic lesion
morphologic, morphological
    m. assessment
    m. data
morphological
    m. characteristic
    m. sex
morphology
    adrenal gland m.
    endometrial m.
    kidney m.
    m. of breast cancer
morphometric
morphometrics
    body m.

M

Morquio
    M. disease
    M. syndrome
Morquio-Brailsford
    M.-B. disease
    M.-B. syndrome
Morquio-Ullrich
    M.-U. disease
    M.-U. syndrome
Morrow
    M. myotomy-myectomy
    M. procedure
morselize (*var. of* morcellize)
mortality
    anesthesia-related maternal m.
    m. data
    fetal m.
    high-altitude perinatal m.
    infant m.
    maternal m.
    morbidity and m.
    neonatal m. (NNM)
    Pediatric Risk of M.
     (PRISM)
    perinatal m. (PM)
    postneonatal m.
    m. predictor
    prenatal m.
    m. rate
    reproductive m.
    m. risk factor
mortiferum
    Fusobacterium m.
mortise view
morula
MOS
    medical optical spectroscopy
mosaic
    m. aneuploidy
    gene m.
    m. pattern
    m. perfusion
    m. tetrasomy 8p syndrome
    m. translocation
    m. trisomy 14
    Turner m.
    m. Turner syndrome
    m. verruca
mosaicism
    chromosomal m.
    erythrocyte m.
    m. for XXX
    germ cell m.
    germ line m.
    gonadal m.
    low-grade m.
    placental m.
    somatic m.
    trisomy 8 m.

    Turner m.
    45,X/46,XY m.
Moschcowitz
    M. culdoplasty procedure
    M. fashion
Moschowitz culdoplasty
MOSF
    multiple-organ system failure
***mos* protooncogene**
moss
    M. classification
    M. tube
mossy fiber sprouting
Mosteller method
mothball
    naphthalene m.
mother
    m. and baby endoscope
    m. burnout
    diabetic m.
    Du-positive m.
    gestational m.
    high-risk m.
    hysteric m.
    infant of diabetic m. (IDM)
    infant of substance-abusing m.
     (ISAM)
    Rh-negative m.
    rubella-immune m.
    rubella-negative m.
    serology-negative m.
    surrogate m.
    m. wort
Mother2Be
    M. breast nourishing cream
    M. nipple restoration cream
mother-child interaction
motherese speech
motherhood
    surrogate gestational m.
mother-infant
    m.-i. bonding
    m.-i. transmission
mother's breast milk (MBM)
moth patch
motif
motile sperm (MS)
motilin receptor agonist
motility
    altered gastric m.
    decreased gastrointestinal m.
    m. disorder
    gut m.
    intestinal m.
    ocular m.
    receptor for hyaluronan-mediated m.
     (RHAMM)
    sperm m.
motility-related dysphagia

motion
    active range of m. (AROM)
    m. artifact rejection system (MARS)
    chest wall m.
    early cardiac m.
    embryonic heart m. (EHM)
    fetal cardiac m. (FCM)
    limb m.
    limited neck m.
    paradoxical chest wall m.
    passive range of m.
    range of m. (ROM)
    scapulothoracic m.
    m. sickness
motion-resistant pulse oximetry
motoneuron (*var. of* motor neuron)
motor
    m. automatism
    m. block
    m. control
    m. cortex
    m. disability
    m. evoked potential (MEP)
    fine m.
    gross m.
    m. hyperactivity
    m. milestone
    m. nerve
    m. neuron
    m. neuron disease
    m. neuron palsy
    m. neuron sign
    oral m.
    m. pattern
    m. perception
    m. perception dysfunction
    m. planning
    m. restlessness
    m. scale
    m. seizure
    m. sensory neuropathy (MSN)
    m. skill
    m. tic
    m. unit action potential (MUAP)
motor-axonal neuropathy
motorized morcellator
motor-sensory neuropathy, X-linked type II, with deafness and mental retardation
Motrin
    Children's M.
    Ibu-Tab Junior Strength M.
    Junior Strength M.
MOTT
    mycobacteria other than tuberculosis
mottled
    m. enamel
    m. retina
mottling of skin

mount
    chest m.
    direct wet m.
    wet m.
mountain sickness
mouse
    peritoneal m.
mousse
    Rid M.
mouth
    m. breathing
    carp m.
    carp-like m.
    downturned m.
    fish-shaped m.
    m. guard
    inverted V m.
    open m.
    purse-string m.
    tapir m.
    trench m.
Mouth-Aid
    Orajel M.-A.
mouth-and-hand synkinesia
mouthing
mouthpiece
mouth-to-mask breathing
mouth-to-mouth resuscitation (MMR)
mouth-to-nose/mouth resuscitation
mouthwash
    magic m.
Movat stain
movement
    adventitious choreiform m.
    angular m.
    athetoid m.
    bicycling m.
    cardinal m.
    chaotic eye m.
    choreic m.
    choreiform m.
    choreoathetoid m.
    choreoathetotic m.
    circumduction m.
    clonic m.
    compensatory m.
    dancing eye m.
    deviant volitional m.
    dissociated m.
    equal ocular m. (EOM)
    extraocular m. (EOM)
    extrapyramidal m.
    eye m.
    fetal body m.
    fetal breathing m. (FBM)
    gliding m.
    hand-to-mouth m.
    hand-wringing m.
    involuntary m.

M

movement (*continued*)
    irregular stereotyped m.
    maternal assessment of fetal m.
    multifocal clonic m.
    nonrapid eye m. (NREM)
    opposition m.
    pedaling m.
    rapid alternating m.
    rapid eye m. (REM)
    rapid succession m.
    reciprocal m.
    respiratory m.
    rotation m.
    sleep with rapid eye m.
    sound-stimulated fetal m.
    stereotypical m.
    swimming m.
    symmetrical m.
    tonic-clonic m.
    unifocal clonic m.
    vibroacoustic-induced
      fetal m.
    volitional m.
moxa herb
moxalactam disodium
moxibustion
moyamoya
    m. disease
    m. syndrome
Moynahan alopecia syndrome
Mozart ear
MP
    menstrual period
MPA
    medroxyprogesterone acetate
MPF
    maturation-promoting factor
    mitosis-promoting factor
MPGN
    membranoproliferative
      glomerulonephritis
    mesangiocapillary glomerulonephritis
    (type I, II)
MPH
    male pseudohermaphroditism
    methylphenidate
    milk protein hydrolysate
M-phase-promoting factor
MPHD
    multiple pituitary hormone
    deficiency
MPIAS
    multiparameter intraarterial sensor
MPJ
    metacarpophalangeal joint
    metatarsophalangeal joint
MPO
    myeloperoxidase
    MPO deficiency

MPQ
    Multidimensional Personality
    Questionnaire
MPR
    multifetal pregnancy reduction
    multiple pregnancy reduction
MPS
    mucopolysaccharide
    mucopolysaccharidosis
    myofascial pain syndrome
MPT
    multipuncture test
MPV
    mean platelet volume
MR
    medial rotation
mR
    milliroentgen
MRA
    magnetic resonance angiography
mrad
    millirad
MRC
    magnetic resonance cholangiography
MRCP
    magnetic resonance
      cholangiopancreatography
      MRCP using HASTE with a
        phased array coil
mrd
    millirad
MRE
    magnetic resonance elastography
MRELD
    mixed receptive-expressive language
    disorder
MRI
    magnetic resonance imaging
      diffuse tensor brain MRI
      functional MRI (fMRI)
      GRASS MRI
      Siemens Vision MRI
      ultrafast MRI
MRM
    magnetic resonance mammography
mRNA
    messenger ribonucleic acid
    messenger RNA
      posttranslational modification of
        mRNA
MRS
    magnetic resonance spectroscopy
      phosphorus MRS
      proton MRS
MRSA
    methicillin-resistant *Staphylococcus aureus*
MRU
    magnetic resonance urography

MS
    mass spectrometry
    motile sperm
    multiple sclerosis
        acute MS
        MS Contin
        MS Contin Oral
MSAF
    meconium-stained amniotic fluid
MSAFP
    maternal serum alpha-fetoprotein
MSBP
    Münchausen syndrome by proxy
MSD
    multiple sulfatase deficiency
        MSD Enteric Coated ASA
MSEL
    Mullen Scales of Early Learning
MSH
    melanocortin-stimulating hormone
MSI
    magnetic source imaging
MSIR Oral
MSK
    musculoskeletal
MSLSS
    Multidimensional Student Life
    Satisfaction Scale
MSLT
    multiple sleep latency test
MSN
    motor sensory neuropathy
        MSN syndrome
MSOAP
    medications, monitors, suction, oxygen,
    airway equipment, personnel
MSP
    Münchausen syndrome by proxy
MSPS
    musculoskeletal pain syndrome
MSPSS
    Multidimensional Scale of Perceived
    Social Support
MSS
    Marshall-Smith syndrome
MSSB
    MacArthur Story Stem Battery
MST
    multiple subpial transection
    multisystemic therapy
M-Style Mushroom vacuum cup
MSUD
    maple syrup urine disease
3M syndrome
MT
     Pancrease MT
MTC
    multilocular thymic cyst
^{99m}Tc-HMPAO leukocyte scan

mtDNA
    mitochondrial deoxyribonucleic acid
    mitochondrial DNA
M.T.E.-4, -5, -6
MTF
    male-to-female
        MTF medical management
MTHFR
    methylene tetrahydrofolate reductase
        MTHFR gene
        MTHFR thermolability
MTMX
    X-linked myotubular myopathy
MTR
    microsurgical tubal reanastomosis
M-tropic
    macrophage tropic
        M-tropic strain
MTS
    mesial temporal sclerosis
    Mohr-Tranebjaerg syndrome
MTT
    medial tibial torsion
MTX
    methotrexate
M-type extractor
MUAP
    motor unit action potential
Mucat
     M. cervical sampling
     M. cervical sampling device
Mucha-Habermann disease
mucin clot test
mucinous
     m. adenocarcinoma
     m. cancer
     m. carcinoma
     m. cystadenocarcinoma
     m. cystadenoma
     m. ovarian neoplasm
     m. patch
     m. tumor
mucociliary
     m. clearance
     m. function
mucocolpos
mucocutaneous
     m. bleeding
     m. candidiasis
     m. junction
     m. leishmaniasis
     m. lymph node
     m. lymph node syndrome (MCLS,
     MLNS)
     m. pigmentation
     skin, eye, m. (SEM)
     m. ulcer
mucoepidermoid carcinoma
Muco-Fen-LA

M

mucoid (m)
   m. myoma degeneration
   m. otitis media (MOM)
   m. sputum
mucolipidosis (ML)
   m. II (ML-II)
   m. III (ML-III)
mucolytic
Mucomyst solution
mucopeptide
mucoperichondrium
mucopolysaccharide (MPS)
   aggregated m.
   m. pattern
   m. protein
   m. storage disease (I–VIII)
   urine m.
mucopolysaccharidoses (*pl. of*
  mucopolysaccharidosis)
mucopolysaccharidosis (MPS), *pl.*
  mucopolysaccharidoses
   beta-glucuronidase deficiency m.
   m. F
   focal m.
   m. II
   m. I, IH, IH/s, IS
   m. IIIA, B, C, D
   m. IVA, B
   m. unclassified type
mucoprotein
   Tamm-Horsfall m.
mucopurulent cervicitis
mucopus
Mucor
mucormycosis
   cutaneous m.
   pulmonary m.
   rhinocerebral m.
mucorrhea
   cervical m.
mucosa, *pl.* **mucosae**
   atrophic vaginal m.
   buccal m.
   cervical m.
   ectopic gastric m.
   endocervical m.
   estrogenized m.
   gastric m.
   genital m.
   hyalinosis cutis et mucosae
   intestinal m.
   necrotic m.
   palatal m.
   rugated vaginal m.
   thin vaginal m.
   unestrogenized vaginal m.
   vaginal m.
mucosa-associated lymphoid tissue (MALT)

mucosae (*pl. of* mucosa)
mucosal
   m. biopsy
   m. bleeding
   m. ganglioneuromatosis
   m. hyperemia
   m. intact laser tonsillar ablation (MILTA)
   m. leishmaniasis
   m. lesion
   m. neuroma syndrome
   m. rosette
   m. sloughing
   m. transudate
mucosalis
   Campylobacter m.
Mucosil
mucositis
mucosotropic
mucosulfatidosis
mucous
   m. discharge
   m. inspissation
   m. membrane
   m. membrane provocation
   m. membrane wart
   m. patch
   m. plug
   m. plugging
   m. retention cyst
mucoviscidosis
MUCP
   maximum urethral closure pressure
mucupolysaccharidosis V-VIII
mucus
   m. aspirator
   cervical m.
   m. cyst
   m. extractor
   inspissated m.
   midcycle cervical m.
   ovulatory m.
   m. plug
mu dimeric protein
MUDPILES
   methanol, uremia, diabetes, paraldehyde, isoniazid, infection, lactic acidosis, ethylene glycol, salicylate
muffled heart sound
MUGA
   multiple gated acquisition
   MUGA scan
mulberry
   m. molar
   m. ovary
   m. spot
   m. tumor

mulibrey
    m. dwarfism
    m. nanism
muliebris
    hydrocele m.
mu-lipotropin
Mullen Scales of Early Learning
  (MSEL)
Müller
    M. syndrome
    M. tubercle
Müller-Hillis 2nd stage labor maneuver
müllerian
    m. abnormality
    m. adenosarcoma
    m. agenesis
    m. cyst
    m. duct
    m. duct anomaly
    m. duct aplasia, renal
      agenesis/ectopia, cervical somite
      dysplasia (MURCS)
    m. duct aplasia, unilateral
      renalagenesis, and cervicothoracic
      somite abnormalities
    m. duct fusion
    m. duct inhibitory factor
    m. dysgenesis
    m. fusion defect
    m. hypoplasia
    m. inhibiting factor (MIF)
    m. inhibiting hormone (MIH)
    m. inhibiting substance (MIS)
    müllerian, renal, cervicothoracic,
      somite abnormalities (MURCS)
    m. sarcoma
    m. tumor
Mullins long transseptal sheath
MultArray headlight
multicelled embryo
Multicenter AIDS Cohort Study
  (MACS)
multicentric
    m. carcinoma
    m. Castleman disease
    m. lower genital tract neoplasia
multichannel
    m. cystometrogram
    m. discrete analyzer (MDA)
    m. recorder
    m. urodynamic testing
multicolor FISH cytogenetic technique
multicore myopathy
multicystic
    m. dysplastic kidney (MDK)
    m. dysplastic kidney disease
      (MCKD)
    m. encephalomalacia
    m. kidney

    m. kidney disease
    m. renal dysplasia
Multidex gel
multidimensional
    M. Personality Questionnaire (MPQ)
    M. Scale of Perceived Social
      Support (MSPSS)
    M. Student Life Satisfaction Scale
      (MSLSS)
multidisciplinary team
multidose activated charcoal (MDAC)
multidrug
    m. chemotherapy
    m. resistance (MDR)
    m. therapy (MDT)
multidrug-resistant tuberculosis
  (MDR-TB)
multi-electrode
    ESA Coulochem m.-e.
multielectrode
multifactorial
    m. disorder
    m. inheritance
    m. trait
multifetal
    m. gestation
    m. pregnancy
    m. pregnancy reduction (MFPR,
      MPR)
multifetation
multifocal
    m. atrial tachycardia
    m. clonic convulsion
    m. clonic movement
    m. clonic seizure
    m. leukoencephalopathy
    m. osteomyelitis
    m. spike
    m. white matter inflammatory lesion
multifollicular ovary
multiforme
    bullous erythema m.
    erythema m. (EM, E-M)
    glioblastoma m.
multigenerational
multigenic disorder
multigravida
multihandicapped
Multiload Cu-375 intrauterine device
multiloba
    placenta m.
multilocal genetics
multilocular
    m. cyst
    m. thymic cyst (MTC)
multilocularis
    Echinococcus m.
multiloculated cyst
multimammae

M

multimodal treatment plan
multinuclearity
    hereditary erythroblastic m.
multinucleate
multinucleated
    m. cell encephalitis
    m. giant cell
multinucleation parakeratosis
multiorgan
    m. dysfunction syndrome (MODS)
    m. system failure
    m. thrombosis
Multi-Pak-4
multipara
    grand m.
    great-grand m.
multiparameter intraarterial sensor (MPIAS)
multiparity
    grand m. (GM)
multiparous
multiplanar display mode
multiplane
    m. endovaginal (MEVA)
    m. intracavitary probe
multiple
    m. acyl-coenzyme A dehydrogenase deficiency (MADD)
    m. alleles
    m. arbitrary amplicon profiling (MAAP)
    m. articular contracture
    m. articular rigidity
    m. basal cell carcinoma syndrome
    m. basal cell nevoid syndrome
    m. benign circumferential skin creases on limb
    m. births
    m. bone enchondromata
    m. carboxylase deficiency
    m. cartilaginous exostoses
    m. cervix
    m. complex developmental disorder (MCDD)
    m. congenital anomalies
    m. cyst
    m. dislocations
    m. endocrine abnormalities (MEA)
    m. endocrine adenomatosis (MEA)
    m. endocrine neoplasia syndrome
    m. endocrine neoplasia (type I, II, III) (MEN)
    m. epiphysial dysplasia
    m. epiphysial dysplasia-early onset diabetes mellitus (MED-IDDM)
    m. epiphysial dysplasia tarda syndrome
    m. exostosis-mental retardation (MEMR)

    m. gastrointestinal polyps
    m. gated acquisition (MUGA)
    m. gated acquisition scan
    m. gestation
    m. hamartoma syndrome
    m. hereditary cutaneomandibular polyoncosis
    m. lentigines syndrome
    m. marker screening
    m. mononeuropathies
    m. myeloma
    m. myofibromatosis
    m. neuroma syndrome
    m. nevoid-basal cell carcinoma (MNBCC)
    m. nevoid-basal cell carcinoma syndrome
    m. nevoid, basal cell epithelioma, jaw cysts, bifid rib syndrome
    multiples of median (MoM)
    m. opportunistic pathogen infection
    m. oral frenula
    m. organ dysfunction syndrome (MODS)
    m. osteomas
    M. Outcomes of Raloxifene evaluation trial
    m. pituitary hormone deficiency (MPHD)
    m. pregnancies
    m. pregnancy reduction (MPR)
    m. pterygium syndrome
    m. resistant cell lines
    m. ring-enhancing mass lesion
    m. sclerosis (MS)
    m. sexual partners (MSP)
    m. sleep latency test (MSLT)
    m. subpial transection (MST)
    m. sulfatase deficiency (MSD)
    m. synostoses
    m. synostoses syndrome
    m. tics
    m. villous infarction
    m. X syndrome
multiple-organ
    m.-o. failure (MOF)
    m.-o. system failure (MOSF)
multiple-punch resection
multiplex
    arthrogryposis m.
    dysostosis m.
    mononeuritis m.
    myodysplasia fibrosa m.
    paramyoclonus m.
    steatocystoma m.
    synostosis m.
multiplexing
multiplicity of infection (MOI)

multipuncture
  m. technique
  m. test (MPT)
multisite
  m. BRACA
  m. lower genital tract involvement
Multispatula cervical sampling device
**multispectral fluorescent in situ
  hybridization (M-FISH)**
multisymptomatic
multisystemic therapy (MST)
multivalent
multivitamin
multivorans
  Burkholderia m.
MultiVysion PB assay test
multocida
  Pasteurella m.
  Prevotella m.
Mulvihill-Smith syndrome
mummified fetus
mummy wrap
mumps
  m. arthritis
  m. encephalitis
  m. leptomeningitis
  m. meningoencephalitis
  m. orchitis
  m. strain
  m. vaccine
  m. virus
Mumpsvax
Münchausen
  M. disease
  M. syndrome
  M. syndrome by proxy (MSBP, MSP)
munching pattern
munity
Munro
  M. and Parker classification for
    laparoscopic hysterectomy
  M. microabscess
  M. point
Munro-Kerr maneuver
Munson sign
mupirocin
mural
  m. endocardium
  m. pregnancy
  m. thrombosis
MURCS
  müllerian duct aplasia, renal
    agenesis/ectopia, cervical somite
    dysplasia
  müllerian, renal, cervicothoracic, somite
    abnormalities
    MURCS syndrome
murine
  M. ear drops

  m. myeloid leukemia cell line
  M. Plus Ophthalmic
  m. typhus
Murless vacuum extractor
murmur
  aortic ejection m.
  apical presystolic m.
  Austin Flint m.
  blowing decrescendo diastolic m.
  cardiac m.
  continuous shunt m.
  crescendo m.
  decrescendo diastolic m.
  diamond-shaped m.
  diastolic m.
  ejection m.
  flow m.
  functional m.
  Gibson m.
  Graham Steell m.
  harsh pansystolic m.
  heart m.
  holosystolic m.
  innocent m.
  machinery m.
  middiastolic m.
  mill wheel m.
  musical m.
  m. of valvulitis
  pansystolic m.
  presystolic m.
  pulmonary ejection m.
  pulmonic m.
  regurgitant m.
  rumbling m.
  Still m.
  systolic continuous m.
  systolic ejection m. (SEM)
  to-and-fro m.
  vibratory m.
muromonab-CD3
Muro 128 Ophthalmic
Muroptic-5
Murphy
  M. hole
  M. sign
muscarinic
  m. action
  m. effect
muscle
  abdominis m.
  absence of rectal m.'s
  accessory m.
  m. actin
  m. adenosine monophosphate
    deaminase deficiency
  airway smooth m.
  antagonistic m.
  m. atrophy

M

muscle *(continued)*
biceps femoris m.
m. biopsy
bulbocavernosus m.
bulbospongiosus m.
m. bulk
m. carnitine palmityltransferase
  deficiency
ciliary m.
coccygeal m.
coccygeus m.
conal m.
concave temporalis m.
m. cylinder
deltoid m.
depressor anguli oris m.
detrusor m.
diarthrodial m.
divergent rectus m.
m. enlargement
m. enzyme test
external oblique m.
external sphincter m.
extraocular m. (EOM)
eyelid m.
m. fasciculation
gastrocnemius m.
genioglossus m.
gluteal m.
gluteus maximus m.
gluteus medius m.
gluteus minimus m.
m. glycogen storage disorder
gracilis m.
Guthrie m.
m. herniation
hypertrophic bundle of smooth m.
hypoplasia of anguli oris depressor
  m. (HAODM)
m. hypotonia
iliococcygeal m.
iliococcygeus m.
internal oblique m.
ipsilateral lateral rectus m.
ischiocavernosus m.
lateral rectus m.
m. lengthening
levator ani m.
levator palpebrae m.
longitudinal m.
lumbar extensor m.
masseter m.
m. necrosis
oblique flank m.
obturator internus m.
papillary m.
m. paralysis
pectoralis major m.
peroneus brevis m.

peroneus longus m.
pharyngeal m.
m. phosphofructokinase deficiency
m. proprioceptor
pubococcygeal m. (PCM)
pubococcygeus m.
puborectal m.
puborectalis m.
pubovisceral m.
pyramidalis m.
quadratus labiae superioris m.
rectus abdominis m.
rectus femoris m.
m. relaxant
m. rigidity
scalene m.
scalloped temporalis m.
SCM m.
semimembranosus m.
semitendinosus m.
smooth m.
m. spasm (MS)
sphincter m.
m. splitting
sternocleidomastoid m.
m. strength grading scale
stretch receptor in detrusor m.
striated circular m.
superficial transperineal m.
superficial transverse
  perineal m.
superior oblique m.
m. surgery
temporalis m.
m. testing
thyroarytenoid m.
m. tone
m. transposition
transverse vaginal m.
transversus abdominis m.
unilateral hypoplastic pectoral m.
urethrovaginal sphincter m.
uterine m.
vastus lateralis m.
vertical m.
zygomatic head of quadratus labii
  superioris m.
muscle-brain
muscle-eye-brain (MEB)
m.-e.-b. disease of Santavuori
m.-e.-b. syndrome (MEBS)
muscular
m. atrophy
m. cuff
m. dystrophy (MD)
m. hypertrophy syndrome
m. hypotonia
m. infantilism
m. injury

m. torticollis
m. ventricular septum
muscularis
musculature
perineal m.
musculoaponeurotic layer
musculocutaneous nerve
musculofascial supply
musculoperitoneal
transverse rectus abdominis m.
(TRAMP)
musculoskeletal (MSK)
m. disorder
m. injury
m. pain syndrome (MSPS)
m. system
musculotropic drug
Muse pellet
mushroom
Amanita m.
m. gyrus
m. poisoning
mushrooming of fimbria
musical murmur
music therapy
mustard
M. atrial switch procedure
l-phenylalanine m. (L-PAM, l-PAM, LPAM)
nitrogen m.
M. operation
M. TGA technique
Mustardé
M. cheek flap
M. cheek flap procedure
M. hypospadias procedure
Mustargen Hydrochloride
musty vaginal odor
mutagen
mutagenesis
insertional m.
mutagenic treatment
Mutamycin
mutans
Streptococcus m.
mutant
m. allele
m. cell
m. gene
m. homoplasmy
Hoxa5 null m.
mutation
Ashkenazi Jewish cancer
susceptibility m.
autosomal recessive m.
BRCA1 gene m.
BRCA2 gene m.
chromosome 17 m.
Drosophila m.

dynamic m.
factor V Leiden m.
frameshift m.
full m.
function-enhancing m.
gene m.
genetic m.
germ-line m.
G-to-T transversion m.
heparin-binding site m.
hew m.
Leiden m.
missense m.
mutator m.
new m.
nonsense m.
point m.
prothrombin gene m.
reactive site m.
RS m.
single gene m.
m. testing
trinucleotide repeat
expansion m.
mutational dysostosis
mutator mutation
Mutchinick syndrome
mute
mutilans
keratoma hereditarium m.
mutilating keratoderma
mutilation
female genital m. (FMG)
female genital tract m. (FGTM)
genital m.
mutism
akinetic m.
cerebellar m.
selective m.
transient m.
muzzled sperm
MV
measles virus
mechanical ventilation
megavolt
mV
millivolt
MVA
manual vacuum aspiration
microvillus atrophy
MVB
manual ventilation bag
MV(c)ELISA
measles virus enzyme-linked
immunosorbent assay
MVP
mitral valve prolapse
MWT
Mallory-Weiss tear

599

MX2-300 xenon quality light source
myalgia
    m. cruris epidemica
    febrile m.
    tension m.
Myambutol
Myapap
myasthenia
    congenital m.
    m. gravis
    juvenile m.
    transient neonatal m.
myasthenia-like syndrome
myasthenic syndrome
Mycelex
mycelium
mycetoma
    renal m.
Myciguent
Mycinettes
Mycitracin Topical
Myclo-Derm
Myclo-Gyne
mycobacteria (pl. of Mycobacterium, mycobacterium)
mycobacterial
    m. disease
    m. organism
mycobacterium, pl. mycobacteria
    M. abscessus
    M. africanum
    atypical mycobacteria
    M. avium
    M. avium complex (MAC)
    M. avium-intracellulare (MAI)
    M. avium-intracellulare complex (MAC, MAIC)
    M. bovis
    M. chelonae
    M. fortuitum
    M. fortuitum complex
    M. kansasii
    M. leprae
    M. malmoense
    M. marinum
    nontuberculous m. (NTM)
    mycobacteria other than tuberculosis (MOTT)
    M. scrofulaceum
    M. tuberculosis
    M. ulcerans
    M. xenopi
Mycobutin
Mycogen II Topical
Mycolog-II Topical
mycophenolate mofetil
mycophenolic acid

mycoplasma
    M. fermentans
    genital m.
    M. genitalium
    M. hominis
    M. penetrans
    M. pneumonia
    M. pneumoniae
    T strain m.
mycoplasmal antibody
mycoses (pl. of mycosis)
mycosis, pl. mycoses
    m. fungoides
    hypopigmented m.
Mycostatin
mycotic
    m. aneurysm
    m. infection
    m. vaginosis
mycotica
    colpitis m.
Myco-Triacet II
Mydfrin
    M. Ophthalmic
    M. Ophthalmic Solution
Mydriacyl
mydriasis
    congenital m.
    unilateral m.
mydriatic
myelencephalon
myelin
    m. lipid
    m. sheath
myelination, myelinization
myelinization (var. of myelination)
myelinoclastic diffuse cerebral sclerosis
myelinolysis
    central pontine m.
myelitis
    acute transverse m.
    transverse m.
    viral m.
    zoster m.
myeloblast cell
myeloblastic leukemia
myelocele
myelocyte cell
myelocytic leukemia, myelogenic leukemia
myelodysplasia
    pediatric m.
myelodysplastic syndrome (MDS)
myelofibrosis
myelogenic
myelogenous leukemia
myelogram
myelograph
myelography

myeloid leukemia
myeloid-to-erythroid (M/E)
myelokathexis
 warts, hypogammaglobulinemia,
 infections, m. (WHIM)
myeloma
 multiple m.
 m. protein
myelomalacia
myelomeningocele
myelomonocytic leukemia
myeloneuropathy
myeloopticoneuropathy
 subacute m.
myelopathy
 compression m.
 craniocervical m.
 delayed m.
 human T-cell lymphotrophic virus
  type I associated m. (HAM)
 postirradiation m.
 schistosomal m.
 tropical spastic paraparesis/HTLV-I
  associated m. (TSP/HAM)
 vacuolar m.
 vascular m.
myeloperoxidase (MPO)
 m. deficiency
myelophthisis
myelopoiesis
 ineffective m.
myeloproliferative
 m. disorder
 m. syndrome
myeloradiculitis
 acute m.
myeloschisis
 dorsal m.
myelosuppression
myelosuppressive agent
myelotoxicity
myenteric
 m. plexus
 m. plexus neuropathy
Myhre syndrome
myiasis
Mykrox
Mylanta Gas
Mylar glove
Myleran
Mylicon drops
Mylocel tablet
myoblastoma
 granular cell m.
myoblast transfer therapy
myocardial
 m. abscess
 m. band (MB)

m. blood flow
m. contusion
m. fiber degeneration
m. function
m. hypertrophy
m. infarction (MI)
m. ischemia
m. muscle creatine kinase
 isoenzyme (CK-MB)
m. phosphodiesterase inhibitor
m. siderosis
m. steal syndrome
m. stunning
myocarditis
 acute interstitial m.
 diphtheritic toxic m.
 enteroviral m.
 eosinophilic m.
 Fiedler m.
 giant cell m.
 granulomatous m.
 infectious m.
 interstitial m.
 lymphocytic m.
 silent m.
 toxic m.
 viral m.
myocardium
 stunned m.
myocellular
Myochrysine
myoclonia
myoclonic
 m. absence
 m. ataxia
 m. convulsion
 m. dystonia
 m. encephalopathy
 m. epilepsy
 m. epilepsy with ragged red fibers
  (MERRF)
 m. jerk
 m. petit mal
 m. seizure
 m. spasm
myoclonic-astatic seizure
myoclonus
 Baltic m.
 benign neonatal m.
 benign neonatal sleep m.
 cortical reflex m.
 m. epilepsy
 epileptic m.
 essential m.
 intention m.
 jaw m.
 Mediterranean m.
 neonatal m.

M

myoclonus (*continued*)
    nocturnal m.
    nonepileptic m.
    ocular m.
    reflex m.
    reticular reflex m.
    sleep m.
    m. syndrome
myocolpitis
myocutaneous
    m. flap
    transverse rectus abdominis m.
      (TRAM)
myocytic hypertrophy
myocytolysis
    coagulative m.
myodysplasia
    m. fetalis deformans
    m. fibrosa multiplex
myodystrophia (*var. of* myodystrophy)
    m. fetalis deformans
myodystrophy, myodystrophia
    Duchenne m.
myoepithelial cell
myofascial
    m. injection
    m. layer
    m. pain
    m. pain syndrome (MPS)
    m. release
    m. release technique
myofiber disarray
myofibril
myofibromatosis
    congenital multiple m.
    infantile m.
    multiple m.
    periorbital infantile m.
    renal m.
    solitary renal m.
myofilament
myogenic
myoglobin
myoglobinuria
    recurrent m.
    sporadic m.
myognathus
myography
myoinositol
myokymia
    interictal m.
myolysis
myoma
    asymptomatic m.
    calcified m.
    cervical m.
    degenerating m.
    m. fixation instrument
    intracavitary m.

    intraligamentous m.
    intramural m.
    parasitic m.
    retained m.
    m. screw
    subendometrial m.
    submucosal m.
    submucous m.
    subserous m.
    subserous pedunculated m.
    m. uteri
    uterine m.
myomatectomy (*var. of* myomectomy)
myomectomy, myomatectomy
    abdominal m.
    hysteroscopic m.
    laparoscopic m.
    vaginal m.
    vaginal birth after m.
myometrial
    m. contraction
    m. coring
    m. fiber
    m. invasion
    m. neurofibroma
    m. protein
myometritis
myometrium
    hypotonic m.
    m. of pregnancy
    uterine m.
myomotomy
myonecrosis
    clostridial m.
myoneural junction disorder
myopathica
    metrorrhagia m.
myopathic limb-girdle syndrome
myopathy
    Batten-Turner congenital m.
    Bethlem m.
    broad A-band m.
    cardioskeletal m.
    central core m.
    centronuclear m. (CNM)
    congenital m.
    dysmaturative m.
    dystrophic m.
    familial visceral m.
    fatal infantile m.
    genetic m.
    hypothyroid m.
    infantile myofibrillar m.
    inflammatory m.
    m., lactic acidosis, sideroblastic
      anemia
    lipid m.
    metabolic m.
    minicore m.

mitochondrial m.
multicore m.
myotonic m.
myotubular m.
nemaline m.
nemaline rod m.
nonfamilial visceral m.
ocular m.
Proteus syndrome m.
ragged red m.
rod m.
Sengers mitochondrial m.
steroid-induced m.
trilaminar m.
visceral m.
X-linked cardioskeletal m.
X-linked centronuclear m.
X-linked myotubular m. (MTMX,
XLMTM)
X-linked recessive centronuclear m.
X-linked recessive myotubular m.
zebra body m.
myopathy-myxedema syndrome
myopericarditis
myophosphorylase deficiency
myopia
high m.
severe m.
myosalpingitis
myosalpinx
myosin
m. filament
m. light-chain kinase
m. light-chain phosphorylation
myosis
myositis
eosinophilic m.
inflammatory m.
intrauterine viral m.
m. ossificans
m. ossificans circumscripta
m. ossificans progressiva
myositis/fasciitis
necrotizing m./f.
myotomy
Heller m.
Livaditis circular m.
myotomy-myectomy
Morrow m.-m.
Myotonachol
myotonia
chondrodystrophic m.

m. chondrodystrophica
cold-induced m.
m. congenita
grip m.
m. neonatorum
percussion m.
spondyloepimetaphysial dysphasia
with m.
myotonic
m. chondrodystrophy
m. dystrophy (MD)
m. muscular dystrophy
m. myopathy
myotonica
chondrodystrophia m.
MyoTrac EMG
myotubular myopathy
Myozyme
Myphetapp
myringitis
bullous m.
myringotomy
laser m.
laser-assisted m. (LAM)
Otoscan laser-assisted m. (OtoLAM)
m. tube
wide-field m.
myrtiform caruncle
myrtiformis
caruncula m.
Mysoline
mystery syndrome
Mytelase
Mytrex F Topical
Mytussin DM
myxedema
m. coma
infantile m.
**myxedema-myotonic dystrophy
syndrome**
myxedematous infantilism
myxoid
m. dysplasia
m. histopathologic subtype
m. liposarcoma
m. matrix
myxoma
familial cardiac m.
myxorrhea
M-Zole
M-Z. 7 combination pack
M-Z. 3 combination pack

M

NA
nosocomially acquired
Na, Na+
sodium
NAA
nucleic acid amplification
NAA technique
NAA test
Nabi-HB hepatitis B immune globulin human
Naboth
N. cyst
N. follicle
N. gland
nabothian
n. cyst
n. follicle
n. gland
n. vesicle
NAC
nipple-areola complex
N-acetylaspartate
N-acetylaspartic acid
N-acetylcysteine
N-acetyl-galactosamine
N-acetylgalactosamine-4-sulfatase deficiency
N-acetyl-glucosamine
N-acetylglutamate
N-a. synthetase
N-a. synthetase deficiency
N-acetylneuraminic
N-a. acid (NANA)
N-a. acid storage disease (NSD)
NaCl
sodium chloride
NACS
Neurologic and Adaptive Capacity Score
nadir of deceleration
Nadler forceps
nadolol
Nadopen-V
Nadostine
NADPH
nicotinamide adenine dinucleotide phosphate
NADPH oxidase
Naegeli
chromatophore nevus of N.
N. syndrome
thrombasthenia of Glanzmann and N.
Naegeli-Franceschetti-Jadasshon (NJF)
Naegleria fowleri

naeslundii
Actinomyces n.
naevoid (*var. of* nevoid)
nafarelin acetate
nafcillin sodium
naftifine hydrochloride
Naftin
Nägele
N. forceps
N. obliquity
N. pelvis
N. rule
Nager
N. anomaly
N. sign
N. syndrome
Nager-de Reynier syndrome
Nager-type acrofacial dysostosis
NaHCO$_3$
sodium bicarbonate
nail
n. bed cyanosis
n. bed telangiectasia
brittle n.
clubbing of n.'s
n. defect
dystrophic n.
n. dystrophy
n. fold telangiectasia
hippocratic n.
hypertrophic n.
hypoplastic n.
n. matrix
n. pitting
n. ringworm
shedding of n.'s
spoon-shaped n.
titanium elastic n.
n. trephination
yellow n.
nail-fold
n.-f. capillary
n.-f. infection
nailing
titanium elastic n. (TEN)
nail-patella syndrome
NAIT
neonatal alloimmune thrombocytopenia
Najjar syndrome
nalbuphine
Nalcrom
NALD
neonatal adrenoleukodystrophy
Nalfon
Nalgest

N

Nal-Glu
nalidixic
    n. acid
    n. acid agar
nalorphine
naloxone hydrochloride
NALS
    neonatal adjuvant life support
NALT
    nasopharyngeal-associated lymphoid
    tissue
naltrexone
NAMCS
    National Ambulatory Medical Care
    Survey
NAME
    nevi, atrial myxoma, myxoid
    neurofibromas, ephelides
    NAME syndrome
naming
    pointing for n.
    n. speed deficit
NANA
    N-acetylneuraminic acid
nana
    pelvis n.
NANBH
    non-A, non-B hepatitis
Nance-Horan syndrome (NHS)
nandrolone
nanism
    mulibrey n.
    Russell n.
    Seckel n.
nanism-constrictive pericarditis syndrome
nanocephalic dwarfism
nanocephaly
Nanoduct sweat test system
nanogram
nanoid
nanomelia
nape nevus
naphazoline
naphthalene mothball
naphthoquinone
NAPI
    Neurodevelopmental Assessment of
    Preterm Infants
NAPNAP
    National Association of Pediatric
    Nurse Associates and Practitioners
nappy test
Naprosyn
naproxen sodium
Naqua
narasin
naratriptan
Narcan
narcissus

narcolepsy
narcoleptic
    n. attack
    n. sleep
narcosis
narcotic
    n. analgesia
    n. analgesic
    n. antagonist
    n. depression
    n. drug
    intrathecal n.
    n. withdrawal syndrome
Nardil
nares (*pl. of* naris)
naris, *pl.* nares
    anteverted n.
Naropin
NARP
    neuropathy, ataxia, retinitis pigmentosa
    NARP syndrome
narrow
    n. band spectrophotometer
    n. bifrontal diameter
    n. complex supraventricular
    tachycardia
    n. foot
    n. hand
    n. mediastinal waist
    n. mediastinum
    n. mesenteric stalk
    n. palate
    n. pubic arch
    n. pulmonary outflow tract (NPOT)
narrow-band instrument
narrowing
    vaginal n.
narrowness
    intermaxillary n.
narrow-spectrum blue light
Narula sinoatrial conduction time
  method
NAS
    neonatal abstinence syndrome
    NAS score
Nasacort AQ
nasal
    n. air emission
    n. ala
    n. alar cartilage cleft
    n. antral window
    n. antrum
    n. aspirator
    Ayr N.
    n. bone
    n. bridge
    n. cannula
    n. cauterization
    n. consonant

n. continuous positive airway pressure (nCPAP)
n. CPAP
n. decongestant
n. diphtheria
n. encephalocele
n. flaring
n. hypoplasia, peripheral dysostosis, mental retardation syndrome
n. lavage
n. mastocytosis
N. Moist
n. obstruction
n. packing
n. polyp
n. polyposis
Privine N.
n. prong continuous positive airway pressure (NP-CPAP)
n. pyriform aperture stenosis
n. regurgitation
n. retractor
n. root
n. septum
n. smear
n. speculum
n. swab
n. swab culture
n. tampon
n. tip thermistor
n. tube intubation
n. turbinate
Tyzine N.
n. ulceration
n. voice
n. wash

NasalCrom

Nasalide
   N. Nasal Aerosol
   N. Nasal Inhaler

Nasarel nasal spray

NASBA
   nucleic acid sequence-based amplification

nascentium
   trismus n.

NASH
   nonalcoholic steatohepatitis

nasi
   ala n.
   flaring of ala n.

nasion

nasoduodenal feeding

nasoendoscopy

nasofrontal suture

nasogastric (NG)
   n. aspirate
   n. decompression
   n. drainage

n. drip feeding
n. tube (NGT)
n. tube feeding (NTF)

nasojejunal (NJ)
   n. tube

nasolabial
   n. fold asymmetry
   n. reflex

nasolacrimal
   n. duct (NLD)
   n. duct obstruction (NLDO)
   n. sac

Nasonex

nasoorbitoethmoid (NOE)

nasopharyngeal
   n. airway obstruction
   n. aspirate (NPA)
   n. carcinoma
   n. fibroma
   n. reflux (NPR)
   n. suction
   n. suctioning
   n. swab
   n. wash

nasopharyngeal-associated lymphoid tissue (NALT)

nasopharyngitis

nasopharyngolaryngoscopy (NPL)

nasopharynx

nasotracheal intubation (NTI)

NASPGN
   North American Society for Pediatric Gastroenterology and Nutrition

NASS
   Neonatal Abstinence Scoring System

nata
   pro re n. (as needed)

natal
   n. cleft
   n. teeth

NatalCare Plus film-coated tablet

natality

NataTab
   N. CFe film-coated tablet
   N. FA film-coated tablet
   N. Rx film-coated tablet

natiform skull

natimortality

nation
   Study of Women's Health Across the N. (SWAN)

national
   N. Acute Spinal Cord Injury Study
   N. Ambulatory Medical Care Survey (NAMCS)
   N. Association of Pediatric Nurse Associates and Practitioners (NAPNAP)

N

national (*continued*)
 N. Asthma Education and
 Prevention Program
 N. Breast and Cervical Cancer
 Early Detection Program
 N. Cancer Database
 N. Cancer Institute (NCI)
 N. Center for Child Abuse and
 Neglect (NCCAN)
 N. Childhood Vaccine Injury Act of
 1986
 N. Clearing House on Child Abuse
 and Neglect (NCCANH)
 N. Collaborative Diethylstilbestrol
 Adenosis Project (DESAD)
 N. Collaborative Perinatal project
 N. Committee for Quality Assurance
 (NCQA)
 N. Educational Longitudinal Survey
 (NELS)
 N. Fertility Clinic
 N. Health and Nutrition
 Examination Survey (NHANES)
 N. Health Interview Survey
 (NHIS)
 N. Hospital Discharge Survey
 (NIDS)
 N. Institute of Child Health and
 Human Development (NICHD)
 N. Institute of Mental Health
 (NIMH)
 N. Institutes of Health (NIH)
 N. Institutes of Health Consensus
 Conference on Ovarian Cancer
 N. Joint Committee on Learning
 Disabilities (NJCLD)
 N. Maternal and Infant Health
 Survey
 N. Organization for Rare Disorders
 (NORD)
 N. Osteoporosis Foundation
 N. Ovarian Cancer Early Detection
 Program
 N. Pediatric Trauma Registry
 (NPTR)
 n. recipient waiting list
 N. Society of Genetic Counselors
 (NSGC)
 N. Surgical Adjuvant Breast Project
 (NSABP)
 N. Vaccine Advisory Committee
 (NVAC)
 N. Wilms Tumor Study (NWTS)
 N. Wilms Tumor Study Group
 (NWTSG)
 N. Women's Health Network
native
 n. ileum
 n. squamous epithelium

NATP
 neonatal alloimmune thrombocytopenic
 purpura
natriuresis
natriuretic peptide
natural
 n. antibody
 n. childbirth (NCB)
 n. child spacing
 n. conception
 n. delivery
 n. environment
 n. family planning
 n. fecundity
 n. hormone replacement therapy
 (NHRT)
 n. killer (NK)
 n. killer cell (NKC)
 n. killer lymphocyte
 n. killer T cell
 n. monozygotic twins
 n. penicillin
 n. resistance
 n. selection
 n. synthetic surfactant
 n. vaccination
naturales
 per vias n.
nature of specimen
Naturetin
naturopath (NP)
naturopathy
nausea
 acute chemotherapy associated n.
 n. and vomiting (N/V, N&V)
 anticipatory chemotherapy
 associated n.
 delayed chemotherapy-
 associated n.
 n. gravidarum
Navajo brainstem syndrome
Navane
NAVEL
 femoral nerve, artery, vein, empty
 space, lymphatics
navel
 blue n.
Navelbine
navicular
 accessory n.
 n. bone
 carpal n.
navicularis
 fossa n.
naviculocuneiform joint
NB
 neuroblastoma
 newborn
 novobiocin

NBAS
  Neonatal Behavioral Assessment Scale
  Newborn Behavior Assessment Scale
NBCC
  nevoid basal cell carcinoma
NBCCS
  nevoid basal cell carcinoma
    syndrome
NBCIE
  nonbullous congenital ichthyosiform
    erythroderma
NBI
  nosocomial bacterial infection
NBIC
  newborn intensive care
NBICU
  newborn intensive care unit
NBRS
  Neurobiologic Risk Scale
    nursery NBRS
NBS
  neonatal Bartter syndrome
  nevoid basal cell carcinoma syndrome
  new Ballard score
  Nijmegen breakage syndrome
NBSCU
  newborn special care unit
NBT
  nitroblue tetrazolium
    NBT dye test
NBTV
  nonbacterial thrombotic vegetation
NCAH
  nonclassic adrenal hyperplasia
NCB
  natural childbirth
NC-CAH
  nonclassic congenital adrenal
    hyperplasia
NCCAN
  National Center for Child Abuse and
    Neglect
NCCANH
  National Clearing House on Child
    Abuse and Neglect
NCCDS
  North American Collaborative Crohn
    Disease Study
NCCPC-R
  Noncommunicating Children's Pain
    Checklist-Revised
NCI
  National Cancer Institute
NCL
  neuronal ceroid lipofuscinosis
    adult NCL
    infantile NCL
    juvenile NCL
    late infantile NCL

nCPAP
  nasal continuous positive airway
    pressure
NCQA
  National Committee for Quality
    Assurance
NCSE
  nonconvulsive status epilepticus
NCV
  nerve conduction velocity
ND
  neonatal death
  neurologic development
NDH
  neurogenic dysplasia of hip
n-diethyl-m-toluamide (*var. of*
  n,n-diethyl-m-toluamide)
ND-Stat
NDT
  neurodevelopment therapy
NDW
  number of different words
Nd:YAG
  neodymium:yttrium-aluminum-garnet
    Nd:YAG laser
    Nd:YAG laser ablation
NE
  neonatal encephalopathy
NE-8000 analyzer
near
  n. drowning
  n. gaze reflex
  n. infrared photoplethysmography
    (NIRP)
  n. infrared spectrophotometry
    (NIRS)
  n. infrared spectroscopy (NIRS)
  n. vision
near-anhydramnios
near-drowning
  freshwater n.-d.
  saltwater n.-d.
  very cold water n.-d.
  warm water n.-d.
near-miss
  n.-m. SIDS
  n.-m. sudden infant death syndrome
    (NMSIDS)
near-myeloablative chemotherapy
nearsightedness
near-term
  n.-t. delivery
  n.-t. infant
  n.-t. pregnancy
near-viable fetus
neat pincer grasp
Nebcin injection
Nebules
  Ventolin N.

N

nebulization
   ipratropium n.
   n. ventilator
nebulized prostacyclin
nebulizer
   Aeroneb n.
   compressed air-driven n.
   DuraNeb portable n.
   Hudson T Up-Draft II disposable n.
   jet n.
   Micro-Mist disposable n.
   Pari LC Plusjet n.
   PulmoMate n.
   Respirgard II n.
   Schuco n.
NebuPent Inhalation
NEC
   necrotizing enterocolitis
   Neurologic Examination for Children
Necator americanus
necessitatis
   empyema n.
neck
   bladder n.
   femoral n.
   n. reflex
   n. response
   short n.
   stiff n.
   thick n.
   twisted n.
   vesical n.
   webbed n.
necklace
   Casal n.
neck-righting reflex
neck-shaft angle (NSA)
necrobiosis
   n. lipoidica
   n. lipoidica diabeticorum (NLD)
necrolysis
   erythema multiforme/toxic epidermal
     n. (EM/TEN)
   toxic epidermal n. (TEN)
necrophorum
   Fusobacterium n.
necropsy, necroscopy
necroscopy (*var. of* necropsy)
necroses (*pl. of* necrosis)
necrosis, *pl.* **necroses**
   acute tubular n. (ATN)
   aseptic n.
   avascular n. (AVN)
   basal ganglion n.
   bone avascular n.
   caseating n.
   centrilobular n.
   cerebral cortical n.
   coagulation n.

   cortical n.
   cystic medial n.
   decidual fibrinoid n.
   excitotoxic n.
   fascial n.
   fat n.
   fibrinoid n.
   full-thickness n.
   hepatic n.
   idiopathic juvenile avascular n.
   intrauterine facial n.
   ischemic decidual n.
   juvenile avascular n.
   liquefactive n.
   medial n.
   medullary n.
   miliary calcified n.
   muscle n.
   neuronal n.
   papillary n.
   periportal hemorrhagic n.
   pituitary n.
   pontosubicular neuron n. (PSN)
   postpartum pituitary n.
   postsurgical fat n.
   posttraumatic fat n.
   progressive outer retinal n. (PORN)
   pulp n.
   radiation n.
   renal cortical n.
   renal tubular n.
   selective neuronal n.
   spotty n.
   subcutaneous fat n.
   superficial n.
   tissue n.
   tubular n.
   tumor n.
   unilateral intrauterine facial n.
   uterine n.
   white matter n.
necrospermia
necrotic
   n. arachnidism
   n. cellular debris
   n. coagulum
   n. facial dysplasia
   n. mucosa
necrotizing
   n. adrenalitis
   n. arteriolitis
   n. arteritis
   n. colitis
   n. encephalopathy
   n. enterocolitis (NEC)
   n. erysipelas
   n. factor
   n. fasciitis
   n. funisitis

n. gingivitis
n. glomerulonephritis
n. granulomatous lymphadenitis
n. granulomatous vasculitis
n. jejunitis
n. myositis/fasciitis
n. pneumonia
n. ulcerating gingivitis (NUG)
necrozoospermia
nedocromil
n. sodium
n. sodium ophthalmic solution
N.E.E. 1/35
need
Carolina Curriculum for Infants and Toddlers with Special N.'s
Children with Special Health Care N.'s (CWSN)
special n.'s
needle
Adair-Veress n.
n. aspiration
Bard Biopty cut n.
Biopty cut n.
butterfly scalp vein n.
Chiba n.
coaxial sheath cut-biopsy n.
Cobb-Ragde n.
n. cricothyroidotomy
n. cricothyrotomy
CT1 n.
CUSALap accessory n.
n. cystourethropexy
Dieckmann intraosseous n.
disposable butterfly n.
D-Tach removal n.
Echotip Norfolk aspiration n.
Echotip percutaneous entry n.
Endopath Ultra Veress n.
Ethiguard n.
Euro-Med FNA-21 aspiration n.
eXcel-DR Glasser laparoscopic n.
n. excision
n. excision of transformation zone
FNA-21 n.
GraNee n.
Hawkins breast localization n.
n. holder
Howell biopsy aspiration n.
insufflation n.
intraosseous n.
J n.
n. localization
n. localization breast biopsy
Nottingham colposuspension n.
Osgood bone marrow n.
Pereyra n.
Potocky n.
scalp vein n.

screw-tipped intraosseous n.
SH n.
short-bevel 21-gauge n.
spinal n.
splittable n.
Stamey n.
stereotactic breast biopsy n.
Sur-Fast n.
n. suspension
n. thoracentesis
n. tip
Tuohy spinal n.
Veress n.
Vim-Silverman n.
Virginia n.
Wolf-Veress n.
needlestick exposure
NEEP
negative end-expiratory pressure
Neer
N. classification
N. view
nefazodone
negative
n. affectivity
n. balance
n. balance of body fluid
catalase n.
n. chemotaxis
n. contraction stress test
n. end-expiratory pressure (NEEP)
n. inspiratory force (NIF)
n. inspiratory pressure
n. interference
polyarthritis, RF n.
n. punch biopsy
n. reinforcement
negative-pressure
n.-p. box
n.-p. respirator
negativism
negevensis
Simkania n.
NegGram
neglect
child abuse and n. (CAN)
National Center for Child Abuse and N. (NCCAN)
National Clearing House on Child Abuse and N. (NCCANH)
suspected child abuse or n. (SCAN)
negligence
negotiation
condom n.
Negri body
Neill-Dingwall syndrome
Neisseria
N. gonorrhea
N. meningitidis

N

neisserial infection
nelfinavir
Nellcor
    N. FS-10 oximeter sensor
    N. FS-14 oximeter sensor
    N. N-499 fetal oxygen saturation
      monitor
    N. N-400/FS system
    N. N-200 home monitor
    N. N-3000 home monitor
    N. N20, N200 pulse oximeter
    N. Puritan Bennett home monitor
    N. Puritan Bennett oxygen
      saturation monitor
NELS
    National Educational Longitudinal Survey
Nelson
    N. sign
    N. syndrome
nemaline
    n. myopathy
    n. rod
    n. rod disease
    n. rod myopathy
nematode endophthalmitis
Nembutal
NEMD
    nonspecific esophageal motility disorder
neoadjuvant
    n. chemotherapy
    n. hormonal therapy (NHT)
neoaneurysm
neoantigen
neoaorta formation
neoaortic valve
neobladder diversion procedure
Neocate One+ formula
Neo-Codema
NeoCure cryoablation system
neocystostomy
neodarwinism
neodymium:yttrium-aluminum-garnet
  (Nd:YAG)
Neo-Estrone
neofetus
neoformans
    Cryptococcus n.
Neo-fradin
neogala
neologism
Neoloid
Neolon surgical glove
neomucosa
neomycin
    n. and polymyxin B
    n., polymyxin B, bacitracin
    n., polymyxin B, hydrocortisone
    n., polymyxin B, prednisolone
    n. sulfate

neomycin-polymycin combination otic
  solution
neonatal
    n. abdominal mass
    N. Abstinence Scoring System
      (NASS)
    n. abstinence sign
    n. abstinence syndrome (NAS)
    n. acne
    n. adjuvant life support (NALS)
    n. adrenoleukodystrophy (NALD)
    n. alloimmune thrombocytopenia
      (NAIT)
    n. alloimmune thrombocytopenic
      purpura (NATP)
    n. amblyogenic stimulus
    n. apnea
    n. asphyxia
    n. assessment
    n. autoimmune neutropenia
    n. autoimmune thrombocytopenia
    n. Bartter syndrome (NBS)
    N. Behavioral Assessment Scale
      (NBAS)
    n. blood volume
    n. brain injury
    N. Brazelton Assessment Scale
    n. breast hyperplasia
    n. bullous dermatitis
    n. candidiasis
    n. cardiomyopathy
    n. chest disease
    n. cholestasis
    n. cholestatic hepatitis
    n. cholestatic jaundice
    n. chronic idiopathic neutropenia
    n. cold injury
    n. condition
    n. conjunctivitis
    n. convulsion
    n. cuff
    n. cyanosis
    n. cyanotic congenital heart
      disease
    n. death (ND, NND)
    n. dermatology
    n. diabetes mellitus
    n. diagnosis
    n. distress
    n. elastin deposition
    n. encephalopathy (NE)
    n. endocrine disorder
    n. erythrocyte
    Exosurf N.
    n. extracorporeal life support
    n. facial coding system (NFCS)
    n. glucose requirement
    n. gonococcal disease
    n. Graves disease

n. Guillain-Barré syndrome
n. Guthrie card
n. gynecomastia
n. hemochromatosis (NH)
n. hepatitis syndrome
n. herpes
n. herpes simplex
n. herpes simplex virus infection
n. HMD
n. HSV-1 encephalitis
n. HSV-2 encephalitis
n. hydronephrosis
n. hyperbilirubinemia
n. hyperparathyroidism
n. hyperthermia
n. hypocalcemia (NHC)
n. hypoglycemia
n. hypomagnesemia
n. hypoxic-ischemic encephalopathy
N. Infant Pain Scale (NIPS)
n. intensive care unit (NICU)
n. intubation
n. iron-storage disease (NISD)
n. isoimmune hemolytic anemia
n. isoimmune thrombocytopenia (NIT)
n. isoimmune thrombocytopenic purpura
n. jaundice (NNJ)
n. leukemoid reaction
n. line
n. listeriosis
n. lupus
n. lupus erythematosus (NLE)
n. lupus syndrome
n. macrosomia
n. Marfan syndrome
n. marker
n. maturity classification of Dubowitz
n. medicine
n. meningitis
n. metabolism
n. midgut volvulus
n. monitor
n. morbidity
n. mortality (NNM)
n. mortality rate (NMR)
n. mortality risk (NMR)
n. myasthenia gravis
n. myasthenic syndrome
n. myoclonus
n. narcotic pack
n. narcotic withdrawal or abstinence syndrome
n. neuroblastoma
n. nongoitrous hypothyroidism
n. ocular prophylaxis
n. OPCA

n. ophthalmia
n. osseous dysplasia
n. outcome
n. pemphigus vulgaris
N. Perception Inventory (NPI)
n. period
n. pneumonia
n. polycythemia
n. progeroid syndrome (NPS)
n. pseudohydrocephalic progeroid syndrome
n. purpura fulminans
n. pustular melanosis
n. pustule
n. RDS
n. respiratory depression
n. respiratory distress syndrome (NRDS)
n. resuscitation
N. Resuscitation Program (NRP)
n. ring
n. scabies
n. scalp abscess
n. screening
n. seborrheic dermatitis
n. seizure
n. sepsis
n. septic arthritis
N. Skin Assessment Score
n. small left colon syndrome
n. stadiometer
n. stress
n. teeth
n. tetanus
n. tetany
n. thymectomy
n. thyrotoxicosis
n. thyrotropin
n. torticollis
n. transport
n. varicella
n. vascular accident
N. Withdrawal Inventory (NWI)

neonate
athyrotic n.
cola-colored n.
dysmature n.
early n.
n. examination
n. gut microflora
N. One Plus
postmature n.
preterm n.
seronegative n.
stress n.
surgical n.

neonatologist
neonatology

N

neonatorum
  acne n. (AN)
  adiponecrosis subcutanea n.
  anemia n.
  anoxia n.
  apnea n.
  asphyxia n.
  diabetes n.
  eczema n.
  edema n.
  erythema toxicum n.
  erythroblastosis n.
  gonococcal ophthalmia n.
  herpes n.
  icterus n.
  icterus gravis n.
  impetigo n.
  keratolysis n.
  mastitis n.
  melena n.
  milia n.
  myotonia n.
  noma n.
  ophthalmia n. (type 1, 2)
  pemphigus n.
  sclerema n.
  sepsis n.
  tetania n.
  tetanus n.
  trismus n.
  volvulus n.

Neopap
neoplasia
  Adjuvant Chemotherapy in Ovarian N.
  anal intraepithelial n. (AIN)
  bowenoid vulvar intraepithelial n.
  cervical epithelial n.
  cervical intraepithelial n. (CIN)
  endometrial n.
  endometrial intraepithelial n. (EIN)
  estrogen-dependent n.
  favor n.
  gestational trophoblastic n. (GTN)
  glandular n.
  hematologic n.
  intraepithelial n.
  invasive n.
  lobular n.
  lymphoreticular n.
  multicentric lower genital tract n.
  multiple endocrine n. (type I, II, III) (MEN)
  syndrome of multiple endocrine n.
  thyroid n.
  trophoblastic n.
  vaginal intraepithelial n. (VAIN)
  vascular n.
  vulvar intraepithelial n. (VIN)

neoplasm
  adrenal n.
  benign ovarian n.
  benign vascular n.
  bilateral ovarian n.
  borderline epithelial ovarian n.
  borderline malignant epithelial n.
  cerebellar n.
  cervix n.
  cystic cerebellar n.
  endometrial n.
  epithelial stromal ovarian n.
  germ cell n.
  germ cell ovarian n.
  gonadal germ cell n.
  hepatic n.
  hormone-producing n.
  indigenous n.
  intracranial n.
  isologous n.
  large intestine n.
  lipid cell n.
  lipoid ovarian n.
  malignant ovarian n.
  mesenchymal n.
  mucinous ovarian n.
  neural n.
  ovarian n.
  ovarian lipid cell n.
  ovarian malignant epithelial n.
  ovarian sex-cord stromal n.
  papillary n.
  posterior fossa n.
  primary intrapulmonary n.
  serous ovarian n.
  sex cord stromal n.
  soft tissue ovarian n.
  squamous cell n.
  testicular n.
  uterine n.
  vulvar n.

neoplastic
  n. cyst
  n. fibrosis
  n. sequela
  n. trophoblastic disease

NeoProfen
neopterin
Neoral
neosalpingostomy
  terminal n.

Neosar
Neo-Sert
  N.-S. umbilical vessel catheter
  N.-S. umbilical vessel catheter insertion set

Neosporin
  N. Cream
  N. GU irrigant

N. Ophthalmic Ointment
N. Topical Ointment
neostigmine
NeoSure nutritional supplement
Neo-Synephrine
N.-S. 12 Hour Nasal Solution
N.-S. Ophthalmic Solution
Neo-Therm neonatal skin temperature probe
Neotrace-4
Neotrend
N. premature infant blood gas/temperature monitor
N. sensor
N. system
neoumbilicus
neourethra
neovagina
gracilis flap n.
reconfiguration for n.
neovascularization of disc (NVD)
neovascular tissue
NephrAmine
nephrectomy
nephrin
nephritic factor
nephritides (*pl. of* nephritis)
nephritis, *pl.* **nephritides**
acute interstitial n.
acute postinfectious n.
Alport syndrome-like n.
autoimmune interstitial n.
diffuse proliferative lupus n.
focal lupus n.
n. gravidarum
hemorrhagic familial n.
hemorrhagic hereditary n.
hereditary familial congenital n.
interstitial n.
lupus n.
membranous lupus n.
mesangial lupus n.
postinfectious n.
proliferative lupus n.
pyoderma-associated n.
shunt n.
tubulointerstitial n. (TINU)
nephritogenic
nephroblastoma
nephroblastomatosis
diffuse n.
Nephro-Calci
nephrocalcinosis
Nephrocaps
Nephro-Fer
nephrogenesis
nephrogenetic (*var. of* nephrogenic)
nephrogenic, nephrogenetic
n. cord

n. diabetes insipidus
n. fibrosing dermopathy
n. rest
nephrolithiasis
uric acid n.
X-linked hypercalciuric n. (XLHN)
X-linked recessive n.
nephrologist
nephroma
congenital mesoblastic n.
cystic n.
mesoblastic n.
nephron
cortical n.
n. loss
Nephronex
nephronophthisis (NPH), nephrophthisis
juvenile n.
n. type 1 (NPH1)
nephropathia (*var. of* nephropathy)
nephropathy, nephropathia
diabetic n.
familial juvenile hyperuricemic n.
HIV-associated n.
immunoglobulin A n.
membranous n.
pediatric lupus n.
reflux n.
renal cortical n.
sickle cell n.
thin basement membrane n.
urate n.
nephrophthisis, nephronophthisis
familial juvenile n. (FJN)
nephrosclerosis
malignant n.
nephrosis
congenital n.
n., microcephaly, hiatus hernia syndrome
nephrosis-microcephaly syndrome
nephrostomy
percutaneous n.
nephrotic syndrome
nephrotoxicity
aminoglycoside n.
nephrotoxin
nephroureterectomy
nepiology
Neptazane
NERICP
New England Regional Infant Cardiac Program
neridronate
nerve
abducens n.
accessory n.
acoustic n.
anterior labial n.'s

nerve (*continued*)
    auditory n.
    n. block
    ciliary n.
    clitoral n.
    n. conduction study
    n. conduction velocity (NCV)
    cranial n. (II–XII)
    n. dysplasia
    facial n.
    femoral n.
    femoral cutaneous n.
    genitofemoral n.
    glioma of optic n.
    glossopharyngeal n.
    n. growth factor (NGF)
    hemorrhoidal n.
    hypoglossal n.
    inferior hemorrhoidal n.
    inferior rectal n.
    infraorbital n.
    n. injury
    interior hemorrhoidal n.
    laryngeal n.
    motor n.
    musculocutaneous n.
    nociceptive sensory n.
    obturator n.
    oculomotor n.
    optic n.
    n. palsy
    n. paralysis
    paralysis of superior laryngeal n.
    parasympathetic n.
    pelvic floor n.
    perineal n.
    phrenic n.
    postauricular n.
    posterior labial n.'
    preauricular n.
    presacral n.
    pudendal n.
    sacral n.
    saphenous n.
    sciatic n.
    sensory n.
    n. sheath tumor
    n. sprouting
    superior laryngeal n.
    n. thickening
    thoracolumbar sympathetic n.
    n. tract
    trigeminal n.
    trochlear n.
    vagus n.
    vestibular n.
    vestibulocochlear n.
nerve-muscle pedicle
nervi (*pl. of* nervus)

Nervine
Nervocaine
nervorum
    vasa n.
nervosa
    anorexia n. (AN)
    bulimia n. (BN)
    mild anorexia n.
nervous
    n. colon
    n. system
    n. system sarcoidosis
    n. tissue nevus
nervus, *pl.* **nervi**
    nervi erigentes
nesidioblastosis
nest
    cancer n.
    crow's n.
    Walthard n.
Nestabs FA
net
    Chiari n.
    n. ultrafiltration pressure
NET-EN
    norethindrone enanthate
Netherton syndrome
netilmicin sulfate
net-like rash
netting
    Baby Air mesh n.
Nettleship-Falls ocular albinism
Nettleship syndrome
network
    American College of Obstetrics
      Gynecology n.
    Cooperative Human Tissue N.
      (CHTN)
    Human Genome Epidemiology N.
      (HuGENET, HuGENet)
    National Women's Health N.
    Pelvic Floor Disorders N.
    SEER n.
    support n.
    trans-Golgi n.
Neubauer
    N. chamber
    N. hemocytometer
Neugebauer-Le Fort colpocleisis procedure
Neuhauser syndrome
neuii
    Actinomyces n.
Neu-Laxova syndrome (NLS)
Neumega
Neupogen
neural
    n. arch
    n. arch joint

n. axis
n. cell adhesion molecule L1 (LICAM)
n. ceroid lipofuscinosis
n. crest
n. crest cell
n. crest-derived cell lineage
n. crest tissue
n. crest tumor
n. discharge
n. groove
n. index
n. mechanism
n. neoplasm
n. plate
n. reflex pathway
n. retina
n. tissue accretion
n. tube
n. tube closure
n. tube defect (NTD)
n. tube disorder
n. tube rupture
neuralgia
mammary n.
postherpetic n. (PHN)
neurally
n. mediated hypotension
n. mediated syncope (NMS)
neuraminic acid
neuraminidase
n. deficiency
n. inhibitor
neuraxial anesthesia
neuraxis tumor imaging
neurectomy, neuroectomy
presacral n.
neurenteric
n. canal
n. cyst
neurepithelium (*var. of* neuroepithelium)
neurilemmoma (*var. of* neurilemoma)
neurilemoma, neurilemmoma, neurolemmoma
malignant n.
neurinoma
neurinomatosis
n. centralis
n. universalis
neuritic cytoplasmic process
neuritis
acute n.
bilateral optic n.
cranial n.
intraocular optic n.
optic n.
peripheral n.

retrobulbar n.
subacute n.
unilateral optic n.
neuritogenesis
neuroacanthocytosis
neuroanatomical
neuroangiomatosis
neuroarthromyodysplasia
neuroaxonal dystrophy
neurobehavioral
n. abnormality
n. disturbance
neurobiologic
n. influence
N. Risk Scale (NBRS)
neurobiological
neuroblastoma (NB)
n. cell
central n.
familial n.
metastatic n.
neonatal n.
occult n.
peripheral n.
neuroborreliosis
Lyme n.
neurocardiogenic syncope
neurochemical
neurocognitive
n. impairment
n. potential
neurocristopathy
neurocutaneous
n. disorder
n. melanosis syndrome
NeuroCybernetic prosthesis
neurocysticercosis
intraventricular n.
neurodermatitis
circumscribed n.
neurodevelopmental
n. assessment
N. Assessment of Preterm Infants (NAPI)
n. complication
n. deficit
n. delay
n. disability
n. disease
n. handicap
n. problem
n. sequela
n. treatment
neurodevelopment therapy (NDT)
neuroectoderm
neuroectodermal
n. hamartoma
n. tumor
neuroectomy (*var. of* neurectomy)

N

neuroendocrine
  n. response
  n. system
neuroendocrinology
neuroepithelioma
  peripheral n.
neuroepithelium, neurepithelium
  telencephalic n.
neurofaciodigitorenal (NFDR)
  n. syndrome
neurofibroma
  abdominal n.
  clitoral n.
  lumbosacral n.
  myometrial n.
  ovarian n.
  plexiform n.
  subcutaneous n.
  vaginal n.
  vulvar n.
neurofibromatosis (NF)
  bilateral acoustic n.
  central type n.
  familial spinal n.
  peripheral n.
  plexiform n.
  segmental n.
  spinal n.
  n. type 1 (NF1)
  n. type 2 (NF2)
  vaginal n.
  von Recklinghausen n.
  n. with Noonan phenotype
neurofibromatosis-Noonan syndrome (NF-NS)
neurofibrosarcoma
neurofilament antibody
neurofunctional
neurogenetic (*var. of* neurogenic)
neurogenic, neurogenetic, neurogenous
  n. atrophy
  n. bladder
  n. bladder dysfunction
  n. bowel
  n. clubfoot
  n. detrusor instability
  n. detrusor overactivity
  n. diabetes insipidus
  n. dysplasia of hip (NDH)
  n. equinus deformity
  n. hip disease
  n. hip dysplasia
  n. polydipsia
  n. pulmonary edema
  n. respiratory failure
  n. sarcoma
  n. shock
  n. stuttering
  n. talipes equinovarus
  n. tumor
neurogenous (*var. of* neurogenic)
neuroglial heterotopia
neurogram
  pudendal n.
neurohormonal
neurohypophysis
neuroichthyosis-hypogonadism syndrome
neuroid
  n. cell
  n. nevus
neuroimaging study
neurolemmoma (*var. of* neurilemoma)
neuroleptic
  n. drug
  n. malignant syndrome (NMS)
  n. medication
neurologic, neurological
  n. abnormality
  n. adverse effect
  N. and Adaptive Capacity Score (NACS)
  n. complication
  n. condition
  n. demyelinating disease
  n. development (ND)
  n. disability
  n. disease syndrome
  n. disorder
  n. dysfunction
  n. examination
  N. Examination for Children (NEC)
  n. factor
  n. impairment
  n. injury
  n. involvement
  n. maturity
  n. sequela
  n. shellfish poisoning
  n. soft signs
  n. status
neurological (*var. of* neurologic)
neurologist
  pediatric n.
neurolysis
  intrathecal n.
  transcutaneous n.
neuroma, neurinoma, *pl.* **neuromata, neuromas**
  acoustic n.
  bilateral acoustic n.'s
  incisional n.
neuromas (*pl. of* neuroma)
neuromata (*pl. of* neuroma)
neuromelanin
neuromelanogenesis
neuromodulator

neuromotor dysfunction
neuromuscular
    n. blockade
    n. blockage
    n. blocking agent
    n. disease
    n. disorder
    n. imbalance
    n. injury
    n. junction (NMJ)
    n. maturity
    n. maturity assessment
    n. scoliosis
    n. scoliosis syndrome
neuromyelitis optica
neuron, neurone
    Cajal-Retzius n.
    hippocampal n.
    motor n.
    oxytocin-secreting n.
    n. palsy
    parasympathetic n.
neuronal
    n. ceroid lipofuscinosis
      (CLN, NCL)
    n. damage
    n. dysplasia
    n. GM1 gangliosidosis
    n. heterotopia
    n. migration disorder
    n. necrosis
neurone (*var. of* neuron)
neuronitis
    vestibular n.
neuronophagia, neuronophagy
neuronophagy
neuronotmesis (*var. of* neurotmesis)
neuron-specific enolase (NSE)
Neurontin
neurooculocutaneous angiomatosis
neuropathic
    n. anhidrosis
    n. bladder
    n. cystinosis
neuropathy
    acute motor-axonal n. (AMAN)
    acute motor-sensory axonal n.
      (AMSAN)
    neuropathy, ataxia, retinitis
      pigmentosa (NARP)
    autonomic n.
    bulbar hereditary motor n. (type I,
      II)
    chronic peripheral n.
    congenital hypomyelinating n.
      (CHN)
    congenital sensory n.
    distal symmetric sensorimotor n.
    familial visceral n.

    femoral n.
    giant axonal n.
    glue-sniffing n.
    hereditary autonomic n.
    hereditary motor-sensory n. (type
      IA, II–VII) (HMSN)
    hereditary sensory autonomic n.
    hereditary sensory radicular n.
    Leber hereditary optic n. (LHON)
    Leber optic n.
    motor-axonal n.
    motor sensory n. (MSN)
    myenteric plexus n.
    nutritional n.
    obstetric n.
    optic n.
    peripheral entrapment n.
    porphyric n.
    postdiphtheritic n.
    pudendal n.
    radicular n.
    reflux n. (RN)
    retractor n.
    sensory n.
    tomaculous n.
    toxic n.
    tropical ataxic n.
    ulnar n.
neuropeptide
    enteric n.
neuropharmacology
neurophysin I, II
neurophysiologic testing
neurophysiology
neuropore
    caudal n.
    rostral n.
neuroprotection
neuropsychiatric
    n. behavior
    n. disorder
    n. syncope
neuropsychiatry
neuropsychologic, neuropsychological
    n. profile
    n. sequela
neuropsychological (*var. of*
  neuropsychologic)
neuropsychology
    clinical assessment in n.
neuropsychopharmacology
neuroradiographic study
neuroretinitis
    optic n.
neuroretinoangiomatosis
neurosarcoidosis
neuroschisis
neurosecretion
neurosecretory

N

neurosensory
  n. deafness
  n. impairment (NSI)
neurosis
  pregnancy n.
neurosonographic
neurospongioblastosis diffusa
neurosteroid
neurostimulation
neurosurgeon
neurosurgical
  n. closure
  n. shunt
neurosyphilis
  congenital paretic n.
  congenital tertiary n.
  tabetic n.
neurotensin
neurotic
neurotmesis, neuronotmesis
neurotoxicity
  methylmercury n.
neurotoxic shellfish poisoning
neurotoxin
  botulinus n.
  tetanus n.
neurotransmission
neurotransmitter
  n. imbalance
  n. precursor
  n. release
  substance P pain n.
neurotrauma
neurotrichocutaneous syndrome
neurotrophic keratitis
neurovascular
  n. compromise
  n. dystrophy
neurovegetative
  n. functioning
  n. functioning or symptom
neurovirulence
neurovisceral lipidosis
neurula
neurulation
neutral
  K-Phos N.
  n. lipid storage disease
  n. pH
  n. pH of vagina
  n. position
  n. protamine Hagedorn
    (NPH)
  n. protamine Hagedorn insulin
  n. rotation
neutralization
neutralize
Neutra-Phos
Neutra-Phos-K

Neutrogena
  N. Acne Mask
  N. T/Derm
neutron
  fast n.
  n. therapy
neutropenia
  alloimmune neonatal n. (ANN)
  autoimmune n. (AIN)
  benign n.
  cardioskeletal n.
  chemotherapy-related n.
  chronic benign n. (CBN)
  chronic idiopathic n.
  congenital n.
  cyclic n.
  drug-induced n.
  idiopathic n.
  immune n.
  immune-mediated n.
  Kostmann n.
  neonatal autoimmune n.
  neonatal chronic idiopathic n.
  peripheral n.
  persistent n.
  severe chronic n. (SCN)
  severe congenital n.
  transient n.
  X-linked cardioskeletal myopathy
    and n.
neutropenic
neutrophile
  n. actin deficiency
  n. actin dysfunction
  n. apoptosis
  band form n.
  n. chemotactic deficiency
  circulating n.'s
  n. egress
  n. G6PD deficiency
  n. granulopoiesis
  hypersegmented n.
  mature n.
  n. protease-3
  segmented n.
  n. transfusion
neutrophile (*var. of* neutrophil)
neutrophilia
  acute acquired n.
neutrophilic
  n. leukocytosis
  n. pleocytosis
  n. rhinitis
NEV
  noninvasive extrathoracic ventilator
nevi (*pl. of* nevus)
Neville-Barnes forceps
nevirapine
nevocellular nevus

nevoid, naevoid
  n. amentia
  n. basal cell carcinoma (NBCC)
  n. basal cell carcinoma syndrome
    (NBCCS, NBS)
  n. hyperkeratosis of nipple and
    areola
nevomelanocyte
Nevo syndrome
nevoxanthoendothelioma
nevus, *pl.* **nevi**
  achromic n.
  acquired melanocytic n. (AMN)
  n. anemicus
  angiomatous involuting n.
  n. araneus
  nevi, atrial myxoma, myxoid
    neurofibromas, ephelides (NAME)
  atypical melanocytic n.
  bathing trunk n.
  Becker n.
  benign n.
  blue rubber bleb n.
  cellular blue n.
  combined n.
  n. comedonicus
  common blue n.
  compound n.
  congenital n.
  congenital hairy n.
  congenital melanocytic n.
  congenital nevomelanocytic n.
  congenital pigmental n.
  conjunctival n.
  connective tissue n.
  cutaneous n.
  depigmented n.
  n. depigmentosus
  dermal n.
  dysplastic n.
  eczematous halo n.
  n. elasticus of Lewandowsky
  epidermal n.
  epithelioid cell n.
  eruptive n.
  faun tail n.
  n. flammeus
  giant congenital pigmented n.
  hairy n.
  halo n.
  intradermal n.
  involuting n.
  Ito n.
  Jadassohn-Tièche n.
  junctional n.
  lentigines, atrial myxomas, cutaneous
    papular myxomas, blue nevi
    (LAMB)
  lentiginous n.

  linear verrucous epidermal n.
  melanocytic n.
  Meyerson n.
  nape n.
  nervous tissue n.
  neuroid n.
  nevocellular n.
  n. of Ito
  n. of Jadassohn
  n. of Ota
  organoid n.
  Ota n.
  pigmented n.
  n. pigmentosus systematicus
  port-wine n.
  rubber bleb n.
  satellite melanocytic n.
  sebaceous n.
  n. sebaceus
  n. sebaceus linearis
  n. sebaceus of Jadassohn (SNJ)
  n. simplex
  speckled lentiginous n.
  spider n.
  n. spilus
  spindle cell epithelioid n.
  Spitz n.
  strawberry n.
  telangiectatic n.
  n. unius lateris
  Unna n.
  vascular n.
  verrucose streaky epidermal n.
  vulvar nevomelanocytic n.
  white sponge n.
  woolly hair n.
  zosteriform lentiginous n.
new
  n. Ballard score (NBS)
  N. England Regional Infant Cardiac
    Program (NERICP)
  n. MacArthur emotion story-stems
  N. Moves obesity-prevention
    program
  n. mutation
  n. variant CJD
  n. variant Creutzfeldt-Jakob disease
    (nvCJD)
  N. York Heart Association (NYHA)
newborn (NB)
  ABO hemolytic disease of the n.
  N. Behavior Assessment Scale
    (NBAS)
  car seat for n.
  congenital anemia of n.
  congenital epulis of n.
  cyanotic n.
  epulis of n.
  n. euglycemia

N

newborn (*continued*)
n. examination
full-term n. (FTNB)
n. genetic screening test
genital crisis of n.
gingival cyst of n.
gonococcal arthritis of n.
hemolytic disease of n. (HDN)
hemorrhage of n. (HN)
hemorrhagic disease of n.
(HDN)
horizontal suspension in n.
hyperthermia in n.
n. intensive care (NBIC, NIC)
n. intensive care unit (NBICU)
jaundice of n. (JNB)
lamellar desquamation of n.
metabolic disease in n.
n. narcotic withdrawal syndrome
nonfollicular pustulosis of n.
n. nursery
Parrot atrophy of n.
n. period
persistent pulmonary hypertension of
n. (PPHN)
physiologic jaundice of n.
n. platelet antigen typing
pulmonary hypertension of n.
n. rehospitalization after early
discharge
n. respiratory distress syndrome
respiratory distress syndrome of
the n.
n. resuscitation
retinopathy of n.
Rh disease of n.
n. screening kit
n. special care unit (NBSCU)
spontaneous gangrene of n.
transient bullous dermolysis of n.
transient tachypnea of n. (TTN,
TTNB)
transient tyrosinemia of n.
transitory fever of n.
new-onset
n.-o. diabetes mellitus
n.-o. hydrocephalus
n.-o. JDM
newport
N. medical instrument
Salmonella n.
N. Wave ventilator
newtonian aberration
Newtrition
N. Isofiber formula
N. Isotonic formula
**NexPill SmartCap medication monitoring
system**
Nezelof syndrome

Nezhat-Dorsey
N.-D. aspirator
N.-D. suction-irrigator
NF
neurofibromatosis
NF1
neurofibromatosis type 1
NF1 gene
NF2
neurofibromatosis type 2
NFAT
nuclear factor of activated T cell
NFCS
neonatal facial coding system
NFDR
neurofaciodigitorenal
NFDR syndrome
NF-NS
neurofibromatosis-Noonan
syndrome
NG
nasogastric
NG tube
NGF
nerve growth factor
NGHD-SS
nongrowth hormone-deficient short
stature
NGT
nasogastric tube
NGT Topical
NH
neonatal hemochromatosis
NHANES
National Health and Nutrition
Examination Survey
NHC
neonatal hypocalcemia
NHIS
National Health Interview Survey
NHL
non-Hodgkin lymphoma
NHRT
natural hormone replacement
therapy
NHS
Nance-Horan syndrome
NHT
neoadjuvant hormonal therapy
niacinamide
niacin poisoning
nialamide
Niaspan
NIBPM
noninvasive blood pressure
measurement
NIC
newborn intensive care
nicardipine

NICHD
National Institute of Child Health and Human Development
niche
ontogenetic n.
Nichols
N. procedure
N. sacrospinous fixation
nicked human chorionic gonadotropin
nickel dermatitis
Nickerson
N. BiGGY vial
N. medium
nick translation
niclosamide
Nico-400
Nicobid
Nicoderm
Nicolas-Favre disease
nicotinamide adenine dinucleotide phosphate (NADPH)
nicotine patch therapy
Nicotinex
nicotinic acid
nicotinyl alcohol
nicoumalone
Nic the Dragon pediatric aerosol mask
NICU
neonatal intensive care unit
nidation
NIDDM
non-insulin-dependent diabetes mellitus
nidi (*pl. of* nidus)
NIDS
National Hospital Discharge Survey
nidulans
Aspergillus n.
nidus, *pl.* **nidi**
Niemann-Pick
N.-P. cell
N.-P. disease type A (NPA)
N.-P. disease type B (NPB)
N.-P. disease type C (NPC)
N.-P. disease (type I, II) (NPD)
NIF
negative inspiratory force
nifedipine
nifurtimox
niger
Aspergillus n.
Peptococcus n.
night
n. blindness
n. pain
n. splint
n. splinting
n. sweat
n. terror
NightForm infant sleep mattress

Nightingale examining lamp
nightmare
nigra
linea n.
lingua n.
substantia n.
nigricans
acanthosis n.
hirsutism, androgen excess, insulin resistance, acanthosis n. (HAIR-AN)
hyperandrogenism, insulin resistance, acanthosis n. (HAIRAN, HAIR-AN)
pseudoacanthosis n.
n. syndrome
nigricans-hyperinsulinemia syndrome
nigripalpus
Culex n.
nigrostriatal tract
NIH
National Institutes of Health
NIHF
nonimmune hydrops fetalis
Niikawa-Kuroki syndrome
Nijmegen breakage syndrome (NBS)
Nikolsky sign
Nilandron
nilutamide
Nimbex
NIMH
National Institute of Mental Health
NIMH global scale
nimodipine
NIMV
noninvasive motion ventilation
nine
rule of n.'s
Niplette device
nipple
accessory n.
adenoma of n.
n. aspiration fluid
n. discharge
n. eczema
erosive adenomatosis of n.
extranumerary n.
n. fed
n. feeding
n. flow rate
n. inversion
inverted n.
McGovern n.
O_2 flowmeter n.
out-of-profile n.
Paget disease of n.
preemie n.
n. retraction
n. shield

N

nipple (*continued*)
    n. soreness
    n. stimulation
    n. stimulation test
    supernumerary n.
nipple-areola complex (NAC)
nipple-fed baby
nipplelike lesion
nippling
Nipride
NIPS
    Neonatal Infant Pain Scale
NIRP
    near infrared photoplethysmography
NIRS
    near infrared spectrophotometry
    near infrared spectroscopy
NIS-2
    Second National Incidence
      Study
NISD
    neonatal iron-storage disease
Nisentil
Nissen fundoplication
Nissl
    N. bodies
    N. granule
NIT
    neonatal isoimmune
      thrombocytopenia
nit
Nitabuch layer
Nite Train-r Alarm
nitidus
    lichen n.
nitrate
    butoconazole n.
    miconazole n.
    silver n.
Nitrazine
    fern-positive N.
    N. paper
    N. test
nitric
    n. oxide (NO)
    n. oxide oxidation
nitrite
    plasma n.
    n. urine test
Nitro-Bid Ointment
nitroblue
    n. tetrazolium (NBT)
    n. tetrazolium dye reduction test
Nitrocap
nitrocellulose
Nitro-Dur Patch
nitrofurantoin
    n. monohydrate
    n. monohydrate macrocrystal

Nitrogard Buccal
nitrogen (N)
    blood urea n. (BUN)
    n. dioxide inhalation
    liquid n.
    n. mustard
    n. partial pressure (PN_2)
    serum urea n. (SUN)
    urea n.
    n. washout
    n. washout test
nitrogenous
    n. base
    n. waste
nitroglycerin (NTG)
    n. paste
    topical n.
Nitroglyn Oral
nitroimidazole compound
Nitrolingual Translingual Spray
Nitrol Ointment
Nitronet
Nitrong
Nitropress
nitroprusside
    n. sodium
    sodium n. (SNP)
nitrosourea
Nitrospan
Nitrostat Sublingual
nitrotyrosine
nitrous oxide (N_2O)
nitrovasodilator
Nivea cream
Nix Creme Rinse
nizatidine
Nizoral
NJ
    nasojejunal
      NJ tube
NJCLD
    National Joint Committee on Learning
      Disabilities
NJF
    Naegeli-Franceschetti-Jadasshon
      NJF syndrome
NK
    natural killer
NKC
    natural killer cell
NKH
    nonketotic hyperglycemia
NKHG
    nonketotic hyperglycemia
NLD
    nasolacrimal duct
    necrobiosis lipoidica diabeticorum
NLDO
    nasolacrimal duct obstruction

NLE
neonatal lupus erythematosus
NLGCLS
Noonan-like giant cell lesion syndrome
N2-L-lysylbradkinin
NLP
no light perception
NLS
Neu-Laxova syndrome
NMGTD
nonmetastatic gestational trophoblastic
disease
NMJ
neuromuscular junction
NMN
Novy-McNeal-Nicolle
NMR
neonatal mortality rate
neonatal mortality risk
nuclear magnetic resonance
NMR spectroscopy
NMS
neurally mediated syncope
neuroleptic malignant syndrome
NMSIDS
near-miss sudden infant death
syndrome
N-Multistix clinical test strip
NND
neonatal death
n,n-diethyl-m-toluamide (DEET),
n-diethyl-m-toluamide
NNJ
neonatal jaundice
NNM
neonatal mortality
NNRTI
nonnucleoside reverse transcriptase
inhibitor
NNS
nonnutritive sucking
N₂O
nitrous oxide
NO
nitric oxide
no
n. light perception (NLP)
n. tears
Noack syndrome
Noble-Mengert perineal repair
Nocardia
N. asteroides
N. brasiliensis
N. caviae
N. farcinica
N. nova
N. otitidiscaviarum
N. transvalensis
nocardiosis

nociception
nociceptive
n. pathway
n. sensory nerve
n. stimulus
nociferous cortex
nocturia, nycturia
nocturnal
n. angina
n. asthma
n. enuresis
n. epilepsy
n. leg cramp
n. micturition
n. myoclonus
n. polyuria syndrome
n. pulse oximetry
n. retrosternal chest pain
n. sweating
nocturnus
pavor n.
nodal
n. involvement
n. tachycardia
nodding spasm
node
anterior pectoral n.
aortic n.
atrioventricular n.
axillary lymph n.
caseous n.
Cloquet n.
deep cervical n.
femoral lymph n.
gluteal lymph n.
Hensen n.
hypogastric lymph n.
iliac n.
infraclavicular n.
inguinal lymph n.
inguinofemoral lymph n.
interpectoral n.
intramammary lymph n.
locoregional n.
lymph n.
mucocutaneous lymph n.
Osler n.
paraaortic n.
parapharyngeal lymph n.
parauterine lymph n.
pelvic lymph n.
peracervical n.
periaortic lymph n.
rectal n.
retroperitoneal n.
retropharyngeal lymph n.
Rotter n.
sacral lymph n.
Schmorl n.

node (*continued*)
    sentinel lymph n. (SLN)
    shotty n.
    signal n.
    sinoatrial n. (SA)
    sternal n.
    subaortic lymph n.
    subclavian n.
    subpectoral axillary n.
    ureteral n.
    vulvar lymph n.

nodosa
    distal trichorrhexis n.
    infantile periarteritis n. (IPN)
    infantile polyarteritis n.
    (IPAN, IPN)
    isthmica n.
    maculopapular n.
    periarteritis n.
    polyarteritis n. (PAN)
    salpingitis isthmica n. (SIN)
    trichorrhexis n.

nodosum
    amnion n.
    erythema n.

nodular
    n. adrenal hyperplasia
    n. blueberry lip
    n. cortical sclerosis
    n. cystic acne
    n. embryo
    n. fasciitis
    n. gastritis
    n. infiltration
    n. lymphoid hyperplasia
    n. melanoma
    n. nerve thickening
    n. nonsuppurative panniculitis
    n. renal blastoma
    n. sclerosing Hodgkin disease
    n. thyroid disease

nodularity
    uterosacral n.

nodule
    Albini n.
    Aschoff n.
    blueberry muffin n.
    Bohn n.
    Brown n.
    Busacca iris n.
    cold n.
    cutaneous n.
    Hoboken n.
    hot n.
    iris Lisch n.
    Koeppe iris n.
    Lisch n.
    Lutz-Jeanselme n.
    palpable n.

    parenchymal n.
    pearly-white n.
    placental site n.
    rheumatoid n.
    Sister Mary Joseph n.
    subcutaneous n.
    subserous n.
    thyroid n.
    vocal n.

nodulocystic lesion
NOE
    nasoorbitoethmoid
    NOE fracture
NOFT
    nonorganic failure to thrive
NOFTT
    nonorganic failure to thrive
Noguchi test
noir
    tache n.
noise
    expiratory n.
    upper airway n.
Nolahist
Nolvadex
noma
    n. neonatorum
    n. pudendi
    n. vulvae
nomenclature
    FIGO n.
    Fisher-Race Rh system n.
    TNM n.
nomogram
    body mass index n.
    Done n.
    gestation-specific n.
    Lubchenco n.
    Rumack-Matthew n.
    Siggaard-Andersen n.
non-A
    n.-A hepatitis
    n.-A, non-B hepatitis (NANBH)
    n.-A, non-B hepatotropic virus
non-ABCDE hepatitis
nonaccidental spiral tibial fracture
nonadjuvant therapy
nonalcoholic steatohepatitis (NASH)
nonalkylating agent
nonallele
nonallergenic
    n. perrenial rhinitis
    n. rhinitis with eosinophilia
nonallergic rhinitis
nonallopathic health care system
nonalpha cell tumor
nonambulatory
nonangiitic vasculopathic condition
nonanion gap metabolic acidosis

nonappendiceal carcinoid
nonatopic wheezer
nonautoimmune myasthenic syndrome
nonautologous reconstruction
nonautonomous attachment
non-B hepatitis
nonbacterial
    n. thrombotic endocarditis
    n. thrombotic vegetation (NBTV)
nonbilious vomiting
nonbranching pseudohypha
non-breath-hold MR cholangiography
nonbronchoscopic bronchoalveolar
  lavage
nonbullous
    n. congenital ichthyosiform
    erythroderma (NBCIE)
    n. impetigo
noncalcific vasculopathy
noncalcified nodular mass
noncalculous
noncarbonic acid
noncardiac pulmonary edema
noncarrier
noncaseating sarcoidlike granuloma
non-casein-based diet
noncategorical placement
nonchylous pleural effusion
noncirrhotic ascitic disease
nonclassic, nonclassical
    n. adrenal hyperplasia (NCAH)
    n. congenital adrenal hyperplasia
    (NC-CAH)
    n. 21-hydroxylase deficiency
nonclassical (var. of nonclassic)
noncleft median face syndrome
noncoiled cord
noncoital
    n. sexual pain
    n. sexual stimulation
noncommunicating
    N. Children's Pain Checklist-Revised
    (NCCPC-R)
    n. cyst
    n. hydrocephalus
    n. uterine horn
noncompliance
    medical n.
noncontact ultrasound
noncontingent scheduling
nonconvulsive
    n. seizure
    n. status epilepticus (NCSE)
noncosmetic panniculectomy
noncovalent
noncyanotic congenital heart
  disease
noncyclic breast pain
nondeciduous placenta

nondeletion
nondepolarizing paralyzing agent
nondiagnostic culdocentesis
nondirective
    n. counseling
    n. supportive psychotherapy
nondisjunction
    chromosomal n.
    n. trisomy 21
nondisplaced lateral condylar fracture
nondysgerminomatous germ cell tumor
nonencephalitogenic cell
nonepileptic
    n. myoclonus
    n. paroxysmal disorder
    n. seizure
nonerythropoietic heme
nonessential amino acid
nonestrogen drug
nonestrogen-regulated growth
nonexercise activity thermogenesis
nonexudative conjunctival injection
nonfamilial
    n. aniridia
    n. hyperinsulinemic hypoglycemia
    n. hyperinsulinism of infancy
    n. visceral myopathy
nonfat milk
nonfenestrated forceps
nonfixing eye
nonfollicular
    n. pustulosis
    n. pustulosis of newborn
nonfrank breech
nonfunctional
    n. pituitary tumor
    n. streak
nongamma Coombs test
nongenetic syndrome
nongenital pelvic organ
nongenotoxic
nongestational choriocarcinoma
nongonococcal
    n. cervicitis
    n. urethritis
nongranulomatous salpingitis
nongrowth hormone-deficient short
  stature (NGHD-SS)
nonhematogenous tumor
nonheme iron
nonhemolytic
    n. aerobic organism
    n. reaction
nonhistone
non-Hodgkin lymphoma (NHL)
nonhomologous chromosome
nonhydropic fetus
nonhyperinsulinemic hypoglycemia
non-IgE-mediated food allergy

N

nonimmune
- n. fetal hydrops
- n. hemolysis
- n. hydrops fetalis (NIHF)

non-insulin-dependent
- n.-i.-d. diabetes
- n.-i.-d. diabetes mellitus (NIDDM)
- n.-i.-d. diabetic

noninvasive
- n. blood pressure measurement (NIBPM)
- n. detection of trisomy 18
- n. extrathoracic ventilator (NEV)
- n. management
- n. motion ventilation (NIMV)
- n. respiratory support
- n. test

nonionic
- n. contrast material
- n. contrast medium

nonionizing nonthermal application
nonirritating
nonisomorphic presentation
nonketotic
- n. hyperglycemia (NKHG)
- n. hyperosmolar coma (NKHC)
- n. hypoglycemia

nonkinesigenic dyskinesia
nonlactating breast
nonlinkage
nonlocking closure
nonlymphoblastic leukemia
nonlymphocytic leukemia
nonmaleficence
nonmaternal death
nonmendelian disorder
nonmetastatic gestational trophoblastic disease (NMGTD)
nonmigrainous headache
nonmonogamous partner
nonmotile sperm
nonmusical wheeze
nonmutogenic
nonmyeloablative stem cell transplant
nonnarcotic abstinence syndrome
Nonne-Milroy-Meige syndrome
nonneoplastic epithelial disorder
nonneural congenital defect
nonneurogenic
- n. dysphagia
- n. neurogenic bladder

nonnucleoside reverse transcriptase inhibitor (NNRTI)
nonnutritional rickets
nonnutritive
- n. sucking (NNS)
- n. sucking opportunity (NSO)

nonobstruction
large-volume n.

nonobstructive
- n. pattern
- n. pyelonephritis

nonoliguric ARF
nonorganic failure to thrive (NOFT, NOFTT)
nonossifying fibroma
nonoxynol-9/octoxynol-9
nonpalpable
- n. abnormality
- n. testis

nonparalytic
- n. hypotonia
- n. poliomyelitis
- n. strabismus

nonparous
nonpathologic fracture
nonpharmacologic anesthesia
nonphotogenic seizure
nonpigmented endometriosis
nonpitting induration
non-PKU phenylalaninemia
nonpolio enterovirus
nonpregnant endometrium
nonprimary
- n. first episode
- n. infection

nonprogressive
- n. cerebellar disorder with mental retardation
- n. hypoplastic syndrome
- n. motor impairment syndrome
- n. ventriculomegaly

nonprolapsed uterus
nonproliferative
- n. diabetic retinopathy
- n. fibrocystic change

nonproteinuric hypertension
nonpsychotic
nonpuerperal
- n. endometritis
- n. mastitis

nonpurging
bulimia nervosa n. (BN-NP)

non-Q-wave AMI
nonradioactive immunoassay
nonrandom mating
nonrapid eye movement (non-REM, NREM)
nonreactive
- n. immunoassay
- n. NST

nonreassuring
- n. fetal heart beat pattern
- n. fetal heart rate pattern
- n. fetal status
- n. fetal testing
- n. FHR

nonrebreather
　　n. face mask
　　high-flow n.
nonreciprocal gait
non-REM
　　nonrapid eye movement
　　non-REM sleep
nonresting energy expenditure (NREE)
nonrhabdomyogenic soft tissue sarcoma
nonrhabdomyomatous sarcoma
nonrhabdomyosarcoma soft tissue
　sarcoma (NRSTS)
non-Rh D/non-ABO hemolytic disease
nonsalt-losing adrenogenital syndrome
nonsecreting pituitary tumor
nonsense mutation
nonseptated
non-sex hormone-binding globulin bound
　testosterone
nonspastic paraparesis
nonspecific
　　n. arrhythmia (NSA)
　　n. encephalopathy
　　n. esophageal motility disorder
　　　(NEMD)
　　n. ileitis
　　n. immunotherapy
　　n. mental retardation
　　n. mesenchyme
　　n. urethritis (NSU)
　　n. vaginitis
　　n. vaginosis
　　n. vulvovaginitis
nonspherical congruent hips
nonspherocytic anemia
nonsteroidal antiinflammatory drug
　(NSAID)
nonstreptococcal pharyngitis
nonstressed fetus
nonstress test (NST)
nonstructural gene
nonsuppurative panniculitis
nonsusceptible
nonsustained ventricular tachycardia
non-syncytium-inducing (NSI)
　　n.-s.-i. strain
　　n.-s.-i. variant of AIDS virus
nonsyndromic
　　n. bile duct paucity
　　n. bile duct paucity syndrome
nontension pneumothorax
nonthyroidal illness (NTI)
nontoxic
nontreponemal
　　n. serology
　　n. test
non-*Treponema* titer
nontubal ectopic pregnancy
nontuberculous

　　n. mycobacterial infection
　　n. mycobacterium (NTM)
nontumoral hyperprolactinemia
nontypeable organism
non-typhi *Salmonella* (NTS)
nontyphoidal *Salmonella*
nontyphoid *Salmonella*
nonulcer dyspepsia
nonunion
nonvalent pneumococcal conjugate
　vaccine (PnCV)
nonvascular
nonverbal
　　n. communication
　　n. developmental index
　　n. learning disability (NVLD)
　　n. perceptual-organization-output
　　　disorder
nonvertex fetus
nonvertex-nonvertex
nonvertex-vertex
nonvertiginous condition
nonvesicular rash
nonviable fetus
nonvolatile acid
nonweightbearing activity
non-Wessel colic
Noonan-Ehmke syndrome
Noonan-like
　　N.-l. giant cell lesion
　　N.-l. giant cell lesion syndrome
　　　(NLGCLS)
Noonan syndrome
noradrenaline
　　plasma n.
noradrenergic
　　n. locus ceruleus
　　n. system
Norcept-E 1/35
Norcuron
NORD
　　National Organization for Rare
　　Disorders
Nordette contraceptive pill
Norditropin Injection
norelgestromin
norepinephrine reuptake inhibitor
Norethin
　　N. 1/35M
　　N. 1/50M
norethindrone
　　n. acetate
　　n. acetate and ethinyl estradiol
　　n. enanthate (NET-EN)
　　ethinyl estradiol and n.
　　mestranol and n.
norethisterone
norethynodrel
　　mestranol and n.

N

Norflex
norfloxacin
norgestimate
    n. and ethinyl estradiol
    ethinyl estradiol and n.
    n. progestin
norgestrel
    ethinyl estradiol and n.
norgestrel/ethinyl estradiol combination
norimbergensis
    Burkholderia n.
Norinyl
    N. 1+35
    N. 1+50
Norisodrine
Norlestrin
    N. 1/50
    N. 2.5/50
    N. Fe
normal
    n. blood loss
    n. blood pressure
    n. female sex chromosome type (XX)
    n. fetal development
    n. flap-valve mechanism
    n. gastroesophageal reflux of infancy
    n. intelligence
    n. male sex chromosome type (XY)
    n. ovariotomy
    n. placentation
    n. pressure hydrocephalus (NPH)
    n. saline (NS)
    n. saline solution (NSS)
    n. spontaneous vaginal delivery (NSVD)
    n. temperature
    n. transformation zone
    n. vaginal delivery (NVD)
normally progressing pregnancy (NPP)
Norman-Landing syndrome
Norman Miller vaginopexy
Norman-Roberts lissencephaly syndrome
Norman-Wood syndrome
Normegon
Nor-Mil
normoactive bowel sounds
normobaric oxygen
normoblast cell
normoblastemia
normocalcemic
normocapnia
normocephalic
normochromic anemia
normocytic anemia
Normodyne
normoglycemia
normogonadotropic anovulation
normophosphatemic

normoprolactinemia
normospermic
normotensive intrauterine growth restriction
Normotest
normothermia
norm-referenced test
Norovirus
Noroxin
Norpace CR
Norplant
    N. implant
    N. system
Norpramin
Nor-QD
Norrbottnian Gaucher disease
Norrie
    N. disease
    N. syndrome
Norrie-Warburg syndrome
nortestosterone
19-nortestosterone derivative
Nor-tet Oral
north
    N. American Collaborative Crohn Disease Study (NCCDS)
    N. American Society for Pediatric Gastroenterology and Nutrition (NASPGN)
    N. Asian tick typhus
northern
    N. blot
    N. blot test
Northway staging
Norton operation
Nortrel 7/7/7
nortriptyline hydrochloride
Nortussin
Norvir
    N. capsule
    N. oral solution
Norwalk
    N. agent
    N. virus
Norwalk-like virus
Norwegian scabies
Norwood
    N. operation
    N. palliation
    N. procedure
    N. stage
Norwood-Fontan procedure
nose
    beaked n.
    bifid n.
    broad flat n.
    flat n.
    prominent n.
    rabbit n.

saddle n.
short beaked n.
nosebleed
nose-breather
obligate n.-b.
nosocomial
n. bacterial infection (NBI)
n. bacterial meningitis
n. diarrhea
n. infection
n. pneumonia
n. sepsis
nosocomially acquired (NA)
nosology
nostril
anteverted n.
N. Nasal Solution
reverse n.'s
Nostrilla
notch
alveolar n.
interarytenoid n.
intercondylar n.
median alveolar n.
N. receptor
sacrosciatic n.
suprasternal n.
notching
rib n.
not delivered
note
hyperresonant calvarial percussion n.
notochord
notogenesis
notomelus
Nottingham
N. breast cancer grading system
N. colposuspension needle
nova
Nocardia n.
N. Rectal
Novafed
Novafil
Novahistine
Novak curette
Novamoxin
Novantrone
Novapren
NovaSaline prefilled breast implant
Novasome
Novasoy soy isoflavone
NovaSure
N. device
N. endometrial ablation
N. endometrial ablation procedure
N. impedance-controlled endometrial ablation system
N. wand
novo

de n.
stress incontinence de n.
Novo-AZT
novobiocin (NB, Nov)
Novo-Cimetidine
Novo-Clobetasol
Novo-Cloxin
Novo-Cromolyn
Novo-Difenac
Novo-Difenac-SR
Novo-Diflunisal
Novo-Dipam
Novo-Doxylin
Novo-Famotidine
Novo-Fibrate
Novo-Flurazine
Novo-Flurprofen
Novo-Hydrazide
Novo-Keto-EC
Novo-Lexin
Novolin
N. 70/30
N. insulin
N. L
N. N
N. N PenFill
N. 70/30 PenFill
N. R
N. R PenFill
Novo-Naprox
Novo-Nidazol
Novo-Pen-VK
Novo-Piroxicam
Novo-Pramine
Novo-Profen
Novopropamide
Novo-Ranidine
Novo-Reserpine
Novo-Ridazine
Novo-Rythro Encap
Novo-Seven
Novo-Soxazole
Novo-Tamoxifen
Novo-Terfenadine
Novo-Tetra
Novo-Trimel
Novy-McNeal-Nicolle (NMN)
N.-M.-N. biphasic blood agar
Now RSV test
noxae
NOxBOXmobile
N. monitor
N. nitric oxide delivery and monitoring system
NOxBOX+ monitor
Nozinan
NPA
nasopharyngeal aspirate
Niemann-Pick disease type A

N

N95 particulate respirator surgical mask

NPB
Niemann-Pick disease type B

NPC
Niemann-Pick disease type C

NP-CPAP
nasal prong continuous positive airway pressure

NPD
Niemann-Pick disease (type I, II)

NPH
nephronophthisis
neutral protamine Hagedorn
normal pressure hydrocephalus
NPH Iletin I, II
NPH insulin
pork NPH

NPH1
nephronophthisis type 1

NPI
Neonatal Perception Inventory

NPL
nasopharyngolaryngoscopy

NPOT
narrow pulmonary outflow tract

NPP
normally progressing pregnancy

NPR
nasopharyngeal reflux

NPTR
National Pediatric Trauma Registry

NR
Organidin NR
Tussi-Organidin DM NR

NRDS
neonatal respiratory distress syndrome

NREE
nonresting energy expenditure

NREM
nonrapid eye movement
NREM arousal parasomnia

NRP
Neonatal Resuscitation Program

NRSTS
nonrhabdomyosarcoma soft tissue sarcoma

NRTI
nucleoside reverse transcriptase inhibitor
thymidine analog NRTI

NS
normal saline
ProctoFoam NS

NSA
neck-shaft angle
nonspecific arrhythmia
NSA of femur

NSABP
National Surgical Adjuvant Breast Project

NSAID
nonsteroidal antiinflammatory drug

NSD
N-acetylneuraminic acid storage disease

NSE
neuron-specific enolase

NSGC
National Society of Genetic Counselors

NSI
neurosensory impairment
non-syncytium-inducing
NSI strain

NSO
nonnutritive sucking opportunity

NSS
normal saline solution

NST
nonmyeloablative stem cell transplant
nonstress test
antepartum fetal NST
fetal NST
nonreactive NST
NST tracing

NSU
nonspecific urethritis

NSVD
normal spontaneous vaginal delivery

NT
N-telopeptide
nuchal translucency

NTD
neural tube defect

N-telopeptide (NT)
N-t. cross-links (NTx)
N-t. test

NTF
nasogastric tube feeding

NTG
nitroglycerin

NTI
nasotracheal intubation
nonthyroidal illness

NTM
nontuberculous mycobacterium

NTS
non-typhi Salmonella

NTT
nuchal translucency thickness

NTx
N-telopeptide
N-telopeptide cross-links
NTx test

Nu-Amoxi

Nu-Ampi

Nubain

Nu-Cephalex
nuchal
- n. arm
- n. cord
- n. cystic hygroma
- n. fold
- n. pad thickening
- n. rigidity
- n. thickness
- n. translucency (NT)
- n. translucency in a fetus
- n. translucency measurement
- n. translucency screening
- n. translucency thickness
(NTT)

nuchal-spinal sign
Nu-Cimet
Nuck
- N. canal
- canal of N.
- N. diverticulum
- N. hydrocele

nuclear
- n. agenesis
- n. antigen
- n. aplasia
- n. atypia
- n. debris
- n. degeneration
- n. dust
- n. factor of activated T cell
(NFAT)
- n. jaundice
- n. magnetic resonance (NMR)
- n. milk
- n. radiation
- n. scintigraphy
- n. sex

nuclease
nucleated red blood cell
nucleatum
- *Fusobacterium* n.

nuclei (*pl. of* nucleus)
nucleic
- n. acid
- n. acid amplification (NAA)
- n. acid hybridization
- n. acid probe
- n. acid sequence-based amplification
(NASBA)

nucleoid
nucleolar chromosome
nucleolus
nucleoside
- n. analog
- n. pair
- n. phosphorylase
- n. reverse transcriptase inhibitor
(NRTI)

nucleosome
nucleotide
- adenine n.
- antisense n.
- cytosine n.
- guanine n.
- thymine n.

nucleotide-fortified formula
nucleotidylexotransferase
- DNA n.

nucleotidyltransferase
- DNA n.
- RNA n.

nucleus *pl.* **nuclei**
- n. accumbens
- arcuate n.
- Béclard n.
- caudate n.
- cerebellar n.
- cranial nerve n.
- dentate n.
- disorganized brainstem nuclei
- Edinger-Westphal n.
- inferior olivary n.
- lentiform n.
- olivary n.
- owl's eye n.
- red n.
- n. reticularis gigantocellularis
- n. retroambiguus
- steroid n.
- superior olivary n.
- n. tractus solitarius
- X-linked congenital recessive muscle
hypotrophy with central nuclei

NucliSens assay
Nu-Cloxi
Nu-Cotrimox
Nu-Diclo
Nu-Diflunisal
Nu-Doxycycline
Nu-Famotidine
Nu-Flurprofen
NUG
- necrotizing ulcerating gingivitis

Nu Gauze dressing
Nu-Gel dressing
Nugent criteria
Nu-Ibuprofen
Nu-Ketoprofen
Nu-Ketoprofen-E
null
- n. cell tumor
- n. zone

nulligravida
nullipara
nulliparity
nulliparous woman
NuLYTELY

number
    fetal n.
    n. of different words (NDW)
    ovulation n.
    Reynolds n.
numbing
Numby Stuff
nummular
    n. dermatitis
    n. eczema
Numorphan
Nu-Naprox
Nu-Pen-VK
Nupercainal cream
Nu-Pirox
Nuprin
Nu-Ranit
Nuromax Injection
nurse
    public health n.
    wet n.
nursemaid's elbow
nurse-midwife
    certified n.-m.
nursery
    intensive care n. (ICN)
    intensive special care n. (ISCN)
    level 1–3 n.
    n. NBRS
    newborn n.
    observation n.
    well-baby n. (WBN)
Nursette prefilled disposable bottle
nursing
    adoptive n.
    Association of Women's Health,
      Obstetrics, and Neonatal N.
      (AWHONN)
nurturant
nurture
Nuss concave chest correction technique
nutans
    eclampsia n.
    spasmus n.
nutcracker
    n. esophagus
    n. syndrome
Nu-Tetra
Nutracort Topical
Nutraderm cream
Nutramigen formula
Nutren
    N. 1.0, 1.5, 2.0 formula
    N. 1.0 with Fiber formula
nutrient
    intraluminal n.
    n. requirement
Nutrilipid
nutrition

    American Society for Parenteral and
      Enteral N.
    central venous n. (CVN)
    diet and n.
    fetal n.
    fluids, electrolytes, n. (FEN)
    home parenteral n. (HPN)
    inadequate maternal n.
    maternal n.
    North American Society for
      Pediatric Gastroenterology and N.
      (NASPGN)
    parenteral n. (PN)
    PediaSure liquid n.
    pediatric n.
    ProBalance liquid n.
    total parenteral n. (TPN)
    total peripheral parenteral n.
      (TPPN)
nutritional
    n. assessment
    n. deprivation syndrome
    n. hepatotoxicity
    n. immunology
    n. milk unit
    n. neuropathy
    n. problem
    n. requirement
    n. rickets
    n. supplement
    n. support
    n. surveillance
nutrition-associated
    parenteral n.-a. (PNAC)
nutritionist
Nutropin AQ Injection
NuvaRing vaginal contraceptive ring
N&V
    nausea and vomiting
N/V
    nausea and vomiting
NVAC
    National Vaccine Advisory Committee
nvCJD
    new variant Creutzfeldt-Jakob disease
NVD
    neovascularization of disc
    normal vaginal delivery
NVLD
    nonverbal learning disability
NWI
    Neonatal Withdrawal Inventory
NWTS
    National Wilms Tumor Study
    National Wilms Tumor Study
NWTSG
    National Wilms Tumor Study Group
NX
    Talwin NX

Nyaderm
nyctalopia
nycturia (*var. of* nocturia)
Nydrazid Injection
NYHA
    New York Heart Association
      NYHA classification of heart
      disease
Nylen maneuver
nylidrin hydrochloride
nylon
    n. suture (ns, NS)
    n. suture material
nympha
nymphectomy
nymphitis
nymphomania
nymphoncus
nymphotomy
NyQuil
    Vicks Children's N.
Nyquist frequency
nystagmus
    acquired n.
    asymmetric n.
    congenital jerky n.
    congenital pendular n.
    convergent n.

    downbeat n.
    fixation n.
    gaze-evoked n.
    gaze-paretic n.
    horizontal n.
    jerk n.
    latent n.
    monocular n.
    optokinetic n.
    pendular n.
    positional n.
    railroad n.
    retractive n.
    n. retractorius
    seesaw n.
    spontaneous n.
    unilateral optokinetic n.
    upbeat n.
    vertical n.
    vestibular n.
nystatin
    n. and triamcinolone cream
    n. and triamcinolone ointment
Nystat-Rx
Nystop topical powder
Nytilax
Nytol
Nytone enuretic control unit

N

O10003
  occipital
  occiput
O²
  oxygen
    O₂ flowmeter nipple
    hood O₂
    O₂ saturation
OA
  occipitoanterior
  occiput anterior
  ocular albinism
  osteoarthritis
OAAS
  Observer Assessment of Alertness and Sedation
OAB
  overactive bladder
OAC
  optic aspirating curette
OAD
  overanxious disorder
OADP-CDS
  Oregon Adolescent Depression Project-Conduct Disorder Screener
OAE
  otoacoustic emission
    OAE test
    OAE testing
OAR
  Ottawa Ankle Rules
oasthouse urine disease
oat cell carcinoma
OATS
  oligoasthenoteratozoospermia syndrome
OAV
  oculoauriculovertebral
    OAV syndrome
OAVS
  oculoauriculovertebral spectrum
obesity
  adolescent o.
  age-adjusted o.
  android o.
  exogenous o.
  experimental o.
  gynecoid o.
  hypotonia, hypopigmentia, hypogonadism, o. (HHHO)
  o. in endometrial sarcoma
  mild-to-moderate o.
  progressive o.
  o. risk
  truncal o.
obesity-hypotonia syndrome

obesity-hypoventilation syndrome
obesity-related hyposomatotropism
Obetrol
Obezine
OB Gees maternity orthotic
OB-GYN, OB/GYN
  obstetrician-gynecologist
  obstetrics and gynecology
obidoxime chloride
object
  o. assembly test
  o. constancy
  o. permanence
  unidentified bright o.
objective probability
obligate
  o. carrier
  o. heterozygote
  o. intracellular parasite
  o. nose-breather
obligatory
  o. heel valgus
  o. primitive reflex
  o. tonic neck reflex
obliqua
  diameter o.
oblique
  o. diameter
  o. flank muscle
  o. fracture
  left anterior o. (LAO)
  o. lie
  o. presentation (OP)
  o. radiograph
  right anterior o. (RAO)
  o. view
obliquity
  antimongoloid o.
  Litzmann o.
  Nägele o.
obliterans
  bronchiolitis o.
obliterated
  o. processus vaginalis
  o. umbilical artery
  o. urachus
  o. vein
obliteration
  cul-de-sac o.
  o. of apophysial space
  vessel o.
obliterative
  o. arachnoiditis
  o. bronchitis
  o. coronary artery disease

O

obliterative (*continued*)
   o. endarteritis
   o. fibroproliferative bronchiolitis
   o. procedure
oblongata
   medulla o.
OB/Mobius elastic abdominal retractor
Obrinsky syndrome
observation
   o. hip
   o. nursery
   prelinguistic autism diagnostic o.
   (PL-ADOS)
Observer Assessment of Alertness and Sedation (OAAS)
obsession
obsessionality
obsessive-compulsive
   o.-c. behavior (OCB)
   o.-c. disorder (OCD)
   o.-c. personality disorder
   (OCPD)
obstetric, obstetrical
   o. accident
   o. analgesia
   o. anesthesia
   o. auscultation
   o. binder
   o. brachial plexus palsy
   o. canal
   o. care
   o. complication
   o. conjugate
   o. conjugate diameter
   o. conjugate of outlet
   o. damage
   o. emergency room
   o. forceps
   o. history
   o. hysterectomy
   o. nerve palsy
   o. neuropathy
   o. operation
   o. outcome
   o. palsy
   o. paralysis
   o. position
   o. risk
   o. risk factor
   o. traction injury
   o. ultrasonography
   o. ultrasound (OUS)
   o. ultrasound examination
obstetrical (*var. of* obstetric)
obstetric-gynecologic care
obstetrician (OB)
   high-risk o.
obstetrician-gynecologist (OB-GYN, OB/GYN)

obstetrics (OB)
   ambulatory o.
   o. and gynecology (OB-GYN, OB/GYN)
   defensive o.
   family-centered o.
   general o.
   International Federation of Gynecology and O. (FIGO)
obstipation
obstructed
   o. bowel loop
   o. calyx
   o. cardiac output
   o. labor
obstructing periureteral fibrosis
obstruction
   airway o.
   arterial o.
   bilateral ureteral o. (BUO)
   bladder neck o. (BNO)
   bowel o.
   cervical stenosis o.
   check valve o.
   closed loop o.
   colonic o.
   congenital gastrointestinal o.
   congenital lacrimal duct o.
   congenital nasolacrimal duct o. (CNLDO)
   congenital urinary tract o.
   distal intestinal o.
   distal tubal o.
   ductal o.
   duodenal o.
   esophageal o.
   extrahepatic portal vein o.
   extrahepatic presinusoidal o.
   extramural upper airway o.
   extrathoracic o.
   fimbrial o.
   functional outlet o.
   gastric outlet o.
   gastrointestinal o.
   genital tract o.
   glottal o.
   hypopharyngeal-glottal o.
   iatrogenic urethral o.
   incomplete bowel o.
   infravesical o.
   intestinal o.
   intrabronchial o.
   intrabronchiolar o.
   intraluminal upper airway o.
   intramural upper airway o.
   intrathoracic airway o.
   intrauterine ureteral o.
   lacrimal duct o.

left ventricular outflow tract o.
   (LVOTO)
left ventricular outlet o.
lymphatic o.
mechanical o.
meconium o.
milk bolus o.
nasal o.
nasolacrimal duct o.
   (NLDO)
nasopharyngeal airway o.
o. of appendix
outflow o.
pelviureteric junction o.
portal vein o. (PVO)
positional airways o.
presinusoidal o.
proximal tubal o.
pseudointestinal o.
pulmonary venous o.
renal o.
right ventricular outflow tract o.
   (RVOTO)
small bowel o.
strangulating o.
o. syndrome
systemic outflow o.
tracheobronchial o.
tubal o.
unilateral ureteral o.
   (UUO)
UPJ o.
ureteral o.
ureterovesical o.
urinary outlet o.
urinary tract o. (UTO)
uterine outflow o.
UVJ o.
valve o.
variable o.
vein o.
venous o.
ventricular outflow o.
obstructive
   o. apnea
   o. atelectasis
   o. azoospermia
   o. dysmenorrhea
   o. hydrocephalus
   o. jaundice
   o. lung disease
   o. malformation
   o. megaloureter
   o. overinflation
   o. respiratory disease
   o. shock
   o. sleep apnea (OSA)
   o. sleep apnea/hypoventilation
      (OSA/H)

o. sleep apnea syndrome (OSAS)
o. symptom
o. uropathy
o. voiding
o. voiding
Obtryx midurethral sling
obtundation
obtunded
obturator
   o. artery
   Endopath Optiview optical
      surgical o.
   o. fascia
   o. foramen
   o. internus
   o. internus muscle
   o. nerve
   o. nerve damage
   Optiview optical surgical o.
   plastic o.
   o. sign
   tension-free vaginal tape o.
   vaginal tape o.
obtuse marginal
OB-View imaging
OC
   oral contraceptive
OCA
   oculocutaneous albinism
   olivopontocerebellar atrophy
      yellow OCA
OCB
   obsessive-compulsive behavior
OCC
   oculocerebrocutaneous
occasional bacteria
occipital
   o. bossing
   o. horn syndrome
   o. osteodiastasis
   o. plagiocephaly
occipitoanterior (OA)
   left o. (LOA)
   o. position
   right o. (ROA)
occipitoatlantal instability
occipitofrontal (OF)
   o. circumference (OFC)
   o. diameter (OFD)
occipitomental
   o. diameter
   o. view
occipitoposterior (OP)
   o. position
   right o.
occipitotransverse (OT)
   left o. (LOT)
   o. position
   right o. (ODT, ROT)

O

occiput
o. anterior (OA)
flattened o.
o. posterior (OP)
o. posterior position
o. presentation
o. transverse (OT)
Occlucort
occludens
zonula o.
occluder
Amplatzer septal o.
occluding spring embolus
occlusal
o. problem
o. radiograph
Occlusal-HP liquid
occlusion
airway o.
o. amblyopia
Angle classification of o.
arteriolar o.
basal arterial o.
cerebral artery o.
coil o.
constant flow end-inspiratory
airway o.
o. dermatitis
distal o.
end-inspiratory airway o.
fetal endoscopic tracheal o.
fetal tracheal o.
fetoscopic laser o.
isthmic o.
mechanical tubal o.
middle cerebral artery o.
(MCAO)
proximal o.
roller o.
salpingitis after previous tubal o.
(SPOT)
surgical tape o.
tracheal o.
tubal o.
tuboovarian abscess after previous
tubal o. (TOAPOT)
occlusive
o. dressing
o. vascular disease
o. vasculitis
occult
o. bacteremia
o. blood
o. cancer
o. cord prolapse
o. focus
o. neuroblastoma
o. neurogenic bladder

o. spinal dysraphism
occulta
spina bifida o.
occultum
cranium bifidum o.
occupational
o. acne
o. history
o. therapy (OT)
occurrence
inconsequential o.
OCD
obsessive-compulsive
disorder
osteochondritis dissecans
Ocean Nasal Mist
Ochoa syndrome
Ochrobactrum anthropi
ochronosis
Ochsner forceps
Ockelbo virus
OCL
oral colonic lavage
O'Connor-O'Sullivan retractor
OCP
oral contraceptive pill
OCPD
obsessive-compulsive personality
disorder
OCR
oculocerebrorenal
OCR syndrome
OCRL
oculocerebrorenal
OCRL syndrome
OCT
oral contraceptive therapy
ornithine carbamoyltransferase
oxytocin challenge test
OCT deficiency
octaploidy
Octocaine Injection
Octostim
octoxynol
o. 3
o. 9
octreotide
o. acetate
o. therapy
OcuClear Ophthalmic
Ocufen Ophthalmic
Ocuflox ophthalmic solution
Ocugram
ocular
o. adnexa
o. albinism (OA)
o. alignment
o. aspergillosis

o. bobbing
o. coloboma
o. coloboma-imperforate anus syndrome
o. erythema
o. flutter
o. hypertelorism
o. hypotelorism
o. hypotony
o. involvement
o. larva migrans
o. lubricant
macrosomia, obesity, macrocephaly, o. (MOMO)
o. malformation
o. manifestation
o. motility
o. motor dysmetria
o. muscular dystrophy
o. myoclonus
o. myopathy
o. nonnephropathic cystinosis
o. oscillation
o. pain
o. paresis
o. prophylaxis
o. prosthesis
o. sarcoidosis
o. toxoplasmosis
oculi (*pl. of* oculus)
oculoauricular dysplasia
oculoauriculofrontonasal syndrome
oculoauriculovertebral (OAV)
o. dysplasia
o. spectrum (OAVS)
oculocephalic reflex
oculocephalogyric reflex
oculocerebral
o. dystrophy
o. hypopigmentation syndrome
oculocerebrocutaneous (OCC)
oculocerebrofacial syndrome
oculocerebrorenal (OCR, OCRL)
o. disease of Lowe
o. dystrophy
o. syndrome of Lowe
oculocutaneous
o. albinism (OCA)
o. lesion
o. telangiectasia
o. tyrosinemia
o. tyrosinosis
oculodental syndrome
oculodentodigital (ODD)
o. dysplasia
o. syndrome
oculodentodigitalis
dysplasia o.

oculodentoosseous dysplasia (ODOD)
oculo-digito-esophagoduodenal (ODED)
oculofacial paralysis
oculogenitolaryngeal syndrome
oculoglandular tularemia
oculogyration
oculogyria
oculogyric crisis
oculomandibular dyscephaly
oculomandibulodyscephaly (OMD)
oculomandibulodyscephaly-hypotrichosis syndrome
oculomandibulofacial (OMF)
oculomelic amyoplasia
oculomotor
o. apraxia
o. dysfunction
o. nerve
oculomuscular
oculopalatoskeletal syndrome
oculopharyngeal muscular dystrophy
oculoplethysmography
oculosympathetic paresis
oculovestibular response
Ocu-Sol
OD$_{450}$
delta OD$_{450}$
ODD
oculodentodigital
oppositional defiant disorder
osteodental dysplasia
ODD syndrome
odd chromosome
odds
logarithm of o.
o. ratio
ODED
oculo-digito-esophagoduodenal
ODED syndrome
od gene
ODN
oligodeoxynucleotide
optokinetic nystagmus
ODOD
oculodentoosseous dysplasia
O'Donnell operation
odontogenesis
odontogenic keratocyst
odontoid
o. process
o. process hypoplasia
odontoideum
os o.
odontolyticus
Actinomyces o.
odontoonychodermal dysplasia
odor
acrid o.

O

odor (*continued*)
    amine o.
    fishy vaginal o.
    fruity breath o.
    musty vaginal o.
odorant
odorous
ODT
    orally disintegrating tablet
    right occipitotransverse
      Orapred ODT
      Zofran ODT
odynophagia
OE
    otitis externa
OEC
    ovarian epithelial cancer
Oedipus complex
Oestrilin
OF
    occipitofrontal
OFC
    occipitofrontal circumference
OFD
    occipitofrontal diameter
    oral-facial-digital
    orofaciodigital
      OFD syndrome, type I–IV, VI–IX
      OFD with tibial dysplasia
offender
    extrafamily o.
    intrafamily o.
office
    o. cystometrics
    o. hysteroscopy
    o. laparoscopy under local anesthesia (OLULA)
    O. of Special Education Programs (OSEP)
officer
    guidance o.
offspring psychopathology
ofloxacin
OG
    orogastric
      OG tube
OGCT
    oral glucose challenge test
Ogen
    O. Oral
    O. Vaginal
Ogino-Knaus rule
Ogita test
OGTT
    oral glucose tolerance test
    oral glucose tolerance testing
Oguchi disease

OH
    hydroxyl radical
Ohdo blepharophimosis syndrome
Ohio
    O. bed
    O. humidifier
    O. warmer
Ohmeda
    O. Care-Plus incubator
    O. Minx pulse oximeter
    O. 3800 pulse oximeter
    O. SoftProbe probe
21-OH nonclassical adrenal hyperplasia
17-OHP
    17-hydroxyprogesterone
17-OH progesterone
OHS
    ovarian hyperstimulation syndrome
OHSS
    ovarian hyperstimulation syndrome
Ohtahara syndrome
OI
    osteogenesis imperfecta (type I–IV)
    oxygenation index
OIA
    optic immunoassay
      BioStar Flu OIA
oil
    algal o.
    BAL in O.
    camphorated o.
    castor o.
    cod liver o.
    o. cyst
    o. enema
    ethiodized o.
    evening primrose o. (EPO)
    fish o.
    fungal o.
    glycerin, lanolin and peanut o.
    immersion o.
    Lorenzo's o.
    MCT o.
    mineral o. (M-O)
    peanut o.
    Progesterone O.
Oilatum soap
ointment
    A and D O.
    Aquaphor healing o.
    Calmoseptine o.
    Centany o.
    Cormax o.
    hydrophilic o.
    Lacri-Lube SOP lubricant eye o.
    LCD o.
    liquor carbonis detergens o.
    Medi-Quick Topical O.

Monistat 1 1-day vaginal o.
Neosporin Ophthalmic O.
Neosporin Topical O.
Nitro-Bid O.
Nitrol O.
nystatin and triamcinolone o.
oxytetracycline/polymyxin o.
Polyphenon E o.
Polysporin o.
Protopic o.
salicylic acid o.
Sutilains O.
tioconazole 6.5% o.
Topicort o.
triamcinolone acetonide o.
Triple Paste o.
Triple Paste medicated o.
undecylenic acid o.
Vusion o.
Whitfield o.
Xylocaine topical o.
zinc oxide o.
OIS
Organ Injury Scaling
Oka
O. strain
O. strain varicella vaccine
Okazaki fragment
Oklahoma ankle joint
OKT3
Orthoclone OKT3
olanzapine
OLB
open lung biopsy
Olean
oleandomycin phosphate
O'Leary technique
oleate-condensate
triethanolamine polypeptide o.-c.
olecranon
o. apophysitis
o. fossa
o. fracture
olestra
olfaction
olfacto-ethmoidohypothalamic dysraphia
olfactogenital
o. dysplasia
o. syndrome
olfactory
o. hallucination
o. placode
oligamnios (*var. of* oligoamnios)
oligemia
oligo
allele specific oligo
oligoamnios, oligamnios
oligoanuria
oligoarthritis

oligoarticular
o. arthritis
o. disease
oligoasthenospermia
oligoasthenoteratozoospermia syndrome (OATS)
oligoclonal band
oligoclonality
oligodactylia (*var. of* oligodactyly)
oligodactyly, oligodactylia
postaxial o.
oligodendrocyte
oligodendroglia
oligodendroglial degeneration
oligodendroglioma
anaplastic o.
oligodeoxynucleotide
antisense o.
oligogalactia
oligogenic inheritance
oligohydramnios
oligomeganephronia
oligomenorrhea
oligomer
oligonucleotide (oligo)
antisense o.
o. probe analysis
oligoovulation
oligophrenia
growth retardation, ocular abnormalities, microcephaly, brachydactyly, o. (GOMBO)
oligophrenia-ichthyosis syndrome
oligosaccharide
oligospermatism (*var. of* oligospermia, oligozoospermia)
oligospermia, oligospermatism
eugonadotropic o.
reversible o.
oligoteratoasthenozoospermia syndrome
oligozoospermatism (*var. of* oligozoospermia)
oligozoospermia, oligospermia, oligospermatism, oligozoospermatism
oligozoospermic
oliguresia (*var. of* oliguria)
oliguresis (*var. of* oliguria)
oliguria, oliguresis, oliguresia
transient o.
oliguric ARF
olivary nucleus
olive
pyloric o.
superior o.
Oliver-McFarlane syndrome
Oliver syndrome
olivopontocerebellar
o. atrophy (OPCA)
o. degeneration

Ollier
O. disease
O. syndrome
Ollier-Klippel-Trenaunay-Weber syndrome
olopatadine hydrochloride
olpadronate
olsalazine sodium
Olshausen
O. sign
O. suspension
O. uterine suspension procedure
OLTx
orthotopic liver transplant
OLULA
office laparoscopy under local
anesthesia
olympian brow
Olympus
O. disposable cannula
O. disposable trocar
O. flexible hysterofiberscope
O. GIF-XP10 video endoscope
O. hysteroscope
OM
otitis media
omalizumab
OMD
oculomandibulodyscephaly
OME
otitis media with effusion
omega fatty acid
omega-3 fatty acid
omega-shaped epiglottis
Omenn syndrome
omenta (*pl. of* omentum)
omental
o. adhesion
o. biopsy
o. cake
o. cyst
omentectomy
partial o.
omentum, *pl.* **omenta**
lymphocyst o.
matted o.
omeprazole
OMF
oculomandibulofacial
OMF syndrome
OMI
oocyte maturation inhibitor
OMM
ophthalmomandibulomelic
Ommaya reservoir
Omnicef oral suspension
OmniCup
Kiwi O.
Omnipaque
Omni-Tract vaginal retractor

omovertebral bone
omphalitis
omphaloangiopagus
omphalocele
omphalocele-cleft palate syndrome
omphalomesenteric
o. artery
o. canal
o. cord
o. cyst
o. duct
o. duct remnant
omphalopagus
omphalorrhagia
omphalorrhea
omphalorrhexis
omphalotomy
omphalotripsy
Omron monitor
Omsk
O. hemorrhagic fever
O. virus
OMS Oral
on
latching o.
onanism
Onat syndrome
Oncaspar
Onchocerca volvulus
onchocerciasis
oncofetal
o. antigen
o. fibronectin
oncogene
Bcl-2 oncogene
c-erb B-2 o.
c-myc o.
o. expression
her 2 neu o.
H-ras o.
human epidermal growth
factor-2 o.
K-ras o.
oncogenous rickets
oncologist
Gynecologic Cancer Foundation -
Society of Gynecologic O.'s
Society of Gynecologic O.'s (SGO)
oncology
American Society of Clinical O.
(ASCO)
gynecologic o.
On-Command catheter
oncoprotein
c-*erb* B-2 o.
OncoScint
O. CR103 monoclonal antibody
O. CR/OV contrast medium
O. test

oncotic
    o. force
    o. pressure
Oncovin
oncychomycosis
    subungual o.
ondansetron HCl
Ondine curse
Ondine-Hirschsprung syndrome
Ondogyne
O'Neil
    O. cup
    O. vacuum extractor
One Step Button gastrostomy device
ONH
    optic nerve hypoplasia
onion
    o. bulb formation
    o. skinning
onion-skin appearance
onlay
    o. island flap
    o. patch anastomosis
onset
    infantile o.
    juvenile o.
    optic atrophy 2 with early o.
ONTD
    open neural tube defect
ontogenesis
ontogenetic, ontogenic
    o. niche
    o. shift
ontogenic (*var. of* ontogenetic)
ontogeny
ontology
onychatrophia, onychatrophy
onychatrophy (*var. of* onychatrophia)
onychia
onychodysplasia
onychodystrophy-congenital deafness syndrome
onycholysis
    distal o.
onychomycosis
    candidal o.
    proximal white subungual o.
    sublingual o.
    superficial o.
    white superficial o.
onychoosteodysplasia
onychophagia
Ony-Clear Spray
o'nyong-nyong virus
Onyx transobturator midurethral sling system
ooblast
oocyesis

oocyte
    aspiration of mature o.
    o. atresia
    o. collection
    o. cryopreservation
    cryopreserved embryo from donor o. (CPEDO)
    o. culture
    o. donation
    o. donor
    donor o.
    o. extrusion
    o. fertilization
    fertilized o.
    GV o.
    o. maturation inhibitor (OMI)
    o. meiosis
    primary o.
    o. production
    o. recovery
    o. retrieval
    sibling o.
    sporulated o.
    X-bearing o.
oogenesis
oolemma
oophoralgia
oophorectomy
    laparoscopic o.
    medical o.
    prophylactic o.
    surgical o.
    unilateral o.
oophoritic cyst
oophoritis
    autoimmune o.
oophorocystectomy
oophorocystosis
oophorohysterectomy
oophoroma
oophoropathy
oophoropeliopexy
oophoropexy
    laparoscopic o.
oophoroplasty
oophororrhaphy
oophorosalpingectomy
oophorosalpingitis
oophorostomy
oophorotomy
oophorrhagia
oophorus
    cumulus o.
ooplasm
oozing
    venous o.
O&P
    ova and parasites
    stool culture for O&P

OP
oblique presentation
occipitoposterior
occiput posterior
Op
osmotic pressure
opacification
corneal o.
opacity
abnormal o.
corneal o.
fine lens o.
lens o.
lenticular o.
punctate lenticular o.
Opalski cell
Opana
opaque white exudate
OPC
oropharyngeal candidiasis
OPCA
olivopontocerebellar atrophy
neonatal OPCA
X-linked OPCA
OPD
otopalatodigital
OPD syndrome
OPDS
otopalatodigital syndrome
open
o. biopsy
o. bite
o. comedo
o. crib
o. dermal sinus
o. endotracheal suction
o. endotracheal suctioning
o. flap drainage
o. fracture
o. gastrostomy tube placement
o. heart surgery
keep vein o. (KVO)
o. lung biopsy (OLB)
o. mouth
o. neural tube defect
(ONTD)
o. pericardial drainage
o. pneumothorax
o. reading frame
o. spina bifida
to keep o. (TKO)
**OpenGene automated DNA sequencing
system**
opening
gland duct o.
glottic o.
high hymenal o.
hymenal o.
Skene duct o.

tentorial o.
urethral o.
vaginal o.
o. wedge osteotomy
open-mouth view
open-tube bronchoscopy
OPERA
outpatient endometrial resection and
ablation
OPERA procedure
OPERA Star morcellator
OPERA Star SL hysteroscope
operant
o. conditioning theory
o. level
operation
Alexander o.
Altemeier o.
arterial switch o.
atrial switch o.
Bacon-Babcock o.
Baldy o.
Ball o.
Band-Aid o.
Baudelocque o.
Blalock-Hanlon o.
Blalock-Taussig o.
Bozeman o.
cesarean o.
Cotte o.
Counsellor-Davis artificial
vagina o.
Damus-Kaye-Stansel pulmonary
artery to ascending aorta
anastomotic o.
Doyle o.
Emmet o.
Estes o.
Falk-Shukuris o.
Fontan o.
Fothergill o.
Fothergill-Donald o.
Fredet-Ramstedt o.
Freund o.
Gigli o.
Gilliam o.
Gilliam-Doleris o.
Giordano suburethral sling o.
Glenn o.
Grant-Ward head and neck o.
Halsted o.
Haultain inverted uterus o.
Heaney o.
Heller-Belsey esophageal o.
Jatene o.
Kasai o.
Kelly o.
Kennedy-Pacey urinary stress
incontinence o.

Ladd o.
Lash o.
Latzko o.
Le Fort craniofacial dysjunction o.
Madlener o.
MAGPI o.
Manchester o.
Marshall-Marchetti-Krantz o.
McDonald o.
McIndoe o.
modified Fontan o.
morcellation o.
Mustard o.
Norton o.
Norwood o.
obstetric o.
O'Donnell o.
partial exenteration o.
Pomeroy o.
Porro o.
Ramstedt o.
Rastelli o.
Récamier o.
Ross o.
Ross-Konno o.
Ross-Konno-Switch o.
Saenger o.
Schauta vaginal o.
Schroeder o.
Schuchardt o.
second-look o.
Senning o.
sex change o.
Shirodkar o.
Sistrunk o.
Spinelli o.
2-stage arterial switch o.
Stamey antiincontinence o.
Strassman o.
Sturmdorf o.
suspensory sling o.
switch o.
TeLinde o.
Tessier craniofacial o.
Thiersch o.
transsphenoidal o.
Urban o.
vaginal switch o.
Vecchietti neovagina o.
Waters o.
Way o.
Webster o.
Wertheim o.
Wertheim-Schauta o.
window o.

operative
o. management
o. site complication
o. vaginal delivery

operator
o. gene
o. locus
opercular syndrome
operculum
operon
OPG
osteoprotegerin
ophiasis
Ophthacet
Ophthalgan
ophthalmia
gonococcal o.
gonorrheal o.
neonatal o.
o. neonatorum (type 1, 2)
ophthalmic
Achromycin O.
Acular O.
Akarpine O.
AK-Con O.
Albalon Liquifilm O.
Atropine-Care O.
Atropisol O.
Collyrium Fresh O.
Dexacidin O.
Dexasporin O.
Econopred Plus O.
Eyesine O.
Geneye O.
o. herpes
Infectrol O.
Inflamase Forte O.
Inflamase Mild O.
Isopto Atropine O.
Isopto Carpine O.
Maxidex O.
Maxitrol O.
Metreton O.
Murine Plus O.
Muro 128 O.
Mydfrin O.
OcuClear O.
Ocufen O.
Optigene O.
Osmoglyn O.
Pilocar O.
Pilopine HS O.
Piloptic O.
Polysporin O.
Pred Forte O.
Pred Mild O.
o. solution (OS)
o. suspension
Timoptic O.
Timoptic-XE O.
Tobrex O.
VasoClear O.
Vira-A O.

O

ophthalmic (*continued*)
Viroptic O.
Visine Extra O.
Visine L.R. O.
Voltaren O.
ophthalmicus
herpes zoster o. (HZO)
ophthalmitis
ophthalmologic
ophthalmologist
ophthalmomandibulomelic (OMM)
o. dysplasia
ophthalmopathy
thyroid o.
thyroid-related o. (TRO)
ophthalmoplegia
chronic progressive external o.
(CPEO)
external o.
fibrotic o.
internal o.
internuclear o.
o. plus
progressive external o. (PEO)
ophthalmoplegic migraine
ophthalmoscope
direct o.
indirect o.
indirect laser o.
ophthalmoscopy
indirect o.
Ophthetic
opiate
endogenous o.
o. poisoning
o. receptor
OPIM
other potentially infectious
material
opioid
o. activity
o. addiction
endogenous o.
epidural o.
o. medication
o. peptide
o. receptor antagonist
opioidergic control impairment
opipramol hydrochloride
opisthorchiasis
Opisthorchis
opisthotonic posturing
opisthotonos, opisthotonus
o. fetalis
opisthotonus (*var. of* opisthotonos)
Opitz
O. BBBG syndrome
O. G/BBB syndrome
O. trigonocephaly syndrome

Opitz-Christian syndrome
Opitz-Frias syndrome
Opitz-Kaveggia syndrome
opium
alcoholic tincture of o.
o. tincture
Opmilas CO_2 laser
opocephalus
opodidymus
Oppenheim
O. congenital hypotonia
O. disease
O. reflex
O. syndrome
opponens splint
opportunistic infection
opportunity
nonnutritive sucking o. (NSO)
opposing wall
opposition
finger o.
o. movement
precise finger o.
oppositional
o. behavior
o. defiant disorder (ODD)
o. disorder
oppositionalism
OPS
orthogonal polarization spectral
osteoporosis-pseudoglioma syndrome
OPS imaging
opsoclonia (*var. of* opsoclonus)
opsoclonus, opsoclonia
o. disorder
transient o.
opsoclonus-myoclonus
o.-m. etiology
syndrome of o.-m.
opsoclonus/myoclonus syndrome
opsomyoclonus
opsonic capacity
opsonin defect
opsonization
poor o.
o. system
opsonophagocytosis
optic, optical
o. aspirating curette (OAC)
o. atrophy-ataxia syndrome
o. atrophy 2 with early onset
o. chiasma
o. density
o. density measurement
o. disc
o. disc hyperemia
o. fundus
o. immunoassay (OIA)
o. nerve

o. nerve aplasia
o. nerve atrophy
o. nerve cupping
o. nerve disease
o. nerve dysplasia
o. nerve edema
o. nerve glioma
o. nerve hypoplasia (ONH)
o. nerve sheath
o. nerve sheath meningioma
o. nerve tumor
o. neuritis
o. neuropathy
o. neuroretinitis
o. pathway glioma
o. pathway tumor
o. prism
o. spectroscopy
o. tomography

optica
neuromyelitis o.
optical (*var. of* optic)
optician
Opticrom
Opti-Flow catheter
Optigene Ophthalmic
optimal
o. debulking
O. Observation Score
o. timing
optimality score
Optimine
Optimox
O. C-500
O. Mag 200
Optimyd
opt-in approach
OptiNate prenatal vitamin
option
alternative reproductive o.
therapeutic o.
Optiview optical surgical obturator
Optivite PMT
Optochin-resistant *Streptococcus pneumoniae* (**ORSP**)
Optochin test
optode
indwelling o.
optokinetic nystagmus
optometrist
opt-out approach
Opus immunoassay system
OPV
oral polio vaccine
oral poliovirus vaccine
Sabin OPV
OPV vaccine
ora, *pl.* **orae**
o. serrata retinae

Orabase
O. gel
O. HCA Topical
Kenalog in O.
Orabase-B
Orabase-O
Oracit
orae (*pl. of* ora)
Oragrafin
Orajel
O. Maximum Strength
O. Mouth-Aid
O. Perioseptic
oral
o. administration
o. allergy syndrome
AllerMax O.
Ansaid O.
o. aphthous ulcer
Apresoline O.
Aquasol E O.
Aristocort O.
Asacol O.
o. attenuated *Salmonella* typhi vaccine
Benadryl O.
Bentyl Hydrochloride O.
o. bronchodilator
Calm-X O.
o. candidiasis
o. cavity (OC)
Ceftin O.
Celestone O.
Chlor-Trimeton O.
Cipro O.
Cleocin HCl O.
Cleocin Pediatric O.
o. colonic lavage (OCL)
o. conjugated estrogen
o. contraception
o. contraceptive (OC)
o. contraceptive efficacy
o. contraceptive pill (OCP)
o. contraceptive therapy (OCT)
o. contraceptive use
Cortef O.
o. Crohn disease
Curretab O.
Cytomel O.
Decadron O.
Delta-Cortef O.
Demadex O.
Dexameth O.
Dilaudid O.
Dormin O.
Doxy O.
Dynacin O.
Edecrin O.
o. enanthem

O

oral (*continued*)
- o. epithelium
- Estrace O.
- Estratest O.
- o. estrone
- o. exploration
- Flagyl O.
- Flumadine O.
- o. gastric tube
- Genahist O.
- o. glucose challenge test (OGCT)
- o. glucose tolerance test (OGTT)
- o. glucose tolerance testing (OGTT)
- Gly-Oxide O.
- o. hairy leukoplakia
- o. hormone replacement therapy
- Hydrocortone O.
- o. hypoglycemic
- Indocin SR O.
- o. intake
- Lasix O.
- o. leukokeratosis
- Levothroid O.
- Loniten O.
- Marmine O.
- Medrol O.
- Mephyton O.
- Mestinon O.
- o. misoprostol
- o. moniliasis
- o. motor (OM)
- MS Contin O.
- MSIR O.
- o. mucosa cyanosis
- o. mucous membrane graft
- Nitroglyn O.
- Nor-tet O.
- Ogen O.
- OMS O.
- Oramorph SR O.
- Ortho-Est O.
- o. osmotic (OROS)
- Panmycin O.
- PediaCare O.
- Pediapred O.
- Pentasa O.
- Phenergan O.
- o. phosphate
- o. play
- o. polio vaccine (OPV)
- o. poliovirus vaccine (OPV)
- Prelone O.
- Proglycem O.
- Provera O.
- Proxigel O.
- o. reflex
- o. rehydration solution (ORS)
- o. rehydration therapy (ORT)
- Rheumatrex O.
- Salagen O.
- o. sex
- Siladryl O.
- Sinequan O.
- Sominex O.
- o. steroid contraceptive
- o. stimulation
- Sumycin O.
- o. suspension
- Synthroid O.
- o. tactile defensiveness
- o. temperature
- o. thrush (OT)
- Toradol O.
- o. transmucosal fentanyl citrate (OTFC)
- o. tube intubation
- Twilite O.
- Ucephan O.
- o. ulceration
- Urolene Blue O.
- Valium O.
- Vancocin O.
- Vasotec O.
- Videx O.
- Vistaril O.
- Voltaren O.
- Voltaren-XR O.
- Xylocaine O.

Oralet lollipop

oral-facial-digital (OFD)
- o.-f.-d. syndrome with retinal abnormalities

oral-genital sex

orally
- o. administered estrogen
- o. disintegrating tablet (ODT)

oral-motor dysfunction

Oramide

Oraminic II

Oramorph
- O. SR
- O. SR Oral

orange
- Agent O.
- o. peel erythema

orange-peel skin

oranienburg
- *Salmonella o.*

Orap

Orapred
- O. ODT
- O. solution

OraQuick rapid HIV-1 antibody test

Orasept

Orasol

OraSure
  O. device
  O. oral HIV-1 antibody testing system
  O. oral HIV test
Orazinc
Orbeli syndrome
Orbenin
orbiculare
  Pityrosporum o.
orbit
  O. blade
  shallow o.
orbital
  o. blowout
  o. blowout fracture
  o. bone hypoplasia
  o. cellulitis
  o. floor
  o. hemorrhage
  o. hypotelorism
  o. inflammation
  o. septum
  o. subperiosteal abscess
  o. tumor
  o. wall fracture
orbitofrontal gyrus
orbitopagus
orchidectomy
orchiditis
orchidoblastoma
orchidoepididymitis
orchidometer, orchiometer
  Prader o.
orchidopexy (*var. of* orchiopexy)
orchidorrhaphy (*var. of* orchiopexy, orchiorrhaphy)
orchiometer (*var. of* orchidometer)
orchiopexy, orchidopexy, orchidorrhaphy
  Fowler-Stephens o.
  scrotal o.
orchiorrhaphy, orchidorrhaphy
orchitis, orchiditis, testitis
  mumps o.
orciprenaline
  o. oral suspension
  o. sulfate
order
  DNR o.
  high fetal o.
  hold clot o.
Ordinal Scales of Intellectual Development
Oregon Adolescent Depression Project-Conduct Disorder Screener (OADP-CDS)
Oregon-type tyrosinemia
oregovomab murine monoclonal antibody

Oretic
organ
  O. Injury Scaling (OIS)
  internal generative o.
  nongenital pelvic o.
  o. of Rosenmüller
  pelvic o.
  reproductive o.
  sensory o.
  o. situs
  o. transplant
  o. transplantation
  Zuckerkandl o.
organelle
organic
  o. acidemia
  o. acid metabolism
  o. acidosis
  o. acid screen
  o. aciduria
  o. arsenical
  o. brain disease
  o. brain lesion
  o. heart disease
  o. hyperkinetic syndrome
  o. lead
  o. mental syndrome
  o. mercury poisoning
  o. tricuspid incompetence
Organidin NR
organism
  antibiotic-resistant gram-negative o. (ARGNO)
  coliform o.
  comma-shaped o.
  gram-negative o.
  gram-positive o.
  mycobacterial o.
  nonhemolytic aerobic o.
  nontypeable o.
  parasitic o.
  transgenic o.
organization
  health maintenance o. (HMO)
  managed care o. (MCO)
  preferred provider o. (PPO)
  World Health O. (WHO)
organized blood clot
organoaxial volvulus
organochlorine pesticide
organogenesis
  fetal o.
organoid
  o. nevus
  o. nevus syndrome
organoleptic characteristic
organomegaly
Organon percutaneous E2 implant

O

organophosphate
    o. ingestion
    o. insecticide
    o. poisoning
organ-specific medication
orgasm
orgasmic, orgastic
    o. disorder
    o. flush
    o. motor response
    o. plateau
orgastic (*var. of* orgasmic)
O'Riain skin wrinkle test
Oriental spotted fever
orientation
    child-centered literary o. (CCLO)
    sexual o.
    spatial o.
Orientia tsutsugamushi
orienting
orifice
    eccentric o.
orificial tuberculosis
origin
    O. balloon
    congenital amaurosis of retinal o.
    fever of undetermined o. (FUO)
    fever of unknown o. (FUO)
    histoimmunological o.
    parental o.
    Somatropin of rDNA o.
    O. Tacker
    O. trocar
original
    O. Doan's
    K-Phos O.
Orimune poliovirus vaccine
oris
    depressor anguli o.
    fetor o.
ORLAU
    Orthotic Research and Locomotor
    Assessment Unit
    ORLAU swivel walker
orlistat
Ornade
ornidazole
ornipressin
ornithine
    o. carbamoyltransferase
    o. decarboxylase
    difluoromethyl o. (DFMO)
    o. to citrulline ratio
    o. transcarbamylase (OTC)
    o. transcarbamylase deficiency
    (OTCD)
ornithine-ketoacid aminotransferase deficiency
ornithosis

orocecal transit time
orocraniodigital syndrome
orodigitofacial
    o. dysostosis
    o. syndrome
orofacial
    o. cleft
    o. dyskinesia
orofaciodigital
orogastric (OG)
orogenital
    o. sexual practices
    o. syndrome
orolabial herpes
oromandibular
    o. dystonia
    o. limb hypoplasia
oromotor
    o. function
    o. sign
oronasal
oropharyngeal
    o. candidiasis (OPC)
    o. colonization
    o. tularemia
oropharynx
OROS
    oral osmotic
    osmotic release oral system
    OROS methylphenidate
    hydrochloride
orotic
    o. acid
    o. acidemia
    o. aciduria
orotracheal intubation
Oroya fever
orphan
    o. drug
    enteric cytopathogenic human o.
    (ECHO)
    enterocytopathogenic human o.
    (ECHO)
    respiratory enteric o.
orphanage
orphenadrine
Orr rectal prolapse repair
ORS
    oral rehydration solution
ORSP
    Optochin-resistant Streptococcus
    pneumoniae
ORT
    oral rehydration therapy
ortho
    O. All-Flex diaphragm
    O. diaphragm kit
    O. Evra
    O. Evra transdermal patch

O. Personal Pak
O. Tri-Cyclen
Ortho-Cept
Orthoclone OKT3
Ortho-Creme
Ortho-Cyclen
orthodeoxia
orthodiagram
Ortho-Dienestrol Vaginal
orthodontic appliance
orthodontist
orthodromic
    o. conduction
    o. reciprocating tachycardia
Ortho-Est Oral
Orthoglass splint
orthognathic surgery
orthogonal
    o. lead system
    o. plane
    o. polarization spectral (OPS)
orthographic
Ortho-Gynol
orthology
orthomolecular therapy
orthomyxovirus
Ortho-Novum
    O.-N. 1/35
    O.-N. 1/50
    O.-N. 10/11
    O.-N. 7/7/7
orthopaedic (*var. of* orthopedic)
orthopaedics (*var. of* orthopedics)
orthopaedist (*var. of* orthopedist)
orthopedic, orthopaedic
    o. anomaly
    o. appliance
    o. condition
orthopedically disabled
orthopedics, orthopaedics
orthopedist, orthopaedist
orthophoria
Orthoplast jacket
orthoplasty
orthopnea
orthopoxvirus
Ortho-Prefest
orthoroentgenogram
orthoses (*pl. of* orthosis)
orthosis *pl.* **orthoses**
    ankle-foot o. (AFO)
    Atlanta Scottish Rite Hospital o.
    Boston o.
    cranial o.
    CranioCap cranial o.
    foot o. (FO)
    hip-knee-ankle-foot o. (HKAFO)
    knee-ankle-foot o. (KAFO)
    lumbosacral o. (LSO)

    reciprocating gait o. (RGO)
    soft Boston o.
    supramalleolar o. (SMO)
    thoracolumbosacral o.
    (TLSO)
orthostasis
orthostatic
    o. dizziness
    o. hypotension
    o. intolerance
    o. proteinuria
    o. proteinuria test
    o. syncope
    o. tachycardia syndrome
    o. test
orthosympathetic
orthotic
    OB Gees maternity o.
    O. Research and Locomotor
    Assessment Unit
orthotonos, orthotonus
orthotonus (*var. of* orthotonos)
orthotopic
    o. heart transplantation
    o. liver transplant (OLTx)
orthovoltage radiation
Orthoxine
Ortolani
    O. click
    O. congenital hip dislocation
    technique
    O. maneuver
    O. sign
    O. test
Orudis KT
Oruvail
os
    cervical os
    external os
    internal os
    os odontoideum
    parous os
    per os
    os pubis
    Scanzoni second os
    os subfibulare
    os trigonum
OSA
    obstructive sleep apnea
OSA/H
    obstructive sleep apnea/hypoventilation
OSAS
    obstructive sleep apnea syndrome
Osborne wave
Os-Cal 500
oscillation
    o. amplitude
    anal sphincter o.
    flutter-like o.

O

oscillation (*continued*)
    high-frequency o. (HFO)
    ocular o.
oscillator
    Babylog 8000 o.
    high-frequency o.
    Infant Star 8000 o.
    Sensormedic 3100A 8000 o.
    Stephanie 8000 o.
oscillatory ventilation
oscillometric
    o. method
    o. technique
oscilloscope
    cathode ray o. (CRO)
OSD
    Osgood-Schlatter disease
Osebold-Remondini syndrome
oseltamivir
OSEP
    Office of Special Education Programs
Osgood bone marrow needle
Osgood-Schlatter
    O.-S. disease (OSD)
    O.-S. syndrome
Osler node
Osler-Weber-Rendu
    O.-W.-R. disease (OWRD)
    O.-W.-R. syndrome (OWRS)
Osler-Weber syndrome
osmiophilic body
Osmitrol Injection
OsmoCyte pillow
Osmoglyn Ophthalmic
osmolality
    morning o.
    plasma o.
    serum o.
osmolarity
Osmolite HN formula
osmoregulation
osmotic
    o. agent
    o. diarrhea
    o. dilator
    o. diuresis
    o. fragility test
    o. gap
    o. laxative
    oral o. (OROS)
    o. pressure (Op)
    o. release oral system (OROS)
    o. UF
Osp
    outer surface protein
OspA
    outer surface protein A
    recombinant OspA
ospemifene

osseous, osteal
    o. BA lesion
    o. coalition
ossicle
    Andernach o.
    anlagen of auditory o.
    auditory ossicles
ossicular
    o. discontinuity
    o. disruption
ossiculum terminale
ossificans
    myositis o.
ossification
    appositional o.
    enchondral o.
    endochondral o.
    extra o.
ossifying fibroma
ossium
    fragilitas o.
osteal (*var. of* osseous)
ostectomy, osteoectomy
osteitis
    acute mastoid o.
    alveolar o.
    o. condensans generalisata
    o. fibrosa
    o. fibrosis cystica
    mastoid o.
    o. pubis
    rarefying o.
OsteoAnalyzer densitometer
osteoarthritis (OA)
    degenerative o.
osteoarthroophthalmopathy
osteoarthropathy
    hypertrophic o.
osteoarthrophthalmopathy
    hereditary o.
osteoblast (OB)
osteoblastic osteosarcoma
osteoblast-like cell
osteoblastoma (OB)
osteocalcin
    serum o.
osteochondral fracture
osteochondritis
    capitellar o.
    o. deformans juvenilis
    o. dissecans (OCD)
    o. ischiopubica
    metatarsal head o.
    o. of capitellum
    radial head o.
    tarsal navicular o.
osteochondrodysplasia
    hereditary o.
    hypertrichotic o.

osteochondrodystrophia deformans
osteochondrodystrophy
    familial o.
osteochondroma
osteochondromuscular dystrophy
osteochondrosis
    o. deformans tibiae
    inflammatory o.
osteochondrotic lesion
osteoclast
osteoclastic
osteoclast-mediated bone resorption
osteoclastogenesis
osteocranium
osteocystoma
osteodental dysplasia (ODD)
osteodiastasis
    occipital o.
osteodysplasia
osteodysplastic primordial dwarfism
osteodystrophia (*var. of* osteodystrophy)
    o. juvenilis
osteodystrophy, osteodystrophia
    Albright hereditary o. (AHO)
    azotemic o.
    renal o.
osteoectomy (*var. of* ostectomy)
osteofibrous dysplasia
osteogenesis
    o. imperfecta congenita syndrome
    o. imperfecta cystica
    o. imperfecta (type I–IV) (OI)
osteogenic sarcoma
osteoglophonic
    o. dwarfism
    o. dysplasia
OsteoGram bone density test
osteohypertrophic varicose syndrome
osteoid
    malignant o.
    o. osteoma
    o. seam
osteoma
    multiple osteomas
    osteoid o.
osteomalacia
    juvenile o.
Osteomark NTx serum test
Osteomeasure computer-assisted image
  analyzer
osteomyelitis
    acute hematogenous o.
    calvarial o.
    chronic o.
    chronic recurrent multifocal o.
     (CRMO)
    diaphysial o.
    hematogenous o.
    meningococcal multifocal o.

    multifocal o.
    Pasteurella multocida o.
    o. pubis
    pyogenic o.
    Salmonella o.
    sclerosing o.
    spinal o.
    subacute o.
    tuberculous o.
    vertebral o.
osteonecrosis
osteoarthropathy
osteo-onchodysostosis
Osteopatch
osteopathia
    o. dysplastica familiaris
    o. striata
    o. striata with cranial sclerosis
osteopathic medicine
osteopedion
osteopenia
    ground-glass o.
    juxtaarticular o.
    relative o.
osteopenic halo
osteopetrosis
    congenital o.
    infantile o.
    malignant infantile o.
    o. tarda
osteopoikilosis
osteopontin
osteoporosis
    corticosteroid-induced o.
    juvenile o.
    postmenopausal o. (PMO)
osteoporosis-pseudoglioma syndrome (OPS)
osteoporotic fracture
osteoprotegerin (OPG)
osteopsathyrosis
osteoradionecrosis
osteorhabdotosis
Osteosal test
osteosarcoma
    chondroblastic o.
    femoral o.
    fibroblastic o.
    osteoblastic o.
    secondary o.
    small cell o.
    telangiectatic o.
osteotabes
osteotomy
    derotation femoral o.
    diaphysial fibular o.
    femoral o.
    fibular o.
    innominate o.
    lengthening o.

O

osteotomy (*continued*)
    opening wedge o.
    pelvic lengthening o.
    plantarflexion o.
    proximal humeral derotation o.
    rotational o.
    Salter o.
    shortening dorsal wedge radial o.
    tibial valgus o.
    transiliac lengthening o.
    valgus o.
    varus o.
    wedge o.
OsteoView
    O. device
    O. 2000 system
ostia (*pl. of* ostium)
ostiomeatal complex
ostium, *pl.* **ostia**
    abdominal o.
    follicular o.
    o. primum
    o. primum ASD
    o. secundum
    o. secundum ASD
    tubal o.
    o. venosus ASD
    vessel o.
ostomy
    intestinal o.
ostrich maneuver
Ostrum-Furst syndrome
O'Sullivan-O'Connor retractor
O'Sullivan screen
OT
    occipitotransverse
    occiput transverse
    occupational therapy
    oral thrush
Ota
    O. nevus
    nevus of O.
otalgia
OTC
    ornithine transcarbamylase
    over-the-counter
    OTC deficiency
OTCD
    ornithine transcarbamylase deficiency
OTFC
    oral transmucosal fentanyl citrate
other
    o. cerebral palsy
    o. potentially infectious material
    (OPIM)
otic
    Acetasol HC o.
    AntibiOtic O.
    Cerumenex O.

    Cipro HC O.
    Cortisporin O.
    Cortisporin-TC o.
    Debrox O.
    O. Domeboro
    Drotic O.
    Floxin O.
    LazerSporin-C O.
    Otic-Care o.
    Otocort O.
    Otomycin-HPN O.
    o. suspension
    VoSol o.
    VoSol HC o.
Otic-Care otic
oticus
    herpes zoster o.
Otis-Lennon Intelligence Test
otitic hydrocephalus
otitidiscaviarum
    Nocardia o.
otitis
    adhesive o.
    Alloiococcus o.
    o. externa (OE)
    external o.
    o. media (OM)
    o. media with effusion (OME)
    o. media without effusion
    o. media with perforated tympanic
    membrane
otitis-conjunctivitis syndrome
otoacoustic emission (OAE)
Otobiotic
Otocalm Ear
Otocort Otic
otocyst
otofaciocervical syndrome
otogenic brain abscess
OtoLAM
    Otoscan laser-assisted myringotomy
otolaryngologist
otolaryngology
    pediatric o.
otologist
otomandibular
    o. dysostosis
    o. facial dysmorphogenesis
    o. syndrome
Otomycin-HPN Otic
otomycosis
otopalatodigital (OPD)
    o. syndrome (OPDS)
otorhinolaryngologist
otorrhea
    CSF o.
Otoscan laser-assisted myringotomy
    (OtoLAM)
otosclerosis syndrome

otoscope
    MacroView o.
    pneumatic o.
    Siegel o.
otoscopy
    pneumatic o.
otospondylomegaepliphysial dysplasia
otospongiosis syndrome
Ototemp 3000 thermometer
ototoxic drug
ototoxicity
Otovent
    O. autoinflation kit
    O. negative pressure treatment
Oto-Wick
    Pope O.-W.
Ottawa Ankle Rules (OAR)
Otto
    O. pelvis
    O. syndrome
ouabain
Oucher scale
ounce (oz)
    calorie per o. (cal/oz)
OUS
    obstetric ultrasound
out
    toeing o.
outbreak
    recurrent herpetic o.
outbreeding
outcome
    adverse o.
    Bayley cognitive o.
    fetal o.
    maternal o.
    neonatal o.
    obstetric o.
    perinatal o.
    poor pregnancy o.
    pregnancy o.
    teratogenic o.
outer
    o. canthus
    o. chorion
    o. ear
    o. surface protein (Osp)
    o. surface protein A (OspA)
outercourse
outflow
    o. obstruction
    o. tract
outlet
    conjugate of pelvic o.
    o. foramina
    o. forceps
    o. forceps delivery
    obstetric conjugate of o.
    parous o.

    pelvic plane of o.
    rule of o.
    o. septum
    vaginal o.
    vulvovaginal o.
outline
    fetal o.
out-of-phase endometrial biopsy
out-of-profile nipple
outpatient
    o. anticoagulation
    o. endometrial resection and
      ablation (OPERA)
    o. fetal nonstress testing
    o. postpartum care
output
    cardiac o.
    decreased urine o.
    elevated cardiac o.
    high o.
    hyperdynamic ventricle with high o.
    intake and o. (I&O, I/O)
    low o.
    obstructed cardiac o.
    urinary o.
    urine o.
    urine acid o. (UAO)
outtoe gait
out-toeing (*var. of* outtoeing)
outtoeing, out-toeing
outward menstrual flow
ova (*pl. of* ovum)
oval
    o. scaling
    o. window
ovale
    foramen o. (FO)
    patent foramen o. (PFO)
    Pityrosporum o.
    Plasmodium o.
ovalis
    fossa o.
ovalocytary anemia
ovalocytosis
    Southeast Asian o. (SAO)
OvaRex
    O. MAb
    O. vaccine
ovaria (*pl. of* ovarium)
ovarialgia
ovarian
    o. ablation
    o. abnormality
    o. abscess
    o. activity
    o. agenesis
    o. amenorrhea
    o. androgen production
    o. androgen secretion

O

ovarian (*continued*)
o. antibody
o. aplasia
o. artery
o. axis dysfunction
o. cancer
o. cancer metastasis
o. carcinoma antigen
o. carcinoma debulking
o. cautery
o. clear cell adenocarcinoma
o. colic
o. cortex
o. cycle
o. cycle change
o. cyst
o. cystadenocarcinoma
o. cystectomy
o. cystic teratoma
o. disorder
o. drilling procedure
o. dwarfism
o. dysfunction
o. dysgenesis
o. dysgenesis-sensorineural deafness syndrome
o. dysgerminoma
o. dysmenorrhea
o. embryonal teratoma
o. endometrioma
o. endometriosis
o. epithelial cancer (OEC)
o. estrogen synthesis
o. excrescence
o. factor
o. failure
o. fibroma
o. fibromatosis
o. follicle exhaustion
o. function
o. gametogenesis
o. germinal epithelium
o. gonadoblastoma
o. hormone
o. hyperandrogenism
o. hyperstimulation
o. hyperstimulation syndrome (OHS, OHSS)
o. hypertrophy
o. leiomyoma
o. ligament
o. lipid cell neoplasm
o. lymphoma
o. malignancy
o. malignant epithelial neoplasm
o. malignant germ cell tumor
o. mass
o. neoplasm
o. neurofibroma

o. plexus
o. pregnancy
o. preservation
o. proliferative cystadenoma
o. remnant syndrome
o. reserve
o. retention
o. retrieval
o. rupture
o. seminoma
o. sex-cord stromal neoplasm
o. short stature syndrome
o. small cell carcinoma
o. sonography
o. steroid
o. steroidogenesis
o. stimulation
o. stroma
o. stromal hyperthecosis
o. thecoma
o. torsion
o. tubular adenoma
o. tumor
o. varicocele
o. vasculitis
o. vein
o. vein syndrome
o. vein thrombosis (OVT)
o. venous plexus
o. vessel
o. wedge resection
ovarian-sparing irradiation
ovarica
fimbria o.
ovaricus
cumulus o.
ovariectomy
ovarii
hydrops o.
hyperthecosis o.
mesoblastoma o.
struma o.
ovarioabdominal pregnancy
ovariocele
ovariocentesis
ovariocyesis
ovariodysneuria
ovariogenic
ovariohysterectomy
ovariolytic
ovariopathy
ovariorrhexis
ovariosalpingectomy
ovariosalpingitis
ovariosteresis
ovariostomy
ovariotomy
Beatson o.
normal o.

ovaritis
ovarium, *pl.* **ovaria**
    o. bipartitum
    o. disjunctum
    o. gyratum
    o. lobatum
ovary
    accessory o.
    autoamputation of o.
    contralateral o.
    cystic teratoma of o.
    dermoid cyst of o.
    o. in inguinal hernia
    JGCT of o.
    mulberry o.
    multifollicular o.
    oyster o.
    palpable postmenopausal o. (PPO)
    polycystic o. (PCO)
    resistant o.
    rete cyst of o.
    sclerocystic disease of the o.
    Stein-Leventhal type of polycystic o.
    streak o.
    strumal carcinoid of o.
    supernumerary o.
    suspensory ligament of o.
    torsion of o.
    transposition of o.
    tubes and ovaries (T&O)
    wandering o.
Ovation falloposcopy system
ovatus
    Bacteroides o.
O-Vax vaccine
Ovcon
    O. 35
    O. 50
over
    crossing o.
overactive bladder (OAB)
overactivity
    detrusor o.
    idiopathic detrusor o.
    neurogenic detrusor o.
overaeration
overanxious
    o. disorder (OAD)
    o. disorder of childhood
overcirculation
    pulmonary o.
overcorrection
overcrowding
overdistension (*var. of* overdistention)
overdistention, overdistension
    lung o.
    o. syndrome
overdose syndrome
overfeeding

overflow
    o. incontinence
    o. proteinuria
    tear o.
overgrowth
    cyclosporine-induced gingival o.
    gingival o.
    phenytoin-induced gingival o.
    small bowel o.
    o. syndrome
overhead warmer
overheating
overhydration
overinflation
    congenital lobar o. (CLO)
    generalized obstructive o.
    obstructive o.
overlap
    criterion o.
overlapping
    o. clones
    o. closure of peritoneum
    o. toe
overload
    diastolic o.
    fluid o.
    iron o.
    o. pattern
    sensory o.
    systolic o.
    volume o.
overloading
    carbohydrate o.
overmature gamete
overpressuring
overprotection
overriding
    o. aorta
    o. finger
    o. of sutures
    o. toe
oversewing placental bed
overshadowing
    diagnostic o.
overstimulated
overt
    o. bilirubin encephalopathy
    o. insulin-dependent diabetes mellitus
    o. loss
over-the-counter (OTC)
    o.-t.-c. drug
    o.-t.-c. medication
over-the-needle catheter
overtraining syndrome
overuse
    o. injury
    o. syndrome
overwhelming infection

O

Oves
- O. Cervical Cap
- O. conception cap

ovicidal

Ovide
- O. lotion
- O. Topical

Ovidrel powder

oviduct
- ampulla of o.
- angiomyoma of o.

ovigenesis

ovoid
- Delclos o.
- Fleming o.
- Manchester o.

ovotestes (*pl. of* ovotestis)

ovotestis, *pl.* **ovotestes**
- dysgenetic o.

Ovral contraceptive pill

Ovrette contraceptive pill

O-V Staticin

OVT
- ovarian vein thrombosis

OvuDate fertility test kit

OvuGen test kit

ovukit
- O. self-test kit
- O. test

ovular transmigration

ovulation
- o. assessment
- contralateral o.
- o. detection kit
- incessant o.
- o. induction
- o. number
- paracyclic o.
- o. rate
- spontaneous o.
- o. stimulation

ovulational sclerosis

ovulation-associated hemoperitoneum

ovulation-inducing drug

ovulatory
- o. age
- o. defect
- o. disturbance
- o. menstrual cycle
- o. mucus

Ovules
- Cleocin Vaginal O.

ovulocyclic porphyria

ovum, *pl.* **ova**
- ova and parasites (O&P)
- blighted o.
- Bryce-Teacher o.
- o. capture

- o. donation
- fertilized o.
- o. forceps
- frozen o.
- Hertig-Rock o.
- holoblastic o.
- o. maturation
- Miller o.
- Peters o.
- o. pickup mechanism
- primitive o.
- primordial o.
- o. transport
- trapped o.

ovum-capture inhibitor

ovumeter

OvuQuick
- O. self-test
- O. self-test kit
- O. self-test ovulation predictor
- O. 1-step ovulation kit

OvuStick

OV-Watch fertility predictor

owl's
- o. eye cell
- o. eye inclusion body
- o. eye nucleus
- o. eye view of hydrocele

OWRD
- Osler-Weber-Rendu disease

Owren disease

OWRS
- Osler-Weber-Rendu syndrome

oxacillin sodium

oxalate

oxaliplatin
- pegylated liposomal doxorubicin and o.

oxalosis
- primary o.

Oxandrin

oxandrolone

oxazepam

oxcarbazepine

Oxepa formula

Oxford
- O. diagnostic criteria
- O. Family Planning Association Contraceptive Study

oxiconazole

6-oxidase
- lysine 6-o.

oxidase
- catechol o.
- cholesterol o.
- monoamine o. (MAO)
- NADPH o.

oxidation
- o. disorder

fatty acid o. (FAO)
nitric oxide o.

oxidative
o. brain injury
o. phosphorylation (OXPHOS)
o. stress

oxidative-reductase activity

oxide
inhalation of nitrous o.
inhaled nitric o. (iNO, INO)
magnesium o.
nitric o. (NO)
nitrous o. (N_2O)
zinc o.

OxiFirst fetal pulse oximetry

oxime
hexamethyl propylene amine o.
(HMPAO)
technetium hexamethylpropyleneamine
o. (Tc HMPAO)

oximeter
Healthdyne o.
Invos 3100 cerebral o.
Nellcor N20, N200 pulse o.
Ohmeda Minx pulse o.
Ohmeda 3800 pulse o.
Oxyshuttle pulse o.
Oxytrak pulse o.
pulse o.
RPO o.
o. sensor

oximetric data

oximetry
cerebral o.
fetal pulse o. (FPO)
Mars pulse o.
Masimo SET signal extraction
pulse o.
motion-resistant pulse o.
nocturnal pulse o.
OxiFirst fetal pulse o.
pulse o.
reflectance pulse o. (RPO)
signal extraction pulse o.
stress o.
transcutaneous o.

Oxistat Topical
5-oxoprolinase deficiency
Ox-Pam
OXPHOS
oxidative phosphorylation
OXPHOS disease

oxprenolol
ox's eye
oxtriphylline
Oxy-10 Advanced Formula for Sensitive Skin
oxybutynin chloride
oxycardiorespirogram

Oxycel
O. cautery
O. gauze

oxycephalia (*var. of* oxycephaly)
oxycephaly, oxycephalia
oxychlorosene sodium
oxycodone
o. and acetaminophen
o. and aspirin

Oxydess II
oxygen (O_2)
blow-by o.
o. consumption
o. consumption per minute (Vo_2)
o. delivery
o. deprivation
o. dissociation curve
o. extraction ratio
fraction of inspired o. (FIO_2)
free-flow o.
helium and o. (heliox)
home o.
hood o.
o. hood
hyperbaric o.
inspired o.
o. mask
normobaric o.
partial pressure o. (PO_2)
partial pressure alveolar o. (PaO_2)
partial pressure arterial o. (PaO_2)
positive pressure o.
o. saturation (SaO_2)
supplemental o.
o. tent
o. therapy
o. toxicity
o. toxicity lung disease
transcutaneous partial pressure of o.
($tCpO_2$)
o. transport parameter

oxygenase
heme o.

oxygenated fetal blood
oxygenation
congenital diaphragmatic
hernia-extracorporeal membrane o.
(CDH-ECMO)
extracorporeal membrane o. (ECMO)
fetal cerebral o.
fetal scalp o.
o. index (OI)
meconium aspiration syndrome
extracorporeal membrane o.
(MAS-ECMO)

oxygenator
Lilliput neonatal o.

oxygen-diffusing capacity
oxygen-free radical

O

oxygen-hemoglobin dissociation curve
Oxygent temporary blood substitute
oxyhemoglobin
    o. saturation
    total o.
Oxyhood oxygen hood
oxymetazoline
oxymetholone
oxymorphone
oxyphenbutazone
oxyphencyclimine
oxyphenonium bromide
Oxyshuttle pulse oximeter
oxytetracycline HCl
oxytetracycline/polymyxin
  ointment
oxytoca
    Klebsiella o.
oxytocia
oxytocic stimulation
oxytocin
    o. administration

o. analog
o. augmentation
o. challenge test (OCT)
intravenous o.
o. secretion
o. stimulation of labor
o. stress test
oxytocinase
oxytocin-secreting neuron
Oxytrak pulse oximeter
Oxy 10 Wash
Oyst-Cal 500
Oystercal 500
oyster ovary
oz
    ounce
ozaenae
    Klebsiella o.
10p
    partial tetrasomy 1.
^{32}P
    phosphorus-32

p
   partial pressure
     P protein
p53
     p53 gene
     p53 tumor suppressor gene
Pa
   arterial partial pressure
   pascal
P&A
   protection and advocacy
PA
   alveolar partial pressure
   pernicious anemia
   plasminogen activator
   posteroanterior
   pulmonary artery
     PA pressure
PAAS
   pediatric acute admission severity
     PAAS classification
PAB
   passenger air bag
Pabanol
PAB-equipped vehicle
PAC
   papular acrodermatitis of
     childhood
pacchionian granulation
PACE-2C DNA probe test
paced auditory serial addition test
pacemaker
   artificial p.
   wandering atrial p.
pachydermatitis
   Malassezia p.
pachygyria
   localized p.
pachyonychia
   p. congenita
   p. congenita syndrome
pachysalpingitis
pachysalpingoovaritis
pachytene
   p. phase of meiosis
   p. stage
pachyvaginitis cystica
Pacific
   P. Islander
   P. yew
pacificus
   Ixodes p.
pacifier
   sucrose p.
   sugar-dipped p.

   sweetened p.
   water p.
pacing
   epicardial p.
   phrenic nerve p.
   transvenous p.
pacinian corpuscle
Pacis
   P. BCG bladder cancer treatment
   P. BCG immunotherapy
pack
   barrier p.
   E-Z Heat hot p.
   Flents breast comfort p.
   Monistat 3 vaginal cream
     combination p.
   M-Zole 3 combination p.
   M-Zole 7 combination p.
   neonatal narcotic p.
   Peri-Cold P.
   Peri-Gel P.
   perineal cold p.
   perineal warm p.
   Peri-Warm P.
   respiratory therapy p.
   vaginal p.
packaging RNA
packed
   p. erythrocyte
   p. RBC transfusion
   p. red blood cells (PRBC)
   p. red blood cell transfusion
packer
   Kitchen postpartum gauze p.
packing
   anterior nasal p.
   impregnated vaginal p.
   iodoform gauze p.
   Kaltostat p.
   nasal p.
   posterior nasal p.
   uterine p.
   vaginal p.
paclitaxel
PACNS
   primary angiitis of CNS
PaCO$_2$
   partial pressure of arterial carbon
     dioxide
PACTG
   pediatrics AIDS clinical group
PAD
   pelvic adhesive disease
pad
   p. and bell technique for enuresis

P

pad (*continued*)
    Aquaflex ultrasound gel p.
    arch insole p.
    blue chux p.
    Breathe Easy foam p.
    buccal fat p.
    Bumpa Bed crib bumper p.
    chux p.
    InSync miniform p.
    laparotomy p.
    malar fat p.
    pronator fat p.
    scaphoid p.
    Sleep Guardian foam p.
    Soothies glycerin gel breast p.
    sucking p.
    suctorial p.
    suprapubic fat p.
    p. test
    Triaz benzoyl peroxide p.
paddle forceps
PadKit sample collection system
Paecilomyces
paediatric (*var. of* pediatric)
paediatrics (*var. of* pediatrics)
PAG
    pictorial anticipatory guidance
Paget
    P. disease
    P. disease of anus
    P. disease of breast
    P. disease of nipple
    P. disease of vulva
pagetic
pagetoid
Pagon syndrome
pagophagia
PAH
    phenylalanine hydroxylase
PAI
    partial androgen insensitivity
    plasminogen activator inhibitor
    PAI deficiency
PAI-1
    plasminogen activator inhibitor type 1
PAI-2
    plasminogen activator inhibitor type 2
PAIDS
    pediatric acquired immunodeficiency syndrome
pain
    abdominal p.
    abdominopelvic p.
    acyclic pelvic p.
    afterbirth p.
    asymbolia for p.
    back p.
    bearing-down p.
    bladder p.

    bone p.
    chest p.
    chronic pelvic p. (CPP)
    colicky abdominal p.
    congenital insensitivity to p. (CIPA)
    p. crisis
    cyclic breast p.
    p. disorder
    epigastric p.
    expulsive p.'s
    facial p.
    false p.'s
    flank p.
    functional abdominal p.
    heel p.
    hypogastric p.
    incapacitating p.
    intermenstrual p.
    intractable p.
    labor p.'s
    lightning p.
    low back p.
    lower abdominal p.
    menstrual p.
    myofascial p.
    night p.
    nocturnal retrosternal chest p.
    noncoital sexual p.
    noncyclic breast p.
    ocular p.
    p., paresthesia, paresis, pallor, pulselessness
    patellofemoral malalignment p.
    pelvic p.
    periumbilical p.
    pleuritic p.
    postoperative p.
    psychogenic pelvic p.
    recurrent abdominal p. (RAP)
    referred pelvic p.
    retrosternal chest p.
    Rome criteria for functional abdominal p.
    round ligament p.
    somatic p.
    splanchnic pelvic p.
    suprapubic p.
    p. threshold
    visceral p.
    vulvar p.
Paine syndrome
painful
    p. bladder syndrome (PBS)
    p. joint
    p. menstruation
painless hematuria
paint
    chromosome p.
    whole chromosome p. (wcp)

whole chromosome 1-22 p.
whole chromosome X, Y p.

PAIR
percutaneous aspiration, instillation of hypertonic saline, respiration

pair
base p.
chromosome p.
kb p.
nucleoside p.
vertex-nonvertex p.
vertex-vertex p.

paired
p. allosome
P. Associate Learning Task (PALT)
p. box
p. crura

pairing
chromosome p.

PAIVS
pulmonary atresia with intact ventricular septum

Pajot maneuver

Pak
Ortho Personal P.
Pedi-Boro Soak P.'s
Trovan/Zithromax Compliance P.

Palant cleft palate syndrome

palatal
p. expansion
p. fistula
p. fistula closure
p. mucosa
p. paresis
p. petechia

palatal-digital-oral syndrome

palate
abnormal p.
cleft p. (CP)
cleft lip and p. (CLP)
conotruncal cardiac defect, abnormal face, thymic hypoplasia, cleft p. (CATCH 22)
high-arched p.
isolated cleft p.
midline cleft p.
narrow p.
p. repair
soft p.
submucous cleft p.

palatine tonsil
palatognathous
palatopharyngeal incompetence
palatorespiratory dysfunction
palatoschisis
paleartica
pale stool
palilalia
palisading granuloma

palivizumab
palliation
Norwood p.
p. of great vessels

palliative
p. care
p. procedure
p. sedation
p. shunt
p. surgery

pallid
p. breath-holding spells
p. complexion

pallida
asphyxia p.

pallidal degeneration
pallidin
pallidotomy
pallidum
Treponema p.

pallidus
globus p.

Pallister
P. mosaic aneuploidy
P. mosaic syndrome
P. W syndrome

Pallister-Hall syndrome
Pallister-Killian syndrome
pallor
blanching p.
circumoral p.
p. of skin
placental p.
white matter p.
yellow-green p.

PALM
premature accelerated lung maturation

palm
p. leaf pattern
tripe p.

palmar
p. and plantar keratosis and keratitis
p. and plantar punctate hyperkeratosis
p. crease
p. erythema
p. grasp
p. grasping reflex
p. grasp reflex
p. hyperlinearity
p. lesion
p. pustulosis
p. xanthoma

palmaris
keratosis p.
pustulosis p.
tinea nigra p.
xanthoma striata p.

P

palmar-plantar sign
palmatae
    plicae p.
Palmaz stent
palm-chin reflex
Palmer ovarian biopsy forceps
palmitate
    colfosceril p.
Palmitate-A 5000
palmitic acid
palmitoyltransferase
    carnitine p. (CPT)
palmomental reflex
palmoplantar
    p. keratoderma
    p. pustulosis
palmoplantaris
    keratosis p.
PalmPump
    Kiwi P.
PalmVue system
palpable
    p. bony abnormality
    p. cord
    p. gonad
    p. kidney
    p. nodule
    p. postmenopausal ovary
    (PPO)
    p. purpura
    p. spongy mass sign
palpably enlarged kidney
palpate
palpation
    spoke-wheel p.
    vaginal p.
palpebral
    p. conjunctiva
    p. conjunctivitis
    p. fissure
    p. reflex
    p. slant
palpebrum
    pediculosis p.
palpitation
PALS
    pediatric advanced life support
palsy
    abducens p.
    abducent p.
    acquired abducens p.
    acquired sixth nerve p.
    ataxic cerebral p.
    athetoid cerebral p.
    atonic cerebral p.
    Bell p.
    brachial birth p.
    brachial plexus p.
    bulbar p.

    cerebellar cerebral p.
    cerebral p. (CP)
    choreoathetoid cerebral p.
    congenital sixth nerve p.
    cranial nerve p.
    diaphragm p.
    double elevator p.
    Duchenne p.
    dyskinetic cerebral p.
    dystonic cerebral p.
    Erb p.
    Erb-Duchenne p.
    Erb-Klumpke p.
    extraocular muscle p.
    extrapyramidal cerebral p.
    facial nerve p.
    familial congenital fourth cranial
    nerve p.
    familial congenital superior oblique
    oculomotor p.
    familial congenital trochlear nerve p.
    fourth nerve p.
    gaze p.
    hemiparetic cerebral p.
    hemiplegic cerebral p.
    hereditary neuropathy with liability
    to pressure p. (HNPP)
    horizontal supranuclear gaze p.
    hypotonic cerebral p.
    Klumpke brachial p.
    Landry p.
    lateral rectus p.
    liability to pressure p.
    lower motor neuron p.
    Lyme-associated peripheral facial
    nerve p.
    mild spastic diplegic cerebral p.
    mixed cerebral p.
    mixed-type cerebral p.
    motor neuron p.
    nerve p.
    neuron p.
    obstetric p.
    obstetric brachial plexus p.
    obstetric nerve p.
    other cerebral p.
    peripheral facial nerve p. (PFNP)
    phrenic nerve p.
    postinfectious abducens p.
    pressure p.
    progressive bulbar p.
    pseudobulbar p.
    pyramidal cerebral p.
    rectus p.
    rigid cerebral p.
    sixth nerve p.
    spastic cerebral p.
    supranuclear p.
    third nerve p.

trochlear nerve p.
vertical gaze p.
PALT
Paired Associate Learning Task
PAM
primary amebic meningoencephalitis
pamabrom
PAME
primary amebic meningoencephalitis
Pamelor
pamidronate
Pamine
pamoate
pyrantel p.
pyrvinium p.
pampiniform plexus
PAN
polyarteritis nodosa
panagglutinin
panamensis
Leishmania p.
pANCA
perinuclear antineutrophil cytoplasmic
antibody
pancarditis
acute p.
pancreas
anular p.
direct stimulation of p.
p. divisum
p. sufficient (PS)
Pancrease MT
pancreatic
p. agenesis
p. duct stent
p. dysfunction
p. enzyme replacement
p. enzyme replacement therapy
(PERT)
p. exocrine deficiency
p. exocrine insufficiency
p. head resection
p. hypoplasia
p. insufficiency syndrome
p. islet cell
p. oncofetal antigen (POA)
p. panniculitis
p. pseudocyst
p. rest
p. ring
p. sequestrum
p. tumor
p. ultrasound
pancreaticobiliary, panreatobiliary,
p. anomaly
p. malunion
pancreaticojejunostomy *(var. of*
pancreatojejunostomy)
pancreatin

pancreatitis
acute hemorrhagic p.
choledochal cyst-induced p.
chronic p.
cyst-induced p.
drug-induced p.
gallstone p.
hereditary p.
idiopathic p.
infectious p.
pancreatoblastoma
pancreatojejunostomy,
pancreaticojejunostomy
Pancrecarb
pancrelipase
panculture
pancuronium bromide
pancytopenia
aplastic p.
Fanconi p.
p. syndrome
PANDAS
pediatric autoimmune neuropsychiatric
disorders associated with
streptococcus
pandemic
Pander island
Pandoraea
P. apista
P. pnomenusa
P. pulmonicola
P. sputorum
panduraformis
placenta p.
panel
American Foundation of Urologic
Disease Consensus P.
streptococcal antigen p.
von Willebrand p.
panencephalitis
progressive rubella p.
rubella p.
sclerosing p.
subacute sclerosing p. (SSPE)
Paneth cell inclusion
Panex
Panhematin
panhypogammaglobulinemia
panhypopituitarism
familial p.
panhysterectomy
panic
p. attack
p. disorder
panlobar disarray
Panmycin Oral
Panner disease
panneuropathy
megalencephaly with hyaline p.

667

panni (*pl. of* pannus)
panniculectomy
    noncosmetic p.
panniculi (*pl. of* panniculus)
panniculitis
    cold p.
    factitial p.
    lobar p.
    nodular nonsuppurative p.
    nonsuppurative p.
    pancreatic p.
    popsicle p.
    poststeroid p.
    relapsing nodular nonsuppurative p.
    septal p.
panniculus, *pl.* **panniculi**
    hanging p.
pannus, *pl.* **panni**
Panogauze
panopacification
panophthalmitis
PanoPlex dressing
panoramic radiograph
Panorex view
PanOxyl-AQ
PanOxyl Bar
panreatobiliary (*var. of* pancreaticobiliary)
Panretin topical gel
pansystolic murmur
pantothenate
    calcium p.
pantothenic acid
pants-over-vest technique
panty spica
panuveitis
PaO₂ — PaO$_2$
    partial pressure alveolar oxygen
    partial pressure arterial oxygen
PAOP
    pulmonary artery occluded pressure
PAP
    pulmonary alveolar proteinosis
    acquired PAP
    primary PAP
    secondary PAP
Pap
    Papanicolaou
    Pap Plus HPV screen
    Pap plus speculoscopy (PPS)
    Pap smear
PAPA
    preschool-age psychiatric assessment
Papanicolaou (Pap)
    P. smear
PAPase
    phosphatidic acid phosphohydrolase
papaverine

paper
    filter p. (FP)
    Nitrazine p.
paper-doll fetus
Papette
    P. cervical collector
    P. device
papG allele
Papile grading
papilla, *pl.* **papillae**
    Bergmeister p.
    columnar epithelium p.
    edematous p.
    fungiform p.
    p. of columnar epithelium
    p. of Vater
papillae (*pl. of* papilla)
papillary, papillate
    p. adenocarcinoma
    p. dermis
    p. endometrial carcinoma
    p. hidradenoma
    p. muscle
    p. muscle dysfunction
    p. necrosis
    p. neoplasm
    p. serous cervical carcinoma
    p. serous cystadenocarcinoma
    p. squamous cell carcinoma
    p. variant
papillate (*var. of* papillary)
papilledema
    chronic p.
papilliferum
    syringocystadenoma p.
papillitis
papillocarcinoma
    choroid plexus p.
papilloma
    choroid plexus p. (CPP)
    ductal p.
    intraductal p.
    laryngeal p.
    pathognomonic p.
    raised raspberry-like p.
    raspberry-like p.
    respiratory p.
    tan p.
papillomacular bundle
papillomatosis
    benign p.
    juvenile p.
    laryngeal p.
    recurrent respiratory p. (RRP)
    respiratory p.
    subareolar duct p.
    vulvar p.
papillomavirus
    human p. (HPV)

p. hybridization
p. infection
p., polyoma virus, simian virus 40 vacuolating virus (PAPOVA)
transcriptionally active human p.
type 16 p.
Papillon-Léage-Psaume syndrome
Papillon-Lefèvre syndrome
Pap-Kaps
Papnet
P. automated cervical cystology system
P. reader
P. test
P. testing
P. testing system
papoose board
PAPOVA
papillomavirus, polyoma virus, simian virus 40 vacuolating virus
PAPP
pregnancy-associated plasma protein
PAPP-A
pregnancy-associated plasma protein A
PAPP-C
pregnancy-associated plasma protein C
PAPPC
pregnancy-associated plasma protein C
PAPP-D
pregnancy-associated plasma protein D
Pap-Perfect
P.-P. plastic spatula
P.-P. supply system
PapSure
papular
p. acrodermatitis
p. acrodermatitis of childhood (PAC)
p. dermatitis of pregnancy (PDP)
p. eruption
p. exanthema
p. lesion
p. rash
p. urticaria
papule
acral keratotic p.
acuminate p.
blue p.
crop of p.'s
erythematous p.
filiform p.
flesh-colored p.
genital p.
Gottron p.
keratinized p.
keratotic p.
lichenoid p.
polygonal p.

pruritic urticarial p.
satellite p.
urticarial p.
verrucose p.
violaceous polygonal p.
white p.
papulonecrotica
tuberculosis p.
papulonecrotic tuberculid
papulonodular lesion
papulosa
deciduas tuberosa p.
papulosis
bowenoid p.
papulosquamous
p. eruption
p. rash
p. skin change
papulovesicle
papulovesicular
p. acrodermatitis
p. lesion
PAPVR
partial anomalous pulmonary venous return
papyraceous fetus
papyraceus
fetus p.
PAQLQ
Pediatric Asthma Quality of Life Questionnaire
PAR
population-attributable risk
para (p, pa)
paraaminosalicylate
paraaminosalicylic acid (PAS)
paraaortic
p. lymphadenectomy
p. node
p. node irradiation
p. positivity
parabasal cell
paraben
parabiosis
dialytic p.
vascular p.
parabola
parabolic twin
paracentesis
paracentric inversion
paracervical
p. anesthesia
p. area
p. block
p. blockade
p. extension
p. injection
p. lymphatics
paracetamol suppository

P

parachute
    p. mitral valve
    p. reflex
    p. response
Paracoccidioides brasiliensis
paracoccidioidin skin testing
paracoccidioidomycosis
paracolic gutter
paracolpitis
paracolpium
paracrine-acting growth factor
paracrine communication
paracrystalline inclusion
paracyclic ovulation
paracyesis
paradoxic (*var. of* paradoxical)
paradoxical, paradoxic
    p. aciduria
    p. breathing
    p. chest wall motion
    p. incontinence
    p. pulse
    p. pupil reaction
    p. respiration
paradoxus
    pulsus p.
paraductal acanthosis
paraduodenal hernia
paraesophageal hiatal hernia
paraesthesia (*var. of* paresthesia)
Parafon Forte DSC
paraganglioma
    gastrointestinal p.
ParaGard
    P. intrauterine copper device
    P. T380A intrauterine copper
      contraceptive
    P. T380 copper IUD
paragonimiasis
    cerebral p.
Paragonimus westermani
parahaemolyticus
    Vibrio p.
parahemophilia
parainfluenza
    p. virus (type 1–4) (PIV)
parainfluenzae
    Haemophilus p.
parakeratosis
    multinucleation p.
Paral
paraldehyde
parallel
    p. circulation
    p. play
    p. speech
    p. study arm
paralogy
paralyses (*pl. of* paralysis)

paralysis, *pl.* **paralyses**
    abducens facial p.
    acute flaccid p.
    anal sphincter p.
    antigenic p.
    birth p.
    bladder sphincter p.
    bulbar p.
    ciliary p.
    congenital abducens facial p.
    congenital oculofacial p.
    congenital unilateral lower lip
      p.
    deltoid p.
    diaphragm p.
    Duchenne p.
    Erb-Duchenne p.
    facial nerve p.
    familial hypokalemic periodic p.
    flaccid p.
    fleeting p.
    hereditary abductor vocal
      cord p.
    hyperkalemic periodic p.
    hypokalemic periodic p.
    hysteric p.
    idiopathic facial p.
    immunologic p.
    infantile p.
    Klumpke p.
    Klumpke-Dejerine p.
    Landry type of p.
    laryngeal abductor p.
    laryngeal adductor p.
    laryngeal nerve p.
    lower lip p.
    mononeuritis with p.
    muscle p.
    nerve p.
    obstetric p.
    oculofacial p.
    p. of conjugate upward gaze
    p. of superior laryngeal nerve
    parturient p.
    phrenic nerve p.
    poliomyelitis-like p.
    postictal p.
    postterm pregnancy-related p.
    pseudohypertrophic muscular p.
    recurrent laryngeal nerve p.
    respiratory ciliary p.
    sleep p.
    spastic spinal p.
    sphincter p.
    p. spinalis spastica
    tick p.
    Todd p.
    total muscle p.
    unilateral lower lip p.

unilateral partial facial p.
vocal cord p.
Werdnig-Hoffmann p.
paralytic
p. hypotonia
p. idiocy
p. ileus
p. poliomyelitis
p. rabies
p. shellfish poisoning
p. strabismus
paramagnetic particle
paramedian incision
paramenia
parameningeal infection
paramesonephric duct
parameter
fetal growth p.
growth p.
hemodynamic p.
oxygen transport p.
paramethadione syndrome
parametrectomy
radical p.
parametrial
p. extension
p. phlegmon
parametritic abscess
parametritis
parametrium
paramyoclonus multiplex
paramyotonia congenita
paramyxovirus
paranasal sinus
paraneoplastic
p. amyloidosis
p. symptom
p. syndrome
paraneoplastica
acrokeratosis p.
paranoid
p. ideation
p. personality disorder
paraovarian
p. adhesion
p. cyst
paraparesis
acute spastic p.
areflexic p.
familial spastic p.
flaccid p.
HTLV-I associated
myelopathy/tropical spastic
p.
nonspastic p.
spastic p.
tropical spastic p. (TSP)
parapertussis
Bordetella p.

parapharyngeal
p. abscess
p. lymph node
paraphasia, paraphrasia
paraphimosis
paraphrasia (*var. of*
paraphasia)
Paraplatin
paraplegia
congenital spastic p.
familial spastic p. (FSP)
flaccid p.
hereditary spastic p.
infantile spastic p.
spastic p. (SP)
p. spastica
paraplegic
paraplegin
parapneumonic pleural effusion
parapodium
Toronto p.
paraprofessional
parapsilosis
Candida p.
parapsoriasis guttata
paraquat
p. ingestion
p. lung
pararectal space
parasagittal
p. cerebral injury
p. cortical infarction
parasalpingitis
parasite
intestinal p.
obligate intracellular p.
ova and p.'s (O&P)
parasitemia
parasitic
p. fetus
p. gastroenteritis
p. infection
p. leiomyoma
p. myoma
p. organism
p. pregnancy
parasiticus
chorioangiopagi p.
dipygus p.
janiceps p.
parasitized cecal pouch
parasomnia
NREM arousal p.
REM p.
paraspadias
paraspinal mass
parasternal
p. lift
p. short-axis view

P

671

parastremmatic dwarfism
parasuicide
parasympathetic
  p. fiber
  p. nerve
  p. nervous system
  p. neuron
  p. tone
parasympatholytic drug
parasympathomimetic drop
paratesticular tumor
parathyroid
  p. adenoma
  p. disease
  p. disorder
  p. gland
  p. gland immaturity
  p. hormone (PTH)
  p. hormone-related peptide (PTH-rP, PTHrPP)
parathyroidectomy
parathyromatosis
Paratrol shampoo
paratropicalis
  Candida p.
paratubal cyst
paratyphi
  Salmonella p.
paratyphoid fever
paraumbilical defect
paraurethral
  p. cyst
  p. duct
  p. gland
parauterine
  p. abscess
  p. lymph node
paravaginal
  p. cystocele
  p. cystocele repair
  p. defect
  p. hysterectomy
  p. repair
  p. soft tissue
  p. suspension
  p. tissue support
paravaginitis
paraventricular tachycardia
paravertebral abscess
paravesical space
paraxial
  p. fibular hemimelia
  p. mesoderm
  p. tibial hemimelia
parched mucous membrane
parchment skin
paregoric
parencephalia
parencephalous

parencephaly
  syndrome of absence of septum pellucidum with p. (SASPP)
parenchyma
  liver p.
  medullary p.
  patchy infiltration of medullary p.
  placental p.
  renal p.
parenchymal
  p. abscess
  p. brain lesion
  p. cyst
  p. lung disease
  p. lung morphogenesis
  p. nodule
parenchymatous, parenchymal
  p. cerebral cysticercosis
  p. congenital syphilis
  p. damage
  p. form
  p. mastitis
parent
  P. and Teacher Conners Scale
  p. child
  consanguineous p.'s
  Coping Health Inventory for P.'s (CHIP)
  p. effectiveness training (PET)
  p. guidance work
  rearing p.'s
  social p.'s
parentage
  coefficient of p.
  p. determination
parental
  p. chromosome rearrangement
  p. consanguinity
  p. inversion
  p. inversion of chromosomes
  p. karyotype
  p. origin
  P. Stress Index (PSI)
parent-child
  p.-c. interaction
  p.-c. interaction problem
parenteral
  p. administration
  p. alimentation
  p. aqueous penicillin G
  p. fluid therapy
  p. hyperalimentation
  p. medication
  p. nutrition (PN)
  p. nutrition-associated (PNAC)
  p. progesterone
Parenti-Fraccaro syndrome
parenting
  attachment p.

parent-professional partnership
Parent's Choice formula
paresis
> apparent p.
> asymmetric palatal p.
> cochleovestibular p.
> congenital suprabulbar p.
> flaccid p.
> horizontal saccadic gaze p.
> laryngeal p.
> ocular p.
> oculosympathetic p.
> palatal p.
> spastic p.
> suprabulbar p.
> Todd p.

paresthesia, paraesthesia
> Berger p.

paresthetica
> meralgia p.

pargyline
Pari
> P. LC Plusjet nebulizer
> P. Proneb Turbo compressor

paricalcitol
parietal
> p. bone
> p. bulge
> p. cell antibody
> p. cell hyperplasia
> p. encephalocele
> p. foramina
> p. foramina, brachymicrocephaly, mental retardation syndrome
> p. pericardiectomy
> p. peritoneum
> p. shunt

parietalis
> decidua p.

parietooccipital region
Parinaud
> P. oculoglandular syndrome
> P. sign

parity
> vaginal p.

park
> hemoglobin M Hyde P.

Parkes Weber-Dimitri syndrome
Parkinson-Cowan dry gas meter
Parkinson disease
parkinsonian
> p. movement disorder
> p. rigidity

parkinsonian-like
parkinsonism
> rapid-onset dystonia, p.

Parkland
> P. formula
> P. Hospital technique

> P. procedure
> P. tubal ligation

Parlodel
Parnate
paromomycin sulfate
paronychia
> candidal p.

paronychial infection
paroophoritis
paroophoron
parotid
> p. enlargement
> p. gland

parotiditis (*var. of* parotitis)
parotitis, parotiditis
> acute p.
> bacterial p.
> epidemic p.
> suppurative p.

parous
> p. introitus
> p. os
> p. outlet
> vaginally p.
> p. woman

parovarian tumor
parovariotomy
parovaritis
parovarium
paroxetine hydrochloride
paroxysm
> febrile p.

paroxysmal
> p. atrial tachycardia (PAT)
> p. blinking
> p. coughing
> p. depolarization shift (PDS)
> p. dyskinesia
> p. dystonia
> p. emotional state
> p. hypercyanotic attack
> p. hypoxic spell
> p. infantile torticollis
> p. kinesigenic choreoathetosis
> p. movement disorder
> p. nocturnal dyspnea (PND)
> p. nocturnal hemoglobinuria (PNH)
> p. tachycardia (PT)
> p. torticollis
> p. vertigo

PARQ
> procedures, alternatives, risk and questions
> PARQ conference

parrot
> P. artery
> P. atrophy
> P. atrophy of newborn

parrot (*continued*)
    p. fever
    p. jaw
    P. pseudoparalysis
    P. sign
    P. syndrome
Parry-Jones vulvectomy
Parry-Romberg syndrome
PaRS
    pararectal space
PARS
    Personal Adjustment and Role Skills
    PARS III questionnaire
    PARS scale
pars, *pl.* **partes**
    p. interarticularis
    p. tuberalis
part
    fetal small p.'s
    p.'s per million (ppm)
    presenting p.
partes (*pl. of* pars)
parthenogenesis
partial
    p. agenesis
    p. agenesis of vermis
    p. androgen insensitivity
    p. anomalous pulmonary venous
      return (PAPVR)
    p. auxiliary orthotopic liver
      transplantation
    p. breech extraction (PBE)
    p. colpectomy
    p. colpocleisis
    p. complex epilepsy
    p. complex seizure
    p. DiGeorge anomaly
    p. DiGeorge syndrome
    p. epileptogenic discharge
    p. exchange transfusion
    p. exenteration operation
    p. exenteration operation class V
      hysterectomy
    p. external biliary diversion
      (PEBD)
    p. gonadal dysgenesis
    p. hepatectomy
    p. hydatidiform mole
    p. linkage
    p. lipodystrophy
    p. liquid ventilation (PLV)
    p. monosomy 1p–22p
    p. monosomy Xp21, Xp22
    p. monosomy Xq
    p. oculocutaneous albinism
    p. omentectomy
    p. pressure (P)
    p. pressure alveolar oxygen (PaO_2)
    p. pressure arterial oxygen (PaO_2)
    p. pressure of arterial carbon
      dioxide
    p. pressure of carbon dioxide
      (PCO_2)
    p. pressure oxygen (PO_2)
    p. previa
    p. rollerball endometrial
      ablation
    p. salpingectomy
    p. sitting position
    p. squatting position
    p. status epilepticus
    p. tetrasomy 10p
    p. thromboplastin time (PTT)
    p. trisomy 1p–22p
    p. trisomy 10q syndrome
    p. trisomy Xq
    p. villus atrophy
    p. vulvectomy
    p. zona dissection (PZD)
partialis
    placenta previa p.
    rachischisis p.
partially
    p. duplicated ureter
    p. sighted
partial-syndrome eating disorder
partial-thickness burn
particle
    alpha p.
    Dane p.
    paramagnetic p.
particulate
    p. matter
    p. radiation
Partington-Anderson syndrome
Partington X-linked mental retardation syndrome (PRTS)
partition of energy metabolism
partner
    p. abuse
    p. gene
    high-risk p.
    intimate p.
    multiple sexual p.'s
    nonmonogamous p.
    p. violence
    P. Violence Screen (PVS)
partnership
    parent-professional p.
2-part nuclear stage
parturient
    p. apoplexy
    p. canal
    p. fever
    p. paralysis
parturifacient
parturiometer
parturition

parvicollis
  uterus p.
Parvolex
parvoviral infection
parvovirus
  p. B19
  p. B19-induced red blood cell
    aplasia
  p. B19 red blood cell
    aplasia
  human p. (HPV)
parvula
  Veillonella p.
parvum
  Corynebacterium p.
  Cryptosporidium p.
PAS
  paraaminosalicylic acid
  periodic acid-Schiff
  PAS stain
pascal (Pa)
Pashayan-Pruzansky syndrome
Pashayan syndrome
Pasini variant
passage
  meconium p.
  p. of meconium
  transplacental p.
passenger
  p. air bag (PAB)
  evaluation of p.
passer
  MetraPass suture p.
passive
  p. head-up tilt test
  p. immunity
  p. immunization
  p. incontinence
  p. range of motion
  p. supination
  p. venous congestion
passivity
Passos-Bueno syndrome
paste
  Bipp p.
  Boudreaux's Butt P.
  Butt P.
  Monsel p.
  nitroglycerin p.
  Triple P.
  zinc oxide p.
Pasteurella
  P. canis
  P. multocida
  P. multocida osteomyelitis
Pasteur pipette
Pastia
  P. line
  P. sign

PAT
  paroxysmal atrial tachycardia
  preventive allergy treatment
Patanol
Patau syndrome
patch
  Alora transdermal p.
  atrophic p.
  blood p.
  bovine pericardium p.
  Climara estradiol transdermal system
    p.
  contraceptive p.
  corporal cavernosal p.
  Dacron p.
  Daytrana p.
  EMLA p.
  Esclim p.
  fentanyl p.
  Gore-Tex Soft Tissue P.
  hair p.
  hairy p.
  herald p.
  MacCallum p.
  Miniguard P.
  Minitran P.
  moth p.
  mucinous p.
  mucous p.
  Nitro-Dur P.
  Ortho Evra transdermal p.
  pericardium p.
  Peyer p.
  salmon p.
  shagreen p.
  spontaneous atrophic p.
  strawberry p.
  ThermaCare menstrual p.
  transdermal fentanyl p.
  transdermal glyceryl trinitrate p.
  transdermal medication p.
  Transderm-Nitro P.
  Trans-Ver-Sal transdermal p.
  p. unroofing
  p. unroofing of outflow tract
patching
patchy
  p. infiltrate
  p. infiltration
  p. infiltration of medullary
    parenchyma
patella, *pl.* **patellae**
  absent p.
  aplastic p.
  bipartite p.
  chondromalacia p.
  congenital dislocation of p.
  dislocated p.
  dislocating p.

675

patella (*continued*)
    hypoplastic p.
    kissing patellae
    sleeve fracture of p.
    subluxating p.
patellae (*pl. of* patella)
patellar
    p. fracture
    p. ligament
    p. reflex
    p. tendinitis
patellofemoral
    p. malalignment
    p. malalignment pain
    p. pain syndrome (PFPS)
    p. stress syndrome
patency
    probe p.
    tubal p.
    ureteral p.
patent
    p. anus
    p. ductus arteriosis coil embolization
    p. ductus arteriosus (PDA)
    p. ductus venosus
    p. foramen ovale (PFO)
    p. omphalomesenteric duct
    p. urachus
paternal
    p. age
    p. factor
    p. history
    p. karyotype
    p. meiosis I (PMI)
    p. meiosis II (PMII)
    p. postnatal depression
    p. status
    p. uniparenteral isodisomy
paternity
path
    migratory p.
pathergy sign
Pathfinder DFA test
pathogen
    blood-borne p.
pathogenesis
pathogenic bacteria
pathogenicity
pathognomic (*var. of* pathognomonic)
pathognomonic, pathognomic
    p. Koplik spot
    p. papilloma
    p. symptom
pathologic, pathological
    p. amenorrhea
    p. apnea
    p. cavus
    p. discharge
    p. finding

    p. fracture
    p. gynecomastia
    p. model
    p. reflex
    p. retraction ring
    p. retraction ring of Bandl
pathological (*var. of* pathologic)
pathologist
    Cancer Committee of College of American P.'s
    International Society of Gynecologic P.'s (ISGYP)
    perinatal/placental p.
    speech-language p. (SLP)
pathology
    American Society for Colposcopy and Cervical P. (ASCCP)
    anaplastic p.
    hilar cell p.
    International Society for Gynecologic P.
    intracranial p.
    perinatal p.
    Society for Pediatric P. (SPP)
    speech p.
    speech-language p.
    surgically treatable p.
    uterine p.
pathophysiologic, pathophysiological
    p. mechanism
pathophysiological (*var. of* pathophysiologic)
pathophysiology
pathotropic
pathway
    COX p.
    Embden-Meyerhof p. (EMP)
    neural reflex p.
    nociceptive p.
    pericardial p.
    postchiasmal visual p.
    reflex p.
    visual p.
PATI
    Penetrating Abdominal Trauma Index
patient
    adolescent-onset p.
    amenorrheal p.
    analbuminemic p.
    anovulatory p.
    antenatal p.
    CMV-seronegative transplant p.
    gynecologic cancer p.
    high-risk p.
    infertile p.
    P. Outcomes Research Team (PORT)
    pregnant cardiac p.
    p. rights

thalassemic p.
transplant p.
Zoladex in premenopausal p.'s (ZIPP)
patient-controlled
p.-c. analgesia (PCA)
patient-triggered ventilation
patter
cocktail party p.
pattern
abnormal respiratory p.
abnormal vasculature flow p.
age-to-dose p.
android p.
apple p.
atypical vessel colposcopic p.
banding p.
behavior p.
bimodal p.
biphasic temperature p.
branching p.
breathing p.
burst-suppression p.
capillary p.
central fat distribution p.
characteristic electroencephalogram p.
chessboard p.
Christmas tree p.
chromosomal p.
complete suppression p.
contraction p.
dermatoglyphic p.
developmental p.
diastolic overload p.
distribution p.
dysfunctional labor p.
eggbeater running p.
extensor thrust p.
fat distribution p.
ferning p.
fern leaf p.
fetal heart rate p.
fleur-de-lis breast reconstruction p.
flow p.
fracture p.
genetic inheritance p.
ground-glass p.
growth p.
gynecoid fat distribution p.
gyral p.
heliotrope p.
herringbone p.
hyperkinetic behavior p.
hypsarrhythmic p.
inactivation p.
interweaving p.
4-leaf clover p.
Le Fort fracture p.
linear branching p.

marking time p.
menstrual p.
mixed p.
mosaic p.
motor p.
mucopolysaccharide p.
munching p.
nonobstructive p.
nonreassuring fetal heart beat p.
nonreassuring fetal heart rate p.
overload p.
palm leaf p.
pear p.
persistent primitive reflex p.
primitive reflex p.
prominent ductal p.
prosodic p.
reflex p.
respiratory p.
restrictive breathing p.
reticulogranular p.
reticulonodular p.
silent fetal heart rate p.
silent oscillatory p.
sinusoidal heart rate p.
skin ridge p.
sleep p.
sleeping p.
snowflake p.
soap bubble gas p.
startle p.
subpleural reticulonodular p.
suckling p.
sun-seeking p.
systolic overload p.
temperature p.
temporospatial p.
tonic neck p.
urinary mucopolysaccharide p.
vasculature flow p.
voiding p.
patterned breathing
patterning therapy
Patterson pseudoleprechaunism syndrome
Patterson-Stevenson-Fontaine syndrome
patty
Cellolite p.
patulous rectal sphincter
pauciarticular
p. JRA
p. juvenile chronic arthritis
pauciarticular-onset
p.-o. JRA
p.-o. juvenile arthritis
paucicellular
pauciimmune glomerulonephritis
paucity
bile duct p.
intrahepatic bile duct p.

paucity (*continued*)
    nonsyndromic bile duct p.
    p. of gas
    p. of interlobular bile duct (PILBD)
    syndromic p.
Paul-Bunnell
    P.-B. antibody test
    P.-B. reaction
Paul-Bunnell-Davidsohn test
Pavacap
Pavacen
Pavatest
Pavlik harness
PAVM
    pulmonary arteriovenous malformation
pavor
    p. diurnus
    p. nocturnus
PAW
    pulmonary artery wedge
Pawlik fold
PAWP
    pulmonary artery wedge pressure
PAX3 gene
Paxil
PBAC
    pictorial blood loss assessment
      chart
PBC
    periodic breathing cycle
    plasma bilirubin concentration
    primary biliary cirrhosis
PBE
    partial breech extraction
PBF
    percent body fat
    placental blood flow
    pulmonary blood flow
PBL
    peripheral blood lymphocyte
PBMC
    peripheral blood mononuclear cell
PBMNC
    peripheral blood mononuclear cell
PBS
    phosphate-buffered saline
      isotonic PBS
PBSC
    peripheral blood stem cell
PCA
    patient-controlled analgesia
    postconceptional age
      epidural PCA
PCC
    Poison Control Center
    postcoital contraception
PCC-R
    Percentage of Consonants
    Correct-Revised

PCD
    primary ciliary dyskinesia
PCDAI
    Pediatric Crohn Disease Activity Index
PCE
    physical capacity evaluation
PCEC
    purified chick embryo cell culture
      PCEC vaccine
4p+ chromosome
PC-IOL
    posterior chamber intraocular lens
PCIOL
    posterior chamber intraocular lens
PCM
    pubococcygeal muscle
PCNSL
    primary central nervous system
      lymphoma
PCO
    polycystic ovary
PCO$_2$
    partial pressure of carbon dioxide
    pressure of CO_2
PCOD
    polycystic ovarian disease
PCOS
    polycystic ovary syndrome
PCP
    phencyclidine
    Pneumocystis carinii pneumonia
    primary care physician
PCR
    polymerase chain reaction
      allele-specific PCR
      PCR assay
      PCR test
PCr
    phosphocreatine
PCS
    pelvic congestion syndrome
    primary cesarean section
PCT
    postcoital test
    procalcitonin
      serum PCT
PCV7
    pneumococcal 7-valent conjugate
      vaccine
PCVC
    percutaneous central venous catheter
PCWP
    pulmonary capillary wedge pressure
PD
    peritoneal dialysis
    personality disorder
    postural drainage
      Bromfenex PD
      Iofed PD

PDA
  patent ductus arteriosus
    bidirectional PDA
P.D. Access with Peel-Away needle introducer
PDD
  pervasive developmental disorder
PDD-NOS
  pervasive developmental disorder not
    otherwise specified
PDE
  personality disorder examination
PdE
  pediatric endocrinology
PDE5
  phosphodiesterase 5
PDHC
  pyruvate dehydrogenase complex
    PDHC deficiency
PDI
  phosphodiesterase inhibitor
  psychiatric diagnostic interview
  psychomotor development index
PDL
  primary dysfunctional labor
PDM
  pregestational diabetes mellitus
PDMS
  Peabody Developmental Motor
    Scale
PDP
  papular dermatitis of pregnancy
  positive distending pressure
PDPH
  postdural puncture headache
PDS
  paroxysmal depolarization shift
PDSC
  placental-derived stem cell
PE
  preeclampsia
  premature ejaculation
  pressure equalization
  pulmonary embolism
    PE tube
Peabody
  P. Developmental Motor Activity
    Card
  P. Developmental Motor Scale
    (PDMS)
  P. picture vocabulary test (PPVT)
  P. Picture Vocabulary Test-Revised
    (PPVT-R)
Peacock bromide
peak
  adaptive p.
  p. admittance
  p. and trough
  p. and trough levels

  Bragg p.
  p. end-expiratory pressure
  p. expiratory flow (PEF, PEFR)
  p. expiratory flow rate (PEFR)
  p. flow measurement
  p. flow meter (PFM)
  p. flow meter monitor
  p. flow rate (PFR)
  p. growth velocity
  p. inspiratory pressure (PIP)
  p. instantaneous gradient
  p. systolic velocity
  Webb-McCall p.
Péan
  P. clamp
  P. forceps
peanut oil
PEARL
  physiologic endometrial
    ablation/resection loop
pearl
  Bohn epithelial p.
  collar of pearls
  epithelial p.
  Epstein pearls
  P. index
  perineal p.
pearly-white nodule
pear pattern
pear-shaped uterus
Pearson marrow-pancreas syndrome
pea soup stool
peau
  p. d'orange
  p. d'orange appearance
  p. d'orange appearance of breast
pebbly skin lesion
PEBD
  partial external biliary diversion
PEC
  protein-induced eosinophilic
    colitis
pecorum
  Chlamydia p.
pectin
  kaolin and p.
pectinate line
pectora (*pl. of* pectus)
pectoralis major muscle
pectoriloquy
  whispered p.
pectoris (*pl. of* pectus)
pectus, *pl.* **pectoris, pectora**
  p. bar
  p. carinatum
  p. excavatum
  p. gallinatum
  p. recurvatum
peculiar facies

P

PED
    pediatric emergency department
    prenatally exposed to drugs
pedaling movement
pedal pulse
Pedameth
Pederson vaginal speculum
PEDI
    Pediatric Evaluation of Disability
    Inventory
PediaCare
    P. Cough-Cold
    P. Fever
    P. Night Rest
    P. Oral
Pediacof
Pediaflor
Pedialyte
    P. formula
    P. oral electrolyte maintenance
    solution
Pediamist
Pediapred Oral
Pediarix
PediaSure
    P. liquid nutrition
    P. with Fiber formula
pediatric, paediatric
    p. acquired immunodeficiency
    syndrome (PAIDS)
    p. acute admission severity
    (PAAS)
    p. advanced life support (PALS)
    pediatrics AIDS clinical group
    (PACTG)
    American Academy of P.'s (AAP)
    American Board of P.'s
    p. anesthesiologist
    p. anticipatory guidance
    p. aphakia
    P. Asthma Quality of Life
    Questionnaire (PAQLQ)
    p. autoimmune neuropsychiatric
    disorders associated with
    streptococcus (PANDAS)
    p. balloon
    behavioral pediatrics
    Benylin P.
    p. bone rongeur
    p. bronchoscopy
    p. bulldog clamp
    p. cataract
    p. cocktail
    Committee on Infectious Diseases of
    the American Academy of
    Pediatrics
    P. Crohn Disease Activity Index
    (PCDAI)
    p. dermatology

    p. dosing information
    p. EKG
    p. emergency department (PED)
    p. emergency medicine (PEM)
    p. endocrinology (PdE)
    P. Evaluation of Disability Inventory
    (PEDI)
    P. Examination at Three (PEET)
    P. Examination of Educational
    Readiness (PEER)
    p. exanthema
    p. exercise physiologist
    p. exercise physiology (PEP)
    p. fever
    p. gonococcal conjunctivitis
    p. gonococcal infection
    p. gynecology
    p. hypertension
    p. infectious disease (PID)
    p. intensive care unit (PICU)
    p. labial agglutination
    P. Liver Transplant-Specific Scale
    (PLTSS)
    p. lung surgery
    p. lupus nephropathy
    p. myelodysplasia
    p. neurocritical care
    p. neurologist
    p. nutrition
    P. Oncology Group (POG)
    p. otolaryngology
    p. ovarian teratoma
    Prostin VR P.
    p. public health
    p. pulmonary medicine
    p. radiologist
    P. Risk of Mortality
    (PRISM)
    Robitussin P.
    Rynatan P.
    p. sedation
    p. sedation unit (PSU)
    p. self-retaining retractor
    p. spectrum of disease (PSD)
    p. surgeon
    P. Symptom Checklist (PSC)
    p. thyroid carcinogenesis
    P. Trauma Score (PTS)
    p. tuberculosis
    p. vaginoscopy
    p. vascular clamp
    Vicks Formula 44 P.
    p. viral diarrhea
    Vivonex P.
    p. vulvovaginitis
Pediatrician infant dietary
supplement
Pediatrix vaccine
Pediazole

Pedi-Bath Salts
Pedi-Boro Soak Paks
Pedi-cap detector
pedicle
    p. clamp
    nerve-muscle p.
    renal p.
    uterosacral ligament p.
Pedicran with Iron
pedicterus
pediculosis
    p. capitis
    p. corporis
    p. corpus
    p. palpebrum
    p. pubis
Pediculus
    P. humanus
    P. humanus capitis
    P. humanus corporis
Pedi-Dri Topical
pedigree
    p. analysis
    CEPH p.
    p. chart
Pediotic
Pedi PEG tube
Pedi-Pro Topical
Pedituss Cough
pedodontist
pedologist
pedometer
Pedric
Pedtrace-4 hyperalimentation
peduncle
    cerebral p.
    inferior p.
    middle cerebellar p.
pedunculated
    p. leiomyoma
    p. lesion
    p. molluscum fibrosum
    p. polyp
PedvaxHIB vaccine
PEEP
    peak end-expiratory pressure
    positive end-expiratory pressure
    PEEP ventilator
PEER
    Pediatric Examination of Educational
    Readiness
peer
    p. conformity inventory
    p. relation
PEET
    Pediatric Examination at Three
pefloxacin
PEFR
    peak expiratory flow rate

PEG
    percutaneous endoscopic gastrostomy
    polyethylene glycol
    PEG tube
PEG-ADA
    pegademase bovine
    polyethylene glycol-modified adenosine
    deaminase
pegademase bovine (PEG-ADA)
Peganone
pegaspargase
pegboard
    grooved p.
peglike teeth
peg-shaped upper central incisor
pegylated
    p. interferon
    p. liposomal doxorubicin and
      oxaliplatin
PEHO
    progressive encephalopathy, edema,
    hypsarrhythmia, optic atrophy
    PEHO syndrome
Peiper reflex
Pel-Ebstein fever
Pelger-Huet anomaly
peliosis
    bacillary p.
    p. hepatis
Pelizaeus-Merzbacher disease (PMD)
pellagra
pellagra-like skin rash
pellet
    Muse p.
    YAG p.
Pelletier-Leisti syndrome
Pellizzi syndrome
pellucida
    agenesis of septa p.
    macula p.
    zona p. (ZP)
pellucidum
    cavum septum p.
    enlarged cavum septum p.
    septum p.
Pelosi
    P. hysterotomy
    P. tenaculum
    P. vaginal hysterectomy
pelves (*pl. of* pelvis)
pelvic
    p. abscess
    p. actinomycosis
    p. adhesion
    p. adhesive disease (PAD)
    p. anatomy
    p. appendicitis
    p. architecture

P

pelvic (*continued*)
- p. arterial embolization
- p. arteriogram
- p. arteriovenous malformation
- p. artery
- p. axis
- p. band
- p. bleeding
- p. boost radiotherapy
- p. brim
- p. Castleman disease
- p. cavity
- p. cellulitis
- p. congestion syndrome (PCS)
- p. connective tissue
- p. contraction
- p. damage
- p. diaphragm
- p. direction
- p. endometriosis
- p. examination
- p. exenteration
- p. exostosis
- p. fibromatosis
- p. floor
- p. floor damage
- P. Floor Disorders Network
- p. floor distress inventory (PFDI)
- p. floor electrical stimulation (PFS)
- p. floor laxity
- p. floor muscle exercise (PFME)
- p. floor muscle training (PFMT)
- p. floor nerve
- p. floor surgery
- p. fluoroscopy
- p. forceps
- p. girdle relaxation (PGR)
- p. gutter
- p. hematocele
- p. inclination
- p. index
- p. infection
- p. inflammation
- p. inflammatory disease (PID)
- p. involvement
- p. irradiation
- p. joint
- p. kidney
- p. laparoscopy
- p. lengthening osteotomy
- p. lymphadenectomy
- p. lymph node
- p. lymphocyst
- p. malignancy in pregnancy
- p. mass
- p. muscle exercise
- p. muscle-strengthening exercise
- p. muscle training
- p. nerve injury
- p. node dissection (PND)
- p. organ
- p. organ prolapse (POP)
- P. Organ Prolapse Quantification (POP-Q)
- P. Organ Prolapse Quantification system
- P. Organ Prolapse-Quantified (POPQ)
- p. organ prolapse quantitation
- p. ovarian vein thrombosis (POVT)
- p. pain
- p. pain assessment form
- p. peritonitis
- p. plane
- p. plane of greatest dimensions
- p. plane of inlet
- p. plane of least dimensions
- p. plane of outlet
- p. plexus
- p. pole
- p. presentation
- p. radial
- p. radiation
- p. reconstruction surgeon
- p. reconstructive surgery
- p. recurrence
- p. relaxation
- p. rest
- p. score
- p. shape
- p. side wall
- p. support defect
- p. support index (PSI)
- p. tenderness
- p. thrombophlebitis
- p. tilt
- p. tuberculosis
- p. tumor
- p. type A, B, C fracture
- p. ultrasound
- p. vein congestion
- p. vein incompetence
- p. vein thrombophlebitis
- p. venous congestion syndrome
- p. version
- p. viscera

pelvicephalography
pelvicephalometry
pelvicocleidocranial dysostosis
pelviectasis
pelvifixation
pelvigraph
PelviLace transobturator biourethral support system
pelvimeter

pelvimetry
    clinical p.
    CT p.
    manual p.
    planographic p.
    radiographic p.
    stereoscopic p.
    x-ray p.
pelvioperitonitis, pelviperitonitis
pelvioplasty
pelvioscopy, pelvoscopy, pelviscopy
pelviperitonitis
pelvis, *pl.* **pelves**
    android p.
    anthropoid p.
    arcus tendineus fasciae p.
    assimilation p.
    axis of p.
    beaked p.
    bifid p.
    bowl of p.
    breech location out of p.
    calcified phleboliths in p.
    p. capsular dysplasia
    concrete p.
    conjugata anatomic p.
    conjugata diagonalis p.
    conjugata externa p.
    conjugata vera p.
    contracted p.
    cordate p.
    Deventer p.
    dilated renal p.
    dwarf p.
    elephant p.
    p. enlargement
    false p.
    flat p.
    flying-T p.
    frozen p.
    funnel-shaped p.
    gynecoid p.
    heart-shaped p.
    inverted p.
    p. justo major
    p. justo minor
    juvenile p.
    Kilian p.
    kyphotic p.
    longitudinal oval p.
    p. major
    masculine p.
    mesatipellic p.
    p. minor
    Nägele p.
    p. nana
    Otto p.
    p. plana

    platypellic p.
    Prague p.
    renal p.
    reniform p.
    Robert p.
    Rokitansky p.
    round p.
    sweep the p.
    transverse oval p.
    trefoil p.
    true p.
    well engaged in p.
pelviscope
pelviscopic intrafascial hysterectomy
pelviscopy (*var. of* pelvioscopy)
pelvis-shoulder dysplasia
pelvitherm
pelviureteric junction obstruction
pelviureteroradiography (*var. of*
  pyelography)
pelvocephalography
pelvoscopy (*var. of* pelvioscopy)
PEM
    pediatric emergency medicine
Pemberton
    P. acetabuloplasty
    P. procedure
pemirolast potassium
pemoline
    P. C-IV
    magnesium p.
pemphigoid
    bullous p.
    childhood cicatricial p.
    cicatricial p.
    p. gestationis
pemphigus
    benign familial chronic p.
    p. foliaceus
    p. neonatorum
    syphilitic p.
    p. vulgaris
pen
    P. A/N
    Epi E-Z P.
    Humalog P.
    Humulin P.
    insulin p.
    P. Kera moisturizing cream
Pena
    P. anorectal malformation corrective
      procedure
    P. midsagittal anorectoplasty
Pena-Shokeir
    P.-S. phenotype
    P.-S. syndrome (I, II)
Penbritin
penciclovir cream

P

683

pencil
>Conmed electrosurgical p.
>Valleylab p.

pencil-handled laryngoscope
pendelluft
Pendred syndrome
pendular nystagmus
pendulous
>p. abdomen
>p. breast

pendulum
>molluscum fibrosum p.

Penecort Topical
penes (*pl. of* penis)
Penetrak test
penetrance
penetrans
>*Mycoplasma p.*

penetrant
>p. gene
>p. trait

penetrating
>P. Abdominal Trauma Index
>(PATI)
>p. brain injury
>p. mole
>p. trauma

penetration
>accidental p.
>anal p.
>cercarial skin p.
>skin p.

Penetrex
PenFill
>Novolin 70/30 P.
>Novolin N P.
>Novolin R P.

penial (*var. of* penile)
penicillamine
penicillin
>antistaphylococcal p.
>aqueous crystalline p.
>benzathine p.
>extended-spectrum p.
>p. G
>p. G benzathine
>natural p.
>penicillinase-resistant p.
>phenoxymethyl p.
>procaine p.
>semisynthetic p.
>p. V potassium
>p. V, VK

penicillinase-producing gonococcus
penicillinase-resistant penicillin
penicillin-nonsusceptible *Streptococcus pneumoniae* (**PNSP**)
penicillin-resistant Streptococcus pneumoniae (**PRSP**)

penicilliosis
Penicillium marneffei
penile, penial
>p. agenesis
>p. chordee
>p. curvature
>p. duplication
>p. dysgenesis
>p. erection
>p. flaccidity
>p. ischemia
>p. Kaposi sarcoma
>p. length
>p. torsion
>p. ulceration
>p. urethra
>p. urethral meatus
>p. zipper entrapment

penis, *pl.* **penes, penises**
>bulbus p.
>buried p.
>concealed p.
>corona of p.
>fracture of p.
>glans p.
>hidden p.
>hypoplastic p.
>inconspicuous p.
>uncircumcised p.
>webbed p.

penischisis
penises (*pl. of* penis)
Pen-Jr
>Epi E-Z P.-J.

Penlon infant resuscitator
Pennington
>P. clamp
>P. forceps

Penn pouch procedure
Pennsaid
penopubic urethral meatus
penoscrotal
>p. hypospadias
>p. Kaposi sarcoma
>p. transposition

Penrose drain
Pentacef
pentaerythritol tetranitrate
pentagastrin
pentalogy
>Fallot p.
>p. of Cantrell
>p. of Fallot

pentamidine isethionate
Pentam-300 Injection
Pentamycetin
pentane
>exhaled p.

Pentasa Oral
pentasomy
    chromosome X p.
    p. X syndrome
pentastarch
pentavalent vaccine
penta-X
    p.-X chromosomal aberration
    p.-X syndrome
Pentax
    P. EG-2430 video endoscope
    P. FG 24-x video endoscope
    P. laryngoscope
Pentazine
pentazocine
pentobarbital
    p. coma
    sodium p.
pentobarbitone
pentosan polysulfate
Pentostam
pentosuria
    essential benign p.
Pentothal Sodium
pentoxifylline
Pentrax
Pentritol
penumbra
Pen-Vee K
PEO
    progressive external ophthalmoplegia
    PEO syndrome
PEP
    pediatric exercise physiology
    postexposure prophylaxis
    progestogen-dependent endometrial
    protein
Pepcid
    P. AC
    P. AC Acid Controller
    P. Complete
    P. RPD
PEPCK
    phosphoenolpyruvate carboxykinase
    PEPCK deficiency
PEPI
    postmenopausal estrogen and progestin
    intervention
    PEPI study
pepper
    monk's p.
    P. syndrome
pepsic (*var. of* peptic)
Peptamen
    P. Jr.
    P. Jr. formula
peptic, pepsic
    p. esophagitis
    p. gastritis

    p. ulcer
    p. ulcer disease (PUD)
peptide
    amino-terminal p.
    atrial natriuretic p. (ANP)
    brain p.
    carboxyl terminal p. (CTP)
    corticotropin-like intermediate
    lobe p.
    endogenous opioid p.
    glucose-dependent insulinotropic p.
    gonadotropin-releasing
    hormone-associated p. (GAP)
    p. growth factor receptor signal
    p. growth factor signaling
    mechanism
    helix termination p.
    p. hormone
    insulinotropic p.
    91kD cytochrome b p.
    mitogenic p.
    natriuretic p.
    opioid p.
    parathyroid hormone-related p.
    (PTH-rP, PTHrP, PTHRP)
    PTH-derived p.
    synthetic gliadin p.
    thrombin receptor-activating p.
    (TRAP)
    trypsin activation p. (TAP)
    vasoactive intestinal p.
    (VIP)
Pepto
    Children's P.
Pepto-Bismol
Peptococcus
    P. anaerobius
    P. asaccharolyticus
    P. niger
Peptostreptococcus
per
    p. os
    p. rectum (p.r.)
    p. square meter method
    p. vaginam
    p. vias naturales
peracervical node
Perative formula
Perceived Stress Scale
percent
    p. body fat (PBF)
    p. fractional shortening
    milligram p.
    p. of ideal body weight
    (%IBW)
percentage
    high oxygen p. (HOPE)
    P. of Consonants Correct-Revised
    (PCC-R)

P

percentile
- head circumference-for-age p.
- length-for-age p.
- weight-for-age p.
- weight-for-length p.

perception
- deficits in attention, motor control, p. (DAMP)
- depth p.
- light p. (LP)
- motor p.
- no light p. (NLP)

perceptual
- p. domain
- p. skill

perchlorate

perchloroethylene

Percocet

Percodan

Percoll sperm preparation technique

percreta
- placenta p.

Percuflex Plus stent

percussion
- abdominal p.
- chest p.
- costovertebral angle tenderness to p.
- dullness to p.
- flatness to p.
- hyperresonance to p.
- p. myotonia
- p. therapy

percutaneous
- p. adductor tenotomy
- p. aspiration, instillation of hypertonic saline, respiration (PAIR)
- p. blood sampling
- p. catheter drainage
- p. central venous catheter (PCVC)
- p. central venous catheterization
- p. cholangiography
- p. cyst aspiration
- p. endoscopic gastrostomy (PEG)
- p. epididymal sperm aspiration (PESA)
- p. femoral venous catheter
- p. fetal transfusion
- p. line
- p. lung tap
- p. multipuncture technique
- p. nephrostomy
- p. nephrostomy catheter
- p. patent ductus arteriosus closure
- p. pin fixation
- p. renal biopsy
- p. retrograde scleroembolization
- p. Seldinger technique

- p. suprapubic telescopy
- p. therapy
- p. tracheostomy
- p. transluminal angioplasty (PTA)
- p. transluminal coronary rotational ablation (PTCRA)
- p. umbilical blood sampling (PUBS)

percutaneously inserted central line catheter (PICC)

Perdiem
- P. Fiber
- P. Plain

perennial
- p. allergic rhinitis
- allergic rhinitis p.
- p. asthma
- p. rye grass

Pereyra
- P. needle
- P. needle suspension
- P. procedure

Perez-Castro forceps

Perez reflex

perfectionism
- rigid p.

Perfectoderm Gel

perflubron emulsion temporary blood substitute

perfluorocarbon (PFC)

perfluorocarbon-assisted gas exchange

perfluorochemical (PFC)
- p. liquid

perfluorodecaline (PFD)

perflutren microsphere

perforated
- p. appendicitis
- p. bowel
- p. eardrum
- p. tympanic membrane
- p. viscus

perforating
- p. collagenosis
- p. granuloma annulare
- p. wound

perforation
- appendiceal p. (AP)
- biliary p.
- eardrum p.
- esophageal p.
- gastric p.
- ileal p.
- small bowel p.
- spontaneous biliary p. (SBP)
- tympanic membrane p.
- uterine p.

perforator
- Baylor amniotic p.
- deep inferior epigastric p. (DIEP)

Performa
- P. Acoustic Imaging system
- P. diagnostic ultrasound imaging system
- P. ultrasound

performance
- cardiovascular p.
- hemodynamic p.
- reproductive p.

perfringens
- *Clostridium p.*

perfused twin

perfusion
- fallopian tube sperm p. (FTSP)
- luxury p.
- mosaic p.
- peripheral p.
- placental p.
- pulmonary p.
- renal p.
- twin reversed arterial p. (TRAP)
- uteroplacental p.

pergolide

Pergonal

Perheentupa syndrome

periadenitis mucosa necrotica recurrens

perianal
- p. abscess
- p. aphthosis
- p. candidiasis
- p. dermatitis
- p. disease
- p. fistula
- p. hypopigmentation
- p. pruritus
- p. skin tag
- p. suture

perianastomotic ulceration

periaortic lymph node

periappendiceal abscess

periaqueductal tumor

periarteritis nodosa

periarticular

periauricular lymphadenitis

periaxial encephalitis

peribronchial
- p. fibrosis
- p. infiltration

peribronchiolar infiltration

pericanalicular fibroadenoma

pericapillary inflammatory cuffing

pericardial
- p. constriction-growth failure syndrome
- p. cyst
- p. effusion
- p. friction rub
- p. knock

- p. pathway
- p. puncture
- p. tamponade

pericardicentesis (*var. of* pericardiocentesis)

pericardiectomy
- parietal p.
- visceral p.

pericardiocentesis, pericardicentesis

pericardiotomy, pericardotomy

pericarditis
- acute fibrinous p.
- bacterial p.
- constrictive p.
- dry p.
- fibrinous p.
- immune complex-mediated p.
- infectious p.
- purulent p.

pericardium patch

pericardotomy (*var. of* pericardiotomy)

pericentric inversion

pericentromeric marker

perichondritis

perichondrium

Peri-Colace

Peri-Cold Pack

pericolpitis

periconceptional rubella

periconceptual intake

pericoronitis
- acute p.

pericranium

pericyte

periderm, periderma

periderma (*var. of* periderm)

Peridex

Peridin-C

Peridol

peridural
- p. analgesia
- p. anesthesia

perifascicular atrophy

perifollicular accentuation

perifolliculitis

Perigee Prolapse Repair System

Peri-Gel Pack

perihepatitis
- gonococcal p.

perihilar
- p. infiltrate
- p. shadow
- p. streaking

periimplantation

perikaryon

perilobular connective tissue

perilymph, perilympha

perilympha (*var. of* perilymph)

perilymphatic fistula (PLF)

P

perimembranous
    p. septum
    p. VSD
perimenopausal woman
perimenopause
perimenstrual tenesmus
perimesencephalic region
perimetritic
perimetritis
perimolysis, perimylolysis
perimortem
    p. cesarean section
    p. delivery
    p. sampling
perimylolysis (*var. of* perimolysis)
perinatal
    p. acidosis
    p. asphyxia
    p. assessment
    p. cerebral hemorrhage
    p. death
    p. distress prediction
    p. effect
    p. grief
    p. herpes
    p. hydronephrosis
    p. hypoxemia
    p. hypoxia
    p. insult
    p. lethal osteogenesis
      imperfecta
    p. medicine
    p. morbidity
    p. mortality (PM)
    p. mortality rate (PMR, PNMR)
    p. outcome
    p. pathology
    p. period
    p. risk factor
    p. stroke
    p. telencephalic leukoencephalopathy
    p. transmission
    p. trauma
perinatally acquired HIV infection
perinatal/placental pathologist
perinate
perinatologist
perinatology
perinea (*pl. of* perineum)
perineal
    p. analgesia
    p. anesthesia
    p. artery
    p. body
    p. body integrity
    p. cold pack
    p. defect
    p. descent
    p. desquamation

    p. fistula
    p. hygiene
    p. hypospadias
    p. infiltration
    p. irritation
    p. itching
    p. laceration
    p. lesion
    p. massage
    p. membrane
    p. musculature
    p. nerve
    p. pearl
    p. raphe
    p. repair
    p. resection
    p. retractor
    p. scar
    p. sphincter disruption
    p. surgical apron
    p. testis
    p. trauma
    p. warm pack
perineometer
perineoplasty
perineorrhaphy
    vaginal p.
perineoscrotal hypospadias
perineotomy
perineovaginal fistula
perinephric
    p. abscess
    p. phlegmon
perinephritis
perineum, *pl.* **perinea**
    central tendon of p.
    dashboard p.
perineuria (*pl. of* perineurium)
perineurium, *pl.* **perineuria**
perinuclear antineutrophil cytoplasmic
  antibody (pANCA)
PerioChip
period
    alveolar p.
    antepartum p.
    blastogenic p.
    canalicular p.
    effective refractory p.
    embryonic p.
    fertile p.
    incubation p. (ICP)
    intrapartum p.
    last menstrual p. (LMP)
    last normal menstrual p. (LNMP)
    latency p.
    menstrual p. (MP)
    missed p.
    neonatal p.
    newborn p.

perinatal p.
postictal p.
postpartum p.
postseizure p.
previous menstrual p. (PMP)
pseudoglandular p.
puerperal p.
rest/sleep p.'s
saccular p.
terminal saccular p.
window p.

periodic
p. acid-Schiff (PAS)
p. auscultation
p. breathing
p. breathing cycle (PBC)
p. breathing in infants
p. fever
p. fever, aphthous stomatitis, pharyngitis, cervical adenitis (PFAPA)
p. movement disorder
p. patient assessment

periodicity

periodontal disease

periodontitis
juvenile p.
localized juvenile p. (LJP)
prepuberal p.

PerioGard

perioophoritis

perioophorosalpingitis

perioperative

perioptic meningioma

perioral
p. cyanosis
p. rash
p. tissue loss

periorbital
p. ecchymosis
p. edema
p. fullness
p. hyperpigmentation
p. infantile myofibromatosis
p. puffiness
p. skin cellulitis
p. violaceous erythema

periorificial
p. dermatitis
p. rhagades

Perioseptic
Orajel P.

periosteal
p. cloaking
p. elevation
p. reaction
p. stripping

periosteitis (*var. of* periostitis)

periosteum

periostitis, periosteitis
pubic symphysis p.

periovaritis

peripad

peripancreatic fluid

peripartal heparin anticoagulation

peripartum
p. cardiomyopathy
p. symphysis separation

peripheral
p. ablative surgery
p. acrocyanosis
p. airway structure
p. androgen activity
p. androgen activity marker
p. arterial cannulation
p. arterial catheter
p. arterial disease
p. arterial line
p. arteriovenous fistula
p. arthritis
p. auditory disorder
p. blood
p. blood lymphocyte (PBL)
p. blood mononuclear cell (PBMC, PBMNC)
p. blood smear
p. blood stem cell (PBSC)
p. cyanosis
p. dysostosis, nail hypoplasia, mental retardation (PNM)
p. entrapment neuropathy
p. eosinophilia
p. facial nerve palsy (PFNP)
p. fractional oxygen extraction (PFOE)
p. hormone level
p. hyperalimentation
p. instantaneous X-ray imager (PIXI)
p. insulin resistance
p. intravenous (PIV)
p. intravenous catheter
p. jaundice
p. mononeuropathy
p. myelin protein (PMP)
p. nerve block
p. nerve injury
p. neuritis
p. neuroblastoma
p. neuroectodermal tumor
p. neuroepithelioma
p. neurofibromatosis
p. neutropenia
p. perfusion
p. placental separation
p. precocious puberty
p. primitive neuroectodermal tumor (PPNET)

P

peripheral (*continued*)
    p. pulmonary stenosis
    p. pulmonic stenosis
    p. stem cell transplantation
    p. thrombophlebitis
    p. vascular resistance
    p. vascular shock
    p. vasodilator
    p. venous catheterization
    p. vertigo
    p. vision
peripherally
    p. inserted catheter (PIC)
    p. inserted central catheter (PICC)
periphery
periportal hemorrhagic necrosis
peripubertal examination
perirectal
    p. abscess
    p. fascia
perirenal abscess
perisalpingitis
perisphincteric factor
perissodactylous
peristalsis
    fallopian tube p.
    intestinal p.
    ureteral p.
    visible p.
peristaltic wave
perisulcal topography
perisylvian
    p. abnormality
    p. syndrome
peritomy
peritonea (*pl. of* peritoneum)
peritoneal
    p. biopsy
    p. button
    p. carcinoma
    p. catheter
    p. cavity
    p. cytology
    p. dialysis (PD)
    p. dissemination
    p. drain
    p. envelope
    p. exudate
    p. fibrosis
    p. fluid
    p. hernia
    p. implant
    p. insufflation
    p. lavage
    p. macrophage
    p. mesothelium
    p. mouse
    p. oocyte sperm transfer (POST)
    p. reflection

    p. seeding
    p. serosa
    p. serous papillary carcinoma
    p. sign
    p. studding
    p. tap
    p. venous shunt
    p. washing
peritonei
    gliomatosis p.
    processus vaginalis p.
    pseudomyxoma p.
peritoneoscopy
peritoneum, *pl.* **peritonea**
    abdominal p.
    Blake closure of p.
    matted p.
    overlapping closure of p.
    parietal p.
    visceral p.
peritonitis
    acute secondary localized p.
    bacterial p.
    bile p.
    chemical p.
    infectious p.
    localized p.
    meconium p.
    pelvic p.
    primary p.
    secondary localized p.
    spontaneous bacterial p. (SBP)
    tuberculous p.
peritonsillar
    p. abscess (PTA)
    p. cellulitis
    p. edema
peritubal adhesion
peritubular fibrosis
periumbilical
    p. artery blood sampling
    p. incision
    p. pain
periungual
    p. avascularity
    p. desquamation
    p. erythema
    p. fibroma
    p. flaking
    p. wart
periurethral
    p. bulk injections
    p. collagen injection
    p. gland
perivaginitis
perivascular
    p. calcification
    p. emphysema
    p. eosinophilic infiltrate

p. inflammatory infiltrate
p. polymorphonuclear infiltrate
p. pseudorosette formation
perivasculitis
granulomatous p.
periventricular
p. echolucency (PVEL)
p. encephalomalacia
p. hemorrhage (grade 1–4) (PVH)
p. infarction
p. leukomalacia (PVL)
p. nodular gray matter heterotopia
periventricular-intraventricular hemorrhage (PIVH)
perivitelline space
Peri-Warm Pack
Perkin
P. Elmer rhodamine dye terminator kit
P. line
perlèche
Perlman nephroblastomatosis syndrome
perlocutionary stage
Perls iron stain
permanence
object p.
permanent
p. dentition
p. hearing loss (PHL)
p. molar
p. posthemorrhagic hydrocephalus
p. sterilization
p. suture
p. teeth
permanganate
potassium p.
Permanone
Permapen Isoject
PermCath catheter
permeability
intestinal p. (IP)
vascular p.
permethrin
p. 5% cream
p. creme rinse
permission, limited information, specific suggestions, intensive therapy (PLISSIT)
permissive hypercapnia
permutation
pernicious
p. anemia (PA)
p. anemia of pregnancy
p. vomiting
pernio
lupus p.
Pernox
perocormus
perodactylia (*var. of* perodactyly)
perodactyly, perodactylia

peromelia, peromely
peromely (*var. of* peromelia)
peroneal
p. atrophy, X-linked recessive
p. dislocation
p. muscular atrophy
p. muscular atrophy, axonal type
p. muscular dystrophy
p. nerve function
p. retinaculum
p. rupture
p. sign
p. spastic flatfoot
peroneus
p. brevis muscle
p. brevis tendon
p. longus muscle
p. longus tendon
peropus
perosplanchnia
peroxidase
p. defect
eosinophil p.
glutathione p.
streptavidin p.
peroxidation
lipid p.
plasma lipid p.
peroxidative enzyme
peroxide
benzoyl p.
carbamide p.
hydrogen p.
lipid p.
zinc p.
peroxisomal
p. congenital disorder
p. deficiency
p. disease
p. ghost
peroxisome import disorder
Peroxyl
peroxynitrite
peroxyoxalate
perphenazine
Per-Q-Cath catheter
PerQ SANS system
Perrault syndrome
Persantine
perseveration
persistence
foramen ovale p.
p. of fetal circulation
persistent
p. alkaline urine
p. anovulation
p. cancer
p. ectopic pregnancy
p. estrogen secretion

P

persistent (*continued*)
    p. fetal circulation (PFC)
    p. gastrocutaneous fistula
    p. gestational trophoblastic disease
    p. hyperinsulinemic hypoglycemia of infancy (PHHI)
    p. hyperplastic primary vitreous (PHPV)
    p. müllerian duct syndrome
    p. neutropenia
    p. occiput posterior fetal position
    p. occiput posterior presentation
    p. ovarian mass
    p. postmolar gestational trophoblastic tumor
    p. primitive reflex pattern
    p. proteinuria
    p. pulmonary hypertension (PPH)
    p. pulmonary hypertension of newborn (PPHN)
    p. pupillary membrane
    p. right umbilical vein
    p. tachycardia
    p. trismus
    p. trophoblastic tissue
    p. urachus
    p. vegetative state (PVS)
    p. ventricular dilation
personal
    P. Adjustment and Role Skills (PARS)
    p. hygiene history
    p. lubricant
    p. probability
personality
    p. change
    p. disorder (PD)
    p. disorder examination (PDE)
    P. Inventory for Children (PIC)
personal-social skill
personnel
    medications, monitors, suction, oxygen, airway equipment, p. (MSOAP)
perstans
    telangiectasia macularis eruptiva p. (TMEP)
persulcatus
    Ixodes p.
Persutte and Lenke study
PERT
    pancreatic enzyme replacement therapy
pertactin
pertechnetate
    technetium-99m p.
pertenue
    Treponema p.

Perthes disease
pertubation
    cardiovascular p.
Pertussin ES
pertussis
    acellular p.
    Bordetella p.
    diphtheria, tetanus toxoid, p. (DTP)
    diphtheria, tetanus toxoid, acellular p. (DTPa)
    diphtheria, tetanus toxoid, whole-cell p. (DTPw)
    diphtheria toxoids-acellular p.
    diphtheria toxoid with p.
    tetanus, diphtheria and p. (TdaP)
    p. toxin (PT)
    p. toxoid (PT)
peruana
    verruca p.
peruviana
pervasive
    p. developmental disorder (PDD)
    p. developmental disorder not otherwise specified (PDD-NOS)
    p. support
perversus
    situs p.
pes
    p. anserina bursitis
    p. anserinus
    p. cavus
    p. cavus deformity
    dorsalis pedis
    p. equinovarus
    p. planus
    tinea pedis
PESA
    percutaneous epididymal sperm aspiration
pessary
    Albert-Smith p.
    blue ring p.
    cube p.
    diaphragm p.
    doughnut p.
    Dumontpallier p.
    Dutch p.
    Findley folding p.
    Gariel p.
    Gehrung p.
    Gellhorn rigid p.
    Hodge with knob p.
    incontinence dish p.
    inflatable ball p.
    p. injection
    Mayer p.
    Menge p.

PGE₂ p.
Prentif p.
Prochownik p.
prostaglandin p.
Regula p.
ring p.
Risser p.
Smith p.
Smith-Hodge p.
Tandem-Cube p.
vaginal p.
pesticide
organochlorine p.
pestis
Yersinia p.
PET
parent effectiveness training
positron emission tomography
postexposure treatment
preeclamptic toxemia
pressure equalization tube
PET scan
petechiae (*pl. of* petechia)
palatal petechia
petechial
p. hemorrhage
p. rash
Peters
P. anomaly
P. anomaly, corneal clouding, growth and mental retardation syndrome
P. anomaly-short limb dwarfism syndrome
P. ovum
Peters-plus syndrome
pethidine
petit
P. canals
P. hernia
P. herniotomy
P. ligament
P. lumbar triangle
p. mal
p. mal attack
p. mal epilepsy
p. mal-like seizure disorder
p. mal seizure
p. mal status
p. mal variant
P. sinus
Petri cast
petrificans
urethritis p.
petrolatum
liquid p.
petroleum
p. distillate poisoning
p. jelly

petrositis
Pettigrew syndrome (PGS)
Peutz-Jeghers
P.-J. polyp
P.-J. syndrome
Peyer patch
Peyronie disease
Pezzer
P. catheter
P. tube
PF
Astramorph PF
Pfannenstiel incision
PFAPA
periodic fever, aphthous stomatitis, pharyngitis, cervical adenitis
Pfaundler-Hurler syndrome
PFC
perfluorocarbon
perfluorochemical
persistent fetal circulation
PFD
perfluorodecaline
polyostotic fibrous dysplasia
PFDI
pelvic floor distress inventory
Pfeiffer syndrome
PFGE
pulsed field gel electrophoresis
PFIC
progressive familial intrahepatic cholestasis
PFK
phosphofructokinase
PFK deficiency
Pflüger law
PFM
peak flow meter
TruZone PFM
PFME
pelvic floor muscle exercise
PFMT
pelvic floor muscle training
PFNP
peripheral facial nerve palsy
PFO
patent foramen ovale
PFOE
peripheral fractional oxygen extraction
PFP
purified fusion protein
PFP vaccine
PFPS
patellofemoral pain syndrome
PFR
peak flow rate
pericardial friction rub
PFS
pelvic floor electrical stimulation

P

PFS (*continued*)
  preservative-free solution
    Adriamycin PFS
    Idamycin PFS
    Vincasar PFS
PFT
  placentofetal transfusion
  pulmonary function test
pfu
  plaque-forming unit
PG
  phosphatidylglycerol
  prostaglandin
    1-hour PG
P/G
  Fulvicin P/G
pg
  picogram
PGD
  preimplantation genetic diagnosis
PGE
  prostaglandin E
PGE$_1$
  prostaglandin E$_1$
PGE$_2$
  prostaglandin E$_2$
    PGE$_2$ pessary
PGF
  placental growth factor
  prostaglandin F
PGF2 alpha
PGG
  prostaglandin G
PGH
  placental growth hormone
  prostaglandin H
PGK
  phosphoglycerate kinase
    PGK deficiency
    PGK hereditary nonspherocytic
      anemia
P-glycoprotein
PGR
  pelvic girdle relaxation
  progesterone receptor
    symptom-giving PGR
PgR
  progesterone receptor
PGS
  Pettigrew syndrome
  prolapse-gastropathy syndrome
PGSI
  prostaglandin synthetase inhibitor
PGWB
  Psychological General Well-Being
    PGWB index
pH
  hydrogen ion concentration
  phase

cord pH
cord blood pH
endoesophageal pH
fetal blood pH
fetal scalp blood pH
intracellular pH (pHi)
intragastric pH
neutral pH
pH probe
scalp pH
umbilical arterial pH
venous pH
PH-1
  primary hyperoxaluria type 1
Ph1
  Philadelphia chromosome
PHA
  phytohemagglutinin
PHACE
  posterior fossa malformations,
    hemangiomas, arterial anomalies,
    coarctation of aorta, cardiac defects,
    eye abnormalities
    PHACE syndrome
phacomatosis, phakomatosis
  fifth p.
  fourth p.
Phaedra complex
phage phenotype
phagocyte
  mononuclear p.
  polymorphonuclear p.
phagocytic
phagocytophila
  Ehrlichia p.
phagocytophilia
  anaplasma p.
phagocytosis
  poor p.
phakoma
phakomatosis
  Jadassohn nevus p.
    (JNP)
phalangectomy
phalanges (*pl. of* phalanx)
phalanx (phal), *pl.* **phalanges**
  delta p.
phalli (*pl. of* phallus)
phalloides
  Amanita p.
phalloidin
phallometric assessment
phalloplasty
phallus, *pl.* **phalli**
Phaneuf
  P. clamp
  P. uterine artery forceps
Phaneuf-Graves enterocele repair
phantasy (*var. of* fantasy)

phantom
    p. limb
    p. pregnancy
    Schultze p.
pharaonic circumcision
Pharmaceutical Research and Manufacturers of America (PhRMA)
pharmacodynamic response
pharmacokinetic
pharmacologic, pharmacological
    p. immunosuppression
    p. intervention
    p. management
    p. treatment
pharmacological (*var. of* pharmacologic)
pharmacologically induced hypomania
pharmacotherapy
    stand-alone p.
pharmacy
    compounding p.
Pharmaflur
Pharmaseal
    P. disposable cervical dilator
    P. disposable uterine sound
Pharsight
    P. Trial Designer
    P. Trial Designer simulation program
pharyngeal
    p. diphtheria
    p. diverticulum
    p. gonococcal infection
    p. gonorrhea
    p. incompetence
    p. mirror
    p. muscle
    p. pouch syndrome
    p. space
pharynges (*pl. of* pharynx)
pharyngitis
    acute lymphonodular p.
    bacterial p.
    exudative p.
    GABHS p.
    group C p.
    lymphonodular p.
    nonstreptococcal p.
    purulent p.
    streptococcal p.
    viral p.
pharyngoconjunctival fever
pharyngoplasty
    sphincter p.
pharyngotonsillitis
pharynx, *pl.* **pharynges**

phase
    acceleration p.
    active p.
    p. advance treatment
    aqueous p.
    beta p.
    deceleration p.
    deep tendon reflex delayed relaxation p.
    p. delay chronotherapy
    delayed relaxation p.
    p. delay treatment
    early proliferative p.
    end-expiratory p. (EEP)
    equilibrium p.
    fertile p.
    follicular p.
    hair growth p.
    hyperprolactinemia-associated luteal p.
    icteric p.
    immune p.
    implantation p.
    inadequate luteal p.
    Korotkoff p.
    late p.
    latent p.
    luteal p.
    menses p.
    menstrual p.
    mitosis p.
    p. of maximum slope of labor
    polyuric p.
    postictal p.
    pre-pulseless p.
    proliferative p.
    prolonged expiratory p.
    prolonged latent p.
    pulseless p.
    resolution p.
    S p.
    secretory p.
    stance p.
    telogen p.
    viremic p.
phase-contrast microscopy
phased array probe
phasic tone
Phazyme infant drops
PHC
    primary hepatocellular carcinoma
PHE
    phenylalanine
        blood PHE
        serum PHE
phenacetin
phenanthrene
phenazocine

P

695

phenazone
phenazopyridine
    p. HCl
    p. hydrochloride
phencyclidine (PCP)
phendimetrazine
phenelzine
Phenergan
    P. injection
    P. Oral
    P. Rectal
phenindamine
phenindione
pheniramine
phenobarbitone
phenocopy
phenogenetics
phenolphthalein
phenolsulfonphthalein test
phenomena (*pl. of* phenomenon)
phenomenology
phenomenon, *pl.* phenomena
    all-or-none p.
    Arias-Stella p.
    clasp-knife p.
    crankshaft p.
    dawn p.
    dissociative p.
    doll's eye p.
    Hata p.
    intrapsychic p.
    Kasabach-Merritt p.
    Katz-Wachtel p.
    Köbner p.
    lip p.
    Marcus Gunn p.
    memory p.
    pseudo-Köbner p.
    Raynaud p. (RP)
    rebound p.
    recall p.
    ritualistic p.
    Rumpel-Leede p.
    Schwartzman p.
    Somogyi p.
    squatting p.
    steal p.
    stuck twin p.
    tension-discharging p.
    trigger p.
    triple-color p.
    Wenckebach phenomena
    X-linked p.
phenothiazine
    p. intoxication
    p. poisoning
phenotype
    body p.
    Bombay erythrocyte p.

    cardiac abnormality, T-cell deficit,
      clefting, hypocalcemia p.
    CATCH 22 p.
    fibroblast growth factor-10 null p.
    hemoglobin SC p.
    hemoglobin SS p.
    hemoglobin S-Thal p.
    Hunter-Hurler p.
    MASS p.
    neurofibromatosis with Noonan p.
    Pena-Shokeir p.
    phage p.
    Potter p.
    Turner p.
    XX and XY Turner p.
phenotypic
    p. female
    p. sex
    p. threshold
    p. variance
phenoxybenzamine
phenoxymethyl penicillin
phenprocoumon
phensuximide
phentermine
phentolamine
phenylacetate
    sodium p.
phenylacetic acid
phenylacetylglutamine
phenylalanine (PHE)
    p. dehydroxylase
    p. hydroxylase (PAH)
    p. 4-monooxygenase
phenylalaninemia
    malignant p.
    non-PKU p.
phenylbutazone
phenylbutyrate
    sodium p.
phenylephrine
    guaifenesin, phenylpropanolamine, p.
    promethazine and p.
phenylethylamine
phenylhydantoin
phenylketonuria (PKU)
    maternal p.
    preconceptionally treated p.
    p. test
phenylpiperazine
phenylpropanolamine
    bromopheniramine and p.
phenylpyruvate
phenylpyruvic acid
phenyl salicylate
phenyltoloxamine
phenytoin
    p. encephalopathy
    p. therapy

phenytoin-associated adenopathy
phenytoin-induced gingival overgrowth
pheochromocytoma
    extrarenal p.
PHH
    posthemorrhagic hydrocephalus
PHHI
    persistent hyperinsulinemic
     hypoglycemia of infancy
PHI
    Prehospital Index
pHi
    intracellular hydrogen ion
     concentration
    intracellular pH
Phialophora
PhiCal fecal calprotectin immunoassay
Philadelphia
    P. chromosome (Ph1)
    P. collar
Philip gland
Philips SensorTouch temple
  thermometer
Phillips' Milk of Magnesia
Phillips phototherapy light
philtra (*pl. of* philtrum)
philtrum, *pl.* **philtra**
    hypoplastic p.
    short p.
    smooth p.
phimoses (*pl. of* phimosis)
phimosis, *pl.* **phimoses**
    p. clitoridis
    secondary p.
    p. vaginalis
phimotic ring
pHisoHex
    p. bath
    p. soap
PHL
    permanent hearing loss
phlebarteriectasis
phlebectasia
    congenital generalized p.
    generalized p.
phlebitis
    infective p.
    puerperal p.
    string p.
    suppurative p.
    syphilitic p.
phlebography
phlebolith
    calcified p.
phlebometritis
phlebothrombosis
phlebotomum
    Bunostomum p.
phlebotomus fever

phlebotomy
phlegmasia
    p. alba dolens
    cellulitic p.
    p. dolens
    thrombotic p.
phlegmon
    parametrial p.
    perinephric p.
    postcesarean p.
phlegmonous mastitis
phlyctenule
PHMB
    polyhexamethyl biguanide
PHN
    postherpetic neuralgia
    public health nurse
phobia
    fever p.
    school p.
    simple p. (SPh)
    social p.
    specific p.
phobic
    p. avoidance
    p. hallucination
Phocas
    P. disease
    P. syndrome
phocomelia syndrome
pholcodine
phonation
    abnormal p.
phoneme segmentation task
phonemic
    p. awareness
    p. awareness task
phonetics
phonocardiography
phonologic (*var. of* phonological)
phonological, phonologic
    p. coding
    p. development
    p. disorder
phonologic-syntactic syndrome
phonology
phonophobia
phorbol ester
phoria
Phos-Flur
phosphatase
    acid p.
    alkaline p. (ALP)
    bone alkaline p. (BAP)
    bone-specific alkaline p.
    placental alkaline p. (PLAP)
    tyrosine p.
5-phosphate
    pyridoxal 5-p.

P

phosphate
    adenosine p.
    calcium p.
    chloroquine p.
    chromic p.
    Cleocin P.
    clindamycin p.
    p. enema
    etoposide p.
    p. leak
    nicotinamide adenine dinucleotide p. (NADPH)
    oleandomycin p.
    oral p.
    plasma p.
    polyestradiol p.
    polyribosylribitol p. (PRP)
    potassium titanyl p. (KTP)
    primaquine p.
    pyridoxal p.
    sodium hydrogen p.
    p. supplement
    p. toxicity
    p. wasting
phosphate-buffered
    p.-b. saline (PBS)
    p.-b. saline solution
phosphatidic acid phosphohydrolase (PAPase)
phosphatidylcholine
    dipalmitoyl p. (DPPC)
    disaturated p.
    unsaturated p.
phosphatidylethanolamine
phosphatidylglycerol (PG)
    p. level
phosphatidylinositol (PI)
phosphaturia
phosphene
5-phospho-alpha-d-ribosyl pyrophosphate (PRPP)
phosphocreatine (PCr)
phosphodiesterase
    p. 5 (PDE5)
    cGMP-specific p.
    cGMP-specific p. 5
    p. inhibitor (PDI)
phosphoenolpyruvate carboxykinase (PEPCK)
phosphofructokinase (PFK)
    congenital defect of p.
    p. deficiency
phosphoglycerate kinase (PGK)
phosphohydrolase
    phosphatidic acid p. (PAPase)
phosphokinase
    creatine p. (CPK)
    creatinine p.

phospholipase (PL)
    p. A_2 (PLA2, PLA_2)
    p. activity
    p. C
phospholipid
    p. antibody
    egg p.
phospholipidosis
phosphoribosylpyrophosphate synthetase superactivity
phosphoribosyltransferase
    adenine p.
phosphorus (P)
    p. metabolism
    p. MRS
phosphorus-32 (^{32}P, P-32)
phosphorus-31 magnetic resonance imaging (^{31}P MRI)
phosphoryl
phosphorylase
    p. kinase deficiency
    nucleoside p.
    purine nucleoside p. (PNP)
phosphorylated drug form
phosphorylation
    mitochondrial oxidative p.
    myosin light-chain p.
    oxidative p. (OXPHOS)
    protein p.
    sperm tail protein p.
Phospho-Soda
    Fleet P.-S.
photic stimulation
photoallergic reaction
photobilirubin
photochemotherapy
photocoagulation
    infrared p. (IRC)
    laser p.
PhotoDerm PL handpiece
photodistributed lesion
photodynamic therapy
Photofrin
photogenic seizure
photometabolism
photometer
    HemoCue hemoglobin p.
    reflectance p.
photometric analysis
photometry
    scanning p.
photomicrograph
photon
photophobia
    ichthyosis, follicularis, atrichia, p. (IFAP)
photophobic iritis
photophoresis

photoplethysmography (PPG)
  near infrared p. (NIRP)
  red p.
Photoplex
photoretinopathy
photoscreening
photosensitive
  p. dermatitis
  p. epilepsy
  p. porphyria
  p. seizure
photosensitivity
photostethoscope
phototesting
phototherapy
  p. bulb
  double-bank p.
  double-blanket p.
  fiberoptic p. (FO-PT)
  halogen spotlight p.
  intensive p.
  maximum-intensive p.
  PUVA p.
  ultraviolet A p.
photothermal sclerosis
photothermolysis
  selective p. (SPTL)
phototoxic reaction
photovaporization
  laser p.
PHPV
  persistent hyperplastic primary vitreous
phrenic
  p. nerve
  p. nerve pacing
  p. nerve palsy
  p. nerve paralysis
phrenoesophageal ligament
PhRMA
  Pharmaceutical Research and
  Manufacturers of America
PHS
  pseudoprogeria-Hallermann-Streiff
  PHS syndrome
phthalate
  dimethyl p.
phthalylsulfacetamide
phthalylsulfathiazole
PHVD
  posthemorrhagic ventricular dilation
PHVM
  posthemorrhagic ventriculomegaly
phycomycosis
pHydrion strip
phygogalactic
Phyllocontin
phyllodes
  cystosarcoma p.
  p. tumor

phylloides
  Demodex p.
phylloquinone, phylloquinone K
phylogenesis
physeal (*var. of* physial)
physial, physeal
  p. arrest
  p. bridge
  p. closure
  p. destruction
  p. fracture
  p. injury
  p. separation
physiatrist
physical
  p. abuse
  p. capacity evaluation (PCE)
  p. intimacy
  p. maneuver
  p. map
  p. maturity
  p. therapy (PT)
  p. victimization
physical-sexual abuse
physician
  medical control p. (MCP)
  p. payment review commission
  (PPRC)
  primary care p. (PCP)
physician-applied force
physician-patient relationship
physiognomy
physiologic, physiological
  p. addiction/abstinence syndrome
  p. amenorrhea
  p. anemia
  p. anemia of infancy
  p. anemia of pregnancy
  p. bowleg
  p. cavus
  p. change
  p. childbirth
  p. delay
  p. delay of puberty
  p. derangement
  p. discharge
  p. endometrial ablation/resection
  loop (PEARL)
  p. flatfoot
  p. follicular regulation
  p. genu valgum
  p. genu varum
  p. gynecomastia
  p. hypogammaglobulinemia
  p. icterus
  p. jaundice
  p. jaundice of newborn
  p. knock-knee
  p. leukorrhea

P

physiologic (*continued*)
    p. neonatal withdrawal bleed
    p. reflex
    p. reflux
    p. regurgitation
    p. replacement dose
    p. retraction ring
    p. saline
    p. salt solution (PSS)
    p. sclerosis
    P. Stability Index (PSI)
    p. third-stage management
    p. transient hypoparathyroidism
    p. tumescence
physiological (*var. of* physiologic)
physiologically corrected transposition
physiologist
    exercise p.
    fetal p.
    pediatric exercise p.
physiology
    Eisenmenger p.
    exercise p.
    fetal p.
    maternal p.
    maternal-fetal p.
    pediatric exercise p. (PEP)
    pregnancy p.
    Score for Neonatal Acute P. (SNAP)
physiopathologic, physiopathological
physiopathological (*var. of* physiopathologic)
physiotherapist
physiotherapy (PT)
    chest p. (CPT)
physis
    bridging p.
    broad p.
    radial p.
    serpiginous cephalad curved p.
physometra
physopyosalpinx
physostigmine
phytanic
    p. acid
    p. acid oxidation disorder
    p. acid storage disease
phytoagglutinin
phytobezoar
phytoestrogen
phytohemagglutinin (PHA, PHY)
phytomenadione
phytonadione
phytophotodermatitis
phytosterol (PS)
pi
    p. cone monochromatism
    p. dimeric protein

PI
    phosphatidylinositol
    ponderal index
    premature infant
    present illness
    protease inhibitor
    pulsatility index
    alpha-1 PI
    PI type
    PI type gene
    PI type 2 gene
    PI type 22 gene
    PI type ZZ gene defect
pial thickening
pia mater
piano-wire adhesion
PIC
    peripherally inserted catheter
    Personality Inventory for Children
PICA
    Pictorial Instrument for Children and Adolescents
    posterior inferior cerebellar artery
pica craving
PICC
    percutaneously inserted central line catheter
    peripherally inserted central catheter
    PICC kit
    PICC line
pickettii
    Burkholderia p.
    Ralstonia p.
pickups
    Adson p.
    rat tooth p.
pickwickian syndrome
picky eater
picogram (pg)
picornavirus
PICP
    carboxyterminal propeptide of type 1 procollagen
picrotoxin
pictorial
    p. anticipatory guidance (PAG)
    p. blood loss assessment chart (PBAC)
    P. Instrument for Children and Adolescents (PICA)
picture
    p. chart
    p. completion test
    postencephalitic parkinsonian p.
pictures of syndromes and undiagnosed malformations (POSSUM)
PICU
    pediatric intensive care unit

PID
  pediatric infectious disease
  pelvic inflammatory disease
  primary immune deficiency
  primary immunodeficiency
PIE
  postinfectious encephalomyelitis
  preimplantation embryo
  pulmonary infiltrate with
    eosinophilia
  pulmonary interstitial emphysema
    PIE Medical ultrasound
    PIE syndrome
piebald
piebaldism
piercing
  cartilage p.
Pierre
  P. Robin malformation
    sequence
  P. Robin syndrome
**Piers-Harris Children's Self-Concept
  Scale**
Piersol point
piezoelectric sensor
PIF
  prolactin inhibiting factor
pigeon
  p. breast
  p. toe
pigeon-toed, pigeontoed
pigeontoed (*var. of* pigeon-toed)
Pigg-O-Stat
pigment
  bile p.
  melanin-like p.
  p. stone
pigmentary stage
pigmentation
  black p.
  contiguous p.
  p. disorder of vulva
  mucocutaneous p.
  reticulated p.
pigmented
  p. lesion
  p. melanocyte
  p. nevus
  p. nodular adrenal hyperplasia
pigmenti
  Block-Sulzberger incontinentia p.
  incontinentia p. (type I, II)
pigmentosa
  autosomal dominant retinitis p.
    (adRP)
  congenital bullous urticaria p.
  congenital retinitis p.
  neuropathy, ataxia, retinitis p.
    (NARP)

  retinitis p.
  urticaria p.
pigmentosa-dysostosis
  dystrophia retinae p.-d.
pigmentosum
  xeroderma p.
pigtail catheter
PIH
  periventricular-intraventricular
    hemorrhage
  pregnancy-induced hypertension
    PIH symptom
pilar cyst
pilaris
  keratosis p.
  pityriasis rubra p. (PRP)
PILBD
  paucity of interlobular bile duct
pileus
pill
  birth control p. (BCP)
  combined birth control p.
  emergency contraception p. (ECP)
  emergency contraceptive p. (ECP)
  Levlen contraceptive p.
  Lo/Ovral contraceptive p.
  morning-after p.
  Nordette contraceptive p.
  oral contraceptive p. (OCP)
  Ovral contraceptive p.
  Ovrette contraceptive p.
  progestin-only p. (POP)
  Seasonale birth control p.
  Tri-Levlen contraceptive p.
  Triphasil contraceptive p.
pillar
  bladder p.
  rectal p.
pill-free week
pillow
  Crescent p.
  OsmoCyte p.
Pilocar Ophthalmic
pilocarpine
  p. iontophoresis
  p. iontophoresis method
pilocytic fibrillary astrocytoma
piloid tumor
pilomatricoma, pilomatrixoma
pilomatrixoma (*var. of* pilomatricoma)
pilonidal
  p. cyst
  p. dimple
  p. sinus
Pilopine HS Ophthalmic
Piloptic Ophthalmic
pilosebaceous
  p. duct
  p. gland

P

pilosebaceous (*continued*)
>   p. gland of Zeis
>   p. unit

pilot
>   P. audiometer
>   P. suturing guide

pimagedine
pimecrolimus cream
pimozide
pin
>   Beath p.
>   Surgin hemorrhage occluder p.
>   p. tract

Pinard
>   P. maneuver
>   P. sign

pincer grasp
pindolol
pineal
>   p. body
>   p. cyst
>   p. germinoma
>   p. gland
>   p. tumor

pinealoblastoma, pineoblastoma
pinealoma
>   ectopic p.

pineoblastoma (*var. of* pinealoblastoma)
ping-pong
>   p.-p. ball deformity
>   p.-p. ball depression
>   p.-p. fracture
>   p.-p. spread of disease

pinguecula, pinguicula
pinguicula (*var. of* pinguecula)
pinhole
>   p. collimated scan
>   p. collimation
>   p. test

pink
>   p. diaper syndrome
>   p. disease
>   p. tetralogy of Fallot

pinked up
pinkeye
pinna
>   anteverted p.
>   displaced p.
>   malformed p.

pinning
>   in situ p.

pinopode
pinpoint hemorrhage
P32 intraperitoneal treatment
pinworm
>   p. infestation
>   p. vaginitis

Pin-X

PIP
>   peak inspiratory pressure

pipecolic acidemia
Pipelle
>   P. biopsy
>   P. endometrial suction curette
>   Unimar P.

piper
>   P. fatigue scale
>   P. forceps

piperacetazine
piperacillin
>   p. and tazobactam
>   p. sodium/tazobactam sodium

piperazine
>   p. dione
>   p. estrone sulfate

piperidolate hydrochloride
piperonyl butoxide
pipestem urethra
pipet (*var. of* pipette)
>   P. Curette

pipette, pipet
>   FemTest endometrial biopsy p.
>   Pasteur p.

pipiens
>   *Culex p.*

PIPP
>   Premature Infant Pain Profile
>   PIPP score

piracetam
pirbuterol
Pirie syndrome
piriform aperture stenosis
piriformis
>   p. muscle spasm
>   p. syndrome

piroxicam
Piskacek sign
Pistofidis cervical biopsy forceps
pit
>   commissural lip p.
>   congenital lip p.
>   lip p.
>   preauricular p.

pitcher's elbow
Pitocin
>   P. augmentation
>   P. induction

Pitressin
Pitrex
pitted
>   p. keratolysis
>   p. teeth

pitting
>   digital p.
>   p. edema
>   nail p.

Pitt-Rogers-Danks syndrome (PRDS)

Pitt syndrome
Pitt-Williams brachydactyly
pituitary
    p. adenoma
    p. axis
    p. cell
    p. desensitization
    p. disorder
    p. dwarfism
    p. forceps
    p. gigantism
    p. gland
    p. gland function
    p. gland gumma
    p. gland transplantation
    p. gland tumor
    p. gonadotropin
    p. gonadotropin effect
    p. gonadotropin inhibition
    p. gonadotropin regulation
    p. gonadotropin secretion
    p. gonadotropin suppression
    p. hormone
    p. hormone release
    p. necrosis
pituitary-adrenal function
pituitary-hypothalamic circulation
pituitary-ovarian function
pityriasis
    p. alba
    p. lichenoides
    p. lichenoides chronica (PLC)
    p. lichenoides et varioliformis acuta
    (PLEVA)
    p. rosea
    p. rotunda
    p. rotunda treatment
    p. rubra pilaris (PRP)
    p. versicolor
Pityrosporum
    P. disease
    P. orbiculare
    P. ovale
    P. yeast
PIV
    parainfluenza virus
    peripheral intravenous
    PIV catheter
pivampicillin
Piver type II procedure
PIVH
    periventricular-intraventricular
    hemorrhage
PIVKA
    protein-induced vitamin K absence
PIVKA-II assay
pivoting
    prone p.
pivot lock

pixel
PIXI
    peripheral instantaneous X-ray imager
    PIXI bone densitometer
Pixie minilaparoscope
PK
    PlasmaKinetic
    pyruvate kinase
    PK activity
    PK deficiency
    PK factor
    Synsorb PK
PKC
    protein kinase C
PKD
    polycystic kidney disease
    infantile PKD
PKDL
    post-kala azar dermal leishmaniasis
PKU
    phenylketonuria
    PKU test
PLA2
    phospholipase A_2
placebo
placebo-controlled study
placement
    categorical p.
    catheter tip p.
    central venous catheter p.
    cerclage p.
    external jugular vein catheter p.
    extraovular p.
    gastrostomy tube p.
    internal jugular vein catheter p.
    intracervical p.
    intraosseous line p.
    intravenous line p.
    irregular tooth p.
    J-wire p.
    line p.
    noncategorical p.
    open gastrostomy tube p.
    prenatal p.
    stent p.
    tooth p.
    tube p.
placenta
    accessory p.
    accessory lobe of p.
    p. accreta
    p. accreta vera
    adherent p.
    anular p.
    battledore p.
    bidiscoidal p.
    p. biloba
    bilobate p.
    bilobed p.

P

placenta (*continued*)
  p. bipartita
  chorioallantoic p.
  chorioamnionic p.
  choriovitelline p.
  circummarginate p.
  p. circumvallata
  circumvallate p.
  cotyledonary p.
  p. creta
  deciduate p.
  diamniotic dichorionic p.
  dichorionic p.
  dichorionic diamniotic p.
  p. diffusa
  p. dimidiata
  disperse p.
  Duncan p.
  p. duplex
  endotheliochorial p.
  epitheliochorial p.
  p. extrachorales
  p. fenestrata
  hemochorial p.
  horseshoe p.
  immature p.
  incarcerated p.
  p. increta
  p. in situ
  labyrinthine p.
  p. marginata
  p. membranacea
  monochorionic diamniotic p.
  monochorionic monoamniotic p.
  p. multiloba
  nondeciduous p.
  p., ovary, uterus (POU)
  p. panduraformis
  p. percreta
  p. previa (PP)
  p. previa centralis
  p. previa creta
  p. previa marginalis
  p. previa partialis
  p. reflexa
  p. reniformis
  retained p.
  Schultze p.
  p. spuria
  Stallworth p.
  succenturiate p.
  supernumerary p.
  p. triloba
  p. tripartita
  p. triplex
  twin p.
  p. velamentosa
  velamentous p.

  villous p.
  zonary p.
placentae
  ablatio p.
  abruptio p. (AP)
  amotio p.
placentaire
  bruit p.
placental
  p. abnormality
  p. abruption
  p. adaptive angiogenesis
  p. alkaline phosphatase (PLAP)
  p. barrier
  p. bed
  p. bleeding
  p. bleeding site
  p. blood flow (PBF)
  p. bruit
  p. cotyledon
  p. damage
  p. disc
  p. dysfunction
  p. dysfunction syndrome
  p. dystocia
  p. edema
  p. extrusion
  p. fragment
  p. function
  p. giant cell
  p. grade
  p. grading
  p. growth
  p. growth factor (PGF, PlGF)
  p. growth hormone (PGH)
  p. hemangioma syndrome
  p. hemorrhage
  p. hormone
  p. hydrops
  p. immunology
  p. implantation
  p. implantation site
  p. infarction
  p. insufficiency
  p. interface
  p. intervillositis
  p. lactogen
  p. leakage
  p. lobule
  p. localization
  p. location
  p. margin
  p. maturity index
  p. membrane
  p. metabolism
  p. metastasis
  p. migration
  p. mosaicism

placental · planographic

p. mosaicism for triploidy
p. oxygen transfer
p. pallor
p. parenchyma
p. perfusion
p. polyp
p. presentation
p. profusion
p. progesterone deficiency
p. protein
p. respiration
p. secretion
p. separation
p. septa
p. sign
p. site gestational trophoblastic disease
p. site nodule
p. site trophoblastic tumor (PSTT)
p. site tumor
p. souffle
p. stage
p. stage of labor
p. steroid
p. sulfatase deficiency
p. surface area
p. thickness
p. thrombosis
p. tissue transplant
p. transfer
p. transfusion
p. transfusion syndrome
p. trophoblastic tissue
p. vascular anastomosis
p. vasopressin
p. villus
p. weight
placental-derived stem cell (PDSC)
placental-to-fetal weight ratio
placentascan
placentation
abnormal p.
p. abnormality
dichorionic p.
fundal p.
monochorionic p.
normal p.
placentitis
coccidioidal p.
placentofetal transfusion (PFT)
placentography
indirect p.
placentology
placentoma
placentotherapy
Placidyl
placing
p. reflex
p. response

placode
olfactory p.
PL-ADOS
prelinguistic autism diagnostic observation
plagiocephalic
plagiocephaly
deformational occipital p.
frontal p.
p. headband
p. helmet
occipital p.
unilateral occipital p.
plague vaccine
plain
p. abdominal radiograph
Perdiem P.
plan
P. Ahead Test
Asthma Action P.
P. B emergency contraceptive
birthing process p.
cleavage p.
exit p.
Individualized Family Service P. (IFSP)
multimodal treatment p.
transition p.
plana
coxa p.
pelvis p.
verruca p.
vertebra p.
planar bone scan
plane
equatorial p.
fat p.
first parallel pelvic p.
fourth parallel pelvic p.
median p.
p. of greatest diameter
p. of least diameter
p. of midpelvis
p. of pelvic canal
orthogonal p.
pelvic p.
sagittal p.
second parallel pelvic p.
soft tissue fat p.
third parallel pelvic p.
wide p.
planning
family p.
motor p.
natural family p. (NFP)
poor motor p.
rhythm method of family p.
planographic pelvimetry

P

705

planovalgus
flexible pes p.
talipes p.
plant
p. alkaloid
anticholinergic p.
p. thorn synovitis
plantar
p. crease
p. dermatosis
p. eccrine bromhidrosis
p. fascia
p. fasciitis
p. grasp
p. grasp reflex
p. imaging
p. response
p. wart
plantarflexion osteotomy
plantaris
keratosis palmaris et p.
pustulosis palmaris et p.
verruca p.
plantarum
Lactobacillus p.
plantigrade
planum temporale
planus
acute eruptive lichen p.
eruptive lichen p.
hypermobile pes p.
lichen p.
lichen ruber p. (LRP)
pes p.
talipes p.
PLAP
placental alkaline phosphatase
plaque
acuminate p.
bacterial p.
calcified bacterial p.
confluent p.
erythematous confluent p.
erythematous cutaneous p.
filiform p.
honey-crusted p.
hyperpigmented lichenified p.
lichenified p.
linear hyperkeratotic p.
p. of nummular eczema
p. of thrush
pruritic urticarial p.
pruritic urticarial papules and p.'s
 (PUPP)
pulmonary p.
p. radiotherapy
sclerose en p.
uncalcified bacterial p.
verrucose p.

white p.
white-yellow p.
plaque-forming unit (pfu)
plaquelike rash
Plaquenil Sulfate
plaque-type psoriasis
Plasbumin
plasm (*var. of* plasma)
plasma, plasm
p. albumin
p. amino acid concentration
p. aminogram
p. ammonia
p. anion gap
p. arginine
p. bicarbonate (PHCO$_3$)
p. bilirubin concentration (PBC)
p. cell
p. cell balanitis
p. cell infiltrate
p. cell mastitis
p. cell pneumonia
p. cell vulvitis
p. cholesterol
p. citrulline
p. coagulation factor VIII, IX
p. cortisol
p. dissector
p. estrogen level
p. exchange
p. fibrinogen
p. fraction
fresh frozen p. (FFP)
frozen p.
p. glucose
p. histamine concentration
p. inorganic pyrophosphate
p. iron-binding capacity
p. iron concentration
p. lactate
p. lactoferrin
p. linoleic acid
p. lipid peroxidation
p. membrane
p. neuropeptide Y
p. nitrite
p. noradrenaline
p. oncotic pressure
p. ornithine level
p. osmolality
p. phosphate
p. phosphate concentration
platelet-poor p. (PPP)
platelet-rich p. (PRP)
postingestion p.
p. prolactin
p. prorenin
p. prorenin increase
p. protein

p. renin activity
p. retinol concentration
seminal p.
p. testosterone
p. theophylline concentration
p. thromboplastin
p. thromboplastin antecedent (PTA)
p. thromboplastin antecedent factor
p. TPO
p. transfusion
p. very long chain fatty acid
p. viral load
p. viremia
p. vitamin A concentration
p. volume
p. volume expansion
p. volume regulation
plasmacellularis
balanitis circumscripta p.
plasmacrit test
plasma-free iron
PlasmaKinetic (PK)
P. instrument
P. tissue management system
Plasmanate
plasmapheresis
plasmatic
progesterone p.
plasmid
p. DNA
p. fingerprinting
plasmin
plasminogen
p. activator (PA)
p. activator inhibitor (PAI)
p. activator inhibitor deficiency
p. activator inhibitor type 1 (PAI-1)
p. activator inhibitor type 2 (PAI-2)
p. level
Plasmodium
P. falciparum
P. malariae
P. ovale
P. vivax
plaster
Mediplast P.
Sal-Acid P.
urea p.
Plastibell circumcision method
plastic
p. blanket
p. bronchitis
p. cup vacuum extractor
p. deformation
p. deformation fracture
p. heat shield
p. obturator
p. pleurisy

plastica
linitis p.
rectal linitis p. (RLP)
plasticity
plastid
plasty
labioscrotal Y-V p.
PLAT C
plate
agar p.
basal p.
breast p.
Brucella agar p.
chocolate agar p.
chorionic p.
cribriform p.
epiphysial growth p.
epithelial p.
p. fracture
growth p.
hemineural p.
levator p.
Mancini p.
neural p.
tarsal p.
trigonal p.
tubularized incised p. (TIP)
urethral p.
vaginal p.
widened growth p.
plateau
p. encephalopathy
orgasmic p.
platelet
p. abnormality
p. adhesion
p. aggregation
p. antigen
p. calmodulin level
p. cofactor I
p. concentrate
p. concentration
p. count
p. cyclooxygenase
p. disorder
p. function test
p. membrane
p. neutralization procedure
p. neutralizing procedure
p. plugging
single donor apheresis p.
p. transfusion
TRAP-activated neonatal p.
p. trapping
platelet-activating factor
platelet-antigen incompatibility
platelet-associated antibody
platelet-derived growth factor
platelet-poor plasma (PPP)

P

platelet-rich plasma (PRP)
platelet-type von Willebrand disease
plate-like atelectasis
Platelin Plus Activator
platform
> Aspen ultrasound p.
> wedge-shaped p.

Platinol
> bleomycin, Eldisine, mitomycin, P. (BEMP)
> bleomycin, etoposide, P. (BEP)
> bleomycin, ifosfamide, P. (BIP)

platinum
platinum-based regimen
platybasia
platypellic, platypelloid
> p. pelvis

platypelloid (*var. of* platypellic)
platypnea
platyspondyly
play
> p. activity
> doll p.
> imitative p.
> oral p.
> parallel p.
> p. therapy
> vocal p.

PLC
> pityriasis lichenoides chronica

pleasure
> sexual p.

Pleatman
> P. pouch
> P. sac

pleconaril
pledget
> cotton p.

pleiotropia
pleiotropic
> p. cytokine
> p. functional defect
> p. gene

pleiotropy, pleiotropia
pleocytosis
> CSF lymphocytic p.
> eosinophilic p.
> lymphocytic p.
> mononuclear p.
> neutrophilic p.

pleomastia, pleomazia
pleomazia (*var. of* pleomastia)
pleomorphic
> p. cellular infiltrate
> p. gram-negative rod
> p. spindle cell tumor

pleomorphism of hepatocyte
pleonosteosis
> Leri p.

Plesiomonas shigelloides
plethora
plethoric
plethysmograph
> face-out, whole-body p.

plethysmography
> finger p.
> impedance p.
> jugular occlusion p.
> respiratory inductive p. (RIP)
> Respitrace inductance p.
> venous occlusion p.

pleura, *pl.* **pleurae**
> stripping of p.

pleuracentesis (*var. of* pleurocentesis)
pleurae (*pl. of* pleura)
pleural
> p. abrasion
> p. biopsy
> p. decortication
> p. effusion
> p. fluid analysis
> p. friction rub

pleurectomy
Pleur-evac chest catheter
pleurisy
> dry p.
> plastic p.
> serofibrinous p.

pleuritic pain
pleuritis
pleuroamniotic shunt
pleurocentesis, pleuracentesis
pleurodesis
> chemical p.
> surgical p.
> tetracycline p.

pleurodynia
> epidemic p.

pleuromelus
pleuropericardial
pleuroperitoneal
> p. fold
> p. foramen
> p. hernia

pleuropulmonary
> p. blastoma (PPB)
> p. involvement

pleuroscopy
pleurosomus
PLEVA
> pityriasis lichenoides et varioliformis acuta

plexectomy
plexiform
> p. neurofibroma
> p. neurofibromatosis

plexopathy
> brachial p.

plexus, *pl.* plexus, plexuses
  Auerbach p.
  brachial p.
  branchial p.
  cavernous p.
  choroid p.
  Frankenhäuser p.
  hypogastric p.
  Kiesselbach p.
  p. lesion
  Meissner p.
  myenteric p.
  ovarian p.
  ovarian venous p.
  pampiniform p.
  pelvic p.
  subareolar p.
  submucosal p.
  superior mesenteric p.
  vaginal venous p.
plexuses (*pl. of* plexus)
PLF
  perilymphatic fistula
PlGF
  placental growth factor
PLH
  pulmonary lymphoid hyperplasia
plica, *pl.* plicae
  plicae palmatae
plicae (*pl. of* plica)
plicamycin
plicata
  lingua p.
plicate
plication
  diaphragmatic p.
  fundal p.
  Kelly p.
  Kelly-Kennedy p.
  laparoscopic uterosacral p.
  p. of diaphragm
  transverse p.
  uterosacral p.
PLISSIT
  permission, limited information, specific
  suggestions, intensive therapy
ploidy
  DNA p.
Plott syndrome
PLP
  proteolipid protein
  pyridoxal phosphate
PLTSS
  Pediatric Liver Transplant-Specific
  Scale
plucked chicken skin lesion
plug
  anorectal p.
  colonic p.

copulation p.
epithelial p.
fentendo p.
intraluminal p.
keratinous p.
meconium p.
mucous p.
mucus p.
silicone p.
p. the lung until it grows (PLUG)
urethral p.
PLUG
  plug the lung until it grows
plugging
  follicular p.
  mucous p.
  platelet p.
plumbism
plume
  electrosurgical p.
  laser p.
  smoke p.
plural pregnancy
pluripotentiality
plus
  Answer P.
  Betadine PrepStick P.
  Cenafed P.
  Duramist P.
  Fact P.
  GentleLASE P.
  P. Jet
  Lorcet P.
  Neonate One P.
  ophthalmoplegia p.
  Riopan P.
PLV
  partial liquid ventilation
PM
  perinatal mortality
PM-60/40
  Similac PM-60/40
PMB
  postmenopausal bleeding
PMD
  Pelizaeus-Merzbacher disease
PMDD
  premenstrual dysphoric disorder
PMF
  protein modified fast
PMI
  paternal meiosis I
PMII
  paternal meiosis II
PML
  premature labor
  progressive multifocal
  leukoencephalopathy

PMN
polymorphonuclear
PMO
postmenopausal osteoporosis
PMP
peripheral myelin protein
previous menstrual period
PMPO
postmenopausal palpable ovary
syndrome
PMR
perinatal mortality rate
PMS
premenstrual syndrome
PMS Escape
Lurline PMS
PMS-Amantadine
Pm-Scl antigen
PMS-Cyproheptadine
PMS-Diazepam
PMS-Erythromycin
PMS-Imipramine
PMS-Ketoprofen
PMS-Lindane
PMS-Methylphenidate
PMS-Nystatin
PMS-Progesterone
PMS-Pseudoephedrine
PMS-Sodium Cromoglycate
PMT
point of maximum tenderness
postmenstrual tension
Optivite PMT
PMTS
premenstrual tension syndrome
PMVP
pulmonary microvascular permeability
to protein
PN
parenteral nutrition
pronucleus
PNAC
parenteral nutrition-associated
PNAC liver disease
PncD
pneumococcal conjugate diphtheria
toxoid
PncD vaccine
PNCRM7 vaccine
PncT
pneumococcal conjugate tetanus protein
PncT vaccine
PnCV
nonvalent pneumococcal conjugate
vaccine
PND
paroxysmal nocturnal dyspnea
pelvic node dissection
postnatal depression

PNET
primitive neuroectodermal tumor
PNET/MB
primitive neuroectodermal tumor
medulloblastoma
pneumatic
p. cell
p. compression
p. compression stocking
p. dilation
p. otoscope
p. otoscopy
pneumatocele formation
pneumatosis
p. cystoides intestinalis
p. intestinalis
pneumocapillary infusion pump
pneumocardiogram
pneumocele
pneumocephalus
tension p.
pneumococcal
p. conjugate diphtheria toxoid
(PncD)
p. conjugate tetanus protein
(PncT)
p. conjugate vaccine
p. facial cellulitis
p. immunization
p. mastoiditis
p. meningitis
p. pneumonia
p. polysaccharide vaccine
p. protein conjugate vaccine
p. sepsis
p. vaccine
p. 7-valent conjugate vaccine
(PCV7)
pneumococcus
cephalosporin-resistant p.
latex test for p.
resistant p.
pneumocystiasis
Pneumocystis
P. carinii
P. carinii pneumonia (PCP)
P. jiroveci
pneumocystography
pneumocystosis
pneumocyte
type II p.
pneumoencephalogram
pneumoencephalography
pneumogram
2-channel p.
pneumography
impedance p.
pneumohydrometra
pneumomediastinum

pneumonia
    acquired p.
    acute interstitial p.
    adenoviral p.
    p. alba
    p. alba of Virchow
    aspiration p.
    bacteremia-associated pneumococcal
      p. (BAPP)
    bacterial p.
    bronchiolitis obliterans organizing p.
      (BOOP)
    chemical p.
    chickenpox p.
    chlamydial p.
    Chlamydia trachomatis p.
    congenital p.
    desquamative interstitial p.
      (DIP)
    early onset neonatal p.
    Enterobacter p.
    eosinophilic p.
    exogenous lipoid p. (ELP)
    fulminant early-onset neonatal p.
    giant cell p.
    gram-negative p.
    group B streptococcal p.
    Hecht p.
    herpes simplex p.
    hydrocarbon p.
    hypostatic p.
    interstitial plasma cell p.
    intrauterine p.
    Kaufman p.
    lipoid p.
    lobar p.
    measles p.
    Mycoplasma p.
    necrotizing p.
    neonatal p.
    nosocomial p. (NP)
    plasma cell p.
    pneumococcal p.
    Pneumocystis carinii p. (PCP)
    postinfluenza p.
    postviral p.
    recurrent aspiration p.
    respiratory syncytial virus p.
    retrocardiac p.
    rheumatic p.
    staphylococcal p.
    streptococcal p.
    Streptococcus p.
    suppurative p.
    thrush p.
    transplacental bacterial p.
    transplacental viral p.
    tuberculous p.
    vaccine-associated p.
    varicella p.
    ventilator-associated p. (VAP)
    viral p.

pneumoniae
    Chlamydia p.
    Diplococcus p.
    drug-resistant *Streptococcus* p.
      (DRSP)
    Klebsiella p.
    Mycoplasma p.
    Optochin-resistant *Streptococcus* p.
      (ORSP)
    penicillin-nonsusceptible *Streptococcus*
      p. (PNSP)
    penicillin-resistant *Streptococcus* p.
      (PRSP)
    Streptococcus p.

pneumonic
    p. consolidation
    p. tularemia

pneumonitis
    acute p.
    aspiration p.
    chemical p.
    desquamative interstitial p. (DIP)
    hypersensitivity p.
    interstitial p.
    lipoid interstitial p. (LIP)
    lymphocytic interstitial p. (LIP)
    lymphoid interstitial p. (LIP)
    radiation p.
    RSV p.
    secondary p.
    varicella p.
    viral p.

pneumonocyte
    type II p.

pneumootoscope

pneumoparotiditis

pneumopericardium

pneumoperitoneum

pneumophila
    Legionella p.

pneumotachography

pneumotachygraph

pneumotaxic center

Pneumotest kit

pneumothoraces (*pl. of* pneumothorax)

pneumothorax (PTX), *pl.*
  pneumothoraces
    catamenial p.
    iatrogenic p.
    nontension p.
    open p.
    simple p.
    spontaneous p.
    tension p.
    traumatic p.

Pneumovax 23

P

Pneumo-Wrap
PNH
    paroxysmal nocturnal hemoglobinuria
PNM
    perinatal mortality
    peripheral dysostosis, nail hypoplasia, mental retardation
    pneumonia
PNMR
    perinatal mortality rate
pnomenusa
        Pandoraea p.
PNP
    purine nucleoside phosphorylase
        PNP deficiency
PNSP
    penicillin-nonsusceptible *Streptococcus pneumoniae*
PNTML
    pudendal nerve terminal motor latency
POA
    pancreatic oncofetal antigen
POADS
    postaxial acrofacial dysostosis syndrome
POAH
    posterior occipitoatlantal hypermobility
POC
    postoperative care
    products of conception
pocket
        amniotic fluid p.
Pocket-Dop 3 monitor
Pocketpeak peak flow meter
POD
    polycystic ovarian disease
podalic
    p. extraction
    p. version
podencephalus
Podocon-25
podocyte
podofilox
podophyllin
    p. resin
    topical p.
podophyllotoxin
    purified p.
POE
    prone on elbows
    POE position
POEMS
    polyneuropathy, organomegaly, endocrinopathy, M protein, skin changes
        POEMS syndrome
POF
    premature ovarian failure
    primary ovarian failure

POG
    Pediatric Oncology Group
Pogosta virus
poikilocyte
    fragmented p.
poikilocytosis
poikiloderma
    p. congenitale
    infantile p.
poikiloploidy
point
    p. A, subspinale
    p. B, supramentale
    cardinal p.
    Halle p.
    hypothalamic set p.
    infection p.
    lead p.
    Legat p.
    McBurney p.
    Munro p.
    p. mutation
    p. of maximal impulse (PMI)
    p. of maximum impulse (PMI)
    p. of maximum tenderness (PMT)
    Piersol p.
    pressure p.
    set p.
    p. tenderness
    trigger p.
2-point discrimination
3-point
    3-p. position
    3-p. technique
pointer
    hip p.
    p. syndrome
pointes
    torsade de p.
pointing for naming
4-point position
point-spread artifact
Poiseuille-Hagen relationship
Poison Control Center (PCC)
poisoning
    accidental p.
    acute iron p.
    aflatoxin p.
    amnesic shellfish p.
    anticholinergic p.
    antidepressant p.
    antimalarial p.
    antinauseant p.
    antipsychotic p.
    antispasmodic p.
    arsenic p.
    barbiturate p.
    carbon monoxide p.
    castor bean p.

ciguatera fish p.
cobalt p.
cyclic antidepressant p.
diarrheal shellfish p.
ethanol p.
fish p.
food p.
heavy metal p.
histamine fish p.
intentional p.
iron p.
lead p.
mercury vapor p.
metal p.
monosodium glutamate p.
mushroom p.
neurologic shellfish p.
neurotoxic shellfish p.
niacin p.
opiate p.
organic mercury p.
organophosphate p.
paralytic shellfish p.
petroleum distillate p.
phenothiazine p.
rodenticide p.
salicylate p.
salt p.
scombroid p.
scopolamine p.
sedative p.
shellfish p.
strychnine p.
tetrodotoxin p.
thallium p.
vapor p.
zinc p.

pokeweed mitogen (PWM)
Poland
P. anomalad
P. anomaly
P. malformation sequence
P. syndrome
polar
p. body
p. body in situ hybridization
p. presentation
Polaris
P. reusable cutter
P. reusable dissector
P. reusable forceps
P. reusable grasper
P. reusable instrument
polarity
polarization
amniotic fluid fluorescence p.
fluorescent p.
pole
caudal p.

cephalic p.
fetal p.
germinal p.
head p.
kidney p.
pelvic p.
police
food p.
polio
poliomyelitis
poliodystrophia cerebri progressiva infantilis
poliodystrophy
polioencephalitis
bulbar p.
poliomyelitis (polio)
abortive p.
bulbar p.
bulbospinal p.
p. immunization
inapparent p.
nonparalytic p.
paralytic p.
pure bulbar p.
spinal paralytic p.
vaccine-associated paralytic p. (VAPP)
poliomyelitis-like
p.-l. paralysis
p.-l. syndrome
poliosis
poliovirus
P. hominis
inactivated p.
p. vaccine
vaccine-acquired p.
polish
Sklar instrument p.
Politano-Leadbetter
P.-L. ureteroneocystostomy
P.-L. ureteroneocystostomy technique
Politzer
method of P.
pollakiuria
pollen
p. allergy
birch tree p.
grass p.
ragweed p.
tree p.
pollen-induced rhinitis
pollenosis (*var. of* pollinosis)
pollical ray
pollicization of index finger
pollination
pollinosis, pollenosis
seasonal p.
Pollitt syndrome
Pollock forceps

P

pollution
  air p.
Poloxamer 407 barrier material
poly
  p. A RNA
  P. CS device
polyacrylamide gel electrophoresis
polyaluminum hydroxide complex
polyamine
polyarteritis
  microscopic p.
  p. nodosa (PAN)
polyarthritis
  juvenile p.
  migratory p.
  p., RF negative
  RF-negative juvenile p.
  p., RF positive
polyarticular
  p. JRA
  p. juvenile chronic arthritis
polybutester
polycarbophil
  calcium p.
polycheiria, polychiria
polychiria (var. of polycheiria)
polychlorinated biphenyl
polychondritis
polychromasia
polychromatophilia
Polycitra K
Polycitra-LC
polyclonal
  p. antiendotoxin anticore antibody
  p. B cell activation
  p. cryoglobulin
  p. hypergammaglobulinemia
polyclonal-monoclonal antibody
Polycose
  P. liquid formula
  P. powder
  P. powder formula
polycyesis
polycystic
  p. encephalomalacia
  p. fibrous dysplasia
  p. kidney
  p. kidney disease (PKD)
  p. ovarian disease (PCOD)
  p. ovarian syndrome (PCOS)
  p. ovary (PCO)
  p. ovary syndrome (PCOS, POS)
  p. renal disease
polycythemia
  neonatal p.
  primary p.
  relative p.
  p. rubra vera
  secondary p.

polycythemia-hyperviscosity syndrome
polydactylism
polydactyly
  Majewski short rib p.
  microcephalus, imperforate anus,
    syndactyly, hamartoblastoma,
    abnormal lung lobulation, p.
    (MISHAP)
  postaxial p.
  preaxial p.
polydactyly-chondrodystrophy syndrome
polydactyly-craniofacial
  p.-c. anomalies syndrome
  p.-c. dysmorphism syndrome
polydactyly-imperforate anus syndrome
polydimethylsiloxane
polydioxanone
polydipsia
  neurogenic p.
  primary p.
  psychogenic p.
polydysplasia
  hereditary ectodermal p.
polydysspondylism
polydystrophic dwarfism
polydystrophy
  pseudo-Hurler p.
polyembryoma
polyembryony
polyester suture material
polyestradiol phosphate
polyethylene
  p. catheter
  p. feeding tube
  p. glycol
  p. glycol-ADA
  p. glycol-electrolyte solution
  p. glycol-modified adenosine
    deaminase (PEG-ADA)
  p. glycol solution
  p. suture material
polygalactia
Polygam S/D
Polygeline colloid solution
polygene
polygenic
  p. disorder
  p. inheritance
  p. mode
polygenic/multifactorial disorder
polyglactin 910 suture
polyglandular
  p. autoimmune disease
    (type I, II)
  p. autoimmune syndrome
polyglutamate
polyglutamation
polyglutamine-expanded Huntington
polyglycolic acid

polyglycol suture
polyglyconate suture
polygnathus
polygonal papule
polygraphy
PolyHeme blood substitute
polyhexamethyl biguanide (PHMB)
Poly-Histine DM
polyhydramnios
polyhypermenorrhea
polyhypomenorrhea
polymastia, polymazia
polymazia (var. of polymastia)
PolyMem dressing
polymenorrhea
polymer
    sodium polyacrylate p.
polymerase
    p. chain reaction (PCR)
    DNA p.
    DNA-directed RNA p.
    RNA p.
    RNA-directed DNA p.
    viral DNA p.
polymeric diet
polymetacarpalia, polymetacarpalism
polymetacarpalism (var. of
  polymetacarpalia)
polymetatarsalia, polymetatarsalism
polymetatarsalism (var. of
  polymetatarsalia)
polymicrobial
    p. bacteremia
    p. coverage
    p. pelvic infection
polymicrogyria
    syndrome of symmetric parasagittal
      parietooccipital p.
polymicrogyric
polymorpha
    Mima p.
polymorphic light eruption of pregnancy
polymorphism
    amplified fragment length p.
    genetic p.
    restriction fragment length p.
      (RFLP)
    single nucleotide p.
    single stranded conformational p.
polymorphonuclear (PMN)
    p. infiltrate
    p. leukocyte
    p. lymphocyte
    p. phagocyte
polymorphonucleocyte
polymorphous
    p. exanthema
    p. light eruption
    p. rash

polymyalgia rheumatica
polymyositis (PM)
    juvenile p.
    primary idiopathic p.
polymyositis/dermatomyositis
polymyxin
    p. B, E
    p. B sulfate
polyneuritiformis
    heredopathia atactica p.
polyneuritis
    acute infectious p.
    infantile p.
    infectious p.
    mixed sensory p.
    purely sensory p.
    relapsing infectious p.
    sensory p.
polyneuropathy
    acute inflammatory demyelinating p.
     (AIDP)
    p., cataract, deafness syndrome
    chronic inflammatory demyelinating
     p. (CIDP)
    erythredema p.
    p., organomegaly, endocrinopathy, M
     protein, skin changes (POEMS)
    spinal p.
polynomial
polynuclear leukocyte
polyomavirus JC
polyonchosis (var. of polyoncosis)
polyoncosis, polyonchosis
    hereditary cutaneomandibular p.
    multiple hereditary cutaneomandibular
     p.
polyostotic, polystotic
    p. fibrous dysplasia
polyotia
polyp
    adenomatous p.
    allergic p.
    antral choanal p.
    aural p.
    cervical p.
    charcoal p.
    cobblestone sessile p.
    colonic p.
    diffuse intestinal p.
    embryonal p.
    endocervical p.
    endometrial p.
    fibrinous p.
    fibroepithelial p.
    fundic gland p.
    gastrointestinal p.
    hydatid p.
    hyperplastic p.
    inflammatory p.

P

polyp (*continued*)
    intestinal p.
    juvenile colonic p.
    multiple gastrointestinal p.'s
    nasal p.
    pedunculated p.
    Peutz-Jeghers p.
    placental p.
    prolapsing p.
    retention p.
    sessile p.
    umbilical p.
    uterine p.
polypectomy
polypeptide
    factor V p.
    gastric inhibitory p. (GIP)
    S-methionine-labeled p.
    vasoactive intestinal p. (VIP)
polyphagia
    Acanthamoeba p.
polypharmacy
Polyphenon
    P. E
    P. E ointment
polyphonic wheeze
polyphosphatidylinositide
polyphosphol inositide
polypiform (*var. of* polypoid)
polyploid
polyploidy
polypoid, polypiform
    p. epithelial tumor
    p. hyperplasia
polyposa
    decidua p.
polyposis
    adenomatous colonic p.
    colonic p.
    familial adenomatous p. (FAP)
    intestinal p.
    nasal p.
    small bowel intestinal p.
    p. syndrome
Poly-Pred Liquifilm
polypropylene
    p. fascial strip
    p. suture material
polyradiculoneuritis
    epidemic motor p.
polyradiculoneuropathy
    chronic inflammatory demyelinating p. (CIDP)
    chronic relapsing p.
    chronic unremitting p.
polyribosylribitol phosphate (PRP)
polysaccharide (PS)
    anti-O-specific p.
    p. group-specific antigen

    meningococcal p.
    purified p.
polyscelia
polyserositis
    idiopathic p.
polysiloxane cast
polysomia
polysomnogram (PSG)
    p. with flow-volume loop
polysomnographic
polysomnography (PSG)
    ambulatory p.
    8-hour p.
polysomy
    sex chromosomal p.
Polysonic ultrasound lotion
Polysorb suture
polyspermia (*var. of* polyspermy)
polyspermism (*var. of* polyspermy)
polyspermy, polyspermia, polyspermism
polyspike discharge
polysplenia syndrome
Polysporin
    P. ointment
    P. Ophthalmic
    P. Topical
polystotic (*var. of* polyostotic)
polysulfate
    pentosan p.
polysymbrachydactyly
polysyndactyly
    crossed p.
polysyndactyly-peculiar skull syndrome
polysynostosis syndrome
Polytar shampoo
polytene chromosome
polytetrafluoroethylene graft
polythelia
polytherapy
polythiazide
polytrauma
Polytrim eye drops
polyunsaturate
polyunsaturated fatty acid (PUFA)
polyurethane
    p. catheter
    p. dressing
polyuria
polyuric phase
polyvalent
    antivenin p.
    p. immunoglobulin therapy
    p. pneumococcal vaccine
Poly-Vi-Flor vitamin
polyvinyl chloride
polyvinylidene fluoride (PVDF)
polyvinylpyrrolidone (PVP)
Poly-Vi-Sol vitamin

PolyWic
POMC
    proopiomelanocortin
Pomeroy
    P. method
    P. operation
    P. tubal ligation
    P. tubal ligation technique
pommel
pomona
    Leptospira p.
Pompe
    P. glycogen storage disease
        (type I, II)
    P. syndrome
pompholyx
POMS
    Profile of Mood States
    POMS score
ponderal index (PI)
pond fracture
Pondocillin
pons
Ponstan
Ponstel
Ponten fasciocutaneous flap
Pontiac fever
pontile, pontine
    p. glioma
    p. hypertrophy
    p. tumor
pontine (*var. of* pontile)
pontis
    basis p.
pontobulbar palsy with neurosensory deafness
Pontocaine
pontocerebellar hypoplasia
pontomedullary junction
pontosubicular neuron necrosis (PSN)
PONV
    postoperative nausea and vomiting
pool
    amniotic fluid p.
    gene p.
    p. test
pooling
    dependent p.
    venous p.
poor
    p. adaptability
    p. attention span
    p. caloric intake
    p. capillary refill
    p. convergence
    p. coordination
    p. dental hygiene
    p. feeding

    p. feeding interaction
    p. head control
    p. linear growth
    p. man's clot test
    p. man's cystometrogram
    p. motor planning
    p. muscle tone
    p. opsonization
    p. oral intake
    p. phagocytosis
    p. pregnancy outcome
    p. suck
    p. weight gain
poorly marginated mass
POP
    pelvic organ prolapse
    progestin-only pill
popcorn
    p. formation
    p. metaphysis
popcorn-like calcification
Pope
    P. night splint
    P. Oto-Wick
popliteal
    p. angle
    p. cyst
    p. pterygium syndrome
    p. space
    p. web syndrome
pop-off valve
popping
    eye p.
    skin p.
POP-Q
    Pelvic Organ Prolapse Quantification
POPQ
    Pelvic Organ Prolapse-Quantified
    POPQ staging system
popsicle
    p. injury
    p. panniculitis
population-attributable risk (PAR)
poractant alfa
Porak-Durante syndrome
porcine
    p. surfactant
    p. valve
porcupine skin
porencephalia (*var. of* porencephaly)
porencephalic, porencephalous
    p. cyst
    p. diverticulum
porencephalous (*var. of* porencephalic)
porencephaly, porencephalia
    central p.
    p. cortical dysplasia
porfimer sodium
Porges-Meier test

P

pork
- p. insulin
- p. NPH
- p. Regular Iletin II
- p. tapeworm

PORN
- progressive outer retinal necrosis

porokeratosis of Mibelli

porphyria
- acute intermittent p. (AIP)
- congenital erythropoietic p. (CEP)
- congenital photosensitive p.
- p. cutanea tarda
- p. cutanea tarda hereditaria
- p. cutanea tarda symptomatica
- cutaneous hepatic p.
- erythrohepatic p.
- erythropoietic p.
- hepatic p.
- hepatoerythropoietic p. (HEP)
- intermittent p.
- mixed p.
- ovulocyclic p.
- photosensitive p.
- South African genetic p.
- Swedish p.
- symptomatic p.
- p. variegata
- variegate p. (VP)

porphyric neuropathy

porphyrin
- p. metabolism disorder
- stool p.

Porphyromanus gingivalis

Porro
- P. cesarean section
- P. hysterectomy
- P. operation

port
- laparoscopy p.
- p. site hernia
- umbilical p.

PORT
- Patient Outcomes Research Team

portable respirator

Port-A-Cath catheter

Portagen formula

Portage project

porta hepatis

portal
- p. fibrosis
- p. hypertension
- p. inflammation
- p. mesenchyme
- p. pyelophlebitis
- p. system
- p. vein obstruction (PVO)
- p. vein sepsis
- p. venous pressure

Porta-Lung noninvasive extrathoracic ventilator

PORTEC
- Post Operative Radiation Therapy in Endometrial Carcinoma

Porteous syndrome

Porter-Silber reaction

Portia

portio, *pl.* **portiones**
- p. supravaginalis
- p. vaginalis

portion
- upper contractile p.

portiones, (*pl. of* **portio**)

Portland
- hemoglobin P.

portoaortal shunt

portocaval shunt

portoenterostomy
- Kasai p.

portosystemic shunt

Portuguese disease

port-wine
- p.-w. hemangioma
- p.-w. mark
- p.-w. nevus
- p.-w. stain
- p.-w. stained angioma

POS
- polycystic ovary syndrome

POSIT
- Problem-Oriented Screening Instrument for Teenagers

position
- Adam p.
- alternative birthing p.
- antigravity p.
- arm p.
- asynclitic p.
- back-up p.
- batrachian p.
- birthing p.
- Bozeman p.
- breech p.
- brow p.
- brow-anterior p.
- brow-down p.
- brow-posterior p.
- brow-up p.
- cervical p.
- chin p.
- coaxial p.
- cock-robin p.
- coital p.
- cross-cradle p.
- dorsal birthing p.
- dorsal lithotomy p.
- dorsal supine p.
- Duncan p.

en face p.
English p.
equinus p.
face-to-pubes fetal p.
fencing p.
fetal head p.
fetal spine p.
Fowler p.
frogleg p.
frontoanterior p.
frontoposterior p.
frontotransverse p.
genucubital p.
genupectoral p.
half-kneeling p.
hands-feet p.
intrauterine p.
jackknife p.
knee-chest p.
knee-elbow p.
kneel-stand p.
Kraske p.
lateral p.
lateral recumbent p.
left frontoanterior p.
left frontoposterior p. (LFP)
left frontotransverse p.
left lateral p.
left lateral decubitus p. (LLDP)
left mentoanterior p.
left mentoposterior p. (LMP)
left mentotransverse p.
left occipitoanterior p.
left occipitoposterior p. (LOP)
left occipitotransverse p.
left sacroanterior p.
left sacroposterior p. (LSP)
left sacrotransverse p.
left scapuloanterior p.
left scapuloposterior p. (LScP)
lithotomy p.
maternal p.
maternal birthing p.
mentum anterior fetal p.
mentum posterior fetal p.
mentum transverse fetal p.
missionary p.
neutral p.
obstetric p.
occipitoanterior p.
occipitoposterior p.
occipitotransverse p.
occiput posterior p.
partial sitting p.
partial squatting p.
persistent occiput posterior fetal p.
POE p.
3-point p.
4-point p.

prone sleep p.
puppy p.
right acromiodorsoposterior fetal p.
right frontoanterior p.
right frontoposterior p.
right frontotransverse p.
right lateral p.
right mentoanterior p.
right mentoposterior p.
right mentotransverse p.
right occipitoposterior p.
right occipitotransverse p.
right sacroanterior p.
right sacroposterior p.
right sacrotransverse p.
right scapuloanterior p.
right scapuloposterior p.
sacroanterior p.
sacroposterior p.
sacrotransverse p.
scissored p.
scrotal p.
semi-Fowler p.
semiprone p.
Simon p.
Sims p.
sitting p.
sleep p.
sleeping p.
sniffing p.
squatting p.
standing p.
supine sleep p.
supranormal scrotal p.
swimming p.
Trendelenburg p.
tripod p.
tripod-supporting p.
tube p.
uterine p.
Valentine p.
vertex p.
waiter's tip p.
Walcher p.
wearing p.
withdrawal p.
W sitting p.

positional
p. airways obstruction
p. cloning
p. clubfoot
p. nystagmus
positioner
head p.
positioning
intrauterine p.
positive
p. airway pressure
p. chemotaxis

P

positive (*continued*)
    p. contraction stress test
    Coombs p.
    p. distending pressure (PDP)
    p. end-expiratory pressure (PEEP)
    false p.
    Hematest p.
    p. interference
    polyarthritis, RF p.
    p. pool test
    p. pressure mechanical ventilation
    p. pressure oxygen
    p. pressure urethrography
    p. reinforcement
    P. Reinforcement in the Menopausal Experience (PRIME)
    smear p.
    p. support reflex
positive-pressure
    high-frequency p.-p. (HFPP)
    p.-p. ventilation (PPV)
positivity
    lymph node p.
    paraaortic p.
positron emission tomography (PET)
posseting
possible migrational abnormality
POSSUM
    pictures of syndromes and undiagnosed malformations
    POSSUM database
post
    p. cordocentesis bradycardia
    p. dates
    P. Operative Radiation Therapy in Endometrial Carcinoma (PORTEC)
POST
    peritoneal oocyte sperm transfer
postabortal
    p. pelvic inflammatory disease
    p. syndrome
postadolescence
postalveolar cleft
postanesthetic apnea
postanginal sepsis
postanoxic dystonic syndrome
postasphyxial
    p. apoptosis
    p. cerebral edema
    p. change
    p. encephalopathy
    p. seizure
postaugmentation
postauricular
    p. ecchymosis
    p. nerve
postaxial
    p. acrofacial dysostosis syndrome (POADS)

    p. hexadactyly
    p. oligodactyly
    p. polydactyly
postcesarean
    p. hemorrhage
    p. phlegmon
postchiasmal visual pathway
postcoartectomy syndrome
postcoital
    p. bleeding
    p. contraception (PCC)
    p. contraceptive medication
    p. douching
    p. estrogen
    p. spotting
    p. test (PCT)
    p. testing
postconceptional age (PCA)
postconcussion syndrome
postconvulsive hemiparesis
postdate pregnancy
postdatism
postdiphtheritic neuropathy
postdose serum
postdouching
    p. bleeding
    p. spotting
postductal
    p. coarctation
    p. oxygen saturation
postdural puncture headache (PDPH)
postdysenteric arthritis
postembolization syndrome
postencephalitic parkinsonian picture
postenteritis arthritis
posterior
    anterior and p. (A&P)
    p. asynclitism
    p. chamber intraocular lens (PC-IOL)
    p. colpoperineorrhaphy
    p. colporrhaphy
    p. column sensory deficit
    p. commissure
    p. cranial fossa
    p. cul-de-sac
    p. cul-de-sac gutter
    dysplasia marginalis p.
    p. embryotoxon
    p. exenteration
    p. fontanelle
    p. fornix
    p. fossa anaplastic ependymoma
    p. fossa arachnoid cyst
    p. fossa arachnoiditis
    p. fossa hemorrhage
    p. fossa malformations, hemangiomas, arterial anomalies, coarctation of aorta, cardiac

defects, eye abnormalities
(PHACE)
p. fossa neoplasm
p. fossa tumor
p. fourchette
p. hypospadias
p. iliac crest
p. inferior cerebellar artery
(PICA)
p. intravaginal slingplasty
p. labial arteries
p. labial nerves
p. lenticonus
p. leukoencephalopathy syndrome
p. lie
p. nasal packing
p. neural tube closure
p. occipitoatlantal hypermobility
(POAH)
occiput p. (OP)
p. pelvic exenteration
p. pharyngeal laceration
p. pharyngeal pseudodiverticulum
p. pharyngeal wall elevation
p. pituitary disorder
p. probability
rachischisis p.
p. rectal wall resection
p. rectus sheath
p. repair
p. rhizotomy
p. sagittal anorectoplasty
p. sagittal diameter
p. segmental fixation instrumentation
p. splenium
p. superior iliac spine
p. synechia
p. talofibular ligament (PTFL)
p. tibial artery cannulation
p. tibial pulse
p. triangle
p. urethra
p. urethral valves, unilateral reflux,
renal dysplasia (VURD)
p. urethral valve [type I-IV]
(PUV)
p. urethritis
p. uterosacral ligament
p. uveitis
p. vagina
p. vaginal cuff
p. vaginal fornix
p. vaginismus
p. wall defect
posteroanterior (PA)
posterolateral fontanelle
posteromedial
p. articular depression
p. bow

p. bow of tibia
p. tibial bowing
postevacuation management
postexchange transfusion syndrome
postexposure
p. prophylaxis (PEP)
p. treatment (PET)
postextubation stridor
postganglionic acetylcholine release
**postgastroenteritis malabsorption
syndrome**
posthemorrhagic
p. hydrocephalus (PHH)
p. ventricular dilation (PHVD)
p. ventriculomegaly (PHVM)
posthepatic aplastic anemia
postherpetic neuralgia (PHN)
posthetomy
posthitis
posthysterectomy
p. infection
p. prolapse
postictal
p. confusion
p. depression
p. lethargy
p. paralysis
p. period
p. phase
p. weakness
posticus
saccus p.
postinfectious
p. abducens palsy
p. arthritis
p. cerebellitis
p. encephalitis
p. encephalomyelitis (PIE)
p. glomerulonephritis
p. ileus
p. immune response
p. nephritis
p. secondary lactase deficiency
postinflammatory
p. adenopathy
p. depigmentation
postinfluenza
p. pneumonia
p. vaccination encephalitis
postingestion plasma
postirradiation
p. destruction
p. myelopathy
p. syndrome
postischemic stenosis
**post-kala azar dermal leishmaniasis
(PKDL)**
postlumbar puncture headache
postlumpectomy

P

postmature
    p. fetus
    p. infant
    p. labor
    p. neonate
postmaturity syndrome
postmeasles encephalitis
postmeiotic segregation
postmembrane
    p. pressure
    p. rupture
postmenarchal
    p. bleeding
    p. cyclicity
postmenopausal
    p. amenorrhea
    p. atrophy
    p. bleeding (PMB)
    p. body mass
    p. bone loss
    p. estrogen replacement therapy
    p. hirsutism
    p. level
    p. osteoporosis (PMO)
    p. palpable ovary syndrome (PMPO)
    p. urogenital symptom
    p. woman
postmenopause
postmenstrual
    p. stress
    p. tension (PMT)
postmicturition dribble
postmigrainous stroke hemiplegia
postmolar persistent gestational trophoblastic tumor
postmortal pregnancy
postmortem
    p. cesarean section
    p. delivery
    p. lividity
    p. sampling
    p. study
postnasal drip
postnatal
    p. age
    p. bacterial meningitis
    p. depression (PND)
    p. factor
    p. gonadotropin surge
    p. management
    p. penicillin prophylaxis (PPP)
    p. septicemia
    p. year
postnatally
post-necrotic (*var. of* postnecrotic)
postnecrotic, post-necrotic
    p. cirrhosis
postneonatal mortality

postoperative
    p. apnea
    p. bladder dysfunction
    p. care
    p. chemotherapy
    p. complication
    p. congestive epididymitis
    p. cuff cellulitis
    p. cystitis
    p. fever
    p. hypertension
    p. ileus
    p. infection
    p. nausea and vomiting (PONV)
    p. pain
    p. pelvic radiation
    p. radiotherapy
    p. sepsis
    p. seroma
    p. shock
    p. sudden death
    p. symptom analysis
    p. voiding dysfunction
postovulatory age
postpartum
    p. amenorrhea
    p. attitude
    p. blues
    p. cardiomyopathy (PPCM)
    p. care
    p. confinement
    p. depression (PPD)
    p. endometritis (PPE)
    p. endomyometritis
    p. evaluation
    p. febrile morbidity
    p. hemodynamic change
    p. hemolytic uremic syndrome
    p. hemorrhage (PPH)
    p. hypertension
    p. incontinence
    p. infection
    p. mastitis
    p. metritis
    p. partial salpingectomy
    p. period
    p. pituitary necrosis
    p. pituitary necrosis syndrome
    p. pleuropulmonary and cardiac disease
    p. psychosis
    p. sterilization (PPS)
    p. tetanus
    p. thyroiditis (PPT)
    p. visit
postperfusion syndrome
postpericardiotomy syndrome (PPS)
postphlebitic syndrome (PPS)
postpill amenorrhea

postpolio syndrome
postponed labor
postponing sexual involvement (PSI)
postprandial
    p. glucose
    p. hyperemia
    p. plasma cholecystokinin
postpuberal, postpubertal
postpubertal (var. of postpuberal)
postpuberty
postpubescent
postrabies vaccine encephalomyelitis
postradiation
    p. cystitis
    p. fistula
    p. periureteral fibrosis
postreduction mammaplasty
postrenal ARF
postrheumatic valve disease
postrubella syndrome
postscabetic syndrome
postseizure period
postseptal cellulitis
postsplenectomy
poststeroid panniculitis
poststreptococcal
    p. glomerulonephritis
    p. reactive arthritis
postsurgical fat necrosis
postsynaptic fiber
postterm
    p. AGA
    p. infant
    p. LGA
    p. pregnancy
    p. pregnancy-related paralysis
    p. SGA
postthoracotomy pulmonary edema
posttransfusion hematocrit
posttranslational
    p. modification
    p. modification of mRNA
posttransplant
    p. lymphoproliferative disease
      (PTLD)
    p. lymphoproliferative disorder
      (PTLD)
posttraumatic
    p. amnesia
    p. epilepsy
    p. fat necrosis
    p. hyperemia
    p. signs or symptoms (PTSS)
    p. stress disorder (PTSD)
    p. stress syndrome
posttreatment
    p. evaluation
    p. surveillance
posttubal ligation syndrome

posttussive
    p. apnea
    p. emesis
postulate
postural
    p. deformity
    p. drainage (PD)
    p. orthostatic tachycardia syndrome
      (POTS)
    p. proteinuria
    p. reaction
    p. reflex
    p. round-back
    p. scoliosis
    p. tachycardia
    p. tone
    p. version
posture
    bipedal p.
    extensor leg p.
    fetal p.
    frogleg p.
    hemiparetic p.
    scissoring p.
    surrender p.
    waiter's tip p.
posturing
    athetotic p.
    decerebrate p.
    decorticate p.
    dystonic p.
    opisthotonic p.
    transient dystonic p.
posturography
    dynamic p.
postvaccinal encephalopathy
postvaginal fusion
postvagotomy dumping syndrome
postviral
    p. encephalitis
    p. pneumonia
    p. subacute thyroiditis
postvoid
    p. residual (PVR)
    p. residual urine test
    p. residual urine volume
potable
potassium
    p. bromide
    p. chloride (KCl)
    p. chloride stain
    p. citrate
    clavulanate p.
    diclofenac p.
    extracellular plasma p.
    p. gluconate
    p. hydroxide (KOH)
    p. hydroxide preparation
    p. iodide

P

potassium (*continued*)
    p. iodide Enseals
    pemirolast p.
    penicillin V p.
    p. permanganate
    p. sensitivity test
    p. supplement
    ticarcillin and clavulanate p.
    p. titanyl phosphate (KTP)
    total body p. (TBK)
potassium-sparing diuretic
potato-like mass
potbelly
potent
potential
    auditory evoked p. (AEP)
    brainstem auditory evoked p. (BAEP)
    brief, small, abundant motor-unit action p. (BSAP)
    compound muscle action p. (CMAP)
    event-related p. (ERP)
    evoked p.
    fetal brainstem auditory evoked p.
    fibrillation p.
    insertion p.
    low malignant p. (LMP)
    motor evoked p. (MEP)
    motor unit action p. (MUAP)
    neurocognitive p.
    p. renal solute load (PRSL)
    resting membrane p
    somatosensory evoked p. (SSEP)
    stage IIIc papillary tumor of low malignant p.
    vertex p.
    visual evoked p. (venostasis, VEP)
Potocky needle
POTS
    postural orthostatic tachycardia syndrome
Pott
    P. disease
    P. puffy tumor
Potter
    P. disease
    P. facies
    P. oligohydramnios sequence
    P. phenotype
    P. syndrome
    P. version
Potts shunt
potty-train
potty-trained
potty-training
POU
    placenta, ovary, uterus
pouce flottant

pouch
    blind vaginal p.
    branchial p.
    Broca p.
    cecal p.
    colon p.
    continent urinary p.
    Denis Browne p.
    Douglas p.
    Florida p.
    Indiana p.
    intravaginal p.
    kangaroo p.
    Kock p.
    Mainz p.
    Marsupial p.
    Morison p.
    parasitized cecal p.
    Pleatman p.
    Rathke p.
    Reality vaginal p.
    rectal p.
    rectouterine p.
    right colon p.
    Rowland p.
    Seessel p.
    sigmoid p.
    vaginal p.
    vulvovaginal p.
    wallaby p.
pouchitis
pouchogram
Poupart ligament
Pourcelot index
poverty of content
povidone-iodine
    p.-i. douche
    p.-i. gel
    p.-i. solution
    p.-i. wipe
POVT
    pelvic ovarian vein thrombosis
Powassan encephalitis
powder
    Bluboro p.
    p. burn spot
    Casec p.
    cocaine hydrochloride p.
    Fiberall P.
    fluticasone propionate inhalation p.
    Lotrimin AF spray p.
    More-Dophilus acidophilus p.
    Nystop topical p.
    Ovidrel p.
    Polycose p.
    p. pseudocalcification
    Questran p.
    salicylic sugar p.
    salmeterol p.

Secretin-Ferring p.
Sklar Kleen p.
talcum p.
Zeasorb p.
Zeasorb-AF p.
zinc stearate p.

powder-burn
p.-b. endometrial lesion
p.-b. visual appearance

powdered
p. casein
p. milk formula

powder-free glove

power
p. Doppler sonography
p. spectral analysis (PSA)

POWER
PTH for osteoporotic women on estrogen replacement

POWSBP
pulse oximetry waveform systolic blood pressure
POWSBP measurement

pox

Poxviridae family

Pozzi procedure

PP
placenta previa
postpartum
precocious pubarche

1p–22p
monosomy 1p–22p
partial monosomy 1p–22p
partial trisomy 1p–22p

PPB
pleuropulmonary blastoma

PPC
primary peritoneal carcinoma

PPCM
postpartum cardiomyopathy

PPD
postpartum depression
primary peritoneal drainage

PPE
postpartum endometritis

PPG
photoplethysmography

PPH
persistent pulmonary hypertension
postpartum hemorrhage
primary postpartum hemorrhage
primary pulmonary hypertension

PPHN
persistent pulmonary hypertension of newborn

PPHP
pseudopseudohypoparathyroidism

PPI
proton pump inhibitor

ppm
parts per million

PPNET
peripheral primitive neuroectodermal tumor

PPO
palpable postmenopausal ovary
preferred provider organization
PPO syndrome

PPP
platelet-poor plasma
postnatal penicillin prophylaxis

PPRC
physician payment review commission

PPROM
preterm premature rupture of membranes
prolonged premature rupture of membranes
PPROM UCI

PPS
Pap plus speculoscopy
postpartum sterilization
postpericardiotomy syndrome
postphlebitic syndrome

PPSH
pseudovaginal perineoscrotal hypospadias

PPT
postpartum thyroiditis

PPTT
prepuberal testicular tumor

PPV
positive-pressure ventilation

PPVT
Peabody picture vocabulary test

PPVT-R
Peabody Picture Vocabulary Test-Revised

PR
progesterone receptor
PR interval

practice
Advisory Committee on Immunization P.'s (ACIP)
orogenital sexual p.'s
P. Parameters for the Assessment and Treatment of Anxiety Disorders
sexual p.

practitioner
general p. (GP)
National Association of Pediatric Nurse Associates and P.'s (NAPNAP)

Prader-Labhart-Willi-Fanconi syndrome

Prader-Labhart-Willi syndrome

Prader orchidometer

P

725

Prader-Willi
  P.-W. syndrome (PWS)
  P.-W. syndrome critical region
    (PWSCR)
praecox
  dentia p.
  familial lymphedema p.
  icterus p.
  lymphedema p.
  macrogenitosomia p.
  pubertas p.
pragmatic and semantic-pragmatic
  deficits
pragmatics
Prague
  P. maneuver
  P. pelvis
pralidoxime chloride
PrameGel
Pramosone
pramoxine
PRAMS
  Pregnancy Risk Assessment Monitoring
    System
Pratt
  P. dilator
  sigmoid pouch of P.
praxis
prazepam
praziquantel
prazosin
PRBC
  packed red blood cells
pRb tumor suppressor gene
PRDS
  Pitt-Rogers-Danks syndrome
preabortion counseling
preadolescent vaginal bleeding
prealbumin
preantral follicle
preaspiration mammography
preauricular
  p. adenopathy
  p. nerve
  p. pit
  p. sinus
  p. tag
preaxial
  p. acrofacial dysostosis
  p. hexadactyly
  p. mandibulofacial dysostosis
  p. polydactyly
precancerous lesion
precapillary
PreCare Conceive
precaution
  airway and cervical spine p.'s
Precef
Prechtl test

precipitable
precipitant
precipitate
  p. labor
  p. labor and delivery
precipitating factor
precipitation
  aragonite p.
precipitin
precipitous
  p. delivery
  p. labor
precise
  P. disposable skin stapler
  p. finger opposition
  P. pregnancy test
Precision Tack transvaginal anchor
  system
preclinical carcinoma
Preclude peritoneal membrane
precocious
  p. adrenarche
  p. menarche
  p. pseudopuberty
  p. pubarche (PP)
  p. puberty
  p. teeth
  p. thelarche
precocity
  complete isosexual p.
  contrasexual p.
  GnRH-independent sexual p.
  isosexual p.
  sexual p.
  true p.
preconception
  p. care
  p. counseling
  p. immunization
  p. risk assessment
  p. visit
preconceptionally treated phenylketonuria
preconceptual workup
precordial
  p. bulge
  p. catch syndrome
  p. thump
precordium
  hyperdynamic p.
  quiet p.
  silent p.
Precose
precursor
  cell p.
  p. lesion
  neurotransmitter p.
Pred
  P. Forte Ophthalmic
  P. Mild Ophthalmic

predecidual
predeciduous teeth
Pred-G
prediction
    perinatal distress p.
    prenatal risk p.
    scar p.
predictive value of test
predictor
    ClearPlan Easy ovulation p.
    Conceive ovulation p.
    First Response ovulation p.
    morbidity p.
    mortality p.
    OvuQuick self-test ovulation p.
    OV-Watch fertility p.
    Q-test ovulation p.
predigested formula
predisposing factor
predisposition
    genetic p.
prednicarbate
prednisolone
    p. and gentamicin
    neomycin, polymyxin B, p.
    p. sodium
Prednisol TBA injection
prednisone
    cyclophosphamide,
      hydroxydaunorubicin, methotrexate,
      p. (CHOP)
predominance
predominant
    lymphocyte p.
preductal coarctation
preeclampsia (PE)
    early-onset p.
    p. headache
    superimposed p.
preeclamptic
    p. state
    p. toxemia (PET)
preembryo
    triploid p.
preemie
  premature infant
    preemie nipple
    preemie Simpson forceps
preexcitation syndrome
preexisting maternal medical
  condition
preference
    hand p.
    sexual p.
preferred provider organization (PPO)
prefilled disposable bottle
preformation
Prefrin Ophthalmic Solution
prefrontal

pregestational
    p. diabetes
    p. diabetes mellitus (PDM)
Pregestimil formula
pregnancy
    abdominal p.
    aborted ectopic p.
    accidental p.
    acute fatty liver of p. (AFLP)
    adolescent p.
    ampullar p.
    anaphylactoid syndrome of p.
    anembryonic p.
    at-risk p.
    Besnier prurigo of p.
    bigeminal p.
    bilateral ectopic p.
    bilateral simultaneous tubal
      pregnancies
    biochemical p.
    broad ligament p.
    p. category A, B, C, D, X
    p. cell
    cervical p.
    cervical ectopic p.
    chemical p.
    cholestatic hepatosis of p.
    clinical p.
    coincident p.
    combined p.
    p. complication
    compound p.
    cornual p.
    p. dating
    diabetogenic effect of p.
    dichorial p.
    direct agglutination p. (DAP)
    dyspnea of p.
    ectopic p. (EP)
    epulis of p.
    euploid p.
    extraamniotic p.
    extrachorial p.
    extramembranous p.
    extrauterine p.
    failed intrauterine p.
    fallopian p.
    false p.
    fatty liver of p.
    p. fear
    fimbrial ectopic p.
    first-cycle clinical p.
    full-term p. (FTP)
    gemellary p.
    glucosuria of p.
    grand p.
    hemolytic uremia syndrome
      associated with p.
    hepatic p.

P

pregnancy (*continued*)
heterotopic p.
heterotropic pregnancies
high-risk p. (HRP)
p. hormone
hydatid p.
iatrogenic multiple p. (IMP)
idiopathic cholestasis of p.
idiopathic recurrent jaundice of p.
inherited thrombophilia in p.
interstitial p.
intrahepatic cholestasis of p. (ICP)
intraligamentary ectopic p.
intramural p.
intraperitoneal p.
intrauterine p. (IUP)
isoimmunization in p.
isthmic p.
IVF-induced abdominal p.
late p.
ligamentous ectopic p.
linear IgM disease of p.
p. loss
p. luteoma
luteoma of p.
macrocytic anemia of p.
p. management
mask of p.
mesometric p.
molar p.
monochorionic twin p.
multifetal p.
multiple pregnancies
mural p.
myometrium of p.
near-term p.
p. neurosis
nontubal ectopic p.
normally progressing p. (NPP)
p. outcome
ovarian p.
ovarioabdominal p.
papular dermatitis of p. (PDP)
parasitic p.
pelvic malignancy in p.
pernicious anemia of p.
persistent ectopic p.
phantom p.
physiologic anemia of p.
p. physiology
plural p.
polymorphic light eruption of p.
postdate p.
postmortal p.
postterm p.
previous p.
primary abdominal p.
prolonged p.

prurigo of p.
pruritic folliculitis of p.
pruritic urticarial papules and plaques of p. (PUPPP)
recurrent jaundice of p.
recurrent molar p.
p. reduction
refractory anemia of p.
renal disease in p.
rhinitis of p.
P. Risk Assessment Monitoring System (PRAMS)
p. risk factor (PRF)
sarcofetal p.
secondary abdominal p.
selective termination of p.
singleton p.
splenic p.
spurious p.
successful p.
SureCell rapid test kit for p.
systolic murmur of p.
term p.
p. termination
p. test
toxemia of p.
toxemic rash of p.
toxemic retinopathy of p.
transient hypertension of p.
treatment-associated p.
treatment-independent p.
triplet p.
tubal p.
tuboabdominal p.
tuboovarian p.
tubouterine p.
p. tumor
twin p.
unplanned p.
unrecognized p.
uterine p.
p., uterine, not delivered (PUND)
uteroabdominal p.
voluntary interruption of p. (VIP)
vomiting of p.
p. wastage
Working Group on Asthma and P.
p. workup
p. zone protein
pregnancy-associated
p.-a. gingivitis
p.-a. globulin
p.-a. hypertension
p.-a. hypoplastic anemia
p.-a. plasma protein (PAPP)
p.-a. plasma protein A (PAPP-A)
p.-a. plasma protein C (PAPPC, PAPP-C)

p.-a. plasma protein D (PAPP-D)
p.-a. thrombosis
p.-a. urinary stasis
pregnancy-induced
p.-i. hypertension (PIH)
p.-i. hypertension symptom
pregnancy-specific protein
pregnane
pregnanediol
glucuronate p.
pregnanetriol
pregnant
p. cardiac patient
p. diabetic
pregnenolone
Pregnosis
Pregnyl
pregranulosa cell
pregravid weight
pre-hCG estradiol
prehension
Prehn sign
Prehospital Index (PHI)
preicteric stage
preimplantation
p. diagnosis
p. embryo (PIE)
p. genetic diagnosis (PGD)
p. HLA testing
preinvasive
p. cervical disease
p. lesion
prekallikrein deficiency
prelabor
p. membrane rupture
p. rupture of membranes (PROM)
preleukemic syndrome
Prelief
prelingual deafness
prelinguistic autism diagnostic observation (PL-ADOS)
preload
LV p.
ventricular p.
Prelone Oral
Prelu-2
PREM
Prematurity Risk Evaluation Measure
PREM score
premalignant
p. disease
p. lesion
premammary abscess
Premarin
premature (preemie, premie)
p. accelerated lung maturation (PALM)
p. adrenarche
p. aging

p. airway closure
p. amnion rupture
p. atrial contraction
p. birth
p. centromere division
p. cervical dilation
p. closure of coronal suture
p. colostrum
p. delivery
p. ductus arteriosus closure
p. ejaculation
p. infant (PI, preemie)
P. Infant Pain Profile (PIPP)
P. Infant Pain Profile score
p. labor (PML)
p. lung
p. luteal regression
p. membrane rupture
p. menarche
p. menopause
p. ovarian failure (POF)
p. placental separation
p. pubarche
p. rupture of membranes (PROM)
p. senility
p. suture synostosis
p. thelarche
p. uterine contraction inhibition
p. ventricular contraction (PVC)
prematurity
anemia of p.
anetoderma of p.
apnea of p. (AOP)
fetal p.
high oxygen percentage in retinopathy of p. (HOPE-ROP)
hypothyroxinemia of p. (HOP)
idiopathic apnea of p.
p. prevention program
pulmonary insufficiency of p.
retinopapillitis of p.
retinopathy of p. (ROP)
P. Risk Evaluation Measure (PREM)
sequelae of extreme p.
spontaneous atrophic patch of p.
Supplemental Therapeutic Oxygen for Prethreshold Retinopathy of P. (STOP-ROP)
premembrane
p. pressure
p. rupture
premenarchal
p. age
p. girl
p. vulvovaginitis
premenopausal
p. bleeding
p. breast cancer

P

premenstrual
    p. dysphoria
    p. dysphoric disorder (PMDD)
    p. edema
    P. Record of Impact and Severity
      of Menstruation
    p. salivary syndrome
    p. symptoms
    p. syndrome (PMS)
    p. tension (PMT)
    p. tension syndrome
      (PMTS)
premenstruum
PremesisRx
premie
    premature
Premphase
Prempro
premutation allele
prenatal
    p. appointment
    p. asphyxia
    p. care
    p. cytogenetic analysis
    p. cytomegalovirus
    p. detection
    p. diethylstilbestrol exposure
    p. embryologic malformation
    p. fibroelastosis
    p. genetic counseling
    p. genetic diagnosis
    p. genetics
    p. growth retardation
    p. history
    p. hydronephrosis
    p. infection
    p. interphase fluorescence in situ
      hybridization
    p. interview
    p. magnetic resonance imaging
    p. mortality
    p. placement
    p. placement of thoracoamniotic
      shunt
    p. risk
    p. risk factor
    p. risk prediction
    p. screen
    p. screening
    p. selection
    p. sex determination
    p. smoking
    p. smoking intervention
    p. stroke
    p. surgery
    p. testing
    p. tocolysis
    p. treatment
    p. ultrasound

    p. visit
    p. vitamin (PNV)
prenatally exposed to drugs (PED)
Prenate
    P. 90
    P. GT delayed-release gel-coated
      tablet
    P. Ultra
Prentif
    P. cavity-rim cervical sap
    P. pessary
prenylamine
preoperational stage
preorthognathic surgery manipulation
preovulatory
    p. follicle
    p. LH surge
Pre-Par
preparation
    aseptic p.
    bowel p.
    P. H
    hemorrhoidal p.
    improper formula p.
    International Reference P. (IRP)
    KOH p.
    LE cell p.
    potassium hydroxide p.
    recombinant FSH p.
    sickle cell p.
    site p.
    Tzanck p.
    wet p.
Preparation-H hydrocortisone cream
PREPARE
    prevent postmenopausal Alzheimer with
    replacement estrogens
prepared semen
**preparticipation sports examination
(PSE)**
prepartum
prepatellar bursitis
Pre-Pen
prepenile testis
preperitoneal fat
Prepidil
    P. Gel cervical ripener
    P. Vaginal Gel
prepregnancy
    p. body mass index
    p. care
    p. level
prepuberal, prepubertal
    p. depression
    p. examination
    p. mania
    p. periodontitis
    p. testicular tumor (PPTT)
    p. vaginal flora

prepuberal-onset bipolarity
prepubertal (*var. of* prepuberal)
   p. vaginal bleeding
   p. vulvovaginitis
prepuberty
prepubescent vagina
prepuce
pre-pulseless phase
preputial
   p. flap
   p. sac
   p. washing
preputiale
   sebum p.
preputii
   smegma p.
prereading stage
prerenal
   p. ARF
   p. azotemia
   p. insufficiency
prereproductive
presacral
   p. fascia
   p. nerve
   p. neurectomy
   p. space
   p. sympathectomy
preschool
preschool-age psychiatric assessment (PAPA)
preschooler
   Miller Assessment for P.'s
prescription (Rx)
   p. drug (Rx)
   P. Strength Desenex
preseizure state
presence
   family member p. (FMP)
present
   p. episode
   p. illness (PI)
presentation
   acromion p.
   arm p.
   breech p. (BP)
   brow p.
   brow-down p.
   cephalic p. (CP)
   complete breech p. (CBP)
   compound p.
   double breech p. (DBP)
   double footling p.
   Duncan p.
   face p.
   face/chin p.
   fetal p.
   foot p.
   footling breech p.

   frank breech p.
   full breech p.
   funic p.
   hand and head p.
   head p.
   incomplete breech p.
   incomplete foot p.
   incomplete knee p.
   isomorphic p.
   knee p.
   longitudinal p.
   mentoanterior p.
   mentoposterior p.
   military p.
   nonisomorphic p.
   oblique p. (OP)
   occiput p.
   p. of cord
   p. of fetus
   pelvic p.
   persistent occiput posterior p.
   placental p.
   polar p.
   right occipitoposterior p.
   shoulder p.
   sincipital p.
   single breech p.
   single footling p.
   singleton breech p.
   torso p.
   transverse p.
   transverse lie p.
   trunk p.
   umbilical p.
   unstable fetal p.
   vertex p.
   vertex-breech twin p.
   vertex-transverse twin p.
   victim p.
presenting part
preseptal cellulitis
preservation
   ovarian p.
preservative-free solution (PFS)
PreservCyt
presinusoidal
   p. hypertension
   p. obstruction
Preslip SCFE
presomite embryo
press-in
   p.-i. bone anchor
   p.-i. bone anchor system
Press-Mate model 8800T blood pressure monitor
pressor
   p. agent
   p. medication
   p. response

P

pressure
  abdominal leak point p. (ALPP)
  airway opening p.
  airway transmural p.
  alveolar partial p.
  ambulatory blood p. (ABP)
  aortic blood p.
  arterial p.
  arterial blood p. (ABP)
  arterial partial p.
  auto-positive end-expiratory p.
    (auto-PEEP)
  bilevel positive airway p.
    (BiPAP)
  bladder p.
  blood p. (BP)
  carotid sinus p.
  central venous p. (CVP)
  cerebral perfusion p. (CPP)
  colloid oncotic p.
  colloid osmotic p. (COP)
  constant positive airway p.
  continuous distending p. (CDP)
  continuous distending airway p.
    (CDAP)
  continuous negative airway p.
    (CNAP)
  continuous negative extrathoracic p.
    (CNEP)
  continuous positive airway p.
    (CPAP)
  p. controlled ventilation
  cricoid p.
  detrusor p.
  diastolic arterial p. (DAP)
  diastolic blood p.
  distending p.
  elevated intracranial p.
  end-expiratory p. (EEP)
  p. equalization
  p. equalization tube (PET)
  erratic blood p.
  esophageal p.
  extrinsic positive end-expiratory p.
  p., facial expression, sleeplessness
  fetal hydrostatic p.
  finger arterial blood p. (FABP)
  fundal p.
  p. gradient
  high bladder p.
  hydrostatic p.
  increased intracranial p.
  inspiratory p.
  intraabdominal p.
  intracranial p. (ICP)
  intraluminal p.
  intraocular p. (IOP)
  intravascular oncotic p.
  intravesical p.

  intrinsic positive and end-
    expiratory p.
  jugular venous p. (JVP)
  leak-point p. (LPP)
  left arterial p.
  LES p.
  p. load
  p. mapping
  maternal abdominal p.
  maximum inspiratory p.
  maximum urethral closure p.
    (MUCP)
  mean airway p. (MAP)
  mean aortic p.
  mean arterial p. (MAP)
  mean arterial blood p. (MABP)
  mean left atrial p.
  mean pulmonary artery p.
  mean right atrial p.
  Monro-Kellie doctrine of
    intracranial p.
  nasal continuous positive airway p.
    (nCPAP)
  nasal prong continuous positive
    airway p. (NP-CPAP)
  negative end-expiratory p. (NEEP)
  negative inspiratory p. (NIP)
  net ultrafiltration p.
  nitrogen partial p. (PN_2)
  normal blood p.
  p. of carbon dioxide
  p. of CO_2
  oncotic p.
  osmotic p. (Op)
  PA p.
  p. palsy
  partial p. (P)
  peak end-expiratory p.
  peak inspiratory p. (PIP)
  plasma oncotic p.
  p. point
  portal venous p.
  positive airway p.
  positive distending p. (PDP)
  positive end-expiratory p. (PEEP)
  postmembrane p.
  premembrane p.
  pulmonary artery occluded p.
    (PAOP)
  pulmonary artery wedge p. (PAWP)
  pulmonary capillary wedge p.
    (PCWP)
  pulse p.
  pulse oximetry waveform systolic
    blood p. (POWSBP)
  rectal p.
  resting anal sphincter p.
  right atrial p. (RAP)
  p. support mode

p. support ventilation
suprapubic p.
systolic arterial p. (SAP)
systolic blood p.
p. transducer
p. transmission
transpulmonary p.
tubal perfusion p. (TPP)
urethral closure p. (UCP)
p. urticaria
vacuum p.
venous p.
wide pulse p.
zero end-expiratory p.
pressure-cycled ventilator
pressured speech
pressure-preset ventilator
pressure-separator tubing
Pressyn
presternal edema
PreSun
presyncope
presystolic
p. murmur
p. thrill
preterm
p. birth
p. delivery (PTD)
p. formula
p. infant
p. labor (PTL)
p. labor arrest
p. milk (PTM)
p. neonate
P. Prediction Study
p. premature rupture of membranes (PPROM)
p. rupture of membranes (PROM)
p. spontaneous rupture of membranes (PSROM)
prethickened formula
pretibial skin dimple
Pretz
Pretz-D
prevaccination
Prevacid SoluTab
prevalence rate
Prevalite
Preven emergency contraception kit
prevention
Centers for Disease Control and P. (CDC)
injury p.
primary p.
secondary prematurity p.
tertiary p.
preventive
p. allergy treatment (PAT)

p. antibiotic
p. antioxidant
prevent postmenopausal Alzheimer with replacement estrogens (PREPARE)
Preveon
prevesical space
Prevex HC
previa
central placenta p.
complete placenta p.
low-lying placenta p.
marginal p.
partial p.
placenta p. (PP)
total p.
total placenta p.
vasa p. (VP)
previable fetus
Prevident
previllous embryo
previous
p. maternal immunity
p. menstrual period (PMP)
p. pregnancy
p. preterm delivery
p. transfundal uterine surgery
Prevnar pneumococcal vaccine
Prevotella
P. bivia
P. disiens
P. multocida
prezygotic
PRF
pregnancy risk factor
prolactin releasing factor
priapism
Pribnow box
prickly heat
prick test
Prieto syndrome (PRS)
prilocaine
lidocaine and p.
Prilosec
Primacor
primaquine phosphate
primary
p. abdominal pregnancy
p. acquired urticaria
p. adrenal insufficiency
p. amebic meningoencephalitis (PAM, PAME)
p. amenorrhea
p. amine
p. anastomosis
p. angiitis of CNS (PACNS)
p. antiphospholipid syndrome
p. aqueductal stenosis
p. atelectasis
p. bile acid malabsorption

733

primary (*continued*)
p. biliary cirrhosis (PBC)
p. bubo
p. bullous disorder
p. cardiac arrhythmia
P. Care Evaluation of Mental Disorders (PRIME-MD)
p. caregiver
p. care physician (PCP)
p. caretaker
p. carnitine deficiency
p. central nervous system lymphoma (PCNSL)
p. cesarean section (PCS)
p. chondrodystrophy
p. ciliary dyskinesia (PCD)
p. circular reaction
p. cleft palate repair
p. closure
p. congenital glaucoma
p. craniosynostosis
p. cytoreductive surgery
p. dentition
p. dysfunctional labor (PDL)
p. dysmenorrhea
p. dystonia
p. EFE
p. embryonic cell
p. empty sella syndrome
p. follicle
p. generalized epilepsy
p. generalized seizure
p. headache
p. hepatocellular carcinoma (PHC)
p. herpetic gingivostomatitis
p. hyperoxaluria
p. hyperoxaluria type 1 (PH-1)
p. hypersomnia
p. hyperuricemia syndrome
p. hypoalphalipoproteinemia
p. hypochondriasis
p. hypogonadism
p. hypomagnesemia
p. hypophosphatemic rickets
p. hypothyroidism
p. idiopathic dermatomyositis
p. idiopathic polymyositis
p. immune deficiency (PID)
p. immunodeficiency (PID)
p. immunodeficiency disorder
p. infection
p. infertility
p. insomnia
p. intraocular tumor
p. intrapulmonary neoplasm
p. lactic acidosis
p. lactose intolerance
p. lung bud formation
p. lymphedema

p. macrodactyly
p. macular atrophy
p. megalencephaly
p. microcephaly
p. molar
p. nasal mastocytosis
p. nephrotic syndrome
p. neuraminidase deficiency
p. nocturnal enuresis
p. oocyte
p. ovarian failure (POF)
p. ovarian insufficiency
p. oxalosis
p. PAP
p. peritoneal carcinoma (PPC)
p. peritoneal drainage (PPD)
p. peritonitis
p. polycythemia
p. polydipsia
p. postpartum hemorrhage (PPH)
p. prevention
p. prophylaxis
p. pulmonary hemosiderosis
p. pulmonary hypertension (PPH)
p. pulmonary tuberculosis
p. radiation therapy
p. repair of esophageal atresia
p. sclerosing cholangitis
p. sex cord
p. snoring
p. syphilis
p. teeth
p. testicular failure
p. testis-determining factor
p. thrombocythemia (PT)
p. tracheal tumor
p. tracheomalacia
p. uterine inertia
p. vesicoureteral reflux
p. writing tremor
p. xanthomatosis
Prima Series LEEP speculum
Primatene Mist
Primaxin
PRIME
Positive Reinforcement in the Menopausal Experience
PRIME patient support program
primed in situ labeling (PRINS)
PRIME-MD
Primary Care Evaluation of Mental Disorders
primer
allele specific associated p.
arbitrarily p.
degenerate consensus p.
degenerate oligonucleotide p. (DOP)
p. pair system
primidone

primigravida (G1)
    elderly p.
priming
    cervical p.
    p. dose
    gastrointestinal p.
primipara
primiparity
primiparous
primitive
    p. aorta
    p. blastoma
    p. cloaca
    p. fetal hemoglobin (HbP)
    p. groove
    p. knot
    p. lipoblastoma
    p. neuroectodermal tumor (PNET)
    p. neuroectodermal tumor
      medulloblastoma (PNET/MB)
    p. ovum
    p. reflex
    p. reflex pattern
    p. streak
primordia (*pl. of* primordium)
primordial
    p. cephalization
    p. dwarfism
    p. follicle
    p. germ cell
    p. ovum
    p. pluripotent stem cell
    vesicourethral p.
primordium, *pl.* **primordia**
    choroid plexus primordia
    esophagotracheal p.
    thymus p.
    uterovaginal p.
Primrose syndrome
Primsol solution
primum
    foramen p.
    ostium p.
    septum p.
Principen
principle
    ALARA p.
    Doppler p.
    Fick p.
    Fontan p.
    Frank-Starling p.
    Mitrofanoff p.
Pringle disease
Prinivil
PRINS
    primed in situ labeling
prion disease
prior
    p. complete mole

    p. low transverse uterine incision
    p. low vertical uterine incision
    p. partial mole
    p. probability
Priscilla White classification of diabetes in pregnancy system (class A, A1, A2, B, C, D, F, R, H, T)
prism
    optic p.
    P. score
PRISM
    Pediatric Risk of Mortality
Pritchard intramuscular regimen
private blood group
Privine Nasal
p.r.n.
    pro re nata (as needed)
PRO
    PRO 2000 Gel
    PRO infusion catheter
proaccelerin
Pro-Amox
Pro-Ampi
proanthocyanidin
probability
    conditional p.
    joint p.
    objective p.
    personal p.
    posterior p.
    prior p.
    subjective p.
Probalan
ProBalance liquid nutrition
proband
probe
    bacterial artificial chromosome p.
    biopsy p.
    biplane intracavitary p.
    bipolar circumactive p. (BICAP)
    bipolar laparoscopic p. (BiLAP)
    blunt p.
    convex p.
    dedicated Doppler p.
    DNA dual color p.
    Doppler p.
    Endopath needle tip electrosurgery p.
    endovaginal p.
    Envision endocavity p.
    gene p.
    in-line p.
    IntraDop p.
    linear p.
    locus-specific p.
    MEVA p.
    multiplane intracavitary p.
    Neo-Therm neonatal skin temperature p.

P

probe (*continued*)
    nucleic acid p.
    Ohmeda SoftProbe p.
    p. patency
    pH p.
    phased array p.
    ribonucleic acid p.
    p. sheath
    Spencer p.
    p. system
    transrectal p.
    transvaginal
      transducer p.
    Universal vaginal p.
    ViraType p.
    V-Probe cryoablation p.
    V33W Endocavity p.
    YSI neonatal temperature p.
probenecid
probiotic
PROBIT
    promotion of breastfeeding intervention
    trial
problem
    acid-base p.
    attention-distractibility p.
    chronic behavior p.
    dietary p.
    feeding p.
    growth p.
    internalizing p.
    intersex p.
    neurodevelopmental p.
    nutritional p.
    occlusal p.
    parent-child interaction p.
    psychosexual p.
    secondary emotional p.
    sensory p.
    sexual p.
    p. solving
    speech p.
    toileting p.
    urologic p.
    V code rational p.'s
Problem-Oriented Screening Instrument
for Teenagers (POSIT)
proboscis
    disruptive p.
    holoprosencephalic p.
    p. lateralis
    lateral nasal p.
    supernumerary p.
Probst
    bundle of P.
procainamide
procaine
    p. penicillin
    p. penicillin G

procalcitonin (PCT)
    cerebrospinal fluid p.
    serum p.
procarbazine
Procardia XL
procaryote (*var. of* prokaryote)
procaterol
procedural sedation and analgesia (PSA)
procedure
    Abbe-McIndoe total endoscopic
      vaginal reconstruction p.
    Abbe-McIndoe-Williams
      vaginoplasty p.
    Abbe-Wharton-McIndoe vaginal
      reconstruction p.
    abdominopelvic p.
    ablative p.
    ACE p.
    ACS p.
    Aldridge urethral sling p.
    Altemeier perineal rectal
      pullthrough p.
    procedures, alternatives, risk and
      questions (PARQ)
    American Cancer Society p.
    antegrade continence enema p.
    anterior cricoid split p.
    Aries-Pitanguy p.
    arterial switch p.
    atrial inversion p.
    atrial septoplasty p.
    atrial septostomy p.
    atrial switch p.
    Baldy-Webster uterine displacement
      repair p.
    Ball-Burch p.
    Barbero-Marcial p.
    bidirectional Glenn p.
    Bishop-Koop p.
    Blair-Brown p.
    Blalock-Hanlon atrial septostomy p.
    Blalock-Park p.
    Blalock-Taussig shunt p.
    Boix-Ochoa p.
    bowel lengthening p.
    Bricker ileoureterostomy p.
    Burch p.
    buried vaginal island p.
    Castaneda tetralogy of Fallot
      repair p.
    Chassar Moir pubovaginal sling p.
    Chassar Moir-Sims urinary fistula
      repair p.
    Chiari p.
    Coblation-Channeling surgical p.
    Cohen p.
    Cole intubation p.
    cricoid split p.
    cyclodestructive p.

Cyclops p.
Dall-Miles cable grip p.
Damus-Fontan p.
Damus-Kaye-Stansel pulmonary
  artery to ascending aorta
  anastomosis p.
Davydov vaginoplasty p.
Delorme rectal prolapse repair p.
diagnostic p.
diverting colostomy with
  pull-through p.
Donald p.
dot-blot p.
double-switch p.
drainage p.
Duckett tubularized neourethra p.
Duhamel abdominoperineal
  pullthrough p.
enema p.
Estes ovarian transfer p.
Evans-Steptoe p.
Everard Williams retropubic
  cystourethropexy suspension p.
excisional p.
EXIT p.
fascial sling p.
female sterilization p.
fetal surgical p.
Fetendo clip p.
Fontan p.
Frank p.
Fredet-Ramstedt extramucosal
  longitudinal myotomy p.
Gittes endoscopic bladder neck
  suspension p.
glans-cavernosal p.
Goebell p.
Goebell-Stoeckel-Frangenheim p.
Halban culdoplasty p.
heel-stick p.
hemi-Fontan p.
Heyman-Herndon clubfoot p.
Hoffer p.
Hood p.
Ilizarov limb-lengthening p.
Ingelman-Sundberg gracilis muscle
  vesicovaginal fistula repair p.
interventional p.
intestinal bypass p.
Jatene arterial switch p.
Jones p.
Kalicinski ureteral folding
  technique p.
Kasai portoenterostomy p.
Kelly-Kennedy p.
Kelly urethrovesical plication p.
Kennedy p.
Kimura p.
Koyanagi p.

Ladd mobilization of intestine p.
laparoscopic unipolar
  coagulation p.
Lash laparoscopic supracervical
  hysterectomy p.
Latzko p.
Leadbetter-Politano
  ureteroneocystostomy p.
LETZ p.
loop electrosurgical excision p.
  (LEEP)
Lyodura sling p.
MAGPI p.
Mantel-Haenszel p.
Marshall-Marchetti p.
Marshall-Marchetti-Krantz retropubic
  cystourethrography suspension p.
Martius labial fat flap urinary
  fistula repair p.
Mayo-Fueth inversion p.
McCall-Schumann enterocele p.
McDonald p.
McIndoe-Hayes p.
McIndoe vaginal construction p.
Meigs-Okabayashi radical
  hysterectomy p.
Mikulicz p.
mini-Pena p.
MMK retropubic cystourethropexy
  suspension p.
modified Fontan p.
Morrow p.
Moschcowitz culdoplasty p.
Mustard atrial switch p.
Mustardé cheek flap p.
Mustardé hypospadias p.
neobladder diversion p.
Neugebauer-Le Fort colpocleisis p.
Nichols p.
Norwood p.
Norwood-Fontan p.
NovaSure endometrial ablation p.
obliterative p.
Olshausen uterine suspension p.
OPERA p.
ovarian drilling p.
palliative p.
Parkland p.
Pemberton p.
Pena anorectal malformation
  corrective p.
Penn pouch p.
Pereyra p.
Piver type II p.
platelet neutralization p.
platelet neutralizing p.
Pozzi p.
psoas hitch p.
pubovaginal sling p.

P

procedure (*continued*)
pull-through p.
Ramstedt p.
Rashkind atrial septostomy p.
Rastelli right ventricle and
pulmonary artery conduit p.
Ravitch pectus excavatum repair p.
Raz-Leach p.
Raz sling p.
Récamier uterine curettage p.
restorative p.
retroperitoneal laparoscopic p.
retropubic needle p.
retropubic suspension p.
retropubic urethropexy p.
Richter and Albrich vaginal
sacrospinous suspension p.
Ross p.
Rotazyme diagnostic p.
Salter p.
Schauffler p.
Schauta-Aumreich radical vaginal
hysterectomy p.
selective embolization p.
selective tubal occlusion p. (STOP)
semidefinitive p.
Senning atrial switch p.
Seton p.
Shirodkar cervix encirclement
suture p.
sling p.
Soave abdominal pull-through p.
SPARC urological sling p.
Spence urethral diverticulum p.
split p.
3-stage Norwood-Fontan p.
Stamey modification of Pereyra
bladder neck suspension p.
Stamm temporary gastrostomy p.
Stanley Way p.
Steele p.
Sting p.
Sugiura p.
surgical sterilization p.
Sutherland p.
Swenson colonic pullthrough p.
tension-free vaginal tape p.
Tompkins p.
Tonnis hip dysplasia p.
Torkildsen p.
triangular vaginal patch sling p.
Uchida p.
UPLIFT p.
urinary undiversion p.
vaginal tubal p.
vaginal wall sling p.
valvulotomy p.
ventricular shunt p.
WAMBA p.

Waterston-Cooley aorto-to-right
pulmonary artery anastomosis p.
Waterston shunt p.
Whipple radical
pancreatoduodenectomy p.
Winter glans-cavernosal p.
W-stapled urinary reservoir p.
procedure-related pyrexia
process
acromion p.
antenatal disease p.
attaching p.
binary p.
birthing p.
cleft premaxillary p.
CytoRich p.
freezing p.
grieving p.
immune p.
inflammatory p.
latching-on p.
lateralization p.
lymphoproliferative p.
mastoid p.
microangiopathic p.
neuritic cytoplasmic p.
odontoid p.
quality assurance p.
short p.
tapering cytoplasmic p.
processed blood product
processing
slow cognitive p.
visuoperceptual/simultaneous
information p.
processor
ThinPrep p.
process-oriented measure
processus, *pl.* **processus**
p. vaginalis
p. vaginalis peritonei
Prochieve
prochlorperazine
Prochownik
P. neonatal resuscitation method
P. pessary
procidentia uteri
procoagulant protein
procollagen
carboxyterminal propeptide of type
1 p. (PICP)
serum type III p.
procollagenase
proconvertin
procreation
assisted medical p. (AMP)
Procrit
proctitis
HSV2 p.

proctocolpoplasty
Proctocort Rectal
ProctoCream-HC
proctoelytroplasty
proctoepisiotomy
ProctoFoam-HC
ProctoFoam NS
proctogram
    defecating p.
proctography
    evacuation p.
proctoscopy
proctosigmoiditis
proctosigmoidoscopy
proctotomy
ProCup
    Kiwi P.
procyclidine
procyonis
    Baylisascaris p.
Procytox
prodromal
    p. illness
    p. labor
    p. symptom
prodromata
prodrome, prodromus
    menstrual p.
    viral p.
prodromus (*var. of* prodrome)
Prodrox
prodrug
product
    P. 80056
    advanced oxidation protein p.
    alpha-1 thymosin p.
    blood p.
    clearance of fetal p.
    fibrin degradation p.
    fibrinogen degradation p.
      (FDP)
    fibrinogen-fibrin degradation p.
    fibrinogen split p.
    fibrin split p. (FSP)
    gene p.
    p.'s of conception
    processed blood p.
    red blood cell p.
    Repliform alternative p.
    unpasteurized milk p.
production
    cyclic hormone p.
    endogenous hormonal p.
    extraglandular testosterone p.
    fetal urine p.
    insufficient milk p.
    in vitro antibody p. (IVAP)
    ketone p.
    milk p.

    oocyte p.
    ovarian androgen p.
    sebum p.
    speech p.
productivity
ProDynamic monitor
prodynorphin
Proellex
proemial breast
proencephalon (*var. of* prosencephalon)
proencephalus
proenkephalin
    p. A
    p. B
proenzyme
Profasi HP
profenamine
Profiber formula
proficiency
    Bruininks-Oseretsky Test of Motor
    P.
profilaggrin
Profilate OSD
profile
    acylcarnitine p.
    Alpern-Boll Developmental P.
    anatomic p. (AP)
    biometric p.
    biophysical p. (BPP)
    coagulation p.
    fatty acid p.
    fetal biophysical p.
    fetal movement p.
    Hawaii Early Learning P. (HELP)
    lung p.
    modified biophysical p. (MBPP)
    neuropsychologic p.
    P. of Mood States (POMS)
    Premature Infant Pain P. (PIPP)
    protein p.
    rectilinear p.
    Sickness Impact P. (SIP)
    torsional p.
    urethral pressure p.
    urethral pressure cough p.
    P. viral probe test
Profile-II
    Developmental P.-II (DP-II)
profiling
    multiple arbitrary amplicon p.
    (MAAP)
Profilnine
    P. Heat-Treated
    P. SD
profilometry
    urethral pressure p. (UPP)
profluens
    hydrops tubae p.
profound mental retardation

P

profunda
    miliaria p.
    tinea p.
profundus
    lupus erythematosus p.
profusa
    lentiginosis p.
profusion
    placental p.
PRO/Gel ultrasound transmission gel
progenitor
    erythroid p.
    fetal erythroid p.
progeny
progeria
    adult p.
    p. syndrome
progeria-like syndrome
progeroid
    p. facies
    p. short stature-pigmented nevi
    syndrome
Progestasert intrauterine device
progestational
    p. activity
    p. agent
    p. challenge
    p. compound
    p. effect
    p. protection
    p. state
    p. therapy
progesterone
    p. antagonist
    p. breakthrough bleeding
    p. challenge test
    p. cream
    p. dermatitis
    first-generation p.
    p. level
    p. metabolism
    micronized p.
    p. myometrial level
    17-OH p.
    P. Oil
    parenteral p.
    p. plasmatic
    P. Radioimmunoassay Kit
    p. receptor (PgR, PR)
    second-generation p.
    p. secretion
    serum p.
    p. synthesis
    third-generation p.
    urinary free p.
    p. withdrawal bleeding
progesterone-releasing T-shaped device
progestin
    C_{21} p.

    norgestimate p.
    p. oral contraceptive
progestin-impregnated vaginal ring
progestin-induced decidualization
progestin-only
    p.-o. implant
    p.-o. injectable contraceptive
    p.-o. "minipill"
    p.-o. oral contraceptive
    p.-o. pill (POP)
progestin-releasing IUD
progestogen
    C_{21} p.
    p. support therapy
progestogen-dependent endometrial protein (PEP)
Proglycem Oral
prognathia (*var. of* prognathism)
prognathism, prognathia
    mandibular p.
    microcephaly, microphthalmia,
    ectrodactyly, p. (MMEP)
prognosis
    clinical p.
prognostic
    p. factor
    p. indicator
    p. scoring system
prognostication
prognosticator
Prograf
program
    antepartum surveillance p.
    bed rest support p.
    behavior modification p.
    Bridge Reading P.
    Childhood Asthma Management P.
    (CAMP)
    Children's Health Insurance P.
    (CHIP)
    chronic hypertransfusion p.
    Early Childhood Special Education
    P.
    early-discharge p.
    early intervention p. (EIP)
    Easy Breathing asthma management
    p.
    Epidemiologic Catchment P.
    EPSDT p.
    expanded food nutrition education p.
    (EFNEP)
    Free to Be Me body image p.
    Fria muscle training device p.
    Individualized Education P. (IEP)
    infant development p.
    InfantSEE vision p.
    infant stimulation p.
    Lovaas p.
    Merrill p.

Metropolitan Atlanta Congenital Defects P. (MACDP)
National Asthma Education and Prevention P.
National Breast and Cervical Cancer Early Detection P.
National Ovarian Cancer Early Detection P.
Neonatal Resuscitation P. (NRP)
New England Regional Infant Cardiac P. (NERICP)
New Moves obesity-prevention p.
Office of Special Education P.'s (OSEP)
Pharsight Trial Designer simulation p.
prematurity prevention p.
PRIME patient support p.
PSI p.
residential p.
Restore p.
Special Supplemental Nutrition P.
State Children's Health Insurance P. (SCHIP)
STEPS p.
The Injury Prevention P. (TIPP)
universal newborn hearing screening p. (UNHSP)
WIC p.

progress
cessation of p.
failure to p.

progression
intraepithelial disease p.
tumor p.

progressiva
fibrodysplasia ossificans p. (FOP)
myositis ossificans p.

progressive
p. biliary cirrhosis
p. bulbar palsy
p. bulbar palsy with epilepsy
p. bulbar palsy with perceptive deafness
p. bulbar paralysis of childhood
p. central nervous system failure
p. deforming osteogenesis imperfecta
p. dystonia
p. encephalitis
p. encephalopathy
p. encephalopathy, edema, hypsarrhythmia, optic atrophy (PEHO)
p. external ophthalmoplegia (PEO)
p. facial hemiatrophy
p. familial intrahepatic cholestasis (PFIC)
p. familial scleroderma

p. granuloma
p. hydronephrosis
p. labyrinthitis
p. multifocal leukoencephalopathy (PML)
p. muscular dystrophy of childhood
p. myoclonic epilepsy
p. obesity
p. obliterative cholangiopathy
p. outer retinal necrosis (PORN)
p. primary pulmonary tuberculosis
p. renal failure
p. rubella panencephalitis
p. systemic sclerosis

proguanil hydrochloride
prohormone
proinflammatory cytokine
project
Breast Cancer Detection P.
Breast Cancer Detection Demonstration P. (BCDDP)
Diana P.
Fort Bragg evaluation p. (FBEP)
genome p.
Human Genome P.
National Collaborative Diethylstilbestrol Adenosis P. (DESAD)
National Collaborative Perinatal p.
National Surgical Adjuvant Breast P. (NSABP)
Portage p.
social interaction and perinatal addiction p. (SIPAP)
P. TEACCH

projectile vomiting
projection
bony p.
red blood cell spiny p.

projective assessment
prokaryote, procaryote
prokaryotic reaction
prokinetic agent
prolactin
p. deficiency
p. inhibiting factor (PIF)
p. level
plasma p.
p. regulation
p. releasing factor (PRF)
p. secretion
serum p.
p. stimulation
p. suppression

prolactinoma
bromocriptine p.
bromocriptine-resistant p.
estrogen-induced p.

prolactin-producing adenoma

P

741

prolactin-secreting
    p.-s. adenoma
    p.-s. macroadenoma
prolapse
    aortic cusp p.
    cervical p.
    complete rectal p.
    concealed rectal p.
    cord p.
    fallopian tube p.
    fimbrial p.
    first-degree p.
    genital p.
    ICS bladder p. (stage I–III)
    incomplete rectal p.
    intrapartum cord p.
    massive genital p.
    mitral valve p. (MVP)
    occult cord p.
    p. of corpus luteum
    p. of umbilical cord
    p. of uterus
    pelvic organ p. (POP)
    posthysterectomy p.
    rectal p.
    p. repair system
    second-degree p.
    stage I–IV p.
    third-degree p.
    total vaginal vault p.
    umbilical cord p. (UCP)
    urethral p.
    uterine p.
    uterovaginal p.
    vaginal stump p.
    vaginal vault p.
    valve p.
    vault p.
prolapsed
    p. cord
    p. ectopic ureterocele
    p. uterus
prolapse-gastropathy syndrome
prolapse-quantified
    Pelvic Organ P.-Q. (POPQ)
prolapsing
    p. apex
    p. apex of intussusception
    p. polyp
Prolastin
Prolene suture
prolidase deficiency
proliferating hemangioma
proliferation
    beta FGF-stimulated cell p.
    endometrial p.
    epithelial cell p.
    mesangial cell p.
    p. of stroma

proliferative, proliferous
    p. change
    p. endometrium
    p. glomerulonephritis
    p. histology
    p. lesion
    p. lupus nephritis
    p. phase
    p. retinitis
    p. vasculopathy
    p. zone (PZ)
proliferous (*var. of* proliferative)
Prolift graft
proligerus
    discus p.
proline
    p. aminopeptidase activity
    p. hydroxyproline
prolinemia
    encephalopathy with p.
Prolixin
prolongation
    excessive QT p.
    QTc p.
prolonged
    p. bradycardia
    p. capillary refill
    p. delivery hospitalization
    p. EEG monitoring
    p. expiratory apnea
    p. expiratory phase
    p. gestation
    p. indirect hyperbilirubinemia
    p. jaundice
    p. labor
    p. latent phase
    p. partial asphyxia
    p. pregnancy
    p. premature rupture of membranes
    (PPROM)
    p. QT interval
    p. QT syndrome
    p. regard
    p. rupture
    p. rupture of membranes
    (PROM)
    p. unconjugated hyperbilirubinemia
    p. variable decelerations
Proloprim
PROM
    prelabor rupture of membranes
    premature rupture of membranes
    preterm rupture of membranes
    prolonged rupture of membranes
Promensil
prometaphase
promethazine
    p. and phenylephrine
    p. hydrochloride

promethazine, phenylephrine, codeine
   P. VC Plain Syrup
Prometrium
prominence
   calcaneal p.
   cephalic p.
   Rokitansky p.
prominent
   p. ductal pattern
   p. ear
   p. heart sound
   p. incisors-obesity-hypotonia
    syndrome
   p. mandible
   p. maxillary incisor
   p. nose
   p. quadrigeminal plate cistern
   p. skin discoloration
ProMod formula
promontorium (*var. of* promontory)
promontory, promontorium
   sacral p.
promoter
   AIRE p.
Promote with Fiber formula
promotion of breastfeeding intervention
  trial (PROBIT)
prompted voiding
promyelocyte cell
promyelocytic leukemia
pronate
pronated foot
pronation
pronator
   p. fat pad
   p. sign
prone
   p. board
   p. extension test
   p. on elbows (POE)
   p. pivoting
   p. sleep position
   p. stander
pronephroi (*pl. of* pronephros)
pronephros, *pl.* **pronephroi**
Pronestyl-SR
prong
   binasal p.'s
   Hudson p.'s
pronormoblast cell
Pronto Shampoo
pronuclear embryo
pronucleate
   p. stage embryo transfer
    (PROST)
   p. stage tubal transfer (PROST)
pronucleus (PN)
proopiomelanocortin (POMC)
prooxyphysin

Propac Plus formula
Propaderm
Propadrine
propagation
propamidine
propantheline bromide
Propaq Encore vital signs monitor
proparacaine
propendens
   venter p.
propeptide
   carboxyterminal p.
proper
   glans p.
properdin
   p. deficiency
   p. factor B
property
   teratogenic p.'s
prophase
prophylactic
   p. antibiotic
   p. antibiotic therapy
   p. anticoagulation
   p. aspirin use
   p. bed rest
   p. cerclage
   p. chemotherapy
   p. culdoplasty
   p. episiotomy
   p. heparin
   p. immunization
   p. isoniazid
   p. mastectomy
   p. medication
   p. oophorectomy
   p. red-cell transfusion
   p. tetracycline
   p. tocolysis
   p. treatment
prophylaxes (*pl. of* prophylaxis)
prophylaxis, *pl.* **prophylaxes**
   antibiotic p.
   antimicrobial p.
   aspiration p.
   Credé p.
   drug p.
   endocarditis p.
   intrapartum antibiotic p. (IAP)
   neonatal ocular p.
   ocular p.
   postexposure p. (PEP)
   postnatal penicillin p. (PPP)
   primary p.
   rabies p.
   SBE p.
   secondary p.
   silver nitrate eye p.
   tetanus p.

P

prophylaxis (*continued*)
    thromboembolic p.
    trimethoprim-sulfamethoxazole p.
    vitamin K p.
propidium iodide
Propine
propionate
    beclomethasone p.
    clobetasol p.
    fluticasone p.
Propionibacterium
    P. acnes
    P. propionicus
propionic acidemia
propionicus
    Propionibacterium p.
propionyl CoA carboxylase deficiency
Pro-Piroxicam
Proplex
    P. SX-T
    P. T
propofol
propositus
propoxyphene and acetaminophen
propping
    bottle p.
    p. reflex
2-propranol
propranolol (PROP)
    p. hydrochloride
propressophysin
propria, *pl.* **propriae**
    lamina p.
    substantia p.
propriae (*pl. of* propria)
proprioception
proprioceptive
    p. input
    p. sensation
proprioceptor
    muscle p.
proptosis
    spinal p.
Propulsid
propulsion
    decreased p.
propylene
    p. glycol
    p. glycol diacetate
propylthiouracil (PTU)
Propyl-Thyracil
prorenin
    plasma p.
prorenin-renin-angiotensin system
Prorex injection
Prosed/DS
prosencephalon, proencephalon
ProSobee formula
prosocial behavior scale

prosodic pattern
prosody
prosopoanoschisis
prosopopagus
prosoposchisis
prosoposternodymus
prosopothoracopagus
ProSound SSD-5500 ultrasound
PROST
    pronucleate stage embryo transfer
    pronucleate stage tubal transfer
prostacyclin
    p. 2 (PGI_2)
    p. assay
    p. deficiency
    nebulized p.
prostacyclin-stimulating factor (PSF)
prostaglandin (PG)
    p. biosynthesis
    p. D_2
    p. E (PGE)
    p. E_1 (PGE_1)
    p. E_2 (PGE_2)
    p. E analog
    p. E_2 gel
    p. endoperoxide synthase
    p. F
    p. F_2
    p. F_2 alpha (PGF2 alpha)
    p. G (PGG)
    p. gel induction
    p. H (PGH)
    1-hour p.
    p. I_2
    intravaginal p.
    p. metabolism
    15-methyl p.
    p. pessary
    serum p.
    p. suppository
    p. synthesis inhibition
    p. synthetase inhibitor (PGSI)
    vaginal p.
    vasoactive p.
prostanoid
    cyclooxygenase-2-derived p.
prostatic utricle
Pro-Step hCG
prostheses (*pl. of* prosthesis)
prosthesis, *pl.* **prostheses**
    Becker breast p.
    breast p.
    Introl bladder neck
     support p.
    NeuroCybernetic p.
    ocular p.
    vaginal prolapse p.
    valvular p.

prosthetic
   p. attachment
   p. graft implantation
   p. patch aortoplasty
prosthodontist
Prostigmin
Prostin
   P. E2 Vaginal Suppository
   P. VR Pediatric
Prostin/15M
protamine
   p. insulin zinc suspension
   p. sulfate
protease
   p. inhibitor (PI)
   p. inhibitor-induced lipodystrophy
   p. inhibitor type
   vitamin K-dependent serine p.
protease-3
   neutrophil p.-3
ProtectaCap cap
Protectaid
   P. contraceptive sponge
   P. contraceptive sponge with F-5 gel
protection
   airway p.
   p. and advocacy (P&A)
   progestational p.
protective
   p. colostomy
   p. extension
   p. protein
   p. service agency
protector
   LATS p.
proteiform syndrome
protein
   accessory p.
   agouti p.
   bactericidal/permeability-increasing p. (BPI)
   Bcl-2 p.
   Bence Jones p.
   p. binding
   binding p.
   p. C
   carrier p.
   cartilage oligomeric matrix p. (COMP)
   p. C coagulation inhibitor
   p. C concentrate
   p. C deficiency
   chimeric p.
   Clara cell 16 p.
   congenital absence of iron-binding p.
   cow's milk p. (CMP)
   C-reactive p. (CRP)

   deficiency of C4-binding p.
   dimeric p.
   E-cadherin p.
   endometrial p.
   eosinophilic cationic p. (ECP)
   fetoneonatal estrogen-binding p.
   FK binding p.
   follicle regulatory p. (FRP)
   fragile X mental retardation p. (FMRP)
   G p.
   glial fibrillary acidic p. (GFAP)
   gonadotropin-releasing hormonelike p.
   growth hormone-binding p. (GHBP)
   H p.
   heat shock p.
   H-*ras* p21 p.
   p. hydrolysate
   p. hydrolysate formula
   hydrolyzed p.
   I IFG-binding p.
   implantation p.
   insulinlike growth factor-binding p. (IGFBP)
   p. intolerance
   intracellular myometrial p.
   iron-binding p.
   KAL p.
   p. kinase C (PKC)
   lipoprotein receptor-related p. (LRP)
   p. loss
   macrophage inflammatory p. (MIP)
   major basic p. (MBP)
   p. marker
   membrane p.
   methyl-CpG-binding p. 2 (MeCP2)
   p. modified fast (PMF)
   mucopolysaccharide p.
   mu dimeric p.
   myeloma p.
   myometrial p.
   outer surface p. (Osp)
   P p.
   peripheral myelin p. (PMP)
   p. phosphorylation
   pi dimeric p.
   placental p.
   plasma p.
   pneumococcal conjugate tetanus p. (PncT)
   pregnancy-associated plasma p. (PAPP)
   pregnancy-associated plasma p. A (PAPP-A)
   pregnancy-specific p.
   pregnancy zone p.
   procoagulant p.
   p. profile

protein (*continued*)

progestogen-dependent endometrial p. (PEP)
protective p.
proteolipid p. (PLP)
pulmonary microvascular permeability to p. (PMVP)
pulmonary surfactant p.
purified fusion p. (PFP)
receptor-associated p. (RAP)
retinol-binding p.
p. S
p. S antithrombin
Schwangerschafts p. 1
p. S coagulation inhibitor
p. S deficiency
p. solder
p. standard
surfactant-associated p. (SAP)
T p.
Tamm-Horsfall p.
theta dimeric p.
thrombus precursor p. (TpP)
thyroxine-binding p. (TBP)
transmembrane conductance regulatory p.
transport-associated p. (TAP)
urinary excretion of p. (UEP)
vimentin p.
vitamin D-binding p.
zona p.

protein-1

sphingolipid activator p.-1 (SAP1)
thyroid-specific enhancer binding p.-1

protein-3

insulinlike growth factor-binding p.-3 (IGFBP-3)

protein-A

surfactant p.-A (SP-A)

proteinaceous subretinal fluid

proteinase

p. factor
p. K
serine p.

protein-B

surfactant p.-B (SP-B)

protein-C

surfactant p.-C (SP-C)

protein-calorie malnutrition
protein-conjugated vaccine
protein-energy malnutrition
protein-induced

p.-i. eosinophilic colitis (PEC)
p.-i. vitamin K absence (PIVKA)

protein-losing enteropathy
proteinosis

alveolar p.
congenital alveolar p.
lipoid p.
pulmonary alveolar p. (PAP)

protein-sparing modified fast (PSMF)
protein-to-urine creatinine ratio
proteinuria

gestational p.
glomerular p.
idiopathic low molecular weight p.
LMW p.
orthostatic p.
overflow p.
persistent p.
postural p.
renal p.
selective p.
transient p.
treatment-resistant p.
tubular p.

proteinuric
Proteobacteria

alpha P.

proteoglycans
proteolipid protein (PLP)
proteolysis

cellular p.

proteolytic enzyme
proteus

P. mirabilis
P. morganii
P. syndrome (PS)
P. syndrome myopathy

prostheses (*pl. of* prosthesis)
prosthesis, *pl.* prostheses
prothrombic tendency
prothrombin (pro)

p. gene mutation
p. time (pro-time, PT)
p. time coagulation test

prothrombokinase
ProTime microcoagulation system
protirelin
protoblast
protocol

AIDS Clinical Trials Group p.
Bagshawe p.
chemotherapy p.
management p.
modified Bagshawe p. (MBP)
rape p.
Reese Clark p.
wean and feed p.

protocoproporphyria
Protocult stool sampling device
protodiastolic gallop
protodyssomnia
protogaster
proton

p. MRS
p. MR spectroscopy

p. pump antagonist
p. pump inhibitor (PPI)
protooncogene
c-*erb* B-2 p.
c-fms p.
fes p.
fgr p.
fyn p.
hck p.
Her 2/neu p.
lck p.
lyn p.
mos p.
raf p.
RET p.
Scr p.
yes p.
Protopic ointment
protoplast
protoporphyria
erythrohepatic p.
erythropoietic p. (EPP)
protoporphyrin
free erythrocyte p.
(FEP)
tin p. (SnPP)
zinc p. (ZnPP)
Protozoa
protracted
p. depressive episode
p. diarrhea
p. diarrhea of infancy
protraction disorder
Pro-Trin
protriptyline
Protropin Injection
protruding tongue
protrusio acetabuli
protrusion
reduction of p.
protuberance
Rokitansky p.
protuberans
dermatofibrosarcoma p.
protuberant step deformity
Proud syndrome
Proval
Proventil HFA
Provera Oral
Providencia rettgeri
provisional calcification
provocation
bronchial p.
epinephrine p.
mucous membrane p.
p. test
provocative
p. bronchial challenge testing
p. stress test

prowazekii
Rickettsia p.
proXeed
proxetil
cefpodoxime p.
Proxigel Oral
proximal
p. bowel
p. convoluted tubule
p. enterostomy
p. femoral epiphysis
p. femoral focal deficiency
p. humeral derotation osteotomy
p. humeral stress fracture
p. jejunum
p. occlusion
p. outflow tract
p. pattern weakness
p. pulmonary artery
p. pulmonary artery banding
p. row carpectomy
p. RTA
p. shaft hypospadias
p. splenorenal shunt
p. tibial epiphysis
p. transverse septum
p. tubal blockage
p. tubal obstruction
p. tubulopathy
p. urethra
p. white subungual onychomycosis
proxy
factitious disorder by p. (FDP)
Münchausen syndrome by p.
(MSBP, MSP)
Prozac
Prozine-50
PRP
pityriasis rubra pilaris
platelet-rich plasma
polyribosylribitol phosphate
PRPP
5-phospho-alpha-d-ribosyl pyrophosphate
PRPP synthetase superactivity
PRS
Prieto syndrome
PRSL
potential renal solute load
PRSP
penicillin-resistant *Streptococcus pneumoniae*
PRTS
Partington X-linked mental retardation syndrome
prune
p. belly
p. belly syndrome
pruning
synaptic p.

P

prurigo
actinic p.
p. gestationis
p. of pregnancy
pruritic
p. folliculitis of pregnancy
p. rash
p. urticarial papule
p. urticarial papules and plaques (PUPP)
p. urticarial papules and plaques of pregnancy (PUPPP)
p. urticarial plaque
p. vesiculopapular eruption
pruritus
anal p.
p. ani
drug reaction p.
genital p.
p. gravidarum
perianal p.
p. vulvae
vulvar p.
PS
pancreas sufficient
phytosterol
polysaccharide
Proteus syndrome
pulmonic stenosis
5 Ps
PSA
physical-sexual abuse
power spectral analysis
procedural sedation and analgesia
PSA test
psammoma body
PSC
Pediatric Symptom Checklist
P450scc
cytochrome P450scc
PSD
pediatric spectrum of disease
PSE
preparticipation sports examination
Pseudallescheria boydii
pseudarthrosis, pseudoarthrosis
clavicular p.
congenital p.
p. of tibia
tibial p.
pseudautonomy
pseudencephalus
pseudoacanthosis nigricans
pseudoacephalus
pseudoachondroplasia syndrome
pseudoachondroplastic dysplasia
pseudoaddiction
pseudoallele
pseudoallergic

pseudoaminopterin syndrome
pseudoaneurysm
uterine artery p.
pseudoappendicitis
pseudoappendicular syndrome
pseudoarthrosis (*var. of* pseudarthrosis)
pseudoautosome
pseudobulbar palsy
pseudocalcification
powder p.
pseudocarcinomatous hyperplasia
pseudocholinesterase deficiency
pseudochromosome
pseudochylous milky fluid
pseudocoagulopathy
pseudocoloboma
macular p.
pseudoconstipation
pseudo-Crouzon disease
pseudocyesis
monosymptomatic delusional p.
pseudocyst
pancreatic p.
pseudodeciduosis
pseudodiastrophic dysplasia
pseudodiverticulum
posterior pharyngeal p.
pseudoencapsulated lesion
pseudoephedrine
carbinoxamine and p.
p. hydrochloride
triprolidine and p.
pseudoepitheliomatous hyperplasia, pseudocarcinomatous hyperplasia
pseudoesotropia
pseudoexstrophy
pseudofemale
hairless p.
pseudogene
pseudo-genu varum
pseudogestational sac
pseudoglandular
p. period
p. stage
p. stage of lung development
p. synovial sarcoma
pseudoglioma congenita
pseudogynecomastia
pseudohermaphrodite
pseudohermaphroditism
female p. (FPH)
male p. (MPH)
pseudo-Hurler
p.-H. deformity
p.-H. polydystrophy
p.-H. syndrome
pseudohypertrophic
p. adult muscular dystrophy

p. muscular paralysis
p. progressive muscular dystrophy
pseudohypertrophy
pseudohypha
nonbranching p.
pseudohypoaldosteronism
pseudohyponatremia
pseudohypoparathyroidism (type I, Ia, II)
pseudohypopyon
pseudoinfarction
pseudointestinal obstruction
pseudointraligamentous
pseudo-Köbner phenomenon
pseudoleukemia
pseudolithiasis
reversible biliary p.
pseudolobular cirrhosis
pseudolymphoma
pseudomallei
Burkholderia p.
Pseudomonas p.
pseudomembrane
adherent p.
pseudomembranous
p. colitis
p. conjunctivitis
p. enterocolitis
p. trigonitis
pseudomenopause
pseudomenstruation
Pseudomonas
P. aeruginosa
P. cepacia
P. exotoxin
P. fluorescens
P. pseudomallei
P. septic arthritis
pseudomonoamniotic cavity
pseudomosaicism
pseudomucinous tumor
pseudomyxoma peritonei
pseudonuchal infantilism
pseudoobstruction
chronic idiopathic intestinal p. (CIIP)
chronic intestinal p.
intestinal p.
pseudopapilledema
pseudoparalysis
Parrot p.
pseudoperoxidation
iron-catalyzed p.
pseudopili anulati
pseudopolyp
pseudoporencephalic cyst
pseudoporphyria
pseudoprecocious puberty
pseudopregnancy

pseudoprogeria-Hallermann-Streiff (PHS)
pseudoprogeria syndrome
pseudopseudohypoparathyroidism (PPHP)
pseudopuberty
precocious p.
pseudorabies
pseudoreaction
pseudo-Roth spot
pseudosarcoma
botryoid p.
pseudoscleroderma
pseudosclerosis
pseudoscurvy
pseudoseizure
pseudostrabismus
pseudosubluxation
pseudothalidomide syndrome
pseudotoxemia
pseudotoxoplasmosis syndrome
pseudotrisomy 13 syndrome
pseudotropicalis
Candida p.
pseudotruncus
pseudotuberculosis
Yersinia p.
pseudotumor
p. cerebri
inflammatory p. (IPT)
retinal p.
trophoblastic p.
pseudo-Turner syndrome
pseudo-Ullrich-Turner syndrome
pseudovagina
pseudovaginal perineoscrotal hypospadias (PPSH)
pseudovertigo
pseudo-von Willebrand disease
pseudo-Wernicke syndrome
pseudoxanthoma elasticum
PSF
prostacyclin-stimulating factor
PSG
polysomnogram
polysomnography
PSI
Parental Stress Index
pelvic support index
Physiologic Stability Index
postponing sexual involvement
PSI program
psittaci
Chlamydia p.
psittacosis
PSMF
protein-sparing modified fast
PSMF diet
PSN
pontosubicular neuron necrosis

P

psoas
- p. abscess
- p. hitch procedure
- p. margin
- p. sign

p55 soluble tumor necrosis factor receptor

p75 soluble tumor necrosis factor receptor

psoralen and ultraviolet A (PUVA)

Psorcon

psoriasiform lesion

psoriasis
- classic plaque p.
- generalized pustular p.
- p. guttata
- guttate p.
- plaque-type p.
- p. vulgaris
- vulvar p.

psoriasis-associated arthritis

psoriatic
- p. arthritis
- p. dermatitis
- p. diaper rash

PsoriGel

PSROM
- preterm spontaneous rupture of membranes

PSS
- physiologic salt solution

P&S Shampoo

PSTT
- placental site trophoblastic tumor

PSU
- pediatric sedation unit

PS23 23-valent polysaccharide vaccine

psychedelic drug

psychiatric
- p. diagnostic interview (PDI)
- p. drug
- p. illness

psychiatrics (*var. of* psychiatry)

psychiatrist
- child and adolescent p.

psychiatry, psychiatrics
- American Academy of Child and Adolescent P. (AACAP)
- child and adolescent forensic p.

psychoactive drug

psychodynamic
- p. psychotherapy
- p. therapy

psychogenetic (*var. of* psychogenic)

psychogenic, psychogenetic
- p. arthralgia
- p. cough
- p. cough tic

- p. impotence
- p. limp
- p. pelvic pain
- p. polydipsia
- p. seizure

psychologic (*var. of* psychological)

psychological, psychologic
- p. abuse
- p. comorbidity
- p. distress
- p. effect
- P. General Well-Being (PGWB)
- P. General Well-Being index
- p. nonneuropathic bladder
- p. sex
- p. stress
- p. trauma

psychologist

psychometric
- p. assessment
- p. test

psychometrics (*var. of* psychometry)

psychometrist

psychometry, psychometrics

psychomotor
- p. development index (PDI)
- p. epilepsy
- p. evaluation
- p. retardation
- p. seizure
- p. status

psychopathology
- offspring p.

psychopharmacogenetic

psychopharmacological intervention

psychopharmacology

psychoprophylaxis

psychoses (*pl. of* psychosis)

psychosexual
- p. dysfunction
- p. problem

psychosine lipidosis

psychosis, *pl.* **psychoses**
- brief reactive p.
- climacteric p.
- gestational p.
- involutional p.
- postpartum p.
- puerperal p.
- reactive p.
- symbiotic p.

psychosocial
- p. adjustment
- p. deprivation
- p. development
- p. dwarfism
- p. factor
- p. support
- p. therapy

psychosomatic
    p. complaint
    p. disease
psychostimulant medication
psychother
   psychotherapy
psychotherapy
    cognitive behavioral p.
    nondirective supportive p.
    psychodynamic p.
    supportive p.
psychotic depression
psychotropic drug (PTD)
psyllium
4p syndrome
5p syndrome
9p syndrome
PT
   pertussis toxin
   pertussis toxoid
   physical therapy
   physiotherapy
   primary thrombocythemia
   prothrombin time
      PT coagulation test
PTA
   percutaneous transluminal angioplasty
   peritonsillar abscess
   plasma thromboplastin antecedent
   pure-tone average
PTC
   pulmonary tissue concentration
PTCRA
   percutaneous transluminal coronary
    rotational ablation
PTD
   preterm delivery
   psychotropic drug
P.T.E.-4, -5
PTEN
   pentaerythritol tetranitrate
    PTEN gene
pteridine ring compound
pterin
    synthetic p.
    urinary p.
pteroylglutamic acid
pterygium
    p. colli
    congenital p.
    p. universale
pterygoarthromyodysplasia congenita
PTFL
   posterior talofibular ligament
PTH
   parathyroid hormone
    PTH for osteoporotic women on
    estrogen replacement (POWER)
PTH-derived peptide

Pthirus pubis
PTH-rP, PTHRP, PTHrP
   parathyroid hormone-related
    peptide
PTK gene
PTL
   preterm labor
PTLD
   posttransplant lymphoproliferative
   disease
   posttransplant lymphoproliferative
   disorder
ptoses (*pl. of* ptosis)
ptosis, *pl.* **ptoses**
    bilateral congenital p.
    congenital p.
    Marcus Gunn jaw-winking p.
    p. of eyelids, diastasis recti, hip
     dysplasia
    unilateral congenital p.
    upside-down p.
ptotic areola
PTS
   Pediatric Trauma Score
   Screening Tool for Early Predictors
    of PTSD (STEPP)
PTSD
   posttraumatic stress disorder
PTSS
   posttraumatic signs or
    symptoms
   posttraumatic stress syndrome
PTT
   partial thromboplastin time
PTU
   propylthiouracil
PTX
   pneumothorax
ptyalism
pubarche
    precocious p. (PP)
    premature p.
puberal, pubertal
    p. aberrancy
    p. arrest
    p. change
    p. delay
    p. growth
    p. gynecomastia
    p. milestone
    p. stage
    p. staging
pubertal (*var. of* puberal)
pubertas praecox
puberty
    abnormal p.
    asynchronous p.
    central precocious p. (CPP)
    complete precocious p.

P

puberty (*continued*)
    constitutional delay of p.
    constitutional precocious p.
    delayed p.
    factitious precocious p.
    familial male precocious p.
     (FMPP)
    gonadotropin-dependent precocious p.
    gonadotropin-independent
     precocious p.
    heterosexual precocious p.
    iatrogenic precocious p.
    idiopathic isosexual precocious p.
    incomplete precocious p.
    p. initiation
    isosexual idiopathic precocious p.
    peripheral precocious p.
    physiologic delay of p.
    precocious p.
    pseudoprecocious p.
    true precocious p.
pubescence, pubescency
pubescency (*var. of* pubescence)
pubescent
pubic
    p. arch
    p. hair
    p. hairline
    p. lice
    p. ramus
    p. ramus stress fracture
    p. symphysis
    p. symphysis periostitis
    p. triangle
    p. tubercle
pubiotomy
pubis
    arcuate ligament of p.
    mons p.
    os p.
    osteitis p.
    osteomyelitis p.
    pediculosis p.
    Pthirus p.
    ruptured symphysis p.
    symphysis p.
    widened symphysis p.
public health nurse (PHN)
pubocervical
    p. fascia
    p. ligament
pubococcygeal muscle
  (PCM)
pubococcygeus muscle
puborectalis
    p. muscle
    p. sling
puborectal muscle
pubourethral

pubovaginal
    p. sling procedure
    p. suspension
pubovesical ligament
pubovesicam
    ligamentum p.
pubovisceral muscle
PUBS
    percutaneous umbilical blood sampling
PUD
    peptic ulcer disease
puddle sign
pudenda (*pl. of* pudendum)
pudendal
    p. anesthesia
    p. apron
    p. area
    p. artery
    p. block
    p. canal
    p. hematocele
    p. injection
    p. nerve
    p. nerve terminal motor latency
     (PNTML)
    p. neurogram
    p. neuropathy
    p. sac
pudendi
    frenulum labiorum p.
    labium majus p.
    labium minus p.
    noma p.
pudendum, *pl.* **pudenda**
Pudenz
    P. reservoir
    P. shunt
puerorum
    hydroa p.
puerpera
puerperal
    p. convulsion
    p. eclampsia
    p. endometritis
    p. febrile morbidity
    p. fever
    p. hematoma
    p. infection
    p. inversion
    p. mastitis
    p. period
    p. phlebitis
    p. psychosis
    p. pyemia
    p. sepsis
    p. septicemia
    p. tetanus
puerperant
puerperia (*pl. of* puerperium)

puerperium, *pl.* **puerperia**
PUFA
    polyunsaturated fatty acid
puffiness
    periorbital p.
puff-of-smoke disease
puffy skin
pug nose-peripheral dysostosis syndrome
Pulec and Freedman congenital ear
  abnormality classification
pullback
    catheter p.
pull-down
    testicular p.-d.
pulled elbow
pulling
    hair p.
pull-through, pullthrough
    endorectal p.-t.
    ileoanal p.-t.
    p.-t. procedure
    retrorectal transanal p.-t.
    p.-t. surgery
pullthrough (*var. of* pull-through)
    p. technique
pull-to-sit reflex
pull-up, pullup
pullup (*var. of* pull-up)
    gastric p.
Pulmicort
    P. Respules
    P. Turbuhaler
Pulmo-Aid ventilator
Pulmocare
    P. diet
    P. formula
PulmoMate nebulizer
pulmonale
    cor p.
pulmonary
    p. acinar aplasia
    p. agenesis
    p. alveolar microlithiasis (PAM)
    p. alveolar proteinosis (PAP)
    p. alveolus
    p. angiography
    p. anthrax
    p. arborization
    p. arterial banding
    p. arterial flow
    p. arterial oxygen content
    p. arterial trunk
    p. arteriogram
    p. arteriole
    p. arteriovenous malformation
    (PAVM)
    p. artery (PA)
    p. artery angioplasty
    p. artery atresia

p. artery banding
p. artery catheterization
p. artery/ductus view
p. artery occluded pressure (PAOP)
p. artery pressure monitoring
p. artery sling
p. artery thermodilution
p. artery wedge (PAW)
p. artery wedge pressure (PAWP)
p. ascariasis
p. aspergillosis
p. aspiration
p. atresia with intact ventricular
  septum (PAIVS)
p. bleb
p. blood flow (PBF)
p. branch stenosis
p. bud
p. capillary wedge pressure (PCWP)
p. compliance
p. complication
p. contusion
p. cryptococcosis
p. cyanosis
p. diffusing capacity
p. disorder
p. distress
p. dysmaturity syndrome
p. dysplasia
p. edema
p. ejection click
p. ejection murmur
p. ELF
p. embolism (PE)
p. embolus
p. endometriosis
p. eosinophilia
p. fat embolism
p. function
p. function test (PFT)
p. function testing
p. gangrene
p. hemangiomatosis
p. hemorrhage
p. hemosiderosis
p. histoplasmosis
p. hypertension
p. hypertension of newborn
p. hyperthyroidism
p. hypoplasia
p. immaturity
p. infarction
p. infiltrate
p. infiltrate with eosinophilia (PIE)
p. infiltrate with eosinophilia
  syndrome
p. injury
p. insufficiency
p. insufficiency of prematurity

P

pulmonary (*continued*)
- p. interstitial emphysema (PIE)
- p. interstitial fibrosis
- p. lavage
- p. leukostasis
- p. lymphangiectasia
- p. lymphoid hyperplasia (PLH)
- p. maturation
- p. medicine
- p. metastasis
- p. microvascular permeability to protein (PMVP)
- p. mucormycosis
- p. outflow tract
- p. overcirculation
- p. parenchymal disease
- p. perfusion
- p. plaque
- p. porcine valve
- p. recurrence
- p. resection
- p. resistance
- p. sequestration
- p. shunt
- p. sound
- p. suppuration
- p. surfactant
- p. surfactant protein
- p. thermodilution catheter
- p. thromboembolism
- p. time constant
- p. tissue concentration (PTC)
- p. toilet
- p. tuberculosis
- p. tularemia
- p. undervascularity
- p. valve disease
- p. valve stenosis
- p. vascular bed
- p. vascular congestion
- p. vascular development
- p. vascular marking
- p. vascular resistance (PVR)
- p. vascular restrictive index (PVRI)
- p. vascular tone
- p. vasodilation
- p. vein
- p. venoocclusive disease
- p. venous drainage
- p. venous obstruction
- p. venous oxygen content
- p. ventilation

pulmonic
- p. murmur
- p. regurgitation
- p. stenosis (PS)
- p. valve

pulmonicola
- Pandoraea p.

Pulmozyme
pulp, pulpa
- digital p.
- p. necrosis

pulpa (*var. of* pulp)
pulpal degeneration
pulpectomy
pulsatile
- p. air jet
- p. discharge
- p. fontanelle
- p. GnRH administration
- p. human menopausal gonadotropin
- p. release

pulsatility
- p. index (PI)
- intrinsic p.

pulsating exophthalmos
pulse
- apical p.
- bounding p.
- cutaneous pressure p.
- p. dexamethasone
- dorsalis pedis p.
- p. frequency
- p. interval
- jugular venous p.
- maternal p.
- p. methylprednisolone
- p. oximeter
- p. oximeter sensor N-25 and I-20
- p. oximetry
- p. oximetry waveform systolic blood pressure (POWSBP)
- paradoxical p.
- pedal p.
- posterior tibial p.
- p. pressure
- sharp p.
- p. steroid therapy
- thready p.
- p. volume
- p. width

pulsed
- p. Doppler ultrasound
- p. electromagnetic wave
- p. field gel electrophoresis (PFGE)
- p. intervention

pulsed-wave
- p.-w. Doppler
- p.-w. ultrasound

pulseless
- p. disease
- p. electrical activity
- p. phase

pulselessness
- pain, paresthesia, paresis, pallor, p. (5 Ps)

pulsion
    p. enterocele
    p. theory
pulsus
    p. alternans
    p. bisferiens
    p. paradoxus
pulvinar
Pulvules
    Seromycin P.
pump
    Advanced Collection breast p.
    Barron p.
    Basis breast p.
    battery-operated breast p.
    bilateral breast p.
    breast p.
    Chicco breast p.
    Chid breast p.
    Clarus model 5169 peristaltic p.
    Egnell breast p.
    electric breast p.
    Elmed peristaltic irrigation p.
    EstroGel p.
    Grafco breast p.
    infusion p.
    P. In Style breast pump
    insulin p.
    Kangaroo enteral feeding p.
    Kangaroo infusion p.
    Kendall McGaw Intelligent p.
    KM-1 breast p.
    Lactina Select breast p.
    low-pressure breast p.
    manual breast p.
    Mary Jane breast p.
    MasterFlex fetal perfusion p.
    Medela Dominant vacuum delivery p.
    Medela manual breast p.
    Medfusion 1001 syringe infusion p.
    Mityvac reusable vacuum p.
    Na^+ p.
    pneumocapillary infusion p.
    Salem p.
    servocontrolled ventilation p.
    suction p.
    p. twin
    Unicare breast p.
    Zyklomat infusion p.
punch
    baby Tischler biopsy p.
    Baker p.
    p. biopsy
    p. biopsy forceps
    Eppendorfer biopsy p.
    Keyes dermatologic p.
    Keyes vulvar p.
    Miltex disposable biopsy p.

    p. skin biopsy
    p. tenderness
    Tischler-Morgan biopsy p.
    Townsend biopsy p.
    Wittner biopsy p.
punched-out lytic lesion
puncta (*pl. of* punctum)
punctata
    chondrodysplasia p.
    chondrodystrophia congenita p.
    dysplasia epiphysealis p.
    recessive X-linked chondrodysplasia p.
    rhizomelic chondrodysplasia p. (RCDP)
punctate
    p. epiphyseal dysplasia
    p. epithelial keratitis
    p. hyperkeratosis
    p. lenticular opacity
    p. wheal
punctation
punctum, *pl.* **puncta**
puncture
    accidental dural p.
    arterial p.
    bone marrow p.
    cisternal p.
    lumbar p. (LP)
    pericardial p.
    p. punch site
    subdural p.
    transparenchymal needle p.
    transvaginal amniotic p. (TAP)
    ventricular p.
PUND
    pregnancy, uterine, not delivered
punishment
    corporal p.
Punnett square
pupil
    Adie p.
    Argyll Robertson p.
    cat's eye p.
    conjugate p.
    keyhole p.
    Marcus Gunn p.
    p. reaction
    white p.
pupillae
    ectopia lentis et p.
pupillary
    p. change
    p. light response
    p. membrane
    p. red reflex
    p. syndrome
PUPP
    pruritic urticarial papules and plaques

P

puppet children
puppetlike
    p. appearance
    p. syndrome
PUPPP
    pruritic urticarial papules and plaques
    of pregnancy
puppy position
pure
    p. bulbar poliomyelitis
    p. esophageal atresia
    p. gonadal dysgenesis
    p. random drift
    p. red blood cell aplasia
pureed diet
Puregene DNA extraction system
Puregon
purely sensory polyneuritis
pure-tone average (PTA)
purging
    anorexia nervosa with binging and
    p. (AN-BP)
    p. rate
Puri-Clens
purified
    p. chick embryo cell culture
    (PCEC)
    p. fusion protein (PFP)
    p. gamma globulin
    p. hormone
    p. human factor IX
    p. podophyllotoxin
    p. polysaccharide
    p. protein derivative (PPD)
    p. urinary FSH
    urofollitropin for injection, p.
purine
    p. metabolism
    p. metabolism disorder
    p. nucleoside phosphorylase (PNP)
Purinethol
Puritan swab
Purkinje
    P. cell
    P. cell tumor
    P. fibers
puromycin
purple
    p. hallux
    p. hue
    p. toes syndrome
Purpose cream
purpura
    alloimmune neonatal
    thrombocytopenic p.
    anaphylactic p.
    anaphylactoid p.
    autoimmune thrombocytopenic p.
    (AITP)

childhood idiopathic
    thrombocytopenic p.
drug-related p.
p. fulminans
p. hemorrhagica
Henoch-Schönlein p. (HSP)
idiopathic thrombocytopenic p. (ITP)
immune thrombocytopenic p. (ITP)
maternal idiopathic thrombocytopenic
    p. (MITP)
neonatal alloimmune
    thrombocytopenic p. (NATP)
neonatal isoimmune
    thrombocytopenic p.
palpable p.
Schönlein-Henoch p.
thrombocytopenic p.
thrombotic p.
thrombotic thrombocytopenic p.
    (TTP)
vascular p.
wet p.
purpuric
    p. light eruption
    p. rash
purse
    shepherd's p.
purse-string
    p.-s. mouth
    p.-s. suture
Purtilo syndrome
Purtscher retinopathy
purulent
    p. arthritis
    p. conjunctivitis
    p. meningitis
    p. nasal discharge
    p. pericarditis
    p. pharyngitis
    p. rhinitis
    p. sputum
    p. venous thrombosis
purulenta
    lochia p.
pus
    p. burrow
    sterile p.
    p. tube
pusher
    Endo-Assist endoscopic knot p.
    knot p.
    MetraTie knot p.
    Ranfac knot p.
pustular
    p. melanosis
    p. varicella
pustule
    neonatal p.
    satellite p.

pustulosa
    miliaria p.
    varicella p.
pustulosis
    infantile p.
    Malassezia furfur p.
    nonfollicular p.
    palmar p.
    p. palmaris
    p. palmaris et plantaris (PPP)
    palmoplantar p. (PPP)
    staphylococcal p.
    p. vacciniformis acuta
putamen
putrefaciens
    Alteromonas p.
putrescence
putrescine
PUV
    posterior urethral valve [type I-IV]
PUVA
    psoralen and ultraviolet A
    PUVA phototherapy
Puzo endoscopic cancer findings method
PVC
    premature ventricular contraction
P.V. Carpine Liquifilm
PVDF
    polyvinylidene fluoride
PVEL
    periventricular echolucency
PVH
    periventricular hemorrhage (grade 1–4)
PVL
    periventricular leukomalacia
    plasma viral load
        cystic PVL
PVO
    portal vein obstruction
PVP
    penicillin V potassium
    polyvinylpyrrolidone
    PVP solution
PVR
    postvoid residual
    pulmonary vascular resistance
PVRI
    pulmonary vascular restrictive index
PVS
    Partner Violence Screen
    persistent vegetative state
P-wave axis
PWM
    pokeweed mitogen
PWS
    Prader-Willi syndrome
PWSCR
    Prader-Willi syndrome critical region

pycnodysostosis
Pycnogenol
pyelectasia (*var. of* pyelectasis)
pyelectasis, pyelectasia
    fetal p.
pyelitis
pyelocaliectasis
pyelogram, pyeloureterogram
    dragon p.
    intravenous p. (IVP)
    limited-exposure intravenous p.
    retrograde p.
    single-shot intravenous p.
    washout p.
pyelography, pelviureteroradiography
    intravenous p. (IVP)
    retrograde p.
pyelonephritis
    acute p.
    antepartum p.
    hereditary interstitial p.
    p. in exenteration
    nonobstructive p.
    xanthogranulomatous p.
pyelophlebitis
    portal p.
pyeloplasty, pelvioplasty
pyelostomy
    cutaneous p.
pyeloureterogram (*var. of* pyelogram)
pyemia
    puerperal p.
pygoamorphus
pygodidymus
pygomelus
pygopagus
pyknocyte
pyknocytosis
    infantile p.
pyknodysostosis syndrome
pyknoepilepsy, pyknolepsy
pyknolepsy (*var. of* pyknoepilepsy)
pyknotic cell
Pyle
    bone age standard of Greulich and P.
    P. disease
    P. syndrome
pylephlebitis
pylori (*pl. of* pylorus)
pyloric
    p. atresia
    p. mass
    p. nitric oxide synthase
    p. olive
    p. sphincter relaxation
    p. stenosis
    p. string sign

P

pyloromyotomy
> Ramstedt p.
> Ramstedt-Fredet p.

pyloroplasty
> Heineke-Mikulicz p.

pylorospasm

pylorus, *pl.* **pylori**
> *Campylobacter pylori*
> congenital double p.
> double p.
> *Helicobacter pylori*
> PYtest for *Helicobacter pylori*

pyocolpocele

pyocolpos

pyoderma
> p. alopecia
> blastomycosis-like p.
> p. gangrenosum
> streptococcal p.
> p. vegetans

pyoderma-associated nephritis

pyogenes
> *Actinomyces p.*
> *Staphylococcus p.*
> *Streptococcus p.*

pyogenetic (*var. of* pyogenic)

pyogenic, pyogenetic, pyogenous
> p. abscess
> p. arthritis
> p. bacteria
> p. granuloma
> p. infection
> p. lymphadenitis
> p. mediastinitis
> p. meningitis
> p. osteomyelitis
> p. salpingitis

pyogenicum

pyogenous (*var. of* pyogenic)

pyogranulomatous response

pyometra

pyometritis

pyomyoma
> uterine p.

pyomyositis
> tropical p.

pyoovarium

Pyopen

pyophysometra

pyopneumothorax
> iatrogenic p.

pyosalpingitis

pyosalpingo-oophoritis

pyosalpingo-oothecitis

pyosalpinx

pramid
> Food Guide P.

pyramidal
> p. cerebral palsy

> p. lesion
> p. tract
> p. tract disease
> p. tract sign

pyramidalis muscle

pyrantel pamoate

pyrazinamide

pyrethrins and piperonyl butoxide

pyrethroid

pyrethrum extract

pyrexia
> maternal p.
> procedure-related p.

Pyribenzamine

Pyridiate

pyridinoline

Pyridium

pyridostigmine bromide

pyridoxal
> p. 5-phosphate
> p. phosphate

pyridoxine
> p. deficiency
> p. dependency

pyridoxine-dependency syndrome

pyridoxine-dependent seizure

pyridoxine-refractory sideroblastic anemia

pyridoxine-responsive anemia

pyrilamine maleate

Pyrilinks-D assay

pyrimethamine
> sulfadoxine and p.

pyrimethamine-sulfadoxine

pyrimidine

Pyrinex Pediculicide Shampoo

Pyrinyl
> P. II Liquid
> P. Plus Shampoo

pyrogen
> endogenous p.

pyrogenicity

pyroglutamic acidemia

Pyronema domesticum

pyrophosphate
> 5-phospho-alpha-d-ribosyl p. (PRPP)
> plasma inorganic p.

pyrophosphorylase

pyropoikilocytosis
> hereditary p. (HPP)

pyrosis

pyrroloporphyria

pyruvate
> p. decarboxylase
> p. dehydrogenase
> p. dehydrogenase complex (PDHC)
> p. dehydrogenation
> p. kinase (PK)
> p. kinase deficiency

pyruvic acid
6-pyruvoyl tetrahydropteridine
  synthetase
pyrvinium pamoate
PYtest for *Helicobacter pylori*
pyuria

amicrobic p.
sterile p.

PZ
  proliferative zone
PZD
  partial zona dissection

P

q
    long arm of chromosome
Q
    quotient
        Q angle
        Q band
        Q fever
21q
    tetrasomy 21q
Q10, Q-10
    coenzyme Q_{10} (CoQ_{10})
22q11
    microdeletion of chromosome
        22q11
QCT
    quantitative computed tomography
22q11.2 deletion syndrome
QDR
    quantitative digital radiography
QDR-1500 bone densitometer
qEEG
    quantitative electroencephalography
Qf
    rate of fluid filtration
QIAamp Tissue kit
QNS
    quantity not sufficient
QOL
    quality of life
qr
    quadriradial
QS complex
Qs/Qt
    intrapulmonary shunt ratio
    right-to-left shunt ratio
QT
    cardiac output
        QT interval
QTc prolongation
Q-test ovulation predictor
QTest Strep test
Q-tip
    Q-t. test
    Q-t. test for determining urethral
        mobility
QTL
    quantitative trait locus
QT-Watch messaging wristwatch
quadrant
    q. assessment
    left lower q. (LLQ)
    left upper q. (LUQ)
    right lower q. (RLQ)
    right upper q. (RUQ)
4-quadrant assessment

quadrantectomy, axillary dissection,
  radiation therapy (QUART)
quadrate hepatic lobe
quadratum
    caput q.
quadratus labiae superioris muscle
quadriceps femoris muscle biopsy
quadrigemina
    corpora q.
quadripara
quadriparesis
    flaccid q.
    spastic q.
quadriplegia
    spastic q.
    transient q.
quadriplegic
quadriradial (qr)
quadrivalent human papillomavirus
  type 6, 11, 16, 18
quadruped
quadruple-contrast study
quadruple screen
quadruplet
qualitative
    q. detection kit
    q. developmental assessment
    q. disorder
    q. urine screen
quality
    q. assurance process
    q. of life (QOL)
    q. of life in persons with urinary
        incontinence (I-QOL)
    q. of life issue
    Q. of Upper Extremities Test
        (QUEST)
Quan-Smith syndrome
quantification
    q. of fetal activity
    Pelvic Organ Prolapse Q. (POP-Q)
Quantikine
    Q. human IL-6 Immunoassay
    Q. IVD
quantitation
    amniotic fluid q.
    pelvic organ prolapse q.
quantitative
    q. analysis of fat content
    q. beta hCG level
    q. Bethesda assay
    q. computed tomography (QCT)
    q. digital radiography (QDR)
    q. disorder
    q. electroencephalography (qEEG)

quantitative (*continued*)
    q. immunoglobulin
    q. inheritance
    q. insulin sensitivity check index
      (QUICKI)
    q. intradermal skin test
    q. serum drug assay
    q. sudomotor axon-reflex test
    q. trait locus (QTL)
    q. ultrasound (QUS)
quantity
    q. not sufficient (QNS)
    sufficient q.
Quantum 2000 electrosurgical system
quarantine
QUART
    quadrantectomy, axillary dissection,
    radiation therapy
quarternary ammonium ion
quarter-strength formula
quartipara
Quarzan
quasicontinuous inheritance
quasidiploid
quasidominance
Queckenstedt test
Queensland
    Q. fever
    Q. tick typhus
Quelicin
query fever
QUEST
    Quality of Upper Extremities Test
question
    HEADS q.
    procedures, alternatives, risk and q.'s
      (PARQ)
questionnaire
    Achenbach q.
    Ages and Stages Q. (ASQ)
    attitude behavior q. (ABQ)
    autism spectrum screening q.
      (ASSQ)
    BFLUTS q.
    child health q. (CHQ)
    childhood trauma q. (CTQ)
    Conners Abbreviated Parent Q.
    Denver Home Screening Q.
    Dominic-R q.
    Q. for Identifying Children with
      Chronic Conditions (QuICCC)
    Harter self-esteem q.
    HRQOL q.
    human health and behavior q.
      (HBQ)
    Incontinence Impact Q. (IIQ)
    Incontinence Stress Q. (ISQ)
    Inflammatory Bowel Disease Q.
      (IBDQ)

    King's Health Q.
    Multidimensional Personality Q.
      (MPQ)
    PARS III q.
    Pediatric Asthma Quality of Life Q.
      (PAQLQ)
    Reynolds suicide ideation q.
    Seasonal Pattern Assessment Q.
      (SPAQ)
    SF-36 Health Status q.
    Terry q.
    Wolraich q.
questionnaire-revised
    Incontinence Impact Q.-R.
      (IIQ-R)
Questran
    Q. Light
    Q. powder
Quetelet body mass index
quetiapine fumarate
Queyrat
    Q. erythroplasia
    erythroplasia of Q.
Quibron-T
Quibron-T/SR
QuICCC
    Questionnaire for Identifying Children
      with Chronic Conditions
quickening
QUICKI
    quantitative insulin sensitivity check
    index
quick-relief medication
Quick test
Quickvue
    Q. A+B differentiated flu test
    Q. *Chlamydia* test
    Q. In-Line one-step Strep A test
    Q. one-step hCG-Combo pregnancy
      test
    Q. one-step hCG-urine test
    Q. *One-Step H. pylori* test
    Q. UrinChek 10+ urine test strip
Quidel group B strep test
quiescence
    uterine q.
quiescent endometrium
quiet
    q. alertness
    q. and alert state
    q. precordium
    q. sleep
QuietTrak monitor
Quik Connect fetal monitor
Quikheel lancet
QuikPac-II OneStep hCG pregnancy test
quinacrine
    q. banding
    q. hydrochloride

Q

Quinaglute Dura-Tabs
quinalbarbitone sodium
quinate
quinestrol
quinethazone
quingestanol acetate
Quinidex Extentabs
quinidine gluconate
quinine
    q. dihydrochloride
    q. sulfate
quinolinic acid
quinolone
Quinones uterine-grasping forceps
quinquefasciatus
    Culex q.
Quinsana Plus Tropical
quinsy
quintana
    Bartonella q.

quintessence
quintipara
Quinton dual-lumen catheter
quintuplet
quintuple-X syndrome
quinupristin
Quips genetic imaging system
quivering
    chin q.
quotidian fever
quotient
    developmental q. (DQ)
    developmental motor q. (DMQ)
    Griffith General Q.
    intelligence q. (IQ)
    mean developmental q.
    respiratory q.
    ventilation/perfusion q.
QUS
    quantitative ultrasound

R
  radius
  roentgen
    R band
RA
  rheumatoid arthritis
^{226}**Ra**
  radium-226
RAA
  right aortic arch
Raaf catheter
RAB
  remote afterloading brachytherapy
RABA
  radioantigen-binding assay
rabbit nose
rabeprazole
rabies
  r. immunoglobulin (RIG)
  paralytic r.
  r. prophylaxis
  r. vaccine
  r. vaccine, absorbed (RVA)
Rabson-Mendenhall syndrome
raccoon eyes
racemic
  r. ephedrine
  r. epinephrine
racemose form
Racephedrine
rachiopagus, rachipagus
rachipagus (*var. of* rachiopagus)
rachischisis
  craniospinal r.
  r. partialis
  r. posterior
  thoracolumbar r.
  r. totalis
rachitic
  r. bone deformity
  r. change
  r. metaphysis
  r. rosary
rachitis fetalis
racial difference
RAD
  reactive airways disease
radial
  r. aplasia-thrombocytopenia syndrome
  r. arterial catheter
  r. arterial line
  r. artery
  r. artery catheter
  r. artery catheterization
  r. clubhand

  r. curettage
  r. digital grasp
  r. dysplasia
  r. epiphysis
  r. head dislocation
  r. head fracture
  r. head osteochondritis
  r. head subluxation (RHS)
  r. jaw biopsy forceps
  r. neck fracture
  r. nerve block
  r. palmar grasp
  pelvic r.
  r. physis
  r. ray aplasia
  r. ray defect
  renal, ear, anal, r. (REAR)
  r. scar
  r. sclerosing lesion
radial-femoral delay
radial-renal syndrome
radiant warmer
radiata
  corona r.
radiation
  r. absorbed dose (rad)
  adaptive r.
  r. carcinogenesis
  r. cystitis
  r. danger
  diagnostic r.
  r. dose
  r. dose limit
  r. dysplasia
  electromagnetic r.
  r. encephalopathy
  r. exposure
  external photon beam r.
  IF r.
  intraoperative r.
  intrauterine r.
  intravaginal r.
  involved-field r.
  ionizing r.
  r. necrosis
  nuclear r.
  r. of discomfort
  orthovoltage r.
  particulate r.
  pelvic r.
  r. pneumonitis
  postoperative pelvic r.
  state-of-the-art r.
  supervoltage r.
  r. syndrome

radiation (*continued*)
r. therapy (RT)
tissue tolerance to r.
r. tolerance
whole abdominal r.
radiation-induced
r.-i. heart disease (RIHD)
r.-i. physial injury
radical
r. abdominal hysterectomy
r. excision
free r.
free hydroxyl r.
hydroxyl r. (OH)
intrarenal venous r.
r. local excision
r. mastectomy
oxygen-free r.
r. parametrectomy
r. posteromedial and plantar release
(RPMPR)
superoxide r.
r. surgery
r. surgical therapy
r. vaginal trachelectomy
r. vulvectomy
radicular neuropathy
radiculitis
dorsal r.
radiculomyelitis
acute ascending r.
ascending r.
radiculoneuritis
Lyme r.
radii (*pl. of* radius)
radioactive
r. applicator
r. cobalt
r. colloid
r. element
r. gold
r. immunoassay
r. implant
r. iodine ablation
r. isotope
r. microsphere
r. ribbons
r. seed
r. seed implantation
r. substance
r. tracer
r. uptake
radioallergosorbent test (RAST)
radioantigen-binding assay (RABA)
radiobiology
radiocisternography
radiocontrast material
radiocurable
radiodermatitis

radiofibrinogen uptake scan
radiofrequency
r. ablation (RFA)
r. catheter ablation (RFCA)
r. interstitial tissue ablation system
(RITA)
radiogram
sinus r.
radiograph
abdominal r.
cephalometric r.
chest r.
flat abdominal r.
frogleg lateral r.
intercondylar r.
lateral r.
Lauenstein lateral r.
oblique r.
occlusal r.
panoramic r.
plain abdominal r.
scout r.
serial r.
single-exposure r.
sinus r.
skyline view r.
stress view r.
upright abdominal r.
radiographic
r. absorptiometry
r. bone strength index (RBSI)
r. density
r. pelvimetry
radiography
chest r.
digital r.
quantitative digital r. (QDR)
stereotactic r.
tunnel-view r.
radioimmunoassay (RIA)
Raji cell r.
solid-phase r.
radioimmunodetection (RAID)
**radioimmunoprecipitation assay
(RIPA)**
radioimmunosorbent test (RIST)
radioiodination
radioiodine ablative therapy
radioisotope
r. angiography
r. cisternography
r. milk scan
**radioisotopic reperfusion and excretion
study**
radiolabeled
r. fibrinogen
r. white blood cell scan
radiological examination
radiologic stigmata

radiologist
 pediatric r.
radiology
 American College of R.
 (ACR)
radiolucent
 r. circular shadow in bladder
 r. line
radiomutation
radionuclide
 r. bone scan
 r. cineangiography
 r. heart scan
 r. imaging
 r. scanning
 r. scintigraphy
 r. venography
 r. voiding cystography
 (RVC)
radiopaque
 r. guidewire
 r. marker
radioreceptor assay
radioreceptor-guided surgery
radio-reno-ocular syndrome
radioresistant yolk sac tumor
radiosensitivity
radiosensitization
radiosurgery
 stereotactic r.
radiotherapy
 abdominal strip r.
 adjuvant r.
 fractionated sterotactic r.
 hyperfractionated r.
 pelvic boost r.
 plaque r.
 postoperative r.
 split-course hyperfractionated r.
radiotracer
radioulnar synostosis
radium
 r. implant
 intracavitary r. (ICR)
radium-226 (^{226}Ra)
radius (R), *pl.* **radii**
 absent r.
 hypoplastic r.
 thrombocytopenia absent r.
 (TAR)
RADIUS
 routine antenatal diagnostic imaging
 with ultrasound
 RADIUS trial
radon-222 (^{222}Rn)
Radovici
 R. reflex
 R. sign
raf protooncogene

RAG
 recombinase activating gene
 RAG deficiency
rage
 violent r.
ragged
 r. red fiber (RRF)
 r. red myopathy
ragweed pollen
RAID
 radioimmunodetection
railroad
 r. nystagmus
 r. track line
Raimondi catheter
Raine syndrome
raised
 r. lesion
 r. raspberry-like papilloma
 r. red-black telangiectasia
Raji
 R. cell
 R. cell assay
 R. cell radioimmunoassay
rale
 coarse r.
 crackling r.
 crepitant r.
 wet r.
raloxifene
 Study of Tamoxifen and R. (STAR)
RALPH
 renal, anus, lung, polydactyly,
 hamartoblastoma
 RALPH syndrome
Ralstonia pickettii
Rambam-Hasharon syndrome
rami (*pl. of* ramus)
ramipril
Ramon syndrome
ramosum
 Clostridium r.
Ramsay Hunt syndrome (I–III)
Ramses Condom
Ramstedt
 R. disease
 R. operation
 R. procedure
 R. pyloromyotomy
Ramstedt-Fredet pyloromyotomy
ramus, *pl.* **rami**
 infrapubic r.
 ischiopubic r.
 pubic r.
 superior r.
rancid butter syndrome
Randall
 R. stone forceps
 R. suction curette

random · rash

random
- r. mating
- r. regression model
- r. sampling
- r. X inactivation

randomization
randomized
randomly amplified polymorphic DNA
Ranfac knot pusher
range
- cervical tissue impedance r.
- chromatofocusing pH r.
- r. loss
- r. of motion (ROM)

range-gated Doppler (RGD)
ranitidine hydrochloride
RANS
- retinal arterial narrowing and straightening

Ranson criteria
RANTES
- regulated upon activation, normal T-cell expressed and secreted

ranula
RAO
- right anterior oblique

RAP
- receptor-associated protein
- recurrent abdominal pain
- right atrial pressure

rapamycin
rape
- r. crisis evaluation
- date r.
- r. evidence
- r. evidence kit
- r. kit use
- marital r.
- r. protocol
- statutory r.
- stranger r.
- r. trauma syndrome
- r. treatment

raphe, rhaphe
- anococcygeal r.
- fused r.
- median r.
- r. of scrotum
- perineal r.

rapid
- r. acquisition with resolution enhancement (RARE)
- r. alternating movement
- r. antigen detection test
- r. blinking
- r. bone loss
- r. descent
- r. dissolution formula
- r. eye movement (REM)

- r. eye movement sleep (REMS)
- r. filter testing
- r. filter testing for bacteriuria
- r. Giemsa test
- r. plasma reagin (RPR)
- r. plasma reagin card test
- r. rehydration
- r. sequence induction
- r. sequence intubation (RSI)
- r. shallow breathing index (RSBI)
- r. slide test
- R. Strep screen
- r. strep test
- r. succession movement
- r. UF

rapidly
- first abarelix depot study for treating endometriosis r. (FASTER)
- r. progressive glomerulonephritis

rapid-onset dystonia, parkinsonism
Rapirun test
rapist
Rapp-Hodgkin
- R.-H. ectodermal dysplasia
- R.-H. ectodermal dysplasia syndrome

RARE
- rapid acquisition with resolution enhancement

rare-cutter enzyme
rarefaction
rarefying osteitis
RARS
- refractory anemia with ring sideroblasts

RA27/3 rubella strain
RAS
- renin-angiotensin system

rasa
- tabula r.

rash
- allergic diaper r.
- ampicillin r.
- angiectatic skin r.
- atopic diaper r.
- blueberry muffin r.
- butterfly r.
- candidal diaper r.
- collarette of r.
- r. crop
- diaper r.
- diffuse morbilliform r.
- discoid r.
- drug-induced r.
- ECM r.
- eczematoid skin r.
- eczematous r.
- erythematous r.
- evanescent maculopapular r.
- friction diaper r.

R

heliotrope r.
irritation diaper r.
macular r.
maculopapular r.
malar r.
monilial diaper r.
morbilliform skin r.
net-like r.
nonvesicular r.
papular r.
papulosquamous r.
pellagra-like skin r.
perioral r.
petechial r.
plaquelike r.
polymorphous r.
pruritic r.
psoriatic diaper r.
purpuric r.
roseola r.
salmon-pink r.
sandpaper r.
scarlatiniform r.
seborrheic diaper r.
skin r.
slapped cheek r.
truncal r.
Rashkind
R. atrial septostomy procedure
R. balloon
R. balloon atrial septostomy
Rasmussen
R. encephalitis
R. syndrome
raspberry
r. spot
r. tongue
raspberry-like papilloma
RAST
radioallergosorbent test
Rastelli
R. operation
R. right ventricle and pulmonary
artery conduit procedure
R. transposition of great arteries
repair
rat-bite fever
rate
aldosterone excretion r. (AER)
basal metabolic r. (BMR)
baseline fetal heart r.
baseline variability of fetal heart r.
beat-to-beat variability of fetal
heart r.
birth r.
cerebral metabolic r.
contraceptive failure r.
cumulative conception r. (CCR)
detection r.

erythrocyte sedimentation r. (ESR)
fertility r.
fetal death r.
fetal heart r. (FHR)
flow r.
glomerular filtration r. (GFR)
glucose production r. (GPR)
growth r.
heart r. (HR)
infant mortality r. (IMR)
maternal death r.
maternal mortality r. (MMR)
metabolic clearance r. (MCR)
monthly fecundity r. (MFR)
mortality r.
neonatal mortality r. (NMR)
nipple flow r.
r. of fluid filtration
ovulation r.
peak expiratory flow r. (PEFR)
peak flow r. (PFR)
perinatal mortality r. (PMR, PNMR)
prevalence r.
purging r.
recurrence r.
resting metabolic r. (RMR)
sedimentation r.
seroprevalence r.
sinusoidal fetal heart r.
sinusoidal heart r. (SHR)
stillbirth r. (SBR)
survival r.
ventricular response r.
Rathke pouch
rating
Apgar r.
sexual maturity r. (SMR)
Tanner sex maturity r.
ratio
arterial to alveolar oxygen tension
r.
Ca/Cr r.
calcium-creatinine r.
cardiothoracic r.
CD4/CD8 r.
cerebral-placental r.
corpus-to-cervix r.
cough pressure transmission r.
crude risk r.
estrogen-progesterone r.
expiratory-to-inspiratory r.
HC/AC r.
intensity-duration r.
intensity-time r.
international normalized r. (INR)
intrapulmonary shunt r. (Qs/Qt)
I-to-E r.
lecithin/sphingomyelin r.
L/S r.

ratio (*continued*)
    lung-to-head r.
    milk-plasma r.
    odds r.
    ornithine to citrulline r.
    oxygen extraction r.
    placental-to-fetal weight r.
    protein-to-urine creatinine r.
    right-to-left shunt r. (Qs/Qt)
    risk-benefit r.
    S/D r.
    sex r.
    standardized incidence r. (SIR)
    testosterone/dihydrotestosterone r.
    triene-to-tetraene r.
    umbilical artery pulsatility index to middle cerebral artery pulsatility index r.
    umbilical velocity r.
    upper body segment to lower body segment r.
    urinary lactate-creatinine r.
    variance r.
    ventilation/perfusion r.
    waist-hip r.
    zinc protoporphyrin to heme r.
rationalize
rattle
    death r.
rat tooth pickups
Rauber layer
raven
    R. IQ
    R. Progressive Matrices (RPM)
Ravitch pectus excavatum repair procedure
RAW
    airway resistance
raw score
ray
    beta r.
    gamma r.
    intercalary defect of pollical r.
    pollical r.
Rayleigh-Tyndall scattering
Raynaud
    R. disease
    R. phenomenon (RP)
    R. sign
    R. syndrome
Ray-Tec sponge
Raz
    R. bladder neck suspension
    R. sling procedure
Raz-Leach procedure
Razoxane
RBBB
    right bundle branch block

RBC
    red blood count
        RBC adenosine deaminase level
        RBC P antigen
RBF
    renal blood flow
RBM **gene**
RBSI
    radiographic bone strength index
RCC
    renal cell carcinoma
RCCA
    right common carotid artery
RCDP
    rhizomelic chondrodysplasia punctata
        RCDP syndrome
RCF
    Ross carbohydrate-free
        RCF formula
RCM
    restrictive cardiomyopathy
RCMAS
    Revised Children's Manifest Anxiety Scale
RCS
    repeat cesarean section
RD
    respiratory distress
RDA
    recommended daily allowance
    recommended dietary allowance
    right ductus arteriosus
RDEB
    recessive dystrophic epidermolysis bullosa
RDF
    rapid dissolution formula
        Adriamycin RDF
RDFC
    recurring digital fibroma of childhood
RD1000 resuscitator
RDS
    respiratory distress syndrome
        neonatal RDS
RDW
    red blood cell distribution width
REA
    rollerball endometrial ablation
reabsorption
reactant
    acute-phase r.
Reactine
reaction
    acetowhite r.
    acrosome r.
    acute transfusion r.
    adverse drug r. (ADR)
    adverse food r.

anaphylactic r.
anaphylactoid r.
anorectic r.
arbitrarily primed polymerase
  chain r.
Arthus r.
association r.
automatic movement r.
balance r.
biphasic anaphylactic r.
bullous r.
chain r.
*Chlamydia trachomatis ligase*chain r.
circular r.
coccidioidin r.
conversion r.
cortical r.
decidual r.
delayed transfusion r.
dermatophytid r.
diazo r.
dysphoric r.
dystonic r.
early asthmatic r.
equilibrium r.
febrile nonhemolytic transfusion r.
Felix-Weil r. (FWR)
ferric chloride r.
fetomaternal transfusion r.
fungal id r.
gliotic r.
Gomori trichrome r.
harlequin r.
hypersensitivity r.
id r.
immediate hypersensitivity r.
immunologic r.
insect sting r.
intrusive stress r.
inverse polymerase chain r.
Jarisch-Herxheimer r.
Köbner r.
laser r.
late asthmatic r.
leukemoid r.
ligase chain r. (LCR)
linear Koebner r.
Mitsuda r.
mixed agglutination r. (MAR)
modified Gomori trichrome r.
neonatal leukemoid r.
nonhemolytic r.
paradoxical pupil r.
Paul-Bunnell r.
periosteal r.
photoallergic r.
phototoxic r.
polymerase chain r. (PCR)
Porter-Silber r.

postural r.
primary circular r.
prokaryotic r.
pupil r.
reverse transcription polymerase
  chain r. (RT-PCR)
righting r.
secondary circular r.
serum sickness-like r.
Shwartzman r.
single primer amplification r.
startle r.
Staudinger r.
stranger r.
stress r.
transfusion r.
twin-to-twin transfusion r.
urine ligase chain r.
vagal r.
van den Bergh r.
Weil-Felix r.
wheal and flare r.
zona r.

reactivation tuberculosis
reactive
  r. adenopathy
  r. airway
  r. airways disease (RAD)
  r. arthritis
  r. attachment disorder of infancy or
    early childhood
  cold r.
  r. epilepsy
  r. fibrosis
  r. nonstress test
  r. oxygen species (ROS)
  r. perforating collagenosis (RPC)
  r. psychosis
  r. site (RS)
  r. site mutation
  warm r.
reactivity
  fetal heart rate r.
  skin test r. (STR)
  substance P immune r.
  vascular r.
reactogenicity
reader
  AutoPap r.
  Papnet r.
readiness
  fetal lung r.
  Pediatric Examination of Educational
    R. (PEER)
reading
  r. disability
  r. frame
reagent
  antiimmunoglobulin r.

reagent (*continued*)
    r. strip
    TRIzol r.
reagin
    rapid plasma r. (RPR)
reality
    R. condom
    R. vaginal pouch
real-time
    r.-t. B-scanner
    r.-t. echocardiography
    r.-t. imaging on ultrasound
    r.-t. sonography
    r.-t. ultrasonography
reanastomosis
    microsurgical tubal r. (MTR)
    tubal r.
    tubocornual r.
REAR
    renal, ear, anal, radial
    REAR syndrome
rearfoot
    r. valgus
    r. varus
rearing parents
rearrangement
    balanced chromosome r.
    balanced parental chromosome r.
    de novo balanced chromosome r.
    parental chromosome r.
reassignment
    gender r.
rebelliousness
rebound
    behavioral r.
    bromocriptine r.
    r. dermatitis
    r. edema
    r. hyperglycemia
    r. hypertension
    r. phenomenon
    r. tenderness
recalcitrant condyloma
recall phenomenon
Récamier
    Ré. operation
    Ré. uterine curettage procedure
recanalization
    tubal r.
receiver operating characteristic (ROC)
receptive
    r. aphasia
    r. language
    r. language development
receptive-expressive
    R.-E. Emergent Language Scale (REEL)
    R.-E. Emergent Language Scale, 2nd Edition (REEL-2)

receptivity
    vaginal r.
receptor
    activated estrogen r.
    adrenergic r.
    alpha-adrenergic r.
    alpha-chemokine r.
    androgen r.
    r. assay
    AT1 r.
    AT2 r.
    beta r.
    beta-adrenergic r.
    beta-chemokine r.
    calcitonin r.
    complement r.
    cough r.
    r. coupling
    r. cross talk
    endogenous opiate r.
    endometrial r.
    epidermal growth factor r. (EGFR)
    E-rosette r.
    estradiol r.
    estrogen r. (ER)
    fibroblast growth factor r. (FGFR)
    fibroblast growth factor r. 3
    fibronectin r.
    r. for hyaluronan-mediated motility
    G-protein-coupled r.
    granulocyte colony-stimulating factor r. (G-CSF-R)
    growth hormone r. (GHR)
    H1 r.
    hormone complex r.
    human EP1 r.
    iC3b r.
    r. internalization
    intracellular progesterone r.
    irritant r.
    J pulmonary r.
    keratinocyte growth factor r. (KGFR)
    leptin r.
    ligand r.
    Notch r.
    opiate r.
    progesterone r. (PgR, PR)
    p55 soluble tumor necrosis factor r.
    p75 soluble tumor necrosis factor r.
    soluble tumor necrosis factor r.
    steroid hormone r.
    testosterone r.
    transferrin r. (TfR)
    type A IL-8 r.
    type B IL-8 r.
    tyrosine kinase r.
    vitamin D r. (VDR)

receptor-associated protein (RAP)
receptor-mediated endocytosis
recess
    epitympanic r.
    suprapineal r.
recession
    sternal r.
recessive
    r. allele
    autosomal r. (AR)
    r. deafness-onychodystrophy
      syndrome
    r. disorder
    r. disorder defect
    r. dystrophic epidermolysis bullosa
      (RDEB)
    r. enhanced S-cone syndrome
    r. gene
    r. inheritance
    r. Leber congenital amaurosis
    peroneal atrophy, X-linked r.
    r. trait
    r. Usher syndrome
    X-linked r. (XLR)
    r. X-linked chondrodysplasia
      punctata
rechallenge
recidivism, recidivity
recidivity (*var. of* recidivism)
recipient twin
reciprocal
    r. cross
    r. gene
    r. movement
    r. translocation
reciprocating
    r. gait
    r. gait orthosis (RGO)
recirculation
    enterohepatic r.
Recklinghausen
    R. disease (type I, II)
    R. tumor
Reclomide
Reclus disease
recognition
    facial affect r.
recognizable viral syndrome (RVS)
recoil
    arm r.
Recombigen assay
recombinant
    r. antihemophilic factor
    r. chromosome 8 syndrome
    r. clone
    r. DNA
    r. DNA technique
    r. DNA technology
    r. enzyme

    r. enzyme replacement therapy
    r. factor VIIa
    r. follicle stimulating hormone
      (rFSH)
    r. FSH preparation
    r. hepatitis B immunization series
    r. hepatitis B vaccine
    r. human erythropoietin (r-EPO,
      rHuEPO)
    r. human growth hormone (rhGH)
    r. human insulin-like growth factor-1
      (rhIGF-1)
    r. human MIP-1 alpha
    r. human superoxide dismutase
      (rhSOD)
    r. immunosorbent assay (RIBA)
    r. inbred strain
    r. interleukin 2 (rIL-2)
    r. OspA
    r. outer surface protein A
      (rOspA)
    r. substitution line
    r. tissue type plasminogen activator
      (rt-PA)
recombinase activating gene (RAG)
Recombinate
recombination
    r. fraction
    r. frequency
    homologous r.
    r. map
Recombivax
    R. HB
    R. HB immunization
recommendation
    diet r.
    exercise r.
    Rotterdam consensus r.
    screening r.
    treatment r.
recommended
    r. daily allowance (RDA)
    r. dietary allowance (RDA)
reconfiguration for neovagina
reconstitute
reconstitution
reconstruction
    Abbe-McIndoe vaginal r.
    autologous r.
    cleft lip-nasal r.
    Dibbell cleft lip-nasal r.
    fascial r.
    laryngotracheal r.
    nonautologous r.
    right ventricular outflow tract r.
    transvaginal ultrasound-guided
      urethral r.
    umbilicus r.
    uterine r.

reconstruction (*continued*)
    ventricular outflow tract r.
    Young-Dees-Leadbetter bladder
      neck r.
reconstructive
    r. mammaplasty
    r. pelvic surgery
record
    antenatal r.
    daily fetal movement r.
      (DFMR)
    delivery r.
    Infant Behavior R. (IBR)
    medical r. (MR)
    women-held antenatal r.
recorder
    Digitrapper portable pH r.
    multichannel r.
    VitaGuard 1000 event r.
recording
    closed-circuit video r.
    gastroesophageal reflux-reflex
      apnea r.
recovered memory
recovery
    bacterial r.
    fluid-attenuated inversion r.
      (FLAIR)
    labor, delivery, and r. (LDR)
    oocyte r.
    r. score
    r. time
    ultrasonic egg r.
recreational drug
recrudescence of fever
recrudescent typhus
recruitment
    alveolar r.
    lung r.
recta (*pl. of* rectum)
rectal
    r. administration
    r. balloon manometry
    r. canal
    r. cancer
    r. compliance testing
    r. examination
    r. fissure
    Fleet Babylax R.
    r. fourchette fistula
    Hemet R.
    r. injury
    r. linitis plastica (RLP)
    R. Medicone
    r. node
    Nova R.
    Phenergan R.
    r. pillar
    r. polyethylene tube

    r. pouch
    r. pressure
    Proctocort R.
    r. prolapse
    RMS R.
    Rowasa R.
    r. sensation
    r. sphincter
    r. stump
    r. suppository
    r. swab
    r. temperature
    Tigan R.
    r. vault (RV)
    r. wall resection
recti
    diastasis r.
rectilinear profile
rectoabdominal examination
rectoanal inhibitory reflex
rectocele repair
rectocolonic saline enema
rectolabial fistula
rectopexy
    abdominal r.
    anterior resection r.
    anterior sling r.
    Frykman-Goldberg resection r.
rectosacral space
rectoscopic endometrial ablation
rectoscopy
rectosigmoid
    r. carcinoma
    r. colon
    r. colon endometriosis
rectosigmoidectomy
    Altemeier perineal r.
rectosphincteric reflex
rectourethral fistula
rectouterine
    r. cul-de-sac
    r. fold
    r. pouch
rectovaginal (RV)
    r. examination
    r. fascia defect repair
    r. fistula
    r. septum
    r. space
rectovaginalis
    arcus tendineus fascia r.
    fascia r.
rectovestibular fistula
rectovulvar fistula
rectum, *pl.* **rectums, recta**
    aganglionic r.
    by way of r. (p.r.)
    per r.
rectums (*pl. of* rectum)

rectus
    r. abdominis
    r. abdominis muscle
    r. femoris
    r. femoris muscle
    r. hematoma
    r. palsy
    r. sheath
recumbent infant board
recurrence
    pelvic r.
    pulmonary r.
    r. rate
    r. risk
recurrens
    periadenitis mucosa necrotica r.
recurrent
    r. abdominal pain (RAP)
    r. abdominal pain of childhood
    r. abortion
    r. ADEM
    r. affective disorder
    r. anaphylaxis
    r. aneuploidy
    r. angioedema
    r. aphthous stomatitis
    r. aspiration pneumonia
    r. bacterial meningitis
    r. blister
    r. Candida
    r. carcinoma
    r. cervical cancer
    r. cholangitis
    r. coarctation
    r. convulsive seizure
    r. disease
    r. early pregnancy loss (REPL)
    r. epistaxis
    r. euploidic abortion
    r. fungal meningitis
    r. genital aphthous ulcer
    r. gross hematuria (RGH)
    r. headache
    r. hemolytic uremia syndrome
    r. hernia formation
    r. herpetic outbreak
    r. ITP
    r. Japanese encephalitis virus
    r. jaundice of pregnancy
    r. laryngeal nerve paralysis
    r. lymphoma
    r. miscarriage (REMIS)
    r. molar pregnancy
    r. myoglobinuria
    r. nonconvulsive seizure
    r. otitis media
    r. pregnancy loss (RPL)
    r. purulent meningitis
    r. pyogenic lymphadenitis

    r. respiratory papillomatosis (RRP)
    r. sinusitis
    r. spontaneous abortion (RSA)
    r. staphylococcal infection
    r. stillbirth
    r. vaginitis
    r. vulvovaginal candidiasis (RVVC)
recurrentis
    Borrelia r.
recurring digital fibroma of childhood (RDFC)
recurvatum
    r. deformity
    genu r.
    pectus r.
recycling
    medullary r.
red
    r. blood cell (RBC)
    r. blood cell antigen
    r. blood cell cast
    r. blood cell distribution width (RDW)
    r. blood cell enzyme deficiency
    r. blood cell membrane
    r. blood cell membrane defect
    r. blood cell phosphoglycerate kinase deficiency
    r. blood cell product
    r. blood cell sickling
    r. blood cell spiny projection
    r. blood cell tagged scan
    r. blood cell transfusion
    r. blood cell volume
    r. blood count (RBC)
    r. clover
    r. degeneration
    r. desaturation
    r. fundus
    r. glass test
    r. nucleus
    r. photoplethysmography
    r. reflex (RR)
    r. reflex test
    r. rubber catheter
    r. strawberry tongue
red-black telangiectasia
Reddick-Saye forceps
Redi-kit
    LEEP R.-k.
redirection
    intraatrial r.
RediTab
    Claritin R.
Redi+Wash cleansing system
reduced
    r. bladder capacity
    r. hemoglobin
    r. liver transplant (RLT)

R

reduced-size liver transplant (RSLT)
reducer
>Axid AR Acid R.

reducible hernia
reducing substance
reductase
>5-alpha r.
>dihydrofolate r.
>dihydropteridine r.
>isomerase r.
>methylene tetrahydrofolate r. (MTHFR)

reduction
>air r.
>chromosome r.
>embryo r.
>failed r.
>fetal r.
>fracture r.
>funic r.
>hydrostatic r.
>in utero r.
>Lejour-type modified breast r.
>limb r.
>r. mammaplasty
>manual r.
>multifetal pregnancy r. (MFPR, MPR)
>multiple pregnancy r. (MPR)
>r. of protrusion
>pregnancy r.
>selective pregnancy r.
>selective transvaginal embryo r.
>sexual risk r.
>weight r.

redundant
>r. hymen
>r. skin

REE
>resting energy expenditure

Reed-Sternberg cell
Reed syndrome
REEL
>Receptive-Expressive Emergent Language Scale

REEL-2
>Receptive-Expressive Emergent Language Scale, 2nd Edition

reel foot
ReEND
>reproductive endocrinology

reentrant supraventricular tachycardia
re-equilibration
Reese Clark protocol
Reese-Ellsworth classification
Reese's Pinworm Medicine
refeeding
reference
>ambiguous r.

referential cohesion
referred pelvic pain
Refetoff syndrome
refill
>capillary r.
>poor capillary r.
>prolonged capillary r.

reflectance
>r. photometer
>r. pulse oximetry (RPO)

reflection
>bladder r.
>corneal light r.
>peritoneal r.

reflectometry
>acoustic r.
>spectral gradient acoustic r. (SGAR)

reflex
>acoustic blink r.
>anal wink r.
>anocutaneous r.
>r. anoxic seizure
>asymmetric tonic neck r. (ATNR)
>automatic r.
>autonomic walking r.
>axon r.
>Babinski r.
>Babkin r.
>Bezold-Jarisch r.
>biceps r.
>bite r.
>blink r.
>bowing r.
>brachioradialis r.
>bregmocardiac r.
>Breuer-Hering inflation r.
>bulbocavernosus r.
>cat's eye r.
>chemosensitive r.
>cochleopalpebral r.
>conditioned orientation r. (COR)
>cremasteric r.
>crossed adductor r.
>crossed extension r.
>darkened r.
>darwinian r.
>dazzle r.
>deep tendon r. (DTR)
>delayed deep tendon r.
>diving r.
>doll's eye r.
>ear-cough r.
>ejection r.
>embrace r.
>r. epilepsy
>extrusion r.
>fencing r.
>Ferguson r.
>flexion r.

forced grasp r.
forced grasping r.
gag r.
Gallant r.
Gamper bowing r.
gastrocolic r.
Gordon r.
grasp r.
Grünfelder r.
Head r.
Hering-Breuer inflation r. (HBIR)
Hoffmann r.
r. HPV test
r. incontinence
inhibitory r.
r. irritability
knee jerk r.
labial r.
labyrinthine r.
Landau r.
laryngeal adductor r. (LAR)
laryngeal vagal r.
letdown r.
r. ligament
lip r.
macular light r.
Magnus and de Kleijn tonic
  neck r.
markedly decreased r.
McCarthy r.
mechanosensitive r.
milk ejection r.
Moro r.
r. myoclonus
nasolabial r.
near gaze r.
neck r.
neck-righting r.
obligatory primitive r.
obligatory tonic neck r.
oculocephalic r.
oculocephalogyric r.
Oppenheim r.
oral r.
palmar grasp r.
palmar grasping r.
palm-chin r.
palmomental r.
palpebral r.
parachute r.
patellar r.
pathologic r.
r. pathway
r. pattern
Peiper r.
Perez r.
physiologic r.
placing r.
plantar grasp r.

positive support r.
postural r.
primitive r.
propping r.
pull-to-sit r.
pupillary red r.
Radovici r.
rectoanal inhibitory r.
rectosphincteric r.
red r. (RR)
rhinobronchial r.
righting r.
rooting r.
Rossolimo r.
sacral r.
snout r.
startle r.
stepping r.
r. stepping
sucking r.
suckling r.
support r.
swallow r.
swallowing r.
swimming r.
symmetrical tonic neck r. (STNR)
r. sympathetic dystrophy (RSD)
r. syncope
tendon stretch r.
tongue protrusion r.
tonic labyrinthine r.
tonic neck r. (TNR)
triceps r.
truncal incurvation r.
vagal r.
walking r.
white pupillary r.
reflexa
placenta r.
reflexology
reflex-placing response
reflux
acid r.
alkaline r.
complicated gastroesophageal r.
contralateral r.
dilating r.
esophageal r.
r. esophagitis
extraesophageal r. (EER)
gastroesophageal r. (GER)
gastrointestinal r.
intrarenal r.
menstrual r.
nasopharyngeal r. (NPR)
r. nephropathy
r. neuropathy (RN)
r. of air
physiologic r.

R

reflux (*continued*)
- primary vesicoureteral r.
- secondary vesicoureteral r.
- silent gastroesophageal r.
- ureterovesical r.
- urinary r.
- vesicoureteral r. (grade 1–4)

refractile body
refraction
refractive error
refractory
- r. anemia of pregnancy
- r. anemia with ring sideroblasts (RARS)
- r. ascites
- r. Crohn disease
- r. depressive symptom
- r. dyserythropoietic anemia
- r. epistaxis
- r. hypoglycemia
- r. sprue
- r. status epilepticus (RSE)

Refsum
- R. disease
- R. syndrome

refusal to bear weight
Regan-Lowe medium
regard
- prolonged r.
- visual r.

Regenbogen-Donnai syndrome
regeneration
- aberrant r.
- tissue r.

regimen
- add-back r.
- COMP drug r.
- conditioning r.
- downregulation r.
- feeding r.
- gonadotropin r.
- hypertransfusion r.
- monophasic r.
- platinum-based r.
- Pritchard intramuscular r.
- Zuspan r.

region
- anogenital r.
- breakpoint cluster r. (bcr)
- flanking r.
- hilar r.
- parietooccipital r.
- perimesencephalic r.
- Prader-Willi syndrome critical r. (PWSCR)
- regulatory r.
- sequence characterized amplified r.
- sex-determining r. (SRY)
- subependymal r.
- subpial r.
- zygomaticofrontal r.

regional
- r. analgesia
- r. block anesthesia
- r. enteritis
- r. gas exchange (R_{AW})
- r. ileitis
- r. lymphadenitis
- r. nerve block
- r. perinatal intensive care center (RPICC)
- r. wall motion abnormality

register
- high-risk r. (HRR)
- r. linkage study

registry
- cord blood r. (CBR)
- Herbst r.
- National Pediatric Trauma R. (NPTR)
- Teratogen R.

Reglan
Regonol Injection
regression
- change-point r.
- Galton law of r.
- premature luteal r.
- trophoblast in r. (TIR)
- tumor r.

regressive infantilism
Regula pessary
regular
- R. Iletin I, II
- r. immunoglobulin
- r. purified pork insulin

regulated upon activation, normal T-cell expressed and secreted (RANTES)
regulation
- arginine vasopressin r.
- Baby Doe r.'s
- cellular r.
- fetal thermal r.
- gonadotropin r.
- menstrual cycle r.
- molecular r.
- physiologic follicular r.
- pituitary gonadotropin r.
- plasma volume r.
- prolactin r.
- serotonin r.

regulator
- autoimmune r. (AIRE)
- cystic fibrosis transmembrane r. (CFTR)
- r. gene
- Medela membrane r.

regulatory
- r. region

r. sequence
steroidogenic acute r. (StAR)
Reguloid
regurgitant
r. fraction
r. murmur
regurgitate
regurgitation
aortic r.
effortless r.
gastric r.
mitral r.
nasal r.
physiologic r.
pulmonic r.
tricuspid r.
rehabilitate
Rehydralyte formula
rehydration
rapid r.
Reichel cloacal duct
Reid sleeve
Reifenstein syndrome
Reiki
Reilly granule
reimplant
common sheath r.
reimplantation
extravesical ureteral r.
r. of ureter
ureteral trigonal r.
Reiner-Beck snare
Reiner-Knight forceps
reinforcement
contingent r.
negative r.
positive r.
reinfusion
autologous bone marrow r.
Reinke crystalloids
reinsemination
Reissner membrane
**Reis-Wertheim vaginal
  hysterectomy**
Reiter syndrome
reject
zero r.
rejection
accelerated r.
acute r.
allograft r.
chronic r.
fetal r.
hyperacute r.
ReJuveness
relactation
relapse
bone marrow r.
testicular r.

relapsing
r. fever
r. infectious polyneuritis
r. iridocyclitis
r. nodular nonsuppurative panniculitis
related
alcohol r. (AR)
r. services
relation
peer r.
relationship
antecedent-behavior-consequence r.
avuncular r.
bisexual r.
blood r.
depth r.
Frank-Starling r.
gay r.
heterosexual r.
lesbian r.
physician-patient r.
Poiseuille-Hagen r.
same-sex r.
sexual r.
spatial r.
relative
r. afferent defect
blood r.
r. macroglossia
r. osteopenia
r. polycythemia
r. risk
r. shunt
r. sterility
r. vascular resistance (RVR)
relaxant
muscle r.
relaxation
isovolumic r. (IVR)
pelvic r.
pelvic girdle r. (PGR)
pyloric sphincter r.
r. technique
uterine r.
r. volume
relaxin
intracervical purified porcine r.
r. serum level
vaginal recombinant human r.
release
Acutrim Precision R.
antioxidant r.
antioxidant r.
R. catheter
colonoscopic r.
complete subtalar r. (CSTR)
counterregulatory hormone r.
extended r. (ER, XL, XR, XT)
GnRH-facilitated FSH r.

release (*continued*)
  GnRH-facilitated LH r.
  growth hormone r.
  hip adduction r.
  increased renin r.
  myofascial r.
  neurotransmitter r.
  pituitary hormone r.
  postganglionic acetylcholine r.
  pulsatile r.
  radical posteromedial and plantar r. (RPMPR)
  Sever r.
  shear stress-mediated nitric oxide r.
  soft tissue r.
Relenza
reliability
Reliance urinary control insert catheter
relief
  Fleet Pain R.
ReliefBand device
religiosity
REM
  rapid eye movement
  REM latency
  REM parasomnia
  REM PolyHesive II patient return electrode
  REM sleep
  REM sleep behavior disorder
remedy
  soy-based r.
Remifemin Menopause tablet
remifentanil
remineralization
REMIS
  recurrent miscarriage
  REMIS study
remission
  complete r.
  induced r.
  spontaneous r.
remnant
  branchial cleft r.
  omphalomesenteric duct r.
  tracheobronchial r.
remodeling
  bone r.
  fracture r.
remote
  r. afterloading brachytherapy (RAB)
  r. tocodynamometry
removal
  extracorporeal CO_2 r. (ECOR)
  hysteroscopic r.
  surgical r.
REMS
  rapid eye movement sleep
remyelination, remyelinization

remyelinization (*var. of* remyelination)
Renaissance spirometry system
renal
  r. acidification
  r. agenesis
  r. aminoaciduria
  r., anus, lung, polydactyly, hamartoblastoma (RALPH)
  r. artery stenosis
  r. biopsy
  r. blastema
  r. blood flow (RBF)
  r. calculus
  r. calyx
  r. candidiasis
  r. cell carcinoma (RCC)
  r. clearance test
  r. colic
  r. cortex
  r. cortex cyst
  r. cortical necrosis
  r. cortical nephropathy
  r. cystic disease
  r. disease in pregnancy
  r. duplication
  r. dysfunction
  r. dysgenesis
  renal, ear, anal, radial (REAR)
  r. ectopia
  r. electrolyte wasting
  r. failure
  r. Fanconi syndrome
  r. fistula
  r. function test
  r. fungus ball
  r. glycosuria
  r. hypercalciuria
  r. hyperechogenicity
  r. hypertension
  r. hypodysplasia
  r. impairment
  r. infarction
  r. insufficiency
  r. insufficiency rickets
  r. interstitium
  r. loss
  r. malrotation
  r. manifestation
  r. medullary carcinoma
  r. medullary dysplasia
  r. mesangial sclerosis-eye defects syndrome
  r. mycetoma
  r. myofibromatosis
  r. obstruction
  r. osteodystrophy
  r. parenchyma
  r. pedicle
  r. pelvis

r. perfusion
r. plasma flow
r. proteinuria
r. reserve filtration capacity (RRFC)
r. rickets
r. salt wasting
r. scarring
r. scintigraphy
r. solute load (RSL)
r. stone
r. tract
r. transplantation
r. tuberculosis
r. tubular acidosis (RTA)
r. tubular bicarbonate wasting
r. tubular crystalluria
r. tubular epithelial cell
r. tubular Fanconi syndrome
r. tubular function
r. tubular necrosis
r. tubular pituitary syndrome
r. tubule
r. ultrasound
r. vascular resistance
r. vascular thrombosis
r. vasculitis
r. vein
r. vein thrombosis
vertebral (defects), (imperforate)
  anus, tracheoesophageal (fistula),
  radial and r. (dysplasia) (VATER)
Rendu-Osler-Weber
R.-O.-W. disease
R.-O.-W. syndrome
Renese
reniformis
placenta r.
reniform pelvis
renin
elevated r.
r. substrate
renin-angiotensin-aldosterone system
renin-angiotensin system (RAS)
Renografin
renogram
MAG-3 diuretic r.
renography
diuretic r.
renovascular hypertension
Renpenning syndrome
rent
uterine r.
reossification
reossify
Reoviridae
Reovirus (type 1–3)
reoxygenation
repair
abdominal paravaginal r.

anterior and posterior r.
A&P r.
Cantwell-Ransley r.
CDH r.
clawhand deformity r.
cleft palate r.
cystocele r.
Danus-Stanzel r.
defect-specific r.
delayed r.
enterocele r.
episiotomy r.
Fothergill-Hunter uterine
  prolapse r.
hypospadias r.
imperforate anus r.
intraatrial r.
Marckwald cervical os r.
Noble-Mengert perineal r.
Orr rectal prolapse r.
palate r.
paravaginal r.
paravaginal cystocele r.
perineal r.
Phaneuf-Graves enterocele r.
posterior r.
primary cleft palate r.
Rastelli transposition of great
  arteries r.
rectocele r.
rectovaginal fascia defect r.
Richardson paravaginal r.
Senning transpostion of great
  arteries r.
Snodgrass hypospadias r.
sphincter r.
staged r.
surgical r.
Tennison-Randall r.
transannular patch r.
vaginal wall r.
vesicovaginal r.
York-Mason rectourinary fistula r.
Zancolli clawhand deformity r.
repeat
r. cesarean section (RCS)
r. curettage
inverted r.
simple sequence r.
tandem r.
repeated
r. abortion
r. complete mole
r. partial seizure
r. pregnancy loss (RPL)
repeat-loop excision
repellent
insect r.
reperfusion injury

repetitive
    r. DNA
    r. pregnancy loss
REPL
    recurrent early pregnancy loss
replacement
    cephalic r.
    cortisol r.
    electrolyte r.
    esophageal r.
    estrogen r.
    fascial r.
    fluid r.
    frozen embryo r. (FER)
    gamma globulin r.
    heart valve r.
    pancreatic enzyme r.
    PTH for osteoporotic women on estrogen r. (POWER)
    r. therapy
    volume r.
replenishment
Replens lubricant
replicate
replication
    DNA r.
    r. fork
replicon
Repliform alternative product
Replogle
    R. suction catheter
    R. sump tube
r-EPO
    recombinant human erythropoietin
repolarization
report
    Janus r.
    Walton r.
reporter
    mandated r.
repositioning
    scapular r.
representation
    internal r.
    symbolic r.
representative section
repressed gene
repressor gene
reproduction
    assisted r.
    vegetative r.
reproductive
    r. age
    r. axis
    r. cycle
    r. disorder
    r. endocrinology (ReEND)
    r. endocrinology-infertility

    r. failure
    r. function
    r. genetics
    r. history
    r. liberty
    r. mortality
    r. organ
    r. performance
    r. system
    r. system development
    r. technology
    r. toxin
    r. tract
    r. tract abnormality
    r. tract embryology
    r. wastage
Repronex
reptilase time
requirement
    increased resting oxygen r.
    iron r.
    mineral r.
    minimum daily r. (MDR)
    neonatal glucose r.
    nutrient r.
    nutritional r.
    resting oxygen r.
    sodium r.
    vitamin r.
Rescriptor
rescue
    abdominal r.
    ablative therapy with bone marrow r.
    r. breathing
    r. cervical cerclage
    r. dose
    r. medication
    r. surfactant
    r. therapy
    trisomic r.
research
    American Pediatric Society/Society for Pediatric R.
    HIV Epidemiology R. (HER)
    International Committee for Contraceptive R. (ICCR)
resectability
resecting intrapartum uterine wall
resection
    abdominoperineal r. (APR)
    atretic extrahepatic bile duct r.
    bile duct r.
    bowel loop r.
    bowel segment r.
    cornual r.
    cystoscopic transurethral tumor r.
    dilated bowel loop r.
    distal dilated bowel segment r.

duodenal r.
en bloc r.
endocervical r. (ECR)
endometrial r.
endomyometrial r. (EMR)
extrahepatic bile duct r.
gallbladder r.
hysteroscopic septum r.
in utero r.
laparoscopic multiple-punch r.
laparoscopic ureterosacral ligament r.
  (LUSLR)
laterally extended endopelvic r.
late uterine wedge r.
liver lobe r.
low rectal r.
multiple-punch r.
ovarian wedge r.
pancreatic head r.
perineal r.
posterior rectal wall r.
pulmonary r.
rectal wall r.
segmental r.
subtotal colon r.
surgical r.
Torpin cul-de-sac r.
transcervical r.
transsphenoidal microsurgical r.
wedge r.
Resectisol Irrigation Solution
resectoscope
specialized tissue aspirating r.
  (STAR)
USA Elite System gynecologic
  rotating continuous flow r.
Wallach colposcope and r.
reseeding
Resercen
reserpine
reservatus
coitus r.
reserve
coronary flow r. (CFR)
ovarian r.
r. zone (RZ)
reservoir
Camey r.
catheter r.
double-bubble flushing r.
ileal r.
Mainz pouch urinary r.
Ommaya r.
Pudenz r.
sperm r.
subcutaneous ventricular catheter r.
ventricular r.
residential program
residua (*pl. of* residuum)

residual
r. coarctation
r. ductal tissue
r. hearing
r. in situ
r. ovary syndrome
postvoid r. (PVR)
r. urine
r. vision
r. volume (RV)
residue
gastric r.
methanol extraction r. (MER)
residuum, *pl.* **residua**
resin
acid-binding r.
cholestyramine r.
podophyllin r.
resistance
activated protein C r. (APCR)
airway r. (RAW)
androgen r.
antibiotic r.
antiretroviral r.
bromocriptine r.
dicumarol r.
differential vascular r.
fetal pulmonary vascular r.
increased vascular r.
r. index (RI)
insulin r.
intrinsic flow r.
in vitro r.
lithium r.
multidrug r. (MDR)
natural r.
peripheral insulin r.
peripheral vascular r. (PVR)
pulmonary r.
pulmonary vascular r. (PVR)
relative vascular r. (RVR)
renal vascular r.
respiratory system r. (R_{rs})
systemic vascular r. (SVR)
thyroid hormone r.
tissue insulin r.
total peripheral r. (TPR)
total pulmonary r.
vascular r.
resistant
ampicillin r.
r. condyloma
drug r.
r. ovary
r. ovary syndrome
r. pneumococcus
resisted abduction
resolution
axial r.

resolution (*continued*)
    clot r.
    lateral r.
    r. phase
resonance
    nuclear magnetic r. (NMR)
resorption
    r. atelectasis
    bone r.
    fetal r.
    osteoclast-mediated bone r.
    tooth root r.
resource
    R. Just for Kids with Fiber
      formula
    R. Plus formula
    r. specialist
    R. Standard formula
Respa-DM
Respa-GF
Resp-EZ piezoelectric sensor
RespiGam
Respihaler
    Decadron R.
Respinol-G
respiration
    activity, pulse, grimace, appearance,
      r. (Apgar)
    agonal r.'s
    artificial r.
    Bouchut r.
    Cheyne-Stokes r.
    gasping r.
    grunting r.
    internal r.
    Kussmaul r.
    paradoxical r.
    percutaneous aspiration, instillation
      of hypertonic saline, r. (PAIR)
    placental r.
    sighing r.
    vicarious r.
respirator, ventilator
    Ambu r.
    BABYbird r.
    Babylog 8000 r.
    Bath r.
    Bear r.
    Bennett r.
    Bird Mark 8 r.
    Bourns infant r.
    Bragg-Paul r.
    Breeze r.
    Clevedon positive pressure r.
    cuirass r.
    Drinker r.
    Emerson r.
    Engstrom r.
    Gill r.

    Huxley r.
    mechanical r.
    Med-Neb r.
    Merck r.
    Monaghan r.
    Morch r.
    negative-pressure r.
    portable r.
    Sanders jet r.
    Stephan HF 300 r.
respiratory
    r. acidosis
    r. alkalosis
    r. arrest
    r. burst assay
    r. chamber
    r. ciliary paralysis
    r. complication
    r. compromise
    r. cycle
    r. depression
    r. distress (RD)
    r. distress syndrome (RDS)
    r. distress syndrome of the newborn
    r. drive
    r. effort
    r. embarrassment
    r. enteric orphan
    r. enteric orphan virus
    r. epithelium
    r. failure
    r. hippus
    r. index score (RIS)
    r. inductive plethysmography (RIP)
    r. infection
    r. insufficiency
    r. movement
    r. papilloma
    r. papillomatosis
    r. pattern
    r. quotient
    r. sinus arrhythmia
    r. suction
    r. suctioning
    r. support
    r. syncytial virus (RSV)
    r. syncytial virus antigen
    r. syncytial virus bronchiolitis
      (RSVB)
    r. syncytial virus immunoglobulin
      (RSV-IG, RSVIG)
    r. syncytial virus immunoglobulin
      intravenous (RSV-IGIV)
    r. syncytial virus pneumonia
    r. system
    r. system elastance (E_{dyn})
    r. system resistance (R_{rs})
    Taiwan acute r. (TWAR)
    r. therapist

r. therapy
r. therapy pack
r. toilet
r. tract
r. tract infection (RTI)
r. tree
Respirgard II nebulizer
respite care
Respitrace inductance plethysmography
Respivir
response
abnormal r.
acute insulin r.
age-related pharmacodynamic r.
allergic inflammatory r.
amnesic r.
anamnestic immune r.
antibody r.
asthmatic r.
auditory brainstem r. (ABR, ABSR)
auditory evoked r. (AER)
automated auditory brainstem r.
  (AABR)
automated brainstem auditory evoked
  r. (ABAER)
Babinski r.
baroreflex r.
Basson model of female sexual r.
biphasic r.
Bobath r.
brainstem auditory evoked r.
  (BAER, BSAER)
brainstem evoked r. (BSER)
buttress r.
characteristic emotional r.
chronotropic r.
clasp-knife r.
clinical r.
cortisol r.
r. cost
cremasteric r.
CTL r.
cytotoxic lymphocyte r.
doll's eye r.
early asthmatic r. (EAR)
emotional r.
esophago-deglutition r.
evoked r.
fall-away r.
female sexual r.
fetal inflammatory r.
fetal startle r.
fight-and-flight r.
glabellar r.
hemodynamic r.
immune r.
infantile breath-holding r.
inflammatory r.
r. inhibition

insulin r.
Köbner r.
lactation letdown r.
Landau r.
late asthmatic r. (LAR)
r. latency
light r.
local inflammatory r.
maternal immune r.
maternal inflammatory r.
maternal vascular r.
menstrual cycle hemodynamic r.
metabolic r.
Moro r.
neck r.
neuroendocrine r.
oculovestibular r.
orgasmic motor r.
parachute r.
pharmacodynamic r.
placing r.
plantar r.
postinfectious immune r.
pressor r.
pupillary light r.
pyogranulomatous r.
reflex-placing r.
Rh immune r.
righting r.
sexual r.
sound-field r.
staircase r.
startle r.
stepping r.
stress r.
sympathetic skin r.
target organ r.
thermogenic r.
thermoregulatory r.
tonic neck r.
treppe r.
vagally mediated r.
vascular r.
visual evoked r. (VER)
Respules
Pulmicort R.
rest
antepartum bed r.
antepartum hospital bed r.
bed r.
cystic Walthard r.
ectopic pancreatic r.
gut r.
hospitalized bed r.
r., ice, compression, elevation
  (RICE)
intralobar r.
Marchand r.
mesonephric r.

R

rest (*continued*)
    nephrogenic r.
    pancreatic r.
    PediaCare Night R.
    pelvic r.
    prophylactic bed r.
    Walthard cell r.
    wolffian r.

resting
    r. anal sphincter pressure
    r. calorimetry
    r. energy expenditure (REE)
    r. membrane potential
    r. metabolic rate (RMR)
    r. oxygen requirement

restless
    r. legs syndrome
    r. sleep

restlessness
    motor r.

restorative procedure
Restore program
Restoril
restraint
    child r.

restriction
    asymmetric growth r.
    at-home activity r.
    r. endonuclease
    r. endonuclease analysis
    r. enzyme
    r. enzyme cutting site
    fetal growth r. (FGR)
    fluid r.
    r. fragment
    r. fragment length polymorphism
    (RFLP)
    intrauterine growth r. (IUGR)
    r. landmark genomic scanning
    r. map
    maternal activity r.
    normotensive intrauterine
    growth r.
    salt r.
    sodium r.
    symmetric growth r.

restrictive
    r. breathing pattern
    r. cardiomyopathy (RCM)
    r. dermopathy
    r. lung disease
    r. respiratory disease

restructuring
rest/sleep periods
result
    Surveillance, Epidemiology and End
    R.'s (SEER)

resumption
    menstrual cycle r.

resuscitate
    do not r. (DNR)

resuscitation
    bag and mask r.
    cardiopulmonary r. (CPR)
    cerebral r.
    fluid r.
    intrauterine r.
    mouth-to-mouth r. (MMR)
    mouth-to-nose/mouth r.
    neonatal r.
    newborn r.

resuscitator
    Ambu infant r.
    Fisher and Paykel RD1000 r.
    Laerdal r.
    Penlon infant r.
    RD1000 r.

Resyl
RET
    retention
    retina
    return
    RET protooncogene

RETA
    rete testis aspiration

retained
    r. bladder syndrome
    r. fetal lung fluid (RFLF)
    r. foreign body (RFB)
    r. hygroscopic cervical dilator
    r. membrane
    r. menstruation
    r. myoma
    r. placenta
    r. placental fragment
    r. products of conception (RPC)

retardate
    Screening Tests for Young Children
    and R.'s
    Sheridan Tests for Young Children
    and R.'s

retardation
    alopecia-mental r. (AMR)
    alopecia universalis with mental r.
    alpha-thalassemia/mental r.
    American Association on Mental R.
    (AAMR)
    aniridia, ambiguous genitalia, mental
    r. (AGR)
    basal ganglion disorder-mental r.
    (BGMR)
    Belgian type mental r.
    Buenos Aires type mental r.
    cataract, hypertrichosis, mental r.
    (CAHMR)
    Charcot-Marie-Tooth syndrome,
    X-linked type II with deafness
    and mental r.

congenital progressive muscular dystrophy with mental r.
fetal growth r.
fragile site mental r. 1 (FMR1)
fragile site mental r. 2 (FMR2)
FRAXE-associated mental r.
growth r.
HbH related mental r.
head-sparing intrauterine growth r.
ichthyosiform erythroderma, hair abnormality, mental and growth r.
infantile spasms with mental r.
intrauterine growth r. (IUGR)
linear growth r.
mental r.
mild mental r. (MMR)
moderate mental r.
motor-sensory neuropathy, X-linked type II, with deafness and mental r.
multiple exostosis-mental r. (MEMR)
nonprogressive cerebellar disorder with mental r.
nonspecific mental r.
r. of growth and deafness
peripheral dysostosis, nail hypoplasia, mental r. (PNM)
prenatal growth r.
profound mental r.
psychomotor r.
severe mental r.
Wilms tumor, aniridia, genitourinary malformations, mental r. (WAGR)
Wilms tumor, aniridia, gonadoblastoma, r. (WAGR)
X-linked alpha-thalassemia/mental r. (ATRX)
X-linked mental r. (1-47)

retarded
r. fetal growth
specific reading r. (SRR)

retching, vomiturition

rete, *pl.* **retia**
r. cord
r. cyst of ovary
r. peg
r. ridge elongation
r. testis
r. testis aspiration (RETA)

retention
carbon dioxide r.
r. enema
fetal r.
fluid r.
ovarian r.
r. polyp
sodium r.
stool r.
r. suture

transitory urinary r.
urinary r.

Rethoré syndrome
rethrombosis
retia (*pl. of* rete)
reticula (*pl. of* reticulum)
reticular, reticulated
r. dermis
r. dysgenesis
r. reflex myoclonus
reticulare
magma r.
reticularis
adrenal r.
livedo r.
zona r.
reticulata
substantia nigra pars r.
reticulated
r. hyperpigmentation
r. pigmentation
r. platelet count
reticulocyte count
reticulocytopenia
reticulocytosis
reticuloendothelial
r. cell
r. sequestration
r. system
reticuloendotheliosis
reticulogranular pattern
reticulonodular pattern
reticulum, *pl.* **reticula**
endoplasmic r. (ER)
rough endoplasmic r. (RER)
sarcoplasmic r.
stellate r.
Retin-A
retina
dragging of r.
embryonic neural r.
macula of r.
mottled r.
neural r.
retinacula (*pl. of* retinaculum)
retinaculum, *pl.* **retinacula**
peroneal r.
retinae
commotio r.
macula r.
ora serrata r.
retinal
r. angioma
r. aplasia
r. arterial narrowing and straightening (RANS)
r. change
r. detachment
r. dysplasia

R

retinal (*continued*)
r. edema
r. hamartoma
r. hemorrhage
r. infiltrate
r. pigmentary degeneration
r. pigment epithelium (RPE)
r. pseudotumor
r. vasculitis
r. venous dilation and tortuosity (RVDT)
r. vessel telangiectasia
retinitis
CMV r.
gravidic r.
indolent granular CMV r.
r. pigmentosa
r. pigmentosa-congenital deafness syndrome
proliferative r.
salt-and-pepper r.
toxoplasmosis r.
retinoblast
retinoblastoma
bilateral r.'s
hereditary r.
rhabdomyosarcoma r.
trilateral r.
retinoblastoma-mental retardation syndrome
retinoic
r. acid
r. acid embryopathy
retinoid therapy
retinol
retinol-binding protein
retinopapillitis of prematurity
retinopathy
diabetic r.
eclamptic r.
gravidic r.
Keith-Wagener r.
nonproliferative diabetic r.
r. of newborn
r. of prematurity (ROP)
r. punctata albescens
Purtscher r.
retinopathy-mental retardation syndrome
retinoschisis
congenital hereditary r. (CHRS)
hereditary r.
juvenile X-linked r. (JXRS)
X-linked r.
retractile testis
retraction
accessory muscle r.
intercostal r. (ICR)
nipple r.

r. ring
skin r.
subcostal r.
substernal r.
supraclavicular r.
r. syndrome
retractive nystagmus
retractor
abdominal r.
Airlift balloon r.
Allport r.
Army-Navy r.
Aufricht nasal r.
Balfour r.
balloon r.
Berkeley-Bonney r.
bladder r.
Bookwalter r.
Breisky-Navratil vaginal r.
Brewster r.
Brown uvula r.
Cer-View lateral vaginal r.
Cottle-Neivert r.
Deaver r.
DeLee Universal r.
Desmarres r.
elastic abdominal r.
Ferris Smith-Sewall r.
Gelpi perineal r.
Gott malleable r.
Guardian vaginal r.
Haight baby r.
Harrington r.
Heaney hysterectomy r.
Heaney-Simon r.
Iron Intern r.
Jackson right-angle r.
Kelly r.
lateral wall r.
long atraumatic r.
Luer r.
malleable r.
Mobius r.
nasal r.
r. neuropathy
OB/Mobius elastic abdominal r.
O'Connor-O'Sullivan r.
Omni-Tract vaginal r.
O'Sullivan-O'Connor r.
pediatric self-retaining r.
perineal r.
Richardson r.
right-angle r.
Roberts thumb r.
Schuknecht r.
self-retaining r.
Senn-Dingman r.
Shambaugh r.
Sims r.

thumb r.
vaginal r.
Weitlaner r.
Wullstein r.
retractorius
nystagmus r.
retraining
bladder r.
r. diary
retransposition
arterial r.
retrieval
egg r.
oocyte r.
ovarian r.
transvaginal ultrasound-directed
oocyte r. (TUDOR)
ultrasonographically guided oocyte
r.
ultrasound-directed egg r.
retriever
Endopouch r.
retroambiguus
nucleus r.
retroauricular
retrobulbar neuritis
retrocallosal
retrocardiac pneumonia
retrocaval ureter
retrocecal hernia
retrocerebellar arachnoidal cyst
retrocervical
retrocession
retrochiasmatic
retrocollis
retroconversion
chemotherapeutic r.
retrodeviation
retrodisplacement
retroesophageal abscess
retroflection (*var. of* retroflexion)
retroflexion, retroflection
uterine r.
retrognathism
retrograde
r. amnesia
r. axoplasmic flow
r. ejaculation
r. intussusception
r. menstrual flow
r. menstruation
r. pyelogram
r. pyelography
r. ureteral dye injection
retrolental fibroplasia (RLF)
retromammary mastitis
retroorbital lymphoma
retroperitoneal
r. dissection

r. drain
r. endometriosis
r. fetus
r. fibrosis
r. hematoma
r. infection
r. laparoscopic procedure
r. lymphadenectomy
r. node
r. soft tissue
r. soft tissue sarcoma
retroperitoneum
retropharyngeal
r. abscess
r. cellulitis
r. lymph node
retroplacental
r. clot
r. hematoma
r. hemorrhage
retroposed
retroposition
retropubic
r. colpourethrocystopexy
r. cystourethropexy
(RPCV)
r. fibrosis
r. needle procedure
r. sling
r. space
r. suspension procedure
r. urethrocystopexy (RPU)
r. urethropexy procedure
r. vesicourethrolysis
retrorectal
r. space
r. transanal pull-through
retrosternal
r. chest pain
r. hernia
retrotonsillar abscess
retrotorsion
retrovaginal
r. septum
r. space
retroversioflexion
retroversion
femoral r.
uterine r.
retroverted uterus
Retrovir
retroviral
r. disease
r. syndrome
retrovirus
retrusion
Rett
R. disorder
R. syndrome

R

rettgeri
    Providencia r.
return
    partial anomalous pulmonary venous
      r. (PAPVR)
    supracardiac total anomalous
      pulmonary venous r.
    systemic caval r.
    total anomalous pulmonary venous
      r. (TAPVR)
returning-soldier effect
Retzius
    space of R.
Reuter tube
revascularization
Reveal HIV-1 antibody test
revenge fantasy
reversal
    dosage-sensitive sex r.
      (DSS)
    gender r.
    hyperandrogenism r.
    r. of tubal ligation
    role r.
    sex r.
    tubal r.
    vasectomy r.
reverse
    r. banding
    r. chylous syndrome
    r. dot blot hybridization
    r. dot blot sequence-specific
      oligonucleotide method
    r. FISH cytogenetic technique
    r. form McRoberts maneuver
    r. last shoe
    r. Marcus Gunn sign
    r. nostrils
    r. 3 sign
    r. transcriptase
    r. transcriptase inhibitor (RTI)
    r. transcription
    r. transcription polymerase chain
      reaction (RT-PCR)
    r. triiodothyronine
reversed end-diastolic flow
reversible
    r. biliary pseudolithiasis
    r. obstructive airway
    r. oligospermia
    r. posterior leukoencephalopathy
      syndrome (RPLS)
Reversol
ReVia
review
    annual r.
    Cochran Database of
      Systemic R.'s
    r. of systems (ROS)

revised
    R. Children's Manifest Anxiety
      Scale (RCMAS)
    Gesell Adaptive and Personal
      Behavior Domain, R.
    Gesell Developmental Schedules, R.
    Gesell Gross Motor Domain, R.
    R. Gesell Language Domain
    r. Jones criteria
    r. Jones criteria for diagnosis of
      acute rheumatic fever
    R. Tests of Cognitive Ability
    R. Trauma Score (RTS)
revision
    Dibbell cleft lip-nasal r.
    lip scar r.
    shunt r.
rewarming
    extracorporeal r.
Reyataz
Reye
    R. hepatic encephalopathy
    R. syndrome
Reye-like syndrome
Reynell
    R. Language Development Scale
      (RLDS)
    R. Verbal Comprehension Test
Reynolds
    R. Child Depression Scale
    R. number
    R. suicide ideation questionnaire
RF
    rheumatoid factor
RFA
    radiofrequency ablation
    right femoral artery
    right frontoanterior position
RFB
    retained foreign body
RFCA
    radiofrequency catheter ablation
RFLF
    retained fetal lung fluid
RFLP
    restriction fragment length
      polymorphism
      RFLP analysis
RF-negative juvenile polyarthritis
RF-seropositive
rFSH
    recombinant follicle stimulating
      hormone
RFT
    right frontotransverse position
RGD
    range-gated Doppler
RGH
    recurrent gross hematuria

RGO
  reciprocating gait orthosis
Rh
  rhesus
    Rh antibody
    Rh antigen
    Rh blood group
    Rh blood group system
    Rh complex
    Rh D disease
    Rh disease of newborn
    Rh factor
    Gamulin Rh
    Rh hemolytic disease
    Rh immune response
    Rh immunization
    Rh immunoglobulin
    Rh immunoglobulin (RhIg)
    Rh incompatibility
    Rh isoimmune hemolytic disease
    Rh isoimmunization
    Rh null cell
    Rh sensitization
rhabdoid tumor
rhabdomyoblast
rhabdomyolysis
  copper-induced r.
  hyperthermic r.
  malignant hyperthermic r.
rhabdomyoma
  cardiac r.
  fetal cardiac r.
rhabdomyosarcoma (RMS),
rhabdosarcoma
  embryonal r.
  r. retinoblastoma
  undifferentiated r.
rhabdosarcoma (*var. of*
  rhabdomyosarcoma)
rhabdosphincter
rhagas
  periorificial rhagades
RHAMM
  receptor for hyaluronan-mediated
  motility
rhamnosus
  Lactobacillus r.
rhaphe (*var. of* raphe)
RhC
  rhesus antigen C
RhCE
  rhesus gene CE
    RhCE gene
RhD
  rhesus antigen D
    RhD immunoglobulin
RhE
  rhesus antigen E
rhegmatogenous detachment

rheometer
rhesus (Rh)
  r. antibody
  r. antigen
  r. antigen C (RhC)
  r. antigen D (RhD)
  r. antigen E (RhE)
  r. factor
  r. gene CE (RhCE)
  r. gene D
  r. isoimmunization
  r. rotavirus tetravalent vaccine
rheumatic
  r. carditis
  r. exanthema
  r. fever
  r. heart disease
  r. pneumonia
  r. valvular heart disease
rheumatica
  polymyalgia r.
rheumaticosis
rheumatism
  desert r.
  European League Against R.
    (EULAR)
  International League Against R.
rheumatogenic
  r. strain
  r. streptococcus
rheumatoid
  r. arthritis (RA)
  r. factor (RF)
  r. granuloma
  r. nodule
  r. spondylitis
  r. vasculitis
rheumatologic disorder
rheumatology
  International League of Associations
    for R. (ILAR)
Rheumatrex Oral
rhGH
  recombinant human growth hormone
RhIg
  Rh immunoglobulin
rhIGF-1
  recombinant human insulin-like growth
    factor-1
Rhinall Nasal Solution
rhinencephalon
rhinitis
  allergic r.
  eosinophilic nonallergic r.
  erosive r.
  infectious r.
  r. medicamentosa
  neutrophilic r.
  nonallergenic perrenial r.

R

rhinitis (*continued*)
  nonallergic r.
  r. of pregnancy
  perennial allergic r.
  pollen-induced r.
  purulent r.
  seasonal allergic r.
  serosanguineous r.
  r. sicca
  syphilitic r.
  vasomotor r.
rhinobronchial reflex
rhinobronchitis
rhinocephalia (*var. of* rhinocephaly)
rhinocephaly, rhinocephalia
rhinocerebral
  r. infection
  r. mucormycosis
rhinoconjunctivitis
  allergic r.
Rhinocort
  R. Aqua nasal spray
  R. Turbuhaler
rhinorrhea
  CSF r.
rhinoscopy
rhinosinusitis
  bacterial r.
  chronic r.
Rhinosyn-DMX
Rhino Triangle brace
rhinovirus
rhizomelia syndrome
rhizomelic
  r. brachymelia
  r. chondrodysplasia
  r. chondrodysplasia punctata
    (RCDP)
  r. dwarfism
  r. limb shortening
rhizotomy
  dorsal r.
  functional posterior r.
  posterior r.
  selective dorsal r. (SDR)
  selective posterior r.
Rh-negative
  Rh-n. antibody
  blood group D variant equivalent to
    Rh-n. (Du)
  Rh-n. mother
Rh-null syndrome
rhod-2
  calcium indicator r.-2
  r.-2 imaging
rhodamine
rhodamine-auramine stain
Rhodesian trypanosomiasis
Rho(D) immunoglobulin (RhoGAM)

Rhodis-EC
Rhodococcus equi
RhoGAM
  Rho(D) immunoglobulin
rhombencephalitis
rhombencephalosynapsis
rhombomere segmentation
rhonchi (rh)
rhonchorous cough
Rhophylac
Rhoprolene
Rhoprosone
Rh-positive
  Rh-p. antibody
  Rh-p. infant
  Rh-p. red cell stroma
RHS
  radial head subluxation
Rh-sensitized fetus
rhSOD
  recombinant human superoxide
  dismutase
rHuEPO
  recombinant human erythropoietin
rhus
  r. dermatitis
  R. javanica
rhusiopathiae
  Erysipelothrix r.
rhysodes
  Acanthamoeba r.
rhythm
  circadian r.
  diurnal r.
  escape r.
  gallop r.
  irregular r.
  junctional r. (JR)
  r. method
  r. method of contraception
  r. method of family planning
rhythmic movement disorder
RI
  resistance index
RIA
  radioimmunoassay
  Insulin RIA 100
rib
  cervical r.
  r. fracture
  r. hump
  r. notching
  r. notching sign
  r. rotation
  r. splitting
  supernumerary r.
  wavy r.
RIBA
  recombinant immunosorbent assay

ribavirin
    aerosolized r.
    intraventricular r.
Ribbing
    R. disease
    R. skeletal abnormality
ribbon
    radioactive r.'s
ribbonlike stool
rib-gap defect-micrognathia
  syndrome
riboflavin deficiency
ribonuclease (RNase)
ribonucleic
    r. acid (RNA)
    r. acid probe
ribonucleoprotein antigen
ribonucleotide
ribosomal RNA
ribosome
ribosuria
ribotide
    succinyl aminoimidazole carboxamide
      r. (SAICAR)
rib-polydactyly
    Saldino-Noonan short r.-p.
    short r.-p. (type I, II)
RICE
    rest, ice, compression, elevation
    RICE sequence
Ricelyte
rich
    calcium r.
    Rolaids Calcium R.
Richardson
    R. paravaginal repair
    R. retractor
Richards-Rundle syndrome
Richner-Hanhart syndrome
Richner syndrome
Richter
    R. and Albrich vaginal sacrospinous
      suspension procedure
    R. hernia
ricin
ricinus
    Ixodes r.
rickets
    familial hypophosphatemic r.
    hypophosphatemic r.
    nonnutritional r.
    nutritional r.
    oncogenous r.
    primary hypophosphatemic r.
    renal r.
    renal insufficiency r.
    type I r.
    type II r.
    vitamin D-dependent r.

    vitamin D-resistant r.
    X-linked hypophosphatemic r.
     (XLHR)
rickettsemia
Rickettsia
    R. africae
    R. akari
    R. australis
    R. conorii
    R. felis
    R. honei
    R. japonica
    R. prowazekii
    R. rickettsii
    R. siberica
    R. typhi
rickettsial
    r. agglutination
    r. disease
    r. infection
rickettsialpox
rickettsii
    Rickettsia r.
rickettsiosis
rid
    R. gel
    R. liquid
    R. Mousse
    R. shampoo
Rid-A-Pain
Ridaura
Ridenol
ride-on toy
ridge
    alveolar r.
    apical ectodermal r.
    cervicovaginal r.
    ectodermal r.
    genital r.
    germ r.
    gonadal r.
    hyperkeratotic r.
    mesonephric r.
    transverse r.
    urogenital r.
    wolffian r.
ridging
    metopic r.
Riechert-Mundinger stereotactic system
Riedel lobe
Rieger
    R. anomaly
    R. malformation
    R. syndrome
rifabutin
Rifadin
rifampicin (*var. of* rifampin)
rifampin, rifampicin
rifamycin

rifapentine
    25-desacetyl r.
Rift Valley fever
RIG
    rabies immunoglobulin
Riga-Fede disease
right
    r. acromiodorsoposterior fetal
        position
    r. anterior oblique (RAO)
    r. aortic arch (RAA)
    r. atrial hypertrophy
    r. atrial pressure (RAP)
    r. axis deviation
    Breathe R.
    r. bundle branch block (RBBB)
    r. colon pouch
    r. common carotid
    r. common carotid artery (RCCA)
    r. ductus arteriosus (RDA)
    r. femoral artery (RFA)
    r. frontoanterior position (RFA)
    r. frontoposterior position (RFP)
    r. frontotransverse position (RFT)
    r. hepatectomy
    r. lateral position
    left to r. (L-R)
    R. Light examination light
    r. lower quadrant (RLQ)
    r. lung hypoplasia
    r. mentoanterior position (RMA)
    r. mentoposterior position (RMP)
    r. mentotransverse position (RMT)
    r. middle lobe syndrome
    r. occipitoanterior (ROA)
    r. occipitoposterior (ROP)
    r. occipitoposterior position
    r. occipitoposterior presentation
    r. occipitotransverse (ODT, ROT)
    r. occipitotransverse position
    r. ovarian vein syndrome
    patient r.'s
    r. sacroanterior position
    r. sacroposterior position
    r. sacrotransverse position
    r. scapuloanterior position (RScA)
    r. scapuloposterior position (RScP)
    r. sit
    termination of parental r.'s
    r. to be well-born
    r. upper quadrant (RUQ)
    r. ventricle (RV)
    r. ventricular dysplasia
    r. ventricular ejection fraction
        (RVEF)
    r. ventricular end-diastolic volume
        (RVEDV)
    r. ventricular hypertrophy (RVH)
    r. ventricular hypoplasia

    r. ventricular infundibulum
    r. ventricular outflow tract
        (RVOT)
    r. ventricular outflow tract
        obstruction (RVOTO)
    r. ventricular outflow tract
        reconstruction
    r. ventricular stroke work index
        (RVSWI)
right-angle
    r.-a. retractor
    r.-a. scissors
    r.-a. suture
righting
    head r.
    r. reaction
    r. reflex
    r. response
right-left discrimination
right-sided
    r.-s. heart failure
    r.-s. lesion
    r.-s. stomach
right-to-left
    r.-t.-l. shunt
    r.-t.-l. shunting
    r.-t.-l. shunt ratio (Qs/Qt)
rigid
    r. bronchoscopy
    r. cerebral palsy
    r. clubfoot
    r. cystoscopy
    r. metatarsus
    r. open-tube endoscope
    r. perfectionism
    r. spine syndrome
    r. supination deformity
rigidity
    chest wall r.
    congenital articular r.
    decerebrate r.
    multiple articular r.
    muscle r.
    nuchal r.
    parkinsonian r.
rigidus
    hallux r.
Rigiflex balloon
RigiScan instrument
rigor
RIHD
    radiation-induced heart disease
rIL-2
    recombinant interleukin 2
Riley-Day syndrome
Riley-Shwachman syndrome
Riley-Smith syndrome
Rimactane
rimantadine

ring
- amnion r.
- r. applicator
- Bandl r.
- combined estrogen and progesterone vaginal r.
- r. constriction
- constriction r.
- continence r.
- contraceptive r.
- Cook balloon-inflated continence r.
- division of pancreatic r.
- double r.
- Estrace VR intravaginal r.
- estradiol-releasing silicone vaginal r.
- Estring estradiol vaginal r.
- Falope r.
- r. finger (RF)
- r. forceps
- gestational r.
- Graefenberg r.
- hymenal r.
- Imlach r.
- Kayser-Fleischer r.
- Milex incontinence r.
- neonatal r.
- NuvaRing vaginal contraceptive r.
- pancreatic r.
- pathologic retraction r.
- r. pessary
- phimotic r.
- physiologic retraction r.
- progestin-impregnated vaginal r.
- retraction r.
- r. sideroblast (RS)
- silastic r.
- Suarez r.
- r. 1–22 syndrome
- trigonal r.
- T-shaped constriction r.
- tubal r.
- vaginal contraceptive r.
- vascular r.
- visual tracking of red r.
- Waldeyer r.
- Wimberger r.
- Yoon r.
- zipper r.

Ringer
- heparinized lactated R.
- R. lactate
- lactated R.
- R. solution

ringworm
- beard r.
- black dot r.
- body r.

- groin r.
- nail r.
- scalp r.

Rinne test

rinse
- Nix Creme R.
- permethrin creme r.

Riopan Plus

RIP
- respiratory inductive plethysmography

RIPA
- radioimmunoprecipitation assay

ripener
- cervical r.
- Prepidil Gel cervical r.

ripening
- Bishop score of cervical r.
- cervical r.
- Cervidil r.
- flow r.
- spontaneous cervical r.
- vertical flow r.

rippling muscle disease

RIS
- respiratory index score

risedronate

risk
- age-related r.
- r. assessment
- r. behavior
- biologic r.
- direct suicide r. (DSR)
- elevated obstetric r.
- environmental r.
- established r.
- r. factor
- fetal r.
- first and second trimester evaluation of r. (FASTER)
- haplotype relative r. (HRR)
- high r.
- r. management
- maternal age-related r.
- neonatal mortality r. (NMR)
- obesity r.
- obstetric r.
- population-attributable r. (PAR)
- prenatal r.
- recurrence r.
- relative r.
- r. stratification
- teratogenic r.

risk-benefit
- r.-b. analysis
- r.-b. ratio

risk-taking behavior

risky behavior

Risperdal

risperidone

R

Risser
    R. brace
    R. classification
    R. curve
    R. localizer cast
    R. pessary
    R. sign
RIST
    radioimmunosorbent test
ristocetin
    r. cofactor
    r. cofactor activity
    r. cofactor assay
risus sardonicus
RITA
    radiofrequency interstitial tissue
      ablation system
Ritalin
Ritalin-SR
Rite Time
Ritgen maneuver
ritodrine hydrochloride
ritonavir
Ritscher-Schinzel syndrome
Ritter disease
ritualism
ritualistic phenomenon
Rivotril
rizatriptan
RLDS
    Reynell Language Development Scale
RLF
    retrolental fibroplasia
RLP
    rectal linitis plastica
RLQ
    right lower quadrant
RLT
    reduced liver transplant
RMR
    resting metabolic rate
RMS
    rhabdomyosarcoma
      alveolar RMS
      embryonal RMS
      RMS Rectal
      RMS Uniserts
RMSF
    Rocky Mountain spotted fever
RMSS
    Ruvalcaba-Myhre-Smith syndrome
RN
    reflux neuropathy
^{222}Rn
    radon-222
RNA
    ribonucleic acid
      complementary RNA
      RNA electrophoresis

      messenger RNA
      RNA nucleotidyltransferase
      packaging RNA
      poly A RNA
      RNA polymerase
      ribosomal RNA
      serum HCV RNA
      soluble RNA
      RNA splicing
      transfer RNA (tRNA)
RNA-directed DNA polymerase
RNAse
    ribonuclease
ROA
    right occipitoanterior
Robafen
    R. AC
    R. DM
Robaxin
Robert pelvis
Roberts
    R. pseudothalidomide syndrome
    R. tetraphocomelia syndrome
    R. thumb retractor
robertsonian
    r. fusion
    r. translocation
Roberts-SC phocomelia syndrome
Robidrine
Robimycin
Robin
    R. anomalad
    R. syndrome
Robinow
    R. dwarfism
    R. mesomelic dysplasia
    R. syndrome
Robinow-Silverman-Smith syndrome
Robinow-Sorauf syndrome
Robins and Guze validation
    strategy
Robinul Forte
RoBi rotating bipolar forceps and
    scissors
Robitussin
    R. Cough Calmers
    R. Pediatric
Robitussin-DM infant drops
Robomol
ROC
    receiver operating characteristic
    ROC XS suture fastener
Rocaltrol
Rocephin
Rochalimaea henselae
Roche
    R. Amplicor Monitor assay
    R. Diagnostics
Rocher-Sheldon syndrome

Rochester
    R. criteria
    R. HKAFO
Rochester-Ochsner forceps
Rochester-Péan forceps
rocker-bottom (*var. of* rockerbottom)
rockerbottom, rocker-bottom
    r. foot
rocket dilator
Rockey-Davis incision
rocking
    body r.
Rock-Mulligan hood
Rocky
    R. Mountain spotted fever
    (RMSF)
    R. Mountain wood tick
rocuronium
rod
    gram-negative r.
    gram-positive r.
    Harrington r.
    hygroscopic r.
    intramedullary r.
    Küntscher r.
    r. myopathy
    nemaline r.
    pleomorphic gram-negative r.
Rodeck method
rodenticide poisoning
Rodriguez lethal acrofacial dysostosis
Roeder
    R. knot
    R. loop slipknot
    modified R.
Roenigk
    R. classification scale
    R. grade
roentgen
roentgenogram
roentgenograph
roentgenographic examination
roentgenography
    chest r.
rofecoxib
Roferon-A
Rogaine Topical
Roger
    R. forceps
    maladie de R.
rogletimide
Rohrer index
Rohr stria
Rohypnol
Rokitansky
    R. pelvis
    R. prominence
    R. protuberance

    R. tubercle
Rokitansky-Küster-Hauser syndrome
Rolaids Calcium Rich
rolandic
    r. epilepsy
    r. seizure
    r. sharp wave
role
    gender r.
    r. reversal
roll
    therapy r.
Rolland-Desbuquois syndrome
Rollator
rollerball
    r. electrode
    r. endometrial ablation (REA)
    r. technique
RollerBar electrode
rollerbar-loop-rollerbar ablation
roller-barrel electrode
RollerLoop vaporizing loop electrode
roller occlusion
rolling
    segmental r.
rollover test
ROM
    range of motion
Romaña sign
Romano-Ward long QT syndrome
Romazicon Injection
Romberg test
Rome
    R. criteria for functional abdominal pain
    R. II criteria for functional bowel disorder
Rondec
    R. drops
    R. Filmtab
    R. Syrup
Rondec-DM
Rondec-TR
rongeur
    pediatric bone r.
    Tobey ear r.
roof
    acetabular r.
    flat acetabular r.
rooftop incision
room
    r. air
    birthing r.
    delivery r.
    emergency r. (ER)
    LDR r.
    obstetric emergency r.
    r. temperature
rooming in, rooming-in

rooming-in (*var. of* rooming in)
root
    aortic r.
    broad nasal r.
    mesenteric r.
    nasal r.
    valerian r.
rooting reflex
ROP
    retinopathy of prematurity
    right occipitoposterior
ropelike filum terminale
rope sign
ropivacaine
    r. HCl
    r. hydrochloride
Rorschach test
ROS
    reactive oxygen species
    review of systems
rosacea
    acne r.
Rosai-Dorfman disease
rosary
    rachitic r.
    scorbutic r.
Rosch-Thurmond fallopian tube
  catheterization set
rosea
    pityriasis r.
Rosenberg Self-Esteem Scale
  (RSES)
Rosenmüller
    organ of R.
Rosenthal fiber
Rosenthal-Kloepfer syndrome
roseola
    r. infantum
    r. rash
roseolalike illness
rose spot
rosette
    Homer Wright r.
    mucosal r.
    r. test
rosettelike blister
Rosewater syndrome
ROSNI
    round spermatid nuclei injection
rOspA
    recombinant outer surface protein A
    rOspA Lyme disease vaccine
Ross
    R. carbohydrate-free (RCF)
    R. growth chart
    R. operation
    R. procedure
    R. pulmonary porcine valve
    R. River virus

Ro/SSA
    Ro/SSA antigen
    Ro/SSA autoantigen
Rossavik growth model
Rosselli-Gulienetti syndrome
Ross-Konno operation
Ross-Konno-Switch operation
Rossolimo reflex
rostral
    r. direction
    r. neuropore
    r. ventromedial medulla
    (RVMM)
rostrocaudal
rostrum
ROT
    right occipitotransverse
Rotacaps
    Ventolin R.
Rotadisk
    Flovent R.
Rotamune
rotary
    r. atlantoaxial luxation
    r. chewing
    r. subluxation
RotaTeq
rotation
    r. and descent
    external r.
    flexion, adduction, internal r.
    (FADIR, fadir)
    forceps r.
    hip r.
    internal r.
    Kjelland r.
    lateral r. (LR)
    lateral hip r.
    manual r.
    medial r. (MR)
    medial hip r.
    r. movement
    neutral r.
    r. of spine
    rib r.
    trunk r.
    upward r.
rotational
    r. delivery
    r. malalignment
    r. osteotomy
rotationplasty
rotatory
    r. displacement
    r. subluxation
rotavirus
    r. enteritis
    r. gastroenteritis
    infantile diarrhea r.

r. vaccination
r. vaccine
Rotazyme
R. diagnostic procedure
R. test
rote memory
Rothmann-Makai syndrome
Rothmund syndrome
Rothmund-Thomson cancer predisposition syndrome
Rothmund-Werner syndrome
Roth spot
Roticulator 55 stapler
Rotor disease
Rotter
R. node
R. Sentence Completion Test
Rotterdam
R. consensus on polycystic ovarian syndrome
R. consensus recommendation
rotunda
pityriasis r.
Roubac
Rouget bulb
rough endoplasmic reticulum (RER)
rough-feeling skin
round
r. back deformity
r. cell tumor
r. iliac bone
r. ligament
r. ligament pain
r. ligament syndrome
r. moon face
r. pelvis
r. spermatid nuclei injection (ROSNI)
r. window electrocochleography (RWECochG)
round-back
postural r.-b.
round-headed acrosomeless spermatozoa
roundworm
Rous sarcoma virus
Roussy-Lévy
R.-L. disease
R.-L. syndrome
route of delivery
routine
r. antenatal diagnostic imaging with ultrasound (RADIUS)
daily r.
r. postoperative care
r. prenatal testing
r. prenatal visit
r. preoperative test
r. screening

r. screening cervical examination
r. wound management
Roux-en-Y
R.-e.-Y anastomosis
R.-e.-Y choledochojejunostomy
Rovamycine
Rovsing
R. sign
R. test
Rowasa
R. enema
R. Rectal
Rowden uterine manipulator-injector (RUMI)
Rowland pouch
Roxanol SR
Roxicet 5/500
Roxicodone
Roxilox
roxithromycin
Royal College of General Practitioners' Oral Contraception Study
RP
Raynaud phenomenon
RP with progressive sensorineural hearing loss
RPC
reactive perforating collagenosis
retained products of conception
RPCV
retropubic cystourethropexy
RPD
Pepcid RPD
RPE
retinal pigment epithelium
RPICC
regional perinatal intensive care center
RPL
recurrent pregnancy loss
repeated pregnancy loss
RPLS
reversible posterior leukoencephalopathy syndrome
RPM
Raven Progressive Matrices
RPMPR
radical posteromedial and plantar release
RPO
reflectance pulse oximetry
RPO oximeter
RPR
rapid plasma reagin
RPR titer
RPRCT
rapid plasma reagin card test
RPU
retropubic urethrocystopexy

R

799

RR
   red reflex
RRF
   ragged red fiber
RRFC
   renal reserve filtration capacity
RRP
   recurrent respiratory papillomatosis
RS
   reactive site
   ring sideroblast
      RS mutation
RS-61443
   mycophenolate mofetil
RSA
   recurrent spontaneous abortion
   respiratory sinus arrhythmia
RSBI
   rapid shallow breathing index
RSD
   reflex sympathetic dystrophy
RSE
   refractory status epilepticus
RSES
   Rosenberg Self-Esteem Scale
RSH/SLO syndrome
RSH/Smith-Lemli-Opitz syndrome
RSH syndrome
RSI
   rapid sequence intubation
RSL
   renal solute load
RSLT
   reduced-size liver transplant
RSV
   respiratory syncytial virus
      RSV antigen
      RSV bronchiolitis
      RSV immunoglobulin for intravenous
         administration
      RSV monoclonal antibody
      RSV nasal wash
      RSV pneumonitis
RSV-associated wheeze
RSVB
   respiratory syncytial virus
      bronchiolitis
RSV-IG, RSVIG
   respiratory syncytial virus
      immunoglobulin
RSV-IGIV
   respiratory syncytial virus
      immunoglobulin intravenous
RT
   radiation therapy
RTA
   renal tubular acidosis
      distal RTA
      hyperkalemic RTA

mineralocorticoid-deficiency RTA
      proximal RTA
      type IV RTA
RTI
   respiratory tract infection
   reverse transcriptase inhibitor
rt-PA
   recombinant tissue type plasminogen
      activator
RT-PCR
   reverse transcription polymerase chain
      reaction
RTS
   Revised Trauma Score
RTUS
   real-time ultrasonography
RTV
   ritonavir
RTx
   radiation therapy
   renal transplantation
Ru
   ruthenium
RU 486
rub
      friction r.
      pericardial friction r.
      pleural friction r.
rubber bleb nevus
rubella
      congenital r.
      r. embryopathy
      r. factor testing
      r. immune
      r. immunization
      r. infection
      maternal r.
      measles, mumps, r. (MMR)
      r. panencephalitis
      periconceptional r.
      r. scarlatinosa
      r. strain
      r. syndrome
      r. titer assessment
      r. vaccine
      r. virus
rubella-immune mother
rubella-negative mother
Rubens flap
rubeola
      r. immunization
      r. scarlatinosa
      r. titer
      r. virus
Rubex
Rubin
      R. cannula
      R. criteria
      R. shoulder dystocia maneuver

R. test
R. tube
Rubinstein syndrome
Rubinstein-Taybi syndrome
Rubivirus
rubor
rubra
    lochia r.
    miliaria r.
rubrum
    tinea r.
    Trichophyton r.
ruddy
Rudiger syndrome
rudimentary
    r. testis syndrome
    r. uterine horn
    r. vagina
rudimentary-type digit
Rud syndrome
rue
    goat's r.
ruga, *pl.* **rugae**
    rugae of vagina
    rugae vaginales
rugae (*pl. of* ruga)
rugal fold
rugated vaginal mucosa
rugation
rugger jersey spine
rule
    10% r.
    Arey r.
    Budin r.
    7-day r.
    Haase r.
    His r.
    4-hour r.
    informed consent disclosure r.'s
    Lossen r.
    McDonald r.
    Mittendorf-Williams r.
    Nägele r.
    r. of nines
    r. of outlet
    r. of 60s
    r. of threes
    Ogino-Knaus r.
    Ottawa Ankle R.'s (OAR)
    Trauma Triage R. (TTR)
    Van Praagh loop r.
    Weinberg r.
10% rule
Rumack-Matthew nomogram
rumble
    middiastolic r.
rumbling murmur
RUMI
    Rowden uterine manipulator-injector

rumination disorder
Rum-K
Rumpel-Leede phenomenon
Runeberg anemia
running
    r. imbricating stitch
    r. locked stitch
runoff
    aortic r.
runt disease
runting
rupture
    amnion r.
    angiomyolipoma r.
    aortic arch r.
    arterial r.
    cardiac r.
    esophageal r.
    follicle aspiration, sperm injection, assisted r. (FASIAR)
    hepatic r.
    marginal sinus r.
    membrane r.
    neural tube r.
    r. of chorioamniotic membrane
    ovarian r.
    peroneal r.
    postmembrane r.
    prelabor membrane r.
    premature amnion r.
    premature membrane r.
    premembrane r.
    prolonged r.
    splenic r.
    testicular r.
    total perineal r.
    tubal r.
    ureteral r.
    uterine r.
ruptured
    r. appendicitis
    r. bronchiole
    r. capsule
    r. cerebral aneurysm
    r. corpus luteum
    r. endometrioma
    r. episiotomy
    r. globe
    r. sinus of Valsalva aneurysm
    r. symphysis pubis
    r. uterus
RUQ
    right upper quadrant
Rusch bag
Rusconi
    anus of R.
rush immunotherapy
Russell
    R. diencephalic syndrome (I, II, III)

Russell (*continued*)
R. dwarf
R. nanism
R. sign
R. traction
R. viper venom time
Russell-Silver
R.-S. dwarfism
R.-S. dwarf syndrome
Russian
R. spring-summer encephalitis
R. tissue forceps
rust-colored sputum
ruthenium
Rutherfurd syndrome
Rutledge
R. classification of extended hysterectomy
R. lethal multiple congenital anomalies syndrome
Rutter mean score
Ruvalcaba-Myhre-Smith syndrome (RMSS)
Ruvalcaba-Myhre syndrome
Ruvalcaba-Reichert-Smith syndrome
Ruvalcaba syndrome
RV
rectal vault
rectovaginal
residual volume
right ventricle
Rv
rotavirus
Rv vaccine
RVA
rabies vaccine, absorbed
RVC
radionuclide voiding cystography

RVDT
retinal venous dilation and tortuosity
RVEDV
right ventricular end-diastolic volume
RVEF
right ventricular ejection fraction
RVH
right ventricular hypertrophy
RVOT
right ventricular outflow tract
RVOTO
right ventricular outflow tract obstruction
RVPaque cream
RVR
relative vascular resistance
RVS
recognizable viral syndrome
RVSWI
right ventricular stroke work index
RVVC
recurrent vulvovaginal candidiasis
RWECochG
round window electrocochleography
Rx
prescription
Rx medibottle
Mission Prenatal Rx
RxFISH DNA probe and analysis system
Ryan agar
Rye classification
Ryna-C
Rynacrom
Ryna-CX
Ryna Liquid
Rynatan Pediatric
RZ
reserve zone

S

S phase
S phase fraction

SA

sacroanterior
sinoatrial node

S-A

sinuatrial
sinoatrial node

SAB

spontaneous abortion

saber

S. BT blunt-tip surgical
trocar
s. cut incision
s. shin
s. shin deformity

Sabin

S. OPV
S. vaccine

Sabinas brittle hair syndrome
Sabin-Feldman dye test
sabot

coeur en s.

Sabouraud medium
sabre

S. FreeHand high-intensity medical
pocket light
scleroderma en coup de s.

Sabril
sac

abnormal gestational s.
allantoic s.
aortic s.
chorionic s.
cystic s.
embryonic s.
fetal s.
gestational s. (GS)
hernia s.
intrauterine s.
Lap S.
monoamniotic s.
nasolacrimal s.
Pleatman s.
preputial s.
pseudogestational s.
pudendal s.
vitelline s.
widened thecal s.
yolk s.

SACA

Service Assessment for Children and
Adolescents

saccade

saccharate

dextroamphetamine s.

Saccharomyces

S. boulardii
S. cerevisiae

saccharopinuria
saccular

s. aneurysm
s. dilation
s. period
s. stage
s. stage of lung development

sacculated
sacculation of uterus
saccus

s. anticus
s. medius
s. posticus
s. superior

sacra, *pl. of* **sacrum**
sacral

s. agenesis
s. colpopexy
s. dimple
s. lymph node
s. meningomyelocele
s. nerve
s. nerve root stimulation
s. neural tube defect
s. promontory
s. reflex

sacroanterior (SA)

left s. (LSA)
s. position

sacrococcygeal teratoma
sacrocolpopexy

abdominal s.
s. graft
laparoscopic s.

sacroiliac (SI)

s. dysfunction
s. joint

sacroiliitis
sacropexy

abdominal s.

sacroposterior (SP)

s. position

sacrosciatic notch
sacrosidase
sacrospinous

s. colpopexy
s. ligament
s. ligament fixation (SSLF)
s. ligament suspension
s. vaginal vault suspension

S

sacrotransverse
    left s. (LST)
    s. position
sacrotuberous ligament
sacrum, *pl.* **sacra**
    hollow of s.
    hypoplastic s.
SAD
    seasonal affective disorder
    separation anxiety disorder
    source-to-axis distance
saddle
    s. block
    s. block anesthesia
    s. nose
saddleback
    s. fever
    s. temperature curve
saddlebag flap
saddle-nose deformity
S-adenosylhomocysteine (SAH)
sadness
Saenger
    S. operation
    S. ovum forceps
Saethre-Chotzen syndrome
SAFE
    sexual assault forensic evidence
safe
    S. kit
    S. Tussin 30
safety
    infant s.
    system for thalidomide education
      and prescription s. (STEPS)
Safil synthetic absorbable surgical
 suture
Saf-T-Coil IUD
saginata
    Taenia s.
sagittal
    s. craniosynostosis
    s. fontanelle
    s. plane
    s. septum of rectus sheath
    s. sinus
    s. sinus thrombosis
    s. suture
    s. suture line
    s. synostosis
sagrada
    cascara s.
SAH
    S-adenosylhomocysteine
Sahara DryEar ear dryer
SAICAR
    succinyl aminoimidazole carboxamide
     ribotide
sail sign

Saint (St.) (*see also* **St.**)
Saizen Injection
Sakati-Nyhan syndrome
SAL
    suction-assisted lipoplasty
salaam
    s. convulsion
    infantile s.
    s. seizure
Sal-Acid Plaster
Salagen Oral
Salazopyrin
salbutamol
Saldino-Noonan
    S.-N. dwarfism
    S.-N. short rib-polydactyly
    S.-N. syndrome
Salem pump
SalEst
    S. immunoassay
    S. preterm labor test system
    S. system test
Salflex
salicylate
    choline s.
    s. intoxication
    magnesium s.
    methanol, uremia, diabetes,
     paraldehyde, isoniazid, infection,
     lactic acidosis, ethylene glycol, s.
     (MUDPILES)
    phenyl s.
    s. poisoning
    sodium s.
    s. toxicity
salicylic
    s. acid
    s. acid ointment
    s. sugar powder
salicylism
salicylsalicylic acid
saline
    s. abortion
    s. cathartic
    s. drop method
    s. drop test
    Dulbecco phosphate buffered s.
    extrarenal s.
    heparinized s.
    hypertonic s.
    hypotonic s.
    iced s.
    s. implant
    s. infusion sonography (SIS)
    s. infusion sonohysterography (SIS)
    isotonic s.
    s. lavage
    s. microscopy
    normal s. (NS

s. nose drops
phosphate-buffered s.
    (PBS)
physiologic s.
s. solution
tris[hydroxymethyl]aminomethane-
    buffered s.
s. wet smear
SalineX
salivarius
    Streptococcus s.
salivary
s. adenitis
s. amylase
s. cortisol
s. cortisol assay
s. estriol
s. estriol test
s. estriol testing
s. gland
salivation, lacrimation, urination, defecation, gastrointestinal distress, emesis (SLUDGE)
Salk
S. IPV
S. vaccine
Salla disease
salmeterol
s. powder
s. xinafoate
salmon
calcitonin s.
s. patch
S. sign
salmonella
S. bacteria
S. choleraesuis
S. dublin
S. enteritidis
S. gastroenteritis
S. heidelberg
S. hirschfeldii
S. meningitis
S. newport
non-typhi *S.* (NTS)
nontyphoid *S.*
nontyphoidal *S.*
S. oranienburg
S. oranienburg sepsis
S. osteomyelitis
S. paratyphi
S. schottmuelleri
S. typhi
S. typhimurium
salmonellosis
salmon-pink rash
Salonen-Herva-Norio syndrome
salpingectomy
laparoscopic s.

partial s.
postpartum partial s.
salpingemphraxis
salpinges (*pl. of* salpinx)
salpingioma
salpingitic
salpingitis
s. after previous tubal occlusion
    (SPOT)
chronic interstitial s.
foreign body s.
gonorrheal s.
granulomatous s.
s. in previously occluded tubes
    (SPOT)
s. isthmica nodosa
    (SIN)
leprous s.
nongranulomatous s.
pyogenic s.
tuberculous s.
salpingocele
salpingocentesis
salpingocyesis
salpingography
transcervical selective s.
salpingolysis
salpingoneostomy
salpingo-oophorectomy
abdominal s.-o.
bilateral s.-o. (BSO)
unilateral s.-o. (USO)
salpingo-oophoritis
salpingo-oophorocele
salpingoovariectomy
salpingoovariolysis
salpingoperitonitis
salpingopexy
salpingoplasty
salpingorrhagia
salpingorrhaphy
salpingoscopy
salpingostomatomy
salpingostomy
linear s.
salpingotomy
abdominal s.
salpinx, *pl.* **salpinges**
salsalate
salt
bile s.
calcium s.
s. craving
s. frosting of skin
gold s.
guanidine s.
inorganic mercury s.
Pedi-Bath S.'s
s. poisoning

S

salt (*continued*)
    s. restriction
    s. wasting
salt-and-pepper
    s.-a.-p. appearance
    s.-a.-p. fundus
    s.-a.-p. retinitis
Salter
    S. osteotomy
    S. procedure
Salter-Harris
    S.-H. classification
    S.-H. classification of epiphysial
      plate injury
    S.-H. classification of fracture
    S.-H. epiphysial fracture
    S.-H. fracture (type I–V)
**salt-losing adrenogenital syndrome
(SLAS)**
salt-wasting
    s.-w. adrenogenital syndrome
    s.-w. congenital adrenal hyperplasia
      (SW-CAH)
saltwater near-drowning
salutary effect
salute
    allergic s.
salvage
    s. cesarean
    s. chemotherapy
    s. intervention
    s. laparotomy
    limb s.
    s. therapy
same-sex relationship
sample
    arterial blood s. (ABS)
    blood s.
    citrate blood s.
    clean-catch midstream urine s.
    cord blood s.
    endocervical s.
    exocervical s.
    midstream urine s.
    urine s.
    venous blood s. (VBS)
sampler
    Cervex-Brush cervical cell s.
    Cordguard umbilical cord s.
    Cytobrush Plus endocervical cell s.
    Endocell endometrial cell s.
    Milex syringe s.
    SelectCells Mini endometrial s.
    Wallach Endocell endometrial cell s.
sampling
    axillary node s.
    biologic s.
    blood s.
    capillary blood gas s.

    cerebrospinal fluid s.
    chemical s.
    chorion s.
    chorionic villus s. (CVS)
    endocervical s.
    endometrial s.
    fetal scalp blood s.
    fetal scalp platelet s.
    fetal skin s.
    hair s.
    heel capillary s.
    histologic s.
    Mucat cervical s.
    percutaneous blood s.
    percutaneous umbilical blood s.
     (PUBS)
    perimortem s.
    periumbilical artery blood s.
    postmortem s.
    random s.
    scalp blood s.
    tissue s.
    transabdominal chorionic villus s.
    transcervical chorionic villus s.
    trophoblast s.
    ultrasound-directed percutaneous
     umbilical blood s.
    umbilical blood s.
    urine s.
    venous blood s.
Sampson
    artery of S.
    S. cyst
    S. theory
    S. theory of endometriosis
San
    S. Joaquin fever
    S. Luis Valley syndrome
Sanchez-Cascos syndrome
Sanchez-Corona syndrome
Sanchez-Salorio syndrome
sandal sign
Sanders jet respirator
Sandhoff
    S. disease
    S. GM2 gangliosidosis (type I, II)
    S. syndrome
Sandifer syndrome
Sandimmune
Sandoglobulin
Sandostatin LAR Depot
sandpaper rash
sandwich
    s. assay
    solid-phase s.
Sanfilippo disease A, B, C, D
Sanger incision
sanguinis
    Gemella s.

sanguinolenta
    lochia s.
sanguinolentis
    fetus s.
sanguinopurulent
Sani-Spec vaginal speculum
Sani-Supp Suppository
Sanjad-Sakati syndrome
SANS
    schedule for assessment of negative
    symptoms
Sansert
Santavuori
    S. disease
    muscle-eye-brain disease of S.
    S. syndrome
Santavuori-Haltia syndrome
S-100 antibody
Santulli enterostomy
SAO
    Southeast Asian ovalocytosis
SaO2
    oxygen saturation
Sao Paulo MCA/MR syndrome
SAP
    surfactant-associated protein
    systolic arterial pressure
sap
    cervical s.
    Prentif cavity-rim cervical s.
SAP1
    sphingolipid activator protein-1
saphenous
    s. nerve
    s. nerve entrapment
    s. vein
    s. vein catheter insertion
saponification
Sapporo virus
saprophytic
saprophyticus
    Staphylococcus s.
SAPS
    schedule for assessment of positive
    symptoms
    simplified acute physiology score
saquinavir
Sarafem
sarcofetal pregnancy
sarcoid
    alveolar s.
sarcoid-like
sarcoidosis
    nervous system s.
    ocular s.
    subcutaneous s.
sarcolemma
sarcoma
    adenosquamous s.

    alveolar soft part s.
    blue-cell s.
    s. botryoid
    botryoid s.
    Burkitt s.
    cervical s.
    chordoid s.
    clear cell s.
    embryonal s.
    endometrial s.
    endometrial stromal s.
    (EES, ESS)
    Ewing s.
    extraosseous Ewing s.
    granulocytic s.
    heterologous uterine s.
    homologous uterine s.
    immunoblastic s.
    Kaposi s. (KS)
    Kaposi varicelliform s.
    mesodermal s.
    mixed mesodermal s. (MMS)
    mixed müllerian s.
    mixed ovarian mesodermal s.
    müllerian s.
    neurogenic s.
    nonrhabdomyogenic soft
      tissue s.
    nonrhabdomyomatous s.
    nonrhabdomyosarcoma soft tissue s.
    (NRSTS)
    obesity in endometrial s.
    osteogenic s.
    penile Kaposi s.
    penoscrotal Kaposi s.
    pseudoglandular synovial s.
    retroperitoneal soft tissue s.
    secretory s.
    soft tissue s.
    synovial s.
    tenosynovial s.
    testicular Kaposi s.
    uterine müllerian s.
    vaginal s.
    vulvar s.
sarcomatous
    s. myoma degeneration
    s. tumor
sarcomere shortening
sarcomeric filament
sarcoplasmic reticulum
Sarcoptes scabiei
sarcoptic mange
sarcosinemia
sardonic smile
sardonicus
    risus s.
sargramostim
Sarna lotion

S

Sarnat
> S. encephalopathy
> S. score

SARS
> severe acute respiratory syndrome

SART
> Sexual Assault Response Team
> Society for Assisted Reproductive Technology

sartorial elegance

Saskatoon
> hemoglobin M S.

SASPP
> syndrome of absence of septum pellucidum with parencephaly

Sassone score

Sastid plain therapeutic shampoo and acne wash

satellite
> s. DNA
> s. lesion
> s. melanocytic nevus
> s. papule
> s. pustule

satellitosis

satiety
> early s.

satisfaction
> sexual s.

sativa
> *Cannabis s.*

Sato syndrome

satumomab pendetide imaging agent

saturated solution of potassium iodide (SSKI)

saturation
> s. analysis
> fetal arterial oxygen s. (FS_pO_2)
> fetal oxygen s.
> O_2 s.
> oxygen s. (SaO_2)
> oxyhemoglobin s.
> postductal oxygen s.
> s. strip
> transferrin s.

satyr ear

satyriasis

Sauflon PW contact lens

Saunders
> S. disease
> S. sign

sausage digit

sausage-shaped bulla

Savage syndrome

Savant Speed-Vac drier

Save-A-Tooth

saver
> Cell S.

saw
> Gigli s.

saw-toothed flutter wave

Saxtorph forceps delivery maneuver

Say-Gerald syndrome

Say-Meyer syndrome

Say syndrome

SB-6 antiserum

SBE
> self-breast examination
> subacute bacterial endocarditis
> > SBE prophylaxis

SBHC
> school-based health center

SBI
> serious bacterial infection

SBM
> selective broth medium

SBP
> spontaneous bacterial peritonitis
> spontaneous biliary perforation

SBPI
> sun protection behavior index

SBR
> stillbirth rate

SBS
> shaken baby syndrome
> short bowel syndrome

SBT
> serum bactericidal titer

S&C
> suction and curettage

SC
> hemoglobin SC
> SC phocomelia syndrome

ScA
> scapuloanterior

scabicide

scabiei
> *Sarcoptes s.*

scabies
> animal s.
> canine s.
> crusted s.
> human s.
> s. mite
> neonatal s.
> Norwegian s.
> s. scraping

SCAD
> short-chain acyl coenzyme A dehydrogenase
> > SCAD deficiency

scala tympani

scalded skin syndrome (SSS)

scalding injury

scale
> Abnormal Involuntary Movement S. (AIMS)

Acute Illness Observation S. (AIOS)
Alberta Infant Motor S. (AIMS)
Albert Einstein Neonatal
  Developmental S. (AENNS)
Anger Expression S.
anxiety-withdrawal s.
Apgar s.
Attention Deficit Disorders
  Evaluation S.
attrition rate s.
BAMO s.
Barnes Akathisia S. (BAS)
Bayley Mental S.
Behavioral and Emotional Rating S.
  (BERS)
Behavior Rating S. (BRS)
Bieri s.
Borg Perceived Exertion S.
Borg Physical Activity S.
Brazelton Neonatal Behavioral
  Assessment S. (BNAS, BNBAS)
broad-band s.
Canadian Acute Respiratory Illness
  and Flu S. (CARIFS)
Capute s.
Carey Temperament S.
Cattell Infant Intelligence S.
  (CIIS)
CGI s.
Child Abuse Trauma S. (CATS)
Child and Adolescent Functional
  Assessment S. (CAFAS)
Childhood Autism Rating S.
  (CARS)
Children's Depression S. (CDS)
Children's Global Assessment S.
  (CGAS)
Children's Manifest Anxiety S.
  (CMAS)
Clinical Adaptive Test/Clinical
  Linguistic and Auditory Milestone
  S. (CAT/CLAMS)
Clinical Linguistic and Auditory
  Milestone S. (CLAMS)
color analog s.
Columbia Impairment S.
Conners Rating S. (CRS)
Cooke-Medley Hostility S.
Cranley Maternal-Fetal
  Attachment S.
CRIES postoperative pain s.
depression rating s.
Depression Self-Rating S.
Disruptive Behavior Disorder S.
Dissociative Experience S. (DES)
Dyadic Adjustment S.
Dyskinesia Identification System:
  Condensed User S. (DISCUS)
Early Language Milestone s.

early neonatal neurobehavioral s.
Edinburgh Postnatal Depression S.
  (EPDS)
Einstein Neonatal Neurobehavioral
  Assessment S. (ENNAS)
electronic s.
ELM s.
Emotionality Activity Sociability S.
  (EAS)
Externalizing Behavior S.
Family Adaptability and Cohesion
  Evaluation S. (FACES)
Family Environment S. (FES)
Female Sexual Distress S. (FSDS)
FLACC s.
Flint Infant Security S. (FISS)
Functional Assessment S. (FAS)
Gesell Child Development Age S.
  (GCDAS)
Gesell Developmental S. (GDS)
Gesell Infant S.
Glasgow coma s. (GCS)
Graham-Rosenblith s.
gray s.
Green climacteric s.
Griffith Mental Developmental S.
  (GMDS)
Hamilton Depression S. (HAMD)
HITS s.
HOME s.
HSC S.
Impact of Events S. (IES)
infant face s.
Internalizing Behavior S.
IPAT Depression S.
Kent Infant Development S. (KIDS)
Leiter International Performance S.
Likert s. (LS)
linear visual analog s.
Locus of Control S.
Maternal Attitude S. (MAS)
McCarthy Memory S.
McGrath s.
mental s.
motor s.
Multidimensional Student Life
  Satisfaction S. (MSLSS)
muscle strength grading s.
Neonatal Behavioral Assessment S.
  (NBAS)
Neonatal Brazelton Assessment S.
Neonatal Infant Pain S. (NIPS)
Neurobiologic Risk S. (NBRS)
Newborn Behavior Assessment S.
  (NBAS)
NIMH global s.
Oucher s.
Parent and Teacher Conners S.
PARS s.

S

scale (*continued*)

Peabody Developmental Motor S. (PDMS)
Pediatric Liver Transplant-Specific S. (PLTSS)
Perceived Stress S.
Piers-Harris Children's Self-Concept S.
Piper fatigue s.
prosocial behavior s.
Receptive-Expressive Emergent Language S. (REEL)
Revised Children's Manifest Anxiety S. (RCMAS)
Reynell Language Development S. (RLDS)
Reynolds Child Depression S.
Roenigk classification s.
Rosenberg Self-Esteem S. (RSES)
shyness s.
Simpson-Angus rating s.
sperm progression s. (0–4)
standardized observation s.
Stanford-Binet intelligence s.
Tanner Developmental S. (stage 1–5)
Toddler Temperament S.
Toronto Alexithymia S. (TAS)
Urge Impact S. (URIS)
verbal analog pain s. (VAPS)
Vineland Adaptive Behavior S.'s
Vineland Social Maturity S.
visual analog s. (VAS)
Wechsler Memory S.
Wender Utah Rating S. (WURS)
Wong-Baker faces pain rating s.
Yale-Brown Obsessive Compulsive S. (YBOCS)
Yale Global Tic Severity S. (YGTSS)
Yale Observation S.
York Incontinence Perceptions S. (YIPS)

scale-III

Family Adaptability and Cohesion S.-III (FACES-III)

scalene muscle
scale-revised

Children's Depression Rating S.-R.

scaling

brawny s.
s. bulla
keratotic s.
Organ Injury S. (OIS)
oval s.

scalloped temporalis muscle
scalloping

frontal bones s.

scalp

s. blood sampling
cutis aplasia of s.
s. electrode
s. intravenous
s. IV
s. laceration
s. pH
s. pH determination
s. ringworm
s. seborrheic dermatitis
s. vein
s. vein catheter
s. vein catheterization
s. vein needle

scalpel

Bowen double-bladed s.
Endo-Assist retractable s.
Harmonic s.
Harmonic Ace s.
Shaw I, II s.

Scalpicin Topical
scaly dermatitis
scan

abdominopelvic s.
abdominopelvic CT s.
bleeding s.
bone s.
CAT s.
CT s.
DEXA s.
double-contrast CT s.
DTPA radionuclide s.
dual-energy x-ray absorptiometry s.
expiratory s.
gallium s.
gallium-67 s.
helical s.
indium-labeled leukocyte s.
iodine 125-labeled fibrinogen s.
longitudinal s.
Meckel s.
MIBG s.
milk s.
^{99m}Tc-HMPAO leukocyte s.
MUGA s.
multiple gated acquisition s.
PET s.
pinhole collimated s.
planar bone s.
radiofibrinogen uptake s.
radioisotope milk s.
radiolabeled white blood cell s.
radionuclide bone s.
radionuclide heart s.
red blood cell tagged s.
serial growth s.'s
spiral s.

technetium bone s.
technetium-99m bone s.
testicular flow s.
time position s.
transverse s.
S. ultrasound gel
ventilation/perfusion s.
V̇/Q̇ s.
xenon CT s.
Scandishake
Scanlon Assessment
scanner
Aloka 650 s.
Aloka SSD-720 real-time s.
BladderManager portable
  ultrasound s.
EUB-405 ultrasound s.
Sonos 5500 echocardiographic s.
scanning
CAT s.
CT s.
Doppler s.
duplex s.
s. electron microscopy (SEM)
gated blood pool s.
iodomethyl-norcholesterol s.
isotope s.
MEVA Probe for endovaginal s.
s. photometry
radionuclide s.
restriction landmark genomic s.
spectrophotometric s.
ultrasound s.
white cell s.
Scanzoni
S. forceps
S. maneuver
S. second os
Scanzoni-Smellie forceps delivery maneuver
scaphocephalism
scaphocephaly
scaphoid
s. abdomen
s. fontanelle
s. pad
s. scapula
scapula, *pl.* scapulae
congenital elevation of s.
scaphoid s.
scapulae (*pl. of* scapula)
scapular
s. fracture
s. repositioning
s. winging
scapularis
Ixodes s.
scapuloanterior (ScA)
left s. (LScA)

scapulohumeral muscular dystrophy
scapuloperoneal dystrophy
scapuloposterior (ScP)
scapulothoracic motion
scar
depressed s.
endometriosis of s.
hypertrophic s.
lower segment s.
perineal s.
s. prediction
radial s.
s. tissue
scare
vaccine-autism s.
SCARED
Screen for Child Anxiety-Related
  Emotional Disorders
SCARF
skeletal abnormalities, cutis laxa,
  craniostenosis, psychomotor
  retardation, facial abnormalities
scarf
s. maneuver
s. sign
scarification
scarlatina antitoxin
scarlatiniform
s. eruption
s. erythema
s. rash
scarlatinoides
scarlatinosa
rubella s.
rubeola s.
scarlet
s. fever
s. fever exanthema
SCARMD
severe childhood autosomal recessive
  muscular dystrophy
Scarpa fascia
scarred womb
scarring
corneal s.
renal s.
scatoma (*var. of* fecaloma)
scattered
s. echo
s. scores
scattering
Rayleigh-Tyndall s.
SCC
squamous cell carcinoma
SCCA
squamous cell carcinoma
SCCD
Schnyder crystalline corneal
  dystrophy

SCCMS
slow-channel congenital myasthenic syndrome
SCD
sickle cell disease
Scepter system
SCF
somatic cell-derived growth factor
SCFA
short-chain fatty acid
SCFE
slipped capital femoral epiphysis
acute-on-chronic SCFE
chronic SCFE
Preslip SCFE
SCH
supracervical hysterectomy
SCHAD
short-chain hydroxyacyl-coenzyme A dehydrogenase
Schafer syndrome
Schatz fetal position maneuver
Schauffler procedure
Schaumann body
Schauta-Aumreich radical vaginal hysterectomy procedure
Schauta vaginal operation
ScheBo pancreatic elastase kit
schedule
agglomeration s.
Autism Diagnostic Observation S. (ADOS)
child assessment s. (CAS)
S. for Affective Disorders and Schizophrenia for School-Age Children (K-SADS)
S. for Affective Disorders and Schizophrenia for School-Age Children-Epidemiologic Version (K-SADS-E)
S. for Affective Disorders and Schizophrenia for School-Age Children-Present Episode (K-SADS-P)
s. for assessment of negative symptoms (SANS)
s. for assessment of positive symptoms (SAPS)
Gesell Developmental S.'s
life events and difficulties s. (LEDS)
scheduled
s. feeding
s. voiding
scheduling
noncontingent s.
Scheibe
S. anomaly
S. aplasia

Scheie syndrome
schema, scheme, *pl.* **schemata**
TNM s.
schemata (*pl. of* schema)
scheme (*var. of* schema)
schenckii
Sporothrix s.
Scheuermann
S. disease
S. juvenile kyphosis (SJK)
Scheuer score
Scheuthauer-Marie-Sainton syndrome
Schick
S. sign
S. test
Schiff test
Schilder
S. disease
S. encephalitis
Schiller
S. solution
S. test
S. tumor
Schiller-Duvall body
Schilling test
Schimke immunoosseous dysplasia
Schimmelbusch
S. disease
S. syndrome
Schimmelpenning-Feuerstein-Mims syndrome
Schindler disease
Schinzel acrocallosal syndrome
Schinzel-Giedion
S.-G. midface-retraction syndrome
S.-G. syndrome (SGS)
SCHIP
State Children's Health Insurance Program
SCHIP evaluation tool
Schirmer syndrome
schistocelia
schistocephalus
schistocormia
schistocystis
schistocyte, schizocyte
schistocytic hemolytic anemia
schistoglossia
schistomelia
schistoprosopia
Schistosoma
S. haematobium
S. intercalatum
S. japonicum
S. mansoni
S. mekongi
schistosomal myelopathy
schistosomia

schistosomiasis
 acute s.
 cerebral s.
 chronic s.
schistosomula
schistosternia
schistothorax
schistotrachelus
schizencephalic cleft
schizencephaly
schizoaffective disorder
schizocyte (*var. of* schistocyte)
schizocytosis
schizoid personality disorder
schizont
schizophasia
schizophrenia
 childhood s.
 childhood-onset s. (COS)
 early-onset s. (EOS)
 very early onset s. (VEOS)
schizophrenic
schizophreniform disorder
schizotypal
schizotypy
Schlemm canal
Schlesinger solution
Schmid-Fraccaro syndrome
Schmidley syndrome
Schmid metaphysial dysplasia
Schmidt-Lantermann incisure
Schmidt syndrome
Schmorl
 S. jaundice
 S. node
Schneckenbecken dysplasia
Schnyder crystalline corneal dystrophy (SCCD)
Schober test
Schofield weight- and height-based resting energy expenditure prediction equation
Scholz
 S. disease
 S. sclerosis
Schönlein-Henoch purpura
school
 s. avoidance
 s. failure hypothesis
 s., home, activities, depression/self-esteem, substance abuse, sexuality, safety assessment
 s. phobia
 S. Sleep Habits Survey
school-based
 s.-b. health center (SBHC)
 s.-b. intervention
schottmuelleri
 Salmonella s.

Schroeder
 S. operation
 S. tenaculum forceps
 S. tenaculum loop
 S. uterine tenaculum
 S. vulsellum forceps
Schubert uterine biopsy forceps
Schuchardt
 S. incision
 S. operation
Schuco nebulizer
Schüffner dot
Schuknecht
 S. age-related hearing loss classification
 S. classification of congenital aural atresia (type A–D)
 S. retractor
Schultze
 S. mechanism
 S. phantom
 S. placenta
Schwangerschafts protein 1
Schwann cell
schwannian differentiation
schwannoma
 acoustic s.
 malignant s.
Schwartz-Jampel
 S.-J. disease
 S.-J. syndrome
Schwartz-Jampel-Aberfeld syndrome
Schwartzman phenomenon
Schwartz syndrome
Schwarz measles strain
sciatic nerve
SCID
 severe combined immunodeficiency
scimitar syndrome
scintigram
scintigraphy
 cortical s.
 dipyridamole myocardial s.
 hepatobiliary s.
 HMPAO leukocyte s.
 nuclear s.
 radionuclide s.
 renal s.
 somatostatin receptor s.
 thyroid s.
 ventilation s.
scintillating scotoma
scintillation
scintimammography (SMM)
 s. prone breast cushion
scintography
 gallium s.
scirrhous carcinoma
scissored position

S

scissoring posture
scissors
    Adson ganglion s.
    Aslan endoscopic s.
    bandage s.
    Braun episiotomy s.
    curved Mayo s.
    electrified s.
    Electroscope disposable s.
    episiotomy s.
    Evershears bipolar laparoscopic s.
    fine Metzenbaum s.
    hysterectomy s.
    Jorgenson s.
    laparoscopic s.
    Lister s.
    Mayo s.
    Metzenbaum s.
    Microline Re-New II 5-mm modular
      laparoscopic s.
    right-angle s.
    RoBi rotating bipolar forceps and s.
    Smellie s.
    Spencer stitch s.
    straight s.
    umbilical s.
    Waldman episiotomy s.
    Yankauer s.
    Z-Scissors hysterectomy s.
SCIWORA
    spinal cord injury without radiographic
      abnormality
      SCIWORA syndrome
SCJ
    squamocolumnar junction
sclera, *pl.* **sclerae**
    blue s.
sclerae (*pl. of* sclera)
scleral
    s. hemorrhage
    s. icterus
scleredema
    s. adultorum
    s. of Buschke
sclerema neonatorum
scleroatonic muscular dystrophy
sclerocornea
    microphthalmia, dermal aplasia, s.
      (MIDAS)
sclerocystic disease of the ovary
sclerodactylia (*var. of* sclerodactyly)
sclerodactyly, sclerodactylia
scleroderma
    s. en coup de sabre
    focal s.
    limited systemic s.
    linear s.
    localized s.
    progressive familial s.

    s. renal crisis
    secondary s.
    systemic s.
scleroderma-like syndrome
sclerodermatomyositis antigen
scleroembolization
    percutaneous retrograde s.
scleromyxedema
sclero-oophoritis
sclerosant
sclerose en plaque
sclerosing
    s. adenitis
    s. adenosis
    s. adenosis of breast
    s. agent
    s. cholangitis
    s. lesion
    s. osteomyelitis
    s. panencephalitis
sclerosis
    Ammon horn s.
    amyotrophic lateral s. (ALS)
    arterial fibrosing s.
    bone s.
    centrolobal s.
    cerebral s.
    childhood progressive systemic s.
    concentric s.
    cranial s.
    diffuse globoid body s.
    diffuse globoid cell cerebral s.
    diffuse glomerular s.
    diffuse mesangial s. (DMS)
    disseminated s.
    dominant choroidal s.
    endocardial s.
    familial centrolobal s.
    focal segmental glomerular s.
    globoid body s.
    globoid cell cerebral s.
    glomerular s.
    hippocampal s.
    isolated diffuse mesangial s. (IDMS)
    juvenile amyotrophic lateral s.
    lobar s.
    mantle s.
    Marburg variant multiple s.
    menstrual s.
    mesangial s.
    mesial temporal s. (MTS)
    metaphysial s.
    multiple s. (MS)
    myelinoclastic diffuse cerebral s.
    nodular cortical s.
    osteopathia striata with cranial s.
    ovulational s.
    photothermal s.
    physiologic s.

progressive systemic s.
Scholz s.
sudanophilic cerebral s.
sudanophilic diffuse s.
systemic s. (SS)
s. tuberosa
tuberous s.
sclerosis-hyalinosis
focal and segmental glomerular s.-h.
sclerosteosis
sclerosus
lichen s.
sclerotherapy
endoscopic s.
endoscopic variceal s. (EVS)
injection s.
sclerotic skin disease
sclerotome
SCM
split cord malformation
sternocleidomastoid
SCM muscle
SCMC
sperm-cervical mucus contact
SCMI
single central maxillary incisor
SCN
severe chronic neutropenia
scoliosis
Adams test for s.
adolescent s.
adolescent idiopathic s. (AIS)
compensatory s.
congenital thoracic s.
Dwyer correction of s.
s. film
idiopathic s.
infantile idiopathic s.
juvenile idiopathic s. (JIS)
mild s.
neuromuscular s.
postural s.
secondary s.
s. with dural ectasia
scombroid
s. intoxication
s. poisoning
scooter board
Scōp
Transderm S.
Scopette device
scopolamine
s. methylbromide
s. poisoning
scorbutic rosary
score
abstinence s.
Apgar s.
Ashworth s.

Asthma Severity S. (ASS)
Attia s.
Ballard s.
Ballard Assessment S. (BAS)
Bayley Motor S.
BDI s.
Berlin s.
BIND s.
biophysical profile s.
birth weight Z s.
Bishop s.
Boix-Ochoa GER s. (BOS)
BPP s.
cervical s.
CRIB s.
Croup s.
developmental assessment s.
Downes s.
Dubowitz s.
Euler and Byrne s.
expanded Ballard s.
externalizing s.
Ferriman-Gallwey hirsutism s.
S. for Neonatal Acute Physiology
S. for Neonatal Acute
   Physiology-Perinatal Extension
Glasgow Meningococcal Septicemia
   S.
global seasonality s.
Herson-Todd s.
home cognitive s.
I antigen s.
injury severity s. (ISS)
internalizing s.
Johnson s. 1–10
Kaufman Factor S.
lower triceps skinfold Z s.
MECA T s.
Methods for the Epidemiology of
   Child and Adolescent Disorders s.
Modified Injury Severity S.
   (MISS)
NAS s.
Neonatal Skin Assessment S.
Neurologic and Adaptive Capacity
   S. (NACS)
new Ballard s. (NBS)
optimality s.
Optimal Observation S.
Pediatric Trauma S. (PTS)
pelvic s.
PIPP s.
POMS s.
PREM s.
Premature Infant Pain Profile s.
PRISM s.
raw s.
recovery s.
respiratory index s. (RIS)

S

score (*continued*)
  Revised Trauma S. (RTS)
  Rutter mean s.
  Sarnat s.
  Sassone s.
  scattered s.'s
  Scheuer s.
  Shwachman s.
  Shwachman-Kulczycki s.
  Silverman s.
  simplified acute physiology s.
    (SAPS)
  standard deviation s. (SDS)
  Stanford-Binet s.
  T bone density s.
  trauma-related injury severity s.
    (TRISS)
  Vineland standard s.'s
  WDL asthma s.
  WISC III factor s.'s
  Wood-Downes asthma s.
  Yale Optimal Observation S.
  Z bone density s.
scoring
  fibrosis s.
  follicular s.
SCOT
  succinyl CoA:3-ketoacid CoA
    transferase
  SCOT deficiency
Scotch tape slide test
scotoma, *pl.* **scotomata**
  facultative s.
  scintillating s.
scotomata (*pl. of* scotoma)
scotopic sensitivity syndrome
SCOT-ROC
  Scottish Gynecological Cancer Trials
    Group
Scott
  S. cannula
  S. craniodigital syndrome
Scottish Gynecological Cancer Trials
  Group (SCOT-ROC)
Scot-Tussin DM Dough Chasers
scotty dog sign
scout radiograph
ScP
  scapuloposterior
SC-pseudothalidomide syndrome
SCPUFA
  short-chain polyunsaturated fatty
    acid
scrape
  s. and smear
  s. cytology
scrapie
scraping
  conjunctival s.

scabies s.
skin s.
scream
  hurt, insult, threat, s. (HITS)
screaming
screen
  abuse assessment s. (AAS)
  antigen s.
  S. for Child Anxiety-Related
    Emotional Disorders (SCARED)
  Glucola s.
  HPV s.
  maternal serum triple s.
  Monospot s.
  organic acid s.
  O'Sullivan s.
  Pap Plus HPV s.
  Partner Violence S. (PVS)
  prenatal s.
  quadruple s.
  qualitative urine s.
  Rapid Strep s.
  serum lysosomal enzyme s.
  suicide risk s. (SRS)
  supplemental newborn s.
  TORCH s.
  toxicology s.
  triple s.
  triple-biochemical s.
  triple-marker s.
  universal bilirubin s.
  universal hearing s.
  urine toxicology s.
screener
  Algo newborn hearing s.
  Oregon Adolescent Depression
    Project-Conduct Disorder S.
    (OADP-CDS)
screening
  AABR hearing s.
  amino acid s.
  AmnioStat-FLM maturity s.
  antenatal s.
  antibody s.
  breast cancer s.
  carrier s.
  colposcopic s.
  s. culture
  cytologic s.
  Denver II s.
  depression s.
  developmental s.
  FA s.
  first trimester s.
  genetic s.
  hearing s.
  hepatitis s.
  iFind handheld device for breast
    cancer s.

immunologic s.
s. laboratory test
mammographic s.
s. mammography
maternal age s.
maternal serum s.
multiple marker s.
neonatal s.
nuchal translucency s.
prenatal s.
s. recommendation
routine s.
sickle cell s.
s. sonogram
S. Tests for Young Children and
  Retardates
S. Tool for Early Predictors of
  PTSD (STEPP)
triple-marker s.
triple serum marker s.
s. ultrasound
ultrasound s.
universal newborn hearing s.
  (UNHS)
uterine s.
vision s.
Screenoscope
Topcon S.
screw
cannulated s.
myoma s.
screwdriver teeth
screw-tipped intraosseous needle
scrofula
scrofulaceum
Mycobacterium s.
scrofuloderma, scrofulodermia
scrofulodermia (*var. of* scrofuloderma)
scrofulosorum
lichen s.
scroll ear
scrota (*pl. of* scrotum)
scrotal
s. edema
s. hypospadias
s. mass
s. orchiopexy
s. position
s. swelling
s. testis
s. tongue
scrotum, *pl.* **scrota, scrotums**
bifid s.
raphe of s.
shawl s.
scrotums (*pl. of* scrotum)
Scr protooncogene
scrub
Sklar s.

Tecnu Extreme poison ivy s.
s. typhus
SCT
stem cell transplantation
SCTAT
sex cord tumor with anular tubule
Scully tumor
sculptatus
hymen s.
Scultetus binder
scurvy
hemorrhagic s.
infantile s.
scybala
SD
standard deviation
AlphaNine SD
SD disease
Profilnine SD
S/D
systolic/diastolic
Gammagard S/D
Polygam S/D
S/D ratio
SDAP
single donor apheresis platelet
SDAT
senile dementia of Alzheimer type
SDF
WinRho SDF
SDH
subdural hematoma
SDR
selective dorsal rhizotomy
SDS
standard deviation score
SDYS
Simpson dysmorphia syndrome
SE
signed English
status epilepticus
SEA
seronegativity, enthesopathy, arthropathy
spinal epidural abscess
spondylitis, enthesitis, arthritis
SEA syndrome
seabather's eruption
sea-blue
s.-b. histiocyte
s.-b. histiocyte syndrome
Seabright bantam syndrome
sealer/divider
LigaSure V s./d.
seal fingers
seal-like cough
seam
osteoid s.
urethral s.
SeaMist

S

searching toe
seasonal
    s. affective disorder (SAD)
    s. allergic rhinitis
    s. asthma
    S. Pattern Assessment Questionnaire (SPAQ)
    s. pollinosis
Seasonale
    S. birth control pill
    S. oral contraceptive
Seasonique
seat
    bath s.
    belt-position booster s.
    s. belt sign
    s. belt syndrome
    Hospital Recliner s.
    Ingram bicycle s.
    lobster s.
SEB
    staphylococcal enterotoxin B
sebaceous
    s. collar
    s. cyst
    s. duct
    s. gland
    s. gland hyperplasia
    s. gland lobule
    s. miliaria
    s. nevus
    s. nevus syndrome
sebaceum
    adenoma s.
sebaceus
    nevus s.
seborrhea
    adolescent s.
    infantile s.
seborrheic
    s. blepharitis
    s. dermatitis
    s. diaper rash
    s. eczema
    s. keratosis
seborrheica
seborrheic-like facies
seborrheic-looking skin lesion
Sebulex
sebum
    s. preputiale
    s. production
    s. secretion
Sebutone shampoo
Sechrist neonatal ventilator
Seckel
    bird-headed dwarf of S.
    S. bird head syndrome
    S. dwarfism
    S. nanism
secobarbital
Seconal
second
    s. bicuspid
    s. branchial cleft cyst
    cycle per s. (cps)
    forced expiratory volume in 1 s. (FEV$_1$)
    s. heart sound
    s. impact syndrome
    S. International Standard (SIS)
    s. messenger
    S. National Incidence Study (NIS-2)
    s. parallel pelvic plane
    s. permanent molar
    s. primary molar
    s. stage of labor
    s. trimester
    s. twin
secondary
    s. abdominal pregnancy
    s. adrenal cortical insufficiency
    s. adrenal hypoplasia
    s. allergic vulvitis
    s. alopecia
    s. amenorrhea
    s. amine
    s. amyloidosis
    s. apnea
    s. arrest
    s. arrest of dilation
    s. atelectasis
    s. carnitine deficiency
    s. circular reaction
    s. closure
    s. craniosynostosis
    s. dysmenorrhea
    s. dystonia
    s. emotional problem
    s. enuresis
    s. epilepsy
    s. headache
    s. hematoma
    s. hyperoxaluria
    s. hypochondriasis
    s. hypothyroidism
    s. infertility
    s. intention
    s. localized peritonitis
    s. lymphedema
    s. macrodactyly
    s. macular atrophy
    s. microcephaly
    s. moyamoya disease
    s. nail dystrophy
    s. nephrotic syndrome

s. osteosarcoma
s. PAP
s. phimosis
s. pneumonitis
s. polycythemia
s. postpartum hemorrhage
s. prematurity prevention
s. prophylaxis
s. scleroderma
s. scoliosis
s. seizure
s. sex characteristic
s. sexual maturation
s. solar urticaria
s. syphilis
s. teeth
s. tracheomalacia
s. uterine inertia
s. vesicoureteral reflux
s. vestibular dyspareunia
s. viremia
second-degree
s.-d. burn
s.-d. descent
s.-d. episiotomy
s.-d. heart block
s.-d. hypospadias
s.-d. laceration
s.-d. prolapse
second-generation progesterone
second-hand
s.-h. smoke
s.-h. smoking
second-line
s.-l. chemotherapy
s.-l. measure
second-look
S.-L. computer-aided detection
system
s.-l. laparoscopy
s.-l. laparotomy
s.-l. operation
second-trimester
s.-t. acute gestosis
s.-t. amniocentesis
s.-t. termination
secretagogue
secrete
secreted
regulated upon activation, normal
T-cell expressed and s.
secretin
Secretin-Ferring powder
secretion
abnormal cortisol s.
adrenal androgen s.
androgen s.
breast s.
cervicovaginal s.

dysregulated insulin s.
excessive acid s.
excessive insulin s.
follicular phase gonadotropin s.
FSH s.
gonadotropin s.
hypothalamic GnRH s.
impaired s.
inappropriate antidiuretic
hormone s.
inspissation of breast s.
insulin s.
luteinizing hormone s.
melatonin s.
ovarian androgen s.
oxytocin s.
persistent estrogen s.
pituitary gonadotropin s.
placental s.
progesterone s.
prolactin s.
sebum s.
steroid s.
surfactant s.
syndrome of inappropriate
antidiuretic hormone s.
vaginal s.
secretively
secretory
s. adenocarcinoma
s. calcification
s. carcinoma
s. diarrhea
s. disease
s. endometrium
s. IgA
s. leukocyte protease inhibitor
s. otitis media
s. phase
s. sarcoma
section
cesarean s. (CS, C-section)
classical cesarean s.
cut s.
elective cesarean s.
emergency cesarean s.
frozen s. (FS)
lower segment transverse cesarean s.
(LSTCS)
lower segment vertical cesarean s.
(LSVCS)
LUST cesarean s.
perimortem cesarean s.
Porro cesarean s.
postmortem cesarean s.
primary cesarean s.
(PCS)
repeat cesarean s. (RCS)
representative s.

S

sectioning
    clot s.
    serial s.
Sectral
Sectra MicroDose mammography system
secundigravida (G2)
secundina
secundines
secundipara
secundum
    foramen s.
    ostium s.
    septum s.
secundum-type
secure attachment
SED
    serious emotional disturbance
    spondyloepiphysial dysplasia
    late-onset SED
sedation
    chloral hydrate s.
    conscious s.
    ketamine s.
    Observer Assessment of Alertness and S. (OAAS)
    palliative s.
    pediatric s.
sedative
    s. effect
    s. poisoning
sedentary
sediment
    spun urine s.
    urinary s.
    urine s.
sedimentation rate
Sedlacková syndrome
sedlakii
    Citrobacter s.
SEE
    signed exact English
seed
    gold s.
    radioactive s.
    vitreous s.
seeding
    hematogenous s.
    peritoneal s.
    single tumor with s.
    tumor s.
    vitreous s.
seeking
    food s.
Seemanová syndrome (type 1, 2)
SEER
    Surveillance, Epidemiology and End Results
    SEER network

seesaw
    s. breathing
    s. nystagmus
Seessel pouch
SEF
    spectral edge frequency
segment
    chromosomal s.
    lower uterine s. (LUS)
    mesodermal dysgenesis of anterior s.
    upper body s.
    uterine s.
segmental
    s. amyoplasia
    s. aneuploidy
    s. dystonia
    s. edema
    s. epidural analgesia
    s. hypoplasia
    s. mesangial hypercellularity
    s. neurofibromatosis
    s. resection
    s. rolling
    s. spinal instrumentation
segmentation
    rhombomere s.
segmentectomy
segmented neutrophil
segregation
    s. distortion
    postmeiotic s.
SEH
    subependymal hemorrhage
Seip-Lawrence syndrome
Seip syndrome
Seitelberger disease
Seitzinger
    S. device
    S. tripolar cutting forceps
seizure
    absence s.
    afebrile s.
    akinetic s.
    anoxic s.
    apneic s.
    astatic s.
    atonic s.
    atypical absence s.
    atypical febrile s.
    atypical petit mal s.
    autonomic s.
    benign familial neonatal s.
    bicuculline-induced s.
    brief tonic s.
    clonic s.
    complex febrile s.
    complex partial s. (CPS)
    s. control

convulsive s.
diffuse-onset s.
s. disorder
drop s.
eclamptic s.
epilepsy s.
epileptic s.
familial neonatal s.
febrile s.
fetal s.
focal clonic s.
focal motor s.
focal-onset s.
gelastic s.
generalized tonic-clonic s.
grand mal s.
hypocalcemic s.
hypoglycemic s.
hyponatremic s.
hysteric s.
hysteric s.
idiopathic s.
infantile monoclonic s.
infantile myoclonic s.
jackknife s.
jacksonian s.
lightning s.
local s.
localization-related
  epilepsy s.
major motor s.
minor motor s.
monoclonic s.
motor s.
multifocal clonic s.
myoclonic s.
myoclonic-astatic s.
neonatal s.
nonconvulsive s.
nonepileptic s.
nonphotogenic s.
partial complex s.
petit mal s.
photogenic s.
photosensitive s.
postasphyxial s.
primary generalized s.
psychogenic s.
psychomotor s.
pyridoxine-dependent s.
recurrent convulsive s.
recurrent nonconvulsive s.
reflex anoxic s.
repeated partial s.
rolandic s.
salaam s.
secondary s.
sensory s.
severe s.

simple febrile s.
simple partial s. (SPS)
subtle s.
sylvian s.
symptomatic s.
temporal lobe s.
tetanic s.
tonic s.
tonic-clonic s.
typical absence s.
unprovoked s.
versive s.
vertiginous s.
vestibular s.
vestibulogenic s.
Seldinger technique
SelectCells Mini endometrial sampler
selection
bulk s.
family s.
fecundity s.
gametic s.
insertion site s.
natural s.
prenatal s.
truncate s.
selective
s. abortion
s. angiography
s. aplasia
s. aplasia of vermis
s. arterial embolization
s. broth medium (SBM)
s. dorsal rhizotomy (SDR)
s. embolization procedure
s. estrogen receptor modulator
  (SERM)
s. feticide
s. IgA deficiency
s. inguinal node dissection
s. intrapartum chemoprophylaxis
  (SIC)
s. mutism
s. neuronal necrosis
s. no-fault system
s. photothermolysis (SPTL)
s. posterior rhizotomy
s. pregnancy reduction
s. proteinuria
s. pulmonary arteriography
s. reading disability
s. renal vein renin determination
s. serotonin reuptake inhibitor
  (SSRI)
s. termination
s. termination of pregnancy
s. transvaginal embryo reduction
s. tubal assessment to refine
  reproductive therapy (STARRT)

selective (*continued*)
    s. tubal occlusion procedure (STOP)
    s. tubal occlusion procedure system
Select joint
selenium sulfide
Sele-Pak
Selepen
self-breast examination (SBE)
self-catheter
    Mentor female s.-c.
self-catheterization
    clean intermittent s.-c.
    intermittent s.-c.
self-comforting behavior
self-deprecation
self-esteem
self-examination
    BD Sensability breast s.-e.
    breast s.-e. (BSE)
self-harm
    self-reported s.-h. (SRSH)
self-harming act
self-help domain
self-incompatibility
self-induced vomiting
selfing
self-injectable epinephrine
self-injurious behavior (SIB)
self-injury
    S.-I. and Self-Restraint checklist
    (SISRC)
    S.-I. Grid (SIG)
self-limited bleeding
self-loathing
self-monitoring
self-mutilating behavior
self-mutilation
    compulsive s.-m.
self-obtained vaginal swab
self-priming action
self-report
    youth s.-r. (YSR)
self-reported self-harm (SRSH)
self-retaining retractor
self-statement
    coping s.-s.
self-sterility
self-stimulation
self-test
    OvuQuick s.-t.
self-worth
sella
    J-shaped s.
    tuberculum s.
    s. turcica
sellar enlargement
Sellheim incision
Sellick maneuver
Selsun Blue Shampoo

selvagem
    fogo s.
SEM
    scanning electron microscopy
    skin, eye, mucocutaneous
    systolic ejection murmur
        SEM infection
semantic memory
semantic-pragmatic disorder
SEMD
    spondyloepimetaphysial dysplasia
semen
    s. analysis
    frozen s.
    s. liquefaction
    prepared s.
    viscous s.
    s. volume
SEMG
    surface electromyogram
    surface electromyography
semiallogenic
Semicid
semicircular canal
semicircularis
    linea s.
semiconservative
semidefinitive procedure
semielemental casein hydrolysate
  formula
semifluid diet
semi-Fowler position
semilobar holoprosencephaly
semilunar
    s. fold of Douglas
    s. line of rectus sheath
semimembranosus muscle
seminal
    s. fluid
    s. fluid analysis (SFA)
    s. plasma
    s. vesicle
semination
seminiferous
    s. tubule
    s. tubule dysgenesis
seminoma
    ovarian s.
semiprone position
semisolid
semisynthetic
    s. penicillin
    s. surfactant
semitendinosus muscle
Semken forceps
Semm
    S. hysterectomy
    S. uterine vacuum cannula
senescent red cell

Sengers
   S. cardiomyopathy
   S. mitochondrial myopathy
   S. syndrome
Sengstaken-Blakemore tube
senile
   s. dementia of Alzheimer type
    (SDAT)
   s. urethritis
   s. vaginitis
senilis
   vaginitis s.
senility
   premature s.
Senior-Loken syndrome
senna
   s. concentrate/docusate sodium
   S. X-Prep
Senna-Gen
Senn-Dingman retractor
sennetsu
   Ehrlichia s.
Senning
   S. atrial switch procedure
   S. operation
   S. transpostion of great arteries
   repair
Senokot-S
senology
SenoScan full-field digital mammography system
Sensability breast self-examination aid
sensation
   falling-out s.
   genital s.
   impaired rectal s.
   integrate s.
   proprioceptive s.
   rectal s.
sense
   vibration s.
Sensenbrenner-Dorst-Owens syndrome
Sensenbrenner syndrome
SensiCare surgical glove
sensitive skin
sensitivity
   assay s.
   chemoreceptor s.
   clitoral s.
   culture and s. (C&S)
   gluten s.
   insulin s.
   microbial s.
sensitization
   anti-Kell s.
   contact s.
   food-antigen s.
   in utero s.
   Kell s.

   latex s.
   Rh s.
sensitizer
   hypoxic cell s.
sensor
   acoustic respiratory motion s.
   (ARMS)
   anal EMG PerryMeter s.
   BreastAlert differential temperature s.
   differential temperature s. (DTS)
   intraarterial s.
   MiniGuard CO_2 s.
   multiparameter intraarterial s.
   (MPIAS)
   Nellcor FS-10 oximeter s.
   Nellcor FS-14 oximeter s.
   Neotrend s.
   oximeter s.
   piezoelectric s.
   Resp-EZ piezoelectric s.
   temperature s.
Sensorcaine
Sensorcaine-MPF
sensorimotor integration
sensorineural
   s. change
   s. deafness
   s. hearing impairment
   s. hearing loss (SNHL)
sensorium
   altered s.
   clouding of s.
   depressed s.
Sensormedic 3100A 8000 oscillator
SensorMedics Horizon metabolic cart
sensory
   s. apraxia
   s. arthropathy
   s. deficit
   s. impairment
   s. information
   s. integration
   s. integration therapy
   s. loss
   s. nerve
   s. nerve conduction velocity
   s. neuropathy
   s. organ
   s. overload
   s. polyneuritis
   s. problem
   s. seizure
   s. stimulation
   s. threshold
sensory-motor stage
sentence
   5-word s.
Senter syndrome

sentinel
>   s. loop
>   s. lymph node (SLN)
>   s. lymph node biopsy (SLNB)

SEPA
>   superficial external pudendal artery

separation
>   amnion-chorion s.
>   s. anxiety
>   s. anxiety disorder (SAD)
>   blastomere s.
>   commissural s.
>   decreased commissural s.
>   ischiopagus tripus s.
>   peripartum symphysis s.
>   peripheral placental s.
>   physial s.
>   placental s.
>   premature placental s.
>   sperm s.
>   spontaneous placental s.
>   symphysial s.
>   uterine scar s.

separation-reunion experience

separator
>   Benson baby pylorus s.

Sephadex binding test

Sephardic Jew

Sepharose
>   CNBr activated S.

Sep-Pak

Seprafilm bioresorbable membrane

sepses (*pl. of* sepsis)

sepsis, *pl.* **sepses**
>   bacterial s.
>   catheter s.
>   *Chlamydia* s.
>   early-onset s.
>   *Escherichia coli* s.
>   fulminant s.
>   fungal s.
>   group B streptococcal s.
>   late-onset s.
>   *Listeria monocytogenes* s.
>   neonatal s.
>   s. neonatorum
>   nosocomial s.
>   pneumococcal s.
>   portal vein s.
>   postanginal s.
>   postoperative s.
>   puerperal s.
>   *Salmonella oranienburg* s.
>   s. syndrome
>   viral s.
>   s. workup

sepsis-pneumonia syndrome

sepsis/shock syndrome

septa (*pl. of* septum)

septal
>   s. defect
>   s. deviation
>   s. hypertrophy
>   s. panniculitis

Septata intestinalis

septate
>   s. hymen
>   s. uterus
>   s. vagina

septation
>   aorticopulmonary s.
>   cardiac s.
>   internal s.
>   tracheoesophageal s.
>   ventricular s.

septectomy
>   atrial s.
>   surgical s.

septic
>   s. abortion
>   s. arthritis
>   s. bursitis
>   s. embolus
>   s. encephalitis
>   s. joint
>   s. meningitis
>   s. pelvic thrombophlebitis (SPT)
>   s. pelvic vein thrombophlebitis
>   s. shock

septicemia
>   clostridia s.
>   gonococcal s.
>   meningococcal s.
>   postnatal s.
>   puerperal s.
>   streptococcal s.

septicum
>   *Clostridium* s.

septimetritis

septooptic-pituitary dysplasia

septophilic

septostomy
>   atrial s.
>   balloon s.
>   balloon atrial s. (BAS)
>   catheter s.
>   echo-guided balloon atrial s.
>   Rashkind balloon atrial s.

Septra DS

septum (S, sept), *pl.* **septa**
>   anterior nasal s.
>   aortopulmonary s.
>   atrioventricular s.
>   conotruncal s.
>   deviated s.
>   enlarged cavum s.
>   interventricular s.

membranous s.
midvaginal transverse s.
muscular ventricular s.
nasal s.
orbital s.
outlet s.
s. pellucidum
s. pellucidum agenesis
perimembranous s.
placental septa
s. primum
proximal transverse s.
pulmonary atresia with intact
  ventricular s. (PAIVS)
rectovaginal s.
retrovaginal s.
s. secundum
supravaginal s.
Swiss cheese s.
trabecular muscular s.
tracheoesophageal s.
transverse vaginal s.
s. transversum
urogenital s.
uterine s.
vaginal s.
ventricular s.
vesicovaginal s.

septuplet
septus
uterus s.
sequel
sequela, *pl.* **sequelae**
cardiovascular s.
delayed neuropsychological s.
  (DNS)
long-term sequelae
neoplastic s.
neurodevelopmental s.
neurologic s.
neuropsychologic s.
sequelae of extreme prematurity
subtle neurologic s.
sequelae (*pl. of* sequela)
Sequels
Diamox S.
sequence
amniotic band disruption s.
autonomous replication s.
base s.
blepharophimosis s.
breech deformation s.
cephalocaudal s.
s. characterized amplified region
cleaved amplified polymorphic s.
complementary s.
consensus s.
conserved s.
DiGeorge malformation s.

DNA s.
fetal akinesia deformation s.
  (FADS)
fetal brain disruption s.
FLAIR s.
Goldenhar s.
HASTE s.
insertion s.
laterality s.
malformation s.
mental retardation-overgrowth s.
Möbius s.
Pierre Robin malformation s.
Poland malformation s.
Potter oligohydramnios s.
regulatory s.
RICE s.
sirenomelia s.
Sotos s.
s. tagged microsatellite
s. tagged site
tandem repeat s.
TRAP s.
X-linked hydrocephalus-stenosis of
  aqueduct of Sylvius s.
Y chromosome-specific DNA s.
sequencing
chromosome s.
gene s.
temporal s.
verbal s.
sequential
s. administration
s. compression device
s. delivery
s. hormone therapy
s. memory
s. multiple analysis (SMA)
s. oral contraceptive
s. peak flow measurement
sequestered
s. lobe
s. lung
sequestra (*pl. of* sequestrum)
sequestration
acute splenic s.
bile acid s.
bronchopulmonary s. (BPS)
s. crisis
extralobar s.
fetal pulmonary s.
intralobar pulmonary s.
pulmonary s.
reticuloendothelial s.
splenic s.
sequestrative
sequestrum, *pl.* **sequestra**
s. formation
pancreatic s.

S

Sequoia
  S. Acuson system
  S. C256 echocardiographic system
sera (*pl. of* serum)
Serax
Sereen
Serentil
Serevent Diskus
serial
  s. casting
  s. digital examinations
  s. fetal assessment
  s. growth scans
  s. maternal serum fibrinogen
  s. neurologic examinations
  s. radiograph
  s. sectioning
series
  acute abdominal s.
  8-drugs-in-1-day treatment s.
  gastrointestinal s.
  Kell s.
  recombinant hepatitis B
    immunization s.
  treatment s.
  upper gastrointestinal s.
serine
  s. protease inhibitor (SERPIN)
  s. proteinase
serine-threonine kinase
seriography
  biplane s.
serious
  s. bacterial infection (SBI)
  s. emotional disturbance
    (SED)
SERM
  selective estrogen receptor modulator
sermorelin acetate
seroconversion illness
seroconverting
serofibrinous pleurisy
serogroup B meningococcus
serologic
  s. marker
  s. test
  s. test for syphilis (STS)
  s. testing
serology
  C-urea s.
  nontreponemal s.
  treponemal s.
serology-negative mother
seroma
  auricular s.
  postoperative s.
Seroma-Cath system
seromuscular intestinal patch graft
Seromycin Pulvules

seronegative
  s. enthesopathy and arthropathy
    syndrome
  s. neonate
  s. spondyloarthropathy
seronegativity, enthesopathy, arthropathy
Serono SR1 FSH analyzer
Serophene
seropositive
  ANA s.
  cytomegalovirus s.
seroprevalence rate
Seroquel
seroreverter
serosa
  lochia s.
  peritoneal s.
  vesicouterine s.
serosal
  s. adhesion
  s. surface
serosanguineous
  s. fluid
  s. rhinitis
serositis
serostatus
Serostim Injection
serotonergic
  s. dysfunction
  s. function
  s. reuptake blockade
  s. system
serotonin
  s. deficiency
  s. hypothesis
  s. receptor antagonist
  s. receptor blockade
  s. regulation
  s. reuptake blocker
  s. reuptake inhibitor (SRI)
  s. syndrome
  s. transporter 5-HTT
serotype
serous
  s. adenocarcinoma
  s. carcinoma
  s. cystadenocarcinoma
  s. cystadenoma
  s. form
  s. form of tuberculous meningitis
  s. otitis media (SOM)
  s. ovarian neoplasm
  s. retinal detachment
  s. tumor
serovar-specific
  s.-s. IgG
  s.-s. IgM
serpiginosa
  elastosis perforans s.

serpiginous
    s. border
    s. cephalad curved physis
SERPIN
    serine protease inhibitor
Serratia
    S. marcescens
    S. marcescens infection
Sertoli
    S. cell
    S. cell tumor
Sertoli-cell-only syndrome
Sertoli-Leydig
    S.-L. cell
    S.-L. cell tumor
sertraline
    s. HCl
    s. hydrochloride
serum, *pl.* **serums, sera**
    s. acetaminophen level
    acute sera
    s. albumin
    s. albumin concentration
    s. amino acid
    s. amino acid concentration
    s. aminotransferase
    s. ammonia
    s. amylase
    s. amylase level
    s. analyte
    s. antibody
    s. anticonvulsant level
    s. antienterocyte antibody
    s. anti-GQ1b antibody
     test
    antilymphocyte sera
    antirabies s.
    s. apolipoprotein
    s. assay
    s. bactericidal titer (SBT)
    s. bile salt level
    s. bilirubin
    s. bilirubin-binding capacity
    s. calcium
    s. carotene level
    s. complement
    convalescent s.
    s. copper
    s. copper level
    s. cortisol level
    s. digoxin level
    s. enzyme-linked
     immunoelectrotransfer
     blot
    s. erythropoietin
    s. estrogen
    s. ferritin
    s. ferritin concentration
    fetal s.

    s. free hemoglobin
    s. glucose
    s. glutamic-oxaloacetic transferase
     (SGOT)
    s. glutamic-pyruvic transaminase
     (SGPT)
    s. HCV RNA
    s. hepatitis
    hereditary erythroblastic
     multinuclearity with positive
     acidified s. (HEMPAS)
    s. hexosaminidase A
    s. hexosaminidase assay
    s. histamine level
    s. *immunoglobulin G*
     anti-Toxoplasma
    s. inhibitory titer (SIT)
    s. iron
    s. ketoacid
    s. lactate dehydrogenase
     concentration
    s. lead level
    s. leptin
    s. leptin level
    s. lithium concentration
    s. lysosomal enzyme screen
    maternal s.
    s. melatonin concentration
    s. müllerian inhibiting substance
    s. osmolality
    s. osteocalcin
    s. parathyroid hormone
    s. PCT
    s. PHE
    postdose s.
    s. pregnancy assay cartridge
    s. procalcitonin
    s. progesterone
    s. prolactin
    s. prostaglandin
    s. protease inhibitor
    s. protein concentration
    s. sickness
    s. sickness-like reaction
    s. sickness-like syndrome
    stored sera
    s. test
    s. testosterone
    s. thyrotropin
    s. transaminase
    s. type III procollagen
    s. urea nitrogen (SUN)
    s. uric acid
    s. zinc
serums (*pl. of* serum)
Serutan
service
    S. Assessment for Children and
     Adolescents (SACA)

service (*continued*)
    child, adolescent, and family mental health s. (CAFMHS)
    Child Protective S.'s (CPS)
    children's s.
    s. coordinator
    Crippled Children's S.'s (CCS)
    Department of Children and Family S.'s (DCFS)
    Department of Children and Youth S.'s
    Department of Children's S.'s (DCS)
    Department of Public Social S.'s (DPSS)
    Guidelines for Adolescent Preventive S.'s (GAPS)
    home care s.
    Hysterectomy Educational Resources and S.'s
    related services
    social s.
    support s.'s
    S. Utilization and Risk Factors (SURF)

servocontrolled
    s. homeothermy
    s. ventilation pump

Servo 900C ventilator

servomechanism

sessile polyp

SEST
    supine empty stress test

sestamibi

set
    Embryon GIFT transfer catheter s.
    Fuhrman pleural drainage s.
    haploid s.
    Health Plan Employer Data and Information S.
    H/S Elliptosphere catheter s.
    Karl Storz rigid TTTS fetoscopy instrument s.
    Mi-Mark endocervical curette s.
    Mi-Mark endometrial curette s.
    Neo-Sert umbilical vessel catheter insertion s.
    s. point
    Rosch-Thurmond fallopian tube catheterization s.

Setleis syndrome

Seton procedure

set-point theory

setting
    fire s.

setting-sun sign

Sever
    S. disease
    S. release

severe
    s. acute respiratory syndrome (SARS)
    s. childhood autosomal recessive muscular dystrophy (SCARMD)
    s. chronic neutropenia (SCN)
    s. combined immunodeficiency (SCID)
    s. congenital neutropenia
    s. dehydration
    s. gastrointestinal bleeding (SGIB)
    s. growth failure
    s. ketoacidosis
    s. megaloblastic anemia
    s. mental retardation
    s. micrognathia
    s. myoclonic epilepsy
    s. myoclonic epilepsy in infancy (SMEI)
    s. myopia
    s. ovarian hyperstimulation syndrome (SOHS)
    s. refractory hypoglycemia
    s. respiratory compromise
    s. seizure

severity
    pediatric acute admission s. (PAAS)

sevoflurane

sex
    s. addict
    s. assignment
    s. cell
    s. change operation
    s. chromatin
    chromosomal s.
    s. chromosomal anomaly
    s. chromosomal polysomy
    s. chromosome
    s. chromosome aberration
    s. chromosome abnormality
    s. cord
    s. cord mesenchymal tumor
    s. cord stromal germ cell tumor
    s. cord stromal neoplasm
    s. cord tumor with anular tubule (SCTAT)
    s. determination
    endocrinologic s.
    genetic s.
    gonadal s.
    high-risk s.
    s. hormone
    s. hormone-binding globulin (SHBG)
    illicit s.
    morphological s.
    nuclear s.
    oral s.

oral-genital s.
phenotypic s.
psychological s.
s. ratio
s. reversal
social s.
s. steroid
s. steroid add-back therapy
s. steroid modulation
s. surrogate
s. therapist
sexarche
sex-conditioned gene
sex-determining region (SRY)
sex-influenced gene
sex-limited gene
sex-linked
s.-l. chromosome
s.-l. disorder
s.-l. gene
s.-l. heredity
s.-l. inheritance
sex-related trauma
sex-specific CDC growth chart
sextuplet
sexual
s. abuse
s. activity
s. addiction
s. ambiguity
s. arousal
s. arousal disorder
s. asphyxia
s. assault
s. assault forensic evidence
(SAFE)
S. Assault Nurse Evaluation
S. Assault Response Team (SART)
s. assault victim
s. aversion disorder
s. behavior
s. contact
s. debut
s. derivation
s. desire
s. deviation
s. differentiation
s. dimorphism
s. dwarfism
s. dysfunction
s. enjoyment
s. excitement
s. function
s. habit
s. hair
s. history
s. infantilism
s. initiation
s. intercourse

s. issue
s. maturation
s. maturation index
s. maturity rating (SMR)
s. molestation
S. Opinion Survey
s. orientation
s. pain disorder
s. pleasure
s. practice
s. precocity
s. preference
s. problem
s. relationship
s. response
s. response curve
s. response cycle
s. risk reduction
s. satisfaction
s. stimulation
s. transmission
s. victimization
sexuality
sexualization
traumatic s.
sexually
s. transmitted disease (STD)
s. transmitted infection (STI)
SF-1
steroidogenic factor-1
SFA
seminal fluid analysis
subclavian flap aortoplasty
SF-36 Health Status questionnaire
S-F Kaon
SFMS
Smith-Fineman-Myers syndrome
SGA
small for gestational age
SGA infant
postterm SGA
term SGA
SGAR
spectral gradient acoustic
reflectometry
SGB
Simpson-Golabi-Behmel
SGBS
Simpson-Golabi-Behmel syndrome
SGH
subgaleal hematoma
SGIB
severe gastrointestinal bleeding
SGLT1 gene
SGO
Society of Gynecologic Oncologists
SGO classification of cancer
SGOT
serum glutamic-oxaloacetic transferase

S

SGPT
  serum glutamic-pyruvic transaminase
SGS
  Schinzel-Giedion syndrome
  short gut syndrome
SH
  sitting height
  sulfhydryl
shadow
  acoustic s.
  cardiothymic s.
  double-bubble gas s.
  heart s.
  perihilar s.
  thymic s.
shaft
  clavicular s.
shaggy heart border
shagreen
  s. patch
  s. spot
Shah permanent tube
Shah-Waardenburg syndrome
shake
  Ensure Healthy Mom s.
  s. test
shaken
  s. baby syndrome (SBS)
  s. impact syndrome
  s. infant syndrome
shaking wrist
shallow
  s. acetabular fossae
  s. acetabulum
  s. orbit
  s. ulcer
  s. ulceration
Shambaugh retractor
shampoo
  A-200 S.
  Exsel s.
  Ionil-T s.
  lindane s.
  Paratrol s.
  Polytar s.
  Pronto S.
  P&S S.
  Pyrinex Pediculicide S.
  Pyrinyl Plus S.
  R&C S.
  Rid s.
  Sebutone s.
  Selsun Blue S.
  T/Gel s.
  Tisit S.
  Triple X s.
shape
  pelvic s.
Shapleigh curette

sharing
  United Network for Organ S.
  (UNOS)
sharp
  s. curettage
  s. dissection
  s. facial features
  s. pulse
Sharplan USA ultrasonic surgical aspirator
sharp-wave
  s.-w. discharge
  s.-w. transient
Shaw I, II scalpel
shawl
  s. scrotum
  s. scrotum syndrome
SHBG
  sex hormone-binding globulin
Shea forceps
shear
  s. fracture
  s. stress
  s. stress-mediated nitric oxide release
Shearer forceps
shearing
  s. force
  s. of catheter
shears
  ADC Medicut s.'s
  LaparoSonic coagulating s.'s (LCS)
shear-strain deformation
sheath
  abdominal s.
  anterior rectus s.
  Bakelite cystoscopy s.
  ERA resectoscope s.
  fibrin s.
  Hemaflex s.
  MicroSpan s.
  Mullins long transseptal s.
  myelin s.
  optic nerve s.
  posterior rectus s.
  probe s.
  rectus s.
  sagittal septum of rectus s.
  semilunar line of rectus s.
Sheathes ultrasound probe cover
shedding
  asymptomatic viral s.
  s. domain
  endometrial s.
  s. endometrium
  fecal s.
  s. of nails
  s. syndrome
  vaccine strain s.

vaccine virus s.
viral s.
Sheehan syndrome
Sheehy syndrome
sheep cell agglutinin titer
sheepskin glove
sheet
amniotic s.
impervious s.
Ioban 2 cesarean s.
sheeting
silicon gel s.
shelf, *pl.* **shelves**
Blumer s.
shell
body s.
s. shock
s. vial culture
shellfish poisoning
shelter
shelves (*pl. of* shelf)
Shenton line
shepherd's
s. crook deformity
s. purse
Shereshevskii-Turner syndrome
Sheridan-Gardiner visual acuity card
Sheridan Tests for Young Children and Retardates
SHG
sonohysterography
Shiatsu therapeutic massage
shield
Bard Cap Sure Continence S.
CapSure continence s.
Dalkon s.
Fuller s.
Lea's S.
nipple s.
plastic heat s.
Surety S.
shield-shaped chest
shift
biobehavioral s.
Doppler s.
luteoplacental s.
midline s.
ontogenetic s.
paroxysmal depolarization s. (PDS)
shifting
s. dullness
weight s.
shiga
S. lipopolysaccharide
S. toxin (Stx)
S. toxin-producing Escherichia coli (STEC)
Shiga-like toxin

Shigella
S. bacteria
S. dysenteriae
S. dysentery
S. flexneri
S. sonnei
S. vaginitis
shigelloides
Plesiomonas s.
shigellosis
Shimada
S. criteria
S. histology
Shimada-Chatten histology
Shimadzu
S. SDU-400 ultrasound
S. ultrasound system
shin
saber s.
s. splint
shiner
allergic s.
shingles
shinsplints
shipyard conjunctivitis
Shirley wound drain
Shirodkar
S. cervical cerclage
S. cervix encirclement suture procedure
S. operation
SHMF
Similac human milk fortifier
shock
anaphylactic s.
anaphylactoid s.
bacteremic s.
cardiogenic s.
cardiovascular s.
compensated s.
cool s.
decompensated s.
distributive s.
endotoxic s.
gram-negative endotoxic s.
gram-negative endotoxin-induced s.
hemorrhagic s.
hypovolemic s.
insulin s.
s. liver
s. lung
neurogenic s.
obstructive s.
peripheral vascular s.
postoperative s.
septic s.
shell s.
spinal s.
s. stage

S

shock (*continued*)
    toxic s.
    uncompensated s.
    warm s.
shoe
    s. contact dermatitis
    reverse last s.
    straight last s.
    s. wedge
shoelace technique
Shohl solution
Shokeir syndrome
Shone
    S. anomaly
    S. syndrome
Shorr stain
SHORT
    short stature, hyperextensibility of joints or hernia, ocular depression, Rieger anomaly, teething
    S. syndrome
short
    s. arm of chromosome (p)
    s. attention span
    s. axis
    s. beaked nose
    s. bowel syndrome (SBS)
    s. cervix
    s. course
    s. frenulum linguae
    s. gut syndrome (SGS)
    s. leg walking cast
    s. limb
    s. maxilla
    s. metacarpal bone
    S. Michigan Alcoholism Screening Test (SMAST)
    s. neck
    s. philtrum
    s. PR interval
    s. process
    s. process of malleus
    s. rib-polydactyly syndrome (SRPS)
    s. rib-polydactyly (type I, II)
    s. small-bowel (SSB)
    s. stature (SS)
    s. stature homeobox (SHOX)
    s. stature, hyperextensibility of joints or hernia, ocular depression, Rieger anomaly, teething (SHORT)
    s. tandem repeat typing
    s. vagina
short-acting beta-2 agonist bronchodilator
short-axis view
short-bevel 21-gauge needle
short-chain
    s.-c. acyl coenzyme A dehydrogenase (SCAD)
    s.-c. fatty acid (SCFA)
    s.-c. hydroxyacyl-coenzyme A dehydrogenase (SCHAD)
    s.-c. polyunsaturated fatty acid (SCPUFA)
shortened cervix
shortening
    acromelic s.
    s. dorsal wedge radial osteotomy
    s. fraction
    fractional s. (FS)
    mesomelic s.
    metacarpal s.
    metatarsal s.
    percent fractional s.
    rhizomelic limb s.
    sarcomere s.
    uterosacral s.
    vaginal s.
shorthand vertical mattress stitch
short-increment sensitivity index (SISI)
short-limb
    s.-l. dwarfism
    s.-l. dystrophy
short-rib dwarfism
short-segment stenosis
Shoshin beriberi
shotgun method
shotty
    s. breast
    s. cervical lymphadenopathy
    s. node
shoulder
    s. dystocia
    Little League s.
    s. presentation
    s. sign
    s. subluxation
    swimmer's s.
show
    bloody s.
SHOX
    short stature homeobox
    SHOX gene
Shprintzen-Goldberg craniosynostosis syndrome
Shprintzen velocardiofacial syndrome
SHR
    sinusoidal heart rate
SHS
    Sutherland-Haan syndrome
shuddering
    s. attack
    s. spell
shuffling gait
Shug male contraceptive device
Shulman syndrome
shunt
    absolute s.
    anatomic s.

aortic-to-pulmonary s.
aortopulmonary s.
arteriovenous s.
atrial s.
atrioventricular s.
bidirectional Glenn s.
Blalock-Taussig s.
s. blockage
central s.
congenital portosystemic venous s.
Cordis-Hakim s.
corpora cavernosa to spongiosa s.
cutaneous s.
cystoperitoneal s.
Delta s.
Denver hydrocephalus s.
distal splenorenal s.
double-bubble ventriculoperitoneal s.
Drapanas mesocaval s.
ductal s.
end-to-side portocaval s.
enterohepatic s.
extracardiac s.
fetoamniotic s.
Glenn s.
intracardiac s.
intrapulmonary s.
jugular s.
Kasai peritoneal venous s.
left-to-right s.
LeVeen s.
lumboperitoneal s.
s. malfunction
mesocaval s.
modified Blalock-Taussig s.
s. nephritis
neurosurgical s.
palliative s.
parietal s.
peritoneal venous s.
pleuroamniotic s.
portoaortal s.
portocaval s.
portosystemic s.
Potts s.
prenatal placement of
  thoracoamniotic s.
proximal splenorenal s.
Pudenz s.
pulmonary s.
relative s.
s. revision
right-to-left s.
side-to-side portocaval s.
side-to-side splenorenal s.
single-reservoir, single-pump s.
splenorenal s.
subdural-peritoneal s.
systemic-to-pulmonary s.

s. tap
thoracoamniotic s.
transjugular intrahepatic
  portosystemic s. (TIPS)
VA s.
ventricular s.
ventriculoamniotic s.
ventriculoatrial s.
ventriculojugular s.
ventriculoperitoneal s. (VPS)
ventriculoperitoneal s.
ventriculopleural s.
ventriculovascular s.
vesicoamniotic s.
VP s.
Warren s.
Waterston s.
Y s.
shunt-dependent hydrocephalus
shunted hydrocephalus
shunting
  bidirectional s.
  ductal s.
  enterohepatic s.
  intrapulmonary s.
  left-to-right s.
  right-to-left s.
  Y s.
Shur-Clens
Shur-Seal
Shur-Strip
shuttle
  cortisol-cortisone s.
Shutt suture punch system
Shwachman
  S. score
  S. syndrome
Shwachman-Bodian syndrome
Shwachman-Diamond syndrome
Shwachman-Kulczycki score
Shwartzman reaction
Shy-Drager syndrome
shy-inhibited temperament
Shy-Magee syndrome
shyness scale
SI
  sacroiliac
  syncytium inducing
SIADH
  syndrome of inappropriate secretion of
    antidiuretic hormone
sialadenitis, sialoadenitis
sialadenosis
sialic
  s. acid
  s. acid storage disease
sialidase
sialidosis
sialoadenitis (*var. of* sialadenitis)

sialoglycoprotein
  glomerular s.
sialogram
sialography
sialomucin
sialophorin
sialorrhea
sialuria, Finnish type
sialyl
  s. Lewis X
  s. Lewis X determinant
  s. Tn antigen
sialylated Lewis A antigen
Siamese twins
SIB
  self-injurious behavior
siberica
  Rickettsia s.
sibling oocyte
SIC
  selective intrapartum
    chemoprophylaxis
sicca
  s. complex
  keratitis s.
  keratoconjunctivitis s.
  rhinitis s.
  s. syndrome
sicchasia
sick
  s. euthyroid syndrome
  s. sinus node syndrome
sickle
  s. beta-thalassemia
  s. cell
  s. cell and beta thalassemia
  s. cell anemia
  s. cell associated hematuria
  s. cell crisis
  s. cell dactylitis
  s. cell disease (SCD, SSD)
  s. cell hemoglobin (HbS)
  s. cell hemoglobin C (HbSC)
  s. cell-hemoglobin C, D disease
  s. cell hemoglobinopathy
  s. cell nephropathy
  s. cell preparation
  s. cell screening
  s. cell sludging
  s. cell-thalassemia disease
  s. cell trait
  s. hepatopathy
Sickledex test
sicklemia
sickling
  s. crisis
  s. disorder
  intravascular s.
  red blood cell s.

sickness
  acute mountain s. (AMS)
  car s.
  falling s.
  S. Impact Profile (SIP)
  Jamaican vomiting s.
  morning s.
  motion s.
  mountain s.
  serum s.
  sleeping s.
SID
  sudden infant death
side
  s. effect
  s. lyer
  s. sitting
side-port adapter
sideroachrestic
  sideroachrestic anemia
sideroblast
  refractory anemia with ring s.'s
    (RARS)
  ring s. (RS)
sideroblastic anemia
siderophagic cyst
siderophilic
siderosis
  myocardial s.
side-to-end anastomosis
side-to-side
  s.-t.-s. portocaval shunt
  s.-t.-s. splenorenal shunt
sidewall
  convergent s.'s
sideways walking
SIDS
  sudden infant death syndrome
  sulfoiduronate sulfatase deficiency
    near-miss S.
Siegel otoscope
Siegert sign
Siemens
  S. Servo 300, 900C ventilator
  S. SI 400 ultrasound
  S. Sonoline SI-400 ultrasound
    system
  S. Vision MRI
Siemens-Bloch pigmented dermatosis
Siemens-Elema Servo 900C ventilator
Siemerling-Creutzfeldt syndrome
Sierra-Sheldon tracheotome
SieScape imaging
sievert (Sv)
SIFT
  transvaginal intrafallopian sperm
    transfer
sift
  fluid s.

SIG
   Self-Injury Grid
Siggaard-Andersen nomogram
sighing respiration
sighted
   partially s.
SigmaStat software
sigma tumor marker
sigmoid
   s. colon
   s. pouch
   s. pouch of Pratt
   s. sinus
sigmoiditis
sigmoidoscopy
sign
   3 s.
   abdominal free-fluid s.
   Ahlfeld s. (I, II)
   Alström s.
   apprehension s.
   Auspitz s.
   Babinski s.
   banana s.
   Barlow s.
   Barré s.
   Battle s.
   Beccaria s.
   Biederman s.
   bilateral pyramidal tract s.'s
   blue dot s.
   Blumberg s.
   Borsieri s.
   Braxton Hicks s.
   brim s.
   Brudzinski s.
   Calkins s.
   candlestick s.
   Carnett s.
   Chadwick s.
   chandelier s.
   cherub s.
   Chvostek s.
   cock-robin s.
   Coopernail s.
   Corrigan s.
   cracked-pot s.
   cranial s.
   crenation s.
   Crowe s.
   Cullen s.
   curtsey s.
   cutoff s.
   Dalrymple s.
   Dance s.
   Danforth s.
   Darier s.
   double-bleb s.
   double-bubble s.

double decidual sac s. (DDSS)
double-tract s.
dovetail s.
dragon s.
E s.
extrapyramidal s.
eye-of-the-tiger s.
fadir s.
false localizing s.
falx s.
figure-of-3 s.
flag s.
fontanelle s.
Gage s.
Galeazzi s.
Gauss s.
Goodell s.
Gottron s.
Gowers s.
Granger s.
Grey Turner s.
Grisolle s.
groove s.
harlequin s.
Hartmann s.
Hawkins s.
Hegar s.
Hellendall s.
Hennebert s.
Hertoghe s.
Higoumenakis s.
Hoehne s.
Homans s.
Hutchinson s.
Hymenoptera s.
iliopsoas s.
Jacquemier s.
Kantor s.
Kergaradec s.
Kernig s.
Kernohan s.
Kleppinger envelope s.
Kussmaul s.
Küstner s.
Ladin s.
lambda s.
s. language
lateralizing s.
lemon s.
Lhermitte s.
localizing s.
long-tract s.
Macewen s.
Marcus Gunn s.
Marfan s.
Mayer s.
McMurray s.
meningeal s.
Metenier s.

S

sign (*continued*)
  milkmaid's s.
  motor neuron s.
  Munson s.
  Murphy s.
  Nager s.
  Nelson s.
  neonatal abstinence s.
  neurologic soft s.'s
  Nikolsky s.
  nuchal-spinal s.
  obturator s.
  Olshausen s.
  oromotor s.
  Ortolani s.
  palmar-plantar s.
  palpable spongy mass s.
  Parinaud s.
  Parrot s.
  Pastia s.
  pathergy s.
  peritoneal s.
  peroneal s.
  Pinard s.
  Piskacek s.
  placental s.
  Prehn s.
  pronator s.
  psoas s.
  puddle s.
  pyloric string s.
  pyramidal tract s.
  Radovici s.
  Raynaud s.
  reverse 3 s.
  reverse Marcus Gunn s.
  rib notching s.
  Risser s.
  Romaña s.
  rope s.
  Rovsing s.
  Russell s.
  sail s.
  Salmon s.
  sandal s.
  Saunders s.
  scarf s.
  Schick s.
  scotty dog s.
  seat belt s.
  setting-sun s.
  shoulder s.
  Siegert s.
  silk s.
  Simon s.
  snowman s.
  soft s.
  Spalding s.
  square window s.

  steeple s.
  Stellwag s.
  Sternberg s.
  string s.
  Tenney-Parker s.
  thumb s.
  Thurston Holland s.
  thymic wave s.
  Toriello-Carey s.
  Trendelenburg s.
  Tresilian s.
  tripod s.
  Trousseau s.
  turtle s.
  twin peak s.
  Uhthoff s.
  umbrella s.
  upper motor neuron s.
  Vipond s.
  vital s.'s (VS)
  von Fernwald s.
  von Graefe s.
  W s.
  Wartenberg s.
  water lily s.
  Weill s.
  Wimberger s.
  wrist s.
  Zaufal s.
SignaDRESS dressing
signal
  abnormal feedback s.
  centromeric s.
  drug reaction with eosinophilia and
    systemic s.
  extracellular matrix s.
  s. extraction pulse oximetry
  s. node
  peptide growth factor receptor s.
  specific growth factor s.
signaling
signed
  s. English (SE)
  s. exact English (SEE)
signet ring cell carcinoma
significance
  atypical glandular cells of uncertain
    s. (AGCUS)
  atypical glandular cells of
    undetermined s.
    (AGCUS, AGUS)
  atypical squamous cells of
    undetermined s. (ASCUS)
  atypical squamous cells of
    undetermined significance/atypical
    glandular cells of undetermined s.
signing
SIL
  squamous intraepithelial lesion

Siladryl Oral
Silafed
Silapap
SIL/ASCUS lesion
silastic
  s. band
  s. catheter
  s. cup extractor
  s. ring
  s. silo reduction of gastroschisis
  s. spring-loaded silo
  s. tube intubation
sildenafil citrate
silence
  electrocortical s.
silent
  s. allele
  s. amnionitis
  s. carrier
  s. celiac disease
  s. congenital CMV infection
  s. DVT
  s. fetal heart rate pattern
  s. gastroesophageal reflux
  s. gene
  s. myocarditis
  s. oscillatory pattern
  s. pelvic inflammatory disease
  s. precordium
  s. stroke
Silfedrine
  Children's S.
silhouette
  cardiac s.
silibinin
silica
silicon
  arsenic nickel s.
  s. gel sheeting
  s. rubber catheter
silicone
  s. band application
  s. catheter
  s. implant
  s. implant leakage
  s. injection
  s. microimplant
  s. plug
silicosis
silk
  s. sign
  s. suture
  s. tie
Sil-K OB barrier
SILL
  subischial leg length
Sillence classification of osteogenesis imperfecta (type I, IA, IB, II, III, IV, IVA, IVB)

silliness
  hebephrenic s.
silo
  s. decompression
  s. filler's disease
  silastic spring-loaded s.
Silon
  S. tent
  S. wound dressing
Silphen
  S. Cough
  S. DM
Silsoft extended wear contact lens
Siltussin DM
Silvadene
silver
  s. cell
  S. dwarfism
  s. fork deformity
  s. nitrate
  s. nitrate administration
  s. nitrate conjunctivitis
  s. nitrate drops
  s. nitrate eye prophylaxis
  s. nitrate solution
  s. nitrate stick
  s. stain
  s. sulfadiazine
  s. sulfadiazine cream
  S. syndrome
  s. thermal hat
  s. wire suture
Silverman
  S. and Nelles Anxiety Disorders Interview Schedule for Children
  S. score
Silverman-Anderson index
Silverman-Handmaker dyssegmental dysplasia
Silver-Russell
  S.-R. dwarfism
  S.-R. syndrome
Silverskiöld syndrome
silver-wire appearance
simethicone
simian
  s. B virus
  s. crease
  s. immunodeficiency virus (SIV)
  s. line
Similac
  S. 2 Advance formula
  S. Alimentum Advance formula
  S. human milk fortifier (SHMF)
  S. human milk fortifier formula
  S. Isomil Advance 2 formula
  S. Isomil DF formula
  S. Lactose Free Advance formula
  S. Natural Care Advance formula

Similac *(continued)*
    S. NeoSure Advance formula
    S. PM 60/40
    S. PM 60/40 formula
    S. Special Care 20, 24, 40 formula
    S. with iron formula
Similac-20
similarities test
similar twins
Simkania
    S. negevensis
    S. negevensis strain Z
Simmonds
    S. disease
    S. syndrome
Simon
    S. focus
    S. position
    S. sign
Simonton biofeedback technique
simple
    s. central anisocoria
    s. coarctation
    s. colloid goiter
    s. cyst
    s. ectopia lentis
    s. epispadias
    s. febrile seizure
    s. hyperplasia
    s. mastectomy
    s. meconium ileus
    s. metatarsus adductus
    s. motor tic
    s. partial seizure (SPS)
    s. phobia (SPh)
    s. pneumothorax
    s. sequence repeat
    s. squamous blepharitis
    s. syndactyly
    s. TGA
    s. ureterocele
    s. urethritis
    s. virilizing congenital adrenal
    hyperplasia (SV-CAH)
    s. vocal tic
    s. vulvectomy
simplex
    Dowling-Meara epidermolysis
    bullosa s.
    epidermolysis bullosa s.
    herpes s. (HS)
    herpetiformis epidermolysis
    bullosa s.
    s. infection
    Köbner epidermolysis bullosa s.
    lentigo s.
    lichen s.
    neonatal herpes s.
    nevus s.

    toxoplasmosis, other agents, rubella,
    cytomegalovirus, herpes s.
    (TORCH)
    Weber-Cockayne epidermolysis
    bullosa s.
simplified acute physiology score
  (SAPS)
Simplirix
simplistic method
Simpson
    S. dysmorphia syndrome (SDYS)
    S. dysplasia syndrome
    S. forceps
    S. uterine sound
Simpson-Angus rating scale
Simpson-Golabi-Behmel (SGB)
    S.-G.-B. fetal overgrowth syndrome
    S.-G.-B. syndrome (SGBS)
Simron
Sims
    S. curette
    S. position
    S. retractor
    S. uterine sound
    S. vaginal speculum
Sims-Huhner test
simultaneous
    s. preductal-postductal PO_2
    S. Technique for Acuity and
    Readiness Testing (STAR)
SIMV
  synchronized intermittent mandatory
  ventilation
SIN
  salpingitis isthmica nodosa
Sinai System
Sinarest 12 Hour Nasal Solution
sincipital presentation
Sindbis virus
Sinding-Larsen-Johansson syndrome
Sinding-Larsen lesion
sinensis
    Clonorchis s.
Sinequan Oral
Sinex Long-Acting
single
    s. breech presentation
    s. cell biopsy
    s. central maxillary incisor (SCMI)
    s. collecting system
    s. donor apheresis platelet (SDAP)
    s. fetal demise
    s. footling presentation
    s. gene defect
    s. gene mutation
    s. intrauterine death
    s. kidney
    s. nucleotide polymorphism
    s. primer amplification reaction

s. ring-enhancing mass lesion
s. rod implant
s. shot fast spin echo (SSFSE)
s. site BRACA
s. stranded conformational
polymorphism
s. transverse palmar crease
s. tumor
s. tumor with seeding
s. ventricle
single-channel urodynamic testing
single-dose methotrexate therapy
single-energy photon absorptiometry
single-exposure radiograph
**single-field hyperthermia combined with
radiation therapy**
single-film cholangiography
single-gene
s.-g. abnormality
s.-g. disorder
single-isotope tracer technique
single-photon
s.-p. absorptiometry
s.-p. emission computed tomography
(SPECT)
s.-p. emission tomography
single-reservoir, single-pump shunt
single-shot intravenous pyelogram
single-suture craniosynostosis
singleton
breech s.
s. breech presentation
s. fetus
s. infant
s. pregnancy
single-tooth tenaculum
single-twin demise
single-use diagnostic system (SUDS)
single-walled incubator
Singley forceps
Singulair
singultus, *pl.* **singultus**
sinistrocardia
sinistrocerebral
sinistrotorsion
Sin Nombre virus
sinoatrial
s. conduction time
s. node
sinobronchitis
Sinografin
sinopulmonary tract infection
sinovaginal bulb
sinuatrial, sinoatrial
s. block
s. node artery
Sinubid
Sinufed
Sinumist-SR caplet

sinus
s. abruption
s. arrest
s. arrhythmia
s. bradycardia
branchial cleft s.
cavernous s.
cervical s.
complex unroofed coronary s.
(CUCS)
coronary s.
s. cycle length
dermal s.
dermoid s.
endodermal s.
ethmoid s.
external branchial s.
s. fistula
high urogenital s.
s. histiocytosis
internal branchial s.
lumbosacral s.
marginal s.
maxillary s.
s. node dysfunction
s. node function
s. of Valsalva
open dermal s.
paranasal s.
Petit s.
pilonidal s.
preauricular s.
s. radiogram
s. radiograph
sagittal s.
sigmoid s.
s. solitus
straight s.
superior sagittal s.
s. surgery
s. tachycardia
s. thrombophlebitis
s. thrombosis
s. tract
s. tumor
unroofed coronary s.
urogenital s.
uterine s.
uteroplacental s.
Valsalva s.
s. venosus
s. venosus defect
sinusitis
acute s.
allergic s.
anterior ethmoidal s.
bacterial s.
cavernous s.
chronic s.

S

sinusitis (*continued*)
  idiopathic cavernous s.
  invasive s.
  recurrent s.
sinusoid
  coronary s.
  hepatic s.
  lacunar s.
sinusoidal
  s. channel
  s. fetal heart rate
  s. heart rate
  s. heart rate pattern
Sinusol-B
SIP
  Sickness Impact Profile
SIPAP
  social interaction and perinatal
    addiction project
siphon effect
Sipple syndrome
Sippy diet
SIR
  standardized incidence ratio
**Sirecust 404N neonatal monitoring
  system**
sireniform fetus
sirenomelia, symmelia
  s. sequence
  s. syndrome
sirenomelic fetus
Siri body fat percentage formula
sirolimus
SIRS
  systemic inflammatory response
    syndrome
SIS
  saline infusion sonography
  saline infusion sonohysterography
  Second International Standard
SISI
  short-increment sensitivity index
SISI test
SISRC
  Self-Injury and Self-Restraint checklist
sister
  s. chromatid
  s. chromatid exchange
  S. Mary Joseph nodule
Sistrunk operation
SIT
  serum inhibitory titer
sit
  right s.
site
  antibody reaction s.
  antigen binding s.
  axillary vein insertion s.
  binding s.

  bleeding s.
  episiotomy s.
  fragile chromosome s. (FRA, fra)
  Luer lock s.
  placental bleeding s.
  placental implantation s.
  s. preparation
  puncture punch s.
  reactive s. (RS)
  restriction enzyme cutting s.
  sequence tagged s.
  transcription start s.
  venipuncture s.
4-site skinfold test
site-specific familial ovarian cancer
sitosterol
sitosterolemia
sitting
  s. height (SH)
  long leg s.
  s. position
  side s.
  tailor s.
situ
  adenocarcinoma in s. (ACIS, AIS)
  carcinoma in s. (CIS)
  ductal carcinoma in s. (DCIS)
  in s.
  lobular carcinoma in s. (LCIS)
  placenta in s.
  residual in s.
  vulvar carcinoma in s.
situated learning
situs
  s. abnormality
  s. ambiguus
  s. indeterminus
  s. inversus
  s. inversus indeterminus
  s. inversus totalis
  s. inversus totalis syndrome
  s. inversus viscerum
  organ s.
  s. perversus
  s. solitus
  s. transversus
  visceral s.
sitz bath
Sitzmarks study
SIUD
  sudden intrauterine unexplained death
SIV
  simian immunodeficiency virus
sivelestat
sixth
  s. disease
  s. nerve palsy
size
  abnormal head s.

appropriate blood pressure
    cuff s.
blood pressure cuff s.
body s.
cardiac s.
corpus luteum s.
focal spot s.
gestational sac s. (GSS)
head s.
infant s. (IS)
maternal s.
small body s.
small head s.
tongue s.
tumor s.
uterine s.

size-date discrepancy
SJK
    Scheuermann juvenile kyphosis
Sjögren-Larsson syndrome
Sjögren syndrome
SJS
    Schwartz-Jampel syndrome
    Stevens-Johnson syndrome
    Swyer-James syndrome
SK-Amitriptyline
skate-flap technique
skeletal
    s. abnormalities, cutis laxa,
    craniostenosis, psychomotor
    retardation, facial abnormalities
    (SCARF)
    s. abnormality
    s. anomaly
    s. arthrogryposis
    s. calcium deficiency
    cerebral, ocular, dental, auricular, s.
    (CODAS)
    s. defect
    s. dysplasia
    s. growth
    s. infection
    s. maturation
    s. mineralization
    s. muscle biopsy
    s. muscle layer
    s. survey
    s. traction
skeleton
    gill arch s.
skeleton-skin-brain syndrome
Skene
    Bartholin, urethral, S. (BUS)
    S. duct
    S. duct cyst
    S. duct opening
    S. gland
skewfoot
skier's thumb

skill
    attending s.
    basic s.
    decreased attending s.
    fine motor-adaptive s.
    gross motor s.
    Kaufman Survey of Early Academic
        and Language S.'s (K-SEALS)
    language s.
    meal-time s.
    motor s.
    perceptual s.
    Personal Adjustment and Role S.'s
        (PARS)
    personal-social s.
    thinking s.

skin
    alligator s.
    s. atrophy
    s. biopsy
    s. breakdown
    s. calcification
    cigarette-paper s.
    collodion s.
    congenital localized absence of s.
        (CLAS)
    crocodile s.
    s. cyst
    s. defect
    s. discoloration
    s. disease
    doughy s.
    dry s.
    dusky s.
    s. end-point titration
    s., eye, mucocutaneous (SEM)
    fish s.
    s. flora
    s. fold
    gelatinous s.
    s. graft
    hyperextensile s.
    hyperkeratotic dry s.
    s. hyperlaxity
    India rubber s.
    s. lesion
    meconium-stained s.
    mitral valve, aorta, skeleton, s.
        (MASS)
    mottling of s.
    orange-peel s.
    Oxy-10 Advanced Formula for
        Sensitive S.
    pallor of s.
    parchment s.
    s. penetration
    s. popping
    porcupine s.
    s. prick test

S

skin (*continued*)
 puffy s.
 s. rash
 redundant s.
 s. retraction
 s. ridge pattern
 rough-feeling s.
 salt frosting of s.
 s. scraping
 sensitive s.
 staphylococcal scalded s.
 s. staple
 s. suture
 s. tag
 s. temperature
 s. tenting
 s. test conversion
 s. test reactivity (STR)
 s. thickening
 thin vulvar s.
 s. traction
 s. trigger theory
 vagabond s.
 s. vesicle
 vulvar s.
skin-covered lipomyelomeningocele
skin-eye-brain syndrome
skin-eye-mouth disease
skinfold
 s. caliper technique
 infarction of s.
 s. thickness
skinning
 s. colpectomy
 onion s.
 s. vulvectomy
skinny-needle biopsy
skin-sparing mastectomy
skin-to-skin
 s.-t.-s. care
 s.-t.-s. contact
skip
 s. area
 s. lesion
Sklar
 S. aseptic germicidal cleaner
 S. aseptic germicidal disinfectant
 S. cream
 S. foam
 S. instrument polish
 S. Kleen liquid
 S. Kleen powder
 S. lube
 S. scrub
skull
 cloverleaf s.
 coronal suture line of s.
 s. fracture
 hot cross bun s.
 lacunar s.
 maplike s.
 natiform s.
 strawberry-shaped s.
 sutures of s.
 thickened base of s.
 tower s.
SKY
 spectral karyotyping
 SKY epidural pain control system
Sky-Boot stirrup system
skyline view radiograph
S/L
 sublingual
 A-Spas S.
SLA
 superficial linear array
 SLA transducer
slant
 antimongoloid eye s.
 down s.
 eye s.
 mongoloid s.
 palpebral s.
slapped
 s. cheek appearance
 s. cheek disease
 s. cheek rash
 s. cheek syndrome
slapping storklike gait
SLAS
 salt-losing adrenogenital syndrome
slate-gray cyanosis
Slavianski membrane
SLE
 St. Louis encephalitis
 systemic lupus erythematosus
 SLE 2000 ventilator
sleep
 active s.
 s. apnea
 s. apnea syndrome
 s. architecture
 s. attack
 s. bruxism
 s. cystogram
 s. debt
 deep s.
 delta s.
 s. disturbance
 s. efficiency
 s. epoch
 S. Guardian foam pad
 hour of s.
 s. hygiene
 indeterminate s.
 s. latency
 s. myoclonus
 narcoleptic s.

non-REM s.
s. paralysis
s. pattern
s. position
quiet s.
rapid eye movement s. (REMS)
REM s.
restless s.
s. start
s. state
s. study
s. talking
s. terror
s. terror disorder
transitional s.
twilight s.
s. with rapid eye movement
sleep-disordered
s.-d. breathing
s.-d. breathing syndrome
Sleepinal
sleep-induced dyskinesia
sleeping
difficulty s.
excessive s.
s. habit
s. pattern
s. position
s. sickness
sleepless
crying, requires oxygen, increased vital signs, expression, s. (CRIES)
sleeplessness
facial expression and s.
pressure, facial expression, s.
sleep-related headache
sleeptalking
sleep-wake transition disorder
sleepwalking disorder
sleepy infant
sleeve
s. fracture
s. fracture of patella
Reid s.
SLI
subdermal levonorgestrel implant
slick-gut syndrome
slide
Testsimplets prestained s.
sliding
s. hiatal hernia
s. lock
sling
Advantage midurethral s.
Aldridge rectus fascia s.
s. anomaly
s. arm
s. baby

fascia lata suburethral s.
I-Stop midurethral s.
levator s.
Lynx midurethral s.
Martius flap and fascial s.
Mersilene mesh s.
midurethral s.
modified s.
Obtryx midurethral s.
s. procedure
puborectalis s.
pulmonary artery s.
retropubic s.
Stratasis urethral s.
suburethral s.
2-team s.
transobturator midurethral s.
TVTO s.
urethral s.
vascular s.
slingplasty
posterior intravaginal s.
slip
capital femoral epiphysis s.
slipknot
Duncan s.
Roeder loop s.
Weston s.
slipped
s. capital femoral epiphysis (SCFE)
s. epiphysis
s. upper femoral epiphysis (SUFE)
slipping rib syndrome
slit-lamp, slitlamp
s.-l. biomicroscopy
slitlamp (*var. of* slit-lamp)
slit ventricle syndrome
SLN
sentinel lymph node
SLNB
sentinel lymph node biopsy
SLO
Smith-Lemli-Opitz
SLO syndrome
Slo-Niacin
Slo-Phyllin Gyrocaps
Slosson Oral Reading Test-Revised (SORT-R)
Slotnick-Goldfarb syndrome
sloughed urethra syndrome
sloughing
cyclic s.
mucosal s.
slow
s. cognitive processing
S. Fe
S. Fe with folic acid
s. growth
s. rate of learning

slow-channel congenital myasthenic syndrome (SCCMS)
slowing
> bilateral s.
> generalized s.

Slow-Mag
slow-release sodium fluoride
Slow-Trasicor
SLP
> speech-language pathologist

SLUDGE
> salivation, lacrimation, urination, defecation, gastrointestinal distress, emesis

sludging
> sickle cell s.

slurry
Sly
> S. disease
> S. syndrome

SMA
> sequential multiple analysis
> spinal muscular atrophy

small
> s. body size
> s. bowel atresia
> s. bowel biopsy
> s. bowel dysmotility
> s. bowel endometriosis
> s. bowel enteroscopy
> s. bowel injury
> s. bowel intestinal polyposis
> s. bowel obstruction
> s. bowel overgrowth
> s. bowel perforation
> s. bowel strangulation
> s. bowel transit
> s. bowel transplantation
> s. cell carcinoma
> s. cell cleaved lymphoma
> s. cell osteosarcoma
> s. chromosome
> s. for dates
> s. for gestational age (SGA)
> s. head size
> s. intestine
> s. intestine decompression
> s. intestine stasis
> s. jaw
> s. left colon syndrome
> s. maxillary bone
> s. noncleaved cell lymphoma (SNCCL)
> s. patella syndrome
> s. premature infant
> s. round blue cell tumor of childhood
> s. single copy
> s. stature

small-bowel
> short s.-b.

smallpox vaccine
Sm antigen
SMART
> surgical myomectomy as reproductive therapy

smart
> street s.

SMAST
> Short Michigan Alcoholism Screening Test

SMC
> supernumerary marker chromosome

Smead-Jones closure of peritoneum and fascia
smear
> acid-fast sputum s.
> anal Pap s.
> ASCUS s.
> blood s.
> cervical s.
> cytologic s.
> low-grade positive s.
> LSIL Pap s.
> nasal s.
> Papanicolaou s.
> peripheral blood s.
> s. positive
> saline wet s.
> scrape and s.
> sputum s.
> squash and s.
> thick blood s.
> ThinPrep s.
> Tzanck s.
> vaginal irrigation s. (VIS)
> wet s.
> Wright-stained s.

smegma
> s. clitoridis
> s. embryonum
> s. preputii

SMEI
> severe myoclonic epilepsy in infancy

Smellie
> S. method
> S. scissors

Smellie-Veit method
S-methionine-labeled polypeptide
SMG22
> chromosome 22 supernumerary marker
> SMG22 syndrome

smile
> Cheshire cat s.
> sardonic s.

smiling incision

Smith
- S. pessary
- S. syndrome

Smith-Fineman-Myers syndrome (SFMS)

Smith-Hodge pessary

Smith-Lemli-Opitz (SLO)
- S.-L.-O. syndrome

Smith-Magenis syndrome (SMS)

Smith-McCort dwarfism

Smith-Theiler-Schachenmann syndrome

SMM
- scintimammography

SMO
- supramalleolar orthosis

smoke
- environmental tobacco s. (ETS)
- s. evacuator
- s. inhalation
- s. plume
- s. removal tube (SRT)
- second-hand s.

smokeless tobacco

smoking
- s. cessation
- maternal s.
- prenatal s.
- second-hand s.

smooth
- s. chorion
- s. muscle
- s. muscle cell
- s. muscle contraction
- s. muscle hamartoma
- s. muscle tumor
- s. philtrum
- s. tongue

SMR
- sexual maturity rating

SMS
- Smith-Magenis syndrome

smudged border

SMZ-TMP
- trimethoprim-sulfamethoxazole

snakebite envenomation

SNAP
- Score for Neonatal Acute Physiology

Snaplets-FR

SNAP-PE
- Score for Neonatal Acute Physiology-Perinatal Extension

snapping
- s. hip
- s. knee syndrome

snapshot GRASS technique

snare
- Reiner-Beck s.

SNCCL
- small noncleaved cell lymphoma

SND
- sinus node dysfunction

Snellen
- S. acuity chart
- S. test

SNHL
- sensorineural hearing loss

sniffing
- s. position
- toluene s.

SNIPPV
- synchronized nasal intermittent positive-pressure ventilation

S-nitrosoglutathione

SNJ
- nevus sebaceus of Jadassohn

Sn-mesoporphyrin (SnMP)

SnMP
- Sn-mesoporphyrin
- tin mesoporphyrin

Snodgrass hypospadias repair

snoring
- habitual s. (HS)
- primary s.

snout reflex

snow
- S. Mountain agent
- S. Mountain virus

snowflake pattern

snowman sign

snowstorm appearance

SNP
- sodium nitroprusside

SnPP
- tin protoporphyrin

Sn-protoporphyrin

snuffbox tenderness

snuffles

Snyder-Robinson syndrome (SRS)

soak
- Barrow solution s.
- Cidex s.

soap
- Alpha Keri s.
- Basis s.
- s. bubble gas pattern
- Lowila s.
- Oilatum s.
- pHisoHex s.
- TLC antiseptic s.

soap-bubble appearance

soapsuds enema

Soave abdominal pull-through procedure

sober

SOC
- surgical overhead canopy

sociability

social
- s. anxiety disorder

S

social (*continued*)
  s. assessment
  s. behavior
  s. deprivation
  s. development
  s. drinking
  s. drug
  s. factor effect
  s. interaction and perinatal addiction project (SIPAP)
  s. isolation
  s. issue
  s. maturity
  s. milestone
  s. parents
  s. phobia
  S. Security Disability Insurance (SSDI)
  s. service
  s. sex
  S. Support Scale for Children (SSSC)
  s. withdrawal
  s. worker
social-adaptive milestone
social-emotional
  s.-e. developmental area
  s.-e. domain
  s.-e. learning disability
social-evaluative fear
social-occupational dysfunction
society
  American Cancer S. (ACS)
  American Fertility S. (AFS)
  American Urogynecologic S.
  S. for Assisted Reproductive Technology (SART)
  S. for Pediatric Pathology (SPP)
  International Continence S. (ICS)
  S. of Gynecologic Oncologists (SGO)
sociobiologic
sociocultural stressor
sociodemographic data
socioeconomic
  s. issue
  s. status
sock
  verruca s.
socket
  dry s.
sodium (Na)
  s. acetate
  alendronate s.
  ampicillin sodium/sulbactam s.
  aqueous penicillin s.
  s. balance
  s. bicarbonate (NaHCO$_3$)
  Brevital S.

  s. bromide
cefazolin s.
cefoperazone s.
cefotaxime s.
cefoxitin s.
ceftriaxone s.
cefuroxime s.
cephalothin s.
s. channelopathy
s. chloride (NaCl)
s. citrate with citric acid
colistimethate s.
s. cromoglycate
cromolyn s.
s. cyclamate
dantrolene s.
s. diatrizoate
diclofenac s.
dicloxacillin s.
divalproex s.
s. docusate
docusate s.
s. equilin sulfate
ertapenem s.
estramustine phosphate s.
s. estrone sulfate
s. etidronate
s. excess
s. excretion
fluorescein s.
s. fluoride
fractional excretion of s. (FENa)
heparin s.
s. hydrogen phosphate
s. hydroxide
s. hyposulfite
ibandronate s.
imipenem-cilastatin s.
s. iodide
s. iodide I-125, I-131
iothalamate s.
ipodate s.
methicillin s.
metrizoate s.
mezlocillin s.
nafcillin s.
naproxen s.
nedocromil s.
nitroprusside s.
s. nitroprusside (SNP)
olsalazine s.
oxacillin s.
oxychlorosene s.
s. pentobarbital
Pentothal S.
s. phenylacetate
s. phenylacetate and sodium benzoate

s. phenylbutyrate
piperacillin sodium/tazobactam s.
s. polyacrylate polymer
s. polystyrene sulfonate
porfimer s.
prednisolone s.
quinalbarbitone s.
s. requirement
s. restriction
s. retention
s. salicylate
senna concentrate/docusate s.
s. serum level
S. Sulamyd
tazobactam s.
s. tetradecyl sulfate
thiopental s.
s. thiosulfate
total body s.
tyropanoate s.
s. valproate
s. wasting
zomepirac s.
sodium-free formula
sodium/glucose
s./g. co-transporter-1
s./g. co-transporter gene
sodomize
sodomy
Soehendra dilator
soft
s. Boston orthosis
s. cup vacuum delivery
s. hands syndrome
s. palate
s. seal catheter
s. sign
s. spot
s. tissue
s. tissue abnormality
s. tissue balancing
s. tissue density
s. tissue fat plane
s. tissue ovarian neoplasm
s. tissue release
s. tissue sarcoma
s. tissue syndactyly
S. Torque uterine catheter
Soft-Cell catheter
soft-cup extractor
softener
stool s.
softness
variable s. (VS)
Softpatch
Impress S.
SoftScan laser mammography system
SoftSpec disposable vaginal speculum

Soft-Wand atraumatic tissue manipulator balloon
software
Babe ultrasound report s.
EsopHogram s.
Medical Manager s.
SigmaStat s.
SOHS
severe ovarian hyperstimulation syndrome
Sohval-Soffer syndrome
soilage
bacterial s.
solar
S. Beam medical examination light
s. urticaria
Solarcaine Topical
solder
protein s.
sole crease
Solenopsis
S. invecta
S. xyloni
soleus
accessory s.
Solganal
solid
s. food
s. organ transplantation (SOT)
s. rod segmental construct
s. tumor
solid-phase
s.-p. enzyme immunoassay
s.-p. enzyme-linked immunospot (ELISpot)
s.-p. enzyme-linked immunospot assay
s.-p. radioimmunoassay
s.-p. sandwich
solitarii (*pl. of* solitarius)
solitarius, *pl.* **solitarii**
nucleus tractus s.
solitary
s. bone cyst
s. bone lesion
s. dilated duct
s. kidney
s. renal myofibromatosis
solitus
sinus s.
situs s.
solium
Taenia s.
Solomon-Fretzin-Dewald syndrome
Solomon syndrome
Solos
S. disposable cannula
S. disposable trocar
Soltamox

847

soluble
- s. antigen excess
- s. gas technique
- s. intercellular adhesion molecule 1
- s. RNA
- s. tumor necrosis factor receptor

Solu-Cortef Injection
Solumbra 30+ SPF fabric
Solu-Medrol injection
Soluprick skin prick test
Solurex LA Injection
Soluspan
- Celestone S.

SoluTab
- Prevacid S.

solute diuresis
solution
- Alamast ophthalmic s.
- aluminum acetate s.
- Anestacon Topical S.
- arterial line flush s.
- Atrovent Inhalation S.
- balanced s.
- Bouin s.
- Burow s.
- cardioplegic s.
- chlorhexidine s.
- cleansing s.
- clindamycin phosphate topical s.
- colloid s.
- Condylox s.
- Cornoy s.
- crystalloid s.
- Dakin antibacterial s.
- Denhardt s.
- Dey-Drop Ophthalmic S.
- Dianeal dialysis s.
- Domeboro s.
- DuraPrep surgical s.
- Duration Nasal S.
- Earle balanced salt s.
- Formula EM oral s.
- Freezone S.
- Fungoid AF Topical S.
- gum arabic rehydration s.
- Hank's balanced salt s. (HBSS)
- Hartmann s.
- hetastarch s.
- hypertonic saline s.
- Intergel irrigating s.
- iodine povidone s.
- irrigation s.
- isotonic electrolyte s.
- lacmoid staining s.
- lactated Ringer s. (LRS)
- Locke s.
- Lugol iodine s.
- Melanex topical s.
- modified Ham F-10 s.

- Monsel s.
- Mucomyst s.
- Mydfrin Ophthalmic S.
- nedocromil sodium ophthalmic s.
- neomycin-polymycin combination otic s.
- Neo-Synephrine 12 Hour Nasal S.
- Neo-Synephrine Ophthalmic S.
- normal saline s. (NSS)
- Norvir oral s.
- Nostril Nasal S.
- Ocuflox ophthalmic s.
- ophthalmic s. (OS)
- oral rehydration s. (ORS)
- Orapred s.
- Pedialyte oral electrolyte maintenance s.
- phosphate-buffered saline s.
- physiologic salt s. (PSS)
- polyethylene glycol s.
- polyethylene glycol-electrolyte s.
- Polygeline colloid s.
- povidone-iodine s.
- Prefrin Ophthalmic S.
- preservative-free s. (PFS)
- Primsol s.
- PVP s.
- Resectisol Irrigation S.
- Rhinall Nasal S.
- Ringer s.
- saline s.
- Schiller s.
- Schlesinger s.
- Shohl s.
- silver nitrate s.
- Sinarest 12 Hour Nasal S.
- sperm viability staining s.
- tobramycin s.
- Transeptic cleansing s.
- trimethoprim HCl oral s.
- Twice-A-Day Nasal S.
- Tyrode s.
- Vigamox s.
- 4-Way Long Acting Nasal S.
- Xopenex inhalation s.
- Xylocaine Topical S.
- Zenker s.

solvent
solving
- means-end problem s. (MEPS)
- problem s.

SOM
- serous otitis media
- suppurative otitis media

SomaSensor
somatic
- s. afferent
- s. cell
- s. cell-derived growth factor (SCF)

s. chromosome
s. complaint
s. differentiation
s. growth measurement
s. hybrid
s. mosaicism
s. nerve block
s. nervous system feedback loop
s. pain
s. sensory innervation
s. symptom
somatization disorder
somatoform disorder
somatoliberin
somatomammotropin
somatomedin
s. C
s. level
Somatom Plus computed tomography
somatopagus
somatoschisis
somatosensory
s. aura
s. evoked potential (SSEP)
s. impairment
somatostatinergic
somatostatin receptor scintigraphy
somatotridymus
somatotrope
somatotrophic (*var. of* somatotropic)
somatotropic, somatotrophic
somatotropinoma
Somatrem growth hormone
Somatropin
S. growth hormone
S. of rDNA origin
Somer uterine elevator
Sominex Oral
somite
s. embryo
s. formation
Sommer syndrome
somnambulance (*var. of* somnambulism)
somnambulism, somnambulance
somni
hora s. (h.s.)
somniloquy
somnolence syndrome
somnolent
somnolescent
Somogyi phenomenon
Somophyllin
Somophyllin-CRT
Sones catheter
Sonic Hedgehog
Sonksen-Silver visual acuity card
sonnei
Shigella s.

SonoAce
S. 6000 II ultrasound
S. 8000 Live ultrasound
Sonoclot
S. coagulation analyzer
S. test
Sonoda syndrome
sonogram
S. fetal ultrasound image card
screening s.
sonographic
s. abdominal circumference
s. assessment
s. evaluation
s. finding
sonography
Acuson computed s.
s. blood dyscrasia
color Doppler s. (CDS)
endovaginal s.
laparoscopic s.
ovarian s.
power Doppler s.
real-time s.
saline infusion s. (SIS)
transvaginal s. (TVS)
transvaginal color Doppler s. (TV-CDS)
vaginal s.
sonohysterogram
sonohysterography (SHG)
saline infusion s. (SIS)
transvaginal s.
Sonoline
S. Prima ultrasound
S. Sienna ultrasound system
sonolucency
sonolucent tissue
sonometer
sonomicroscopy
SonoMix ultrasound gel
Sonopsy ultrasound-guided breast biopsy system
Sonos 5500 echocardiographic scanner
SonoSite 180
Soothies glycerin gel breast pad
S.O.P.
Genoptic S.O.P.
Sopher ovum forceps
sorbitol
Actidose with S.
Sorbitrate
sore
canker s.
s. throat
soreness
nipple s.
Sorensen Transpac transducer
Soriatane

S

sorivudine
Sorsby syndrome
sorter
    fluorescence-activated cell s. (FACS, FACScan)
    magnetically activated cell s. (MACS)
sorting
    cell s.
SORT-R
    Slosson Oral Reading Test-Revised
SOS Bakri tamponade balloon
SOT
    solid organ transplantation
sotalol
Sotos
    S. cerebral gigantism
    S. sequence
    S. syndrome
Sotradecol
souffle
    fetal s.
    funic s.
    funicular s.
    mammary s.
    placental s.
    umbilical s.
    uterine s.
Soules intrauterine insemination catheter
sound
    abnormally wide splitting of second heart s.
    active bowel s.'s
    adventitious breath s.'s
    ambient s.
    bilabial speech s.
    bowel s.'s (BS)
    breath s.'s (BS)
    bronchial breath s.'s
    bronchovesicular breath s.'s
    cracked-pot s.
    decreased breath s.
    fetal heart sounds
    first heart s.
    first Korotkoff s.
    fourth heart s.
    grating s.
    heart s.'s
    high-pitched bowel s.'s
    hyperactive bowel s.'s
    hypoactive bowel s.'s
    Korotkoff s.
    labiodental speech s.
    muffled heart s.
    normoactive bowel s.'s
    Pharmaseal disposable uterine s.
    prominent heart s.

    pulmonary s.
    second heart s.
    Simpson uterine s.
    Sims uterine s.
    speech s.
    speed of s. (SOS)
    third heart s.
    tibial speed of s.
    urethral s.
    uterine s.
    vesicular breath s.'s
    vowel s.
    Waring blender s.
sound-field response
sound-stimulated fetal movement
soup kid facies
source
    cesium s.
    dummy s.
    MX2-300 xenon quality light s.
source-to-axis distance (SAD)
source-to-skin distance (SSD)
south
    S. African genetic porphyria
    S. African tick fever
    S. American blastomycosis
southeast Asian ovalocytosis (SAO)
southern
    S. blot
    S. blot technique
    S. blot test
SOX9 gene
soy
    s. milk
    s. protein intolerance
Soyacal IV fat emulsion
soy-based
    s.-b. protein isolate formula
    s.-b. remedy
soy-protein allergy
SP
    sacroposterior
    spastic paraplegia
    Cordran SP
SP-A
    surfactant protein-A
    SP-A of lung
SPA
    sperm penetration assay
    subperiosteal abscess
space
    anechoic s.
    antecubital s.
    apophysial s.
    s. blanket
    Bogros s.
    Bowman s.
    cranial s.

dead s.
extraembryonic celomic s. (EECS)
intercostal s.
intersphincteric s.
interstitial s.
intervillous s.
intracranial cystic s.
lymphovascular s.
mechanical dead s.
obliteration of apophysial s.
s. of Retzius
s. of Retzius bleeding
pararectal s.
paravesical s.
perivitelline s.
pharyngeal s.
popliteal s.
presacral s.
prevesical s.
rectosacral s.
rectovaginal s.
retropubic s.
retrorectal s.
retrovaginal s.
subaponeurotic cranial s.
subchorial s.
surgical s.
vesicocervical s.
vesicovaginal s. (VVS)
Virchow-Robin s.
volume of dead s.
yolk s.

space-occupying lesion
spacer
dummy s.
spaciness
spacing
natural child s.
third s.
Spalding sign
span
arm s.
attention s.
fertilizable life s.
liver s.
s. of liver dullness
poor attention s.
short attention s.
Spanish fly
SPAQ
Seasonal Pattern Assessment
Questionnaire
SPARC urological sling procedure
sparfloxacin
Sparine
sparing
brain s.
fetal brain s.
Sparlon

sparse hair
spasm
adductor s.
arterial s.
bladder s.
carpopedal s.
ciliary s.
cryptogenic infantile s.
diffuse esophageal s.
esophageal s.
flexion s.
glottic s.
greeting s.
hemifacial s.
infantile s. (IS)
jackknife s.
laryngeal s.
levator ani s.
mixed infantile s.
muscle s. (MS)
myoclonic s.
nodding s.
piriformis muscle s.
symptomatic s.
tetanic s.
tubal s.
urethral s.
vascular s.
X-linked infantile s.
spasmodic
s. croup
s. dysmenorrhea
s. dysphonia
s. torticollis
spasmus nutans
spastic
s. abductor hallucis
s. ataxia
s. cerebral palsy
s. colon
s. diplegia
s. dysphonia
s. hemiparesis
s. hemiplegia
s. levator ani
s. monoplegia
s. paraparesis
s. paraplegia (SP)
s. paresis
s. quadriparesis
s. quadriplegia
s. spinal paralysis
s. synergy
spastica
paralysis spinalis s.
paraplegia s.
spasticity
Ashworth score of s.
bilateral s.

S

spatial
- s. cognition
- s. memory
- s. orientation
- s. relationship

spatula
- Ayre s.
- Cytobrush s.
- s. foot
- Milex s.
- Pap-Perfect plastic s.

SP-B
- surfactant protein-B
- SP-B of lung

SP-C
- surfactant protein-C
- SP-C of lung

SPEA
- streptococcal exotoxin-A

spearing

Spearman-Brown prediction formula

spear tackling

special
- s. education
- s. needs
- S. Supplemental Nutrition Program

specialist
- development s.
- infant development s.
- mobility s.
- resource s.

specialized
- s. prenatal care
- s. tissue aspirating resectoscope (STAR)

speciation

species
- *Klebsiella-Enterobacter s.*
- reactive oxygen s. (ROS)

species-specific antibody

specific
- s. growth factor signal
- s. immunoglobulin
- s. immunotherapy
- s. phobia
- s. phosphodiesterase inhibitor
- s. reading disability
- s. reading retarded (SRR)
- s. transcription factor
- s. urethritis

specificity
- assay s.

specified
- eating disorder not otherwise s. (EDNOS)
- pervasive developmental disorder not otherwise s. (PDD-NOS)

specimen
- catherized urine s.

- catheter s.
- clean-catch urine s.
- cord blood s.
- forensic s.
- hemolyzed s.
- lost surgical s.
- maxillary sinus mucosal s.
- midstream urine s.
- nature of s.
- unspun catheterized urine s.
- urine s. (US)
- vaginal pool s.
- xanthochromic s.

speckled
- s. irides
- s. lentiginous nevus

SPECT
- single-photon emission computed tomography

spectacle
- s. correction
- s. treatment

Spectazole

spectinomycin

spectophotometrical analysis

spectra (*pl. of* spectrum)

Spectra-Diasonics ultrasound

spectral
- s. Doppler
- s. edge frequency (SEF)
- s. gradient acoustic reflectometry (SGAR)
- s. karyotype (SKY)
- s. karyotyping (SKY)
- orthogonal polarization s. (OPS)
- s. power analysis

Spectranetics catheter

spectrin

spectrofluorometric

spectrometer
- atomic absorption s.
- Digilab FTS 40A s.
- mass s.
- Varian Spectra AA40 s.

spectrometry
- electrospray ionization mass s. (ESIMS)
- gas chromatography-mass s. (GC-MS)
- mass s. (MS)
- tandem mass s.

spectrophotometer
- narrow band s.

spectrophotometric scanning

spectrophotometry
- atomic absorption s.
- near infrared s. (NIRS)

spectroscopy
- atomic absorption s.

gas chromatography-mass s. (GC-MS)
infrared s.
longitudinal proton MR s.
magnetic resonance s. (MRS)
medical optical s. (MOS)
near infrared s. (NIRS)
NMR s.
optic s.
proton MR s.
spectrum, *pl.* **spectra, spectrums**
Doppler shift spectra
electromagnetic s.
Spectra 400 extended surveillance and alert system
facioauriculovertebral s. (FAVS)
fortification s.
oculoauriculovertebral s. (OAVS)
S. stethoscope
spectrums (*pl. of* spectrum)
specula (*pl. of* speculum)
specular echo
Speculite chemiluminescent light
speculoscopy
Pap plus s. (PPS)
speculum, *pl.* **specula**
Auvard s.
bivalve s.
blackened s.
Cusco s.
disposable s.
duckbill s.
ear s.
endocervical s.
s. examination
Graves bivalve s.
Halle infant nasal s.
Holinger infant esophageal s.
Huffman adolescent s.
Huffman vaginal s.
illuminated vaginal s.
Kogan endocervical s.
LeeSpec disposable vaginal s.
long weighted s.
nasal s.
Pederson vaginal s.
Prima Series LEEP s.
Sani-Spec vaginal s.
Sims vaginal s.
SoftSpec disposable vaginal s.
vaginal s.
Vu-Max vaginal s.
weighted s.
s. withdrawal
Spee
curve of S.
S. embryo
speech
cued s.

s. delay
s. development
s. disorder
dysarthritic s.
dysfluent s.
hypernasal s.
hyponasal s.
s. lesson
motherese s.
parallel s.
s. pathology
pressured s.
s. problem
s. production
s. reception threshold (SRT)
s. recognition threshold (SRT)
s. sound
s. therapist
s. therapy
speech-language
s.-l. pathologist (SLP)
s.-l. pathology
speechreading
speed
s. of sound (SOS)
tibial s.
Speed-Vac
spell
A&B s.
blue s.
breath-holding s.
cyanotic breath-holding s.
hypercyanotic s.
hypoxic s.
pallid breath-holding s.'s
paroxysmal hypoxic s.
shuddering s.
staring s.
syncopal s.
spelt wheat
Spemann induction
Spence
S. and Duckett marsupialization
S. axillary tail
axillary tail of S.
S. urethral diverticulum procedure
Spencer
S. probe
S. stitch scissors
sperm, spermatozoon
acrosome-intact s.
s. agglutination test
s. allergy
anonymous donor s. (ADS)
artificial insemination with donor s.
s. aspiration
s. attrition
s. bank

sperm (*continued*)
   s. capacitation
   s. capacitation medium
   s. chromatin decondensation
   s. count
   s. donation
   s. donor
   donor s.
   ductal s.
   epididymal s.
   frozen s.
   s. function test
   s. generation time
   s. granuloma
   haploid s.
   s. immobilization test
   microsurgical extraction of ductal s. (MEDS)
   motile s. (MS)
   s. motility
   muzzled s.
   nonmotile s.
   s. penetration assay (SPA)
   s. progression scale (0–4)
   s. reservoir
   s. retrieval technique
   S. Select sperm recovery system
   s. separation
   subzonal injection of s.
   s. surface antibody
   s. tail protein phosphorylation
   s. transport
   s. viability staining solution
   washed s.
   s. washing insemination method (SWIM)
   X-bearing s.
   Y-bearing s.
Spermac stain
spermagglutination
sperm-aster
spermatic
   s. cord
   s. venous complex
spermaticide (*var. of* spermicide)
spermatid
spermatin
spermatocele, spermatocyst
   artificial s.
spermatocide, spermicide
spermatocyst (*var. of* spermatocele)
spermatogenesis
spermatogonia
spermatotoxic
spermatotoxin (*var. of* spermatoxin)
spermatoxin, spermatotoxin, spermotoxin

spermatozoa
   round-headed acrosomeless s.
   washed s.
spermatozoon (*var. of* sperm)
   haploid s.
sperm-cervical
   s.-c. mucus contact (SCMC)
   s.-c. mucus interaction
sperm-containing cyst
sperm-counting fluid
sperm-egg adhesion
sperm-free ejaculate
spermicide, spermaticide
   vaginal s.
spermidine
spermine
spermiogenesis
SpermMar mixed antiglobulin reaction test
sperm-mediated
sperm-oocyte interaction
spermotoxin (*var. of* spermatoxin)
sperm-zona pellucida binding
SPh
   simple phobia
sphenocephaly
sphenoid
   s. bone
   s. dysplasia
   s. fontanelle
sphenopagus
spherical congruent hips
spherocytic
   s. HE
   s. hereditary elliptocytosis
   s. red blood cell
spherocytosis
   congenital s.
   hereditary s.
sphincter
   aganglionic s.
   AMS 800 artificial urethral s.
   anal s.
   artificial anal s.
   artificial urethral s. (AUS)
   artificial urinary s.
   s. deficiency
   esophageal s.
   external anal s. (EAS)
   genitourinary s. (GUS)
   incompetent lower esophageal s.
   internal anal s. (IAS)
   lower esophageal s. (LES)
   s. muscle
   s. paralysis
   patulous rectal s.
   s. pharyngoplasty
   rectal s.
   s. repair

s. tone
upper esophageal s. (UES)
urethral s.
urinary s.
urogenital s.
vertiginous external anal s.
voluntary urinary s.

sphincteric incompetence
sphincteroplasty
sphingolipid
s. activator protein-1 (SAP1)
s. activator protein deficiency
s. storage disease

sphingolipidoses (*pl. of* sphingolipidosis)
sphingolipidosis, sphingolipodystrophy, *pl.*
sphingolipidoses
infantile cerebral s.

sphingolipodystrophy
Sphingomonas
sphingomyelin
sphingosine
sphygmomanometer, sphygmometer
aneroid s.
Tycos aneroid s.

sphygmometer (*var. of*
sphygmomanometer)

spica
s. cast
panty s.
s. splint

spiculated
s. lesion
s. red blood cell

spider
s. angioma
s. bite
black widow s.
brown recluse s.
s. finger
s. nevus
vascular s.

Spiegel
S. criteria
S. method

Spiegelberg criteria
Spielberger State Anxiety
Inventory
Spielmeyer-Vogt
S.-V. disease
S.-V. neural ceroid lipofuscinosis
S.-V. type of late infantile and
juvenile amaurotic idiocy

spigelian hernia
spike
s. and wave complex
benign partial epilepsy with
centrotemporal s. (BPEC)
centrotemporal s.
interictal s.

multifocal s.

spillage
tumor s.

spilled
filled and s.

spilus
nevus s.

spina, *pl.* **spinae**
s. bifida
s. bifida aperta
s. bifida cystica
s. bifida occulta

spinae (*pl. of* spina)
spinal
s. analgesia
s. anesthesia
s. angioma
s. apoptosis
s. arachnoiditis
s. blockade
s. bone loss
s. column
s. column closure defect
s. compression fracture
s. concussion
s. cord
s. cord compression
s. cord dysfunction
s. cord glioma
s. cord injury
s. cord injury without radiographic
abnormality (SCIWORA)
s. cord tethering
s. cord tumor
s. cord wind-up
s. dysraphism
s. epidural abscess (SEA)
s. fusion
s. headache
s. meningocele
s. metastasis
s. muscle atrophy
s. muscular atrophy (SMA)
s. muscular atrophy-mental
retardation syndrome
s. muscular dystrophy
s. needle
s. neurofibromatosis
s. osteomyelitis
s. paralytic poliomyelitis
s. polyneuropathy
s. proptosis
s. shock
s. subarachnoid block
s. tap
s. tuberculosis
s. tumor

spinal-epidural
combined s.-e. (CSE)

S

spindle
  s. cell
  s. cell epithelioid nevus
  s. cell tumor
spine
  anterior superior iliac s.
  bamboo s.
  cleft s.
  cloven s.
  curvature of s.
  dysraphia of s.
  iliac s.
  ischial s.
  lateral curvature of s.
  posterior superior iliac s.
  rotation of s.
  rugger jersey s.
  superior iliac s.
spin-echo
  half-Fourier acquisition single-shot turbo s.-e. (HASTE)
Spinelli operation
Spinhaler
spinigerum
  Gnathostoma s.
spinnbarkeit
spinning-top deformity
spinocerebellar
  s. ataxia-dysmorphism syndrome
  s. ataxia (type 1–7)
  s. degeneration
  s. degenerative disease
spinosa
  ichthyosis s.
spinothalamic sensory deficit
spinulosus
  lichen s.
spiral
  s. computed tomography
  Curschmann s.
  s. electrode
  s. endometrial artery
  s. scan
  s. tibial fracture
spiralis
  Trichinella s.
spiramycin
spirillary rat-bite fever
Spirillum minus
spiritual issue
spirochetal infection
spirochete
spiroforme
  Clostridium s.
spirometric test
spirometry
  incentive s.
Spironazide

spironolactone
  hydrochlorothiazide and s.
Spirozide
spit fistula
Spitz-Holter valve
Spitz nevus
splanchnic
  s. blood flow
  s. fold
  s. hypoperfusion
  s. pelvic pain
splanchnocystica
  dysencephalia s.
splanchnopathy
splanchnopleuric
splash burn
SPLATT
  split anterior tibial tendon transfer
splayfoot
spleen
  accessory s.
  fetal s.
splenectomized
splenectomy
splenic
  s. artery aneurysm
  s. flexure
  s. injury
  s. pregnancy
  s. rupture
  s. sequestration
  s. sequestration crisis
  s. sequestration syndrome
  s. tissue
  s. torsion
  s. vein
splenium
  absent s.
  posterior s.
splenocyte
splenomegalia (*var.* of splenomegaly)
splenomegaly (SM), splenomegalia
splenoportography
splenorenal shunt
splenorrhaphy
splenosis
splicing
  gene s.
  RNA s.
splint
  abduction s.
  acrylic s.
  ankle stirrup s.
  clubfoot s.
  Denis Browne clubfoot s.
  Denis Browne night s.
  dorsal extension s.
  dynamic s.
  Fillauer night s.

Frejka pillow s.
Lorenz night s.
malleable s.
night s.
opponens s.
Orthoglass s.
Pope night s.
shin s.
spica s.
static s.
sugar-tong s.
talipes hobble s.
thumb spica s.
triangular s.
volar s.
splinter hemorrhage
splinting
night s.
splint/stent
kidney internal s./s. (KISS)
split
anterior cricoid s. (ACS)
s. anterior tibial tendon transfer (SPLATT)
s. cord malformation (SCM)
cricoid s.
s. flexor hallucis longus tendon
s. hand/foot syndrome
s. procedure
s. sheath catheter
s. speculum examination
s. spinal cord malformation (SSCM)
split-course hyperfractionated radiotherapy
split-flap technique
split-foot deformity
splittable needle
split-thickness graft
splitting
blastocyst s.
embryo s.
fixed s.
muscle s.
rib s.
split-virus vaccine
spoke-wheel palpation
sponastrime dysplasia
spondylar changes-nasal anomaly-striated-metaphyses
spondylitis
ankylosing s.
s., enthesitis, arthritis (SEA)
juvenile ankylosing s. (JAS)
rheumatoid s.
tuberculous s.
spondyloarthritis
spondyloarthropathy
ankylosing s.

juvenile s.
seronegative s.
spondylocostal dysplasia syndrome
spondyloepimetaphyseal (*var. of* spondyloepimetaphysial)
spondyloepimetaphysial, spondyloepimetaphyseal
s. dysphasia with myotonia
s. dysplasia (SEMD)
spondyloepiphyseal (*var. of* spondyloepiphysial)
spondyloepiphysial, spondyloepiphyseal
s. dysplasia (SED)
s. dysplasia congenita
s. dysplasia congenita syndrome
s. dysplasia tarda
spondylohumerofemoral hypoplasia
spondylolisthesis
spondylolysis
spondylometaphyseal (*var. of* spondylometaphysial)
spondylometaphysial, spondylometaphyseal
s. dysplasia
s. dysplasia, X-linked
spondyloperipheral dysplasia
spondylothoracic
s. dysplasia
s. dysplasia syndrome
sponge
absorbable gelatin s.
s. bath
bupivacaine collagen s.
contraceptive s.
s. forceps
intravaginal s.
Protectaid contraceptive s.
Ray-Tec s.
s. stick
Today vaginal contraceptive s.
vaginal s.
Weck-cel s.
sponge-holding forceps
spongiform encephalopathy
spongioblastoma
spongiosa
zona s.
spongiosis
intraepidermal s.
white matter s.
spongiosum
corpus s.
stratum s.
spongiosus
status s.
spongy
s. degeneration
s. degeneration of infancy
s. degeneration of white matter
s. mass

spontaneous
- s. abortion (SAB)
- s. abortion material
- s. amputation
- s. anaphylaxis
- s. apoptosis
- s. atrophic patch
- s. atrophic patch of prematurity
- s. bacterial peritonitis (SBP)
- s. biliary perforation (SBP)
- s. breech
- s. breech extraction
- s. cephalic delivery
- s. cervical ripening
- s. descent
- s. descent of testis
- s. evolution
- s. gangrene of newborn
- s. hyperstimulation
- s. labor
- s. menstrual cycle
- s. miscarriage
- s. nystagmus
- s. ovulation
- s. periodic breathing
- s. placental separation
- s. pneumothorax
- s. preterm birth (SPTB)
- s. preterm delivery
- s. preterm labor with intrapartum demise
- s. remission
- s. rupture of membranes (SROM)
- s. thymic involution
- s. vaginal delivery (SVD)
- s. version
- s. vertex

spoon forceps
spoon-shaped nail
sporadic
- s. aniridia
- s. Burkitt lymphoma
- s. chromosome abnormality
- s. Creutzfeldt-Jakob disease
- s. myoglobinuria
- s. nonfamilial clear cell carcinoma

Sporanox
spore
- mold s.

Sporothrix schenckii
sporotrichoid appearance
sporotrichosis
- cutaneous s.
- extracutaneous s.

sport
- wheelchair s.

sports-related injury
sporulated oocyte

sporulation enterotoxin
SPOT
- salpingitis after previous tubal occlusion
- salpingitis in previously occluded tubes

spot
- ash-leaf s.
- Bitot s.
- black s.
- blood s.
- blue s.
- blueberry muffin s.
- Brushfield s.
- café au lait s.
- cherry-red macular s.
- coast of California café au lait s.
- coast of Maine café au lait s.
- s. compression
- s. compression film
- s. compression view
- cotton-wool s. (CWS)
- Forchheimer s.
- Fordyce s.
- Graefenberg s. (G-spot)
- hyperirritant s.
- Koplik s.
- macular cherry-red s.
- s. magnification
- money s.
- mongolian s.
- mulberry s.
- pathognomonic Koplik s.
- powder burn s.
- pseudo-Roth s.
- raspberry s.
- rose s.
- Roth s.
- shagreen s.
- soft s.
- strawberry s.
- s. test

spotlight
- KDC-Healthdyne nonfluorescent s.

spotted
- s. fever
- s. fever group

spotting
- midcycle s.
- postcoital s.
- postdouching s.

spotty necrosis
S-pouch
spousal abuse
SPP
- Society for Pediatric Pathology

sprain
Spranger-Wiedemann syndrome
spray
- Astelin Nasal S.

Atrovent Nasal S.
butorphanol tartrate nasal s.
Caldecort Anti-Itch Topical S.
DDAVP nasal s.
desmopressin acetate nasal s.
hair s.
intranasal s.
ipratropium bromide nasal s.
Itch-X s.
Merthiolate s.
Miacalcin Nasal S.
midazolam nasal s.
mometasone furoate aqueous nasal
  s. (MFNS)
Nasarel nasal s.
Nitrolingual Translingual S.
Ony-Clear S.
Rhinocort Aqua nasal s.
sumatriptan nasal s.
Tri-Nasal S.
vaginal feminine s.
Xylocaine Topical S.
SprayGel adhesive barrier
  system
spread
centripetal s.
fecal-oral s.
halstedian concept of tumor s.
hematogenous s.
lymphatic s.
transcoelomic s.
vessel s.
spreading factor
Sprengel
S. anomaly
S. deformity
spring clip application
sprinkle
Depakote s.
Sprintec
sprout
syncytial s.
sprouting
mossy fiber s.
nerve s.
sprue
celiac s.
refractory s.
tropical s.
Spry Infant tooth gel
SPS
simple partial seizure
SPT
septic pelvic thrombophlebitis
SPTB
spontaneous preterm birth
SPTL
selective photothermolysis
SPTL vascular lesion laser

spud dissector
spun
s. glass hair
s. hematocrit
s. urine
s. urine sediment
spur
bony s.
spuria
melena s.
placenta s.
spurious pregnancy
spurium
corpus luteum s.
spurt
growth s.
Spurway syndrome
sputa (*pl. of* sputum)
sputorum
Campylobacter s.
Pandoraea s.
sputum, *pl.* **sputa**
carbonaceous s.
clear mucoid s.
cloudy s.
s. culture
s. cytology
s. eosinophilia
mucoid s.
purulent s.
rust-colored s.
s. smear
squalamine
squama, *pl.* **squamae**
squamae (*pl. of* squama)
squame
fetal s.
squamocolumnar junction (SCJ)
squamous
s. cell
s. cell carcinoma (SCC, SCCA)
s. cell hyperplasia
s. cell neoplasm
s. dysplasia
s. epithelium
s. intraepithelial lesion (SIL)
s. metaplasia
s. metaplasia of amnion
square
s. knot
s. matrix
Punnett s.
s. window
s. window sign
squash and smear
squatting
s. phenomenon
s. position
squeeze technique

S

squeezing
    eyelid s.
SQUIDS
    superconducting quantum interference device susceptometer
squint
    convergent s.
squirming Valsalva
SR
    Calan SR
    Cardizem SR
    Indocin SR
    Isoptin SR
    Mag-Tab SR
    Oramorph SR
    Roxanol SR
Sr.
    EpiPen Sr.
Srb syndrome
SRI
    serotonin reuptake inhibitor
    SRI automated immunoassay analyzer
SROM
    spontaneous rupture of membranes
SRPS
    short rib-polydactyly syndrome
SRR
    specific reading retarded
SRS
    Snyder-Robinson syndrome
    suicide risk screen
SRSH
    self-reported self-harm
SRT
    smoke removal tube
    speech reception threshold
    speech recognition threshold
SRY
    sex-determining region
SS
    short stature
    systemic sclerosis
    hemoglobin SS (HbSS)
SSB
    short small-bowel
SSCM
    split spinal cord malformation
SSCVD
    sterile, spontaneous, controlled vaginal delivery
SSD
    sickle cell disease
    source-to-skin distance
    SSD AF
    SSD cream
SSDI
    Social Security Disability Insurance

SSE
    sterile speculum examination
SSEP
    somatosensory evoked potential
SSFSE
    single shot fast spin echo
S-shaped curve
SSI
    Supplemental Security Income
SSKI
    saturated solution of potassium iodide
SSLF
    sacrospinous ligament fixation
SSNS
    steroid-sensitive idiopathic nephrotic syndrome
SSPE
    subacute sclerosing panencephalitis
SSRI
    selective serotonin reuptake inhibitor
SSS
    scalded skin syndrome
    SSS syndrome
SSSC
    Social Support Scale for Children
SSSS
    staphylococcal scalded skin syndrome
SSVD
    sterile, spontaneous vaginal delivery
SSW
    staggered spondaic word
ST
    syncytiotrophoblast
    ST and T-wave abnormality
    ST change
St. (see also Saint)
    Saint
        St. Anthony's fire
        St. Clair-Thompson curette
        St. John's wort
        St. Joseph Aspirin-Free Cold Tablets for Children
        St. Joseph Cough Suppressant
        St. Jude Children's Research Hospital staging system
        St. Jude Research Hospital
        St. Louis encephalitis (SLE, STLE)
        St. Mark electrode
        St. Vitus dance
STA analyzer
stability
    ankle s.
    collateral ligament s.
    joint s.
stabilization
    cardiovascular s.
    hospital s.
stabilizer
    mast cell s.

stabilizing bar
STABLE
    sugar, temperature, artificial breathing, blood pressure, lab work, emotional support
stable
    s. access cannula
    s. factor
    s. microbubble test
staccato
    s. cough
    s. voiding
staccato-like cough
Stachybotrys
    S. atra
    S. chartarum
stacked coin appearance
Staclot test
stadiometer
    Harpenden s.
    Holtain height s.
    neonatal s.
Stadol
stage
    s. A, B, C, N infection
    acceptance s.
    alveolar s.
    anger s.
    band s.
    bargaining s.
    canalicular s.
    Carnegie s.
    cleavage s.
    cortical supremacy s.
    decoding s.
    delayed first s.
    denial s.
    depression s.
    developmental s.
    diakinesis s.
    dictyate s.
    germinal vesicle s.
    hemolymphatic s.
    hyperirritable s.
    s. IIIc papillary tumor of low malignant potential
    s. I–IV prolapse
    illocutionary s.
    indifferent gonadal s.
    Stages in Reproductive Aging Workshop (STRAW)
    intermediate dystonic s.
    Jirasek gestation s.
    leptotene s.
    locutionary s.
    Marshall-Tanner pubertal s. (1–5)
    meningoencephalitic s.
    Norwood s.
    stages of labor

    pachytene s.
    2-part nuclear s.
    perlocutionary s.
    pigmentary s.
    placental s.
    preicteric s.
    preoperational s.
    prereading s.
    pseudoglandular s.
    puberal s.
    saccular s.
    sensory-motor s.
    shock s.
    Tanner s.
    Tanner developmental s. (1–5)
    Tanner genital s. (1–5)
    Tanner maturation s. (1–5)
    Theiler s.
    transitional reader s.
    trophectoderm s.
    zygotene s.
2-stage arterial switch operation
staged repair
3-stage Norwood-Fontan procedure
Stagesic
staggered spondaic word (SSW)
staging
    clinical s.
    FIGO s.
    genital prolapse s.
    Marshall-Tanner pubertal s. (1–5)
    Northway s.
    puberal s.
    surgical s.
    Tanner grade 1–5 s.
stagnant loop syndrome
stagnation mastitis
STAI
    State-Trait Anxiety Inventory
STAIC
    State-Trait Anxiety Inventory for Children
STAI-I
    State-Trait Anxiety Index-I
stain
    acetylcholinesterase histochemical s.
    acid-fast s.
    acridine orange s.
    auramine-rhodamine s.
    Betke s.
    blood pigment s.
    Brown-Hopp tissue Gram s.
    Bryan-Leishman s.
    calcofluor white s.
    Csaba s.
    DA-DAPI s.
    DFA s.
    Dieterle s.
    eosin s.

stain (*continued*)
  eosin-4 s.
  Feulgen s.
  fluorescein s.
  Giemsa s.
  Golgi s.
  Gomori methenamine-silver s.
  Gomori trichrome s.
  Gram s.
  Gram-Weigert s.
  Grimelius s.
  Hansel s.
  H&E s.
  immunoperoxidase s.
  India ink s.
  iodine s.
  Kinyoun acid-fast s.
  Kinyoun carbol fuchsin s.
  Kleihauer s.
  Kleihauer-Betke s.
  KOH s.
  Leder s.
  Lugol iodine s.
  Luna-Parker acid fuscin s.
  macular s.
  Masson-Fontana s.
  meconium s.
  methenamine silver s.
  modified Dieterle s.
  modified Kinyoun acid-fast s.
  modified trichrome s.
  Movat s.
  PAS s.
  Perls iron s.
  port-wine s.
  potassium chloride s.
  rhodamine-auramine s.
  Shorr s.
  silver s.
  Spermac s.
  Sudan s.
  supravital s.
  toluidine blue s.
  trichrome s.
  TUNEL s.
  Warthin-Starry silver s.
  Wayson s.
  Wright s.
  Ziehl-Neelsen s.
stained
  meconium s.
staining
  acid-Schiff s.
  corneal s.
  DFA s.
  direct immunofluorescent s.
  direct immunohistochemical s.
  endomysial s.
  meconium s.

stainless steel suture
staircase
  s. approach
  s. response
stalk
  allantoic s.
  body s.
  infundibular s.
  mesenteric s.
  narrow mesenteric s.
  yolk s.
stalking
  celery s.
Stallworth placenta
Stamey
  S. antiincontinence operation
  S. catheter
  S. modification of Pereyra bladder
    neck suspension procedure
  S. needle
Stamey-Malecot catheter
Stamey-Pereyra needle suspension
Stamm
  S. gastrostomy
  S. temporary gastrostomy procedure
stammering bladder
stance
  Buddha s.
  horse-riding s.
  s. phase
stand
  warming s.
  s. x-ray
stand-alone pharmacotherapy
standard
  best interests s.'s
  s. curve
  s. deviation (SD)
  s. deviation score (SDS)
  MapMarkers fluorescent DNA sizing
    s.
  protein s.
  Second International S. (SIS)
standardization
standardized
  s. incidence ratio (SIR)
  s. observation scale
  s. reading inventory
  s. test
stander
  prone s.
standing position
standstill
  cardiac s.
Stanford-Binet
  S.-B. intelligence scale
  S.-B. Intelligence Scale for Children
  S.-B. Intelligence Scale, 4th Edition
  S.-B. Intelligence Test

S.-B. Memory Scale, 4th Edition
S.-B. score
Stanford Diagnostic Reading Test
Stanley Way procedure
stanozolol
STAN S-21 fetal heart rate system
stapedes (*pl. of* stapes)
stapes, *pl.* **stapes, stapedes**
staphylococcal
s. blepharitis
s. enterotoxin B (SEB)
s. furuncle
s. furunculosis
s. impetigo
s. infection
s. pneumonia
s. pustulosis
s. scalded skin
s. scalded skin syndrome (SSSS)
s. scarlet fever
s. toxic shock syndrome
s. vulvovaginitides
staphylococcus
s.
S. aureus
S. aureus molluscum
coagulase-negative *S.*
coagulase-positive *S.*
S. epidermidis
S. epidermidis folliculitis
S. intermedius
S. pyogenes
S. saprophyticus
staple
absorbable s.
s. anastomosis
ligate, divide, s.
s. line leak
metallic skin s.
skin s.
titanium s.
stapler
Auto Suture Multifire Endo
GIA s.
Endo GIA 30 suture s.
Endopath endoscopic articulating s.
GIA 60, 80 s.
Precise disposable skin s.
Roticulator 55 s.
TL-90 Ethicon s.
30-V-3 s.
Vista disposable skin s.
stapling
epiphysial s.
gastric s.
unilateral s.
STAR
Simultaneous Technique for Acuity
and Readiness Testing

specialized tissue aspirating
resectoscope
Study of Tamoxifen and
Raloxifene
StAR
steroidogenic acute regulatory
star
s. chart
s. effect
S. ventilator
starch malabsorption
STARFlex device
Stargardt disease
staring spell
Starling
S. equation
S. equilibrium
S. force
S. law of transcapillary exchange
S. mechanism
STARRT
selective tubal assessment to refine
reproductive therapy
start
Head S.
sleep s.
startle
s. disease
s. epilepsy
s. pattern
s. reaction
s. reflex
s. response
starvation
accelerated s.
s. ketoacidosis
s. ketosis
stases (*pl. of* stasis)
stasis, *pl.* **stases**
bile s.
bowel s.
colonic s.
gallbladder s.
large bowel s.
pregnancy-associated urinary s.
small intestine s.
urinary s.
state
accompanying mood s.
active and intense crying s.
awake and active s.
behavioral s.
S. Children's Health Insurance
Program (SCHIP)
chronic pain s.
disseminated intravascular
coagulation s.
emotional s.
fugue s.

S

state (*continued*)

gradient recalled acquisition in the steady s. (GRASS)

gradient refocused acquisition in steady s. (GRASS)

hyperammonemic s.

hypercoagulable s.

hypernatremic s.

hyperosmolar s.

hyponatremic s.

intense emotional s.

menstrual s.

mood s.

s. of alertness

paroxysmal emotional s.

persistent vegetative s. (PVS)

preeclamptic s.

preseizure s.

Profile of Mood S.'s (POMS)

progestational s.

quiet and alert s.

sleep s.

steady s.

transient insulinopenic s.

uremic s.

vegetative s. (VS)

state-of-the-art radiation

State-Trait

S.-T. Anxiety Index-I (STAI-I)

S.-T. Anxiety Inventory (STAI)

S.-T. Anxiety Inventory for Children (STAIC)

static

s. admittance

s. B-scanner

s. deformity

s. elastance (E_{st})

s. encephalopathy

s. immersion

s. splint

Staticin

O-V S.

station

complete/complete/+ s.

fetal s.

zero s.

stationary cycle

statistical model

stature

brittle hair, intellectual impairment, decreased fertility, short s. (BIDS)

constitutional short s.

deafness, hypogonadism, hypertrichosis, short s.

ear, patella, short s. (EPS)

familial short s.

goniodysgenesis, mental retardation, short s. (GMS)

ichthyosis, brittle hair, impaired intelligence, decreased fertility, short s. (IBIDS)

idiopathic short s. (ISS)

maternal s.

nongrowth hormone-deficient short s. (NGHD-SS)

short s. (SS)

small s.

status

absence s.

acid-base s.

s. asthmaticus

circumcision s.

s. dysmyelinisatus

s. epilepticus (SE)

fetal s.

fetal acid-base s.

health s.

Karnofsky performance s.

s. loss

s. lymphaticus

s. marmoratus

neurologic s.

nonreassuring fetal s.

paternal s.

petit mal s.

psychomotor s.

socioeconomic s.

s. spongiosus

s. thymicolymphaticus

s. thymicus

visceral protein s.

statutory rape

Staudinger reaction

stavudine

S-T Cort Topical

STD

sexually transmitted disease

steady state

steal

s. phenomenon

subclavian s.

stearin-lanolin cream

stearrhea (*var. of* steatorrhea)

steatocystoma multiplex

steatohepatitis

nonalcoholic s. (NASH)

steatorrhea, stearrhea

idiopathic s.

steatosis

liver s.

microvesicular s.

STEC

Shiga toxin-producing *Escherichia coli*

Steele procedure

steely-hair syndrome

steeple sign

Steiner
    S. canal
    S. electromechanical morcellator
    S. tumor
Steinert
    S. disease
    S. myotonic dystrophy
    S. syndrome
Steinfeld syndrome
Stein-Leventhal
    S.-L. syndrome
    S.-L. type of polycystic ovary
Stelactiv diaper rash cream
Stelatopia moisturizing cream
Stelazine
stellate
    s. cell
    s. ganglion ablation
    s. iris
    s. laceration
    s. mass
    s. reticulum
    s. wound
stellatoides
    Candida s.
Stellwag sign
stem
    s. cell
    s. cell assay
    s. cell bone marrow transplantation
    s. cell therapy
    s. cell transplantation (SCT)
Stemetil
stenogyria
    agenesis of corpus callosum with s.
stenoses (*pl. of* stenosis)
stenosis, *pl.* **stenoses**
    acute subglottic s.
    anal s.
    anorectal s.
    antral s.
    anular s.
    aortic valve s.
    aqueductal s.
    bile duct s.
    bladder neck s.
    cervical s.
    choanal s.
    cholestasis-peripheral pulmonary s.
    chronic subglottic s.
    congenital aortic s.
    congenital esophageal s.
    congenital hypertrophic pyloric s.
    congenital nasal pyriform aperture s. (CNPAS)
    congenital tracheal s.
    congenital tubular s.
    critical aortic s.
    critical pulmonic s.

discrete subaortic s. (DSS)
duodenal s.
dynamic subaortic s.
esophageal s.
fixed s.
fixed subvalvular s.
hypertrophic s.
hypertrophic pyloric s. (HPS)
idiopathic hypertrophic subaortic s. (IHSS)
infantile hypertrophic pyloric s. (IHPS)
infundibular pulmonic s.
lacrimal duct s.
laryngeal s.
laryngotracheal s. (LTS)
long-segment congenital tracheal s. (LSCTS)
meatal s.
mild pulmonic s.
mitral s.
nasal pyriform aperture s.
s. of esophagus
s. of trachea
peripheral pulmonary s.
peripheral pulmonic s.
piriform aperture s.
s. post intubation
postischemic s.
primary aqueductal s.
pulmonary branch s.
pulmonary valve s.
pulmonic s. (PS)
pyloric s. (PS)
renal artery s.
short-segment s.
subaortic s.
subglottic s.
supravalvular aortic s.
supravalvular pulmonary s.
tracheal s.
tricuspid s.
tubular s.
urethral s.
vaginal s.
valvular pulmonic s.
variable s.
X-linked aqueductal s. (XLAS)
stenotic
    s. hymen
    s. nasolacrimal duct
Stenotrophomonas
    S. maltophilia
    S. maltophilia infection
Stensen duct
stent
    Aboulker s.
    double-J s.
    endoluminal s.

stent (*continued*)
    expandable esophageal s. (EES)
    Lubri-Flex ureteral s.
    Palmaz s.
    pancreatic duct s.
    Percuflex Plus s.
    s. placement
    urinary s.
stenting
    endoluminal s.
stepdown
    s. cannula
    s. therapy
Stephan HF 300 respirator
Stephanie 8000 oscillator
Step laparoscopic trocar
stepoff
STEPP
    Screening Tool for Early Predictors of PTSD
stepping
    s. reflex
    reflex s.
    s. response
STEPS
    system for thalidomide education and prescription safety
    STEPS program
2-step testing
stepwise antiinflammatory therapy
Sterapred
stercoralis
    Strongyloides s.
stercoroma
stereoacuity
stereocolpogram
stereocolposcope
stereognosis
stereomicroscope
stereoscopic pelvimetry
stereotactic, stereotaxic
    s. breast biopsy
    s. breast biopsy needle
    s. core needle biopsy
    s. radiography
    s. radiosurgery
    s. thalamotomy
stereotaxic (*var. of* stereotactic)
stereotaxis, stereotaxy
stereotaxy (*var. of* stereotaxis)
stereotypical
    s. movement
    s. movement disorder
stereotypic behavior
stereotypy
Steri-Drape 2 incise drape
sterile
    s. isolation bag
    s. pus

    s. pyuria
    s. pyuria syndrome
    s. specimen trap
    s. speculum examination (SSE)
    s., spontaneous, controlled vaginal delivery (SSCVD)
    s., spontaneous vaginal delivery (SSVD)
    s. vaginal examination (SVE)
    s. water gastric drip (SWGD)
sterility
    absolute s.
    adolescent s.
    1-child s.
    relative s.
sterilization
    Collaborative Review of S. (CREST)
    Essure micro-insert method of female s.
    female s.
    intermittent s.
    involuntary s.
    male s.
    microlaparoscopic s.
    permanent s.
    postpartum s. (PPS)
    surgical s.
    tubal s.
    voluntary s. (VS)
sterilize
Steri-Strip skin closure
sternal
    s. fracture
    s. node
    s. recession
Sternberg sign
sternochondral junction
sternocleidomastoid (SCM)
    s. fibroma
    s. hemorrhage
    s. muscle
sternodymus
sternomastoid
    s. foramen
    s. tumor
sternopagus
sternoschisis
sternotomy
sternum
    fissure of s.
    fractured s.
steroid
    s. acne
    adrenal s.
    adrenocortical s.
    anabolic androgenic s.
    androgenic s.
    antenatal s.

s. biosynthesis
s. cell
s. concentration
s. conjugate hydrolysis
s. contraceptive
s. cream
endogenous s.
exogenous s.
gonadal s.
s. hormone
s. hormone receptor
inhaled s.
s. inhaler
17-ketogenic s.
long-acting contraceptive s.
low-dose s.
s. metabolism
s. metabolite
s. nucleus
ovarian s.
placental s.
s. secretion
s. secretion inhibition
sex s.
stress dose s.'s
s. sulfatase
s. sulfatase deficiency
s. sulfate
systemic s.
s. therapy
s. treatment
steroid-dependent colitis
steroid-induced myopathy
steroidogenesis
adrenal s.
adrenocortical s.
fetal-placental s.
follicle s.
ovarian s.
testicular s.
steroidogenic
s. aberration
s. acute regulatory (StAR)
s. factor-1 (SF-1)
steroid-sensitive idiopathic nephrotic syndrome (SSNS)
stertor
humid s.
stethoscope
Allen fetal s.
bell s.
Doptone fetal s.
MedaSonics first beat ultrasound s.
Spectrum s.
ultrasound s.
Stevens-Johnson syndrome
Stewart-Treves syndrome
STH
subtotal hysterectomy

STI
sexually transmitted infection
stick
arterial s.
glucose reagent s.
silver nitrate s.
sponge s.
Universal indicator s.
Sticker disease
Stickler
S. dysplasia
S. syndrome
sties (*pl. of* sty)
stiff
s. neck
s. ventricle
stiff-baby syndrome
stiff-man syndrome
stiffness
lead pipe s.
stigma, *pl.* **stigmas, stigmata**
Down stigmata
radiologic stigmata
Ulrich-Turner stigmata
stigmas (*pl. of* stigma)
stigmasterol
stigmata (*pl. of* stigma)
stigmatization
stilbestrol
still
S. disease
S. murmur
stillbirth
s. rate (SBR)
recurrent s.
stillborn infant
Stilling-Türk-Duane syndrome
Stillman cleft
Stilphostrol
Stimate
Stimmler syndrome
stimulant
s. drug
s. laxative
stimulation
ACTH s.
cervical carcinoma s.
contingent vestibular s.
cranial electrical s. (CES)
direct s.
electrical s.
electrophrenic s.
endogenous estrogenic s.
endometrial s.
enterochromaffin cell s.
exogenous estrogenic s.
exogenous gonadotropin s.
fetal scalp s.
follicle maturation s.

S

stimulation (*continued*)
  functional bladder s. (FES)
  functional electrical s. (FES)
  labyrinthine s.
  laryngopharyngeal sensory s. (LPSS)
  nipple s.
  noncoital sexual s.
  oral s.
  ovarian s.
  ovulation s.
  oxytocic s.
  pelvic floor electrical s. (PFS)
  photic s.
  prolactin s.
  sacral nerve root s.
  sensory s.
  sexual s.
  sympathetic s.
  tactile s.
  s. test
  transcranial magnetic s. (TMS)
  transcutaneous electrical nerve s.
    (TENS)
  vagal nerve s.
  vestibular s.
  vibratory acoustic s. (VAS)
  vibroacoustic s. (VAS)
  visual s.
stimulator
  adrenergic s.
  alpha-adrenergic s.
  hemopoietic system s.
  Innova pelvic floor s.
  long-acting thyroid s. (LATS)
  luteinization s.
stimuli (*pl. of* stimulus)
stimulus, *pl.* **stimuli**
  amblyogenic s.
  antigenic s.
  click s.
  congenital amblyogenic s.
  high-intensity click s.
  neonatal amblyogenic s.
  nociceptive s.
  tactile s.
stimulus-response (S-R)
sting
  hornet s.
  S. procedure
stinging insect allergy
stippled epiphysis
stippling
  basophilic s.
  bone s.
  corneal s.
  s. of epiphyses
stirrup
  Allen laparoscopic s.'s
  candy-cane s.'s

  hanging s.
  high s.'s
  Lloyd-Davies s.
stitch
  s. abscess
  baseball s.
  imbricating s.
  inverting baseball s.
  Lembert s.
  McCall s.
  running imbricating s.
  running locked s.
  shorthand vertical mattress s.
  s. tie
STNR
  symmetrical tonic neck reflex
Stocco dos Santos syndrome
stockinette
  s. cap
  impervious s.
stocking
  antiembolism s.
  compression s.
  elastic s.
  Juzo-Hostess 2-way stretch
    compression s.
  leg-compression s.
  pneumatic compression s.
  TED s.
stocking-glove sensory loss
Stock-Spielmeyer-Vogt syndrome
Stokes-Adams
  S.-A. attack
  S.-A. syndrome
Stoll syndrome
Stolte forceps
stoma, *pl.* **stomas, stomata**
  ileal s.
stomach
  s. ache
  s. bubble
  s. cancer metastasis
  herniated s.
  infarction of herniated s.
  leather-bottle s.
  right-sided s.
stomachache (*var. of* stomach
  ache)
Stomahesive
stomas (*pl. of* stoma)
stomata (*pl. of* stoma)
stomatitis
  angular s.
  aphthous s.
  fusospirillary gangrenous s.
  gangrenous s.
  herpes s.
  herpetic s.
  recurrent aphthous s.

vesiculoulcerative s.
Vincent s.
stomatocyte
stomatocytosis
hereditary s.
stomatomy
stomatoschisis
stomatotomy
stomocephalus
stone
cholesterol s.
cystine s.
s. debris
hemolysis-derived black pigment s.
kidney s.
pigment s.
renal s.
struvite s.
uric acid s.
womb s.
stool
acholic s.
s. antigen test
s. colonization
s. culture for O&P
currant jelly s.
electron microscopy of s.
s. examination
greasy s.
grossly bloody s.
guaiac-negative s.
guaiac-positive s.
heme-negative s.
heme-positive s.
s. impaction
s. loss
milk s.
pale s.
pea soup s.
s. porphyrin
s. retention
ribbonlike s.
s. softener
transition s.
s. withholding
stooling
stool-reducing substance
stool-withholding activity
STOP
selective tubal occlusion procedure
STOP nonsurgical permanent
contraception device
stopcock
3-way s.
STOP-ROP
Supplemental Therapeutic Oxygen for
Prethreshold Retinopathy of
Prematurity
STOP-ROP trial

storage
abnormal glucosylceramide s.
s. disease
s. disorder
STORCH test
stored sera
storiform-pleomorphic histologic subtype
stork bite
stork's beak mark
storm
affective s.
thyroid s.
story-stems
new MacArthur emotion s.-s.
Storz
S. disposable cannula
S. disposable trocar
S. endoscope
S. infant bronchoscope
S. laparoscope
Stoxil
STR
skin test reactivity
STR typing
strabismic amblyopia
strabismus
comitant s.
constant s.
s. convergens alternans
convergent s.
divergent s.
incomitant s.
intermittent s.
nonparalytic s.
paralytic s.
s. syndrome
straddle injury
straddling atrioventricular valve
straight
s. back syndrome
s. catheter test
inferior s.
s. last shoe
s. scissors
s. sinus
straightening
retinal arterial narrowing and s.
(RANS)
Straight-In surgical system
straight-leg immobilizer
strain
compression-rarefaction s.
s. down
Enders Edmonston measles s.
s. gauge
impetigo s.
Jeryl Lynn mumps s.
macrophage-tropic s.
measles s.

S

strain (*continued*)
    M-tropic s.
    mumps s.
    non-syncytium-inducing s.
    NSI s.
    Oka s.
    RA27/3 rubella s.
    recombinant inbred s.
    rheumatogenic s.
    rubella s.
    Schwarz measles s.
    T-cell-tropic syncytium-inducing s.
    T-trophic SI s.

strait
    inferior s.
    superior s.

strand
    antisense s.

stranger
    s. anxiety
    s. rape
    s. reaction

strangulated hernia
strangulating obstruction
strangulation
    clitoral s.
    small bowel s.

stranguria (*var. of* strangury)
strangury, stranguria
S-transferase
    glutathione S-t.

strap
    figure-of-8 clavicle s.
    Montgomery s.

strapping
    figure-of-8 s.

Strassman
    S. bicornual uterus metroplasty
      technique
    S. metroplasty
    S. operation
    transverse fundal incision of S.

strata (*pl. of* stratum)
Stratasis urethral sling
StrataSorb dressing
strategy
    maladaptive coping s.
    Robins and Guze validation s.

stratification
    risk s.

stratified squamous epithelium
Stratton-Parker syndrome
stratum, *pl.* **strata**
    s. basale
    s. compactum
    s. corneum
    s. functionale
    s. spongiosum

Strauss method

STRAW
    Stages in Reproductive Aging
      Workshop

strawberry
    s. appearance
    s. cervix
    s. hemangioma
    s. mark
    s. nevus
    s. patch
    s. spot
    s. tongue

strawberry-shaped skull
streak
    s. gonad
    gonadal s.
    intraabdominal s.
    marbled hypopigmented s.
    nonfunctional s.
    s. ovary
    primitive s.

streaking
    perihilar s.

streaky infiltrate
streblodactyly
street
    Great Ormond S. (GOS)
    s. smart

Streeter
    S. band
    S. dysplasia
    S. horizon
    S. syndrome

Strema
strength
    Allerest Headache S.
    Allerest Maximum S.
    Anbesol Maximum S.
    Biotin Forte Extra S.
    Clocort Maximum S.
    double s. (DS, XX)
    extra s. (ES, E.X.)
    Kaopectate Maximum S.
    Orajel Maximum S.
    Tums Extra S.
    Tylenol Extra S.
    Vanceril Double S.

strep
    streptococcus
    s. breath
    s. throat

Streptase
streptavidin peroxidase
Streptex rapid strep test
Streptobacillus moniliformis
streptococcal
    s. antibody
    s. antigen panel
    s. bacteremia

s. cellulitis
s. exotoxin-A (SPEA)
s. gangrene
s. group
group A s.
s. infection
s. meningitis
s. pharyngitis
s. pneumonia
s. pyoderma
s. septicemia
s. tonsillitis
s. tonsillopharyngitis
s. toxic shock syndrome
s. vaginitis
streptococci (*pl. of* streptococcus)
streptococcosis
streptococcus, *pl.* **streptococci**
S. *agalactiae*
anaerobic s.
S. *aureus*
S. *bacteria*
beta-hemolytic s.
S. *bovis*
S. *constellates*
fecal streptococci
group A s. (GAS)
group A beta-hemolytic s. (GABHS)
group B s. (GBS)
group B beta-hemolytic s.
group C s.
group D s.
group G s.
S. *milleri*
S. *mitis*
S. *mutans*
pediatric autoimmune
  neuropsychiatric disorders
  associated with s. (PANDAS)
S. *pneumonia*
S. *pneumoniae*
S. *pyogenes*
s. rapid antigen detection test
rheumatogenic s.
S. *salivarius*
S. *viridans*
viridans s.
streptogramin
streptokinase factor
streptokinase-urokinase
Streptomyces griseus
streptomycin
streptozocin, streptozotocin
streptozocin-induced diabetes
streptozotocin (*var. of* streptozocin)
Streptozyme test
stress
adrenocortical s.
antepartum s.

behavioral s.
clastogenic s.
cold s.
s. dose steroids
end-systolic s. (ESS)
end-systolic wall s.
s. erythrocytosis
s. erythropoiesis
s. fracture
s. incontinence
s. incontinence de novo
s. injury
life s.
maternal s.
neonatal s.
s. neonate
oxidative s.
s. oximetry
postmenstrual s.
psychological s.
s. reaction
s. reaction in exenteration
s. response
shear s.
s. test
thermal s.
s. urinary incontinence (SUI)
s. view radiograph
visual analog scale for s.
stress-associated ulcer
stressed fetus
stress-induced syncope
stressor
sociocultural s.
stress-related peptic ulcer disease
stretch
s. mark
s. receptor in detrusor muscle
s. syncope
stretched
s. penile length
s. phallic length
stretching
bladder s.
brachial plexus s.
stria, *pl.* **striae**
abdominal s.
striae atrophicae
striae cutis distensae
striae gravidarum
Haab s.
Langhans s.
Rohr s.
s. vascularis
Wickham s.
striae (*pl. of* stria)
striata
osteopathia s.
striatal toe

striate
>s. body
>s. hyperkeratosis

striated circular muscle

striation
>dense s.
>hyperostosis generalisata with s.
>longitudinal dense s.
>transverse dense s.
>vertical s.

striatothalamic junction

striatum

striatus
>lichen s.

stricto
>*Borrelia burgdorferi sensu s.*

stricture
>colonic s.
>esophageal s.
>midureteral s.

stricturoplasty

stride

stridor
>audible s.
>biphasic s.
>congenital laryngeal s.
>expiratory s.
>inspiratory s.
>laryngeal s.
>postextubation s.

stridulous breathing

strike
>heel s.

string
>egg on a s.
>s. phlebitis
>s. sign

Stringer technique

strip
>clinical test s.
>ColorpHast Indicator S.'s
>Cover-Strip wound closure s.
>Dextrostix reagent s.
>DiaScreen reagent s.
>fascial s.
>fetal monitoring s.
>leucocyte detection s.
>lung s.
>Mersilene fascial s.
>N-Multistix clinical test s.
>pHydrion s.
>polypropylene fascial s.
>QuickVue UrinChek 10+ urine test s.
>reagent s.
>saturation s.
>s. test
>test s.
>urine test s.

stripe
>endometrial s.
>thickened endometrial s.

stripping
>apical pleural s.
>capsular s.
>membrane s.
>s. of pleura
>periosteal s.

Stroganoff method

stroke
>mitochondrial encephalopathy, lactic acidosis, s.
>perinatal s.
>prenatal s.
>silent s.
>s. volume
>s. volume index (SVI)

strokelike episode

stroma, *pl.* **stromata**
>cellular desmoplastic s.
>cervical s.
>endometrial s.
>fibromuscular cervical s.
>fibromyxoid s.
>gonadal s.
>malignant mesenchymal s.
>ovarian s.
>proliferation of s.
>Rh-positive red cell s.
>uterine endolymphatic s.
>uterine endometrial s.
>uterine epithelial s.

stromal
>s. adenomyosis
>s. cell
>s. development
>s. endometriosis
>s. hyperplasia
>s. hyperthecosis
>s. luteoma
>s. microinvasion
>s. tumor

stromal-epithelial interaction

stromata (*pl. of* stroma)

stromatosis

stromelysin

strong virilization

Strongyloides stercoralis

strongyloidiasis, strongyloidosis

strongyloidosis (*var. of* strongyloidiasis)

strontium bromide

Stroop test

strophocephaly

strophulus

structural
>s. airway change
>s. anomaly
>s. brain defect

s. gene
s. heart defect
s. integration

structure
appendiceal s.
erectile s.
genetic fine s.
hypoechoic s.
limbic s.
peripheral airway s.

Strudwick syndrome

struma, *pl.* **strumae**
s. ovarii

strumae (*pl. of* struma)

strumal carcinoid of ovary

Strumpell-Lorrain disease

struvite stone

strychnine poisoning

STS
serologic test for syphilis
STS deficiency

ST-segment
ST-s. abnormality
ST-s. elevation

Stuart
S. factor
S. index
S. Prenatal vitamin

StuartNatal

Stuart-Prower factor

stub thumb

stuck
s. twin
s. twin gestation
s. twin phenomenon
s. twin syndrome

studding
peritoneal s.

study
acoustic stimulation s.
acute-phase serum s.
ASCUS/LSIL Triage S.
barium s.
biochemical s.
Bogalusa Heart S. (BHS)
bone density s.
breath hydrogen s.
CASH s.
child behavioral s. (CBS)
Childhood Cancer Survivor S.
(CCSS)
chromosomal s.
ciliary function s.
clinical cohort s.
coagulation s. (coag)
cohort s.
Collaborative Perinatal S.
(CPS)
colonic transit s.

controlled bronchoprovocation
challenge s.
cytogenetic s.
cytologic s.
Diabetes in Early Pregnancy S.
Diagnostic Interview for Genetic S.
(DIGS)
DONALD s.
Doppler flow s.
double-blind s.
Dunedin longitudinal s.
electroencephalographic sleep s.
embryonic organ culture s.
epidemiologic s.
fetal blood s.
gene s.
genetic s.
Heart and Estrogen/Progestin
Replacement S. (HERS)
HER S.
histopathological s.
HOPE-ROP s.
immunofluorescence s.
immunologic s.
Iowa bone development s.
Iowa Women's Health S.
large-volume blood s.
longitudinal s.
low birth weight-maternal
employment s. (LBW-MES)
MacArthur Longitudinal Twin S.
MECA s.
methodology s.
mineral balance s.
molecular genetic s.
Multicenter AIDS Cohort S.
(MACS)
National Acute Spinal Cord
Injury S.
National Wilms Tumor S.
(NWTS)
nerve conduction s. (NCS)
neuroimaging s.
neuroradiographic s.
North American Collaborative Crohn
Disease S. (NCCDS)
S. of Tamoxifen and Raloxifene
(STAR)
S. of Women's Health Across the
Nation (SWAN)
Oxford Family Planning Association
Contraceptive S.
PEPI s.
Persutte and Lenke s.
placebo-controlled s.
postmortem s.
Preterm Prediction S.
PRISM s.
quadruple-contrast s.

S

study (*continued*)
    radioisotopic reperfusion and
      excretion s.
    register linkage s.
    REMIS s.
    Royal College of General
      Practitioners' Oral
      Contraception S.
    Second National Incidence S.
      (NIS-2)
    Sitzmarks s.
    sleep s.
    tissue s.
    transesophageal electrophysiologic s.
    videofluoroscopic swallowing s.
      (VFSS)
    videourodynamic s.
    water-deprivation s.
    Women and Infants Transmission S.
      (WITS)
    Women's Health Initiative Memory
      S. (WHIMS)
    Women's HOPE s.
    women's interagency HIV s.
      (WIHS)
    women's intervention nutrition s.
      (WINS)
stuff
    Numby S.
stump
    appendiceal s.
    cervical s.
    inverted appendiceal s.
    rectal s.
    umbilical s.
stun
    cardiac s.
stunned myocardium
stunning
    myocardial s.
stunted
    s. embryo
    s. fetus
stunting
    growth s.
stupor
stuporous
Sturge-Kalischer-Weber
  syndrome
Sturge-Weber
    S.-W. angiomatosis
    S.-W. anomalad
    S.-W. disease
    S.-W. syndrome (SWS)
Sturge-Weber-Dimitri syndrome
Sturge-Weber-Krabbe syndrome
Sturmdorf
    S. hemostatic suture
    S. operation

stuttering
    medication-induced s.
    neurogenic s.
Stüve-Wiedemann syndrome (SWS)
Stx
    Shiga toxin
sty, stye, *pl.* **sties, styes**
stye (*var. of* sty)
styes (*pl. of* sty)
style
    learning s.
stylomastoid foramen
stylopodium
stype
styptic
Suarez ring
subacute
    s. anterior uveitis
    s. bacterial endocarditis
      (SBE)
    s. combined degeneration
    s. encephalitis
    s. fetal hypoxia
    s. myeloopticoneuropathy
    s. necrotizing encephalomyopathy
    s. necrotizing encephalopathy
    s. neuritis
    s. neuronopathic Gaucher disease
    s. osteomyelitis
    s. sclerosing panencephalitis
      (SSPE)
    s. thyroiditis
    s. tracheitis
subaortic
    s. conus
    s. hypertrophic cardiomyopathy
    s. lymph node
    s. membrane
    s. stenosis
    s. stenosis-short stature syndrome
subaponeurotic cranial space
subarachnoid
    s. analgesia
    s. block
    s. bolt
    s. hemorrhage
subareolar
    s. abscess
    s. duct papillomatosis
    s. plexus
    s. tissue
subaverage intelligence
subcapsular
    s. cyst
    s. hepatic hematoma
    s. hepatic hemorrhage
subchorial
    s. lake
    s. space

subchorionic
- s. hematoma
- s. hemorrhage

subclass
- immunoglobulin A s. 1
- immunoglobulin A s. 2

subclavian
- s. artery
- s. artery defect
- s. flap aortoplasty (SFA)
- s. node
- s. steal

subclinical hypothyroidism
subconjunctival hemorrhage
subcoronal hypospadias
subcortical
- s. band heterotopia
- s. laminar heterotopia

subcostal
- s. incision
- s. retraction
- s. view

subcutanea
- lipogranulomatosis s.

subcutaneous
- s. calcification
- s. catheter tunnel formation
- s. desferrioxamine therapy
- s. emphysema
- s. fat necrosis
- s. granuloma annulare
- s. layer
- s. mastectomy
- s. neurofibroma
- s. nodule
- s. sarcoidosis
- s. supply
- s. suspensory ligament
- s. tunnel
- s. ventricular catheter reservoir

subcutaneum
subdermal
- s. contraceptive system
- s. implant
- s. levonorgestrel implant (SLI)

subdiaphragmatic air
subdural
- s. abscess
- s. effusion
- s. empyema
- s. hematoma (SDH)
- s. hemorrhage
- s. puncture
- s. tap

subdural-peritoneal shunt
subendocardial
subendometrial myoma

subependymal
- s. bleeding
- s. cryptic angioma
- s. germinal matrix hemorrhage
- s. germinolysis
- s. hemorrhage (SEH)
- s. heterotopia
- s. region
- s. tuber

subepidermal, subepidermic
- s. blister
- s. keratin cyst

subepidermic (*var. of* subepidermal)
subfascial hammock
subfecundity
subfertility
subfibulare
- os s.

subgaleal
- s. hematoma (SGH)
- s. hemorrhage

subglottic
- s. edema
- s. erosion
- s. stenosis

subhyaloid hemorrhage
subiculum
subinvolution
subischial leg length (SILL)
subitum
- exanthema s.

subjective probability
sublamina densa
sublethal gene
Sublimaze injection
sublingual (S/L)
- s. gland
- s. hematoma
- Nitrostat S.
- s. onychomycosis
- s. thyroid

subluxating patella
subluxation
- atlantoaxial rotary s.
- cervical spine s.
- s. dislocation
- habitual shoulder s.
- radial head s. (RHS)
- rotary s.
- rotatory s.
- shoulder s.

subluxed hip
submammary mastitis
submaxillary gland
submental
- s. hematoma
- s. lymphadenitis
- s. lymphadenopathy

submentovertex view

S

submersion
    iced saline s.
    s. injury
submetacentric chromosome
submucosa
submucosal
    s. arterial malformation
    s. leiomyoma
    s. mass
    s. myoma
    s. plexus
    s. urethral augmentation
submucous, submucosal
    s. cleft
    s. cleft palate
    s. fibroid
    s. leiomyoma
    s. myoma
subnormal
    s. growth velocity
    s. temperature
subnormality
    mental s.
suboccipital craniectomy
suboccipitobregmatic diameter
suboptimal surgery
suborbital edema
subpannicular area
subparta
    ileus s.
subpectoral
    s. axillary node
    s. implant
subperiosteal
    s. abscess (SPA)
    s. aspiration
subphrenic
    s. abscess
    s. gas collection
subpial region
subpleural
    s. bleb
    s. reticulonodular pattern
subpulmonic area
Sub-Q-Set
subretinal
    s. exudate
    s. fluid
subsalicylate
    bismuth s.
subscale
subscapular skinfold thickness
subsegmental atelectasis
subseptate uterus
subseptus
    hymen s.
    uterus s.
subsequent fertility

subserosal (*var. of* subserous)
subserous, subserosal
    s. fascia
    s. fibroid
    s. myoma
    s. nodule
    s. pedunculated myoma
subset
    T-cell s.
subspinale
    point A, s.
substance
    s. abuse
    acid-reacting s.
    illegal s.
    müllerian inhibiting s. (MIS)
    s. P immune reactivity
    s. P pain neurotransmitter
    radioactive s.
    reducing s.
    serum müllerian inhibiting s.
    stool-reducing s.
    thiobarbituric acid-reacting s.
      (TBARS)
    urine-reducing s.
    s. use
    s. use disorder (SUD)
    vasoactive s.
    s. X
substance-induced psychotic disorder
substantia, *pl.* **substantiae**
    s. gelatinosa
    s. nigra
    s. nigra pars reticulata
    s. propria
substantiae (*pl. of* substantia)
substernal retraction
substitute
    blood s.
    s. care
    Oxygent temporary blood s.
    perflubron emulsion temporary
      blood s.
    PolyHeme blood s.
    temporary blood s.
substrate
    renin s.
subsyndromal depressive symptom
subtalar facet
subtest
    Digit Span S.
subthalamicum
    corpus s.
subtilis
    Bacillus s.
subtle
    s. neurologic sequela
    s. seizure

subtotal
  s. colon resection
  s. hysterectomy (STH)
subtrigonal injection
subtype
  Estren-Dameshek s.
  histologic s.
  histopathologic s.
  myxoid histopathologic s.
  storiform-pleomorphic
    histologic s.
subungual, subunguial
  s. exostosis
  s. fibroma
  s. oncychomycosis
subunguial (*var. of* subungual)
subunit
  beta s.
  inhibin s.
  inhibin A s.
subureteric Teflon injection
suburethral
  s. diverticulitis
  s. sling
subvalvular
subxiphoid
subzonal
  s. injection (SUZI)
  s. injection of sperm
  s. insemination (SUZI)
  s. insertion (SUZI)
succedaneum
  caput s.
succenturiate placenta
successful pregnancy
succimer
succinate
  s. dehydrogenase
  hydrocortisone sodium s.
  sumatriptan s.
succinyl
  s. aminoimidazole carboxamide
    ribotide (SAICAR)
  s. CoA:3-ketoacid CoA transferase
  s. CoA:3-oxoacid CoA
    transferase
succinylcholine
succinylsulfathiazole
succumb
suck
  poor s.
  weak s.
sucking
  s. blister
  s. cushion
  nonnutritive s. (NNS)
  s. pad
  s. reflex

suckle
suckling
  s. pattern
  s. reflex
Sucraid
sucralfate
sucrase-isomaltase deficiency
Sucrets
  S. Cough Calmers
  S. Sore Throat
sucrose
  concentrated oral s.
  s. gradient
  s. hemolysis test
  s. pacifier
sucrose-free formula
sucrosuria
suction
  airway s.
  s. and curettage (S&C)
  s. aspiration
  bulb s.
  s. catheter
  s. curette
  s., dilation, and
    curettage
  s. drainage
  endometrial s.
  endotracheal s. (ETS)
  nasopharyngeal s.
  open endotracheal s.
  s. pump
  respiratory s.
  Tis-u-Trap endometrial s.
  Trach Care s.
  Vabra s.
  vacuum s.
  wall s.
suction-assisted lipoplasty
suctioning
  bulb s.
  chest s.
  closed endotracheal tube s.
  DeLee s.
  nasopharyngeal s.
  open endotracheal s.
  respiratory s.
  tracheal s.
suction-irrigator
  Nezhat-Dorsey s.-i.
suctorial pad
SUD
  substance use disorder
  sudden unexpected death
Sudafed 12 Hour
sudamen, *pl.* **sudamina**
  miliary sudamina
sudamina (*pl. of* sudamen)

S

sudanophilic
  s. cerebral sclerosis
  s. diffuse sclerosis
  s. leukodystrophy
Sudan stain
sudden
  s. infant death (SID)
  s. infant death syndrome (SIDS)
  S. Infant Death Syndrome
    Alliance
  s. infant death unexplained by
    history
  s. intrauterine unexplained death
    (SIUD)
  s. unexpected death (SUD)
Sudeck atrophy
sudomotor dysfunction
sudoral miliaria
Sudrin
SUDS
  single-use diagnostic system
    SUDS HIV-1 antibody test
SUFE
  slipped upper femoral epiphysis
Sufenta injection
sufentanil citrate
sufficient
  pancreas s. (PS)
  s. quantity
  quantity not s. (QNS)
suffocation
  infant s.
  mechanical s.
suffusion
  conjunctival s.
sugar
  blood s.
  s. diabetes
  fasting blood s.
  s. intoxication
  low blood s.
  mannose-type s.
  s., temperature, artificial breathing,
    blood pressure, lab work,
    emotional support (STABLE)
sugar-dipped pacifier
Sugarman
  S. brachydactyly
  S. syndrome
sugar-tong splint
Sugiura procedure
SUI
  stress urinary incontinence
suicidal ideation
suicidality
suicide
  attempted s.
  s. gene
  s. gene therapy

  hospitalized attempted s. (HAS)
  s. risk screen (SRS)
suid herpesvirus
suis
  Brucella s.
suit
  MAST s.
Sulamyd
  Sodium S.
sulbactam
  ampicillin and s.
sulci (*pl. of* sulcus)
sulconazole
sulcus, *pl.* **sulci**
  coronal s.
  Harrison s.
Sulf-10
sulfa
sulfabenzamide
sulfacarbamide
sulfacetamide
sulfacytine
sulfadiazine
  silver s.
sulfadimethoxine
sulfadimidine
sulfadoxine and pyrimethamine
sulfaethidole
sulfafurazole, sulphafurazole
sulfaguanidine
Sulfair
sulfalene
sulfamerazine
sulfameter
sulfamethazine
sulfamethizole
Sulfamethoprim
sulfamethoxazole and trimethoprim
sulfamethoxazole/phenazopyridine
  hydrochloride
sulfamethoxydiazine
sulfamethoxypyridazine
Sulfamylon cream
sulfaphenazole
sulfapyridine
sulfasalazine
sulfatase
  iduronate s. (IDS)
  steroid s.
sulfate, sulphate
  amikacin s.
  amphetamine s.
  anhydrous magnesium s.
  atropine s.
  bleomycin s.
  chondroitin s.
  dehydroepiandrosterone s. (DHEAS)
  dehydroisoandrosterone s.
  dermatan s.

dextran s.
dextrin s.
dextroamphetamine s.
DHEA s.
ephedrine s.
estrone s.
ferric s.
ferrous s. (FeSO$_4$)
gentamicin s.
heparan s.
hexoprenaline s.
hydrazine s.
hydroxychloroquine s.
hyoscyamine s.
keratan s.
magnesium s. (MgSO$_4$)
metaproterenol s.
morphine s.
neomycin s.
netilmicin s.
orciprenaline s.
paromomycin s.
piperazine estrone s.
Plaquenil S.
polymyxin B s.
protamine s.
quinine s.
sodium equilin s.
sodium estrone s.
sodium tetradecyl s.
steroid s.
terbutaline s.
trimethoprim s.
vincristine s.
zinc s.
sulfathiazole
sulfathiourea
sulfatide
sulfatidosis
juvenile s.
Sulfatrim DS
Sulfa-Trip
sulfaturia
keratan s.
sulfhydryl (SH)
sulfide
selenium s.
sulfisomidine
sulfisoxazole
**sulfisoxazole/phenazopyridine
hydrochloride**
sulfite oxidase deficiency
Sulfizole
**sulfoiduronate sulfatase deficiency
(SIDS)**
sulfonamide
sulfonate
2-mercaptoethane s. (mesna)
sodium polystyrene s.

sulfonylurea
sulfotransferase
estrogen s.
sulfoxide
dimethyl s. (DMSO)
sulfur, sulphur
s. and salicylic acid
s. dioxide
s. granule
sulfur-deficient brittle hair syndrome
sulindac
sulphafurazole (*var. of* sulfafurazole)
sulphate (*var. of* sulfate)
sulphur (*var. of* sulfur)
sulpiride
sulprostone
Sultrin
Sumacal formula
sumatriptan
s. nasal spray
s. succinate
summation gallop
Sumycin Oral
SUN
serum urea nitrogen
sun protection behavior index
sunburn
blistering s.
sunburst appearance
sunflower
s. cataract
s. oil challenge test
sunken anterior fontanelle
Sunlight Omnisense ultrasound
Sunna circumcision
Sunnex Tri-Star lamp
sunny-side up delivery
sunrise view
sun-seeking pattern
sunset eyes
sunstroke, sun stroke
super
s. blue light
S. Duper Diaper Doo
s. female
s. syringe
superabsorbent
superactivity
phosphoribosylpyrophosphate
synthetase s.
PRPP synthetase s.
**superconducting quantum interference
device susceptometer (SQUIDS)**
superfamily
transforming growth factor B s.
superfecundation
superfetation
superficial
s. circumflex iliac artery

superficial (*continued*)
   s. compartment
   s. compartment of vulva
   s. ectopic testis
   s. epigastric artery
   s. external pudendal artery
    (SEPA)
   s. linear array (SLA)
   s. necrosis
   s. onychomycosis
   s. spreading melanoma
   s. thrombophlebitis
   s. thrombus
   s. transperineal muscle
   s. transverse perineal muscle
superfluous
superimposed
   s. eclampsia
   s. preeclampsia
superimpregnation
superinfection
superinvolution
superior
   s. epigastric artery
   s. fascia
   s. iliac crest
   s. iliac spine
   s. laryngeal nerve
   s. mediastinal syndrome
   s. mesenteric angiogram
   s. mesenteric artery
   s. mesenteric artery syndrome
   s. mesenteric plexus
   s. mesenteric vein
   s. oblique muscle
   s. olivary nucleus
   s. olive
   s. ramus
   saccus s.
   s. sagittal sinus
   s. strait
   s. vena cava (SVC)
   s. vena cava syndrome
   s. venous system
   s. vesical fissure
superlactation
supernatant
   amniotic fluid s.
supernumerary
   s. breast
   s. chromosome
   s. digit
   s. kidney
   s. mamma
   s. marker chromosome
    (SMC)
   s. nipple
   s. ovary
   s. placenta

   s. proboscis
   s. rib
superovulation induction
superoxide
   s. dismutase-1
   s. radical
supersaturation of bile
SuperVent
supervoltage radiation
supinate
supination
   passive s.
supine
   s. empty stress test (SEST)
   s. hypotensive syndrome
   s. length
   s. pressor test
   s. sleep position
Suplena formula
supplement
   Aminosyn-PF s.
   Boost nutritional s.
   calcium s.
   dietary s.
   EleCare nutritional s.
   enzyme s.
   Expecta Lipil s.
   Fer-In-Sol s.
   infant dietary s.
   iron s.
   Lactaid Ultra lactase enzyme s.
   LifePak nutritional s.
   magnesium s.
   NeoSure nutritional s.
   nutritional s.
   Pediatrician infant dietary s.
   phosphate s.
   potassium s.
   vitamin s.
   zinc s.
supplemental
   s. newborn screen
   s. oxygen
   S. Security Income (SSI)
   S. Therapeutic Oxygen for
    Prethreshold Retinopathy of
    Prematurity (STOP-ROP)
supplementary
   s. gene
   s. menstruation
supplementation
   calcium s.
   folate s.
supply
   arterial s.
   iodine s.
   milk s.
   musculofascial s.
   subcutaneous s.

support
advanced cardiac life s. (ACLS)
advanced life s. (ALS)
advanced pediatric life s. (APLS)
advanced trauma life s. (ATLS)
Baby Halo cushioned head s.
basic life s. (BLS)
bone anchor s.
s. catheter
extensive s.
extracorporeal life s. (ECLS)
s. group
Gynemesh PS polypropylene
  mesh s.
inotropic s.
intermittent s.
life s.
limited s.
luteal phase s.
medial longitudinal arch s.
Multidimensional Scale of Perceived
  Social S. (MSPSS)
neonatal adjuvant life s. (NALS)
neonatal extracorporeal life s.
s. network
noninvasive respiratory s.
nutritional s.
paravaginal tissue s.
pediatric advanced life s. (PALS)
pervasive s.
psychosocial s.
s. reflex
respiratory s.
s. services
sugar, temperature, artificial
  breathing, blood pressure, lab
  work, emotional s. (STABLE)
s. trust
urethral s.
urethrovesical angle s.
uterine s.
vaginal vault s.
ventilator s.
ventilatory s.
supportive
s. care
s. group therapy
s. psychotherapy
suppository
Anusol-HC S.
AVC s.
bisacodyl s.
Cort-Dome High Potency S.
Dilaudid S.
First-Progesterone VGS 50
  vaginal s.
First-Progesterone VGS 100
  vaginal s.
glycerin s.

intravaginal s.
Monistat 3 vaginal s.
paracetamol s.
prostaglandin s.
Prostin E2 Vaginal S.
rectal s.
Sani-Supp S.
Terazol vaginal s.
triple sulfa s.
vaginal s.
Supprelin
Supprelin-LA 12-month implant
suppressant
St. Joseph Cough S.
suppressed menstruation
suppression
adrenal s.
antibody-mediated immune s.
  (AMIS)
bone marrow s.
s. burst
endogenous gonadotropin
  activity s.
estradiol s.
fetal parathyroid s.
follicle-stimulating hormone s.
gonadal steroid s.
immunologic s.
pituitary gonadotropin s.
prolactin s.
testosterone s.
Suppress lozenge
suppressor
s. gene
s. T cell
Supprettes
Aquachloral S.
suppurate
suppurating sinus tract
suppuration
intracranial s.
joint s.
pulmonary s.
suppurativa
hidradenitis s. (HS)
vulvar hidradenitis s.
suppurative
s. appendicitis
s. arthritis
s. bursitis
s. cholangitis
s. infection
s. labyrinthitis
s. lymphadenitis
s. mastitis
s. mediastinitis
s. otitis media (SOM)
s. parotitis
s. phlebitis

S

suppurative (*continued*)
   s. pneumonia
   s. thyroiditis
suprabasal blister
suprabulbar paresis
supracardiac total anomalous pulmonary
  venous return
supracervical hysterectomy
  (SCH)
supraciliary tap
supraclavicular
   s. indrawing
   s. retraction
supracondylar humeral fracture
supracristal ventricular septal
  defect
supraglottic
   s. aperture
   s. web
supraglottitis
supralevator
   s. abscess
   s. imperforate anus
supramalleolar orthosis (SMO)
supramentale
   point B, s.
supranormal scrotal position
supranuclear palsy
supraorbital nerve block
suprapineal recess
suprapubic
   s. aspiration of urine
   s. bladder aspiration
   s. catheter
   s. cystostomy
   s. cystotomy
   s. discomfort
   s. fat pad
   s. mass
   s. pain
   s. pressure
   s. stab wound
   s. trocar
   s. urethrovesical suspension
suprasellar
   s. arachnoid cyst
   s. meningioma
suprasternal
   s. notch
   s. notch thrill
   s. view
supratentorial
   s. anaplastic ependymoma
   s. white matter
supratip nasal tip deformity
supraumbilical incision
supravaginalis
   portio s.
supravaginal septum

supravalvular
   s. aortic stenosis
   s. pulmonary stenosis
supraventricular
   s. tachyarrhythmia (SVT)
   s. tachycardia (SVT)
   s. tachydysrhythmia
supraventricularis
   crista s.
supravital
   s. stain
   s. stain test
Suprax
suprofen
sural nerve biopsy
SureCell
   S. chlamydia test kit
   S. herpes test
   S. rapid test kit for pregnancy
SurePath liquid-based Pap test
SurePress
   S. dressing
   S. wrap
SureSite dressing
767 SureTemp 4 oral thermometer
Surety Shield
SURF
   Service Utilization and Risk Factors
surface
   adaptive s.
   amniotic-chorionic s.
   s. antigen
   antimesenteric s.
   decreased mucosal s.
   denuded s.
   s. electromyogram (SEMG)
   s. electromyography (SEMG)
   s. epithelium
   s. epithelium vascular channel
   external s.
   s. furrowing
   s. furrowing of tongue
   s. immunoglobulin
   s. irradiation
   lingual s.
   serosal s.
   s. tension
surfactant
   s. administration
   beractant s.
   bovine s.
   bovine lavage extract s.
    (BLES)
   Curosurf s.
   s. deficiency syndrome
   exogenous s.
   heterologous s.
   homologous s.
   Human Surf s.

Infasurf s.
s. lavage
natural synthetic s.
porcine s.
s. protein-A (SP-A)
s. protein-B (SP-B)
s. protein-C (SP-C)
s. protein deficiency
pulmonary s.
s. replacement therapy
s. replacement trial
rescue s.
s. secretion
semisynthetic s.
Survanta s.
synthetic s.

surfactant-associated
s.-a. protein (SAP)
s.-a. protein C enhancer

surfactant-deficient lung
Surfak
Sur-Fast needle
Surfaxin
dilute S.

surge
estrogen s.
gonadotropin s.
LH s.
midcycle s.
postnatal gonadotropin s.
preovulatory LH s.
TSH s.

surgeon
American College of S.'s
pediatric s.
pelvic reconstruction s.

surgeon's knot
surgery
ablative s.
bladder neck s.
bypass s.
conservative s.
corrective s.
cytoreductive s.
definitive s.
emergency s.
endoscopic sinus s.
extirpative s.
extraocular muscle s.
feminizing s.
fetal s.
gamma knife s.
gastric reduction s.
hysteroscopic s.
inferior turbinate s.
intraabdominal s.
laser s.
lung s.
muscle s.

open heart s.
orthognathic s.
palliative s.
pediatric lung s.
pelvic floor s.
pelvic reconstructive s.
peripheral ablative s.
prenatal s.
previous transfundal uterine s.
primary cytoreductive s.
pull-through s.
radical s.
radioreceptor-guided s.
reconstructive pelvic s.
sinus s.
suboptimal s.
thoracic s.
transfundal uterine s.
tubal reconstruction s.
vaginal s.
video-assisted thoracic s. (VATS)
video-assisted thoracoscopic s. (VATS)
zero gravity s.

surgical
s. abortion
s. asplenia
s. containment
s. correction
s. cricothyrotomy
s. debulking
s. disruption
s. drainage
s. emergency
s. enucleation
s. evacuation
s. excision
s. hemostasis
s. infection
s. management
s. mastoiditis
s. myomectomy as reproductive therapy (SMART)
s. neonate
s. oophorectomy
s. overhead canopy
s. pleurodesis
s. removal
s. repair
s. resection
s. scarlet fever
s. septectomy
s. space
s. staging
s. sterilization
s. sterilization procedure
s. tape occlusion
s. termination

surgical (*continued*)
    s. therapy
    s. trauma
    s. weight loss
surgically
    s. induced abortion
    s. treatable pathology
Surgicel
Surgicenter 40 CO₂ laser
surgicopathologic staging system
Surgidac suture
Surgilase 55W laser
Surgilene
Surgin hemorrhage occluder pin
Surgi-Prep
Surgiview laparoscope
Surmontil
surrender posture
surrogacy
    gestational s.
    traditional s.
surrogate
    gestational s.
    s. gestational motherhood
    s. mother
    sex s.
Survanta surfactant
surveillance
    antepartum fetal s.
    s. colonoscopy
    developmental s.
    S., Epidemiology and End Results (SEER)
    fetal s.
    immune s.
    immunologic s.
    maternal s.
    nutritional s.
    posttreatment s.
    s. technique
    s. tracheal aspirate
    ultrasound s.
survey
    irrigation s.
    Juvenile Wellness and Health S. (JWHS)
    Kids Eating Disorder S. (KEDS)
    National Ambulatory Medical Care S. (NAMCS)
    National Educational Longitudinal S. (NELS)
    National Health and Nutrition Examination S. (NHANES)
    National Health Interview S. (NHIS)
    National Hospital Discharge S. (NIDS)
    National Maternal and Infant Health S.
    School Sleep Habits S.

Sexual Opinion S.
skeletal s.
Urge-IIQ s.
youth risk behavioral s. (YRBS)
survival
    actuarial s.
    allograft s.
    decreased red blood cell s.
    disease-free s. (DFS)
    event-free s. (EFS)
    life table s.
    long-term s.
    s. rate
    transient fetal s.
survivor guilt
susceptibility
    genetic s.
    s. hypothesis
susceptible
susceptometer
    superconducting quantum interference device s. (SQUIDS)
suspected
    s. child abuse or neglect (SCAN)
    s. pituitary adenoma
suspension
    Aldridge-Studdefort urethral s.
    Alexander-Adams uterine s.
    AMS Apogee vault s.
    Apogee vaginal vault s.
    Baldy-Webster uterine s.
    bladder neck s.
    budesonide inhalation s. (BIS)
    Children's Motrin S.
    Ciprodex otic s.
    Coffey s.
    Cortisporin Ophthalmic S.
    Cortisporin Otic S.
    Cortisporin-TC otic s.
    Curosurf intratracheal s.
    DisperMox oral s.
    Donald-Fothergill uterine s.
    endoscopic bladder neck s. (EBNS)
    Gilliam-Doleris uterine s.
    Gittes endoscopic bladder neck s.
    Gittes urethral s.
    high uterosacral ligament s.
    horizontal s.
    iliococcygeus fascia s.
    Infasurf intratracheal s.
    inhalation s.
    intratracheal s.
    laparoscopic s.
    laparoscopic vault s.
    Manchester-Fothergill uterine s.
    Michigan 4-wall sacrospinous s.
    minimal-incision pubovaginal s.
    needle s.
    Olshausen s.

Omnicef oral s.
ophthalmic s.
oral s.
orciprenaline oral s.
otic s.
paravaginal s.
Pereyra needle s.
protamine insulin zinc s.
pubovaginal s.
Raz bladder neck s.
sacrospinous ligament s.
sacrospinous vaginal vault s.
Stamey-Pereyra needle s.
suprapubic urethrovesical s.
transvaginal bladder neck s.
urethral s.
uterine s.
uterosacral ligament s.
vaginal vault s.
ventral s.
Yachia incisionless bladder s.

suspensory
s. ligament laxity
s. ligament of clitoris
s. ligament of ovary
s. ligaments of Cooper
s. sling operation

Sustacal Plus formula
Sustagen formula
sustained
s. autonomic hypoarousal
s. clonus
s. ventricular tachycardia
(SVT)

sustained-release
s.-r. albuterol
s.-r. medication
s.-r. theophylline

Sustiva
Sutherland-Haan syndrome (SHS)
Sutherland procedure
Sutilains Ointment
sutural calcification
suture
absorbable s.
apposition of skull s.
B-Lynch uterine compression s.
buried s.
Caprosyn monofilament s.
catgut s.
coated Vicryl Rapide s.
compression s.
continuous running monofilament s.
corner s.
coronal s. (CS)
cranial s.
Davis-Geck Softgut s.
Dexon II s.
Dexon Plus s.

Endoloop s.
Ethibond polybutilate-coated
polyester s.
frontal s.
Gambee s.
s. grasper forceps
gut s.
half-buried s.
Heaney s.
interrupted s.
inverted subcuticular s.
Investa s.
Kelly s.
left-angle s.
s. ligated
s. ligation
s. ligature
s. line
lower-angle s.
lynch s.
s. material
Maxon delayed absorbable s.
Mersilene s.
Monocryl s.
nasofrontal s.
nylon s. (ns, NS)
sutures of skull
overriding of s.'s
s. penile laceration
perianal s.
permanent s.
polyglactin 910 s.
polyglycol s.
polyglyconate s.
Polysorb s.
premature closure of coronal s.
Prolene s.
purse-string s.
retention s.
right-angle s.
Safil synthetic absorbable surgical s.
sagittal s.
silk s.
silver wire s.
skin s.
stainless steel s.
Sturmdorf hemostatic s.
Surgidac s.
upper-angle s.
Vicryl Rapide s.
wide cranial s.

Suture-Mate
suxamethonium
SUZI
subzonal injection
subzonal insemination
subzonal insertion
Sv
sievert

S

SVC
superior vena cava
SV-CAH
simple virilizing congenital adrenal
hyperplasia
SVD
spontaneous vaginal delivery
SVE
sterile vaginal examination
SVI
stroke volume index
SVR
systemic vascular resistance
SVT
supraventricular tachyarrhythmia
supraventricular tachycardia
sustained ventricular tachycardia
fetal reentrant SVT
swab
calcium alginate s.
cotton-tipped s.
s. examination
nasal s.
nasopharyngeal s.
Puritan s.
rectal s.
self-obtained vaginal s.
s. test
throat s.
umbilical s.
vaginal s.
swallow
barium s.
modified barium s. (MBS)
s. reflex
s. syncope
swallowed
s. blood syndrome
s. maternal blood
swallowing
air s.
s. difficulty
fetal s.
s. reflex
SWAN
Study of Women's Health Across the
Nation
Swan-Ganz catheter
sway
lateral shoulder s.
swayback
SW-CAH
salt-wasting congenital adrenal
hyperplasia
sweat
s. chloride
s. chloride concentration
s. chloride determination
s. chloride iontophoresis

s. chloride level
s. chloride test
s. duct
s. gland
night s.
s. testing
sweating
anhidrotic s.
eccrine s.
excessive s.
hypohidrotic s.
nocturnal s.
sweaty feet syndrome
Swedish
S. national growth chart
S. porphyria
Sween Cream
sweep
s. gas
The Cell S.
s. the pelvis
sweetened pacifier
Sweet syndrome
swelling
brain s.
cerebral s.
diffuse brain s. (DBS)
focal axonal s.
global brain s.
hydrocephalic brain s.
hypoosmotic s. (HOS)
labioscrotal s.
scrotal s.
**Swenson colonic pullthrough
procedure**
SWGD
sterile water gastric drip
Swift disease
SWIM
sperm washing insemination method
Swim-Ear water drying aid
swimmer's
s. ear
s. itch
s. shoulder
swimming
s. movement
s. pool granuloma
s. position
s. reflex
swim-up technique
swine-flu influenza vaccine
swinging
blanket s.
s. flashlight test
Swiss
S. cheese endometrium
S. cheese hyperplasia
S. cheese septum

switch
  adaptive s.
  genetic s.
  s. operation
  venous s.
swivel
  s. arm system
  s. walker
swollen
  s. glomerular tuft
  s. joint
swordfish test
SWS
  Sturge-Weber syndrome
  Stüve-Wiedemann syndrome
Swyer-James-Macleod syndrome
Swyer-James syndrome
Swyer syndrome
SX-T
  Proplex SX-T
sycosis barbae
Sydenham
  S. chorea
  S. chorea criteria
Sydney
  S. crease
  S. line
Syed-Neblett dedicated vulvar plastic template
Syllact
sylvatic typhus
sylvian
  s. aqueduct syndrome
  s. epilepsy
  s. seizure
Sylvius
  aqueduct of S.
Symadine
symbiotic psychosis
symblepharon
symbolic representation
symbrachydactyly
Syme amputation
symmelia
symmetric, symmetrical
  s. communicating uterus
  s. demyelination
  s. growth restriction
  s. IUGR
  s. progressive erythrokeratodermia
symmetrical
  s. conjoined twins
  s. movement
  s. tonic neck reflex (STNR)
sympathectomy, sympathetectomy, sympathicectomy
  presacral s.
sympathetectomy (*var. of* sympathectomy)

sympathetic
  s. adrenergic function
  s. blockade
  s. chain
  s. ganglion
  s. innervation
  s. nervous system
  s. skin response
  s. stimulation
  s. tissue
sympathicectomy (*var. of* sympathectomy)
sympatholytic drop
sympathomimetic amine
sympathovagal
symphalangism, symphalangy
symphalangy (*var. of* symphalangism)
symphyseal (*var. of* symphysial)
symphyseotome (*var. of* symphysiotome)
symphyseotomy (*var. of* symphysiotomy)
symphyses (*pl. of* symphysis, symphysis)
symphysial, symphyseal
  s. separation
  s. wall
symphysiotome, symphyseotome
symphysiotomy, symphyseotomy
symphysis, *pl.* **symphyses, symphyses**
  pubic s.
  s. pubis
  s. pubis diastasis
symphysis-fundus height
symphysodactyly
sympodia
symptom
  B s.'s
  Bristol Female Lower Urinary Tract S.'s (BFLUTS)
  s. contagion
  depressive s.
  dissociative s.
  duration of s.'s
  intrusion s.
  neurovegetative functioning or s.
  obstructive s.
  paraneoplastic s.
  pathognomonic s.
  PIH s.
  postmenopausal urogenital s.
  posttraumatic signs or s.'s (PTSS)
  pregnancy-induced hypertension s.
  premenstrual s.'s
  prodromal s.
  refractory depressive s.
  schedule for assessment of negative s.'s (SANS)
  schedule for assessment of positive s.'s (SAPS)
  somatic s.
  subsyndromal depressive s.
  tic s.

symptom (*continued*)
  Uhthoff s.
  vegetative s.
  vertiginous s.
symptomatic
  s. chronic empyema
  s. dystonia
  s. epilepsy
  s. infection
  s. porphyria
  s. primary immunodeficiency
   disorder
  s. progressive hydrocephalus
  s. seizure
  s. spasm
  s. status epilepticus
symptomatica
  porphyria cutanea tarda s.
symptomatology
symptom-giving PGR
symptothermal
  s. method
  s. method of contraception
symptothermic contraceptive method
sympus
Synacort Topical
synactive theory
synadelphus
Synagis
Synalar Topical
Synalgos-DC
synangiosis
synapse
synapsis
synaptic pruning
synaptogenesis
synaptonemal complex
synaptophysin
Synarel
syncephalus
  s. asymmetros
  craniothoracopagus s.
syncheilia, synchilia
synchilia (*var. of* syncheilia)
synchondrosis disruption
synchondrotomy
synchronic
synchronized
  s. DC cardioversion
  s. intermittent mandatory ventilation
   (SIMV)
  s. nasal intermittent positive-pressure
   ventilation (SNIPPV)
synchronous breathing
synchronously
syncinesis (*var. of* synkinesis)
synclitic
synclitism

syncopal
  s. episode
  s. spell
syncope
  adolescent stretch s.
  arrhythmogenic s.
  cardiac s.
  cardioinhibitory s.
  cerebral s.
  cough s.
  hair groomer's s.
  hysteric s.
  infantile s.
  micturition s.
  neurally mediated s. (NMS)
  neurocardiogenic s.
  neuropsychiatric s.
  orthostatic s.
  reflex s.
  stress-induced s.
  stretch s.
  swallow s.
  vasopressor s.
  vasovagal s.
syncytial
  s. bud
  s. cell
  s. knot
  s. sprout
syncytiotrophoblast (ST)
  malignant s.
syncytiotrophoblastic tumor giant cell
syncytium inducing (SI)
syndactylia (*var. of* syndactyly)
syndactylism
syndactylization
syndactyly, syndactylia, syndactylism
  s., cataracts, mental retardation
   syndrome
  Cenani-Lenz s.
  complete s.
  complex s.
  digit s.
  incomplete s.
  s., microcephaly, mental retardation
   syndrome
  simple s.
  soft tissue s.
  toe s.
syndactyly-anophthalmos syndrome
syndesis
syndesmosis
  tibiofibular s.
syndet cleaning bar
syndrome
  AAA s.
  AADH s.
  Aagenaes s.
  Aarskog s.

Aarskog-Scott s. (ASS)
Aase s.
Aase-Smith s.
abdominal compartment s. (ACS)
abdominal muscle deficiency s.
abdominal musculature aplasia s.
abducted thumbs s.
Aberfeld s.
ablepharon-macrostomia s. (AMS)
absence of abdominal muscle s.
absent pulmonary valve s.
abstinence s.
Abt-Letterer-Siwe s.
abuse dwarfism s.
Accutane dysmorphic s.
ACD mental retardation s.
ACF s.
achalasia-microcephaly s.
Achard s.
Achard-Thiers s.
achondrogenesis s.
achondroplasia s.
acid aspiration s.
acquired immune deficiency s.
  (AIDS)
acquired immunodeficiency s.
  (AIDS)
acquired inflammatory Brown s.
acral-renal-mandibular s.
acrocallosal s. (ACS)
acrodysgenital s.
acrodysostosis s.
acrodysplasia-dysostosis s.
acrofacial dysostosis with postaxial
  defects s.
acromegaloid-cutis verticis
  gyrata-leukoma s.
acroosteolysis s.
acrorenal s.
acrorenomandibular s.
acrorenoocular s.
acute aseptic meningitis s.
acute chest s. (ACS)
acute meningoencephalitis s.
acute radiation s.
acute respiratory distress s.
  (ARDS)
acute retroviral s.
acute traumatic compartment s.
acute urethral s.
Adair-Dighton s.
Adams-Oliver s.
Adams-Stokes s.
Addison disease-cerebral sclerosis s.
Addison disease-spastic paraplegia s.
addisonian s.
Addison-Schilder s.
adducted thumb-clubfoot s.
adducted thumbs s.

adducted thumbs-mental
  retardation s.
Adie chronic pupillary s.
adiposogenital s.
ADR s.
adrenal virilizing s.
adrenocortical atrophy-cerebral
  sclerosis s.
adrenogenital s. (AGS)
adult-onset polyglandular s.
adult respiratory distress s. (ARDS)
AEC s.
AFA s.
afebrile pneumonia s.
AFFN dysostosis s. 1
agenesis of corpus callosum-mental
  retardation-osseous lesions s.
aglossia-adactylia s.
agonadism, mental retardation, short
  stature, retarded bone age s.
AGR s.
agyria-pachygyria s.
Aicardi s.
Aicardi-Goutières s.
air leak s.
airway obstruction s.
Alagille s.
Alagille-Watson s. (AWS)
Alajouanine s.
Albers-Schönberg s.
albinism-deafness s.
Albright s.
ALCAPA s.
aldosteronism-normal blood
  pressure s.
Aldred s.
Aldrich s.
Alexander s.
Alice in Wonderland s.
Allan-Herndon s.
Allan-Herndon-Dudley s. (AHDS)
Allemann s.
Allen-Masters s.
Allgrove s.
Alpers s.
Alport s.
Alström s.
Alström-Hallgren s.
Ambras s.
AMC s.
ameloonychohypohidrotic s.
amenorrhea-galactorrhea s.
aminopterin embryopathy s.
aminopterin-like embryopathy s.
Amish brittle hair s.
amniotic band s.
amniotic fluid embolism s.
amniotic fluid embolus s.
amniotic infection s.

S

syndrome (*continued*)

amotivational s.
AMR s.
anal-ear-renal-radial malfunction s.
Andermann s.
Andersen s.
Andogsky s.
androgen insensitivity s.
androgen resistance s.
anemia s.
Angelman s.
angiomatosis-oculo-orbito-thalamo-
  encephalic s.
angioosteohypertrophy s.
aniridia, cerebellar ataxia-
  oligophrenia s.
aniridia, Wilms tumor
  association s.
aniridia, Wilms tumor,
  gonadoblastoma s.
ankyloblepharon, ectodermal
  dysplasia, clefting s.
ankyloglossia superior s.
anophthalmia, hand-foot defects,
  mental retardation s.
anophthalmia-limb anomalies s.
anophthalmia-syndactyly s.
anophthalmia-Waardenburg s.
anorectal s.
anterior chamber cleavage s.
anterior chamber dysgenesis s.
anterior cord s.
anticonvulsant hypersensitivity s.
antiphospholipid s. (APS)
antiphospholipid antibody s.
  (APAS)
Antley-Bixler s.
anus-hand-ear s.
aortic arch anomaly, peculiar facies,
  mental retardation s.
aortic stenosis, corneal clouding,
  growth and mental retardation s.
Apert s.
Apert-Crouzon s.
aplastic abdominal muscle s.
apraxia-ataxia-mental deficiency s.
apraxia-oculomotor contracture-muscle
  atrophy s.
aprosencephaly s.
aprosencephaly-atelencephaly s.
Arakawa s.
Argonz-Del Castillo s.
arhinia, choanal atresia,
  microphthalmia s.
Arkless-Graham s.
Arnold-Chiari s.
arteriomesenteric duodenal
  compression s.
arthritis-dermatitis s.

arthrogryposis, ectodermal dysplasia,
  cleft lip/palate developmental
  delay s.
Arts s.
ASB s.
Ascher s.
aseptic meningitis s.
Asherman s.
Asperger s. (AS)
asphyxiating thoracic dysplasia s.
asphyxiating thoracic dystrophy s.
aspiration s.
asplenia s.
asymmetric short stature s.
ataxia-deafness s.
ataxia, myoclonic encephalopathy,
  macular degeneration, recurrent
  infections s.
ataxia-telangiectasia s.
atelencephalic s.
Atkin-Flaitz s.
Atkin-Flaitz-Patil s.
ATRX s.
atypical hemolytic uremia s.
Austin s.
autism, dementia, ataxia, loss of
  purposeful hand use s.
autism-fragile X s. (AFRAX)
autistic s.
auto-brewery s.
autoimmune lymphoproliferative s.
  (ALPS)
autoimmune polyendocrine s.
autoimmune polyglandular s.
autosomal dominant macrocephaly s.
autosomal dominant Opitz s.
  (ADOS)
autosomal recessive ocular
  Ehlers-Danlos s.
AWTA s.
Axenfeld s.
Axenfeld-Rieger s.
Babinski-Fröhlich s.
baby bottle s.
bacterial overgrowth s.
Ballantyne-Runge s.
Ballantyne-Smith s.
Baller-Gerold s. (BGS)
Ballinger-Wallace s.
Bamforth s.
Banki s.
Bannayan s.
Bannayan-Riley-Ruvalcaba s.
  (BRRS)
Bannayan-Zonana s. (BZS)
Bannwarth s.
Banti s.
Baraitser-Burn s.
Baraitser-Winter s.

Barber-Say s.
Bardet-Biedl s. (BBS)
bare lymphocyte s.
Barlow s.
Bart s.
Barth s.
Bartholin-Patau s.
Bartsocas-Papas s.
Bartter s. (BS)
basal cell nevus s. (BCNS)
Bassen-Kornzweig s.
battered buttock s.
battered child s. (BCS)
battered fetus s.
battered wife s.
Bazex s.
Bazex-Dupré-Christol s.
BBB s.
BCD s.
BD s.
Beare s.
Beare-Stevenson cutis gyrata s.
Beckwith s.
Beckwith-Wiedemann s. (BWS)
Beemer-Langer s.
Beemer lethal malformation s.
Begeer s.
Behçet s.
Behr s.
Benjamin s.
Berardinelli s.
Berardinelli-Seip s.
Berardinelli-Seip-Lawrence s.
Berdon s.
Bergia s.
Berlin breakage s.
Bernard-Soulier s. (BSS)
Berry s.
Berry-Kravis and Israel s.
Berry-Treacher Collins s.
Bertini s.
Beuren s.
BGMR s.
Bianchine-Lewis s.
Bickers-Adams s.
BIDS s.
Bielschowsky s.
Biemond s. 1, 2
bile acid defect s.
bile plug s.
Binder s.
binge eating s.
biopsychosocial s.
bird-headed dwarf s.
birdlike face s.
bitemporal forceps marks s.
Bixler s.
Björnstad s.
Blackfan-Diamond s.

black locks with albinism and
  deafness s. (BADS)
bladder outlet s.
Bland-Garland-White s.
blepharocheilodontic s.
blepharonasofacial malformation s.
blepharophimosis, ptosis, epicanthus
  inversus s. (BPEIS)
blepharophimosis, ptosis, epicanthus
  inversus, primary amenorrhea s.
blepharophimosis, ptosis, syndactyly,
  short stature s.
blepharoptosis, blepharophimosis,
  epicanthus inversus, telecanthus s.
blind loop s.
Blizzard s.
Bloch-Siemens s.
Bloch-Sulzberger s.
Bloodgood s.
Bloom s.
Blount s.
blue baby s.
blueberry muffin s.
blue diaper s.
blue dome s.
blue histiocyte s.
blue rubber bleb nevus s. (BRBNS)
bobble-head doll s.
BOD s.
Bohring s.
Bonneau s.
Bonnet-Dechaume-Blanc s.
Bonnevie-Ullrich s.
Boom s.
boomerang s.
BOR s.
Börjeson s.
Börjeson-Forssman-Lehmann s.
Bosma Henkin Christiansen s.
Bourneville s.
Bourneville-Pringle s.
Bowen-Conradi s.
Bowen Hutterite s.
Brachmann-Cornelia de Lange s.
  (BCDLS)
brachycephaly, deafness, cataract,
  microstomia, mental retardation s.
brachydactyly-distal
  symphalangism s.
brachydactyly, dwarfism, hearing
  loss, microcephaly, mental
  retardation s.
brachydactyly, mesomelia, mental
  retardation, aortic dilation, mitral
  valve prolapse, characteristic
  facies s.
brachydactyly, nystagmus, cerebellar
  ataxia s.
brachymesomelia-renal s.

S

syndrome (*continued*)
brachymetacarpalia, cataract,
  mesiodens s.
brachymorphism, onychodysplasia,
  dysphalangism s.
bradycardia-tachycardia s.
Brailsford s.
brain death s.
branchial arch s.
branchial clefts-lip pseudocleft s.
branchiooculofacial s. (BOFS)
branchiootic s.
Brandt s.
breast/ovarian familial cancer s.
Brett s.
Briard-Evans s.
bright thalamus s.
Brissaud s.
brittle hair-mental deficit s.
broad ligament tear s.
broad thumb-hallux s.
broad thumb-mental retardation s.
bronze baby s.
Brooks s.
Brooks-Wisniewski-Brown s.
brown baby s.
Brown-Séquard s.
Brown superior oblique tendon
  sheath s.
Brown vertical retraction s.
Brown-Vialetto-van Laere s.
Bruck-de Lange s.
Brugada s.
Brunner s.
Brusa-Torricelli s.
Brushfield-Wyatt s.
BSG s.
bubbly lung s.
Budd-Chiari s.
bulldog s.
burning vulva s.
Burn-McKeown s.
Buschke-Ollendorf s.
Byler s.
C s.
3C s.
Caffey pseudo-Hurler s.
Caffey-Silverman s.
CAHMR s.
Calabro s.
Calvé-Legg-Perthes s.
CAMAK s.
CAMFAK s.
camptomelic s.
Camurati-Engelmann s.
cancer family s.
cancer predisposition s.
Cantrell s.
Cantú s.

capillary leak s. (CLS)
carbohydrate-deficient glycoprotein s.
  (type I, II)
carcinoid s.
cardiac, abnormal facies, thymic
  hypoplasia, cleft palate,
  hypocalcemia s.
cardiac-limb s.
cardiocranial s.
cardiofacial s.
cardiogenital s.
cardiovascular/central nervous
  system s.
cardiovertebral s.
Carey-Fineman-Ziter s.
Carmi s.
Carnevale s.
Carney s.
Caroli s.
carpal tunnel s.
Carpenter s.
Cast s.
cataract-dental s.
cataract-oligophrenia s.
catatonic s.
CATCH 22 s.
Catel-Manzke s.
cat's cry s.
cat's eye s. (CES)
cat's urine s.
cauda equina s.
caudal dysplasia s.
caudal regression s. (CRS)
cavernous sinus s.
cavum septum pellucidum, cavum
  vergae, macrocephaly, seizures,
  mental retardation s.
Cayler cardiofacial s.
CCC s.
celiac s.
central anticholinergic s. (CAS)
central cord s.
central hypoventilation s.
central nervous system/
  cardiovascular s.
centromeric
  instability-immunodeficiency s.
cephalopolysyndactyly s.
cerebral dysfunction s.
cerebroarthrodigital s.
cerebrocostomandibular s. (CCMS)
cerebrohepatorenal s. (CHRS)
cerebrooculomuscular s. (COMS)
cerebrooculonasal s.
CFA s.
CFC s.
Chanarin-Dorfman s.
Char s.
Charcot-Marie-Tooth s. (CMTS)

Charcot-Marie-Tooth-Hoffmann s.
CHARGE s.
Charlevois-Saguenay s.
Cheadle s.
Chédiak-Higashi s.
Chemke s.
Cheney s.
cherry-red spot myoclonus s.
cherubism, gingival fibromatosis,
 epilepsy, mental deficiency s.
chest s.
Chiari-Arnold s.
Chiari-Frommel s.
Chilaiditi s.
CHILD s.
CHIME s.
Chinese restaurant s.
cholestatic s.
chondrodysplasia-
 pseudohermaphrodism s.
chondroectodermal dysplasia-like s.
Chotzen s.
Christian s. (1, 2)
Christian-Andrews-Conneally-
 Muller s.
Christian-Opitz s.
Christ-Siemens-Touraine s.
chromosomal
 breakage-immunodeficiency s.
chromosome diploid/tetraploid
 mixoploidy s.
chromosome GI deletion s.
chromosome 9 inversion s.
chromosome 1–22 monosomy s.
chromosome 1p–22p deletion s.
chromosome 1q–22q deletion s.
chromosome 1q–22q duplication s.
chromosome 1q–22q tetrasomy s.
chromosome 1q–22q triplication s.
chromosome 8 recombinant s.
chromosome 1–22 ring s.
chromosome tetraploidy s.
chromosome triploidy s.
chromosome 1–22 trisomy s.
chromosome 14 uniparental
 disomy s.
chromosome X autosome
 translocation s.
chromosome X fragility s.
chromosome X inversion s.
chromosome XO s.
chromosome Xp21 deletion s.
chromosome Xp22 deletion s.
chromosome Xq deletion s.
chromosome Xq duplication s.
chromosome XXX s.
chromosome 47,XXX s.
chromosome XXXXX s.
chromosome XXXXY s.

chromosome XXY s.
chromosome Y;18 translocation s.
chronic aspiration s.
chronic biopsychosocial s.
chronic compartment s.
chronic fatigue s. (CFS)
chronic pupillary s.
Chudley s. (1, 2)
Chudley-Lowry-Hoar s.
Churg-Strauss s.
chylomicronemia s.
Cianchetti s.
circumferential skin
 creases-psychomotor retardation s.
Clarke-Hadfield s.
clasped thumbs-mental retardation s.
cleavage s.
cleidocranial dysplasia s.
cleidorhizomelic s.
Clifford s.
climacteric s.
clitoris tourniquet s. (CTS)
clomiphene-resistant polycystic
 ovary s.
Clouston s.
Clover s.
cloverleaf skull s.
clumsy child s.
COACH s.
Cobb s.
Cockayne s. (A, B)
cocktail party s.
CODAS s.
COD-MD s.
Coffin s. (1, 2)
Coffin-Lowry s.
Coffin-Siris fifth digit s.
Coffin-Siris-Wegienka s.
COFS s.
Cogan s.
Cohen s.
Cole s.
Cole-Carpenter s.
Cole-Hughes macrocephaly-mental
 retardation s.
Cole-Rauschkolb-Toomey s.
coloboma-anal atresia s.
compartment s.
compensatory antiinflammatory s.
complete androgen insensitivity s.
 (CAIS)
complete androgen resistance s.
complete DiGeorge s.
complete feminizing testes s.
complex regional pain s.
 (CRPS)
concussion s.
congenital acromicria s.
congenital anemia s.

S

syndrome (*continued*)

congenital anosmia-hypogonadotropic hypogonadism s.

congenital arthromyodysplastic s.

congenital bone marrow failure s.

congenital cataracts, sensorineural deafness, Down syndrome facial appearance, short stature, mental retardation s.

congenital central hypoventilation s. (CCHS)

congenital clasped thumbs-mental retardation s.

congenital emphysema, cryptorchidism, penoscrotal web, deafness, mental retardation s.

congenital Guillain-Barré s.

congenital heart defect s.

congenital high airway obstruction s. (CHAOS)

congenital hydantoin s.

congenital hypertrichosis-osteochondrodysplasia-cardiomegaly s.

congenital hypocupremia s.

congenital hypothyroidism s.

congenital ichthyosis-mental retardation-spasticity s.

congenital ichthyosis-trichodystrophy s.

congenital LCMV s.

congenital long QT s.

congenital microcephaly, hiatus hernia, nephrotic s.

congenital muscular hypertrophy-cerebral s.

congenital nephrotic s.

congenital pseudohydrocephalic progeroid s.

congenital rubella s. (CRS)

congenital thrombocytopenia, Robin sequence, agenesis of corpus callosum, distinctive facies, developmental delay s.

congenital varicella s.

congenital warfarin s.

congestive cardiomyopathy-hypergonadotropic hypogonadism s.

conjunctivitis-otitis s.

Conn s.

conotruncal anomaly face s. (CTAF)

conotruncal facial s.

Conradi s.

Conradi-Hünermann s.

constriction band s.

constrictive pericarditis-dwarfism s.

contiguous gene deletion s.

contractural arachnodactyly s.

contracture, muscle atrophy, oculomotor apraxia s.

conus medullaris s.

Cooks s.

Cooper s.

Cornelia de Lange s. (CDLS)

corpus luteum deficiency s.

Costello s.

coumarin s.

Cowchock s.

Cowchock-Fischbeck s.

Cowden s.

coxoauricular s.

CPLS s.

Crandall ectodermal dysplasia s.

Crane-Heise s.

cranioacrofacial s.

craniocarpotarsal s.

craniocerebellocardiac s.

craniofacial dysmorphism-polysyndactyly s.

craniofrontonasal s. (CFNS, CNFS)

cranioorodigital s.

craniosynostosis-lid anomalies s.

craniosynostosis-radial aplasia s.

craniosynostotic s.

CRASH s.

CREST s.

cretinism-muscular hypertrophy s.

Creutzfeldt-Jakob s.

cri-du-chat s.

Crigler-Najjar s. (type I, II)

Crisponi s.

Crome s.

Cronkhite-Canada s.

crooked fingers s.

Cross s.

Cross-McKusick-Breen s.

Crouzon s.

CRST s.

crying cat s.

cryptomicrotia-brachydactyly s.

cryptophthalmos s.

cryptophthalmos-syndactyly s.

CSW s.

Curran s.

Curry-Jones s.

Curtis s.

Cushing s.

cushingoid s.

cyclic vomiting s.

Cypress facial neuromusculoskeletal s.

cytomegaly s.

dancing eye s.

Dandy-Walker s. (DWS)

Dandy-Walker-like s.

Dandy-Walker malformation-basal ganglia disease-seizures s.

Danlos s.
Darrow-Gamble s.
Davidenkow s.
David-O'Callaghan s.
4-day s.
dead fetus s.
deafness-craniofacial s.
deafness-nephritis s.
Deal s.
Debré-Sémélaigne s.
De Crecchio s.
defective abdominal wall s.
de Grouchy s. 1, 2
Dejerine-Klumpke s.
Dejerine-Sottas s.
de Lange s.
de Lange s. 1, 2
delay s.
delayed sleep phase s. (DSPS)
del Castillo s.
deletion 1–22 s.
deletion 1p–22p s.
deletion 1q–22q s.
deletion Xp21 s.
deletion Xp22 s.
deletion Xq s.
Delleman s.
Demons-Meigs s.
de Morsier s.
de Morsier-Gauthier s.
dengue shock s.
Dennie-Marfan s.
Denys-Drash s.
depressor anguli oris muscle
  hypoplasia s.
dermotrichic s.
Derry s.
De Sanctis-Cacchione s.
Desbuquois s.
descending perineum s.
Desmons s.
de Toni-Fanconi s.
de Toni-Fanconi-Debré acute s.
developmental delay-multiple
  strawberry nevi s.
dextrocardia/situs inversus s.
diabetes-deafness s.
diabetes mellitus, mental retardation,
  lipodystrophy, dysmorphic traits s.
Diamond-Blackfan s.
diaper s.
diarrhea-associated hemolytic
  uremic s.
diarrhea-malnutrition s.
Dickinson s.
DIDMO s.
DIDMOAD s.
diencephalic s. (DS)
DiFerrante s.

diffuse mesangial sclerosis-ocular
  abnormalities s.
DiGeorge microdeletion s.
Dighton-Adair s.
digitorenocerebral s. (DRC)
Dilantin s.
DiSala s.
disequilibrium s.
distal intestinal obstruction s.
  (DIOS)
distal limb deficiency-mental
  retardation s.
disturbed equilibrium s.
disuse s.
Donahue s.
Donohue s.
DOOR s.
double cortex s.
Down s. (DS)
Drash s.
DRD s.
dry eye s.
Duane retraction s.
Dubin-Johnson s.
Dubowitz s.
Duchenne s.
Duchenne-Griesinger s.
dumping s.
Duncan s.
duplication-deficiency s.
duplication 1p–22p s.
duplication 1q–22q s.
duplication Xq s.
dup (10p)/del (10q) s.
dup (1p)–(22p) s.
dup (9q)/del(9p) s.
dup (1q)–(22q) s.
dup (Xq) s.
dwarf s.
dwarfism, congenital medullary
  stenosis s.
dwarfism, onychodysplasia s.
dwarfism, pericarditis s.
dwarfism, polydactyly, dysplastic
  nails s.
Dyggve-Melchior-Clausen s.
Dyke-Davidoff s.
dyscephaly, congenital cataract,
  hypotrichosis s.
dysfibronectinemic Ehlers-Danlos s.
dysgenesis s.
dysmaturity s.
dysmorphic s.
dysmotile cilia s.
dysmotility s.
dysplasia s.
dysplastic nevus s.
dystocia-dystrophia s.
dystonia-deafness s.

S

syndrome (*continued*)

dystrophia retinae-dysacousis s.
dysuria-pyuria s.
dysuria-sterile pyuria s.
Eagle-Barrett s.
early-onset diabetes
  mellitus-epiphysial dysplasia s.
early-onset parkinsonism-mental
  retardation s.
Eastman-Bixler s.
Eaton-Lambert myasthenic s.
ecchymotic Ehlers-Danlos s.
ectodermal dysplasia, cleft lip and
  palate, hand and foot deformity,
  mental retardation s.
ectodermal dysplasia, cleft lip and
  palate, mental retardation,
  syndactyly s. (I, II)
ectodermal dysplasia, mental
  retardation, syndactyly s.
ectrodactyly-cleft lip/palate s.
ectrodactyly, ectodermal dysplasia
  and cleft lip/palate s.
ectrodactyly, mandibulofacial
  dysostosis s.
Eddowes s.
Edinburgh malformation s.
Edwards s.
Edwards-Gale s.
EEC s.
Ehlers-Danlos s. (EDS)
Eisenmenger s.
Elejalde s.
elfin facies hypercalcemia s.
Ellis-Sheldon s.
Ellis-van Creveld s.
ElSahy-Waters s.
embryofetal alcohol s. (EFAS)
embryonic testicular regression s.
Emery-Dreifuss s.
EMG s.
empty scrotum s.
empty sella s.
encephalotrigeminal s.
endovascular hemolytic-uremic s.
Engman s.
enterocolitis s.
eosinophilia-myalgia s.
epicomus s.
epidermal nevus s.
epileptic s.
epiphysial s.
episodic dyscontrol s.
EPS s.
Erb s.
Erb-Charcot s.
Erb-Goldflam s.
Erlacher-Blount s.
Eronen s.

Escalante s.
Escobar s.
ethmocephaly s.
euthyroid sick s.
Evans s.
extended rubella s.
extraordinary urinary frequency s.
extrapyramidal-pyramidal s.
eye defects-diffuse renal mesangial
  sclerosis s.
facet s.
facial-digital-genital s.
facial dysmorphia s.
facial dysplasia, hyperextensibility of
  joints, clinodactyly, growth
  retardation, mental retardation s.
faciocardiorenal s.
faciodigitogenital s.
faciogenital s.
Fadhil s.
FAE s.
Fairbank-Keats s.
Fallot s.
familial aortic ectasia s.
familial ataxia-hypogonadism s.
familial atypical multiple mole
  melanoma s.
familial cardiac myxoma s.
familial chylomicronemia s.
familial endocrine-neuroectodermal
  abnormalities s.
familial insomnia s.
familial macroglossia-omphalocele s.
familial polysyndactyly-craniofacial
  anomalies s.
familial pterygium s.
familial pyridoxine-dependency s.
familial third and fourth pharyngeal
  pouch s.
familial Turner s.
Fanconi-Albertini Zellweger s.
Fanconi-Bickel s.
Fanconi pancytopenia s.
Fanconi-Prader s.
Fanconi-Schlesinger s.
Farber s.
fast channel s.
fatigue s.
FCS s.
Feingold s.
Feinmesser-Zelig s.
Felty s.
female pseudo-Turner s.
feminization s. (FS)
feminizing testes s.
femoral-facial s.
fetal Accutane s.
fetal akinesia s.
fetal alcohol s. (FAS)

fetal aminopterin s.
fetal aminopterin-like s.
fetal anticoagulant s.
fetal aspiration s.
fetal cocaine s.
fetal Dilantin s.
fetal distress s. (FDS)
fetal dysmaturity s.
fetal facies s.
fetal gigantism, renal hamartoma, nephroblastomatosis s.
fetal hydantoin s. (FHS)
fetal inflammatory response s.
fetal isotretinoin s.
fetal methotrexate s.
fetal nutritional deprivation s.
fetal overgrowth s.
fetal paramethadione-trimethadione s.
fetal phenytoin s.
fetal rubella s.
fetal tobacco s. (FTS)
fetal transfusion s.
fetal trimethadione s.
fetal valproate s. (FVS)
fetal varicella s. (FVS)
fetal warfarin s. (FWS)
fetofetal transfusion s.
Feuerstein-Mims s.
Fèvre-Languepin s.
FFU s.
FG s.
FHUF s.
fibrinogen-fibrin conversion s.
fibromyalgia s. (FMS, FS)
fifth digit s.
Filippi s.
Fine-Lubinsky s.
first and second branchial arch s.
Fishman s.
Fitz-Hugh-Curtis s.
Fitzsimmons s.
Floating-Harbor s. (FHS)
floppy infant s.
flulike s.
FOAR s.
focal dermal hypoplasia s.
follicular atrophoderma, basal cell carcinoma s.
Fontaine s.
food-induced enterocolitis s.
Forbes-Albright s.
formiminotransferase deficiency s.
Fountain s.
FPO s.
fragile X s. (FXS)
fragile X mental retardation s.
fragile Xq s.
Franceschetti s.
Franceschetti-Goldenhar s.

Franceschetti-Jadassohn s.
Franceschetti-Klein s.
Franceschetti-Zwahlen s.
Franceschetti-Zwahlen-Klein s.
François dyscephalic s.
Fraser s.
Fraser-François s.
Fraser-like s.
fra(X) s.
FRAXq27 s.
Freeman-Sheldon s.
frequency dysuria s.
Fried s.
Friend s.
Fritsch s.
Fritsch-Asherman s.
Fröhlich s.
frontodigital s.
Fryns s. (1–3)
Fryns-Moerman s.
Fryns-van den Berghe s.
FTT s.
Fuhrmann s.
Fukuyama s.
Fuller Albright s. 1
functional prepuberal castrate s.
Funston s.
G s.
Gaillard s.
galactorrhea-amenorrhea s.
Galloway s.
Galloway-Mowat s.
Gamble-Darrow s.
Garcia-Lurie s.
Gardner s.
Gardner-Silengo-Wachtel s.
Gareis-Mason s.
Gasser s.
gastrointestinal s.
gender dysphoria s.
Genée-Wiedemann s.
genetic s.
genital anomaly-cardiomyopathy s.
genital ulcer s.
genitopalatocardiac s.
Genoa s.
Gerhardt s.
German s.
Gerstmann s.
Gerstmann-Sträussler-Scheinker s.
Gianotti-Crosti s.
giant platelet s.
Gilbert s.
Gilbert-Dreyfus s.
Gilbert-Lereboullet s.
Gilles de la Tourette s.
Gillespie s.
gingival hypertrophy-corneal dystrophy s.

S

syndrome (*continued*)
Gitelman s.
Glanzmann s.
Glanzmann-Riniker s.
glossopalatine ankylosis s.
gloves and socks s.
glutaric aciduria s. (type I, II)
GMS s.
goiter-deafness s.
Golabi-Ito-Hall s.
Golabi-Rosen s. (GRS)
Goldberg s.
Goldenhar-Gorlin s.
Goldenhar microphthalmia s.
Goldston s.
Goltz s.
Goltz-Gorlin s.
Goltz-Peterson-Gorlin-Ravitz s.
GOMBO s.
Gomez and López-Hernández s.
gonadal agenesis s.
gonadal dysgenesis s.
gonadal failure, short stature, mitral
  valve prolapse, mental
  retardation s.
gonadotropin-resistant ovary s.
goniodysgenesis, mental retardation,
  short stature s.
Goodman s.
Goodpasture s.
Gordon s.
Gorlin s. (1, 2)
Gorlin-Goltz s.
Gorlin-Psaume s.
Gougerot-Carteaud s.
Gradenigo s.
Graefe-Usher s.
Graham s.
granddad s.
Grant s.
gravis type Ehlers-Danlos s.
gray baby s.
gray platelet s.
Greig s.
Greig cephalopolysyndactyly s.
Griscelli s.
Grisel s.
growth failure-pericardial
  constriction s.
Grubben s.
Gruber s.
grunting baby s.
Guerin-Stein s.
Guillain-Barré s. (GBS)
Guillain-Barré-Landry s.
Gurrieri s.
Gustavson s.
HAIR-AN s.
hair-brain s.

Hajdu-Cheney s.
Hakim s.
Hakim-Adams s.
Halban s.
Halbrecht s.
Hall s. (1, 2)
Hallermann s.
Hallermann-Streiff s.
Hallermann-Streiff-François s.
Hallervorden-Spatz s.
Hallopeau-Siemens s.
Hall-Pallister s.
Hall-Riggs s.
Halpern s.
hamartoneoplastic s.
hamartopolydactyly s.
Hamel s.
Hamman-Rich s.
hand-foot s.
hand-foot-genital s.
hand-foot-mouth s.
hand-foot-uterus s.
Hand-Schüller-Christian s.
Hanhart s.
hantavirus cardiopulmonary s.
  (HCPS)
hantavirus pulmonary s.
happy puppet s.
HARD s.
HARD+/-E s.
Hardikar s.
HARP s.
Harrod s.
Hart s.
Haw River s.
Hay-Wells s.
HbH disease-mental retardation s.
hearing-loss-nephritis s.
heart defect s.
heart-hand s.
Heerfordt s.
Heiner s.
HELLP s.
hemangioma-thrombocytopenia s.
hemangiomatous branchial clefts/lip
  pseudocleft s.
hematophagocytic s.
hematuria-dysuria s. (HDS)
hematuria, nephropathy, deafness s.
hemignathia and microtia s.
hemoglobin Bart hydrops fetalis s.
hemolytic uremic s. (HUS)
hemophagocytic s.
hemopoietic s.
hemorrhagic fever with renal s.
  (HFRS)
hemorrhagic shock s.
hemorrhagic shock and
  encephalopathy s. (HSES)

Hennekam lymphangiectasia-lymphedema s.
hepatic copper overload s.
hepatic ductular hypoplasia-multiple malformations s.
hepatitis B arthritis-dermatitis s.
hepatofacioneurocardiovertebral s.
hepatopulmonary s. (HPS)
hepatorenal s.
hepatotoxic s.
hereditary benign intraepithelial dyskeratosis s.
hereditary dysplastic nevus s.
hereditary hematuria s.
hereditary nephritis, deafness, abnormal thrombogenesis s.
hereditary nonpolyposis colorectal cancer s.
Hermansky-Pudlak s.
Hernandez s.
heterotaxia s.
heterotaxy s.
HHH s.
HHHO s.
hiatus hernia, microcephaly, nephrosis s.
high airway obstruction s.
Hinman s.
hirsutism, skeletal dysplasia, mental retardation s.
HMC s.
H2O s.
Holt-Oram s.
Holzgreve s.
Hootnick-Holmes s.
Hopkins s.
Horner s.
Hoyeraal-Hreidarsson s. (HHS)
Hughes s.
Hünermann-Happle s.
Hunter s.
Hunter-Fraser s.
Hunter-MacMurray s.
Hunter-McAlpine craniosynostosis s.
Hurler s.
Hurler-like s.
Hurler-Pfaundler s.
Hurler-Scheie s.
Hurst s.
Hutchinson s.
Hutchinson-Gilford progeria s.
hyaline membrane s.
hydantoin s.
Hyde-Förster s.
hydrocephalus-cerebellar agenesis s.
hydrocephalus, skeletal anomalies, mental disturbances s.
hydrolethalus s.

hydronephrocolpos-postaxial polydactyly-congenital heart disease s.
17-hydroxylase deficiency s.
21-hydroxylase deficiency s.
hyperammonemic s.
hyperandrogenemic chronic anovulation s.
hypercalcemia elfin-facies s.
hypercalcemia/Williams-Beuren s.
hypereosinophilic s.
hyper-IgD s.
hyper-IgE s.
hyper-IgM s.
hyperimmunoglobulin E s.
hyperinsulinism hyperammonemia s.
hyperkinetic child s.
hyperlucent lung s.
hypermobile Ehlers-Danlos s.
hypermobility s.
hyperphosphaturic s.
hyperplastic right heart s.
hyperprostaglandin E_2 s.
hyperprostaglandinuric tubular s.
hypertelorism-hypospadias s.
hypertelorism, microtia, clefting s.
hypertensive xiphoid s.
hypertrichosis, coarse face, brachydactyly, obesity, mental retardation s.
hyperventilation s.
hyperviscosity s.
hypocalcemia and microdeletion 22q11 s.
hypocalcemia, dwarfism, cortical thickening s.
hypochondroplasia s.
hypocomplementemic urticarial vasculitis s.
hypogenital dystrophy with diabetic tendency s.
hypoglossia-hypodactyly s.
hypogonadism-anosmia s.
hypopituitary s.
hypoplastic congenital anemia s.
hypoplastic left heart s. (HLHS)
hypoplastic right heart s. (HRHS)
hypospadias-dysphagia s.
hypospadias-mental retardation s.
hypothalamic hamartoblastoma s.
hypothyroidism s.
hypothyroid-large muscle s.
hypoventilation s.
IADH s.
IBIDS s.
ICE s.
ICF s.
ichthyosis with keratitis and deafness s.

S

syndrome (*continued*)
Idaho s.
idiopathic hemolytic uremia s.
idiopathic hypercalcemia-supravalvular
aortic stenosis s.
idiopathic infantile hypercalcemia s.
idiopathic long QT s.
idiopathic minimal lesion nephrotic
s. (IMLNS)
idiopathic nephrotic s. (INS)
idiopathic primary renal hematuric
proteinuric s.
idiopathic respiratory distress s.
(IRDS)
idiopathic steroid-resistant
proteinuria/nephrotic s.
IFAP s.
IgE s.
iliotibial band friction s.
Illum s.
Imerslünd s.
Imerslünd-Grasbeck s.
immotile cilia s.
immunodeficiency, centromeric
heterochromatin instability, facial
anomalies s.
impingement s.
incontinentia pigmenti s.
infancy-onset diabetes mellitus,
multiple epiphysial dysplasia s.
infantile bilateral striatal necrosis s.
(IBSN)
infantile optic atrophy-ataxia s.
infantile respiratory distress s.
infantile spasms, hypsarrhythmia,
mental retardation s.
infantile tremor s.
infant respiratory distress s.
(IRDS)
infection-associated hemophagocytic
s. (IAHS)
inferior vena cava s.
inflammatory Brown s.
influenza-like s.
inherited hemolytic uremia s.
insensitive ovary s.
insomnia s.
inspissated bile s.
inspissated milk s.
intraepithelial dyskeratosis s.
intrahepatic cholestatic s.
intrauterine growth retardation,
microcephaly, mental retardation s.
intrauterine parabiotic s.
inversion 9 s.
inversion duplication (15)
chromosome s.
inversion duplication (8p) s.
Ionasescu s.

iris, coloboma, ptosis, hypertelorism,
mental retardation s.
irritable bowel s. (IBS)
Isaac s.
Isaac-Merton s.
isochromosome 10p s.
isochromosome 12p s.
isolated autosomal dominant s.
isotretinoin dysmorphic s.
isotretinoin teratogenic s.
Ito s.
Ivemark s.
Jabs s.
Jackson-Weiss s. (JWS)
Jacob s.
Jacobsen s.
Jadassohn-Lewandowski s.
Jaeken s.
Jaffe-Campanacci s.
Jaffe-Lichtenstein s.
Jahnke s.
Jakob-Creutzfeldt s.
Jaksch s.
James s.
Jancar s.
Jansen s.
Jansky-Bielschowsky s.
Janus s.
Janz s.
Jarcho-Levin s.
JC s.
Jensen s.
Jervell and Lange-Nielsen long
QT s.
Jessner-Cole s.
Jeune s.
Job s.
Johanson-Blizzard s.
Johnson-McMillin s.
Johnson neuroectodermal s.
Joseph s.
Josephs-Diamond-Blackfan s.
Joubert s.
Juberg-Hayward s.
Juberg-Marsidi s. (JMS)
jumping Frenchmen of Maine s.
Junius-Kuhnt s.
juvenile cataract, cerebellar atrophy,
mental retardation, myopathy s.
juvenile hyperuricemia s.
juxtaglomerular hyperplasia s.
Kabuki s. (KS)
Kabuki makeup s. (KMS)
Kalischer s.
Kallmann s.
Kallmann-de Morsier s.
Kanner s.
Kaplan s.
Kapur-Toriello s.

Kartagener s.
Kasabach-Merritt s.
Kaufman-McKusick s.
Kaufman oculocerebrofacial s.
Kaveggia s.
Kawasaki s. (KS)
Kaznelson s.
KBG s.
Kearns-Sayre s. (KSS)
Keipert s.
Keller s.
Kelley-Seegmiller s.
Kelly s.
Kenny s.
Kenny-Caffey s.
Kenny-Linarelli s.
Kenny-Linarelli-Caffey s.
keratosis palmaris et
  plantaris-corneal dystrophy s.
keratosis palmoplantaris-corneal
  dystrophy s.
ketoaciduria-mental deficiency s.
Keutel s. (1, 2)
KID s.
Killian s.
Kimmelstiel-Wilson s.
kinky-hair s.
Kinsbourne s.
kleeblattschädel s.
Kleine-Levin s.
Klein-Waardenburg s.
Klinefelter s.
Klinefelter-Reifenstein s.
Klinefelter-Reifenstein-Albright s.
Klippel-Feil s.
Klippel-Trenaunay s.
Klippel-Trenaunay-Parkes-Weber s.
Klippel-Trenaunay-Weber s.
Kloepfer s.
Klotz s.
Klüver-Bucy s.
Kniest s.
Kobberling-Dunnigan s.
Koby s.
Kocher-Debré-Sémélaigne s.
Koerber-Salus-Elschnig s.
Kostmann s.
Kowarski s.
Krabbe s.
Kramer s.
Krause s.
Krause-Kivlin s.
Krause-van Schooneveld-Kivlin s.
Laband s.
lacrimoauriculodentodigital s.
Ladd s.
LAMB s.
Lambert s.
Lambert-Eaton s.

Lambotte s.
Landau-Kleffner s. (LKS)
Landing s.
Landry-Guillain-Barré s.
Lange-Nielsen s.
Langer s.
Langer-Giedion s.
Langer-Saldino s.
Laron s.
Larsen s.
laryngeal atresia s.
late embryonic testicular
  regression s.
late luteal phase s.
late-onset local junctional
  epidermolysis bullosa-mental
  retardation s.
Laugier-Hunziker s.
Launois s.
Launois-Cléret s.
Laurence-Moon s.
Laurence-Moon-Biedl s.
Laurence-Moon-Biedl-Bardet s.
  (LMBBS)
Lawford s.
Lawrence s.
Lawrence-Seip s.
lazy bladder s.
lazy colon s.
lazy leukocyte s. (LLS)
LCMV s.
Leigh s.
Leiner s.
Lejeune s.
Lemierre s.
Lemli-Opitz s.
Lennox s.
Lennox-Gastaut s.
Lenz dysmorphogenic s.
Lenz-Majewski s.
Lenz microphthalmia s.
LEOPARD s.
Leri s.
Leri-Weill s.
Leroy s.
Leschke s.
Lesch-Nyhan s. (LNS)
lethal multiple pterygium s.
leukoencephalopathy s.
leukoerythroblastic s.
levator ani s.
Levin s.
Levy-Hollister s.
lexical-syntactic s. (LSS)
Lhermitte-Duclos s.
LHON s.
Liddle s.
Li-Fraumeni s. (LFS)
Li-Fraumeni cancer s.

S

syndrome (*continued*)
Lightwood-Albright s.
Lignac s.
limb abnormality s.
limb girdle s. (LGS)
limp infant s.
linear nevus sebaceus s.
linear sebaceous nevus s.
Lin-Gettig s.
lipodystrophy-acromegaloid
  gigantism s.
lip-palate s.
lip pseudocleft-hemangiomatous
  branchial cyst s.
Lison s.
LMB s.
Lobstein s.
lobster-claw with ectodermal
  defects s.
lobulation-polydactyly s.
Löffler s.
Löfgren s.
long Q-T s. (LQTS)
Lorain-Lévi s.
Louis-Bar s.
low cardiac output s.
Lowe s. (LS)
Lowe oculocerebrorenal s.
Lowe-Terry-MacLachlan s.
Lown-Ganong-Levine s.
Lowry s.
Lowry-MacLean s.
Lowry-Wood s. (LWS)
low-sodium s.
low T3 s.
Lub s.
Lucey-Driscoll s.
Lujan-Fryns s.
lupus anticoagulant s.
lupus-like s.
lupus obstetric s.
luteinized unruptured follicle s.
  (LUFS)
Lutembacher s.
Lyell s.
lymphoproliferative s.
Lynch s.
Lynch 2 s.
lysine malabsorption s.
3M s.
MacDermot-Winter s.
Machado-Joseph s.
Macleod s.
macrocephaly-hamartomas s.
macroglossia-omphalocele s.
macroglossia-omphalocele-
  visceromegaly s.
macrophage activation s. (MAS)
macrosomia-mental retardation s.

Maestre de San Juan-Kallmann-de
  Morsier s.
Mafucci s.
Majewski s.
malabsorption s.
malalignment s.
male Turner s.
malformation s.
Mallory-Weiss s.
Malouf s.
Malpuech facial clefting s.
Marañón s.
Marden-Walker s.
Marfan s.
marfanoid craniosynostosis s.
Marie s.
Marie-Sainton s.
Marinesco-Garland s.
Marinesco-Sjögren s.
Marinesco-Sjögren-Garland s.
Marinesco-Sjögren-like s.
marker X s.
Maroteaux-Lamy s.
Maroteaux-Malamut s.
Marshall s.
Marshall-Smith s. (MSS)
Martin-Bell s. (MBS)
Martin-Bell-Renpenning s.
Martsolf s.
MASA s.
masquerade s.
Masters-Allen s.
maternal Bernard-Soulier s.
maternal deprivation s.
maternal hydrops s.
maternal rubella s.
Mauriac s.
Mayer-Rokitansky-Küster-Hauser s.
McCune-Albright s.
McDonough s.
McKusick-Kaufman s.
McLeod s.
Meadows s.
Meckel s.
Meckel-Gruber s.
meconium aspiration s. (MAS)
meconium blockage s.
meconium plug s.
medial collateral ligament s.
medial snapping hip s.
median facial cleft s.
megacystis-megaureter s.
megalocornea-mental retardation s.
Meier-Gorlin s.
Meigs s.
Meigs-Kass s.
MELAS s.
Melkersson s.
Melkersson-Rosenthal s.

Melnick-Fraser s.
Melnick-Needles s.
MEMR s.
mendelian s.
Mendelson s.
Mendenhall s.
Mengert shock s.
Ménière s.
meningoencephalitis s.
meningovascular s.
Menkes s.
Menkes-Kaplan s.
Menkes kinky-hair s. (MKHS)
menopausal s.
mental and growth
  retardation-amblyopia s.
mental retardation-adducted
  thumbs s.
mental retardation-clasped thumb s.
mental retardation-distal
  arthrogryposis s.
mental retardation,
  macroorchidism s.
mental retardation-overgrowth s.
mental retardation-psoriasis s.
mental retardation-sparse hair s.
MERRF s.
mesiodens-cataracts s.
mesoaxial hexadactyly-cardiac
  malformation s.
mesomelic dwarfism-small
  genitalia s.
metabolic acidosis s.
methionine malabsorption s.
Meyer-Schwickerath and Weyers s.
Michelin-tire baby s.
Michels s.
microangiopathic hemolytic
  uremic s.
microcephalic primordial
  dwarfism-cataracts s.
microcephaly-cardiomyopathy s.
microcephaly-chorioretinopathy s.
microcephaly-deafness s.
microcephaly-digital anomalies s.
microcephaly-spastic diplegia s.
microdeletion s.
micrognathia-glossoptosis s.
microphthalmia-mental deficiency s.
microtia, absent patellae,
  micrognathia s.
MIDAS s.
midfetal testicular regression s.
midline cleft s.
Miescher s.
Mietens s.
Mietens-Weber s.
migraine s.
Mikity-Wilson s.

Mikulicz s.
Miles s.
Miles-Carpenter s. (MCS)
milk-alkali s.
Miller s.
Miller-Dieker s.
Miller-Dieker lissencephaly s.
  (MDLS)
Miller-Fisher variant of
  Guillain-Barré s.
MIMyCA s.
minimal change nephrotic s.
  (MCNS)
minimal lesion nephrotic s. (MLNS)
Minkowski-Chauffard s.
Minot-von Willebrand s.
Mirhosseini-Holmes-Walton s.
mirror s.
MISHAP s.
mitis type Ehlers-Danlos s.
mixed antiinflammatory s. (MARS)
MLASA s.
MMEP s.
MMIH s.
MMT s. (MMT)
MNBCC s.
Möbius s.
Mohr s.
Mohr-Claussen s.
Mohr-Tranebjaerg s. (MTS)
Mollica s.
Mollica-Pavone-Anterer s.
MOMO s.
MOMX s.
mononucleosis-type s.
monosomy 7 s.
monosomy G s.
monosomy 1p36 s.
monosomy 22q13,3 deletion s.
Montefiore s.
Moore-Federman s.
Morgagni-Adams-Stokes s.
Morgagni-Turner s.
Morgagni-Turner-Albright s.
morning glory s.
Morquio s.
Morquio-Brailsford s.
Morquio-Ullrich s.
mosaic tetrasomy 8p s.
mosaic Turner s.
moyamoya s.
Moynahan alopecia s.
MSN s.
mucocutaneous lymph node s.
  (MCLS, MLNS)
mucosal neuroma s.
Müller s.
multiorgan dysfunction s. (MODS)
multiple basal cell carcinoma s.

S

syndrome (*continued*)

multiple basal cell nevoid s.
multiple endocrine neoplasia s.
multiple epiphysial dysplasia
    tarda s.
multiple hamartoma s.
multiple lentigines s.
multiple neuroma s.
multiple nevoid-basal cell
    carcinoma s.
multiple nevoid, basal cell
    epithelioma, jaw cysts, bifid rib s.
multiple organ dysfunction s.
    (MODS)
multiple pterygium s.
multiple synostoses s.
multiple X s.
Mulvihill-Smith s.
Münchausen s.
MURCS s.
muscle-eye-brain s. (MEBS)
muscular hypertrophy s.
musculoskeletal pain s. (MSPS)
Mutchinick s.
myasthenia-like s.
myasthenic s.
myelodysplastic s. (MDS)
myeloproliferative s.
Myhre s.
myocardial steal s.
myoclonus s.
myofascial pain s. (MPS, MPS II,
    MPS VII)
myopathic limb-girdle s.
myopathy-myxedema s.
mystery s.
myxedema-myotonic dystrophy s.
Naegeli s.
Nager s.
Nager-de Reynier s.
nail-patella s.
Najjar s.
NAME s.
Nance-Horan s. (NHS)
nanism-constrictive pericarditis s.
narcotic withdrawal s.
NARP s.
nasal hypoplasia, peripheral
    dysostosis, mental retardation s.
Navajo brainstem s.
near-miss sudden infant death s.
    (NMSIDS)
Neill-Dingwall s.
Nelson s.
neonatal abstinence s. (NAS)
neonatal Bartter s. (NBS)
neonatal Guillain-Barré s.
neonatal hepatitis s.
neonatal lupus s.

neonatal Marfan s.
neonatal myasthenic s.
neonatal narcotic withdrawal or
    abstinence s.
neonatal progeroid s.
neonatal pseudohydrocephalic
    progeroid s.
neonatal respiratory distress s.
    (NRDS)
neonatal small left colon s.
nephrosis-microcephaly s.
nephrosis, microcephaly, hiatus
    hernia s.
nephrotic s.
Netherton s.
Nettleship s.
Neuhauser s.
Neu-Laxova s. (NLS)
neurocutaneous melanosis s.
neurofaciodigitorenal s.
neurofibromatosis-Noonan s. (NF-NS)
neuroichthyosis-hypogonadism s.
neuroleptic malignant s. (NMS)
neurologic disease s.
neuromuscular scoliosis s.
neurotrichocutaneous s.
Nevo s.
nevoid basal cell carcinoma s.
    (NBCCS, NBS)
newborn narcotic withdrawal s.
newborn respiratory distress s.
Nezelof s.
NFDR s.
nigricans s.
nigricans-hyperinsulinemia s.
Niikawa-Kuroki s.
Nijmegen breakage s. (NBS)
Noack s.
nocturnal polyuria s.
nonautoimmune myasthenic s.
noncleft median face s.
nongenetic s.
nonnarcotic abstinence s.
Nonne-Milroy-Meige s.
nonprogressive hypoplastic s.
nonprogressive motor impairment s.
nonsalt-losing adrenogenital s.
nonsyndromic bile duct paucity s.
Noonan s.
Noonan-Ehmke s.
Noonan-like giant cell lesion s.
    (NLGCLS)
Norman-Landing s.
Norman-Roberts lissencephaly s.
Norman-Wood s.
Norrie s.
Norrie-Warburg s.
nutcracker s.
nutritional deprivation s.

OAV s.
obesity-hypotonia s.
obesity-hypoventilation s.
Obrinsky s.
obstruction s.
obstructive sleep apnea s. (OSAS)
OCC s.
occipital horn s.
Ochoa s.
OCR s.
OCRL s.
ocular coloboma-imperforate anus s.
oculoauriculofrontonasal s.
oculocerebral hypopigmentation s.
oculocerebrofacial s.
oculodental s.
oculodentodigital s.
oculogenitolaryngeal s.
oculomandibulodyscephaly-
  hypotrichosis s.
oculopalatoskeletal s.
ODD s.
ODED s.
s. of absence of septum pellucidum
  with parencephaly (SASPP)
s. of acute hemiplegia
s. of cerebral atrophy
s. of crocodile tears
s. of inappropriate antidiuretic
  hormone secretion
s. of inappropriate secretion of
  antidiuretic hormone (SIADH)
s. of median longitudinal fasciculus
s. of multiple endocrine neoplasia
s. of opsoclonus-myoclonus
s. of symmetric parasagittal
  parietooccipital polymicrogyria
s. of uncal herniation
Ohdo blepharophimosis s.
Ohtahara s.
olfactogenital s.
oligoasthenoteratozoospermia s.
  (OATS)
oligophrenia-ichthyosis s.
oligoteratoasthenozoospermia s.
Oliver s.
Oliver-McFarlane s.
Ollier s.
Ollier-Klippel-Trenaunay-Weber s.
Omenn s.
OMF s.
omphalocele-cleft palate s.
Onat s.
Ondine-Hirschsprung s.
onychodystrophy-congenital
  deafness s.
OPD s.
opercular s.
Opitz BBBG s.

Opitz-Christian s.
Opitz-Frias s.
Opitz G/BBB s.
Opitz-Kaveggia s.
Opitz trigonocephaly s.
Oppenheim s.
opsoclonus/myoclonus s.
optic atrophy-ataxia s.
oral allergy s.
Orbeli s.
organic hyperkinetic s.
organic mental s.
organoid nevus s.
orocraniodigital s.
orodigitofacial s.
orogenital s.
orthostatic tachycardia s.
Osebold-Remondini s.
Osgood-Schlatter s.
Osler-Weber s.
Osler-Weber-Rendu s. (OWRS)
osteogenesis imperfecta congenita s.
osteohypertrophic varicose s.
osteoporosis-pseudoglioma s. (OPS)
Ostrum-Furst s.
otitis-conjunctivitis s.
otofaciocervical s.
otomandibular s.
otopalatodigital s. (OPDS)
otosclerosis s.
otospongiosis s.
Otto s.
ovarian dysgenesis-sensorineural
  deafness s.
ovarian hyperstimulation s. (OHS,
  OHSS)
ovarian remnant s.
ovarian short stature s.
ovarian vein s.
overdistention s.
overdose s.
overgrowth s.
overtraining s.
overuse s.
4p s.
5p s.
9p s.
pachyonychia congenita s.
Pagon s.
Pai s.
Paine s.
painful bladder s. (PBS)
Palant cleft palate s.
palatal-digital-oral s.
Pallister-Hall s.
Pallister-Killian s.
Pallister mosaic s.
Pallister W s.
pancreatic insufficiency s.

S

syndrome (*continued*)

pancytopenia s.
Papillon-Léage-Psaume s.
Papillon-Lefèvre s.
paramethadione s.
paraneoplastic s.
Parenti-Fraccaro s.
parietal foramina,
  brachymicrocephaly, mental
  retardation s.
Parinaud oculoglandular s.
Parkes Weber-Dimitri s.
Parrot s.
Parry-Romberg s.
partial DiGeorge s.
partial trisomy 10q s.
Partington-Anderson s.
Partington X-linked mental
  retardation s. (PRTS)
Pashayan s.
Pashayan-Pruzansky s.
Passos-Bueno s.
Patau s.
patellofemoral pain s. (PFPS)
patellofemoral stress s.
Patterson pseudoleprechaunism s.
Patterson-Stevenson-Fontaine s.
Pearson marrow-pancreas s.
pediatric acquired immunodeficiency
  s. (PAIDS)
PEHO s.
Pelletier-Leisti s.
Pellizzi s.
pelvic congestion s. (PCS)
pelvic venous congestion s.
Pena-Shokeir s. (I, II)
Pendred s.
pentasomy X s.
penta-X s.
PEO s.
Pepper s.
Perheentupa s.
pericardial constriction-growth failure
  s.
perisylvian s.
Perlman nephroblastomatosis s.
Perrault s.
persistent müllerian duct s.
Peters anomaly, corneal clouding,
  growth and mental retardation s.
Peters anomaly-short limb
  dwarfism s.
Peters-plus s.
Pettigrew s. (PGS)
Peutz-Jeghers s.
Pfaundler-Hurler s.
Pfeiffer s.
PHACE s.
pharyngeal pouch s.

Phocas s.
phocomelia s.
phonologic-syntactic s.
PHS s.
physiologic addiction/abstinence s.
pickwickian s.
PIE s.
Pierre Robin s.
pink diaper s.
Pirie s.
piriformis s.
Pitt s.
Pitt-Rogers-Danks s. (PRDS)
placental dysfunction s.
placental hemangioma s.
placental transfusion s.
Plott s.
POEMS s.
pointer s.
Poland s.
poliomyelitis-like s.
Pollitt s.
polycystic ovarian s. (PCOS)
polycystic ovary s. (PCOS,
  POS)
polycythemia-hyperviscosity s.
polydactyly-chondrodystrophy s.
polydactyly-craniofacial anomalies s.
polydactyly-craniofacial
  dysmorphism s.
polydactyly-imperforate anus s.
polyglandular autoimmune s.
polyneuropathy, cataract, deafness s.
polyposis s.
polysplenia s.
polysyndactyly-peculiar skull s.
polysynostosis s.
Pompe s.
popliteal pterygium s.
popliteal web s.
Porak-Durante s.
Porteous s.
postabortal s.
postanoxic dystonic s.
postaxial acrofacial dysostosis s.
  (POADS)
postcoartectomy s.
postconcussion s.
postembolization s.
posterior leukoencephalopathy s.
postexchange transfusion s.
postgastroenteritis malabsorption s.
postirradiation s.
postmaturity s.
postmenopausal palpable ovary s.
  (PMPO)
postpartum hemolytic uremic s.
postpartum pituitary necrosis s.
postperfusion s.

postpericardiotomy s. (PPS)
postphlebitic s. (PPS)
postpolio s.
postrubella s.
postscabetic s.
posttraumatic stress s.
posttubal ligation s.
postural orthostatic tachycardia s.
  (POTS)
postvagotomy dumping s.
Potter s.
PPO s.
Prader-Labhart-Willi s.
Prader-Labhart-Willi-Fanconi s.
Prader-Willi s. (PWS)
precordial catch s.
preexcitation s.
preleukemic s.
premenstrual s. (PMS)
premenstrual salivary s.
premenstrual tension s. (PMTS)
Prieto s. (PRS)
primary antiphospholipid s.
primary empty sella s.
primary hyperuricemia s.
primary nephrotic s.
Primrose s.
progeria s.
progeria-like s.
progeroid short stature-pigmented
  nevi s.
prolapse-gastropathy s. (PGS)
prolonged QT s.
prominent incisors-obesity-
  hypotonia s.
proteiform s.
Proteus s. (PS)
Proud s.
prune belly s. (PBS)
pseudoachondroplasia s.
pseudoaminopterin s.
pseudoappendicular s.
pseudo-Hurler s.
pseudoprogeria s.
pseudothalidomide s.
pseudotoxoplasmosis s.
pseudotrisomy 13 s.
pseudo-Turner s.
pseudo-Ullrich-Turner s.
pseudo-Wernicke s.
pug nose-peripheral dysostosis s.
pulmonary dysmaturity s.
pulmonary infiltrate with
  eosinophilia s.
pupillary s.
puppetlike s.
purple toes s.
Purtilo s.
pyknodysostosis s.

Pyle s.
pyridoxine-dependency s.
22q11.2 deletion s.
Quan-Smith s.
quintuple-X s.
Rabson-Mendenhall s.
radial aplasia-thrombocytopenia s.
radial-renal s.
radiation s.
radio-reno-ocular s.
Raine s.
RALPH s.
Rambam-Hasharon s.
Ramon s.
Ramsay Hunt s. (I–III)
rancid butter s.
rape trauma s.
Rapp-Hodgkin ectodermal
  dysplasia s.
Rasmussen s.
Raynaud s.
RCDP s.
REAR s.
recessive deafness-onychodystrophy s.
recessive enhanced S-cone s.
recessive Usher s.
recognizable viral s. (RVS)
recombinant chromosome 8 s.
recurrent hemolytic uremia s.
Reed s.
Refetoff s.
Refsum s.
Regenbogen-Donnai s.
Reifenstein s.
Reiter s.
renal Fanconi s.
renal mesangial sclerosis-eye
  defects s.
renal tubular Fanconi s.
renal tubular pituitary s.
Rendu-Osler-Weber s.
Renpenning s.
residual ovary s.
resistant ovary s.
respiratory distress s. (RDS)
restless legs s.
retained bladder s.
Rethoré s.
retinitis pigmentosa-congenital
  deafness s.
retinoblastoma-mental retardation s.
retinopathy-mental retardation s.
retraction s.
retroviral s.
Rett s.
reverse chylous s.
reversible posterior
  leukoencephalopathy s. (RPLS)
Reye s.

S

syndrome (*continued*)

Reye-like s.
rhizomelia s.
Rh-null s.
rib-gap defect-micrognathia s.
Richards-Rundle s.
Richner s.
Richner-Hanhart s.
Rieger s.
right middle lobe s.
right ovarian vein s.
rigid spine s.
Riley-Day s.
Riley-Shwachman s.
Riley-Smith s.
ring 1–22 s.
Ritscher-Schinzel s.
Roberts pseudothalidomide s.
Roberts-SC phocomelia s.
Roberts tetraphocomelia s.
Robin s.
Robinow s.
Robinow-Silverman-Smith s.
Robinow-Sorauf s.
Rocher-Sheldon s.
Rokitansky-Küster-Hauser s.
Rolland-Desbuquois s.
Romano-Ward long QT s.
Rosenthal-Kloepfer s.
Rosewater s.
Rosselli-Gulienetti s.
Rothmann-Makai s.
Rothmund s.
Rothmund-Thomson s.
Rothmund-Thomson cancer
  predisposition s.
Rothmund-Werner s.
Rotterdam consensus on polycystic
  ovarian s.
round ligament s.
Roussy-Lévy s.
RSH s.
RSH/SLO s.
RSH/Smith-Lemli-Opitz s.
rubella s.
Rubinstein s.
Rubinstein-Taybi s.
Rud s.
Rudiger s.
rudimentary testis s.
Russell diencephalic s. (I, II, III)
Russell-Silver dwarf s.
Rutherfurd s.
Rutledge lethal multiple congenital
  anomalies s.
Ruvalcaba s.
Ruvalcaba-Myhre s.
Ruvalcaba-Myhre-Smith s. (RMSS)
Ruvalcaba-Reichert-Smith s.

Sabinas brittle hair s.
Saethre-Chotzen s.
Sakati-Nyhan s.
Saldino-Noonan s.
Salonen-Herva-Norio s.
salt-losing adrenogenital s. (SLAS)
salt-wasting adrenogenital s.
Sanchez-Cascos s.
Sanchez-Corona s.
Sanchez-Salorio s.
Sandhoff s.
Sandifer s.
Sanjad-Sakati s.
San Luis Valley s.
Santavuori s.
Santavuori-Haltia s.
Sao Paulo MCA/MR s.
Sato s.
Savage s.
Say s.
Say-Gerald s.
Say-Meyer s.
scalded skin s. (SSS)
Schafer s.
Scheie s.
Scheuthauer-Marie-Sainton s.
Schimmelbusch s.
Schimmelpenning-Feuerstein-Mims s.
Schinzel acrocallosal s.
Schinzel-Giedion s. (SGS)
Schinzel-Giedion midface-retraction s.
Schirmer s.
Schmid-Fraccaro s.
Schmidley s.
Schmidt s.
Schwartz s.
Schwartz-Jampel s.
Schwartz-Jampel-Aberfeld s.
scimitar s.
SCIWORA s.
scleroderma-like s.
scotopic sensitivity s.
Scott craniodigital s.
SC phocomelia s.
SC-pseudothalidomide s.
SEA s.
sea-blue histiocyte s.
Seabright bantam s.
seat belt s.
sebaceous nevus s.
Seckel bird head s.
secondary nephrotic s.
second impact s.
Sedlacková s.
Seemanová s. (type 1, 2)
Seip s.
Seip-Lawrence s.
Sengers s.
Senior-Loken s.

Sensenbrenner s.
Sensenbrenner-Dorst-Owens s.
Senter s.
sepsis s.
sepsis-pneumonia s.
sepsis/shock s.
seronegative enthesopathy and
  arthropathy s.
serotonin s.
Sertoli-cell-only s.
serum sickness-like s.
Setleis s.
severe acute respiratory s. (SARS)
severe ovarian hyperstimulation s.
  (SOHS)
Shah-Waardenburg s.
shaken baby s. (SBS)
shaken impact s.
shaken infant s.
shawl scrotum s.
shedding s.
Sheehan s.
Sheehy s.
Shereshevskii-Turner s.
Shokeir s.
Shone s.
SHORT s.
short bowel s. (SBS)
short gut s. (SGS)
short rib-polydactyly s. (SRPS)
Shprintzen-Goldberg
  craniosynostosis s.
Shprintzen velocardiofacial s.
Shulman s.
Shwachman s.
Shwachman-Bodian s.
Shwachman-Diamond s.
Shy-Drager s.
Shy-Magee s.
sicca s.
sick euthyroid s.
sick sinus node s.
Siemerling-Creutzfeldt s.
Silver s.
Silver-Russell s.
Silverskiöld s.
Simmonds s.
Simpson dysmorphia s. (SDYS)
Simpson dysplasia s.
Simpson-Golabi-Behmel s. (SGBS)
Simpson-Golabi-Behmel fetal
  overgrowth s.
Sinding-Larsen-Johansson s.
Sipple s.
sirenomelia s.
situs inversus totalis s.
Sjögren s.
Sjögren-Larsson s.
skeleton-skin-brain s.

skin-eye-brain s.
slapped cheek s.
sleep apnea s.
sleep-disordered breathing s.
slick-gut s.
slipping rib s.
slit ventricle s.
SLO s.
Slotnick-Goldfarb s.
sloughed urethra s.
slow-channel congenital myasthenic
  s. (SCCMS)
Sly s.
small left colon s.
small patella s.
SMG22 s.
Smith s.
Smith-Fineman-Myers s. (SFMS)
Smith-Lemli-Opitz s.
Smith-Magenis s. (SMS)
Smith-Theiler-Schachenmann s.
snapping knee s.
Snyder-Robinson s. (SRS)
soft hands s.
Sohval-Soffer s.
Solomon s.
Solomon-Fretzin-Dewald s.
Sommer s.
somnolence s.
Sonoda s.
Sorsby s.
Sotos s.
spinal muscular atrophy-mental
  retardation s.
spinocerebellar ataxia-dysmorphism s.
splenic sequestration s.
split hand/foot s.
spondylocostal dysplasia s.
spondyloepiphysial dysplasia
  congenita s.
spondylothoracic dysplasia s.
Spranger-Wiedemann s.
Spurway s.
Srb s.
SSS s.
stagnant loop s.
staphylococcal scalded skin s.
  (SSSS)
staphylococcal toxic shock s.
steely-hair s.
Steinert s.
Steinfeld s.
Stein-Leventhal s.
sterile pyuria s.
steroid-sensitive idiopathic nephrotic
  s. (SSNS)
Stevens-Johnson s.
Stewart-Treves s.
Stickler s.

S

syndrome (*continued*)

stiff-baby s.
stiff-man s.
Stilling-Türk-Duane s.
Stimmler s.
Stocco dos Santos s.
Stock-Spielmeyer-Vogt s.
Stokes-Adams s.
Stoll s.
strabismus s.
straight back s.
Stratton-Parker s.
Streeter s.
streptococcal toxic shock s.
Strudwick s.
stuck twin s.
Sturge-Kalischer-Weber s.
Sturge-Weber s. (SWS)
Sturge-Weber-Dimitri s.
Sturge-Weber-Krabbe s.
Stüve-Wiedemann s. (SWS)
subaortic stenosis-short stature s.
sudden infant death s. (SIDS)
Sugarman s.
sulfur-deficient brittle hair s.
superior mediastinal s.
superior mesenteric artery s.
superior vena cava s.
supine hypotensive s.
surfactant deficiency s.
Sutherland-Haan s. (SHS)
swallowed blood s.
sweaty feet s.
Sweet s.
Swyer s.
Swyer-James s.
Swyer-James-Macleod s.
sylvian aqueduct s.
syndactyly-anophthalmos s.
syndactyly, cataracts, mental
  retardation s.
syndactyly, microcephaly, mental
  retardation s.
systemic inflammatory response s.
  (SIRS)
systemic vasculitis s.
tachy-brady s.
Takao s.
TAR s.
Tariverdian s.
tarsal-carpal coalition s.
Taussig-Bing s.
Tay s.
Taybi s.
Taybi-Linder s.
Teebi s.
telecanthus-hypospadias s.
Temtamy s.
tenosynovitis-dermatitis s.

teratogenic s.
ter Haar s.
Terry s.
Teschler-Nicola and Killian s.
testicular feminization s.
tethered cord s.
tetrahydrofolate-methyltransferase
  deficiency s.
tetralogy of Fallot s.
tetraphocomelia-cleft lip-palate s.
tetraploidy s.
tetrasomy 15p s.
tetra-X s.
thalidomide teratogenicity s.
Thal intermedia-like s.
thanatophoric dysplasia s.
Thiemann s.
third and fourth pharyngeal
  pouch s.
thoracic compression s.
thrombocytopenia with absent
  radius s.
thymic and parathyroid agenesis
  s.
thymic aplasia s.
thyrohypophysial s.
tibial aplasia-ectrodactyly s.
Tietze s.
tin ear s.
tired housewife s.
Tolosa-Hunt s.
tooth and nail s.
TORCH s.
Toriello s. (1, 2)
Toriello-Carey s.
Torsten Sjögren s.
Tourette s.
Townes s.
Townes-Brocks s.
toxemia s.
toxemic shock s.
toxic oil s.
toxic shock s. (TSS)
tracheal agenesis s.
Tranebjaerg s. (1, 2)
transfusion s.
transient myeloproliferative s.
transient neonatal myasthenic s.
transient respiratory distress s.
  (TRDS)
translocation Down s.
TRAP s.
trapezoidocephaly-synostosis s.
traumatic compartment s.
Treacher Collins s.
Treacher Collins-Franceschetti s.
tremor s.
trichodentoosseous s.
trichorhinophalangeal s.

trichorrhexis nodosa s.
*Trichuris*dysentery s.
Tridione s.
trigonocephaly s.
trilateral retinoblastoma s.
trimethadione s.
triple X s.
triploidy s.
trip 15q s.
trismus-pseudocamptodactyly s.
trisomy 1–22 s.
trisomy C,D,E,G s.
trisomy 18-like s.
trisomy 1p–22p s.
trisomy 1q–22q s.
Troyer s. (TS)
tuberous sclerosis s.
tubulopathy of Lowe s.
tumor lysis s.
Turcot s.
Turner-Albright s.
Turner-Kieser s.
Turner-like s.
Turner mosaic s.
Turner XO s.
twin-peak s.
twin-to-twin transfusion s. (TTS, TTTS)
t Y;18 s.
Ullrich and Fremerey-Dohna s.
Ullrich-Bonnevie s.
Ullrich-Feichtiger s.
Ullrich-Noonan s.
Ullrich-Turner s.
ulnar-mammary s.
umbilical cord s.
uncombable hair s.
unilateral fibular aplastic s.
universal joint s.
Unna-Thost s.
unstable bladder s.
Unverricht-Lundborg s.
upper airway resistance s. (UARS)
upper motor neuron s.
Urban s.
Urban-Rogers-Meyer s.
uremic s.
urethral s.
urgency s.
urgency-frequency s.
urofacial s.
Usher s. (US)
uterine hernia s.
uveomeningoencephalitic s.
uveoparotid fever s.
VACTERL association with hydrocephalus s.
valproic acid s.
Van Buchem s.

van der Hoeve s.
van der Woude s.
vanishing testicle s.
vanishing testis s.
vanishing twin s.
Van Maldergem s.
Váradi s.
Váradi-Papp s.
varicella s.
vascular ring s.
vasculitis s.
VATER s.
velocardiofacial s. (VCFS)
Verner-Morrison s.
viral s.
Virchow-Seckel s.
visceromegaly s.
viscous s.
vitamin B$_6$ dependence s.
Vogt s.
Vogt-Koyanagi s.
Vogt-Koyanagi-Harada s.
Vohwinkel s.
von Hippel-Lindau s.
von Willebrand s.
Voorhoeve s.
vulnerable child s.
vulvar vestibulitis s. (VVS)
vulvovaginal-gingival s.
VURD s.
W s.
Waardenburg-Klein s.
Waardenburg recessive anophthalmia s.
Waelsch s.
Wagner s.
WAGR s.
Waisman s.
Waisman-Laxova s.
Walker-Clodius s.
Walker lissencephaly s.
Walker-Warburg s.
Walton s.
Warburg s.
warfarin s.
Waring blender s.
Warkany s. (1, 2)
wasting s.
Waterhouse-Friderichsen s.
Watson s.
Watson-Alagille s.
Watson-Miller s.
Weaver s.
Weaver-Smith s. (WSS)
Weaver-Williams s.
Weber s.
Weber-Christian s.
Weber-Dimitri s.
Weill-Marchesani s.

S

syndrome (*continued*)
Weismann-Netter s.
Weissenbacher-Zweymuller s.
Werdnig-Hoffmann s.
Wermer s.
Werner s.
Wernicke s.
Wernicke-Korsakoff s.
West s.
wet brain s.
wet lung s.
Weyers oligodactyly s.
Whelan s.
Whipple s.
whistling face s.
whistling face-windmill vane hand s.
WIC s.
Wieacker s.
Wieacker-Wolff s.
Wiedemann s.
Wiedemann-Beckwith s.
Wiedemann-Beckwith-Combs s.
Wiedemann-Rautenstrauch s.
Wildervanck s.
Wildervanck-Smith s.
Wilkins s.
Willebrand-Jurgens s.
Williams s. (WS)
Williams-Barratt s.
Williams-Beuren s.
Williams-Campbell s.
Wilson-Mikity s.
Wilson-Turner s. (WTS)
Winchester s.
Winter s.
Wisconsin s.
Wiskott-Aldrich s. (WAS)
Wittwer s.
Wohlfart-Kugelberg-Welander s.
Wolcott-Rallison s.
Wolf s.
Wolff mental retardation s.
Wolff-Parkinson-White s.
Wolf-Hirschhorn s.
Wolfram s.
Woods s.
Worster-Drought s.
wrinkly skin s. (WSS)
Wyburn-Mason s.
s. X
45,X s.
XK s.
X-linked cataract-dental s.
X-linked congenital cataracts-microcornea s.
X-linked dominant s.
X-linked Ehlers-Danlos s.
X-linked Hurler s.

X-linked hyper-IgM s.
X-linked lymphoproliferative s.
X-linked mental handicap-retinitis pigmentosa s.
X-linked mental retardation with fragile X s.
X-linked Opitz s. (XLOS)
X-linked recessive deafness s.
X-linked recessive skeletal Ehlers-Danlos s.
X-linked severe combined immunodeficiency s.
XO s.
Xq- s.
Xq+ s.
Xq Klinefelter s.
XX male s.
46,XX male s.
47,XXX s.
XXX s.
XXXX s.
XXXXX s.
49, XXXXY s.
XXXXY s.
XXY s.
47,XXY s.
XYY s.
yellow nail s.
yellow vernix s.
Young s.
Young-Hughes s.
Young-Madders s.
Youssef s.
Yunis-Varon s.
YY s.
Zellweger cerebrohepatorenal s.
Zerres s.
Ziehen-Oppenheim s.
Zimmermann-Laband s. (ZLS)
Zinsser s.
Zinsser-Cole-Engman s.
Zinsser-Engman-Cole s.
Ziprokowski-Margolis s.
Zlotogora-Ogür s.
Zollinger-Ellison s.
Zollino s.
Zunich s.
Zwahlen s.
syndromic
s. cleft
s. craniosynostosis
s. paucity
synechia, *pl.* **synechiae**
anterior s.
cleft palate-lateral s. (CPLS)
intrauterine s.
posterior s.
s. vulvae
synechiae (*pl. of* synechia)

912

Synemol Topical
synencephalocele
Synera
Synercid
synergism
synergistic gangrene
synergy
    spastic s.
synesthesia
Synevac vacuum curettage system
Synflex
syngamy
syngeneic
    s. bone marrow transplantation
    s. stem cell
    s. tissue
syngnathia congenita
syngraft
synkinesia
    mouth-and-hand s.
synkinesis, syncinesis, synkinesia
Syn-Minocycline
synophthalmia, synophthalmus,
  synophthalmos
synophthalmos (*var. of* synophthalmia)
synophthalmus (*var. of* synophthalmia)
Synophylate
synorchidism, synorchism
synorchism (*var. of* synorchidism)
synoscheos
synosteosis (*var. of* synostosis)
synostosis, synosteosis
    coronal s.
    cranial s.
    humeroradial s.
    lambdoid s.
    multiple synostoses
    s. multiplex
    premature suture s.
    radioulnar s.
    sagittal s.
    tribasilar s.
    unilambdoid s.
synovectomy
synovial
    s. biopsy
    s. fluid
    s. fluid analysis
    s. hypertrophy
    s. joint
    s. leukocytosis
    s. sarcoma
synoviocyte
    fibroblastoid s.
synovioma
synovitis
    monoarticular s.
    plant thorn s.
    toxic s.

    transient monoarticular s.
    villonodular s.
synovium
Synphasic
Synsorb Pk
syntax
syntenic gene
synteny
synthase
    cystathionine s.
    methionine s.
    prostaglandin endoperoxide s.
    pyloric nitric oxide s.
syntheses (*pl. of* synthesis)
synthesis, *pl.* **syntheses**
    bile acid s.
    cholesterol s.
    decidual prolactin s.
    estrogen s.
    inborn error of bile acid s.
    ovarian estrogen s.
    progesterone s.
    thyroxine s.
    tissue s.
synthesize
synthesizer
    voice s.
synthetase
    carbamoyl phosphate s. (CAPS,
      CPS)
    endothelial nitric oxide s.
    holocarboxylase s.
    N-acetylglutamate s.
    6-pyruvoyl tetrahydropteridine s.
synthetic
    s. conjugated estrogen
    s. DNA
    s. gliadin peptide
    s. prostaglandin E_1
    s. pterin
    s. surfactant
    s. suture material
Synthroid
    S. Injection
    S. Oral
SynVitro Cumulase
syphilis
    biologic false-positive serologic test
      for s. (BF-STS)
    congenital s. (CS)
    early congenital s.
    endemic s.
    s. hereditaria tarda
    late congenital s.
    latent s.
    latent-stage s.
    parenchymatous congenital s.
    primary s.
    secondary s.

S

syphilis (*continued*)
    serologic test for s. (STS)
    tertiary s.
    s., toxoplasmosis, rubella,
      cytomegalovirus, herpes simplex, s.
syphilitic
    s. infection
    s. keratitis
    s. meningitis
    s. pemphigus
    s. phlebitis
    s. rhinitis
syphilotherapy
Syprine
Syracol-CF
syringe
    Asepto s.
    Auto S.
    bulb s.
    s. feeding
    Luer Lok s.
    super s.
    tuberculin s.
    vacuum aspiration s.
syringes (*pl. of* syrinx)
syringobulbia
syringocele
syringocystadenoma papilliferum
syringohydromyelia
syringoma
    eruptive s.
syringomeningocele
syringomyelia
    familial lumbosacral s.
syringomyelic cavity
syringomyelocele
syringopleural drainage
syringosubarachnoid drainage
syrinx, *pl.* **syringes**
syrup
    Bromfed S.
    Claritin s.
    Decofed S.
    ipecac s.
    Karo s.
    s. of ipecac
    Promethazine VC Plain S.
    Rondec S.
    Tusstat S.
    unPromethazine VC Plain S.
    Versed s.
    Zyrtec s.
Sysmex NE8000 cell counter
system
    Abbott LifeCare PCA Plus II
      infusion s.
    ABI model 377 DNA sequencing s.
    ABI model 373 DNA sequencing s.
    ABO blood group s.

    adnexal adhesion classification s.
    Aegis sonography management s.
    Affirm VP microbial identification s.
    Affymetrix GeneChip s.
    AFS adhesion scoring s.
    Aggregate Neurobehavioral Student
      Health Education Review S.
    AI 5200 S Open Color Doppler
      imaging s.
    Aladdin Infant Flow S.
    Aloka SD ultrasound s.
    alternative s.
    American Medical S.'s (AMS)
    American Medical staging s.
    Androderm Transdermal S.
    Ann Arbor staging s.
    Apgar scoring s.
    Apogee 800 ultrasound s.
    Apogee vaginal vault prolapse
      repair s.
    AquaSens FMS 1000 fluid
      monitoring s.
    ascending reticular activating s.
      (ARAS)
    ASG s.
    ATL HDI 3000 ultrasound s.
    Aurora MR breast imaging s.
    AutoCyte S.
    autonomic nervous s. (ANS)
    AutoPap 300 QC s.
    AutoPap Screening S.
    Autoread centrifuge hematology s.
    Auto Suture ABBI s.
    Aviva mammography s.
    Babe OB ultrasound reporting s.
    Baby CareLink s.
    Bactec blood-culturing s.
    Bair Hugger patient warming s.
    Balloon Therapy S.
    basolateral membrane transport s.
    BDProbeTec ET s.
    behavior contract s.
    17-beta-E2 transdermal drug-
      delivery s.
    Bethesda classification s.
    Bethesda II s.
    bicarbonate-carbonic acid s.
    BiliBlanket Plus phototherapy s.
    Biogel Reveal puncture indication s.
    BioMerieux Vitek s.
    Bishop pelvic scoring s.
    Bishop Prelabor Scoring S.
    Blomdahl medical ear piercing s.
    blood group s.
    Breast Cancer S. 2100
    Breast Imaging Reporting and Data
      S. (BIRADS)
    breast leakage inhibitor s. (BLIS)
    Breslow microstaging s.

Bridge extra-support over-the-wire renal stent s.
bursa-dependent s.
CADD-Prizm pain control s.
Capasee diagnostic ultrasound s.
cardiovascular s. (CVS)
CDE blood group s.
Cell Recovery S. (CRS)
central nervous s. (CNS)
centrencephalic s.
cerebellar-vestibular s.
Cineloop image review ultrasound s.
circulatory s.
Clark microstaging s.
Climara estradiol transdermal s.
ColorMate TLc BiliTest S.
ComfortScan imaging s.
Companion 318 nasal CPAP s.
Conceptus fallopian tube catheterization s.
continuous distention irrigation s. (CDIS)
cotyledon perfusion s.
Cre/loxP s.
CRYOcare cryoablation s.
CrystalEyes endoscopic video s.
CS-5 cryosurgical s.
cytochrome *b* s.
Diastat rectal delivery s.
digestive s.
digital mammography s.
DOBI s.
Dolphin hysteroscopic fluid management s.
dopaminergic s.
double collecting s.
drainage s.
drooping lily appearance of lower collecting s.
Duffy s.
Dynamite mattress s.
dysfunctional voiding scoring s. (DVSS)
Eccocee ultrasound s.
Eklund positioning s.
Electroshield monitoring s.
embryonic branchial s.
EMLA disc topical anesthetic adhesive s.
EnAbl thermal ablation s.
Endermologie LPG s.
endocrine s.
Endotek urodynamics s.
ENTec coblator plasma s.
Entree II trocar and cannula s.
Entree Plus trocar and cannula s.
EntriStar gastrostomy s.
enzyme-linked virus-inducible s.'s
Esclim estradiol transdermal s.
Esclim transderm s.
Estraderm transdermal s.
estradiol transdermal s.
EUB-405 ultrasound s.
ExAblate fibroid 2000 s.
Exact-Touch Saccomanno Pap smear collection s.
extrapyramidal nervous s.
EZ-EM Bio-Gun automated biopsy s.
Ferriman-Gallwey hirsutism scoring s.
fibrinolytic and clotting s.
FoamCare cleansing s.
Follistim Pen drug delivery s.
Force GSU argon-enhanced electrosurgery s.
s. for thalidomide education and prescription safety
GE Senographe 2000D digital mammography s.
Glucometer Elite diabetes care s.
Gordon diagnostic s. (GDS)
Guardian DNA s.
Gynecare Thermachoice uterine balloon therapy s.
Gynecare TVT obturator s.
Gynecare TVT Secur s.
HabitEX smoking cessation s.
Halo Sleep S.
haversian s.
hematopoietic s.
HemoCue blood glucose s.
HemoCue blood hemoglobin s.
Her Option uterine cryoablation therapy s.
His-Purkinje s.
Histofreezer portable cryosurgical s.
Hitachi EUB 405 imaging s.
Hitachi UB 420 digital ultrasound s.
humoral immune s.
Hydro ThermAblator endometrial ablation s.
hypothalamic-pituitary s.
iLook 15 handheld ultrasound s.
image recording s.
Imelab vascular diagnostic s.
Imexlab vascular diagnostic s.
immune s.
Infant Flow nCPAP s.
In-Fast bone screw s.
Innova electrotherapy s.
Innova feminine incontinence treatment s.
INOvent delivery s.
International Neuroblastoma Staging S. (INSS)

system (*continued*)

International Staging S.
intrauterine s. (IUS)
intrauterine contraceptive
  progesterone s. (ICPS)
ionKids monitoring s.
JustVision diagnostic ultrasound s.
Kagan staging s.
kallikrein-kinin s.
Kiwi ProCup vacuum delivery s.
KOH colpotomizer s.
Lact-Aid nursing trainer s.
Lancefield streptococcal typing s.
Laparolift s.
Lap-Band adjustable gastric
  banding s.
LATCH s.
LigaSure vessel sealing s.
limbic GABAergic s.
Lone Star retractor s.
lower collecting s.
low-flow oxygen s.
Lumex PT fiberoptic cystometry s.
lymphatic s.
lymphoreticular s.
Macroduct coil s.
male reproductive s.
Mammex TR computer-aided
  mammography diagnosis s.
Mammomat C3 mammography s.
MammoReader computer-aided
  detection s.
MammoScan digital imaging s.
Mammotest breast biopsy s.
Mammotome breast biopsy s.
Maturna bra s.
McAllister grading s.
MEMS 6 TrackCap Monitor
  medication monitoring s.
MicroLap Gold s.
MicroSpan microhysteroscopy s.
MiniArc single incision sling s.
MiniMed continuous glucose
  monitoring s.
mini Vidas automated
  immunoassay s.
mitochondrial glycine cleavage s.
Mityvac vacuum delivery s.
molecular adsorbent recirculating s.
  (MARS)
motion artifact rejection s. (MARS)
musculoskeletal s.
Nanoduct sweat test s.
Nellcor N-400/FS s.
NeoCure cryoablation s.
Neonatal Abstinence Scoring S.
  (NASS)
neonatal facial coding s. (NFCS)
Neotrend s.

nervous s.
neuroendocrine s.
NexPill SmartCap medication
  monitoring s.
nonallopathic health care s.
noradrenergic s.
Norplant s.
Nottingham breast cancer grading s.
NovaSure impedance-controlled
  endometrial ablation s.
NOxBOXmobile nitric oxide delivery
  and monitoring s.
Onyx transobturator midurethral
  sling s.
OpenGene automated DNA
  sequencing s.
opsonization s.
Opus immunoassay s.
OraSure oral HIV-1 antibody
  testing s.
orthogonal lead s.
osmotic release oral s. (OROS)
OsteoView 2000 s.
Ovation falloposcopy s.
PadKit sample collection s.
PalmVue s.
Papnet automated cervical
  cytology s.
Papnet testing s.
Pap-Perfect supply s.
parasympathetic nervous s.
Pelvic Organ Prolapse
  Quantification s.
PelviLace transobturator biourethral
  support s.
Performa Acoustic Imaging s.
Performa diagnostic ultrasound
  imaging s.
Perigee Prolapse Repair S.
PerQ SANS s.
PlasmaKinetic tissue management s.
POPQ staging s.
portal s.
Precision Tack transvaginal
  anchor s.
Pregnancy Risk Assessment
  Monitoring S. (PRAMS)
press-in bone anchor s.
primer pair s.
Priscilla White classification of
  diabetes in pregnancy s. (class A,
  A1, A2, B, C, D, F, R, H, T)
probe s.
prognostic scoring s.
prolapse repair s.
prorenin-renin-angiotensin s.
ProTime microcoagulation s.
Puregene DNA extraction s.
Quantum 2000 electrosurgical s.

Quips genetic imaging s.
radiofrequency interstitial tissue
  ablation s. (RITA)
Redi+Wash cleansing s.
Renaissance spirometry s.
renin-angiotensin s. (RAS)
renin-angiotensin-aldosterone s.
reproductive s.
respiratory s.
reticuloendothelial s.
review of s.'s (ROS)
Rh blood group s.
Riechert-Mundinger stereotactic s.
RxFISH DNA probe and analysis s.
SalEst preterm labor test s.
Scepter s.
Second-Look computer-aided
  detection s.
Sectra MicroDose mammography s.
selective no-fault s.
selective tubal occlusion
  procedure s.
SenoScan full-field digital
  mammography s.
Sequoia Acuson s.
Sequoia C256 echocardiographic s.
Seroma-Cath s.
serotonergic s.
Shimadzu ultrasound s.
Shutt suture punch s.
Siemens Sonoline SI-400
  ultrasound s.
Sinai S.
single collecting s.
single-use diagnostic s. (SUDS)
Sirecust 404N neonatal
  monitoring s.
Sky-Boot stirrup s.
SKY epidural pain control s.
SoftScan laser mammography s.
Sonopsy ultrasound-guided breast
  biopsy s.
Spectra 400 extended surveillance
  and alert s.
Sperm Select sperm recovery s.
SprayGel adhesive barrier s.
STAN S-21 fetal heart rate s.
St. Jude Children's Research
  Hospital staging s.
Straight-In surgical s.
subdermal contraceptive s.
superior venous s.
surgicopathologic staging s.
swivel arm s.
sympathetic nervous s.
Synevac vacuum curettage s.
Technos ultrasound s.
Teratogen Information S. (TERIS)
Testoderm Transdermal S.

Thermachoice uterine balloon
  therapy s.
thermal balloon s.
ThermoChem-HT s.
transdermal therapeutic s. (TTS)
twin-to-twin transfusion s. (TTTS)
Tylok high-tension cerclage
  cabling s.
UD-2000 urodynamic
  measurement s.
Ultramark ultrasound s.
underwater drainage s.
UPS 2020 ambulatory
  measurement s.
urinary s.
Urocyte diagnostic cytometry s.
urogenital s.
UroVive s.
Vaccine Adverse Events Reporting
  S. (VAERS)
Vacutainer s.
Valleylab REM s.
Valley Vac smoke evacuation s.
VersaStep Plus access s.
Vesica press-in suture anchor s.
VestaBlate s.
Vidas automated immunoassay s.
Vidas immunoanalysis testing s.
visual magnocellular s.
Vivelle-Dot estradiol transdermal s.
Wallaby Phototherapy S.
WAVE nucleic acid fragment
  analysis s.

systematicus
  nevus pigmentosus s.
systemic
  s. anesthesia
  s. arteriovenous fistula
  s. azole therapy
  s. behavior family therapy
  s. candidiasis
  s. carnitine deficiency
  s. caval return
  s. disease
  s. fatty acid deficiency
  s. flow
  s. illness
  s. infection
  s. inflammatory response syndrome
    (SIRS)
  s. juvenile chronic arthritis
  s. lupus erythematosus (SLE)
  s. manifestation
  s. mastocytosis
  s. outflow obstruction
  s. scleroderma
  s. sclerosis (SS)
  s. side effect
  s. steroid

systemic (*continued*)
- s. therapy
- s. toxicity
- s. vascular resistance (SVR)
- s. vasculitis
- s. vasculitis syndrome

systemic-active nonspecific immunotherapy

systemic-onset
- s.-o. JRA
- s.-o. juvenile rheumatoid arthritis

systemic-to-pulmonary shunt

systole

systolic
- s. arterial pressure (SAP)
- s. blood pressure
- s. click
- s. component
- s. continuous murmur
- s. ejection murmur (SEM)
- s. murmur of pregnancy
- s. overload
- s. overload pattern

systolic/diastolic (S/D)

Syva test

T

 T band
 T bone density score
 T cell
 T connector
 T extension
 T helper
 T lymphocyte
 T protein
 T strain mycoplasma

T2

 diiodothyronine

T3

 triiodothyronine

T4

 thyroxine

T&A

 tonsillectomy and adenoidectomy

TA

 Takayasu arteritis
 therapeutic abortion
 thoracoabdominal

¹⁸²Ta

 tantalum-182

TAA

 tumor-associated antigen

TAB

 therapeutic abortion

TAb

 therapeutic abortion

tab

 Apo-Doxy T.
 Meda T.

Tabb crura tissue forceps

tabes

 t. dorsalis
 t. infantum
 juvenile t.
 t. mesenterica

tabetic neurosyphilis

table

 Bayley-Pinneau t.
 contingency t.
 cross t.
 cystoscopy t.
 height t.

tablet

 Actifed Allergy T.
 Allerest Children's Tablets
 Aviane-28 t.
 Benadryl decongestant allergy t.
 Bextra t.
 bisacodyl t.
 Bromfed t.
 Cenestin t.

 Coricidin T.
 Coricidin-D T.
 Cryselle t.
 Cyclessa t.
 Dexone T.
 Enpresse t.
 Focalin t.
 Hexadrol T.
 Histalet Forte T.
 hormonal pregnancy test t.
 Levlite t.
 Materna T.
 Metadate ER t.
 Methitest t.
 Mircette t.
 Mylocel t.
 NatalCare Plus film-coated t.
 NataTab CFe film-coated t.
 NataTab FA film-coated t.
 NataTab Rx film-coated t.
 orally disintegrating t. (ODT)
 Prenate GT delayed-release
  gel-coated t.
 Remifemin Menopause t.
 Trivora-28 t.
 Veltane T.
 Whoo-Noz deodorant t.

tabula rasa

TAC

 tetracaine, adrenaline, cocaine
 transient aplastic crisis

tache noir

tachometer

tachyarrhythmia

 atrial t.
 supraventricular t. (SVT)

tachyarrhythmia-bradyarrhythmia

tachycardia

 aberrant supraventricular t.
 accelerated junctional ectopic t.
 atrial t.
 atrioventricular nodal reentrant t.
  (AVNRT)
 atrioventricular reciprocating t.
  (AVRT)
 automatic atrial t.
 AV nodal reentry t.
 baseline fetal t.
 chaotic atrial t.
 congenital paroxysmal atrial t.
 ectopic atrial t.
 fetal t.
 junctional t.
 junctional ectopic t. (JET)
 maternal t.

T

tachycardia (*continued*)
    multifocal atrial t.
    narrow complex supraventricular t.
    nodal t.
    nonsustained ventricular t.
    orthodromic reciprocating t.
    paraventricular t.
    paroxysmal t.
    paroxysmal atrial t. (PAT)
    persistent t.
    postural t.
    reentrant supraventricular t.
    sinus t.
    supraventricular t. (SVT)
    sustained ventricular t. (SVT)
    ventricular t.
    wide complex t.
tachydysrhythmia
    supraventricular t.
tachygastria
tachyphylaxis
tachypnea
    transient t.
tachypneic
tachysystole
    uterine t.
Tac-3 Injection
tacker
    Origin T.
tackling
    spear t.
tacrolimus
tactile
    t. defensiveness
    t. discrimination
    t. fever
    t. fremitus
    t. hallucination
    t. sensory monitoring
    t. stimulation
    t. stimulus
    t. temperature
tadalafil
Taenia
    T. saginata
    T. solium
taeniasis
TAF
    tracheobronchial aspirate fluid
    tumor angiogenesis factor
tag
    cutaneous t.
    expressed sequence t.
    hymenal t.
    perianal skin t.
    preauricular t.
    skin t.
Tagamet-HB
Tago diagnostic kit

TAH
    total abdominal hysterectomy
tail
    axillary t.
    t. bud
    Spence axillary t.
tailgut
tailor sitting
Taiwan acute respiratory (TWAR)
Takao syndrome
Takayasu
    T. arteritis (TA)
    T. disease
TAL
    tendo Achillis lengthening
talar
    t. decancellation
    t. dome fracture
    t. tilt test
    t. to first metatarsal angle
talc
talcum powder
tali (*pl. of* talus)
talipes
    t. calcaneovalgus
    t. calcaneovarus
    t. calcaneus
    t. cavovalgus
    t. cavus
    t. equinovalgus
    t. equinovarus (TEV)
    t. equinovarus deformity
    t. equinus
    t. hobble splint
    t. planovalgus
    t. planus
    t. valgus
    t. varus
talipomanus
talk
    receptor cross t.
talking
    t. down
    sleep t.
talocalcaneal (TC), talocalcanean
    t. angle (TCA)
    t. bar
    t. fusion
talocalcanean (*var. of* talocalcaneal)
talus, *pl.* **tali**
    congenital vertical t.
    vertical t.
Talwin NX
Tambocor
TAME
    tosylarginine methyl ester
Tamm-Horsfall
    T.-H. mucoprotein
    T.-H. protein

Tamofen
Tamone
tamoxifen
>   t. citrate
tampon
>   continence t.
>   Contrelle continence t.
>   nasal t.
>   t. test
>   vaginal t.
tamponade, tamponage
>   balloon t.
>   cardiac t.
>   gastroesophageal balloon t.
>   pericardial t.
tamponage (*var. of* tamponade)
tandem
>   T. Icon II hCG
>   t. mass spectrometry
>   t. repeat
>   t. repeat sequence
>   t. walking
Tandem-Cube pessary
Tandem-R Ostase osteoporosis test
tangential breast field
Tangier disease
Tanner
>   T. classification (1–5)
>   T. Developmental Scale (stage 1–5)
>   T. developmental stage (1–5)
>   T. genital stage (1–5)
>   T. grade 1–5 staging
>   T. maturation stage (1–5)
>   T. sex maturity rating
>   T. stage
>   T. stage of development (1–5)
>   T. staging of genital development (1–5)
Tanner-Whitehouse
>   T.-W. bone age reference value
>   T.-W. II bone/age determination method
tan papilloma
tantalum
tantalum-182 (^{182}Ta)
tantrum
>   temper t.
tanycyte
TAP
>   transport-associated protein
>   transvaginal amniotic puncture
>   trypsin activation peptide
tap
>   bladder t.
>   infant subdural t.
>   lung t.
>   percutaneous lung t.
>   peritoneal t.

>   shunt t.
>   spinal t.
>   subdural t.
>   supraciliary t.
>   ventricular t.
>   VP shunt t.
>   wet t.
Tapanol
Tapar
Tapazole
tape
>   Broselow t.
>   glucose oxidase test t.
>   lap t.
>   Medipore H soft cloth surgical t.
>   tension-free obturator t. (TOT)
>   tension-free vaginal t. (TVT)
>   transobturator t. (TOT)
>   twill t.
tapering cytoplasmic process
tapetoretinal degeneration
tapeworm
>   pork t.
taping
>   buddy t.
tapir
>   levre de t.
>   t. mouth
tapiroid
TAPVC
>   total anomalous pulmonary venous connection
TAPVR
>   total anomalous pulmonary venous return
>   mixed TAPVR
*Taq*I **enzyme**
TAR
>   thrombocytopenia absent radius
>   TAR syndrome
tar
>   Aqua T.
>   coal t.
tarda
>   chondrodystrophia congenita t.
>   *Edwardsiella* t.
>   hypophosphatasia t.
>   lymphedema t.
>   osteopetrosis t.
>   porphyria cutanea t.
>   spondyloepiphysial dysplasia t.
>   syphilis hereditaria t.
tardive
>   t. dyskinesia
>   t. dystonia
target
>   t. cell
>   t. lesion
>   t. organ response

T

targeted
   t. ultrasonographic examination
   t. ultrasound
targeting
   gene t.
targetoid lesion
Tariverdian syndrome
Tarkowski method
Tarnier axis-traction forceps
Taro-Ampicillin
Taro-Cloxacillin
Taro-Sone
tarry cyst
tarsal
   t. coalition
   t. navicular osteochondritis
   t. plate
tarsal-carpal coalition syndrome
tarsalis
   Culex t.
tarsi (*pl. of* tarsus)
tarsometatarsal mobilization
tarsorrhaphy
tarsus, *pl.* **tarsi**
tartrate
   butorphanol t.
   ergotamine t.
   levallorphan t.
   levorphanol t.
   metoprolol t.
   varenicline t.
   zolpidem t.
Tarui disease
TAS
   Toronto Alexithymia Scale
task
   Continuous Performance T.
   t. load
   Paired Associate Learning T.
   (PALT)
   phoneme segmentation t.
   phonemic awareness t.
taste
   t. bud
   impaired t.
TAS/TVS
   transabdominal/transvaginal ultrasound
TAT
   tetanus antitoxin
   tray agglutination test
   tyrosine aminotransferase
TATD
   tyrosine aminotransferase deficiency
taurine
taurodontism
Taussig-Bing
   T.-B. anomaly
   T.-B. disease
   T.-B. syndrome

tautomenial
taxis
   bipolar t.
Taxol
Taxotere
Taybi-Linder syndrome
Taybi syndrome
Taylor dispersion
Tay-Sachs
   T.-S. disease
   T.-S. disease with visceral
   involvement
Tay syndrome
tazarotene
Tazicef
Tazidime
tazobactam
   piperacillin and t.
   t. sodium
TB
   tuberculosis
TBARS
   thiobarbituric acid-reacting
   substance
TBE
   tick-borne encephalitis
TBG
   thyroid-binding globulin
   thyroxine-binding globulin
   TBG deficiency
   TBG excess
TBI
   total body irradiation
   traumatic brain injury
TBK
   total body potassium
TBLC
   term birth, living child
TBMD
   thin basement membrane disease
TBP
   thyroxine-binding protein
TBSA
   total body surface area
   TBSA burn
TBV
   total blood volume
TBW
   total body water
TC
   talocalcaneal
tc
   transcutaneous
TCA
   talocalcaneal angle
   trichloroacetic acid
   tricyclic antidepressant
   topical concentrated TCA
TC7 adhesion barrier

TcB
transcutaneous bilirubin
TCC
transcatheter closure
TCD
transcranial Doppler
TCE
trichloroethanol
T-cell
T-c. activation defect
T-c. antibody induction therapy
T-c. depletion
T-c. dysfunction
T-c. lymphoma
maternal T-c.
T-c. subset
T-c. trophic (T-trophic)
T-cell-depleted
T-c.-d. graft
T-c.-d. haploidentical bone marrow
stem cell
T-cell-mediated disease
T-cell-tropic syncytium-inducing strain
Tc HMPAO
technetium hexamethylpropyleneamine
oxime
Tc HMPAO leukocyte scan
TCI
TCI OcuLook saliva ovulation tester
kit
TCI OvuLook ovulation tester
TCIFTT
transcervical intrafallopian tube transfer
tCpO2
transcutaneous partial pressure of
oxygen
TCT
thrombin clotting time
TCT coagulation test
Tcu-380A intrauterine device
TD
Tourette disorder
traveler's diarrhea
Td
tetanus and diphtheria
Td toxoid vaccine
TdaP
tetanus, diphtheria and pertussis
TdaP vaccine
TDEE
total daily energy expenditure
T/Derm
Neutrogena T/D.
TDF
testis-determining factor
TDI
therapeutic donor insemination
tissue Doppler imaging
Td-IPV vaccine

TDLU
terminal ductal lobular unit
terminal duct lobular unit
tdy gene
TE
thromboembolic event
tea
herbal t.
tea-and-toast diet
TEACCH
treatment and education of autistic
and related communications
handicapped children
Project TEACCH
teacher
infant t.
T. Rating Form (TRF)
T. Report Form (TRF)
tea-colored urine
team
interdisciplinary t.
multidisciplinary t.
Patient Outcomes Research T.
(PORT)
Sexual Assault Response T. (SART)
transdisciplinary t.
2-team sling
tear
absent t.'s
t. film
Mallory-Weiss t. (MWT)
meniscus t.
no t.'s
t. overflow
syndrome of crocodile t.'s
tear-drop vesicle
T4/ebp-1
thyroid-specific enhancer binding
protein-1
Tebrazid
TEC
tetracaine, epinephrine, cocaine
transient erythroblastopenia of
childhood
technetium
t. bone scan
t. hexamethylpropyleneamine oxime
(Tc HMPAO)
technetium-labeled red blood cell
technetium-99m
t.-99m bone scan
t.-99m pertechnetate
technic (*var. of* technique)
technical artifact
technique, technic
agar gel precipitation t.
agar immunoprecipitin t.
automated radiometric t.
Ayre spatula-Zelsmyr Cytobrush t.

T

technique (*continued*)
    balloon catheter t.
    Ball pelvimetry t.
    Barlow mitral regurgitation repair t.
    Beverly-Douglas lip-tongue
      adhesion t.
    biofeedback t.
    B-Lynch t.
    brain imaging t.
    Brockenbrough transseptal
      catheterization t.
    Brown-Wickham urethral pressure
      profilometry t.
    Bruhat neosalpingostomy t.
    buccal feeding t.
    capillary isoelectric focusing t.
    catheter-over-needle t.
    catheter-over-wire t.
    clean-catch t.
    clip t.
    clonogenic t.
    cobalt-60 moving strip t.
    Cobb measurement t.
    Cohen transtrigonal t.
    Colcher-Sussman x-ray
      pelvimetry t.
    contraceptive t.
    Counsellor-Flor modification of
      McIndoe vaginoplasty t.
    dead space t.
    2-diameter pocket t.
    direct insertion t.
    Döderlein hysterectomy t.
    dot-blot t.
    double-catheter t.
    double-freeze t.
    Dufourmentel transposition
      flap t.
    Dyban oocyte fixation t.
    Eklund mammography t.
    enzyme-multiplication immunoassay
      t. (EMIT)
    enzyme-multiplied immunoassay t.
      (EMIT)
    evoked potential t.
    ex utero intrapartum t.
      (EXIT)
    ferning t.
    fetal assessment t.
    fetal surveillance t.
    folklore-based contraceptive t.
    Gittes bladder suspension t.
    Glenn-Anderson ureteric reflux
      repair t.
    Goebell-Frangenheim-Stoeckel
      urethrovesical suspension t.
    Gomco circumcision t.
    gracilis flap t.
    GRASS MRI t.

    Hamou hysteroscopic endometrial
      ablation t.
    Heaney vaginal vault closure t.
    hemisection uterine morcellation t.
    hold t.
    hook traction t.
    hybridoma t.
    hyperglycemic clamp t.
    hyperinsulinemic-euglycemic clamp t.
    immune monitoring t.
    immune separation t.
    immunoperoxidase t.
    insemination swim-up t.
    interrupted-bite t.
    intraluminal electrical impedance t.
    Jones and Jones wedge t.
    Kety-Schmidt cerebral blood flow
      measurement t.
    Kidde cannula
      hysterosalpingogram t.
    Kleihauer fetomaternal hemorrhage
      estimation t.
    labial traction t.
    Lapides vesicourethropexy t.
    Lazarus-Nelson closed peritoneal
      lavage t.
    Leboyer episiotomy t.
    Lich-Gregoire t.
    Lich vesicoureteral reflux repair t.
    Limberg flap t.
    loss-of-resistance t.
    marsupialization t.
    M-FISH cytogenetic t.
    minimally invasive surgical t.
      (MIST)
    Mitrofanoff continent urinary
      diversion t.
    Miyazaki t.
    modified Pomeroy tubal ligation t.
    molecular genetic t.
    multicolor FISH cytogenetic t.
    multipuncture t.
    Mustard TGA t.
    myofascial release t.
    NAA t.
    Nuss concave chest correction t.
    O'Leary t.
    Ortolani congenital hip
      dislocation t.
    oscillometric t.
    pants-over-vest t.
    Parkland Hospital t.
    Percoll sperm preparation t.
    percutaneous multipuncture t.
    percutaneous Seldinger t.
    3-point t.
    Politano-Leadbetter
      ureteroneocystostomy t.
    Pomeroy tubal ligation t.

pullthrough t.
recombinant DNA t.
relaxation t.
reverse FISH cytogenetic t.
rollerball t.
Seldinger t.
shoelace t.
Simonton biofeedback t.
single-isotope tracer t.
skate-flap t.
skinfold caliper t.
snapshot GRASS t.
soluble gas t.
Southern blot t.
sperm retrieval t.
split-flap t.
squeeze t.
Strassman bicornual uterus
  metroplasty t.
Stringer t.
surveillance t.
swim-up t.
thorascopic t.
Tompkins median bivalving t.
toothbrush culture t.
tripod fixation t.
tubal ligation band t.
tube insertion t.
U t.
Wallace ureteroileal anastomosis t.
technology
assisted reproductive t. (ART)
assistive t. (AT)
genetic engineering t.
recombinant DNA t.
reproductive t.
Society for Assisted Reproductive T.
  (SART)
t. transfer
ultrasound t.
Technos ultrasound system
Tecnu Extreme poison ivy scrub
tectal brainstem glioma
tectocephaly
tectocerebellar dysraphia
tectum
mesencephalic t.
TED
thromboembolic disease
TED stocking
teddy-bear gait
TEE
transesophageal echocardiography
Teebi syndrome
Teejel
teenager
Problem-Oriented Screening
  Instrument for T.'s (POSIT)
Teen-Tot Clinic

teeth (*pl. of* tooth)
teething
Babee T.
short stature, hyperextensibility of
  joints or hernia, ocular depression,
  Rieger anomaly, t. (SHORT)
TEF
thermic effect of food
tracheoesophageal fistula
transesophageal fistula
Teflon-coated wire
Teflon periurethral injection
tegmen, *pl.* **tegmina**
tegmentum
tegmina (*pl. of* tegmen)
Tegress urethral implant
Tegretol
Tegretol-XR
Tegrin-HC Topical
teicoplanin
Teilum tumor
telangiectases (*pl. of* telangiectasis)
telangiectasia
ataxia t.
calcinosis, Raynaud phenomenon,
  esophageal dysmotility,
  sclerodactyly, t. (CREST)
calcinosis, Raynaud phenomenon,
  sclerodactyly, t. (CRST)
flat red-black t.
hemorrhagic t.
hereditary hemorrhagic t. (HHT)
intestinal t.
t. macularis eruptiva perstans
nail bed t.
nail fold t.
oculocutaneous t.
raised red-black t.
red-black t.
retinal vessel t.
telangiectasis, *pl.* **telangiectases**
conjunctival t.
cutaneous t.
telangiectatic
t. granuloma
t. nevus
t. osteosarcoma
telangiectatica
cutis marmorata t.
telecanthus
telecanthus-hypospadias syndrome
telecardiology
telemammography
telemedicine
telemetry
telencephalic
t. neuroepithelium
t. subependymal germinal matrix
teleologic theory

T

telepsychiatry
teleradiology
teleroentgenogram
telescopy
    percutaneous suprapubic t.
teletherapy
television epilepsy
TeLinde operation
telocentric chromosome
telogen
    t. effluvium
    t. phase
telomere
telophase
TEM
    therapeutic electromembrane
    transanal endoscopic microsurgery
    transmission electron microscopy
temazepam
Temovate
Temp-a-dot thermometer
temperament
    shy-inhibited t.
temperature
    absolute t.
    ambient t.
    artificial t.
    aseptic t.
    aural t.
    axillary t.
    basal body t. (BBT)
    body t.
    core t.
    critical t.
    t. dysregulation
    ephemeral t.
    erratic t.
    eruptive t.
    maximum t. (T-max)
    normal t.
    oral t.
    t. pattern
    rectal t.
    room t.
    t. sensor
    skin t.
    subnormal t.
    tactile t.
    tympanic t.
temperature-controlled isolette
temper tantrum
template
    Syed-Neblett dedicated vulvar plastic t.
temporal
    t. artery thermometry
    t. balding
    t. lobe
    t. lobe epilepsy
    t. lobe seizure
    t. sequencing
temporale
    planum t.
temporalis muscle
temporary
    t. blood substitute
    t. diverting colostomy
temporomandibular
    t. joint (TMJ)
    t. joint dysfunction
temporospatial pattern
Tempra
Temtamy syndrome
TEN
    titanium elastic nailing
    toxic epidermal necrolysis
tenacious
tenacula (pl. of tenaculum)
tenaculum, pl. tenacula
    Bierer t.
    Braun-Schroeder single-tooth t.
    cervical t.
    double-tooth t.
    Emmett cervical t.
    t. hook
    t. hook loop
    Jacobs t.
    Pelosi t.
    Schroeder uterine t.
    single-tooth t.
    uterine t.
Tenckhoff catheter
tendency
    familial t.
    prothrombic t.
tenderness
    abdominal t.
    cervical motion t. (CMT)
    costovertebral angle t. (CVAT)
    CVA t.
    epigastric t.
    fundal t.
    joint line t.
    lower abdominal t.
    pelvic t.
    point t.
    point of maximum t. (PMT)
    punch t.
    rebound t.
    snuffbox t.
Tender-Touch
    T.-T. extractor
    T.-T. vacuum birthing cup
tendinea
    chordae t.
tendineae
tendines (pl. of tendo)

tendineus
    arcus t.
tendinitis, tendonitis
    patellar t.
    triceps t.
tendinous arch
tendo, *pl.* **tendines**
    t. Achillis
    t. Achillis lengthening (TAL)
tendon
    Achilles t.
    bowstringing of t.
    calcaneal t.
    conjoined t.
    fat flexor hallucis longus t.
    flexor hallucis longus t.
    t. forceps
    t. lengthening
    peroneus brevis t.
    peroneus longus t.
    split flexor hallucis longus t.
    t. stretch reflex
    t. transfer
    t. xanthoma
tendon-bone interface
tendonitis (*var. of* tendinitis)
tendosynovitis (*var. of* tenosynovitis)
tendotomy (*var. of* tenotomy)
tendovaginitis (*var. of* tenosynovitis)
tenesmus
    perimenstrual t.
Tenex
teniposide
Tenney-Parker sign
tennis elbow
Tennison-Randall repair
tenofovir
tenosynovial sarcoma
tenosynovioma
tenosynovitis, tendosynovitis,
  tendovaginitis, tenovaginitis
tenosynovitis-dermatitis syndrome
tenotomy, tendotomy
    percutaneous adductor t.
tenovaginitis (*var. of* tenosynovitis)
TENS
    transcutaneous electrical nerve
    stimulation
tense
    t. ascites
    t. blister
    t. lobule
Tensilon test
tension
    t. cyst
    end-tidal CO_2 t.
    t. headache
    t. hydrothorax
    t. myalgia

    t. pneumocephalus
    t. pneumothorax
    postmenstrual t. (PMT)
    premenstrual t. (PMT)
    surface t.
    vaginal tape t.
    wall t.
tension-discharging phenomenon
tension-free
    t.-f. obturator tape (TOT)
    t.-f. vaginal tape (TVT)
    t.-f. vaginal tape obturator
    t.-f. vaginal tape procedure
tension-type headache
tensor fasciae latae (TFL)
tent
    CAM t.
    face t.
    intracervical t.
    laminaria t.
    mist t.
    oxygen t.
    Silon t.
tenting
    skin t.
tentoria (*pl. of* tentorium)
tentorial
    t. laceration
    t. margin
    t. opening
tentorium, *pl.* **tentoria**
Tenuate
tenuis
    Dirofilaria t.
tenuous
Tenzel calipers
TEOAE
    transient evoked otoacoustic emission
    TEOAE testing
TEOE
    transient evoked otoacoustic emission
tepid
teras, *pl.* **terata**
terata (*pl. of* teras)
teratism
teratoblastoma
teratocarcinoma
teratogen
    environmental t.
    t. exposure
    T. Information System (TERIS)
    T. Registry
teratogenesis
teratogenetic (*var. of* teratogenic)
teratogenic, teratogenetic
    t. agent
    t. effect
    t. exposure
    t. medication

T

teratogenic (*continued*)
 t. outcome
 t. properties
 t. risk
 t. syndrome
teratogenicity
teratogen-induced malformation
teratoid tumor
teratologic dislocation
teratology
teratoma
 atypical t.
 benign cystic t. (BCT)
 benign cystic ovarian t. (BCOT)
 cervical t.
 cystic t.
 germ cell t.
 immature t. (grade 0–3)
 immature malignant t.
 immature ovarian t.
 malignant ovarian t.
 mature t.
 mature cystic t.
 mature cystic ovarian t.
 mediastinal t.
 ovarian cystic t.
 ovarian embryonal t.
 pediatric ovarian t.
 sacrococcygeal t.
teratophobia
teratospermia
teratotoxicity
teratozoospermia
Terazol
 T. Vaginal
 T. 7 vaginal cream
 T. 3 vaginal cream
 T. vaginal suppository
terbinafine
terbutaline
 beta-2 sympathomimetic t.
 caffeine t.
 t. sulfate
terconazole
teres, *pl.* **teretes**
 ligamentum t.
teretes (*pl. of* teres)
terfenadine
Terfluzine
ter Haar syndrome
TERIS
 Teratogen Information System
term
 t. AGA
 t. birth, living child (TBLC)
 t. delivery
 full t. (FT)
 t. gestation
 t. infant

 t. infants, premature infants,
  abortions, living children (TPAL)
 t. LGA
 t. milk
 t. pregnancy
 t. SGA
Term-Guard
terminal
 t. blush
 t. blush formation
 t. bronchiole
 t. cardiotocogram
 t. choledochus
 t. complement component
 t. complement component deficiency
 t. deletion
 t. deoxyribonucleotidyl
  transferase-mediated biotin-16-dUTP
  nick-end labeling (TUNEL)
 t. ductal lobular unit (TDLU)
 t. duct lobular unit (TDLU)
 t. hair
 t. heating method
 t. ileitis
 t. lung differentiation
 t. maturation
 t. motor latency
 t. neosalpingostomy
 t. saccular period
 t. transverse acheiria defect
 t. transverse limb defect
terminale
 filum t.
 ossiculum t.
 ropelike filum t.
terminalis
 lamina t.
 linea t.
termination
 t. codon
 elective t.
 first trimester t.
 medical t.
 t. of parental rights
 pregnancy t.
 second-trimester t.
 selective t.
 surgical t.
terminus
 vaginal t.
Terramycin IM injection
terreus
 Aspergillus t.
terror
 night t.
 sleep t.
Terry
 T. questionnaire
 T. syndrome

Terson disease
tertiary
  t. amine
  t. care center
  t. closure
  t. hypothyroidism
  t. prevention
  t. referral hospital
  t. syphilis
TESA
  testicular sperm aspiration
Teschler-Nicola and Killian
  syndrome
TESE
  testicular sperm extraction
Teslac
Tessier craniofacial operation
test
  Accu-Chek t.
  AccuStat hCG pregnancy t.
  acid elution t.
  acidified serum lysis t.
  acoustic reflex t.
  acoustic stimulation t. (AST)
  ACTH stimulation t.
  activated partial thromboplastin time
    coagulation t.
  Adams forward-bending t.
  Affirm VPIII t.
  agglutination inhibition t.
  air leak t.
  Alcohol Use Disorders Identification
    T. (AUDIT)
  Allen-Doisy t.
  Allen picture t.
  alternate-cover t.
  alternating breath t. (ABT)
  ambulatory uterine contraction t.
  Amiel-Tison t.
  amine t.
  AmnioStat-FLM screening t.
  AmniSure t.
  Amplicor HBV monitor t.
  AneuVysion Assay prenatal
    genetic t.
  anterior drawer t.
  antigen detection t.
  antiglobulin t.
  antitreponemal t.
  Apley compression t.
  apprehension t.
  Apt t.
  APT-Downey t.
  APTT coagulation t.
  arginine-insulin stimulation t.
  arginine-insulin tolerance t.
  arginine tolerance t. (ATT)
  Aschheim-Zondek t.
  automated reagin t. (ART)

  BAER t.
  Ballard t.
  Barlow and Ortolani t.
  Barlow hip dysplasia t.
  BD t.
  Bender Visual Motor Gestalt T.
  Benton Visual Retention T.
  Berens 3-character t.
  Bernstein t.
  Betke-Kleihauer t.
  BH_4 loading t.
  Biocept-G pregnancy t.
  Biocept-5 pregnancy t.
  BioStar Strep A OIA t.
  bitterling pregnancy t.
  bladder muscle stress t.
  bladder neck elevation t.
  block design t.
  blood-type t.
  Bonney blue stress incontinence t.
  Boston Naming T.
  bovine mucus penetration t.
  BRACA mutation t.
  branching snowflake t.
  Bratton-Marshall t.
  breast stimulation contraction t.
    (BSCT)
  breath H_2 t.
  breath hydrogen excretion t.
  Breslow-Day t.
  Brodie-Trendelenburg t.
  bronchial challenge t.
  Bruckner pupillary light reflex t.
  Bruininks-Oseretsky t.
  BTA STAT t.
  bubble stability t.
  Burt Word Reading T.
  buserelin stimulation t.
  BVBLUE t.
  CAGE t.
  cAMP t.
  cancer antigen 125 t.
  Candida skin t.
  caramel t.
  carbon-14 t.
  carbon-13 urea breath t.
  Carnett t.
  Cattell Infant Intelligence T.
  CF t.
  Children of Alcoholics Screening T.
    (CAST)
  Children's Depression Inventory T.
  Children's Eating Attitudes T.
    (ChEAT)
  Chlamydiazyme t.
  chlortetracycline fluorescence t.
  chromosome breakage t.
  Clearview hCG pregnancy t.
  Clinical Adaptive T. (CAT)

T

test (*continued*)

clomiphene citrate challenge t. (CCCT)
coagulation t.
cocaine t.
Colaris genetic susceptibility t.
Collins t.
Color Trails T.
complement t.
complementation t.
complement fixation t.
Concise Plus hCG urine t.
Conners continuous performance t.
Constitutional Genetic Array T. (CGAT)
continuous performance t. (CPT)
contraction stress t. (CST)
Coombs t.
cord blood hemoglobinopathy screening t.
corneal light reflex t.
Corner-Allen t.
Corsi block tapping t.
Cortrosyn stimulation t.
cosyntropin stimulation t.
cotton swab t.
cough t.
cover t.
cover-uncover eye t.
criterion-referenced t.
cuff t.
C-urea breath t.
cyclic adenosine monophosphate t.
cytochrome oxidase t.
DAP t.
deferoxamine challenge t.
dehydroepiandrosterone sulfate loading t.
Denver Developmental Screening T. (DDS, DDST)
dexamethasone suppression t.
DFA t.
Dick t.
DIF t.
differential agglutination t.
Digene HPV t.
Digene Hybrid Capture II HPV T.
diiodothyronine t.
dipstick t.
direct antiglobulin t. (DAT)
direct Coombs t.
direct treponemal t.
D-mire t.
DNA probe t.
dot-blot HPV hybridization t.
dot ELISA t.
Draw-a-Person T.
Duncan t.
dye decolorization t.

dye disappearance t.
Eagle t.
early pregnancy t. (EPT)
Eastern blot t.
Eating Attitudes T.
edrophonium t.
Einstein screening t.
Elek t.
ELISA t.
ELISpot t.
Endtz t.
enzyme-linked antiglobulin t.
epicutaneous t.
estrogen-progestin t.
E-tegrity t.
expressive one-word picture vocabulary t.
factor V Leiden mutation t.
Fact Plus Pro pregnancy t.
family-based t.
Farber t.
Farr t.
FAST blood t.
fern t.
ferric chloride t.
ferritin level t.
fetal acoustic stimulation t.
fetal activity t.
fetal fibronectin t.
fetal surveillance t.
figure-of-4 t.
finger-nose-finger t.
finger-tapping t.
fingertip number writing t.
finger-to-nose t.
flat tire t.
FLM t.
fluorescein-conjugated monoclonal antibody t.
fluorescein treponema antibody t.
fluorescence actin staining t.
fluorescence spot t.
fluorescent antimembrane antibody t.
fluorescent treponemal antibody absorption t.
foam stability t. (FST)
food challenge t.
Fortel ovulation t.
forward-bending t.
Franklin-Dukes t.
Free Running Asthma T. (FRAST)
Frei t.
Friberg microsurgical agglutination t.
Friedman rabbit t.
fructose intolerance t.
FTA t.
galactose breath t.
gelatin agglutination t.
GeneAmp PCR t.

genetic t.
Gen-Probe amplified CT t.
geometric design t.
germ tube t.
Gesell Preschool T.
Gesell School Readiness T.
Gilmore Oral Reading T. (GORT)
glucose challenge t.
glucose tolerance t. (GTT)
Goldmann perimeter visual field t.
gonadotropin agonist stimulation t.
  (GAST)
Gonozyme t.
Goodenough-Harris Drawing T.
Gordon Distractibility T.
granulocyte immunofluorescence t.
  (GIFT)
Gravindex t.
Gray Oral Reading T. (GORT)
growth hormone stimulation t.
  (GHST)
guaiac t.
Guthrie t.
HABA binding t.
hair bulb incubation t.
halo t.
hanging-drop t.
HealthCheck One-Step One Minute
  pregnancy t.
heel-to-shin t.
Heller t.
hemagglutination t.
hemagglutination treponemal t.
  (HATT)
Hematest t.
Hemoccult II t.
HemoCue glucose t.
HemoCue hemoglobin t.
hemoglobin S solubility t.
HEMPAS t.
heparan sulfate urine t.
heparin challenge t.
Heritage Panel genetic screening t.
Herp-Check t.
heterophil t.
Hinton t.
hip rotation t.
Hirschberg corneal reflex t.
Hirschberg light reflex t.
HIV t.
HIVAGEN t.
Hogben t.
home pregnancy t.
homocysteine loading t.
5-hop t.
1-hour glucose challenge t.
1-hour glucose tolerance t.
5-hour glucose tolerance t.
Huhner t.

Huhner-Sims t.
Human Figure Drawing T.
human ovum fertilization t.
hydrogen breath t.
hyperoxia t.
hyperventilation provocative t.
ICD-p24 t.
Icon serum pregnancy t.
Icon strep B t.
Icon urine pregnancy t.
IDI-Strep B t.
IFA t.
IgA AGA t.
IgA HIV antibody t.
IgG-IFA t.
IgM-IFA t.
IgM indirect fluorescent antibody t.
IHA t.
immunobead t. (IBT)
ImmunoCap specific IgE blood t.
immunofluorescent *Chlamydia* t.
immunologic pregnancy t.
impingement t.
India ink t.
Indiclor t.
indirect Coombs t.
inhibin t.
insulin sensitivity t.
insulin tolerance t.
intelligence t.
intradermal t.
inversion stress tilt t.
ischemic exercise t.
Isojima t.
IVA visual consistency t.
Jadassohn t.
Kahn t.
Kapeller-Adler t.
Kell t.
Kibrick t.
Kinyoun acid-fast staining t.
Kleihauer t.
Kleihauer-Betke t.
Kodak hCG serum t.
Kodak SureCell Chlamydia T.
Kodak SureCell hCG-Urine T.
Kodak SureCell Herpes T.
Kodak SureCell LCH in-office
  pregnancy t.
Kodak SureCell Strep A t.
KOH t.
KOH whiff t.
Kolmer t.
Korotkoff t.
Kremer penetration t.
Kupperman menopausal distress t.
Kurzrok-Miller t.
Kurzrok-Ratner t.
Kveim t.

T

test (*continued*)
KW t.
laboratory t.
Lachman t.
lactose breath hydrogen t.
lactose tolerance t.
Landau t.
Lange t.
latex agglutination inhibition t.
  (LAIT)
latex fixation t.
latex particle agglutination t.
LCx Probe System t.
leak-point pressure t.
Letter-R intelligence t.
leucine tolerance t.
leukocyte histamine release t.
levothyroxine t.
LH color t.
Liddle t.
limulus lysate t.
liver function t.'s
Locke-Wallace Marital Adjustment t.
Lumadex-FSI t.
Lundh t.
lysis t.
lysoPC diagnostic ovarian cancer t.
Macherey-Nagel strep t.
Mantoux tuberculin skin t.
MAR t.
Marchetti t.
Marshall t.
Matritech NMP22 bladder cancer t.
Mazzini t.
McCaman-Robins t.
McMurray t.
McNemar t.
mental arithmetic t.
metabolic t.
methemoglobin reduction t.
Metopirone t.
metyrapone t.
Michigan Alcoholism Screening T.
Micral urine dipstick t.
microhemagglutination t.
microimmunofluorescence t.
microscopic agglutination t. (MAT)
MicroTrak t.
MIF t.
Miraluma t.
Miyazaki-Bonney t.
monoclonal antibody
  coagglutination t.
MonoPrep Pap t.
Monospot t.
Monosticon Dri-Dot t.
Mono-Vacc T.
Montenegro skin t.
mucin clot t.

multiple sleep latency t. (MSLT)
multipuncture t. (MPT)
MultiVysion PB assay t.
muscle enzyme t.
NAA t.
nappy t.
NBT dye t.
negative contraction stress t.
newborn genetic screening t.
nipple stimulation t.
Nitrazine t.
nitrite urine t.
nitroblue tetrazolium dye
  reduction t.
nitrogen washout t.
Noguchi t.
nongamma Coombs t.
noninvasive t.
nonstress t. (NST)
nontreponemal t.
norm-referenced t.
Northern blot t.
Now RSV t.
N-telopeptide t.
NTx t.
OAE t.
object assembly t.
t. of linkage disequilibrium
T. of Variables of Attention
t. of variables of attention deficit
  disorder
Ogita t.
OncoScint t.
Optochin t.
oral glucose challenge t. (OGCT)
oral glucose tolerance t. (OGTT)
OraQuick rapid HIV-1 antibody t.
OraSure oral HIV t.
O'Riain skin wrinkle t.
orthostatic t.
orthostatic proteinuria t.
Ortolani t.
osmotic fragility t.
OsteoGram bone density t.
Osteomark NTx serum t.
Osteosal t.
Otis-Lennon Intelligence T.
OvuKit t.
oxytocin challenge t. (OCT)
oxytocin stress t.
PACE-2C DNA probe t.
paced auditory serial addition t.
T. PackChlamydia test
T. Pack hCG
pad t.
Papnet t.
passive head-up tilt t.
Pathfinder DFA t.
Paul-Bunnell antibody t.

Paul-Bunnell-Davidsohn t.
PCR t.
Peabody picture vocabulary t.
(PPVT)
Penetrak t.
phenolsulfonphthalein t.
phenylketonuria t.
picture completion t.
pinhole t.
PKU t.
Plan Ahead T.
plasmacrit t.
platelet function t.
pool t.
poor man's clot t.
Porges-Meier t.
positive contraction stress t.
positive pool t.
postcoital t. (PCT)
postvoid residual urine t.
potassium sensitivity t.
Prechtl t.
Precise pregnancy t.
predictive value of t.
pregnancy t.
prick t.
Profile viral probe t.
progesterone challenge t.
prone extension t.
prothrombin time coagulation t.
provocation t.
provocative stress t.
PSA t.
psychometric t.
PT coagulation t.
pulmonary function t. (PFT)
QTest Strep t.
Q-tip t.
Quality of Upper Extremities T.
(QUEST)
quantitative intradermal skin t.
quantitative sudomotor axon-reflex t.
Queckenstedt t.
Quick t.
QuickVue A+B differentiated flu t.
QuickVue *Chlamydia* t.
QuickVue In-Line one-step
Strep A t.
QuickVue one-step hCG-Combo
pregnancy t.
QuickVue one-step hCG-urine t.
QuickVue *One-Step H. pylori* t.
Quidel group B strep t.
QuikPac-II OneStep hCG
pregnancy t.
radioallergosorbent t. (RAST)
radioimmunosorbent t. (RIST)
rapid antigen detection t.
rapid Giemsa t.

rapid plasma reagin card t.
rapid slide t.
rapid strep t.
Rapirun t.
reactive nonstress t.
red glass t.
red reflex t.
reflex HPV t.
renal clearance t.
renal function t.
Reveal HIV-1 antibody t.
Reynell Verbal Comprehension T.
Rinne t.
rollover t.
Romberg t.
Rorschach t.
rosette t.
Rotazyme t.
Rotter Sentence Completion T.
routine preoperative t.
Rovsing t.
Rubin t.
Sabin-Feldman dye t.
SalEst system t.
saline drop t.
salivary estriol t.
Schick t.
Schiff t.
Schiller t.
Schilling t.
Schober t.
Scotch tape slide t.
screening laboratory t.
Sephadex binding t.
serologic t.
serum t.
serum anti-GQ1b antibody t.
shake t.
Short Michigan Alcoholism
Screening T. (SMAST)
Sickledex t.
similarities t.
Sims-Huhner t.
SISI t.
4-site skinfold t.
skin prick t.
Snellen t.
Soluprick skin prick t.
Sonoclot t.
Southern blot t.
sperm agglutination t.
sperm function t.
sperm immobilization t.
SpermMar mixed antiglobulin
reaction t.
spirometric t.
spot t.
stable microbubble t.
Staclot t.

T

test (*continued*)

    standardized t.
    Stanford-Binet Intelligence T.
    Stanford Diagnostic Reading T.
    stimulation t.
    stool antigen t.
    STORCH t.
    straight catheter t.
    Streptex rapid strep t.
    streptococcus rapid antigen
        detection t.
    Streptozyme t.
    stress t.
    strip t.
    t. strip
    Stroop t.
    sucrose hemolysis t.
    SUDS HIV-1 antibody t.
    sunflower oil challenge t.
    supine empty stress t.
        (SEST)
    supine pressor t.
    supravital stain t.
    SureCell herpes t.
    SurePath liquid-based Pap t.
    swab t.
    sweat chloride t.
    swinging flashlight t.
    swordfish t.
    Syva t.
    talar tilt t.
    tampon t.
    Tandem-R Ostase osteoporosis t.
    TCT coagulation t.
    Tensilon t.
    tetraiodothyronine t.
    Thayer-Martin gonorrhea t.
    therapeutic pulmonary function t.
    ThinPrep Pap t.
    Thorn t.
    thrombin clot t.
    thrombin clotting time coagulation t.
    Thrombostat platelet function t.
    Thrombo-Wellco t.
    thrombus precursor protein t.
    thymol turbidity t.
    thyroid function t. (TFT)
    thyrotropin-releasing hormone
        stimulation t. (TRH-ST)
    thyroxine t.
    tilt t.
    tilt-table t.
    tine t.
    tissue thromboplastin-inhibition t.
    Titmus stereoacuity t.
    TOH t.
    TOL t.
    toluidine blue t.
    TPI t.

    TpP t.
    Trail Making T.
    transglutaminase antibody t.
    transmission disequilibrium t. (TDT)
    transmission/disequilibrium t.
    tray agglutination t. (TAT)
    Trendelenburg t.
    Treponema pallidum
        immobilization t.
    triiodothyronine t.
    triple screen t.
    triple swab t.
    tuberculin t.
    tuberculin skin t. (TST)
    Tuttle t.
    TWEAK t.
    Tzanck t.
    UCG-Slide T.
    Uni-Gold Recombine HIV t.
    urea breath t. (UBT)
    urinary concentration t.
    urinary dipstick t.
    urine CIE t.
    urine ferric chloride t.
    urine latex t.
    Uriscreen urine t.
    vaginal cornification t.
    vaginal mucification t.
    van den Bergh t.
    VDRL t.
    Venning-Brown t.
    ViraPap HPV DNA t.
    ViraType t.
    visual-motor integration t.
    visual-perceptual t.
    Vysis PathVysion genomic disease
        management t.
    Wada t.
    Wampole t.
    Wasserman t.
    water t.
    Watson-Schwartz t.
    Weber t.
    Wepman Auditory Discrimination T.
    Western blot t.
    wet mount t.
    wheat sperm agglutination t.
    whiff amine t.
    Whitaker t.
    Wide Range Assessment of Memory
        and Learning T.
    Wisconsin Card Sorting T. (WCST)
    withdrawal bleeding t.
    Woman Abuse Screening T.
        (WAST)
    Woodcock-Johnson reading t.
    WRAML t.
    Xenopus t.
    Ziehl-Neelsen t.

zona-free hamster egg penetration t.
ZstatFlu t.

test/assay

Berkson-Gage t./a.

tester

TCI OvuLook ovulation t.

testes (*pl. of* testis)

testicle

undescended t.

testicular

t. absence
t. appendage
t. appendage torsion
t. atrophy
t. attachment
t. cancer
t. descent
t. differentiation
t. dislocation
t. dysfunction
t. dysgenesis
t. failure
t. feminization (TF)
t. feminization syndrome
t. flow scan
t. growth
t. hematoma
t. hypertrophy
t. Kaposi sarcoma
t. leukemia
t. neoplasm
t. pull-down
t. relapse
t. rupture
t. sperm aspiration (TESA)
t. sperm extraction (TESE)
t. steroidogenesis
t. tumor
t. volume

testing

airway reactivity t.
ambulatory t.
antenatal t.
antepartum t.
antepartum fetal t.
antimicrobial susceptibility t.
audiological t.
audiometric t.
breath t.
bronchial provocation t.
carrier t.
couple t.
cranial nerve t.
dexamethasone suppression t. (DST)
DNA t.
DNA-based t.
DNA methylation t.
dynamic t.
dynamic exercise t.

fecal occult blood t. (FOBT)
fetal maturity t.
fetal surveillance t.
FP blood lead t.
genetic t.
inhalation bronchial challenge t.
Institute of Personality and Ability
   T. (IPAT)
invasive t.
laryngopharyngeal sensory
   stimulation t.
ligase chain reaction t.
LPSS t.
manual muscle t.
methacholine provocation t.
multichannel urodynamic t.
muscle t.
mutation t.
neurophysiologic t.
nonreassuring fetal t.
OAE t.
oral glucose tolerance t. (OGTT)
outpatient fetal nonstress t.
Papnet t.
paracoccidioidin skin t.
postcoital t.
preimplantation HLA t.
prenatal t.
provocative bronchial challenge t.
pulmonary function t.
rapid filter t.
rectal compliance t.
routine prenatal t.
rubella factor t.
salivary estriol t.
serologic t.
Simultaneous Technique for Acuity
   and Readiness T. (STAR)
single-channel urodynamic t.
2-step t.
sweat t.
TEOAE t.
thermoregulatory sweat t.
thyrotropin t.
tuberculin t.
upright tilt-table t.
urodynamic t.
urodynamics t.
Weil-Felix antibody t.

testis, *pl.* **testes**

absent t.
acquired ascending undescended t.
adenocarcinoma of infantile t.
anular t.
appendix t.
canalicular t.
contralateral hypertrophy of testes
cryptorchid t.
t. determination

T

testis (*continued*)
    dislocated t.
    testes down
    dysgenetic t.
    ectopic t.
    endocrine nonfunctional t.
    femoral t.
    gonadotropin-resistant t.
    hidden t.
    high anular t.
    high scrotal t.
    intraabdominal t.
    t. migration defect
    nonpalpable t.
    perineal t.
    prepenile t.
    rete t.
    retractile t.
    scrotal t.
    spontaneous descent of t.
    superficial ectopic t.
    torsion of t.
    transverse scrotal t.
    true undescended t.
    t. tumor
    undescended t.
    vanished testes
    t. within superficial inguinal pouch
      of Denis Browne
    yolk sac tumor of t.
testis-determining factor (TDF)
testitis (*var. of* orchitis)
testitoxicosis
Testoderm
    T. Transdermal System
    T. TTS
    T. with Adhesive
test-of-cure culture
testolactone
testosterone
    17-alpha-ethinyl t.
    bound t.
    circulating t.
    t. cypionate
    t. enanthate
    ethinyl t.
    free t.
    t. index
    micellar nanoparticle t.
    micronized t.
    non-sex hormone-binding globulin
      bound t.
    plasma t.
    t. propionate cream
    t. receptor
    serum t.
    t. suppression
    topical t.
    total t.

testosterone/dihydrotestosterone ratio
testosterone-estrogen-binding globulin
testosterone-secreting adrenal adenoma
testotoxicosis
Testred
test-revised
    Gardner Expressive One-Word
      Vocabulary T.-R.
    Gray Oral Reading T.-R.
    Peabody Picture Vocabulary T.-R.
    Slosson Oral Reading T.-R.
    Wide Range Achievement T.-R.
Testsimplets prestained slide
test-tube baby
TET
    tubal embryo transfer
tetani
    Clostridium t.
tetania
    t. gravidarum
    t. neonatorum
tetanic
    t. seizure
    t. spasm
    t. uterine contraction
    t. uterus
tetanism
tetanospasmin
tetanus
    t. and diphtheria (Td)
    t. and diphtheria toxoids vaccine
    t. antiserum
    t. antitoxin (TAT)
    cephalic t.
    tetanus, diphtheria and pertussis
      (TdaP)
    diphtheria, pertussis, t. (DPT)
    generalized t.
    t. immunoglobulin (TIg, TIG)
    neonatal t.
    t. neonatorum
    t. neurotoxin
    postpartum t.
    t. prophylaxis
    puerperal t.
    t. toxin
    t. toxoid (TT)
    t. toxoid and diphtheria
    t. toxoid and diphtheria
      vaccine
    t. toxoid booster
    uterine t.
tetanus-diphtheria immunization
tetany
    hypocalcemic t.
    hypomagnesemic t.
    infantile t.
    neonatal t.
    t. of vitamin D deficiency

tethered
    t. catheter
    t. conus medullaris
    t. cord syndrome
    t. spinal cord
tethering
    spinal cord t.
tetrabenazine
tetrabrachius
tetracaine
    t., adrenaline, cocaine (TAC)
    t., epinephrine, cocaine (TEC)
    lidocaine, adrenaline, t.
    lidocaine, epinephrine, t. (LET)
tetrachirus
tetrachloride
    carbon t.
tetracycline
    t. analog
    t. hydrochloride
    t. pleurodesis
    prophylactic t.
tetracycline-induced esophagitis
Tetracyn
tetrad
tetradactyly
tetraethyl lead
tetrahydrobiopterin
    t. cofactor (BH$_4$)
    t. deficiency
tetrahydrocannabinol (THC),
  9-tetrahydrocannabinol
9-tetrahydrocannabinol (*var. of*
  tetrahydrocannabinol)
tetrahydrocortisol
tetrahydrofolate (THF)
tetrahydrofolate-methyltransferase
  deficiency syndrome
tetrahydrogestrinone
tetrahydrozoline
tetraiodothyronine test
tetralogy
    t. of Fallot (TF, TOF)
    t. of Fallot syndrome
tetramastia
tetramelus
tetranitrate
    erythrityl t.
    pentaerythritol t.
tetraotus
tetraparesis
tetraphocomelia-cleft lip-palate syndrome
tetraplegia
    flaccid t.
tetraploid
    t. distribution
    t. embryo
tetraploidy syndrome
tetrascelus

tetrasomy
    chromosome 8p mosaic t.
    t. 15p syndrome
    t. 21q
tetravalent
tetra-X
    t.-X chromosomal aberration
    t.-X syndrome
tetrazolium
    t. dye assay
    nitroblue t. (NBT)
tetrodotoxin poisoning
TEV
    talipes equinovarus
TEWL
    transepidermal water loss
Texas Scottish Rite Hospital (TSRH)
Texidor twinge
TF
    testicular feminization
    tetralogy of Fallot
Tf
    transferrin
TFA
    thigh-foot angle
tFA
    trans fatty acid
TFCC
    triangular fibrocartilaginous
    complex
TFL
    tensor fasciae latae
TFM
    total fat mass
TFP
    trifunctional protein deficiency
TFPI
    tissue factor pathway inhibitor
TfR
    transferrin receptor
TFT
    thyroid function test
TG
    transglutaminase
TGA
    transposition of great arteries
    isolated TGA
    simple TGA
T/Gel shampoo
T-Gesic
TGF
    transforming growth factor
TGF-1
    transforming growth factor-1
TGF-alpha
    transforming growth factor alpha
TGF-beta
    transforming growth factor beta
      TGF-beta birth defect gene

T

TGV
  thoracic gas volume
  transposition of great vessels
T&H
  type and hold
TH
  total hydroperoxide
Thal
  T. fundoplication
  T. intermedia-like syndrome
thalami (*pl. of* thalamus)
thalamostriatal artery
thalamostriate vasculopathy (TSV)
thalamotomy
  stereotactic t.
thalamus, *pl.* **thalami**
thalassanemia (*var. of* thalassemia)
thalassemia, thalassanemia
  alpha t.
  beta t.
  t. facies
  hemoglobin S t. (HbS-Thal)
  homozygous t.
  t. intermedia
  Lepore t.
  t. major
  t. minor
  sickle cell and beta t.
  t. trait
  transfusion-dependent t.
thalassemic patient
thalidomide
  t. embryopathy
  fetal t.
  t. teratogenicity syndrome
thallium
  t. imaging
  t. intoxication
  t. poisoning
thallium-201
thanatophoric
  t. dwarfism
  t. dysplasia
  t. dysplasia syndrome
thawing
  embryo t.
Thayer-Martin
  T.-M. agar
  T.-M. gonorrhea test
  T.-M. medium
THbO2
  total oxyhemoglobin
THC
  tetrahydrocannabinol
the
  T. Cell Sweep
  T. Female Condom
  T. Injury Prevention Program (TIPP)

theca
  t. cell tumor
  t. externa
  t. interna
  lumbar t.
  t. lutein cell
  t. lutein cyst
theca-granulosa cell cooperativity
thecal interstitial cell
thecoma
  luteinized t.
  ovarian t.
Theiler stage
thelarche
  idiopathic premature t.
  precocious t.
  premature t.
theleplasty
theloncus
thelorrhagia
T-helper cell
thenar
Theo-24
Theochron
Theolair
Theon
theophyllinate
  choline t.
theophylline
  t. level
  sustained-release t.
  t. toxicity
theory
  birth trauma t.
  Cartesian t.
  clonal selection t.
  crowding t.
  endorphin, dopamine, prostaglandin t.
  Freud t.
  ganglion trigger t.
  gate-control t.
  grandmother t.
  implantation t.
  Lamarck t.
  t. of mind
  operant conditioning t.
  pulsion t.
  Sampson t.
  set-point t.
  skin trigger t.
  synactive t.
  teleologic t.
  traction t.
  Trivers-Willard t.
Thera-Flur
Thera-Flur-N
TheraGym exercise ball

therapeutic
- t. abortion (TA, TAb, TAB)
- t. anticoagulation
- t. blood level
- t. donor insemination (TDI)
- t. electromembrane (TEM)
- t. heparinization
- t. insemination
- t. insemination, husband (TIH)
- t. option
- t. pulmonary function test
- t. pulmonary lavage
- t. touch
- t. window

therapeutics
- biofield t.

therapist
- respiratory t.
- sex t.
- speech t. (ST)
- vision t.

therapy
- ablation t.
- add-back t.
- adjunctive radiation t.
- adjuvant chemoradiation t.
- aerosol t.
- afterload reduction t.
- aldosterone replacement t.
- alkali t.
- alternative t.
- ambulatory anticoagulation t.
- amnioinfusion t.
- androgen replacement t.
- animal-assisted t. (AAT)
- antenatal corticosteroid t.
- antepartum steroid t.
- antiangiogenic t.
- antibacterial t.
- antibiotic infusion t.
- antibody induction t.
- antibody replacement t.
- anticoagulation t.
- anticysticercal t.
- anti-D t.
- antidepressant t.
- antiemetic t.
- antifungal drug t.
- antihelminthic t.
- antihypertensive t.
- anti-IgE t.
- antiinflammatory t.
- antileukemic t.
- antimicrobial t.
- antioxidant t.
- antiparasitic drug t.
- antiplatelet t.
- antipyretic t.
- antiretroviral t.
- antithyroid drug t.
- antituberculous t.
- antiviral t.
- axillary irradiation t.
- azole t.
- balloon heating t.
- behavioral t. (BT)
- behavioral family systems t. (BFST)
- belly bath t.
- BEP t.
- beta mimetic t.
- biofeedback t.
- biologic t.
- bisphosphonate t.
- bladder installation t.
- blood component t.
- Bobath physical t.
- bolus fluid t.
- breast conservation t. (BCT)
- breast-conserving t. (BCT)
- breast-preserving t.
- broad-spectrum antibiotic t.
- bromocriptine t.
- budesonide t.
- butyrate t.
- caffeine t.
- cancer t.
- chelation t.
- chest physical t. (CPT)
- chest wall radiation t.
- cognitive t.
- cognitive behavioral t. (CBT)
- colloid t.
- colposcopically directed laser t.
- combined hormone t. (CHT)
- conservative t.
- constraint-induced movement t.
- corticosteroid t.
- deficit t.
- definitive t.
- desferrioxamine t.
- dexamethasone t.
- dinitrochlorobenzene t.
- directly observed t. (DOT)
- DNCB t.
- drainage, irrigation, fibrinolytic t. (DRIFT)
- ego-oriented individual t. (EOIT)
- electroconvulsive t. (ECT)
- electrolyte t.
- electroshock t.
- embolization t.
- empiric t.
- endocavitary radiation t.
- enterostomal t.
- enzyme replacement t.
- eradication t.
- estrogen add-back t. (EABT)
- estrogen-progestin replacement t.

T

therapy (*continued*)

estrogen replacement t. (ERT)
exogenous surfactant t.
extended field irradiation t.
external beam radiation t.
external radiation t.
external x-ray t.
ex vivo liver-directed gene t.
eye salvage t.
family t.
fetal drug t.
fibrinolytic t.
flashlamp-pulsed laser t.
fluid replacement t.
frappage t.
Functional Assessment of Cancer T. (FACT)
gene t.
genetic t.
glucocorticosteroid t.
gold t.
group problem-solving t.
growth hormone t.
helmet-molding t.
high-dose t.
highly active antiretroviral t. (HAART)
highly active retroviral t.
home antibiotic infusion t.
hormonal antineoplastic t.
hormone t.
hormone replacement t. (HRT)
HS-tk gene t.
human gene t.
humidification t.
hyperbaric oxygen t. (HOBT)
hyperfractionated radiation t.
immunosuppressive t.
induction t.
inhaled nitric oxide t.
inotropic t.
interactive play t.
interferon t.
internal radiation t.
InterStim t.
interstitial t.
intracisternal t.
intralesional steroid t.
intraperitoneal radiation t.
intravaginal physical t.
intravenous fluid t.
intraventricular fibrinolytic t.
in utero stem cell t.
in vivo gene t.
iodide t.
iron chelation t.
IV anti-D t.
laser t.
LH-RH agonist t.

light t.
l-thyroxine t.
Lupron add-back t.
macrolide t.
maintenance t.
marital t.
massage t.
maternal blood clot patch t.
megavitamin t.
menopausal estrogen replacement t.
milieu t.
mind-body t.
mist t.
monoclonal antibody t.
multidrug t. (MDT)
multisystemic t. (MST)
music t.
myoblast transfer t.
natural hormone replacement t. (NHRT)
neoadjuvant hormonal t. (NHT)
neurodevelopment t. (NDT)
neutron t.
nicotine patch t.
nonadjuvant t.
occupational t. (OT)
octreotide t.
oral contraceptive t. (OCT)
oral hormone replacement t.
oral rehydration t. (ORT)
orthomolecular t.
oxygen t.
pancreatic enzyme replacement t. (PERT)
parenteral fluid t.
patterning t.
percussion t.
percutaneous t.
permission, limited information, specific suggestions, intensive t. (PLISSIT)
phenytoin t.
photodynamic t.
physical t. (PT)
play t.
polyvalent immunoglobulin t.
postmenopausal estrogen replacement t.
primary radiation t.
progestational t.
progestogen support t.
prophylactic antibiotic t.
psychodynamic t.
psychosocial t.
pulse steroid t.
quadrantectomy, axillary dissection, radiation t. (QUART)
radiation t. (RT)
radical surgical t.

radioiodine ablative t.
recombinant enzyme replacement t.
replacement t.
rescue t.
respiratory t.
retinoid t.
t. roll
salvage t.
selective tubal assessment to refine
  reproductive t. (STARRT)
sensory integration t.
sequential hormone t.
sex steroid add-back t.
single-dose methotrexate t.
single-field hyperthermia combined
  with radiation t.
speech t.
stem cell t.
stepdown t.
stepwise antiinflammatory t.
steroid t.
subcutaneous desferrioxamine t.
suicide gene t.
supportive group t.
surfactant replacement t.
surgical t.
surgical myomectomy as
  reproductive t. (SMART)
systemic t.
systemic azole t.
systemic behavior family t.
T-cell antibody induction t.
Thermachoice uterine balloon t.
thiamin t.
thrombolytic t.
tocolytic t.
topical heat t.
transdermal hormone
  replacement t.
transfusion t.
triple-drug t.
uterine balloon t. (UBT)
vaginal estrogen t.
vasopressin t.
vision t.
vitamin t.
xanthochromia t.
x-ray t.
zinc t.
Theratope vaccine
Therex
ThermAblator
Hydro T. (HTA)
ThermaCare menstrual patch
Thermachoice
T. uterine balloon therapy
T. uterine balloon therapy
  system
Therma Jaw hot urologic forceps

thermal
t. balloon ablation
t. balloon system
t. burn
t. gel gradient electrophoresis
t. hat
t. homeostasis
t. injury
t. neutral environment
t. stress
Thermasonic gel warmer
Thermazene
thermic effect of food (TEF)
thermistor
nasal tip t.
t. thermometer
t. wire
ThermoChem-HT system
thermodilution
t. method
pulmonary artery t.
thermodynamic
thermogenesis
brown fat nonshivering t.
nonexercise activity t.
thermogenic response
thermography
thermolability
MTHFR t.
thermometer
basal body t.
Braun tympanic t.
LighTouch Neonate t.
Ototemp 3000 t.
Philips SensorTouch temple t.
767 SureTemp 4 oral t.
Temp-a-dot t.
thermistor t.
Thermoscan Pro-1-Instant t.
Thermoscan tympanic instant t.
thermometry
temporal artery t.
thermoplasty
balloon t.
thermoregulation
hypothalamic t.
thermoregulatory
t. response
t. sweat testing
Thermoscan
T. Pro-1-Instant thermometer
T. tympanic instant thermometer
thermotherapy
Theroxide Wash
theta dimeric protein
thetaiotaomicron
Bacteroides t.
THF
tetrahydrofolate

THI
transient hypogammaglobulinemia of infancy
thiabendazole
thiacetazone
thiamin
t. deficiency
t. hypovitaminemia
t. therapy
thiaminase
thiamin-response sideroblastic anemia
thiazide diuretic
thick
t. blood smear
t. neck
thickened
t. base
t. base of skull
t. endometrial stripe
thickening
bronchial wall t.
bronchiolar t.
decidual mural t.
fusiform nerve t.
intimal t.
nerve t.
nodular nerve t.
nuchal pad t.
pial t.
skin t.
vaginal t.
thickness
endometrial t.
fetal neck fold t.
fetal nuchal translucency t.
nuchal t.
nuchal translucency t. (NTT)
placental t.
skinfold t.
subscapular skinfold t.
triceps skinfold t. (TSF)
Thiemann
T. disease
T. syndrome
Thiersch-Duplay urethroplasty
Thiersch operation
thiethylperazine
thigh-foot
t.-f. angle (TFA)
t.-f. axis
thigh-leg angle (TLA)
thimerosal-free vaccine
thin
t. basement membrane disease (TBMD)
t. basement membrane nephropathy
t. vaginal mucosa
t. vulvar skin

thinking
abstract t.
auditory integration t. (AIT)
t. skill
thin-layer chromatography (TLC)
thinned dermis
thinness
drive for t.
ThinPrep
T. Pap test
T. processor
T. smear
THINsite dressing
thiobarbituric acid-reacting substance (TBARS)
thioctic acid
thiocyanate
thioglycollate broth medium
thioguanine
thiomalate
gold sodium t.
thiopental sodium
Thioplex
thiopropazate
thiopurine methyltransferase (TPMT)
thioridazine hydrochloride
thiosulfate
t. lotion
sodium t.
Thiosulfil
thiotepa
thiothixene
thiphenamil hydrochloride
third
t. and fourth pharyngeal pouch syndrome
t. disease
t. heart sound
t. nerve palsy
t. parallel pelvic plane
t. permanent molar
t. space loss
t. spacing
t. spacing of fluid
t. stage of labor
t. trimester
t. ventricle fenestration
third-degree
t.-d. AV block
t.-d. burn
t.-d. defect
t.-d. descent
t.-d. episiotomy
t.-d. hypospadias
t.-d. laceration
t.-d. prolapse
third-generation progesterone
third-line measure

third-trimester
    t.-t. bleeding (TTB)
    t.-t. measurement
thistle
    milk t.
THL
    true histiocytic lymphoma
thlipsencephalus
Thomas
    T. curette
    T. heel
Thomas-Gaylor biopsy forceps
Thomsen
    T. disease
    T. myotonia congenita
Thomsen-Friedenreich
    T.-F. antigen
    T.-F. antigen assay
thonzonium
thoracentesis
    needle t.
thoraces (*pl. of* thorax)
thoracic
    t. aortogram
    t. asphyxiant dystrophy
    t. cavity
    t. clamp
    t. compression syndrome
    t. duct drainage
    t. duct ligation
    t. gas volume (TGV)
    t. kyphosis
    t. malformation
    t. spine fracture
    t. surgery
    t. trauma
    t. wall excursion
thoracic-pelvic-phalangeal dystrophy
thoracoabdominal (TA)
    t. ectopia cordis
thoracoacromial artery
thoracoamniotic shunt
thoracoceloschisis, thoracogastroschisis
thoracodelphus, thoradelphus
thoracodidymus
thoracodorsal artery
thoracogastrodidymus
thoracogastroschisis
thoracolumbar
    t. gibbus
    t. kyphosis
    t. kyphotic curvature
    t. rachischisis
    t. sympathetic nerve
thoracolumbosacral orthosis (TLSO)
thoracomelus
thoracopagus twin
thoracoparacephalus
thoracoplasty

thoracoschisis
thoracoscope
thoracoscopic pleural débridement
thoracoscopy
thoracostomy
    t. tube
    tube t.
thoracotomy
    closed t.
thoradelphus (*var. of* thoracodelphus)
thorascopic technique
thorax, *pl.* thoraces
    Amazon t.
    t. compression
    great vessel of t.
    milk lines of t.
Thorazine
Thorn test
thought
    t. action fusion
    t. disorder
    t. disturbance
threadworm infestation
thready pulse
threatened
    t. abortion
    t. miscarriage
three
    Pediatric Examination at T. (PEET)
3-day
    3-d. fever
    3-d. measles
three-quarter strength formula
threes
    rule of t.
threonine
threshold
    high pain t.
    high sensory t.
    low pain t.
    low sensory t.
    pain t.
    phenotypic t.
    sensory t.
    speech reception t. (SRT)
    speech recognition t. (SRT)
    t. trait
thrill
    diastolic t.
    presystolic t.
    suprasternal notch t.
thrive
    failure to t. (FTT)
    nonorganic failure to t. (NOFT, NOFTT)
throat
    t. clearing
    eyes, ears, nose, t. (EENT)
    sore t.

T

943

throat (*continued*)
    strep t.
    Sucrets Sore T.
    t. swab
thrombasthenia
    Glanzmann t.
    t. of Glanzmann and Naegeli
thrombectomy
thrombi (*pl. of* thrombus)
thrombin
    t. clot test
    t. clotting time (TCT)
    t. clotting time coagulation test
    t. receptor-activating peptide
    (TRAP)
    topical t.
thrombocyte
thrombocythemia
    essential t. (ET)
    primary t. (PT)
thrombocytopenia
    t. absent radius (TAR)
    alloimmune t.
    autoimmune t.
    congenital amegakaryocytic t.
    consumptive t.
    familial dominant t.
    fetal t.
    fetomaternal alloimmune t. (FMAIT)
    gestational t.
    heparin-induced t. (HIT)
    immune t.
    immune-mediated t.
    incidental t.
    isoimmune fetal t.
    maternal t.
    megakaryocytic t.
    neonatal alloimmune t. (NAIT)
    neonatal autoimmune t.
    neonatal isoimmune t. (NIT)
    transfusion-induced t.
    t. with absent radius syndrome
    X-linked t.
thrombocytopenic purpura
thrombocytosis
thromboembolic
    t. complication
    t. disease (TED)
    t. event (TE)
    t. prophylaxis
thromboembolism
    idiopathic venous t.
    pulmonary t.
    venous t. (VTE)
Thrombogen
thrombohemolytic disease
thrombolytic therapy
thrombomodulin
thrombopenia

thrombophilia
    acquired t.
    factor V Leiden t.
    familial t.
    genetic t.
    hereditary t.
thrombophlebitis
    cortical t.
    deep vein t.
    diffuse cortical t.
    pelvic t.
    pelvic vein t.
    peripheral t.
    septic pelvic t. (SPT)
    septic pelvic vein t.
    sinus t.
    superficial t.
    venous sinus t.
thromboplastin
    plasma t.
thrombopoiesis
thrombopoietin (TPO)
thromboprophylaxis
thromboses (*pl. of* thrombosis)
thrombosis, *pl.* **thromboses**
    anal t.
    arterial t.
    cavernosal artery t.
    cavernous sinus t.
    cerebral t.
    coronary t.
    decidual fibrin t.
    deep vein t. (DVT)
    deep venous t. (DVT)
    dural sinus t.
    dural venous t.
    external anal t.
    intracranial venous sinus t.
    jugular vein t.
    lateral sinus t.
    maternal cortical vein t.
    multiorgan t.
    mural t.
    ovarian vein t. (OVT)
    pelvic ovarian vein t. (POVT)
    placental t.
    pregnancy-associated t.
    purulent venous t.
    renal vascular t.
    renal vein t.
    sagittal sinus t.
    sinus t.
    vacular t.
    vascular t.
    venous sinus t.
thrombospondin
Thrombostat platelet function test
thrombotic
    t. endocarditis

t. microangiopathy (TMA)
t. phlegmasia
t. purpura
t. thrombocytopenic purpura (TTP)
Thrombo-Wellco test
thromboxane
t. A2 (TXA2)
t. dominance
thrombus, *pl.* **thrombi**
chorionic vessel t.
endocardial t.
fibrin t.
intervillous t. (IVT)
intramural t.
t. precursor protein (TpP)
t. precursor protein test
superficial t.
thrush
oral t. (OT)
plaque of t.
t. pneumonia
thrust
jaw t.
manual t.
tongue t.
thumb
broad t.
congenital clasped t.'s
deafness, imperforate anus,
 hypoplastic t.'s
floating t.
gamekeeper's t.
hitchhiker's t.
t. hyperabduction
hypoplastic t.
indwelling t.
t. in palm deformity
mental retardation, aphasia, shuffling
 gait, adducted t.
t. retractor
t. sign
skier's t.
t. spica cast
t. spica splint
stub t.
triphalangeal t.
ThumbGuard appliance
thumbing
cortical t.
thumbsucking
thump
precordial t.
Thurston Holland sign
thymectomy
neonatal t.
thymi (*pl. of* thymus)
thymic
t. agenesis
t. alymphoplasia

t. and parathyroid agenesis
 syndrome
t. aphasia
t. aplasia
t. aplasia syndrome
t. asthma
t. dysplasia
t. hypoplasia
t. hypoplasia anomaly
t. lymphocyte antigen (TL)
t. shadow
t. wave sign
thymic-dependent deficiency
thymicolymphaticus
status t.
thymic-parathyroid aplasia
thymicus
status t.
thymidine analog NRTI
thymine nucleotide
thymocyte
thymol turbidity test
thymoma
thymopoietin
thymosin
thymus, *pl.* **thymi, thymuses**
t. gland
t. hyperplasia
t. primordium
t. transplantation
thymuses (*pl. of* thymus)
Thyrel TRH
thyroarytenoid muscle
thyroglobulin
thyroglossal
t. duct
t. duct cyst
t. duct cyst excision
thyrohypophysial syndrome
thyroid
t. and pituitary agenesis
t. aplasia
t. autoantibody
t. cancer
t. carcinoma
t. crisis
t. deficiency
t. disease
t. dysfunction
ectopic t.
t. enzyme defect
t. function
t. function test (TFT)
t. gland
t. gland dysfunction
t. gland malformation
t. hormone
t. hormone resistance
t. hormone unresponsiveness

T

thyroid (*continued*)
    hypothalamic, pituitary, t. (HTP)
    t. index
    t. Lahey clamp
    t. neoplasia
    t. nodule
    t. ophthalmopathy
    t. scintigraphy
    t. storm
    sublingual t.
    t. transcription factor-1 (TTF-1)
thyroid-binding
    t.-b. globulin (TBG)
    t.-b. globulin deficiency
thyroidectomy
thyroiditis
    acute suppurative t.
    autoimmune t.
    chronic lymphocytic t.
    Hashimoto t.
    lymphocytic t.
    postpartum t. (PPT)
    postviral subacute t.
    subacute t.
    suppurative t.
thyroid-related ophthalmopathy (TRO)
thyroid-specific enhancer binding protein-1 (T4/ebp-1)
thyroid-stimulating
    t.-s. hormone (TSH)
    t.-s. hormone assay
    t.-s. immunoglobulin
Thyrolar
thyrolingual cyst
thyrotoxic crisis, thyroid crisis
thyrotoxicosis
    gestational t.
    neonatal t.
thyrotrope
thyrotrophic (*var. of* thyrotropic)
thyrotrophin (*var. of* thyrotropin)
thyrotropic, thyrotrophic
    t. hormone
thyrotropin, thyrotrophin
    chorionic t.
    t. deficiency
    neonatal t.
    t. releasing hormone (TRH)
    serum t.
    t. testing
thyrotropin-releasing hormone stimulation test (TRH-ST), TRH-stimulation test
thyrotropin-secreting pituitary adenoma
thyroxin (*var. of* thyroxine)
thyroxine (T4), thyroxin
    free t.
    t. synthesis
    t. test

thyroxine-binding
    t.-b. globulin (TBG)
    t.-b. globulin deficiency
    t.-b. protein (TBP)
TIA
    transient ischemic attack
tiagabine
Tiamol
Tiazac
TIBC
    total iron-binding capacity
tibia, *pl.* **tibiae**
    congenital longitudinal deficiency of t.
    congenital pseudoarthrosis of t.
    osteochondrosis deformans tibiae
    posteromedial bow of t.
    pseudarthrosis of t.
    t. vara
tibiae (*pl. of* tibia)
tibial
    t. aplasia-ectrodactyly syndrome
    t. bowing
    childhood accidental spiral t. (CAST)
    t. epiphysis
    t. film
    t. hemimelia
    t. metaphysis
    t. pseudarthrosis
    t. shaft fracture
    t. speed
    t. speed of sound
    t. stress fracture
    t. torsion
    t. tubercle
    t. valgus osteotomy
    t. version
tibiofibular syndesmosis
tibolone
TIC
    ticarcillin
tic
    chronic t.
    complex motor t.
    complex vocal t.
    cough t.
    t. disorder
    maladie des t.'s
    motor t.
    multiple t.'s
    psychogenic cough t.
    simple motor t.
    simple vocal t.
    t. symptom
    vocal t.
Ticar
ticarcillin
    t. and clavulanate potassium

t. clavulanate
t. disodium
ticarcillin/clavulanic acid
Tice BCG
tick
t. bite
deer t.
dog t.
t. fever
Lone Star t.
t. paralysis
Rocky Mountain wood t.
wood t.
tick-borne
t.-b. encephalitis (TBE)
t.-b. infection
t.-b. relapsing fever
t.-b. typhus
ticlopidine
ticonazole
Ticon Injection
TID
tubal inflammatory damage
tidal
t. breathing
t. liquid ventilation (TLV)
t. volume (TV, VT)
tide mark dermatitis
tie
free t.
silk t.
stitch t.
Tietze syndrome
TIG
tetanus immunoglobulin
TIg
tetanus immunoglobulin
Tigan
T. Injection
T. Rectal
tight heel cord
tightness
idiopathic heel-cord t.
Tilade Inhalation Aerosol
Tillaux
T. disease
T. fracture
fracture of T.
tilt
head t.
head-up t. (HUT)
lateral head t.
pelvic t.
t. test
ulnar t.
tilted disc
tilt-table test
tiludronate

time
activated clotting t. (ACT)
activated partial thromboplastin t. (APTT)
bleeding t.
capillary filling t.
capillary refill t.
cell generation t.
circulation t.
clotting t.
doubling t.
euglobulin clot lysis t. (ECLT)
euglobulin lysis t. (ELT)
gastric emptying t.
incision-to-clamp t.
incision-to-delivery t.
inspiration t. (I-time)
inspiratory t. (IT)
intestinal transit t.
isovolumic relaxation t. (IVR)
Ivy bleeding t.
kaolin clotting t.
Lee-White clotting t.
orocecal transit t.
partial thromboplastin t. (PTT)
t. position scan
prothrombin t. (pro-time, PT)
recovery t.
reptilase t.
Rite T.
Russell viper venom t.
sinoatrial conduction t.=
sperm generation t.
thrombin clotting t. (TCT)
timed
t. endometrial biopsy
t. intercourse
Timentin
time-of-flight and absorbance (TOFA)
time-out
timer
Apgar t.
time-resolved fluoroimmunoassay
timing
coital t.
optimal t.
Timolide
timolol maleate
Timoptic Ophthalmic
Timoptic-XE Ophthalmic
timothy grass
tin
t. ear syndrome
t. mesoporphyrin (SnMP)
t. protoporphyrin (SnPP)
Tinactin

T

tincture
>alcoholic t.
>t. of iodine
>opium t.

Tindamax

T-independent antigen

tinea
>t. capitis
>t. corpus
>t. cruris
>t. gladiatorum
>t. incognito
>t. manuum
>t. nigra palmaris
>t. pedis
>t. profunda
>t. rubrum
>t. unguium
>t. versicolor

tine test

tinidazole

tinnitus

tinted

TINU
>tubulointerstitial nephritis

tioconazole 6.5% ointment

TIP
>tubularized incised plate

tip
>bulbous nasal t.
>Corometrics Gold Quik Connect
> Spiral electrode t.
>Frazier suction t.
>needle t.

TIPP
>The Injury Prevention Program

TIPS
>transjugular intrahepatic portosystemic
>shunt

tiptoeing

TIR
>trophoblast in regression

tired housewife syndrome

Tischler cervical biopsy forceps

Tischler-Morgan
>T.-M. biopsy punch
>T.-M. uterine biopsy forceps

Tisit
>T. Blue Gel
>T. Liquid
>T. Shampoo

tissue
>accessory ovarian t.
>t. activator-induced fibrinolysis
>adipose t.
>anechoic t.
>t. anoxia
>attenuating t.
>breast biopsy t.

bronchus-associated lymphoid t.
  (BALT)
t. catabolism
choriodecidual t.
conductive t.
t. confirmation
connective t.
contused t.
t. culture-grown attenuated virus
t. Doppler imaging (TDI)
echogenic t.
ectopic endometrial t.
ectopic ovarian t.
embryonic t.
endometriotic t.
epipericardial connective t.
erectile t.
t. expander
t. expansion vaginoplasty
t. factor
t. factor pathway inhibitor (TFPI)
fibroareolar t.
fibrous connective t.
fibrovascular t.
t. forceps
fragile t.
gastrointestinal-associated lymphoid t.
  (GALT)
glandular t.
granulation t.
gut-associated lymphoid t. (GALT)
t. homogeneity
hyperplastic lymphoid t.
hypertrophied t.
t. inhibitors of metalloproteinase
t. insulin resistance
intestine-associated lymphoid t.
  (IALT)
intralobular connective t.
larynx-associated lymphoid t.
  (LALT)
t. link floating ball
t. loss
lymphoid t.
maternal t.
mucosa-associated lymphoid t.
  (MALT)
nasopharyngeal-associated lymphoid
  t. (NALT)
t. necrosis
neovascular t.
neural crest t.
paravaginal soft t.
pelvic connective t.
perilobular connective t.
persistent trophoblastic t.
t. pH monitoring
placental trophoblastic t.
t. plasminogen activator (TPA, t-PA)

t. regeneration
residual ductal t.
retroperitoneal soft t.
t. sampling
scar t.
soft t.
sonolucent t.
t. specific imaging
splenic t.
t. study
subareolar t.
sympathetic t.
syngeneic t.
t. synthesis
t. thromboplastin-inhibition test
t. tolerance to radiation
t. transglutaminase (tTG)
t. transplant
trophoblastic t.
true breast t.
t. typing
xenogeneic t.
tissue-specific antibody
Tis-u-Trap endometrial suction
titanium
t. elastic nail
t. elastic nailing (TEN)
t. staple
titer
ADB t.
AH t.
ANCA t.
antichlamydial antibody t.
anti-DNase B t.
anti-ds DNA antibody t.
antihyaluronidase t.
antimycoplasma t.
anti-Rho(D) t.
Forssman t.
geometric mean t. (GMT)
HI t.
IgG antibody t.
IgM antibody t.
maternal t.
non-*Treponema* t.
t. of anti-ragweed IgE antibody
RPR t.
rubeola t.
serum bactericidal t. (SBT)
serum inhibitory t. (SIT)
sheep cell agglutinin t.
TORCH t.
viral t.
virus t.
Titmus stereoacuity test
Titralac Plus Liquid
titrate
titration
skin end-point t.

titubation
head t.
TIV
trivalent inactivated influenza vaccine
TKO
to keep open
TL
thymic lymphocyte antigen
tubal ligation
TLA
thigh-leg angle
TLC
thin-layer chromatography
total lung capacity
TLC antiseptic soap
TL-90 Ethicon stapler
TLV
tidal liquid ventilation
total liquid ventilation
TMA
thrombotic microangiopathy
transcription-mediated amplification
transmalleolar axis angle
TMA assay
T-max
maximum temperature
TMD
transient myeloproliferative disorder
TMES
transient marrow edema syndrome of hip
TMJ
temporomandibular joint
TMP-SMX
trimethoprim-sulfamethoxazole
TMS
transcranial magnetic stimulation
TND
transient neonatal diabetes
TNDM
transient neonatal diabetes mellitus
TNF
tumor necrosis factor
TNF-alpha
tumor necrosis factor alpha
TNF-alpha converting enzyme
TNM
tumor, node, metastases
TNM classification
TNM nomenclature
TNM schema
TNR
tonic neck reflex
TnT
troponin T
T&O
tubes and ovaries
TOA
tuboovarian abscess

949

to-and-fro
    t.-a.-f. flow
    t.-a.-f. murmur
TOAPOT
    tuboovarian abscess after previous
    tubal occlusion
toast
    bananas, rice, applesauce, tea, t.
    (BRATT)
    bananas, rice cereal, applesauce, t.
    (BRAT)
tobacco
    smokeless t.
Tobey ear rongeur
TOBI
    tobramycin solution for inhalation
Tobin index
TobraDex
tobramycin
    t. solution
    t. solution for inhalation
    (TOBI)
Tobrex Ophthalmic
TOC
    tuboovarian complex
tococardiography
tocodynagraph
tocodynamometer
tocodynamometry
    remote t.
tocograph
tocography
tocology
tocolysis
    acute t.
    prenatal t.
    prophylactic t.
tocolytic
    t. agent
    t. drug
    t. therapy
tocometer
tocopherol deficiency
tocophobia
tocotransducer
Today vaginal contraceptive sponge
Todd
    T. paralysis
    T. paresis
Todd-Hewitt broth
toddler-age nodulocystic acne
toddler's
    t. diarrhea
    t. fracture
Toddler Temperament Scale
toe
    adducted great t.
    broad t.
    catheter t.
    clubbing of fingers and t.'s
    curly t.
    floating great t.
    t. grasp
    great t.
    hammer t.
    mallet t.
    overlapping t.
    overriding t.
    pigeon t.
    searching t.
    striatal t.
    t. syndactyly
    t. walking
toeing
    t. in
    t. out
toe-in gait
toenail
    ingrown t.
toe-off
toe-out gait
Toesen
toe-walking
TOFA
    time-of-flight and absorbance
TOF
    tetralogy of Fallot
    tracheoesophageal fistula
Togaviridae
togavirus
TOH
    Tower of Hanoi
    TOH test
toilet
    pulmonary t.
    respiratory t.
    t. training
toileting problem
to keep open
Tokos monitor
TOL
    Tower of London
    trial of labor
    TOL test
TOLAC
    trial of labor after cesarean
Tolamide
tolazamide
tolazoline hydrochloride
tolbutamide
Tolectin DS
tolerance
    antigen t.
    carbohydrate t.
    glucose t.
    immunologic t.
    impaired glucose t. (IGT)

radiation t.

t., worried, eye opener, amnesia, kut (cut) down (TWEAK)

Tolerex formula

tolfenamic acid

Tolinase

tolmetin

tolnaftate

Tolosa-Hunt syndrome

tolterodine

toluene sniffing

toluidine

t. blue

t. blue stain

t. blue test

Tolu-Sed DM

tomaculous neuropathy

Tom Jones closure

tomogram

tomographic

tomography

automated computerized axial t. (ACAT)

computed t. (CT)

computed axial t. (CAT)

computerized t.

delayed phase computed t.

electron-beam computed t. (EBCT)

focused computed t.

high-resolution chest computed t.

high-resolution computed t. (HRCT)

hypocycloidal t.

optic t.

positron emission t. (PET)

quantitative computed t. (QCT)

single-photon emission t. (SPECT)

single-photon emission computed t. (SPECT)

Somatom Plus computed t.

spiral computed t.

Tompkins

T. median bivalving technique

T. metroplasty

T. procedure

tone

anal sphincter t.

bronchomotor t.

decreased anal t.

decreased sphincter t.

detrusor t.

fetal t.

flaccid t.

flexor t.

fluctuating t.

high t.

low muscle t.

muscle t.

parasympathetic t.

phasic t.

poor muscle t.

postural t.

pulmonary vascular t.

sphincter t.

uterine t.

vagal t.

vascular t.

tongs

Gardner-Wells t.

tongue

t. biting

black hairy t.

chameleon t.

t. crib

crocodile t.

darting t.

t. depressor

t. fasciculation

fern leaf t.

fissured t.

free t.

geographic t.

hairy t.

hypoplastic t.

large t.

protruding t.

t. protrusion reflex

raspberry t.

red strawberry t.

scrotal t.

t. size

smooth t.

strawberry t.

surface furrowing of t.

t. thrust

white strawberry t.

tongue-lip adhesion

tongue-tied

tonic

t. downgaze

t. labyrinthine reflex

t. neck pattern

t. neck reflex (TNR)

t. neck response

t. seizure

tonic-clonic

t.-c. convulsion

t.-c. movement

t.-c. seizure

t.-c. seizure activity

Tonnis hip dysplasia procedure

tonometry

gastric t.

gut t.

tonsil

cerebellar t.

palatine t.

T

tonsillar, tonsillary
    t. edema
    t. exudate
tonsillary (*var. of* tonsillar)
tonsillectomy and adenoidectomy (T&A)
tonsillitis
    acute exudative t.
    acute follicular t.
    adenoviral t.
    exudative t.
    follicular t.
    streptococcal t.
    white t.
tonsillopharyngeal exudate
tonsillopharyngitis
    streptococcal t.
tonsurans
    Trichophyton t.
tonus
    baseline t.
    uterine t.
tool
    Adolescent and Pediatric Pain T. (APPT)
    SCHIP evaluation t.
too-soft voice
tooth, *pl.* **teeth**
    t. and nail syndrome
    baby teeth
    t. bud
    canine t.
    conical teeth
    crowded teeth
    t. decay
    deciduous teeth
    dystrophic t.
    Fournier t.
    Hutchinson teeth
    hypoplastic teeth
    t. loss
    milk t.
    missing teeth
    Moon teeth
    natal teeth
    neonatal teeth
    peglike teeth
    permanent teeth
    pitted teeth
    t. placement
    precocious teeth
    predeciduous teeth
    primary teeth
    t. root resorption
    screwdriver teeth
    secondary teeth
    wisdom t.
    X-linked cataract with hutchinsonian teeth
toothbrush culture technique

Topamax
Topaz-UPS
Topcon Screenoscope
topectomy
tophi (*pl. of* tophus)
tophus, *pl.* **tophi**
    urate t.
Topicaine
topical
    Achromycin T.
    Aclovate T.
    Acticort T.
    Aeroseb-HC T.
    Ala-Cort T.
    Ala-Scalp T.
    Alphatrex T.
    Anusol HC-1 T.
    Anusol HC-2.5% T.
    Aristocort T.
    Aristocort A T.
    A/T/S T.
    Baciguent T.
    Benadryl T.
    Betatrex T.
    Caldecort T.
    Caldesene T.
    Canesten T.
    Carmol-HC T.
    Cetacort T.
    Cloderm T.
    t. concentrated TCA
    CortaGel T.
    Cortaid Maximum Strength T.
    Cortaid with Aloe T.
    Cort-Dome T.
    Cortef Feminine Itch T.
    Cortizone-10 T.
    Cortizone-5 T.
    Cruex T.
    Cyclocort T.
    Delcort T.
    Dermacort T.
    Dermarest Dricort T.
    Derma-Smoothe/FS T.
    Dermolate T.
    Dermtex HC with Aloe T.
    DesOwen T.
    Diprolene AF T.
    Diprosone T.
    Efudex T.
    Eldecort T.
    Eurax T.
    Exelderm T.
    Fluoroplex T.
    Gynecort T.
    t. heat therapy
    Hi-Cor-1.0 T.
    Hi-Cor-2.5 T.
    Hycort T.

Hydrocort T.
Hydro-Tex T.
Hytone T.
t. imidazole
t. iodine application
Kenalog T.
LactiCare-HC T.
Lanacort T.
Locoid T.
Lotrimin T.
Maxivate T.
MetroGel T.
Micatin T.
Monistat-Derm T.
Mycitracin T.
Mycogen II T.
Mycolog-II T.
Mytrex F T.
NGT T.
t. nitroglycerin
Nutracort T.
Orabase HCA T.
Ovide T.
Oxistat T.
Pedi-Dri T.
Pedi-Pro T.
Penecort T.
t. podophyllin
Polysporin T.
Rogaine T.
Scalpicin T.
Solarcaine T.
S-T Cort T.
Synacort T.
Synalar T.
Synemol T.
Tegrin-HC T.
t. testosterone
t. thrombin
t. treatment
Triacet T.
Tridesilon T.
Triple Antibiotic T.
U-Cort T.
Undoguent T.
Uticort T.
Vitec T.
Vytone T.
Westcort T.
Topicort
T. cream
T. ointment
Topicort-LP
Topilene
topiramate
Topisone
topographic cervical
topography
perisulcal t.

topoisomerase-1 inhibitor
Toposar Injection
topotecan hydrochloride
Topsyn
Toradol
T. injection
T. Oral
TORCH
toxoplasmosis, other agents, rubella, cytomegalovirus, herpes simplex
TORCH infection
TORCH screen
TORCH syndrome
TORCH titer
toremifene citrate
Toriello-Carey
T.-C. sign
T.-C. syndrome
Toriello syndrome (1, 2)
Torkildsen procedure
Toronto
T. Alexithymia Scale (TAS)
T. parapodium
torovirus
Torpin cul-de-sac resection
Torpin-Waters-McCall culdoplasty
torque depressor
torr
torrential pulmonary flow
torsade de pointes
torsemide
torsion
adnexal t.
appendage t.
appendix testis t.
cord t.
t. dystonia
external femoral t.
external tibial t.
femoral t.
internal femoral t.
internal tibial t.
intravaginal testicular t.
lateral femoral t. (LFT)
lateral tibial t. (LTT)
medial femoral t. (MFT)
medial tibial t. (MTT)
t. of adnexa
t. of appendix
t. of endometrioma
t. of gut
t. of ovary
t. of testis
ovarian t.
penile t.
splenic t.
testicular appendage t.
tibial t.

T

torsional
- t. alignment
- t. deformity
- t. profile

torso presentation

Torsten Sjögren syndrome

torti
- pili t.

torticollis
- acquired t.
- acute t.
- benign paroxysmal t.
- congenital muscular t.
- idiopathic t.
- infantile muscular t.
- juvenile muscular t.
- muscular t.
- neonatal t.
- paroxysmal t.
- paroxysmal infantile t.
- spasmodic t.

tortuosity
- retinal venous dilation and t. (RVDT)

tortuous capillary

Torulopsis glabrata

torulosis

torus fracture

tosylarginine
- t. methyl ester (TAME)
- t. methyl ester esterase

tosylate
- bretylium t.

TOT
- tension-free obturator tape
- transobturator tape

total
- t. abdominal hysterectomy (TAH)
- t. anomalous pulmonary venous connection (TAPVC)
- t. anomalous pulmonary venous return (TAPVR)
- t. ascertainment
- t. bilirubin
- t. blood volume (TBV)
- t. body iron
- t. body iron content
- t. body irradiation (TBI)
- t. body potassium (TBK)
- t. body sodium
- t. body surface area (TBSA)
- t. body water (TBW)
- t. breech extraction
- t. cavopulmonary anastomosis
- t. cavopulmonary connection
- t. colonic aganglionosis
- t. colpectomy
- t. communication
- t. daily energy expenditure (TDEE)

- T. Eclipse moisturizing skin lotion
- t. energy expenditure
- t. fat mass (TFM)
- t. hemispherectomy
- t. hemolytic complement
- t. hepatectomy
- t. hydroperoxide (TH)
- t. iron-binding capacity (TIBC)
- t. liquid ventilation (TLV)
- t. lung capacity (TLC)
- t. magnesium
- t. mastectomy
- t. mixing lesion
- t. muscle paralysis
- t. oxyhemoglobin
- t. parenteral nutrition (TPN)
- t. parenteral nutrition-associated cholestasis
- t. pelvic exenteration (TPE)
- t. perineal rupture
- t. peripheral parenteral nutrition (TPPN)
- t. peripheral resistance (TPR)
- t. placenta previa
- t. previa
- t. pulmonary resistance
- t. quality management (TQM)
- t. serum bilirubin (TSB)
- t. testosterone
- t. testosterone index
- t. vaginal vault prolapse
- t. villous atrophy
- t. weight gain

totalis
- alopecia universalis t.
- rachischisis t.
- situs inversus t.

totipotent cell

totipotential cell

toto
- in t.

touch
- t. imprint
- therapeutic t.

Tourette
- T. disease
- T. disorder (TD)
- Gilles de la T.
- T. syndrome

tourniquet
- hair t.

TOVA
- Test of Variables of Attention
- TOVA ADD/ADHD assessment

Towako transvaginal-transmyometrial embryo transfer method

towel
- t. clip
- DisCide disinfecting t.

tower
    T. of Hanoi (TOH)
    T. of London (TOL)
    t. skull
Townes-Brocks syndrome
Townes syndrome
Townsend
    T. biopsy punch
    T. endocervical biopsy curette
toxemia, toxicemia
    florid t.
    t. of pregnancy
    preeclamptic t. (PET)
    t. syndrome
toxemic
    t. rash of pregnancy
    t. retinopathy of pregnancy
    t. shock syndrome
toxic
    t. alopecia
    t. appearance
    t. cascade
    t. dynamics
    t. epidermal necrolysis (TEN)
    t. erythema
    t. hepatitis
    t. ingestion
    t. megacolon
    t. myocarditis
    t. neuropathy
    t. oil syndrome
    t. shock
    t. shock syndrome (TSS)
    t. shock syndrome toxin-1 (TSST-1)
    t. synovitis
toxicemia (var. of toxemia)
toxicity
    acetaminophen t.
    alkali t.
    aluminum t.
    bismuth t.
    bone marrow t.
    carbon monoxide t.
    chronic cyanide t.
    citrate t.
    cognitive t.
    cyanide t.
    hematologic t.
    iron t.
    lidocaine t.
    methylmercury t.
    oxygen t.
    phosphate t.
    salicylate t.
    systemic t.
    theophylline t.
    zinc t.
    t. zone
toxicokinetics

toxicologic analysis
toxicology screen
toxicosis
    copper t.
    idiopathic copper t.
toxicum
    erythema neonatorum t.
toxidrome
toxin
    albumin-bound t.
    bacterial t.
    botulinum t.
    botulinum t. A (BTA)
    botulism t.
    clostridial t.
    Clostridium botulinum type A t.
    diphtheria t. (DT)
    environmental t.
    epidermolytic t.
    epsilon t.
    t. exposure
    pertussis t. (PT)
    reproductive t.
    Shiga t. (Stx)
    Shiga-like t.
    tetanus t.
toxin-1
    toxic shock syndrome t.-1 (TSST-1)
toxin-induced scarlet fever exanthema
Toxocara
    T. canis
    T. cati
toxocariasis
toxoid
    pertussis t. (PT)
    pneumococcal conjugate diphtheria t. (PncD)
    tetanus t. (tet_tox, tet tox, TT)
Toxoplasma
    T. antigen
    T. encephalitis
    T. gondii
    T. lymphadenopathy
toxoplasmic
    t. chorioretinitis
    t. encephalitis
toxoplasmosis
    congenital t.
    fetal t.
    ocular t.
    t., other agents, rubella, cytomegalovirus, herpes simplex (TORCH)
    t., other agents, rubella, cytomegalovirus, herpes simplex virus
    t. retinitis
    t., rubella, cytomegalovirus, herpes simplex, syphilis

T

toy
    ride-on t.
TPA, t-PA
    tissue plasminogen activator
TPAL
    term infants, premature infants,
      abortions, living children
TPC
    tympanocentesis
TPE
    total pelvic exenteration
TPH
    transplacental hemorrhage
      TPH test
TPHA
    Treponema pallidum hemagglutination
T-Phyl
TPI
    Treponema pallidum immobilization
    triose phosphate isomerase
      TPI deficiency
      TPI test
TPMT
    thiopurine methyltransferase
      TPMT deficiency
TPN
    total parenteral nutrition
TPO
    thrombopoietin
      plasma TPO
TPP
    tubal perfusion pressure
TpP
    thrombus precursor protein
      TpP test
TPPN
    total peripheral parenteral nutrition
TPR
    total peripheral resistance
TQM
    total quality management
TRA
    traumatic rupture of thoracic aorta
trabectedin
trabecular muscular septum
trabeculate
trabeculodysgenesis
trabeculotomy
Trace-4
trace metal
tracer
    radioactive t.
Trach Care suction
trachea, *pl.* **tracheae**
    blind t.
    stenosis of t.
tracheae (*pl. of* trachea)
tracheal
    t. agenesis syndrome

    t. aspirate
    t. atresia
    t. catheter
    t. compression
    t. intubation
    t. lavage
    t. occlusion
    t. stenosis
    t. suctioning
    t. tube
    t. tumor
    t. web
tracheal-aspirate culture
tracheitis, trachitis
    acute t.
    bacterial t.
    subacute t.
trachelectomy
    radical vaginal t.
trachelitis
trachelobregmatic diameter
trachelopanus
trachelopexia, trachelopexy
trachelopexy (*var. of* trachelopexia)
tracheloplasty
    ex utero intrapartum t. (EXIT)
trachelorrhaphy
tracheloschisis
trachelotomy
tracheobronchial
    t. aspirate
    t. aspirate fluid (TAF)
    t. compression
    t. obstruction
    t. remnant
    t. trauma
    t. tree
    t. tree injury
tracheobronchitis
tracheobronchomalacia
tracheobronchomegaly
tracheocutaneous fistula
tracheoesophageal
    t. atresia
    t. fistula (TEF, TOF)
    t. septation
    t. septum
tracheomalacia
    intrathoracic t.
    primary t.
    secondary t.
tracheostomy
    flap t.
    percutaneous t.
    t. tube
    t. tube flange
tracheotome
    Sierra-Sheldon t.
tracheotomy (trach)

trachitis (*var. of* tracheitis)
trachoma inclusion conjunctivitis (TRIC)
trachomatis
    Chlamydia t. (CT)
tracing
    lead t.
    NST t.
track
    bear t.'s
tracker
    Breath T.
tracking
    J t.
    visual t.
Tracrium
tract
    aerodigestive t.
    anogenital t.
    benign mesothelioma of
      genital t.
    biliary t.
    brainstem auditory t.
    dermal sinus t.
    dermoid sinus t.
    endomesenchymal t.
    extrahepatic biliary t.
    extrapyramidal t.
    female reproductive t.
    gastrointestinal t.
    genital outflow t.
    genitourinary t.
    gooseneck deformity of left
      ventricular outflow t.
    intestinal t.
    left ventricular outflow t. (LVOT)
    Lissauer t.
    lower genital t.
    lower respiratory t.
    mesolimbic dopamine t.
    narrow pulmonary outflow t.
      (NPOT)
    nerve t.
    nigrostriatal t.
    outflow t.
    patch unroofing of outflow t.
    pin t.
    proximal outflow t.
    pulmonary outflow t.
    pyramidal t.
    renal t.
    reproductive t.
    respiratory t.
    right ventricular outflow t. (RVOT)
    sinus t.
    suppurating sinus t.
    upper respiratory t.
    urinary t.
    urogenital t.
    ventricular outflow t.

traction
    t. alopecia
    t. apophysitis
    t. apophysitis of medial epicondyle
    t. atrophy
    axial t.
    axis t.
    Bryant t.
    45-degree skin t.
    distal femoral skeletal t.
    t. enterocele
    halo t.
    t. injury
    Russell t.
    skeletal t.
    skin t.
    t. theory
    t. treatment
tractional retinal detachment
traditional surrogacy
traffic-light diet
tragi (*pl. of* tragus)
tragus, *pl.* **tragi**
    accessory t.
TRAIDS
    transfusion-related AIDS
Trail Making Test
training
    auditory t.
    auditory integration t. (AIT)
    bladder t.
    forced bowel t.
    Lovaas t.
    parent effectiveness t. (PET)
    pelvic floor muscle t. (PFMT)
    pelvic muscle t.
    toilet t.
trait
    autosomal dominant t.
    autosomal recessive t.
    cytoplasmic t.
    dominant lethal t.
    familial t.
    galtonian t.
    hereditary t.
    mendelian t.
    multifactorial t.
    penetrant t.
    recessive t.
    sickle cell t.
    thalassemia t.
    threshold t.
    X-linked t.
TRALI
    transfusion-associated lung injury
TRAM
    transverse rectus abdominis
    myocutaneous
      TRAM flap

T

TRAMP
> transverse rectus abdominis
> musculoperitoneal
>> TRAMP flap

TRAMPE
> trichorhinophalangeal multiple exostoses

Trandate

Tranebjaerg syndrome (1, 2)

tranexamic acid

tranquilizer drug

transabdominal
> t. amnioinfusion
> t. cervicoisthmic cerclage
> t. chorionic villus sampling
> t. needle transfer
> t. thin-gauge embryofetoscopy
> (TGEF)
> t. transducer
> t. ultrasonography
> t. ultrasound
> t. urethrolysis
> t. uterine electromyography

transabdominal/transvaginal ultrasound (TAS/TVS)

transalar sphenoidal encephalocele

transaminase
> alanine t. (ALT)
> aspartate t. (AST)
> elevated t.
> glutamic-pyruvic t.
> hepatic t.
> serum t.
> serum glutamic-pyruvic t. (SGPT)

transanal
> t. endoscopic microsurgery (TEM)
> t. rectal biopsy

transanimation

transannular patch repair

transcapillary
> t. fluid
> t. fluid balance

transcarbamylase
> ornithine t. (OTC)

transcarotid balloon valvuloplasty

transcatheter
> t. closure (TCC)
> t. coil embolization
> t. uterine artery embolization

transcelomic (*var. of* transcoelomic)

Transcendental Meditation

transcephalic impedance

transcervical
> t. balloon tuboplasty
> t. chorionic villus sampling
> t. division
> t. Foley catheter
> t. intrafallopian tube transfer
> (TCIFTT)
> t. obstruction of fallopian tube

> t. resection
> t. selective salpingography
> t. tubal access
> t. tubal access catheter
> (T-TAC)
> t. ultrasound

transcobalamin (I, II) deficiency

transcoelomic, transcelomic
> t. spread

transcortin

transcranial
> t. Doppler (TCD)
> t. Doppler ultrasonography
> t. magnetic stimulation (TMS)

transcript
> X inactive, specific t. (XIST)

transcriptase
> reverse t.

transcription
> gene t.
> helix-loop-helix t.
> reverse t.
> t. start site

transcriptionally active human papillomavirus

transcription-mediated
> t.-m. amplification (TMA)
> t.-m. amplification assay

transcutaneous
> t. bilirubin (TcB)
> t. blood gas monitor
> t. blood gas monitoring
> t. electrical nerve stimulation
> (TENS)
> t. jaundice meter
> t. measurement
> t. neurolysis
> t. oximetry
> t. oxygen tension monitoring
> t. partial pressure of oxygen
> $(tCpO_2)$

transcystoscopic

transdermal
> t. administration
> Alora T.
> Duragesic T.
> Esclim T.
> Estraderm T.
> t. estrogen
> t. fentanyl patch
> t. glyceryl trinitrate patch
> t. hormone replacement therapy
> t. medication patch
> t. therapeutic system (TTS)
> Vivelle T.

Transderm-Nitro Patch

Transderm Scōp

transdiaphragmatic

transdisciplinary team

transducer
- anular-array t.
- blood pressure t.
- endovaginal t.
- pressure t.
- SLA t.
- Sorensen Transpac t.
- transabdominal t.
- ultrasound t.
- Voluson sector t.

transducer-tipped catheter

transduction

transection, transsection
- complete cord t.
- cord t.
- esophageal t.
- lower esophageal t.
- multiple subpial t. (MST)

transepidermal water loss (TEWL)

Transeptic cleansing solution

transesophageal
- t. echocardiography (TEE)
- t. electrophysiologic study
- t. fistula (TEF)

trans fatty acid (tFA)
- transverse

transfection

transfer
- anterior tibialis t.
- antibody transplacental t.
- blastocyst t.
- direct oocyte t. (DOT)
- direct oocyte sperm t. (DOST)
- donor oocyte t.
- embryo t. (ET)
- embryo intrafallopian t. (EIFT)
- embryo thawing with t.
- t. factor
- frozen-thawed embryo t.
- gamete intrafallopian t. (GIFT)
- gas t.
- gene t.
- intrafallopian t.
- in vitro fertilization-embryo t.
- linear energy t.
- t. medium
- peritoneal oocyte sperm t. (POST)
- placental t.
- placental oxygen t.
- pronucleate stage embryo t. (PROST)
- pronucleate stage tubal t. (PROST)
- t. ribonucleic acid (tRNA)
- t. RNA (tRNA)
- split anterior tibial tendon t. (SPLATT)
- technology t.
- tendon t.
- transabdominal needle t.

transcervical intrafallopian tube t. (TCIFTT)
- transplacental allergen t.
- transvaginal intrafallopian sperm t. (SIFT)
- tubal embryo t. (TET)
- tubal embryo stage t. (TEST)
- zygote intrafallopian t. (ZIFT)

transferase
- t. deficient galactosemia
- gamma glutamyl t. (GGT)
- glucuronyl t.
- serum glutamic-oxaloacetic t. (SGOT)
- succinyl CoA:3-ketoacid CoA t.
- succinyl CoA:3-oxoacid CoA t.

transferrin (Tf)
- t. receptor (TfR)
- t. saturation

transformation
- malignant t.
- t. zone (TZ)

transforming
- t. growth factor (TGF)
- t. growth factor-1 (TGF-1)
- t. growth factor alpha (TGF alpha)
- t. growth factor B
- t. growth factor beta (TGF beta)
- t. growth factor B superfamily

transfundal uterine surgery

transfusion
- acute intrapartum t.
- acute perinatal t.
- antenatal fetofetal t.
- autologous blood t.
- blood t.
- chronic t.
- t. controversy
- cryoprecipitate t.
- direct fetal t.
- double-volume exchange t.
- erythrocyte t.
- exchange t. (EXT)
- fetal t.
- fetofetal t.
- fetomaternal t. (FMT)
- fetoplacental t.
- gamma-irradiated cellular products t.
- granulocyte t.
- HLA-matched platelet t.
- intrapartum fetoplacental t.
- intraperitoneal blood t.
- intraperitoneal fetal t.
- intrauterine blood t.
- intrauterine intraperitoneal fetal t.
- intrauterine maternofetal t.
- intravascular t.
- late complication of t.
- leukocyte t.

T

transfusion (*continued*)
    massive t.
    maternofetal t.
    neutrophil t.
    packed RBC t.
    packed red blood cell t.
    partial exchange t.
    percutaneous fetal t.
    placental t.
    placentofetal t. (PFT)
    plasma t.
    platelet t.
    prophylactic red-cell t.
    t. reaction
    red blood cell t.
    t. syndrome
    t. therapy
    t. transmitted (TT)
    t. transmitted virus
    twin-twin t.
    umbilical cord t.
    umbilical vein packed red blood cell t.
    umbilical vein platelet t.
    whole blood t.
transfusion-associated
    t.-a. cytomegalovirus
    t.-a. lung injury (TRALI)
transfusion-dependent thalassemia
transfusion-induced
    t.-i. hemosiderosis
    t.-i. thrombocytopenia
transfusion-related AIDS (TRAIDS)
transgastric window
transgender
transgendered
transgene
transgenerational analysis
transgenesis
    mammalian t.
transgenic organism
transglutaminase (TG)
    t. antibody
    t. antibody test
    t. deficiency
    tissue t. (tTG)
trans-Golgi network
transgrediens
    keratoderma palmoplantaris t.
transgrow bottle
transient
    t. amblyopia
    t. aplastic crisis (TAC)
    t. bilirubin encephalopathy
    t. bullous dermolysis of newborn
    t. candidemia
    t. cerebellar ataxia
    t. congenital hypothyroidism
    t. cortical blindness

    t. dystonia
    t. dystonic posturing
    t. erythroblastopenia
    t. erythroblastopenia of childhood (TEC)
    t. erythroid hypoplasia
    t. evoked otoacoustic emission (TEOAE)
    t. familial neonatal hyperbilirubinemia
    t. fetal distress
    t. fetal survival
    t. hematuria
    t. hemianopia
    t. hyperammonemia
    t. hypertension
    t. hypertension of pregnancy
    t. hyperthyrotropinemia
    t. hypogammaglobulinemia
    t. hypogammaglobulinemia of infancy (THI)
    t. hypoglycemia
    t. hypothyroxinemia
    t. hypotonia
    t. insulinopenic state
    t. ischemic attack (TIA)
    t. keratitis
    t. marrow edema syndrome of hip (TMES)
    t. monoarticular synovitis
    t. mutism
    t. myeloproliferative disorder (TMD)
    t. myeloproliferative syndrome
    t. neonatal cystinuria
    t. neonatal diabetes (TND)
    t. neonatal diabetes mellitus (TNDM)
    t. neonatal myasthenia
    t. neonatal myasthenia gravis
    t. neonatal myasthenic syndrome
    t. neonatal pustular melanosis
    t. neutropenia
    t. oliguria
    t. opsoclonus
    t. pharyngeal muscle dysfunction
    t. protein intolerance
    t. proteinuria
    t. quadriplegia
    t. respiratory acidosis
    t. respiratory distress syndrome (TRDS)
    sharp-wave t.
    t. tachypnea
    t. tachypnea of newborn (TTN, TTNB)
    t. tic disorder
    t. tyrosinemia
    t. tyrosinemia of newborn
    t. vasospasm

transiliac lengthening osteotomy
transilluminate
transillumination
    blood vessel t.
    t. of head
    vessel t.
transit
    abnormal t.
    small bowel t.
transition
    fetal-to-neonatal t.
    FTM t.
    t. plan
    t. stool
    t. zone
transitional
    t. cell tumor
    t. reader stage
    t. sleep
transitory
    t. fever
    t. fever of newborn
    t. hydrocele
    t. urinary retention
transjugular intrahepatic portosystemic shunt (TIPS)
translabial ultrasound
translation
    anterior t.
    nick t.
    vaginal t.
translevator imperforate anus
translocation
    autosome t.
    bacterial t.
    balanced t.
    balanced reciprocal t.
    t. carrier
    centric fusion t.
    chromosomal t.
    de novo balanced t.
    t. Down syndrome
    jumping t.
    mosaic t.
    t. of chromosome 22
    reciprocal t.
    robertsonian t.
    t. trisomy 21
    unbalanced t.
    X 19 t.
    X-autosome t.
translucency
    nuchal t. (NT)
transmalleolar
    t. axis
    t. axis angle (TMA)
transmembrane
    t. conductance regulator gene

    t. conductance regulatory protein
    t. glycoprotein gp41
transmesenteric hernia
transmigration
    ovular t.
transmissible spongiform encephalopathy (TSE)
transmission
    t. disequilibrium
    t. disequilibrium test (TDT)
    t. electron microscopy (TEM)
    horizontal t.
    maternal-fetal t.
    t. medium
    mother-infant t.
    perinatal t.
    pressure t.
    sexual t.
    vertical t.
    vertical HIV t.
    viral t.
transmission/disequilibrium test
transmitted
    transfusion t. (TT)
transmucosal midazolam
transmural inflammation
transnasal administration
transobturator
    t. midurethral sling
    t. tape (TOT)
    transvaginal t. (TVTO)
Transorbent dressing
transparenchymal needle puncture
transparency mode
transparent bulla
transpeptidase
    gamma glutamyl t.
    glutamyl t. (GTP)
transpericardial echocardiography
transperineal
    t. implant
    t. ultrasonography
    t. ultrasound
transperitoneal cesarean
transplacental
    t. allergen transfer
    t. bacterial pneumonia
    t. fetal bleeding
    t. hemorrhage (TPH)
    t. infection
    t. maternal antibody
    t. passage
    t. viral pneumonia
transplant
    autologous ovarian t.
    bone marrow t. (BMT)
    t. coronary artery disease
    fetal tissue t.
    fetus-to-fetus t.

T

transplant (*continued*)
    haploidentical bone marrow t.
    heart t.
    liver t.
    nonmyeloablative stem cell t.
    organ t.
    orthotopic liver t.
    t. patient
    placental tissue t.
    reduced liver t. (RLT)
    reduced-size liver t. (RSLT)
    tissue t.
transplantation
    allogenic bone marrow t.
    allogenic stem cell t.
    t. antigen
    autologous bone marrow t.
    autologous stem cell t.
    auxiliary orthotopic liver t.
    bone marrow t. (BMT)
    cardiac t.
    cord blood t. (CBT)
    cord stem cell marrow t.
    double-lung t.
    fetal stem cell t.
    heart t.
    hemopoietic stem cell t.
    hepatic t.
    heterotopic liver t.
    high-dose chemotherapy with
      autologous bone marrow t.
      (HDC-ABMT)
    t. immunology
    International Society for Heart T.
      (ISHT)
    intestinal t.
    in utero t.
    kidney t.
    liver t.
    lung t.
    marrow t.
    organ t.
    orthotopic heart t.
    partial auxiliary orthotopic liver t.
    peripheral stem cell t.
    pituitary gland t.
    renal t.
    small-bowel t.
    solid organ t. (SOT)
    stem cell t. (SCT)
    stem cell bone marrow t.
    syngeneic bone marrow t.
    thymus t.
    umbilical cord blood t.
transport
    t. disorder
    egg t.
    t. medium
    neonatal t.

    ovum t.
    sperm t.
transport-associated protein (TAP)
transporter
    carbohydrate homeostasis t.
    glucose t. (GLUT)
transposable element
transposase
transposed adnexa
transposition
    aortopulmonary t.
    arterial t.
    complete t.
    lateral ovarian t.
    muscle t.
    t. of great arteries (TGA)
    t. of great vessels (TGV)
    t. of ovary
    t. of viscera
    penoscrotal t.
    physiologically corrected t.
transposon
transpulmonary pressure
transpyloric
    t. enteral feeding
    t. tube feeding
    t. tube insertion
transrectal
    t. approach
    t. probe
    t. surgical treatment
    t. ultrasound (TRUS)
transsection (*var. of* transection)
transsexual
    lesbian, bisexual, gay, t. (LBGT)
transsexualism
transsphenoidal
    t. microsurgical resection
    t. operation
transtelephonic monitoring (TTM)
transtentorial herniation
transthoracic echocardiography
transthyretin (TTR)
transtracheal
    t. aspiration
    t. catheter
    t. ventilation
**transtubular potassium concentration
  gradient (TTKG)**
transudate
    mucosal t.
    vaginal t.
transudation
    vaginal t.
transudative pleural effusion
**transumbilical breast augmentation
  (TUBA)**
transurethral
    t. ablation

t. ablation of valve
t. catheter
t. collagen injection
t. electrocautery
t. marsupialization
t. self-detachable balloon
transvaginal
t. amniotic puncture (TAP)
t. bladder neck suspension
t. color Doppler sonography (TV-CDS)
t. cone
t. fine-needle biopsy
t. hysterectomy
t. implant
t. intrafallopian sperm transfer (SIFT)
t. sacrospinous colpopexy
t. sonography (TVS)
t. sonohysterography
t. transducer probe
t. transobturator (TVTO)
t. treatment
t. tubal catheterization
t. ultrasonography (TVU, TVUS)
t. ultrasound (TVU, TVUS, TV-UST)
t. ultrasound-directed oocyte retrieval (TUDOR)
t. ultrasound-guided urethral reconstruction
t. urethrolysis
transvalensis
Nocardia t.
transvascular
transvenous
t. coil embolization
t. pacing
transversa
diameter t.
transversalis fascia
transversal nasal crease
Trans-Ver-Sal transdermal patch
transverse
t. arch hypoplasia
t. arrest
t. cervical ligament
t. colon
t. dense striation
t. diameter
t. fetal lie
t. fracture
t. fundal incision of Strassman
t. hemimelia
t. incision
t. lie presentation
t. loop colostomy
lower uterine segment t. (LUST)

t. myelitis
t. nail groove
occiput t. (OT)
t. oval pelvis
t. plication
t. presentation
t. rectus abdominis musculoperitoneal (TRAMP)
t. rectus abdominis myocutaneous (TRAM)
t. ridge
t. scan
t. scrotal testis
t. skin incision
t. vaginal muscle
t. vaginal septum
transversion
transversum
septum t.
transversus
t. abdominis muscle
situs t.
transvestite
Tranxene
tranylcypromine
TRAP
thrombin receptor-activating peptide
twin reversed arterial perfusion
T. sequence
T. syndrome
trap
filtered specimen t.
Luekens t.
sterile specimen t.
TRAP-activated neonatal platelet
trapezoidocephaly-synostosis syndrome
trapped ovum
trapping
air t.
ion t.
platelet t.
Trasicor
trastuzumab
Trasylol
trauma
abdominal t.
acoustic t.
American Association for the Surgery of T. (AAST)
birth t.
blunt t.
blunt cardiac t.
blunt chest t.
cardiac t.
central nervous system t.
chemical t.
chest t.
childhood genital t.
closed head t. (CHT)

T

trauma (*continued*)
  corneal t.
  craniocerebral t.
  dehydration, poisoning, t. (DPT)
  dental t.
  diaphragmatic t.
  fetal t.
  Focused Assessment by Sonography for T. (FAST)
  forceps birth t.
  frictional t.
  genital tract t.
  gluteal t.
  head t.
  lap-belt t.
  maternal t.
  penetrating t.
  perinatal t.
  perineal t.
  psychological t.
  T. Score and Injury Severity Score Analysis
  sex-related t.
  surgical t.
  T. Symptom Checklist for Children (TSCC)
  thoracic t.
  tracheobronchial t.
  T. Triage Rule (TTR)
TraumaCal formula
trauma-related
  t.-r. acute pelvic hemorrhage
  t.-r. injury severity score (TRISS)
traumatic
  t. alopecia
  t. amenorrhea
  t. amputation
  t. aortic disruption
  t. aortic injuries in children
  t. birth injury
  t. bowing
  t. brain injury (TBI)
  t. compartment syndrome
  t. delivery
  t. dissection
  t. glaucoma
  t. hematoma
  t. hemobilia
  t. hyphema
  t. idiocy
  t. imagery
  t. labyrinthitis
  t. pneumothorax
  t. rupture of thoracic aorta (TRA)
  t. sexualization
  t. vaginitis
Travamine
Travamulsion IV fat emulsion
traveler's diarrhea (TD)

tray
  t. agglutination test (TAT)
  EZ-EM PercuSet amniocentesis t.
  HSG t.
  Unimar HSG t.
trazodone
TRDS
  transient respiratory distress syndrome
Treacher
  T. Collins-Franceschetti syndrome
  T. Collins mandibulofacial dysostosis
  T. Collins syndrome
treatable
  known, not t.
treatment
  add-back t.
  adjunctive t.
  allergy t.
  ambulatory antibiotic t.
  amoxicillin-clavulanate t.
  t. and education of autistic and related communications handicapped children (TEACCH)
  antenatal corticosteroid t. (ANS)
  antenatal phenobarbital t.
  antibiotic t.
  anticonvulsant t.
  anti-D globulin t.
  antiinflammatory t.
  antimanic t.
  antimicrobial t.
  ART t.
  biologic t.
  brace t.
  continuous/combined t.
  corticosteroid t.
  domestic violence t.
  double diaper t.
  Early and Periodic Screening, Diagnosis, and T. (EPSDT)
  empiric t.
  exogenous thyroxine t.
  ex utero intrapartum t. (EXIT)
  t. failure
  gonadal hormone t.
  hormonal t.
  hyperbaric oxygen t.
  immunomodulatory t.
  infertility t.
  intrapartum t.
  laparoscopic t.
  laser t.
  local t.
  mutagenic t.
  neurodevelopmental t.
  Otovent negative pressure t.
  Pacis BCG bladder cancer t.
  pharmacologic t.
  phase advance t.

phase delay t.
P32 intraperitoneal t.
pityriasis rotunda t.
postexposure t. (PET)
prenatal t.
preventive allergy t. (PAT)
prophylactic t.
rape t.
t. recommendation
t. series
spectacle t.
steroid t.
topical t.
traction t.
transrectal surgical t.
transvaginal t.
updraft t.
ureteral surgical t.
zidovudine t.
treatment-associated pregnancy
treatment-independent pregnancy
treatment-refractory depression
treatment-resistant proteinuria
Trecator-SC
tree
bronchial t.
differentiation of respiratory t.
extrahepatic biliary t.
t. pollen
respiratory t.
tracheobronchial t.
trefoil pelvis
Treitz
ligament of T.
trembling
hereditary chin t.
tremor
coarse t.
essential t.
familial t.
hereditary t.
intention t.
primary writing t.
t. syndrome
tremulousness
trench
t. fever
t. mouth
Trendelenburg
T. gait
T. limp
T. position
T. sign
T. test
Trental
trepanation (*var. of* trephination)
trephination, trepanation
nail t.
trephine

Treponema
T. *carateum*
T. *pallidum*
T. *pallidum* antibody
T. *pallidum* antigen
T. *pallidum hemagglutination* (TPHA)
T. *pallidum* immobilization (TPI)
T. *pallidum* immobilization test
T. *pertenue*
treponemal serology
treponematosis
treppe response
Tresilian sign
tretinoin
Trevor disease
Trexan
TRF
Teacher Rating Form
Teacher Report Form
TRH
thyrotropin releasing hormone
Thyrel TRH
TRH-ST
thyrotropin-releasing hormone stimulation test
TRH-stimulation test
Triacet Topical
triacetyloleandomycin
triad
AGR t.
allergic t.
aspirin t.
atopic t.
Beck t.
Charcot t.
Currarino t.
Cushing t.
female athlete t. (FAT)
Hutchinson t.
t. of head tilt disorder
triage
trial
Bernoulli t.
breast cancer prevention t. (BCPT)
Canadian Crohn Relapse Prevention T.
cervical incompetence prevention randomized cerclage t. (CIPRACT)
chemotherapy phase t.
diabetes control and complications t. (DCCT)
Diabetes Prevention T.
digital mammographic imaging screening t. (DMIST)
t. forceps
high-frequency ventilation t. (HIFT)
International Collaborative Ovarian Neoplasm T. 1 (ICON1)

trial (*continued*)
    labor t.
    Multiple Outcomes of Raloxifene evaluation t.
    t. of labor (TOL)
    t. of labor after cesarean (TOLAC)
    PEPI t.
    promotion of breastfeeding intervention t. (PROBIT)
    RADIUS t.
    STOP-ROP t.
    surfactant replacement t.
    voiding t.
    WAVE t.
Triam-A injection
triamcinolone
    t. acetonide
    t. acetonide ointment
    t. hexacetonide
Triam Forte injection
Triaminic
    T. AM Decongestant Formula
    T. Oral Infant Drops
triamterene
triangle
    Burger t.
    Codman t.
    Einthoven t.
    femoral t.
    Hesselbach t.
    inguinal t.
    Kiesselbach t.
    Petit lumbar t.
    posterior t.
    pubic t.
    Ward t.
triangular
    t. facies
    t. fibrocartilaginous complex (TFCC)
    t. ligament
    t. splint
    t. uterus
    t. vaginal patch sling procedure
triangularis
    uterus t.
triatriatum
    cor t.
Triaz benzoyl peroxide pad
triazolam
Triazole
Triban
tribasilar synostosis
tribrachius
TRIC
    trachoma inclusion conjunctivitis
tricephalus
triceps
    t. reflex

    t. skinfold thickness (TSF)
    t. tendinitis
trichilemmal cyst
trichilemmoma
Trichinella spiralis
trichinelliasis (*var. of* trichinosis)
trichinellosis (*var. of* trichinosis)
trichiniasis (*var. of* trichinosis)
trichinosis (TRICH), trichinelliasis, trichinellosis, trichiniasis
trichiura
    Trichuris t.
Trichlorex
trichlormethiazide
trichloroacetic acid (TCA)
trichloroethanol (TCE)
trichloroethylene
2,4,5-trichlorophenoxyacetic acid, 4, 5-trichlorophenoxyacetic acid
5-trichlorophenoxyacetic acid
trichobezoar
trichodentoosseous syndrome
trichodysplasia
    hereditary t.
trichoepithelioma
trichomegaly
    eyelash t.
trichomonad
trichomonal
    t. infection
    t. vaginitis
Trichomonas
    T. infection
    T. vaginalis
    T. vaginalis vaginitis
trichomoniasis
trichophagia
trichophagy
Trichophyton
    T. mentagrophytes
    T. rubrum
    T. tonsurans
trichopoliodystrophy
trichorhinophalangeal
    t. multiple exostoses (TRAMPE)
    t. multiple exostosis dysplasia
    t. syndrome
trichorino-auriculophalangeal multiple exostoses dysplasia
trichorionic
trichorrhexis
    t. invaginata
    t. nodosa
    t. nodosa syndrome
trichoschisis
Trichosporon beigelii
trichosporonosis
trichothiodystrophy 2 (TTD 2)
trichotillomania

trichrome stain
trichuriasis
Trichuris
    T. dysentery syndrome
    T. trichiura
Tricosal
tricuspid, tricuspidal, tricuspidate
    t. atresia
    t. insufficiency
    t. regurgitation
    t. stenosis
    t. valve
tricuspidal (*var. of* tricuspid)
tricuspidate (*var. of* tricuspid)
Tri-Cyclen
    Ortho T.-C.
tricyclic antidepressant (TCA)
Tridesilon Topical
tridihexethyl chloride
Tridione syndrome
tridymus
triencephalus
triene-to-tetraene ratio
trientine
triethanolamine polypeptide
  oleate-condensate
triethnic
triethylene tetramine
  dihydrochloride
triethylenethiophosphoramide
trifluoperazine hydrochloride
trifluorothymidine
triflupromazine hydrochloride
trifluridine
trifunctional protein deficiency
  (TFP)
trigeminal
    t. herpes zoster
    t. nerve
    t. nerve distribution
trigemino-encephalo-angiomatosis
trigger
    t. digit
    environmental t.
    t. phenomenon
    t. point
triglyceride
    t. hyperlipidemia
    medium-chain t. (MCT)
    milk t.
    t. storage disease
triglycine
    mercaptoacetyl t.
trigona (*pl. of* trigonum)
trigonal
    t. hypertrophy
    t. plate
    t. ring
    t. urothelium

trigone
    urinary t.
trigonitis
    pseudomembranous t.
trigonocephaly syndrome
trigonum, *pl.* trigona
    os t.
Trihexane
trihexose
    ceramide t.
Trihexy
trihexyphenidyl
TriHIBit vaccine
trihydrate
    ampicillin t.
trihydroxycoprostanic acidemia
Tri-Immunol vaccine
triiniodymus
triiodothyronine (T3)
    free t.
    reverse t.
    t. test
Tri-K
Trikacide
trilaminar
    t. blastoderm
    t. embryonic disc
    t. myopathy
trilateral
    t. retinoblastoma
    t. retinoblastoma syndrome
trileaflet aortic valve
Trileptal
Tri-Levlen contraceptive pill
trilineage development
Trilisate
triloba
    placenta t.
trilogy
    Fallot t.
    t. of Fallot
trilostane
Trilucent breast
TriMark marker system for breast
  biopsy
trimegestone
trimeprazine
trimester
    first t.
    second t.
    third t.
trimethadione
    t. embryopathy
    t. syndrome
trimethaphan camsylate
trimethobenzamide hydrochloride
trimethopri
    cotrimoxazole t.
    t. HCl oral solution

T

trimethopri (*continued*)
    sulfamethoxazole and t. (SMX-TMP, SMX/TMP)
    t. sulfate
trimethoprim-sulfamethoxazole (SMZ-TMP, TMP-SMX)
    t.-s. prophylaxis
trimethylaminuria
trimipramine
Trimstat
Trinalin
Tri-Nasal Spray
trinitrate
    glyceryl t. (GTN)
Tri-Norinyl
Trinsicon
trinucleotide repeat expansion mutation
triocephalus
triopathy
triophthalmos
triose
    t. phosphate isomerase (TPI)
    t. phosphate isomerase deficiency
Triostat Injection
triotus
tripartita
    placenta t.
Tripedia vaccine
tripelennamine hydrochloride
tripe palm
triphalangeal thumb
triphasic
    t. oral contraceptive
    t. pattern blastemal cell
Triphasil contraceptive pill
triphenylethylene selective estrogen receptor modulator
triphosphatase
    adenosine t. (ATPase)
triphosphate
    adenosine t. (ATP)
    deoxynucleotide t. (dNTP)
    digoxigenin-labeled deoxyuridine t.
    guanosine t. (GTP)
    lead t.
triplane fracture
triple
    T. Antibiotic Topical
    t. arthrodesis
    t. bromide
    t. diapers
    t. dye
    T. Paste
    T. Paste medicated ointment
    T. Paste ointment
    t. screen
    t. screen test
    t. serum marker screening
    t. sulfa cream

    t. sulfa suppository
    t. swab test
    T. X Liquid
    T. X shampoo
    t. X syndrome
triple-biochemical screen
triple-color phenomenon
triple-drug therapy
triplegia
triple-lumen
    t.-l. catheter
    t.-l. tube
triple-marker
    t.-m. screen
    t.-m. screening
triplet pregnancy
triple-X, triplo-X
    t.-X chromosomal aberration
    t.-X female
triplex
    placenta t.
triplication
    ureteral t.
triploid
    t. embryo
    t. fetus
    t. preembryo
triploidy
    placental mosaicism for t.
    t. syndrome
triplo-X (*var. of* triple-X)
tripod
    t. fixation technique
    t. position
    t. sign
tripodia
tripoding
tripod-supporting position
trip 15q syndrome
triprolidine
    t. and pseudoephedrine
    t. hydrochloride
Triptil
TripTone caplet
triptorelin
tripus
    t. conjoined twins
    t. limb
triradius
    distal t.
trisalicylate
    choline magnesium t.
trisegmentectomy
triseriatus
    Aedes t.
tris[hydroxymethyl]aminomethane-buffered saline
trismus
    t. nascentium

t. neonatorum
persistent t.
trismus-pseudocamptodactyly syndrome
trisomic
t. abortus
t. fetus
t. rescue
trisomy
t. 1–22
autosomal t.
t. C,D,E,G syndrome
chromosome 1–22 t.
chromosome 1p–22p t.
chromosome 1q–22q t.
chromosome Xq t.
t. 18-like syndrome
mosaic t. 14
t. 8 mosaicism
nondisjunction t. 21
noninvasive detection of t. 18
t. 1p–22p syndrome
t. 1q–22q syndrome
t. 1–22 syndrome
translocation t. 21
t. X
X t.
t. Xq
trisphosphate
inositol t.
TRISS
trauma-related injury severity score
Tristar trocar
Trisulfa
trisulfapyrimidine
Trisulfa-S
Trivagizole 3 vaginal cream
trivalent
t. inactivated influenza vaccine (TIV)
t. live cold-adapted influenza vaccine
Trivers-Willard theory
Tri-Vi-Flor vitamin
Tri-Vi-Sol vitamin
Trivora-28 tablet
Trizivir
TRIzol
T. reagent
T. RNA extractor
trizygotic
tRNA
transfer ribonucleic acid
transfer RNA
TRO
thyroid-related ophthalmopathy
Trobicin
trocar
Bluntport disposable t.
Cabot t.

Circon-ACMI t.
Core Dynamics disposable t.
Dexide disposable t.
Endopath bladeless t.
Endopath Tristar t.
Ethicon disposable t.
t. guide
t. hernia
t. implantation metastasis
Jarit disposable t.
laparoscopic t.
Marlow disposable t.
Olympus disposable t.
Origin t.
Saber BT blunt-tip surgical t.
t. site ecchymosis
Solos disposable t.
Step laparoscopic t.
Storz disposable t.
suprapubic t.
Tristar t.
Visiport optical t.
Weck disposable t.
Wisap disposable t.
Wolf disposable t.
trochanter
greater t.
troche
Cēpacol Anesthetic T.
clotrimazole t.
trochlear
t. nerve
t. nerve palsy
trochocephaly
troglitazone
troleandomycin
trombiculiasis
tromethamine
carboprost t.
dinoprost t.
fosfomycin t.
ketorolac t.
lodoxamide t.
Tronolane
TrophAmine hyperalimentation
trophectoderm
t. biopsy
t. stage
trophic
t. feed
T-cell t. (T-trophic)
trophoblast
extravillous t.
t. in regression (TIR)
intermediate t. (IT)
t. sampling
trophoblastic
t. cell
t. disease

trophoblastic (*continued*)
    t. embolus
    t. invasion
    t. neoplasia
    t. neoplastic disease
    t. pseudotumor
    t. tissue
    t. tumor
trophospongia
trophotropism
trophozoite
tropic
    t. hormone
    macrophage t.
tropica
    Leishmania t.
Tropicacyl
tropical
    t. ataxic neuropathy
    t. bubo
    t. pyomyositis
    Quinsana Plus T.
    t. spastic paraparesis (TSP)
    t. spastic paraparesis/HTLV-I
      associated myelopathy (TSP/HAM)
    t. sprue
tropicalis
    Candida t.
tropicamide
tropism, positive tropism, negative
  tropism
tropoelastin
tropomodulin
troponin
    t. C
    t. I
    t. T (TnT)
trough
    peak and t.
    t. tacrolimus level
trousers
    antishock t.
    military antishock t. (MAST)
Trousseau sign
trovafloxacin
Trovan/Zithromax Compliance
  Pak
Troyer syndrome (TS)
true
    t. accessory breast
    t. breast tissue
    t. conjugate
    t. hermaphroditism
    t. histiocytic lymphoma (THL)
    t. incontinence
    t. labor
    t. macroglossia
    t. pelvis
    t. precocious puberty

    t. precocity
    t. twins
    t. undescended testis
    t. uterine inertia
    t. vertigo
trumpet
    t. cannula
    Iowa t.
truncal
    t. acne
    t. asymmetry
    t. ataxia
    t. incurvation reflex
    t. obesity
    t. rash
truncate selection
truncation
    uterine positioning via ligament
      investment fixation t. (UPLIFT)
trunci (*pl. of* truncus)
truncus, *pl.* **trunci**
    t. arteriosus
    t. arteriosus communis
trunk
    t. control
    t. presentation
    pulmonary arterial t.
    t. rotation
TRUS
    transrectal ultrasound
trust
    support t.
Tru-Trax
TruZone PFM
Trypanosoma
    T. brucei
    T. cruzi
trypanosomal chancre
trypanosome
trypanosomiasis
    African t.
    American t.
    cerebral t.
    Cruz t.
    Gambian t.
    Rhodesian t.
trypsin activation peptide
  (TAP)
trypsinization
trypsinogen, trypsogen
    immunoreactive t. (IRT)
trypsogen (*var. of* trypsinogen)
tryptase
tryptophan
    t. ethylester
    t. malabsorption
tryptophanuria
TS
    Troyer syndrome

TSB
  total serum bilirubin
TSC
  tuberous sclerosis complex
TSCC
  Trauma Symptom Checklist for
    Children
TSE
  transmissible spongiform
    encephalopathy
TSF
  triceps skinfold thickness
TSH
  thyroid-stimulating hormone
    TSH surge
T-shaped
    T-s. constriction ring
    T-s. uterus
TSP
  thrombospondin
  tropical spastic paraparesis
TSP/HAM
  tropical spastic paraparesis/HTLV-I
    associated myelopathy
TSRH
  Texas Scottish Rite Hospital
    TSRH cross-link
    TSRH instrumentation
TSS
  toxic shock syndrome
TSST-1
  toxic shock syndrome toxin-1
TST
  tuberculin skin test
TSTA
  tumor-specific transplantation antigen
T-Stat
tsutsugamushi
    t. fever
    Orientia t.
TSV
  thalamostriate vasculopathy
TT
  tetanus toxoid
  transfusion transmitted
    TT virus (TTV)
T-TAC
  transcervical tubal access catheter
    T-TAC system
TTB
  third-trimester bleeding
TTD 2
TTF-1
  thyroid transcription factor-1
tTG
  tissue transglutaminase
TTKG
  transtubular potassium concentration
    gradient

T1–T10 lymphocyte
TTM
  transtelephonic monitoring
TTN
  transient tachypnea of newborn
TTNB
  transient tachypnea of newborn
TTP
  thrombotic thrombocytopenic purpura
TTR
  transthyretin
  Trauma Triage Rule
T-trophic
  T-cell trophic
    T-trophic SI strain
TTS
  transdermal therapeutic system
  twin-to-twin transfusion syndrome
    Estraderm TTS
    TTS fentanyl
    Testoderm TTS
TTTS
  twin-to-twin transfusion syndrome
  twin-to-twin transfusion system
T-tube cholangiogram
T-tubules
TTV
  TT virus
TUBA
  transumbilical breast augmentation
tubage
tubal
    t. abortion
    t. banding
    t. coagulation
    t. colic
    t. damage
    t. distortion
    t. diverticulum
    t. dysmenorrhea
    t. embryo stage transfer (TEST)
    t. embryo transfer (TET)
    t. endometriosis
    t. endometrium
    t. factor
    t. factor infertility
    t. gestation
    t. inflammatory damage (TID)
    t. insufflation
    t. interruption
    t. ligation (TL)
    t. ligation band technique
    t. mass
    t. metaplasia
    t. microsurgery
    t. obstruction
    t. occlusion
    t. ostium
    t. patency

T

tubal (*continued*)
- t. perfusion pressure (TPP)
- t. pregnancy
- t. reanastomosis
- t. recanalization
- t. reconstruction surgery
- t. reversal
- t. ring
- t. rupture
- t. spasm
- t. sterilization

tubatorsion (*var. of* tubotorsion)
tube, tubing
- t.'s and ovaries
- bilateral myringotomy t.'s (BMT)
- bronchial t.
- Cantor t.
- chest t.
- Cole endotracheal t.
- Cole orotracheal t.
- t. connector
- Cryovial t.
- cuffed endotracheal t.
- cuffed ET t.
- dislodged t.
- Dobbhoff nasogastric feeding t.
- double-focus t.
- ear ventilation t.
- embryonic neural t.
- endotracheal t.
- EntriStar Skin Level T.
- ET t.
- eustachian t. (ET)
- fallopian t.
- t. feed
- feeding t. (FT)
- fimbriated end of fallopian t.
- Foley t.
- follicle aspiration t.
- gastrointestinal t.
- gastrostomy t.
- infundibulum of fallopian t.
- t. insertion technique
- Keofeed t.
- knuckle of t.
- laser office ventilation of ears with insertion of t.'s (LOVE IT)
- Linton t.
- Malecot t.
- Miller-Abbott t.
- molybdenum rotating anode x-ray t.
- Moss t.
- myringotomy t.
- nasogastric t. (NGT)
- nasojejunal t.
- neural t.
- NG t.
- NJ t.
- OG t.
- oral gastric t.
- PE t.
- Pedi PEG t.
- PEG t.
- Pezzer t.
- t. placement
- polyethylene feeding t.
- t. position
- pressure equalization t. (PET)
- pus t.
- rectal polyethylene t.
- Replogle sump t.
- Reuter t.
- Rubin t.
- salpingitis in previously occluded t.'s (SPOT)
- Sengstaken-Blakemore t.
- Shah permanent t.
- smoke removal t. (SRT)
- thoracostomy t.
- t. thoracostomy
- tracheal t.
- tracheostomy t.
- transcervical obstruction of fallopian t.
- triple-lumen t.
- tympanostomy t.
- uncuffed endotracheal t.
- uterine t.
- ventilation t.

tubectomy
tuber
- cortical t.
- cryptic t.
- subependymal t.

tuberalis
- pars t.

tubercle
- choroid t.
- genital t.
- Ghon t.
- Montgomery t.
- Morgagni t.
- Müller t.
- pubic t.
- Rokitansky t.
- tibial t.

tuberculid
- papulonecrotic t.

tuberculin
- t. skin test (TST)
- t. syringe
- t. test
- t. testing

tuberculoid
- borderline t.
- t. leprosy

tuberculoma
- infratentorial t.

tuberculoprotein
tuberculosis (TB, TBC)
    abdominal t.
    bovine t.
    cavitary t.
    congenital t.
    cutaneous t.
    disseminated t.
    drug-resistant t.
    endobronchial t.
    endometrial t.
    extrapulmonary t.
    extrathoracic t.
    gastrointestinal t.
    genital t.
    hematogenous primary t.
    infectious pulmonary t.
    intrathoracic t.
    miliary t.
    multidrug-resistant t. (MDR-TB)
    mycobacteria other than t. (MOTT)
    Mycobacterium t.
    orificial t.
    t. papulonecrotica
    pediatric t.
    pelvic t.
    primary pulmonary t.
    progressive primary pulmonary t.
    pulmonary t.
    reactivation t.
    renal t.
    spinal t.
    t. verrucosa cutis
    visceral t.
tuberculous
    t. abscess
    t. adenitis
    t. cervical lymphadenitis
    t. chancre
    t. colitis
    t. dactylitis
    t. enteritis
    t. gumma
    t. keratoconjunctivitis
    t. meningitis
    t. osteomyelitis
    t. peritonitis (TBP)
    t. pleural effusion
    t. pneumonia
    t. salpingitis
    t. spinal arachnoiditis
    t. spondylitis
tuberculum sella
tuberosity
    bicipital t.
tuberous
    t. breast abnormality
    t. mole

    t. sclerosis
    t. sclerosis complex (TSC)
    t. sclerosis syndrome
    t. subchorial hematoma of decidua
Tubex
Tubigrip bandage
tubing
    blow-by through t.
    Mini-Med t.
    pressure-separator t.
tuboabdominal pregnancy
tubocornual
    t. anastomosis
    t. microsurgery
    t. reanastomosis
tubocurarine chloride
tuboendometrial cell
tubo-ovarian (*var. of* tuboovarian)
tuboovarian, tubo-ovarian
    t. abscess (TOA)
    t. abscess after previous tubal occlusion (TOAPOT)
    t. complex (TOC)
    t. pregnancy
    t. varicocele
tuboperitoneal infertility
tuboplasty
    balloon t.
    transcervical balloon t.
    ultrasound-guided transcervical t.
    ultrasound transcervical t.
tubotorsion, tubatorsion
tubouterine
    t. implantation
    t. pregnancy
tubovaginal fistula
tubular
    t. atrophy
    t. bone
    t. breathing
    t. cancer
    t. carcinoma
    t. disruption
    t. dysgenesis
    t. hypoplasia
    t. interstitial fibrosis
    t. necrosis
    t. proteinuria
    t. stenosis
tubularization
    in situ t.
tubularized incised plate (TIP)
tubule
    anular t.
    convoluted t.
    mesonephric t.
    proximal convoluted t.
    renal t.

tubule (*continued*)
    seminiferous t.
    sex cord tumor with anular t.
    (SCTAT)
tubuloglomerular feedback
tubulointerstitial
    t. disease
    t. lesion
    t. nephritis (TINU)
tubulopathy
    hypokalemic salt-losing t.
    t. of Lowe syndrome
    proximal t.
tuck
Tucker-McLane forceps
Tucker-McLane-Luikart forceps
TUDOR
    transvaginal ultrasound-directed oocyte
    retrieval
tuft
    central gliotic t.
    digital t.
    distal t.
    epithelial t.
    gliotic t.
    glomerular t.
    t. of hair
    swollen glomerular t.
tugging at ears
tularemia
    glandular t.
    oculoglandular t.
    oropharyngeal t.
    pneumonic t.
    pulmonary t.
    t. (type A, B)
    typhoidal t.
    ulceroglandular t.
    t. vaccine
tularensis
    Francisella t.
tumbling E chart
tumescence, turgescence
    physiologic t.
tumescent absorbent bandage
tumor
    adenomatoid oviduct t.
    adnexal t.
    adrenal cell rest t.
    adult granulosa cell t. (AGCT)
    androgen-producing t.
    androgen-producing adrenal t.
    androgen-producing ovarian t.
    t. angiogenesis factor (TAF)
    angiomatoid t.
    t. antigen
    t. antigenicity
    t. ascites
    Askin t.

atypical teratoid t.
atypical teratoid/rhabdoid t.
autochthonous t.
autonomic nerve t.
benign t.
benign cystic t.
bladder t. (BT)
t. blush
bone t.
borderline epithelial ovarian t.
brain t
Brenner t.
Brenner cell t.
t. burden
carcinoid t.
central primitive neuroectodermal t.
  (cPNET)
cerebellar t.
cervical cord t.
cervical stump t.
clear cell t.
CNS t.
colorectal t.
craniofacial t.
t. debulking
debulking of t.
desmoid t.
desmoplastic small round cell t.
  (DSRCT)
dumbbell t.
embryonal t.
endocervical sinus t.
endodermal sinus t. (EST)
endometrial t.
endometrioid epithelial cell t.
epithelial liver t.
epithelial serous t.
epithelial stromal t.
Ewing t.
extragonadal germ cell t.
extranodal t.
extrapelvic solid t.
extrarenal rhabdoid t.
eyelid t.
feminizing adrenal t. (FAT)
fibrovascular t.
Frantz t.
functioning t.
gastrointestinal autonomic nerve t.
  (GANT)
gastrointestinal tract t.
genital t.
genital tract t.
germ cell testicular t.
germinal cell t.
gestational trophoblastic t. (GTT)
Glazunov t.
glomus t.
glycoprotein-producing t.

gonadal stromal cell t.
gonadal stromal ovarian t.
t. grading
granulosa cell t.
granulosa-stromal cell t.
granulosa-theca cell t.
hairlike t.
hemispheric t.
hilar cell t.
hilus cell t.
hormonally responsive t.
hormone-secreting t.
hypothalamic t.
t. immunology
t. immunotherapy
infratentorial t.
insulin-secreting pancreatic t.
intracranial t.
intraocular t.
intrapulmonary t.
intrinsic t.
islet cell t.
juvenile granulosa cell t. (JGCT)
juxtaglomerular cell t. (JGCT)
Koenen t.
Krukenberg t.
Leydig cell t.
lipid cell ovarian t.
lipoid ovarian t.
liver t.
t. lysis syndrome
malignant brain t.
malignant epithelial t.
malignant extrarenal rhabdoid t.
malignant germ cell t.
malignant mesodermal t.
malignant mixed müllerian t. (MMMT)
malignant nerve sheath t.
malignant ovarian germ cell t.
t. marker
t. mass
mediastinal t.
mesodermal t.
mesonephroid t.
metastatic gynecologic t.
midline craniofacial t.
mixed germ cell t.
mixed mesodermal t.
mixed müllerian t. (MMT)
mixed müllerian mesodermal t. (MMMT)
mixed uterine t.
monodermal t.
mucinous t.
mulberry t.
müllerian t.
t. necrosis
t. necrosis factor (TNF)

t. necrosis factor alpha (TNF-alpha)
nerve sheath t.
neural crest t.
neuroectodermal t.
neurogenic t.
tumor, node, metastases (TNM)
nonalpha cell t.
nondysgerminomatous germ cell t.
nonfunctional pituitary t.
nonhematogenous t.
nonsecreting pituitary t.
null cell t.
optic nerve t.
optic pathway t.
orbital t.
ovarian t.
ovarian malignant germ cell t.
pancreatic t.
paratesticular t.
parovarian t.
pelvic t.
periaqueductal t.
peripheral neuroectodermal t.
peripheral primitive neuroectodermal t. (PPNET)
persistent postmolar gestational trophoblastic t.
phyllodes t.
piloid t.
pineal t.
pituitary gland t.
placental site t.
placental site trophoblastic t. (PSTT)
pleomorphic spindle cell t.
polypoid epithelial t.
pontile t.
posterior fossa t.
postmolar persistent gestational trophoblastic t.
Pott puffy t.
pregnancy t.
prepuberal testicular t. (PPTT)
primary intraocular t.
primary tracheal t.
primitive neuroectodermal t. (PNET)
t. progression
pseudomucinous t.
Purkinje cell t.
radioresistant yolk sac t.
Recklinghausen t.
t. regression
rhabdoid t.
round cell t.
sarcomatous t.
Schiller t.
Scully t.
t. seeding
serous t.
Sertoli cell t.

tumor (*continued*)
    Sertoli-Leydig cell t.
    sex cord mesenchymal t.
    sex cord stromal germ
      cell t.
    single t.
    sinus t.
    t. size
    smooth muscle t.
    solid t.
    t. spillage
    spinal t.
    spinal cord t.
    spindle cell t.
    Steiner t.
    sternomastoid t.
    stromal t.
    t. suppression gene
    t. suppressor gene
    Teilum t.
    teratoid t.
    testicular t.
    testis t.
    theca cell t.
    tracheal t.
    transitional cell t.
    trophoblastic t.
    ulcerative t.
    uterine corpus t.
    uterine tumor resembling ovarian
      sex-cord t. (UTROSCT)
    ventricular t.
    virilizing adrenal t.
    vitelline t.
    Wilms t. (stage I–V)
    yolk sac t.
tumor-associated antigen (TAA)
tumor-cloning assay
tumorigenesis
tumorigenicity
tumor-limiting factor
tumorous hyperprolactinemia
tumor-specific transplantation antigen (TSTA)
Tums Extra Strength
TUNEL
    terminal deoxyribonucleotidyl
    transferase-mediated biotin-16-dUTP
    nick-end labeling
    TUNEL assay
    TUNEL stain
tungiasis
tunic, tunica
tunica (*var. of* tunic)
    t. albuginea
    t. vaginalis
tunnel
    intracardiac t.
    lateral atrial t. (LAT)

    subcutaneous t.
    t. vision
tunneled
    t. catheter
    t. CVL
tunnel-view radiography
Tuohy spinal needle
turbidity
Turbinaire
    Decadron T.
    Dexacort Phosphate T.
turbinate, turbinated
    t. bone
    nasal t.
turbinated (*var. of* turbinate)
Turbuhaler
    budesonide T.
    Pulmicort T.
    Rhinocort T.
turbulence
turbulent airflow
turcica
    sella t.
Turco posteromedial release of clubfoot
Turcot syndrome
turgescence (*var. of* tumescence)
turgescent
turgor
Turner
    T. mosaic
    T. mosaicism
    T. mosaic syndrome
    T. phenotype
    T. phenotype with normal karyotype
    T. syndrome in female with X
      chromosome
    T. XO syndrome
Turner-Albright syndrome
Turner-Kieser syndrome
Turner-like syndrome
Turner-Warwick urethroplasty
turning
    contralateral head t. (CHT)
turnover
    bone t.
    iron t.
turricephaly
turtle sign
Tuss-DM
Tussin
    Safe T. 30
Tussi-Organidin DM NR
Tusstat Syrup
Tuttle test
TV
    tidal volume
TV-CDS
    transvaginal color Doppler sonography

TVT
tension-free vaginal tape
TVTO
transvaginal transobturator
TVTO sling
TVU
transvaginal ultrasonography
transvaginal ultrasound
TVUS
transvaginal ultrasonography
transvaginal ultrasound
TWAR
Taiwan acute respiratory
TWAR agent
T-wave
T-w. abnormality
T-w. axis
T-w. inversion
TWEAK
tolerance, worried, eye opener,
amnesia, kut (cut) down
TWEAK test
Tween 80
twenty-nail dystrophy
Twice-A-Day Nasal Solution
twilight sleep
Twilite Oral
twill tape
twin
asymmetrical conjoined t.'s
binovular t.'s
t. birth
t. birth weight discordance
breech-first t.
concordant t.'s
conjoined t.'s
t. delivery
t. demise
diamniotic t.'s
dichorionic t.'s
dichorionic-diamniotic t.'s
discordant t.'s
dissimilar t.'s
dizygotic t.
donor t.
1-egg t.'s
2-egg t.'s
enzygotic t.'s
equal conjoined t.'s
fraternal t.'s
t. gestation
growth-discordant t.'s
identical t.'s
impacted t.
incomplete conjoined t.'s
ischiopagus tripus t.'s
locked t.'s
t. method
monoamniotic t.'s

monochorial t.'s
monochorionic t.'s
monochorionic-diamniotic t.'s
monovular t.'s
monozygotic t.'s
natural monozygotic t.'s
parabolic t.
t. peak sign
perfused t.
t. placenta
t. pregnancy
pump t.
recipient t.
t. reversed arterial perfusion (TRAP)
second t.
Siamese t.'s
similar t.'s
stuck t.
symmetrical conjoined t.'s
thoracopagus t.
tripus conjoined t.'s
true t.'s
unequal conjoined t.'s
uniovular t.'s
unlike t.'s
vanishing t.
twinge
Texidor t.
twinning
acardiac t.
cardiac t.
twin-peak syndrome
twin-to-twin
t.-t.-t. transfusion reaction
t.-t.-t. transfusion syndrome (TTS, TTTS)
t.-t.-t. transfusion system (TTTS)
twin-twin transfusion
twisted
t. hair
t. neck
twister cable
twitch
twitching
arrhythmic t.
TwoCal HN formula
TXA2
thromboxane A2
Tycos aneroid sphygmomanometer
Tygon catheter
Tykerb
Tylenol
T. and Codeine Elixir
T. Cold, Children's
T. Extra Strength
T. With Codeine No. 2, 3, 4
Tylok high-tension cerclage cabling system
tylosis ciliaris

Tylox
tympana (*pl. of* tympanum)
tympani
  chorda t.
  scala t.
tympanic
  t. membrane
  t. membrane compliance
  t. membrane perforation
  t. temperature
tympanites
  uterine t.
tympanitic abdomen
tympanocentesis (TPC)
tympanogram
tympanomastoid suture line
tympanometer
tympanometric
  t. gradient
  t. width
tympanometry
  impedance t.
tympanosclerosis
tympanosquamous suture line
tympanostomy tube
tympanum, *pl.* **tympana, tympanums**
tympanums (*pl. of* tympanum)
tympany
Ty-Pap
type
  accelerated skeletal maturation,
    Marshall-Smith t.
  adenovirus t. 3
  t. A IL-8 receptor
  alpha-thalassemia/mental retardation
    syndrome, deletion t.
  alpha-thalassemia/mental retardation
    syndrome, nondeletion t.
  Amsterdam t.
  t. and hold (T&H)
  axonal t.
  Babesia WA1 t.
  Batten-Bielschowsky t.
  t. B IL-8 receptor
  breech t.
  Caldwell-Moloy pelvis t.
  clinical t.
  dementia of Alzheimer t. (DAT)
  t. 1 diabetes mellitus
  t. 2 diabetes mellitus
  D-mosaic blood t.
  dominantly hyperactive impulsive t.
  Du variant blood t.
  epidermolysis bullosa, macular t.
    (EBM)
  facial clefting syndrome, Gypsy t.
  gangliosidosis GM1 juvenile t.
  generalized gangliosidosis GM1
    adult t.

  generalized gangliosidosis juvenile t.
  t. 7 glycogenosis
  hereditary bullous skin dystrophy,
    macular t.
  human astrovirus t. 1
  hydroxysteroid dehydrogenase t. 2
  t. I collagen C-telopeptide
  t. II pneumocyte
  t. II pneumonocyte
  t. II rickets
  t. I rickets
  t. IV RTA
  MALT t.
  mating t.
  mucopolysaccharidosis unclassified t.
  nephronophthisis t. 1
  neurofibromatosis t. 1
  neurofibromatosis t. 2
  normal female sex chromosome t.
    (XX)
  normal male sex chromosome t. (XY)
  t. 16 papillomavirus
  peroneal muscular atrophy, axonal t.
  Pi t.
  plasminogen activator inhibitor t. 1
  plasminogen activator inhibitor t. 2
  primary hyperoxaluria t. 1
  protease inhibitor t.
  quadrivalent human papillomavirus t.
    6, 11, 16, 18
  senile dementia of Alzheimer t.
    (SDAT)
  sialuria, Finnish t.
  wave t.
  wild t.
typhi
  Rickettsia t.
  Salmonella t.
typhimurium
  Salmonella t.
typhlenteritis (*var. of* typhlitis)
typhlitis, typhlenteritis
typhoid
  t. autoantibody
  t. fever
  t. vaccine
typhoidal tularemia
typhus
  t. fever
  flying squirrel t.
  t. group
  louse-borne t.
  murine t.
  North Asian tick t.
  Queensland tick t.
  recrudescent t.
  scrub t.
  sylvatic t.
  tick-borne t.

typical
  t. absence epilepsy
  t. absence seizure
  t. measles
typing
  blood t.
  DNA t.
  HLA t.
  newborn platelet antigen t.
  short tandem repeat t.
  STR t.
  tissue t.
typus degenerativus amstelodamensis
Tyrode solution
tyropanoate sodium
tyrosinase-negative oculocutaneous albinism
tyrosinase-positive oculocutaneous albinism
tyrosine
  t. aminotransferase (TAT)
  t. aminotransferase deficiency (TATD)
  t. kinase
  t. kinase receptor
  t. phosphatase
  t. transaminase deficiency
tyrosinemia
  hepatorenal t.
  hereditary t.
  oculocutaneous t.
  Oregon-type t.
  transient t.
  t. (type 1, 2)
tyrosinosis
  oculocutaneous t.
  t. (type 1, 2)
t Y;18 syndrome
Tyzine Nasal
TZ
  transformation zone
Tzanck
  T. preparation
  T. smear
  T. test

T

U
 U elevator
UA
 umbilical artery
 urinalysis
UAC
 umbilical artery catheter
UAE
 uterine artery embolization
UAL
 umbilical artery line
UALTE
 unexplained apparent life-threatening
 event
UAO
 urine acid output
UARS
 upper airway resistance
 syndrome
UBE3A gene
UC
 umbilical cord
 urethral catheterization
 urinary catheter
 urine culture
 uterine contraction
UCAC
 uterine cornual access catheter
Ucephan Oral
UCG
 urinary chorionic gonadotropin
UCG-Slide Test
Uchida
 U. fimbriectomy
 U. method
 U. procedure
 U. tubal ligation
UCI
 umbilical coiling index
 PPROM UCI
U-Cort
 U-C. cream
 U-C. Topical
UCP
 umbilical cord prolapse
 urethral closure pressure
UDI
 urinary diagnostic index
 Urinary Distress Inventory
 Urogenital Distress Inventory
UDP
 uridine diphosphate
UDP-galactose-4-epimerase (GALE)
UD-2000 urodynamic measurement
system

UE
 upper extremity
UEP
 urinary excretion of protein
UES
 upper esophageal sphincter
UF
 ultrafiltration
 hydraulic UF
 osmotic UF
 rapid UF
U/F
 Fulvicin U/F
UFC
 urinary free cortisol
UFE
 uterine fibroid embolization
UGA
 urogenital atrophy
u-hFSH
 urinary-derived human
 follicle-stimulating hormone
Uhl anomaly
Uhthoff
 U. sign
 U. symptom
UICC
 International Union Against Cancer
ulcer
 aphthous u.
 bearclaw u.
 chancroid u.
 corneal u.
 decubitus u.
 duodenal u.
 genital aphthous u.
 herpetiform aphthous u.
 herpetiform corneal u.
 Hunner u.
 idiopathic u.
 jejunal u.
 kissing u.
 Lipschütz u.
 mucocutaneous u.
 oral aphthous u.
 peptic u.
 recurrent genital aphthous u.
 shallow u.
 stress-associated u.
 vaginal u.
ulcera (*pl. of* ulcus)
ulcerans
 Mycobacterium u.
ulceration
 aphthous u.

U

ulceration (*continued*)
corneal u.
digital u.
esophageal u.
genital u.
nasal u.
oral u.
penile u.
perianastomotic u.
shallow u.
ulcerative
u. blepharitis
u. colitis
u. tumor
u. vulvitis
ulceroglandular
u. disease
u. tularemia
ulcus, *pl.* **ulcera**
u. vulvae acutum
ULE
unilateral laterothoracic exanthema
ulegyria
uLH
urinary luteinizing hormone
ulinastatin
Ullrich
U. and Fremerey-Dohna syndrome
U. disease
Ullrich-Bonnevie syndrome
Ullrich-Feichtiger syndrome
Ullrich-Noonan syndrome
Ullrich-Turner syndrome
ulna (U), *pl.* **ulnae**
ulnae (*pl. of* ulna)
ulnar
u. clubhand
u. collateral ligament
u. nerve block
u. neuropathy
u. palmar grasp
u. styloid fracture
u. tilt
ulnar-mammary syndrome
Ulrich-Turner stigmata
ultra
U. Bright Beginnings Lipids
formula
Prenate U.
Ultracef
ultrafast
u. magnetic resonance imaging
u. MRI
ultrafiltrate
ultrafiltration (UF)
u. membrane
u. virus clearance
Ultrafort prenatal vitamin
Ultramark ultrasound system

ultrasensitive assay
ultrasonic
u. cephalometry
u. egg recovery
u. endovaginal finding
u. fetometry
ultrasonogram
ultrasonographic
u. assessment
u. determination
u. diagnosis
u. guidance
ultrasonographically guided oocyte retrieval
ultrasonography (US)
color Doppler u. (CDU)
compression u.
cranial u.
diagnostic u.
3-dimensional u.
Doppler u.
endoanal u.
endovaginal u.
graded compression u.
gray-scale u.
hepatobiliary u.
high-resolution u.
intravascular u.
level III u.
obstetric u.
real-time u.
transabdominal u.
transcranial Doppler u.
transperineal u.
transvaginal u. (TVU, TVUS)
umbilical artery Doppler u.
ultrasonohysterography
ultrasonologist
ultrasound (US)
abdominal u.
Acuson 128 Doppler u.
Acuson 128XP-10 u.
Advantage u.
Aloka 650 CL u.
Aloka OB/GYN u.
A-mode u.
antenatal u.
u. assessment
ATL Ultramark 4,8,9 u.
Babe u.
B-mode u.
Cineloop U.
cranial u.
3D u.
u. diagnosis
digital u.
3-dimensional u. (3DUS)
Doppler u.
duplex u.

dynamic image on u.
Elscint ESI-3000 u.
endoanal u.
endovaginal u. (EVUS)
fetal u.
u. fetometry
GE RT 3200 Advantage II u.
u. guidance
HDI 3000 u.
head u.
high-resolution u.
Hitachi EUB 420 digital u.
intracoronary u.
intravascular u. (IVUS)
Maggi disposable biopsy needle
  guide for u.
M-mode u.
noncontact u.
obstetric u. (OUS)
pancreatic u.
pelvic u.
Performa u.
Pie Medical u.
prenatal u.
ProSound SSD-5500 u.
pulsed Doppler u.
pulsed-wave u.
quantitative u. (QUS)
real-time imaging on u.
renal u.
routine antenatal diagnostic imaging
  with u. (RADIUS)
u. scanning
screening u.
u. screening
Shimadzu SDU-400 u.
Siemens SI 400 u.
SonoAce 6000 II u.
SonoAce 8000 Live u.
Sonoline Prima u.
Spectra-Diasonics u.
u. stethoscope
Sunlight Omnisense u.
u. surveillance
targeted u.
u. technology
transabdominal u.
transabdominal/transvaginal u.
  (TAS/TVS)
transcervical u.
u. transcervical tuboplasty
u. transducer
translabial u.
transperineal u.
transrectal u. (TRUS)
transvaginal u. (TVU, TVUS,
  TV-UST)
vaginal probe u.
volumetric bladder u.

ultrasound-directed
  u.-d. egg retrieval
  u.-d. percutaneous umbilical blood
    sampling
ultrasound-guided transcervical tuboplasty
Ultravate
ultraviolet (UV)
  u. A, B
  u. A phototherapy
  u. light
umbilical
  u. arterial EDV
  u. arterial pH
  u. artery (UA)
  u. artery catheter (UAC)
  u. artery catheterization
  u. artery Doppler ultrasonography
  u. artery Doppler velocimetry
  u. artery line (UAL)
  u. artery pulsatility index to middle
    cerebral artery pulsatility index
    ratio
  u. artery waveform notching
    abnormality
  u. blood flow
  u. blood sampling
  u. cardiovascular circulation
  u. clamp
  u. coiling index (UCI)
  u. cord (UC)
  u. cord accident
  u. cord anomaly
  u. cord blood bank
  u. cord blood transplantation
  u. cord compression
  u. cord hematoma
  u. cord insertion
  u. cord leptin
  u. cord mass
  u. cord prolapse (UCP)
  u. cord syndrome
  u. cord transfusion
  u. cyst
  u. Doppler flow velocity
  u. fistula
  u. fold
  u. fungus
  u. granuloma
  u. hernia
  u. ligament
  u. line
  u. polyp
  u. port
  u. presentation
  u. scissors
  u. souffle
  u. stump
  u. swab
  u. vein (UV)

U

umbilical (*continued*)
  u. vein catheter (UVC)
  u. vein catheterization
  u. vein packed red blood cell
    transfusion
  u. vein platelet transfusion
  u. vein varix
  u. velocity ratio
  u. venous catheter (UVC)
  u. venous flow
  u. venous line (UVL)
  u. venous plasma amino acid
  u. vessel
  u. vessel catheter
umbilicalis
  arteritis u.
  chorda u.
  funiculus u.
umbilication of lesion
umbilici (*pl. of* umbilicus)
umbilicoplacental vessel
umbilicoplasty
umbilicus, *pl.* **umbilici**
  areola u.
  furrowlike u.
  u. reconstruction
Umbilicutter
umbrella
  Bard PDA U.
  u. device
  u. sign
  vascular u.
Unasyn
unavoidable hemorrhage
unbalanced
  u. AV canal defect
  u. gamete
  u. parental chromosome
    complement
  u. translocation
unborn child
unbound iron
uncalcified
  u. bacterial plaque
  u. bone matrix
uncal herniation
uncinate fit
uncircumcised penis
uncombable hair syndrome
uncompensated
  u. hydrocephalus
  u. respiratory acidosis
  u. shock
uncomplicated
  u. hernia
  u. measles
unconjugated
  u. bilirubin
  u. estriol (E3, uE3)

  u. estriol level
  u. hyperbilirubinemia
unconscious incontinence
uncuffed endotracheal tube
undecapeptide
undecylenic
  u. acid
  u. acid ointment
underdeveloped
  u. chin
  u. mandible
underdevelopment
  face u.
  middle third of face u.
underdose
underfeeding
underinflation
underlying disease
undernourished
undernourishment
  maternal u.
undernutrition
underperfusion
  uterine u.
undervascularity
  pulmonary u.
underwater
  u. delivery
  u. drainage system
  u. weighing
Underwood disease
undescended
  u. testicle
  u. testis
undifferentiated
  u. gonad
  u. rhabdomyosarcoma
Undoguent Topical
Undritz anomaly
undulant fever
unemancipated
unequal
  u. aeration
  u. conjoined twins
  u. visual input
unestrogenized vaginal mucosa
unexplained
  u. apparent life-threatening event
    (UALTE)
  u. fever
  u. infertility
  u. jaundice
  u. recurrent miscarriage
unfavorable cervix
unfortified human milk
unfractionated heparin
UNG
  uracil-N-glycosylase
ungual

unguium
  tinea u.
UNHS
  universal newborn hearing screening
UNHSP
  universal newborn hearing screening
  program
Uni-Ace
unicameral bone cyst
Unicare breast pump
unicellular
unicentric
unicollis
  uterus bicornis u.
unicommisural
unicornis
  uterus u.
unicornuate uterus
unicorn uterus
unidentified bright object
unifactorial disorder
unifocal clonic movement
Uni-Gold Recombine HIV test
unilambdoid synostosis
unilateral
  u. agenesis
  u. bar
  u. congenital ptosis
  u. cryptorchidism
  u. facial microsomia
  u. fibular aplastic syndrome
  u. flank mass
  u. hearing impairment
  u. hemimegalencephaly
  u. hyperlucent lung
  u. hypoplastic pectoral muscle
  u. intrauterine facial necrosis
  u. laterothoracic exanthema (ULE)
  u. lower lip paralysis
  u. mandibulofacial dysostosis
  u. megalencephaly
  u. microtia
  u. mydriasis
  u. neonatal hydronephrosis
  u. occipital plagiocephaly
  u. oophorectomy
  u. optic neuritis
  u. optokinetic nystagmus
  u. partial facial paralysis
  u. renal agenesis
  u. salpingo-oophorectomy (USO)
  u. stapling
  u. ureteral obstruction (UUO)
unilocular
  u. cystic ovarian mass
  u. ovarian cyst
Unimar
  U. HSG tray
  U. Pipelle

uninducible cervix
uninhibited
  u. bladder
  u. detrusor contraction
uninterrupted estrogen
union
  delayed u.
uniovular twins
uniparental
  u. disomy (UPD)
  u. maternal disomy
  u. paternal disomy
Uniphyl
Uniplant
unipolar
  u. depression
  u. electrocautery
  u. electrode
Uniserts
  acetaminophen U.
  bisacodyl U.
  Hemril-HC U.
  RMS U.
Unisom
unit
  Alexander u.
  antenatal testing u.
  antepartum u.
  Bethesda u.
  BiliBed phototherapy u.
  bone collagen equivalent u. (BCE)
  Bovie u.
  bubble isolation u.
  calf compression u.
  colony-forming u. (CFU)
  dentoalveolar u.
  fetal-placental u.
  Flowtron DVT prophylaxis u.
  human *neu* u. (HNU)
  immunizing u. (IU)
  u. inheritance
  intensive special care u. (ISCU)
  International U. (IU)
  lipase u.
  Log-a-Rhythm Signal Acquisition u.
  maternal-fetal medicine u. (MFMU)
  maternal-placental u.
  maternal-placental-fetal u.
  Montevideo u.
  neonatal intensive care u. (NICU)
  newborn intensive care u. (NBICU)
  newborn special care u. (NBSCU)
  nutritional milk u.
  Nytone enuretic control u.
  Orthotic Research and Locomotor
    Assessment U. (ORLAU)
  pediatric intensive care u. (PICU)
  pediatric sedation u. (PSU)
  pilosebaceous u.

U

unit (*continued*)

    plaque-forming u. (pfu)

    terminal ductal lobular u. (TDLU)

    terminal duct lobular u. (TDLU)

    uteroplacental u.

    warming u.

united

    U. Network for Organ Sharing (UNOS)

    U. States Preventive Services Task Force (USPSTF)

units-erythroid

    burst-forming u.-e. (BFU-E)

univariate

univentricular

universal

    u. bilirubin screen

    u. hearing screen

    U. indicator stick

    u. joint syndrome

    u. newborn hearing screening (UNHS)

    u. newborn hearing screening program (UNHSP)

    u. nose of childhood

    U. reducer cap

    U. vaginal probe

universale

    pterygium u.

universalis

    alopecia u.

    neurinomatosis u.

unlike twins

unmalleable

Unna

    U. mark

    U. nevus

Unna-Thost syndrome

unopposed estrogen

UNOS

    United Network for Organ Sharing

unpaired chromosome

unpasteurized milk product

unplanned pregnancy

unPromethazine VC Plain Syrup

unprotected coital event

unprovoked seizure

unrecognized

    u. apnea

    u. pregnancy

unregulated catabolism

unresponsive

    alertness, response to voice, response to pain, u. (AVPU)

unresponsiveness

    ACTH u.

    immunologic u.

    thyroid hormone u.

unrestrictive ventricular septal defect

unroofed coronary sinus

unroofing

    endoscopic u.

    patch u.

unruptured tubal gestation

unsaturated

    u. fat

    u. linolenic acid

    u. phosphatidylcholine

unspun

    u. catheterized urine specimen

    u. urine

unstable

    u. bladder

    u. bladder of childhood

    u. bladder syndrome

    u. fetal presentation

    u. hemoglobin

    u. lie

unusual hunger

Unverricht disease

Unverricht-Lundborg

    U.-L. disease

    U.-L. syndrome

UOAC

    uterine ostial access catheter

up

    pinked u.

UPA

    uteroplacental apoplexy

u-PA

    urokinase plasminogen activator

upbeat nystagmus

UPD

    uniparental disomy

updraft treatment

UPI

    uteroplacental insufficiency

UPJ

    ureteropelvic junction

    UPJ obstruction

UPLIFT

    uterine positioning via ligament investment fixation truncation

    UPLIFT procedure

UPP

    urethral pressure profilometry

upper

    u. airway noise

    u. airway resistance syndrome (UARS)

    u. airway sleep-disordered breathing

    u. body segment

    u. body segment to lower body segment ratio

    u. contractile portion

    u. contractile portion of uterus

    u. esophageal sphincter (UES)

    u. extremity (UE)

u. gastrointestinal (UGI)
u. gastrointestinal series
u. genital tract infection
u. GI lesion
u. humeral epiphysis
u. limb amelia
u. limb deficiency
u. motor neuron disease
u. motor neuron sign
u. motor neuron syndrome
u. respiratory illness
u. respiratory infection (URI)
u. respiratory tract
u. respiratory tract infection
(URTI)
u. urinary tract infection
upper-angle suture
UPPP
uvulopalatopharyngoplasty
upregulation
upright
u. abdominal radiograph
u. chest film
u. tilt-table testing
upsaliensis
Campylobacter u.
UPS 2020 ambulatory measurement system
UPSC
uterine papillary serous carcinoma
upside-down ptosis
upslanting palpebral fissure
upstairs-downstairs heart
upstream
upstroke
uptake
bone mineral u.
maximum oxygen u. (VO$_2$max)
minute oxygen u.
radioactive u.
upward
u. gaze
u. gaze weakness
u. rotation
urachal
u. cyst
u. fistula
urachus
obliterated u.
patent u.
persistent u.
Uracid
Uracil
uracil-N-glycosylase (UNG)
Uraniscochasm (*var. of* uranoschisis)
uranoschisis, Uraniscochasm
uranostaphyloschisis, uranoveloschisis
uranoveloschisis (*var. of* uranostaphyloschisis)

urate
u. calculus
u. clearance
u. crystal
u. nephropathy
u. tophus
Urbach-Wiethe disease
Urban
U. operation
U. syndrome
Urban-Rogers-Meyer syndrome
urea
u. breath test (UBT)
u. clearance
u. cycle
u. cycle disease
u. cycle disorder
u. cycle enzyme defect
u. nitrogen
u. plaster
urealyticum
Ureaplasma u.
Ureaphil
Ureaplasma
U. culture
U. urealyticum
Urecholine
ureidopenicillin
uremia, urinemia
uremic
u. encephalopathy
u. state
u. syndrome
ureter
atretic u.
double u.
duplicated u.
ectopic u.
u. fistula
ileal u.
partially duplicated u.
reimplantation of u.
retrocaval u.
ureteral, ureteric
u. course
u. duplication
u. dysmenorrhea
u. ectopia
u. injury
u. jet
u. node
u. obstruction
u. patency
u. peristalsis
u. rupture
u. surgical treatment
u. trigonal reimplantation
u. triplication
u. valve

U

ureteric (*var.* of ureteral)
    u. bud
ureterocalycostomy
ureterocele
    ectopic u.
    prolapsed ectopic u.
    simple u.
ureterocervical
ureterocystoplasty
    augmentation u.
ureteroileostomy
    Bricker u.
ureteroneocystostomy
    Glen Anderson u.
    Politano-Leadbetter u.
ureteropelvic junction (UPJ)
ureteropelvioneostomy (*var.* of
  ureteropyelostomy)
ureteropyeloneostomy (*var.* of
  ureteropyelostomy)
ureteropyeloscope
    Karl Storz flexible u.
ureteropyelostomy, ureteropelvioneostomy,
  ureteropyeloneostomy
ureteroscope
    AUR-7 flexible u.
ureterosigmoidostomy
ureterostomy
    cutaneous u.
ureterotubal anastomosis
ureteroureteral anastomosis
ureteroureterostomy
ureterouterine
ureterovaginal fistula
ureterovesical (UV)
    u. junction (UVJ)
    u. obstruction
    u. reflux
ureterovesicoplasty
    Leadbetter-Politano u.
urethra
    bulbus urethrae
    compressor u.
    dilated posterior u.
    drain-pipe u.
    fusiform dilation of u.
    imperforate u.
    lead pipe u.
    low-pressure u.
    milking of u.
    penile u.
    pipestem u.
    posterior u.
    proximal u.
urethral
    u. advancement and glanuloplasty
    u. angle
    u. atresia
    u. candle

    u. cap
    u. caruncle
    u. catheterization (UC)
    u. closure pressure (UCP)
    u. coaptation
    u. detachment
    u. discharge
    u. diverticulectomy
    u. diverticulum
    u. duplication
    u. elongation
    u. epithelium
    u. function
    u. gland
    u. hypermobility
    u. lumen
    u. meatus
    u. occlusion insert
    u. opening
    u. plate
    u. plate division
    u. plug
    u. pressure cough profile
    u. pressure profile
    u. pressure profilometry (UPP)
    u. prolapse
    u. seam
    u. sling
    u. sound
    u. spasm
    u. sphincter
    u. stenosis
    u. support
    u. suspension
    u. syndrome
    u. valve
urethralis
    habenula u.
urethritis
    anterior u.
    atrophic u.
    chlamydial u.
    follicular u.
    gonococcal u. (GCU)
    granular u.
    nongonococcal u.
    nonspecific u. (NSU)
    u. petrificans
    posterior u.
    senile u.
    simple u.
    specific u.
    u. venerea
urethrocele
urethrocutaneous fistula
urethrocystometry
urethrocystopexy
    retropubic u. (RPU)
urethrocystoscopy

urethrography
  positive pressure u.
urethrolysis
  transabdominal u.
  transvaginal u.
urethropexy
  Burch retropubic u.
urethroplasty
  Badenoch u.
  Thiersch-Duplay u.
  Turner-Warwick u.
urethroscopy
urethrotome
urethrotomy
  direct vision internal u. (DVIU)
urethrotrigonitis
urethrovaginal
  u. fistula
  u. sphincter muscle
urethrovesical (UV)
  u. angle (UVA)
  u. angle support
Urex
urge
  U. Impact Scale (URIS)
  u. incontinence
Urge-IIQ survey
urgency
  u. syndrome
  urinary u.
urgency-frequency syndrome
URI
  upper respiratory infection
uric
  u. acid
  u. acid infarction
  u. acid lithiasis
  u. acid nephrolithiasis
  u. acid stone
uricosuria
Uricult culture
uridine diphosphate (UDP)
Uridon
uridyltransferase
  galactose-1-phosphate u. (GALT)
urinalysis (UA)
  bagged u.
  clean-catch u. (CCUA)
  enhanced u.
urinary
  u. beta-core fragment
  u. bladder
  u. bladder dysfunction
  u. calculus
  u. cast
  u. catheter (UC)
  u. catheterization
  u. chorionic gonadotropin (UCG)
  u. concentrating capacity

u. concentrating defect
u. concentration test
u. conduit
u. copper
u. coproporphyrin
u. coproporphyrin I
u. diagnostic index (UDI)
u. diary
u. dipstick test
U. Distress Inventory (UDI)
u. diversion
u. diverticulum
u. excreted melatonin
u. excretion
u. excretion of protein (UEP)
u. exertional incontinence
u. fistula
u. free cortisol
u. free progesterone
u. frequency
u. glucose
u. glycosaminoglycan
u. iodine
u. lactate-creatinine ratio
u. luteinizing hormone (uLH)
u. menopausal gonadotropin
u. mucopolysaccharide pattern
u. orotic acid
u. outlet obstruction
u. output
u. ovulation detection kit
u. ovulation predictor kit
u. potassium wasting
u. pterin
u. reflux
u. retention
u. sediment
u. sphincter
u. stasis
u. stent
u. steroid conjugate
u. stress incontinence (USI)
u. system
u. tract
u. tract abnormality
u. tract anomaly
u. tract dilation
u. tract disorder
u. tract dysplasia
u. tract endometriosis
u. tract infection (UTI)
u. tract malformation (UTM)
u. tract obstruction (UTO)
u. trigone
u. trypsin inhibitor
u. undiversion procedure
u. urgency
urinary-derived human follicle-stimulating hormone (u-hFSH)

U

urination
  fetal u.
urine
  u. acid output (UAO)
  u. CIE test
  Coke-colored u.
  cola-colored u.
  concentrated u.
  u. culture (UC)
  u. cytology
  dark u.
  delirium, infection, atrophic
    urethritis/vaginitis, pharmaceuticals,
    psychological, excess u.
  dilute u.
  u. dipstick
  u. ferric chloride test
  fetal u.
  u. flow
  u. ketoacid
  u. latex test
  u. leakage
  u. ligase chain reaction
  malodorous u.
  maple syrup u.
  u. mucopolysaccharide
  u. organic acid
  u. output
  persistent alkaline u.
  residual u.
  u. sample
  u. sampling
  u. sediment
  u. specimen (US)
  spun u.
  suprapubic aspiration
    of u.
  tea-colored u.
  u. test strip
  u. toxicology screen
  unspun u.
  u. vanillylmandelic acid
  vin rosé-colored u.
urinemia (*var. of* uremia)
urine-reducing substance
uriniferous breath
urinoma
URIS
  Urge Impact Scale
Uriscreen urine test
Urised
Urispas
Uristat
Uri-Three urine culture kit
Uri-Two petri dish
urobilinogen excretion
urobilinogenuria
urobilinoid
urocanase deficiency

urocanic
  u. acid
  u. aciduria
Urocit-K
Urocyte diagnostic cytometry system
urocytogram
urodynamic
  u. stress incontinence
  u. testing
urodynamically
urodynamics testing
uroepithelium
urofacial syndrome
uroflowmetry
urofollitropin
  u. for injection
  u. for injection, purified
urogenital
  u. atrophy (UGA)
  u. congenital anomaly
  u. diaphragm
  U. Distress Inventory (UDI)
  u. epithelium
  u. fistula
  u. fold
  u. hiatus
  u. ridge
  u. septum
  u. sinus
  u. sphincter
  u. system
  u. tract
urogenitogram
urogenitography
Urogesic
urogram
  excretory u.
  intravenous u. (IVU)
urography
  intravenous u. (IVU)
  intravenous excretory u.
  magnetic resonance u. (MRU)
urogynecologic
urogynecologist
urogynecology
urokinase
  u. plasminogen activator (u-PA)
Uro-KP-Neutral
Urolene Blue Oral
urolithiasis
urologic, urological
  u. evaluation
  u. history
  u. injury
  u. problem
urological (*var. of* urologic)
urologist
urology
Uro-Mag capsule

uropathogen
uropathy
    bilateral u.
    fetal u.
    lower obstructive u. (LOU)
    obstructive u.
urorectal
urosepsis
urothelium
    trigonal u.
UroVive system
UroVysion bladder cancer kit
Urozide
ursi
    uva u.
Urso
ursodeoxycholic acid
ursodiol
URTI
    upper respiratory tract infection
urticaria
    acquired u.
    acute u.
    cholinergic u.
    chronic idiopathic u.
    cold u.
    contact u.
    cutaneous u.
    idiopathic u.
    papular u.
    u. pigmentosa
    pressure u.
    primary acquired u.
    secondary solar u.
    solar u.
urticarial, urticarious
    u. papule
    u. raised lesion
urticarious (*var. of* urticarial)
urticate
urtication
US
    ultrasonography
    ultrasound
    urine specimen
    Usher syndrome
    US 1005 uroflow meter
USA Elite System gynecologic rotating continuous flow resectoscope
use
    compassionate u.
    conservative drug u.
    drug u.
    illicit drug u.
    intravaginal foreign body u.
    intravenous drug u. (IDU)
    maternal cocaine u.
    Maternal Interview of Substance U. (MISU)

    oral contraceptive u.
    prophylactic aspirin u.
    rape kit u.
    substance u.
U-shaped
    U-s. deceleration
    U-s. vestibulectomy
Usher syndrome (US)
USI
    urinary stress incontinence
USO
    unilateral salpingo-oophorectomy
U.S. Preventive Services Task Force (USPSTF)
USPSTF
    United States Preventive Services Task Force
uterectomy
uteri (*pl. of* uterus)
uterine
    u. abnormality
    u. absence
    u. access
    u. action
    u. activity
    u. activity alteration
    u. activity monitor
    u. agenesis
    u. angiosarcoma
    u. anomaly
    u. arteriovenous malformation
    u. artery
    u. artery embolization (UAE)
    u. artery hemodynamic adaptation
    u. artery ligation
    u. artery pseudoaneurysm
    u. atony
    u. balloon therapy (UBT)
    u. ballottement
    u. blood flow
    u. body
    u. calculus
    u. carcinosarcoma
    u. cast
    u. cavity
    u. chondrosarcoma
    u. colic
    u. compression
    u. contractile agent
    u. contractility
    u. contraction (UC)
    u. coring
    u. cornu
    u. cornual access catheter (UCAC)
    u. corpus
    u. corpus carcinoma
    u. corpus tumor
    u. cough
    u. cramping

U

uterine (*continued*)
u. cry
u. curette
u. decompression
u. displacement
u. dysfunction
u. dysmenorrhea
u. elevator
u. endolymphatic stroma
u. endometrial stroma
u. enlargement
u. epithelial stroma
u. epithelium
u. evacuator
u. evaluation
U. Explora curette
u. exteriorization
u. factor
u. fibroid
u. fibroid carneous degeneration
u. fibroid embolization (UFE)
u. fibroid red degeneration
u. fibromyoma
u. flora
u. fragmentation
u. fundus
u. gland
u. hematoma
u. hemodynamics
u. hemorrhage
u. hernia syndrome
u. horn
u. hyperstimulation
u. hypertonus
u. hypotonia
u. incarceration
u. incision
u. inertia
u. infection
u. insufficiency
u. inversion
u. involution
u. lateral fusion defect
u. leiomyomata
u. lysosome level
u. malposition
u. manipulator
u. mass
u. massage
u. milk
u. morcellation
u. müllerian sarcoma
u. muscle
u. myoma
u. myometrium
u. necrosis
u. neoplasm
u. ostial access catheter (UOAC)
u. outflow obstruction

u. packing
u. papillary serous carcinoma (UPSC)
u. pathology
u. perforation
u. polyp
u. position
u. positioning via ligament investment fixation truncation (UPLIFT)
u. pregnancy
u. prolapse
u. pyomyoma
u. quiescence
u. reconstruction
u. relaxation
u. rent
u. retroflexion
u. retroversion
u. rupture
u. sarcoma metastasis
u. scar dehiscence
u. scar separation
u. screening
u. segment
u. septum
u. sinus
u. size
u. souffle
u. sound
u. support
u. suspension
u. tachysystole
u. tenaculum
u. tenaculum forceps
u. tetanus
u. tone
u. tonus
u. tube
u. tumor resembling ovarian sex-cord tumor (UTROSCT)
u. tympanites
u. underperfusion
u. vein
u. vessel
u. wall
u. window formation
u. withdrawal bleeding
uterinus
vagitus u.
uterismus
uteritis
utero
fetal death in u. (FDIU)
fetal demise in u. (FDIU)
fetal version in u.
in u. (IU)
uteroabdominal pregnancy
Uterobrush endometrial sample collector

uterocystostomy
uterofixation
uterolith
uterometer
uteroovarian
    u. circulation
    u. ligament
    u. varicocele
uteroperitoneal fistula
uteropexy
uteroplacental
    u. apoplexy (UPA)
    u. blood flow
    u. circulation
    u. insufficiency (UPI)
    u. perfusion
    u. sinus
    u. unit
    u. vessel
uteroplasty
uterosacral
    u. complex
    u. ligament
    u. ligament pedicle
    u. ligament suspension
    u. nerve ablation
    u. nerve ligation
    u. nodularity
    u. plication
    u. shortening
uterosalpingography
uteroscope
uteroscopy
uterotomy
uterotonic
uterotubal junction (UTJ)
uterotubography
uterovaginal
    u. canal
    u. primordium
    u. prolapse
uterus, *pl.* uteri
    u. acollis
    adenomyosis uteri
    adnexa uteri
    anomalous u.
    arcuate u.
    u. arcuatus
    AV/AF u.
    benign nonprolapsed u.
    u. bicornis
    u. bicornis unicollis
    bicornuate u.
    bifid u.
    u. bifidus
    biforate u.
    u. biforis
    u. bilocularis
    bipartite u.

u. bipartitus
bivalving of u.
boggy u.
capped u.
communicating u.
cordiform u.
u. cordiformis
cornu uteri
corpus of u.
Couvelaire u.
Credé maneuver of u.
descensus uteri
u. didelphys
double u.
double-mouthed u.
u. duplex
duplex u.
duplicate u.
gliosis uteri
gravid u.
heart-shaped u.
1-horned u.
horn of u.
hourglass u.
hyperdynamia uteri
hypoplastic u.
ichthyosis uteri
impacted u.
incarcerated gravid u.
incudiform u.
u. incudiformis
inversion of the u.
involution of the u.
large-for-dates u.
leiomyoma uteri
midposition u.
myoma uteri
nonprolapsed u.
u. parvicollis
pear-shaped u.
placenta, ovary, u. (POU)
procidentia uteri
prolapsed u.
prolapse of u.
retroverted u.
ruptured u.
sacculation of u.
septate u.
u. septus
subseptate u.
u. subseptus
symmetric communicating u.
tetanic u.
triangular u.
u. triangularis
T-shaped u.
unicorn u.
u. unicornis
unicornuate u.

U

uterus (*continued*)
    upper contractile portion of u.
UTI
    urinary tract infection
    febrile UTI
Uticort Topical
UTJ
    uterotubal junction
UTM
    urinary tract malformation
UTO
    urinary tract obstruction
Utrata forceps
utricle
    prostatic u.
utriculoplasty
UTROSCT
    uterine tumor resembling ovarian sex-cord tumor
utterance
    mean length of u. (MLU)
UUO
    unilateral ureteral obstruction
UV
    ultraviolet
    umbilical vein
    ureterovesical
    urethrovesical

UVA
    urethrovesical angle
uva ursi
UVC
    umbilical vein catheter
    umbilical venous catheter
uveitides (*pl. of* uveitis)
uveitis, *pl.* **uveitides**
    acute anterior u.
    posterior u.
    subacute anterior u.
uveomeningitic disease
uveomeningoencephalitic syndrome
uveoparotid
    u. fever
    u. fever syndrome
UVJ
    ureterovesical junction
    UVJ obstruction
UVL
    umbilical venous line
uvula, *pl.* **uvuli, uvulae**
    bifid u.
uvulae (*pl. of* uvula)
uvuli (*pl. of* uvula)
uvulitis
uvulopalatopharyngoplasty (UPPP)

VA
   venoarterial
   ventriculoatrial
      VA shunt
VAA
   verbal-auditory agnosia
Vabra
   V. aspiration
   V. cannula
   V. catheter
   V. cervical aspirator
   V. suction
   V. suction curette
VACA
   valvuloplasty and angioplasty of
   congenital anomalies
vaccination
   natural v.
   rotavirus v.
   v. varicella
   varicella v.
   yellow fever 17D v.
vaccinatum
   eczema v.
vaccine
   Acel-Imune v.
   acellular pertussis v.
   ActHIB v.
   V. Adverse Events Reporting
      System (VAERS)
   antipregnancy v.
   aP v.
   autogenous v.
   bacille Calmette-Gúerin v.
   bacillus Calmette-Gúerin v.
   BCG v.
   Certiva v.
   chickenpox v.
   cholera v.
   cold-adapted influenza v. (CAIV)
   cold-adapted intranasal influenza v.
   5-component v.
   Comvax v.
   conjugate pneumococcal v.
   Decavac v.
   diphtheria, tetanus, acellular pertussis
      v.
   diphtheria, tetanus, pertussis v.
   diphtheria, tetanus toxoid, acellular
      pertussis v.
   diphtheria, tetanus toxoids,
      whole-cell pertussis v.
   DTP v.
   Edmonston-Zagreb measles v.
   Engerix-B hepatitis B v.

   enhanced inactivated polio v. (eIPV)
   Escherichia coli v.
   FluMist v.
   GBS v.
   Haemophilus influenzae type b
      conjugate v.
   Haemophilus pertussis v. (HPV)
   Havrix v.
   hepatitis A v. (HAV)
   hepatitis B v. (HBV)
   hepatitis B oligosaccharide-CRM197
      v. (HbOC)
   Hib conjugate v.
   Hib polysaccharide v.
   HibTITER v.
   HPV v.
   human diploid cell v.
   human diploid cell rabies v.
      (HDCV)
   inactivated polio v.
   inactivated poliomyelitis v.
   inactivated poliovirus v. (IPV)
   inactivated virus v.
   Infanrix v.
   influenza v.
   intranasal live influenza v.
   Ipol poliovirus v.
   IPV v.
   killed virus v.
   live attenuated influenza v. (LAIV)
   live-attenuated virus v.
   live poliovirus v.
   live-virus v.
   Lovaxin C cancer v.
   Lyme disease v.
   measles v.
   MenCon v.
   meningococcal conjugate v.
   meningococcal polysaccharide v.
      (MENps)
   MENps v.
   mercury-free v.
   MMR v.
   MMR II v.
   mumps v.
   nonvalent pneumococcal conjugate v.
      (PnCV)
   Oka strain varicella v.
   OPV v.
   oral attenuated *Salmonella typhi* v.v.
   oral polio v. (OPV)
   oral poliovirus v. (OPV)
   Orimune poliovirus v.
   OvaRex v.
   O-Vax v.

V

vaccine (*continued*)
PCEC v.
Pediatrix v.
PedvaxHIB v.
pentavalent v.
PFP v.
plague v.
PncD v.
PNCRM7 v.
PncT v.
pneumococcal v.
pneumococcal conjugate v.
pneumococcal polysaccharide v.
pneumococcal protein conjugate v.
pneumococcal 7-valent conjugate v.
  (PCV7)
poliovirus v.
polyvalent pneumococcal v.
Prevnar pneumococcal v.
protein-conjugated v.
PS23 23-valent polysaccharide v.
rabies v.
recombinant hepatitis B v.
rhesus rotavirus tetravalent v.
rOspA Lyme disease v.
rotavirus v.
rubella v.
Rv v.
Sabin v.
V. Safety Datalink (VSD)
Salk v.
smallpox v.
split-virus v.
v. strain shedding
swine-flu influenza v.
TdaP v.
Td-IPV v.
Td toxoid v.
tetanus and diphtheria
  toxoids v.
tetanus toxoid and diphtheria v.
Theratope v.
thimerosal-free v.
TriHIBit v.
Tri-Immunol v.
Tripedia v.
trivalent inactivated influenza v.
  (TIV)
trivalent live cold-adapted influenza
  v. (CAIV-T)
tularemia v.
typhoid v.
7-valent pneumococcal conjugate v.
Vaqta v.
varicella-zoster virus v.
Varivax v.
v. virus shedding
7VPnC v.
VZV v.

whole cell diphtheria-tetanus-
  pertussis v.
whole cell DTP v.
whole virus v.
yellow fever v. (YF-VAX)
vaccine-acquired poliovirus
vaccine-associated
v.-a. paralytic poliomyelitis
  (VAPP)
v.-a. pneumonia
vaccine-autism scare
vaccinia
v. of vulva
v. virus
vacciniforme
hydroa v.
Vaccinium macrocarpon
VACTERL
vertebral anomalies, anal atresia,
  cardiac defects, tracheoesophageal
  fistula, renal anomalies, limb
  anomalies
VACTERL association
VACTERL association with
  hydrocephalus syndrome
Vacu-Irrigator
Vozzle V.-I.
vacular thrombosis
vacuo
hydrocephalus ex v.
vacuolar myelopathy
vacuolated
vacuolation, vacuolization
vacuole
vacuolization (*var. of* vacuolation)
double v.
duodenal v.
Vacurette
Berkeley V.
Vacutainer
EDTA-anticoagulated V.
V. system
vacuum
v. aspiration
v. aspiration syringe
v. aspirator
v. cannula
v. clitoral therapy device
v. cup
v. curettage
Egnell v.
v. extraction
v. extraction delivery
v. extractor
v. extractor delivery
Kiwi v.
v. pressure
v. suction
vacuum-assisted delivery

VAD
  vitamin A deficiency
VAERS
  Vaccine Adverse Events Reporting
  System
vagabond skin
vagal
  v. activity
  v. inhibition
  v. maneuver
  v. nerve stimulation
  v. reaction
  v. reflex
  v. tone
vagally mediated response
Vagifem
vagina, *pl.* **vaginae**
  adenosis vaginae
  anterior v.
  apex of v.
  artificial v.
  atretic v.
  azygos artery of v.
  blind v.
  blind-ending v.
  bulb of vestibule of v.
  bulbus vestibuli vaginae
  distal v.
  dry v.
  duplicated v.
  exstrophic v.
  imperforate v.
  melanosis vaginae
  neutral pH of v.
  posterior v.
  prepubescent v.
  rudimentary v.
  rugae of v.
  septate v.
  short v.
vaginae (*pl. of* vagina)
vaginal
  v. absence
  v. acidification
  v. adenosis
  v. administration
  v. advancement
  v. agenesis
  v. anomaly
  v. apex
  v. artery
  v. atresia
  v. atrophy
  v. birth after cesarean (VBAC)
  v. birth after cesarean trial of labor
    (VBAC-TOL)
  v. birth after myomectomy
  v. bleeding
  v. breech delivery

v. bulb
v. cancer
v. candidiasis
v. candidosis
v. candle
Canesten V.
v. carcinoma
v. celiotomy
v. cellular maturation
v. clear cell adenocarcinoma
v. colonization
v. condom
v. cone
v. contraceptive
v. contraceptive film (VCF)
v. contraceptive ring
v. cornification test
v. cream
v. cuff
v. cuff adhesion
v. cuff cellulitis
v. cyst
v. cystourethropexy
v. cytology
v. decompression
Dienestrol V.
v. dilator
v. dimple
v. discharge
v. disinfection
v. douche
v. drainage
v. dryness
v. dysmenorrhea
v. dysontogenetic cyst
v. ectopic anus
v. embryonic cyst
v. epithelial abnormality
v. estrogen therapy
v. eversion
v. evisceration
v. examination
v. extension
v. feminine spray
v. flora
v. fluid arborization
v. fluid ferning
v. fluid neutrophil defensins
v. foreign body
v. fornix
v. GIFT
Gyne-Lotrimin V.
v. hand
v. hematoma
v. hood
v. hysterectomy (VH)
v. hysterotomy
v. inclusion cyst
v. infection

V

vaginal (*continued*)
v. injury
v. interruption of pregnancy with dilatation and curettage (VIP-DAC)
v. intraepithelial neoplasia (VAIN, VIN)
v. intraepithelial neoplasia grade III (VAIN III)
v. introitus
v. irrigation smear (VIS)
v. laceration
v. lithotomy
v. lubricant
v. lubrication
v. metastasis
v. microflora
v. misoprostol
v. moisture
Monistat V.
v. morcellation
v. mucification test
v. mucosa
v. myomectomy
v. narrowing
v. neurofibroma
v. neurofibromatosis
Ogen V.
v. opening
Ortho-Dienestrol V.
v. outlet
v. pack
v. packing
v. palpation
v. parity
v. perineorrhaphy
v. pessary
v. pH
v. plate
v. pool specimen
v. pouch
v. probe ultrasound
v. prolapse prosthesis
v. prostaglandin
v. receptivity
v. recombinant human relaxin
v. retractor
v. ring contraception
v. sarcoma
v. secretion
v. septum
v. shortening
v. smear intermediate cell
v. smear parabasal cell
v. smear superficial cell
v. soft tissue dystocia
v. sonography
v. speculum
v. speculum loop

v. spermicide
v. sponge
v. squamous metaplasia
v. stenosis
v. stump prolapse
v. suppository
v. surgery
v. swab
v. switch operation
v. tampon
v. tape obturator
v. tape tension
Terazol V.
v. terminus
v. thickening
v. translation
v. transudate
v. transudation
v. tubal procedure
v. ulcer
Vagistat-1 V.
v. vault
v. vault prolapse
v. vault support
v. vault suspension
v. venous plexus
v. wall
v. wall flap
v. wall repair
v. wall sling procedure
v. wash
v. window
v. yeast
vaginales
rugae v.
vaginalis
Corynebacterium v.
Gardnerella v.
Haemophilus v.
obliterated processus v.
phimosis v.
portio v.
processus v.
Trichomonas v.
tunica v.
vaginally parous
vaginam
per v.
vaginapexy
vaginectomy
vaginism (*var. of* vaginismus)
vaginismus, vaginism
posterior v.
vaginitides (*pl. of* vaginitis)
vaginitis, *pl.* **vaginitides**
v. adhesiva
adhesive v.
amebic v.

atrophic v.
bacterial v. (BV)
Candida albicans v.
Candida glabrata v.
candidal v.
Candida tropicalis v.
chemical v.
chlamydial v.
Corynebacterium v.
v. cystica
cytolytic v.
desquamative inflammatory v.
v. emphysematosa
Gardnerella v.
Haemophilus v.
monilial v.
nonspecific v.
pinworm v.
recurrent v.
senile v.
v. senilis
Shigella v.
streptococcal v.
traumatic v.
trichomonal v.
Trichomonas vaginalis v.
yeast v.
vaginocele
vaginodynia
vaginofixation
vaginogram
vaginography
vaginohysterectomy
vaginometer
vaginomycosis
vaginopathy
vaginoperineoplasty
vaginoperineorraphy
vaginoperineotomy
vaginopexy
Norman Miller v.
vaginoplasty
Fenton v.
tissue expansion v.
vaginorectal
v. culture
v. fistula
vaginoscope
Cameron-Myers v.
Huffman v.
vaginoscopy
pediatric v.
vaginosis
anaerobic v.
bacterial v. (BV)
mycotic v.
nonspecific v.
vaginotomy
anterior v.

Vagisil
V. anti-itch medicated wipe
V. intimate moisturizer
Vagistat-1 Vaginal
Vagi-TEST
vagitus uterinus
vagotomy
vagotonia
vagotonic
v. bradycardia
v. maneuver
vagus nerve
VAIN III
vaginal intraepithelial neoplasia
valacyclovir
v. HCl
v. hydrochloride
valdecoxib
Valentine position
7-valent pneumococcal conjugate vaccine
valerate
betamethasone v.
estradiol v. (EV)
hydrocortisone v.
hydroxyprogesterone and estradiol v.
valerian root
Valertest No. 1
valga
coxa v.
valgum
genu v.
physiologic genu v.
valgus
cubitus v.
forefoot v.
hallux v.
heel v.
hindfoot v.
obligatory heel v.
v. osteotomy
rearfoot v.
talipes v.
VALI
ventilatory-associated lung injury
valine
Valium
V. Injection
V. Oral
vallecula, *pl.* **valleculae**
valleculae (*pl. of* vallecula)
valley
V. fever
V. Vac smoke evacuation system
Valleylab
V. ball electrode
V. Force IC electrosurgical generator
V. loop electrode
V. pencil
V. REM system

V

Valorin
valproate
    sodium v.
valproic
    v. acid
    v. acid embryopathy
    v. acid syndrome
valrubicin
Valsalva
    V. maneuver
    V. sinus
    sinus of V.
    squirming V.
Valstar
Valtchev uterine manipulator
Valtrex
value
    acid-base v.
    adaptive v.
    Astrup blood gas v.
    baseline v.
    complement v.
    fetal blood v.
    maturation v.
    Tanner-Whitehouse bone age
      reference v.
valvar
valve
    v. ablation
    aortic v.
    atrioventricular v.
    bicuspid aortic v.
    bleed-back v.
    double-orifice mitral v.
    Hans Rudolph v.
    Heyer-Schulte v.
    Jatene v.
    mitral v.
    neoaortic v.
    v. obstruction
    parachute mitral v.
    pop-off v.
    porcine v.
    posterior urethral v. [type I-IV]
      (PUV)
    v. prolapse
    pulmonary porcine v.
    pulmonic v.
    Ross pulmonary porcine v.
    Spitz-Holter v.
    straddling atrioventricular v.
    transurethral ablation of v.
    tricuspid v.
    trileaflet aortic v.
    ureteral v.
    urethral v.
    1-way v.
    3-way Hans Rudolph v.
valvectomy, valvulectomy

valvoplasty (*var. of* valvuloplasty)
    balloon pulmonary v. (BPV)
valvotomy, valvulotomy
    aortic v.
    balloon v.
valvular
    v. heart disease
    v. insufficiency
    v. prosthesis
    v. pulmonic stenosis
valvulectomy (*var. of* valvectomy)
valvulitis
    murmur of v.
valvuloplasty, valvoplasty
    v. and angioplasty of congenital
      anomalies (VACA)
    transcarotid balloon v.
valvulotomy (*var. of* valvotomy)
    balloon v.
    v. procedure
van
    v. Bogaert disease
    V. Buchem syndrome
    v. den Bergh reaction
    v. den Bergh test
    v. der Hoeve syndrome
    v. der Woude syndrome
    V. Maldergem syndrome
    V. Praagh classification of truncus
      arteriosus
    V. Praagh loop rule
Vancaillie uterine cannula
Vancenase
    V. AQ
    V. Nasal Inhaler
Vanceril
    V. Double Strength
    V. Oral Inhaler
Vancocin
    V. injection
    V. Oral
Vancoled injection
vancomycin
    v. hydrochloride
    v. intermediate-resistant
      Staphylococcus aureus (VISA)
vancomycin-resistant
    v.-r. enterococcus (VRE)
    v.-r. *Staphylococcus aureus* (VRSA)
Vandazole
Vanicream
vanillylmandelic acid (VMA)
Vaniqa
vanished testes
vanishing
    v. bile duct
    v. fetus
    v. testicle syndrome
    v. testis syndrome

v. twin
v. twin syndrome
Vanquin
Vantin
VAP
ventilator-associated pneumonia
vapocoolant
Vapo-Iso
vaporization
bipolar v.
carbon dioxide laser v.
endometrial v.
laser v.
vaporizer
cool-mist v.
water v.
Vaporole
Amyl Nitrate V.
vapor poisoning
VAPP
vaccine-associated paralytic
poliomyelitis
VAPS
verbal analog pain scale
Vaqta vaccine
vara
adolescent tibia v.
coxa v.
idiopathic tibia v.
infantile tibia v.
juvenile tibia v.
tibia v.
Váradi-Papp syndrome
Váradi syndrome
varenicline tartrate
variabilis
Dermacentor v.
erythrokeratodermia v.
variability
beat-to-beat v.
fetal heart rate v. (FHRV)
heart rate v. (HRV)
interpretation v.
variable
v. deceleration
v. obstruction
v. softness (VS)
v. stenosis
variance
additive genetic v.
dominance v.
environmental v.
gender v.
genetic v.
phenotypic v.
v. ratio
Varian Spectra AA40 spectrometer
variant
albopapuloid epidermolysis bullosa v.

deafness-causing allele v.
v. hemoglobin
Hurler v.
hyperammonemia v.
hyperinsulinism with
hyperammonemia v.
Klinefelter v.
Landau-Kleffner syndrome v.
migraine v.
papillary v.
Pasini v.
petit mal v.
variation
continuous v.
varicella
breakthrough v.
v. bullosa
bullous v.
disseminated v.
v. encephalitis
v. gangrenosa
v. immunization
v. infection
neonatal v.
v. pneumonia
v. pneumonitis
pustular v.
v. pustulosa
v. syndrome
vaccination v.
v. vaccination
varicella-zoster
v.-z. encephalomyelitis
v.-z. immune globulin (VZIG)
v.-z. virus (VZV)
v.-z. virus infection
v.-z. virus vaccine
varicelliform
varices (*pl. of* varix)
varicocele
ovarian v.
tuboovarian v.
uteroovarian v.
varicocelectomy
varicose vein (VV)
varicosity
vulvar v.
variegata
porphyria v.
variegate porphyria (VP)
VARig
varicella-zoster immune globulin
variola virus
varioliform
Varivax vaccine
varix, *pl.* **varices**
gelatinous v.
umbilical vein v.
vulvar v.

V

varum
    developmental genu v.
    genu v.
    physiologic genu v.
    pseudo-genu v.
varus
    v. clubfoot
    congenital metatarsus v.
    cubitus v.
    dynamic pes v.
    forefoot v.
    metatarsus v.
    metatarsus primus v.
    v. osteotomy
    rearfoot v.
    talipes v.
VAS
    vibratory acoustic stimulation
    vibroacoustic stimulation
    visual analog scale
vas, *pl.* **vasa, vasorum**
    v. deferens
    v. deferens aplasia
    vasa nervorum
    vasa previa (VP)
    vasa vasorum
vasa (*pl. of* vas)
vasal
Vas-Cath catheter
vascular
    v. anastomoses in multifetal
      gestation
    v. anomaly
    v. bed
    v. birthmark
    v. calcification
    v. cell adhesion molecule (VCAM)
    v. channel
    v. clip applier
    v. communication
    v. complication
    v. compression
    v. congestion
    v. disease
    v. endothelial growth factor (VEGF)
    v. endothelium
    v. engorgement
    v. headache
    v. injury
    v. leiomyoma
    v. malformation
    v. metastasis
    v. myelopathy
    v. neoplasia
    v. nevus
    v. parabiosis
    v. permeability
    v. permeability factor
    v. proliferative lesion

    v. purpura
    v. reactivity
    v. resistance
    v. response
    v. ring
    v. ring syndrome
    v. sling
    v. spasm
    v. spider
    v. thrombosis
    v. tone
    v. umbrella
vascularis
    stria v.
vascularization
    chorionic v.
vascularized appendix
vasculature
    atypical v.
    v. flow pattern
vasculitic
    v. erythema
    v. skin lesion
vasculitis
    asthma with v.
    Churg-Strauss v.
    cutaneous v.
    dermal v.
    disseminated granulomatous v.
    epididymal vessel v.
    fetal v.
    granulomatous v.
    gut v.
    hypersensitivity v.
    immune complex v.
    immune complex-mediated v.
    leukocytoclastic v.
    lymphocytic v.
    necrotizing granulomatous v.
    occlusive v.
    v. of childhood
    ovarian v.
    renal v.
    retinal v.
    rheumatoid v.
    v. syndrome
    systemic v.
vasculogenesis
vasculopathy
    fetal thrombotic v. (FTV)
    noncalcific v.
    proliferative v.
    thalamostriate v. (TSV)
vasectomy reversal
Vaseline-impregnated gauze
vasitis
vasoactive
    v. intestinal peptide (VIP)
    v. intestinal polypeptide (VIP)

v. prostaglandin
v. substance
VasoClear Ophthalmic
vasocongestion
vasoconstriction
cutaneous v.
hypoxic v.
vasoconstrictor
vasodepressor
vasodil
vasodilation
Vasodilan
vasodilatation (*var. of*
vasodilation)
vasodilation, vasodilatation
pulmonary v.
vasodilator
v. cream
peripheral v.
vasogenic edema
vasomotor
v. flush
v. instability
v. rhinitis
vasoocclusion
vasoocclusive
v. crisis
v. episode
vasopathy
calcific v.
vasopressin
v. analog
arginine v.
(AVP)
v. infusion
placental v.
v. therapy
vasopressor syncope
vasoregulation
vasorum (*pl. of* vas)
Vasospan
vasospasm
cerebral v.
coronary v.
transient v.
Vasotec
V. I.V.
V. Oral
vasotocin
arginine v.
vasovagal
v. faint
v. reflex apnea
v. syncope
vasovasostomy
vastus
v. lateralis
v. lateralis muscle
v. medialis

VATER
vertebral (defects), (imperforate) anus,
tracheoesophageal (fistula), radial and
renal (dysplasia)
V. complex
hydrocephalus with features of V.
V. syndrome
vater
ampulla of V.
papilla of V.
VATS
video-assisted thoracic surgery
video-assisted thoracoscopic surgery
vault
v. cap
v. prolapse
rectal v. (RV)
vaginal v.
vaulting
VBAC
vaginal birth after cesarean
VBAC-TOL
vaginal birth after cesarean trial of
labor
VBG
venous blood gas
VBM
vertebral bone mass
vBMD
volumetric bone mineral density
VBS
venous blood sample
VC
vital capacity
VCA
viral capsid antigen
VCAM
vascular cell adhesion molecule
Vcare uterine manipulator
V-Cath catheter
VCD
vocal cord dysfunction
VCF
vaginal contraceptive film
VCFS
velocardiofacial syndrome
V code rational problems
VCP
vocal cord paralysis
VCU
videocystourethrography
VCU examination
VCUG
vesicoureterogram
voiding cystourethrogram
voiding cystourethrograph
voiding cystourethrography
VD
venereal disease

V

VDR
  vitamin D receptor
VDRL
  Venereal Disease Research Laboratory
  CSF VDRL
  VDRL test
Vecchietti
  V. neovagina construction method
  V. neovagina operation
vectis
vector
  cloning v.
vecuronium
  v. bromide
Veda-scope
VEE
  Venezuelan equine encephalitis
Veetids
vegan
vegetable
  cruciferous v.
  v. oil fat-based formula
vegetans
  pyoderma v.
vegetarian diet
vegetarianism
vegetation
  nonbacterial thrombotic v. (NBTV)
vegetative
  v. reproduction
  v. state (VS)
  v. symptom
VEGF
  vascular endothelial growth factor
vehicle
  PAB-equipped v.
Veillonella
  V. atypica
  V. dispar
  V. parvula
vein
  anomalous pulmonary v.
  antecubital v.
  axillary v.
  azygos v.
  bridging v.
  cardinal v.
  cephalic v.
  v. compression
  dilated v.
  dilated collateral v.
  v. flap
  greater saphenous v.
  hypogastric v.
  iliac v.
  inferior mesenteric v.
  innominate v.
  internal jugular v.
  jugular v.

  left renal v.
  left vertical v.
  main renal v.
  maternal cortical v.
  mesenteric v.
  obliterated v.
  v. obstruction
  v. of Galen
  v. of Galen aneurysm
  v. of Galen malformation
  ovarian v.
  persistent right umbilical v.
  pulmonary v.
  renal v.
  saphenous v.
  scalp v.
  splenic v.
  superior mesenteric v.
  umbilical v. (UV)
  uterine v.
  varicose v. (VV)
Veingard dressing
vela (*pl. of* velum)
velamentosa
  placenta v.
velamentous
  v. cord insertion
  v. insertion of cord
  v. placenta
  v. vessel
velamen vulvae
vellus
  v. hair
  v. hypertrichosis
velocardiofacial syndrome (VCFS)
velocimetry
  Doppler v.
  Doppler umbilical artery v.
  fetal aortic Doppler v.
  fetal arterial v.
  umbilical artery Doppler v.
velocity
  bone quantitative ultrasound v.
  cerebral blood flow v. (CBFV)
  end-diastolic v. (EDV)
  growth v. (GV)
  head growth v.
  height v. (HV)
  linear growth v.
  nerve conduction v. (NCV)
  peak growth v.
  peak systolic v.
  sensory nerve conduction v.
  subnormal growth v.
  umbilical Doppler flow v.
velofacial hypoplasia
velopharyngeal incompetence (VPI)
Velosef
Velosulin Human

Velpeau bandage
Veltane Tablet
velum, *pl.* **vela**
vena (v), vein, *pl.* **venae**
    v. cava
    v. caval filter
    v. caval interruption
venae (*pl. of* vena)
venenata
    dermatitis v.
venerea
    urethritis v.
venereal
    v. bubo
    v. collar
    v. disease (VD)
    V. Disease Research Laboratory
      (VDRL)
    v. lymphogranuloma
    v. wart
venereology
venereum
    lymphogranuloma v. (LGV)
veneris
    mons v.
Venezuelan equine encephalitis (VEE)
Venilon human immunoglobulin
venipuncture
    external jugular v.
    v. site
venlafaxine
    v. HCl
    v. hydrochloride
Venning-Brown test
venoarterial (VA)
    v. cannulation
venodilation
Venodyne pneumatic compressive device
Venoglobulin
Venoglobulin-S
venogram
venography
    ascending v.
    contrast v.
    full v.
    hepatic wedged v.
    limited v.
    radionuclide v.
venom
    Hymenoptera v.
venoocclusive disease (VOD)
venostasis
    visual evoked potential
venosum
    ligamentum v.
venosus
    ductus v.
    patent ductus v.
    sinus v.

venous (V)
    v. angioma
    v. bleb
    v. blood gas (VBG)
    v. blood sample (VBS)
    v. blood sampling
    v. catheter
    v. collateral
    v. engorgement
    v. flow
    v. hum
    v. lake
    v. line
    v. malformation (VM)
    v. obstruction
    v. occlusion plethysmography
    v. oozing
    v. pH
    v. pooling
    v. pressure
    v. sinus thrombophlebitis
    v. sinus thrombosis
    v. switch
    v. thromboembolism (VTE)
venovenous (VV)
    v. cannulation
    v. ECMO
venter propendens
ventilation
    alveolar v.
    assist-control v.
    assisted v. (AV)
    asynchronous intermittent mandatory
      v.
    bag and mask v.
    BVM v.
    v. by mask
    controlled mechanical v. (CMV)
    endotracheal intubation and
      mechanical v. (EI/MV)
    hand v.
    HFJ v.
    HFO v.
    HFPP v.
    high-frequency v. (HFV)
    high-frequency jet v. (HFJV)
    high-frequency oscillatory v. (HFOV)
    high-frequency positive-pressure v.
      (HFPPV)
    intermittent mandatory v. (IMV)
    intermittent mechanical v. (IMV)
    intermittent positive-pressure v.
      (IPPV)
    intratracheal pulmonary v. (ITPV)
    inverse ratio v. (IRV)
    jet v.
    liquid v. (LV)
    liquid-assisted high-frequency
      oscillatory v. (LA-HFOV)

V

ventilation (*continued*)
    mask and bag v.
    mechanical v. (MV)
    noninvasive motion v. (NIMV)
    oscillatory v.
    partial liquid v. (PLV)
    patient-triggered v.
    positive-pressure v. (PPV)
    positive pressure mechanical v.
    pressure controlled v.
    pressure support v.
    pulmonary v.
    v. scintigraphy
    synchronized intermittent mandatory v. (SIMV)
    synchronized nasal intermittent positive-pressure v. (SNIPPV)
    tidal liquid v. (TLV)
    total liquid v. (TLV)
    transtracheal v.
    v. tube
    volume-controlled v.

ventilation/perfusion
    v./p. imbalance
    v./p. mismatch
    v./p. quotient
    v./p. ratio
    v./p. scan

ventilator (*var. of* respirator)
    Amsterdam infant v.
    BABYbird II v.
    Bear Cub infant v.
    Bennett PR-2 v.
    Breeze v.
    CPAP v.
    extrathoracic v.
    Healthdyne v.
    HFJ v.
    HFO v.
    HFPP v.
    high-frequency v.
    high-oscillation v.
    humidification v.
    infant Star high-frequency v.
    jet v.
    nebulization v.
    Newport Wave v.
    noninvasive extrathoracic v. (NEV)
    PEEP v.
    Porta-Lung noninvasive extrathoracic v.
    pressure-cycled v.
    pressure-preset v.
    Pulmo-Aid v.
    Sechrist neonatal v.
    Servo 900C v.
    Siemens-Elema Servo 900C v.
    Siemens Servo 300, 900C v.
    SLE 2000 v.
    Star v.
    v. support
    Vix infant v.
    volume-limited v.
    Wave v.

ventilator-associated pneumonia (VAP)
ventilator-induced lung injury (VILI)
ventilatory
    v. drive
    v. failure
    v. support

ventilatory-associated lung injury (VALI)
Ventolin
    V. Nebules
    V. Rotacaps

ventral (V)
    v. hernia
    v. mesentery
    v. pancreatic anlage
    v. suspension
    v. wall
    v. wall defect

ventricle
    common-inlet single right v.
    dilation of v.
    double-inlet left v.
    double-inlet right v.
    double-outlet v.
    double-outlet right v. (DORV)
    hyperdynamic v.
    hypoplastic left v.
    isolated double outlet right v.
    left v. (LV)
    right v. (RV)
    single v.
    stiff v.
    v.'s to atrium
    v.'s to peritoneal cavity

ventricular
    v. afterload
    v. aneurysm
    v. assist device
    v. bypass
    v. catheter
    v. dysplasia
    v. dysrhythmia
    v. filling
    v. fluid
    v. function
    v. hypertrophy
    v. inversion
    left v. (LV)
    v. noncompaction cardiomyopathy
    v. outflow obstruction
    v. outflow tract
    v. outflow tract reconstruction
    v. preload
    v. premature contraction (VPC)

v. premature depolarization
v. puncture
v. reservoir
v. response rate
v. septal defect (VSD)
v. septal defect patch closure
v. septation
v. septum
v. shunt
v. shunt procedure
v. tachycardia
v. tap
v. tumor
ventriculitis
gram-negative v.
ventriculoamniotic shunt
ventriculoarterial
ventriculoatrial (VA)
v. shunt
ventriculocisternostomy
ventriculography
ventriculojugular shunt
ventriculomegaly
bilateral cerebral v.
cerebral v.
fetal v.
nonprogressive v.
posthemorrhagic v. (PHVM)
ventriculoperitoneal (VP)
v. shunt (VPS)
v. shunt
ventriculopleural shunt
ventriculovascular shunt
ventrogluteal
ventroposterior (VP)
ventrosuspension
Venturi mask
venule
Venus
collar of V.
VEOS
very early onset schizophrenia
VEP
visual evoked potential
VEP acuity
flash VEP
VePesid
etoposide
VER
visual evoked response
vera
decidua v.
placenta accreta v.
polycythemia rubra v.
verapamil
Veratrum alkaloid
verbal
v. abuse
v. analog pain scale (VAPS)

v. fluency
v. sequencing
verbal-auditory agnosia (VAA)
verbalize
verbally assaultive
Verelan
Veress needle
vergae
cavum v.
verge
anal v.
vermicularis
Enterobius v.
vermiculation
vermiform
v. appendix
v. lesion
vermilion border of lip
vermis
agenesis of cerebellar v.
cerebellar v.
v. cerebelli
folia of v.
v. hypoplasia
hypoplasia of v.
hypoplastic superior cerebellar v.
partial agenesis of v.
selective aplasia of v.
Vermont-Oxford Neonatal Database
Vermox
vernal conjunctivitis
Verner-Morrison syndrome
vernix
v. caseosa
v. membrane
vero
V. cell
v. cytotoxin
Veronique bra
verotoxin
verruca, *pl.* **verrucae**
mosaic v.
v. peruana
v. plana
v. plantaris
v. sock
v. vulgaris
verrucae (*pl. of* verruca)
Verruca-Freeze
verruciformis
epidermodysplasia v.
verrucose, verrucous
v. endocarditis
v. papule
v. plaque
v. streaky epidermal nevus
verrucous (*var. of* verrucose)
v. carcinoma

V

VersaLab APM2 portable antepartum monitor
VersaLap
VersaStep Plus access system
Versed syrup
Versenate
    Calcium Disodium V.
versicolor
    pityriasis v.
    tinea v.
version
    bimanual v.
    bipolar v.
    Braxton Hicks v.
    California Verbal Learning
      Test-Children's V.
    cephalic v.
    combined v.
    external v.
    external cephalic v. (ECV)
    Hicks v.
    internal podalic v.
    pelvic v.
    podalic v.
    postural v.
    Potter v.
    Schedule for Affective Disorders
      and Schizophrenia for School-Age
      Children-Epidemiologic V.
      (K-SADS-E)
    spontaneous v.
    tibial v.
    Wigand v.
    Wright v.
versive seizure
vertebra (V, vert), *pl.* **vertebrae**
    apical v.
    biconcave v.
    block v.
    butterfly vertebrae
    cleft vertebrae
    codfish v.
    fishmouth v.
    v. plana
    wedge v.
vertebrae (*pl. of* vertebra)
vertebral
    v. anomalies, anal atresia, cardiac
      defects, tracheoesophageal fistula,
      renal anomalies, limb anomalies
      (VACTERL)
    v. arch defect
    v. artery
    v. artery compression
    v. body
    v. bone loss
    v. bone mass (VBM)
    v. column
    v. column defect

    v. compression fracture
    v. (defects), (imperforate) anus,
      tracheoesophageal (fistula), radial
      and renal (dysplasia)
      (VATER)
    v. fracture
    v. laminar arch
    v. microfracture
    v. osteomyelitis
vertebrodidymus
vertex, *pl.* **vertices**
    v. delivery
    external cephalic version and
      spontaneous v.
    instrumental v.
    v. position
    v. potential
    v. presentation
    spontaneous v.
vertex-breech twin presentation
vertex-nonvertex pair
vertex-transverse twin presentation
vertex-vertex pair
vertical
    v. flow ripening
    v. gaze palsy
    v. HIV transmission
    v. hymen
    v. incision
    v. lie
    v. muscle
    v. nystagmus
    v. pocket depth
    v. striation
    v. talus
    v. transmission
vertically
    v. acquired infection
    v. infected
vertices (*pl. of* vertex)
verticillata
    cornea v.
vertiginous
    v. condition
    v. external anal sphincter
    v. seizure
    v. symptom
vertigo
    benign paroxysmal v. (BPV)
    epidemic v.
    Ménière v.
    paroxysmal v.
    peripheral v.
    true v.
verum
    corpus luteum v.
very
    v. cold water near-drowning
    v. early onset schizophrenia (VEOS)

v. long chain acyl-CoA
dehydrogenase (VLCAD)
v. long chain fatty acid (VLCFA)
v. low birth weight (VLBW)
v. low birth weight child
v. low birth weight infant
v. low density lipoprotein (VLDL)
Vesica
V. press-in suture anchor system
V. sling kit
vesical neck
vesicle
brain v.
chorionic v.
football-shaped v.
germinal v. (GV)
graafian v.
nabothian v.
seminal v.
skin v.
tear-drop v.
vesicoamniotic shunt
vesicobullous
v. disorder
v. eruption
v. skin lesion
vesicocele
vesicocentesis
vesicocervical space
vesicocervicovaginal fistula
vesicocutaneous fistula
vesicofixation
vesicomyectomy
vesicomyotomy
vesicopustular lesion
vesicostomy
cutaneous v.
vesicotomy
vesicoureteral reflux (grade 1–4)
vesicoureterogram (VCUG)
vesicourethral
v. canal
v. primordial
vesicourethrolysis
retropubic v.
vesicouterine
v. fistula
v. serosa
vesicovaginal
v. fistula
v. repair
v. septum
v. space (VVS)
vesicovaginorectal fistula
vesicular
v. breath sounds
v. exanthema
v. mole
v. palmar lesion

v. skin lesion
v. stomatitis virus (VSV)
vesiculation
intraepidermal v.
vesiculopapular eruption
vesiculopustular dermatitis
vesiculoulcerative
v. lesion
v. stomatitis
vespid allergy
vessel
afferent v.
blood v.
brachiocephalic v.
chorioallantoic v.
chorioangiopagus placental v.
complete transposition of great v.'s
corkscrew conjunctival blood v.
dilated optic v.
engorged v.
fetoscopic laser occlusion of
chorioangiopagus v.'s (FLOC)
ghost v.
great v.
hairpin v.
infundibulopelvic v.
v. injury
iris v.
laser photocoagulation of
communicating v.'s (LPCV)
v. obliteration
v. ostium
ovarian v.
palliation of great v.'s
v. spread
v. transillumination
transposition of great v.'s (TGV)
umbilical v.
umbilicoplacental v.
uterine v.
uteroplacental v.
velamentous v.
2-vessel cord
3-vessel cord
vest
EZ-On V.
VestaBlate system
vestibular
v. adenitis
v. anus
v. apparatus
v. board
v. bulb
v. cyst
v. damage
v. duct
v. dyspareunia
v. fistula
v. gland

V

vestibular (*continued*)
　　v. input
　　v. nerve
　　v. neuronitis
　　v. nystagmus
　　v. seizure
　　v. stimulation
vestibule
vestibulectomy
　　U-shaped v.
　　Woodruff v.
vestibulitis
　　vulvar v.
vestibulocochlear nerve
vestibulodynia
vestibulogenic
　　v. epilepsy
　　v. seizure
vestibulovaginal bulb
vestigial
VFSS
　　videofluoroscopic swallowing study
VH
　　vaginal hysterectomy
viability
　　fetal v.
viable
　　v. endometrial cell
　　v. fetus
　　v. infant
vial
　　Nickerson BiGGY v.
Viasorb dressing
Viasys Doppler and antepartum monitor
Vibracare
Vibramycin
Vibra-Tabs
vibration sense
vibrator
vibratory
　　v. acoustic stimulation (VAS)
　　v. murmur
Vibrio
　　V. cholerae
　　V. fetus
　　V. parahaemolyticus
　　V. vulnificus
vibriocidal antibody
vibroacoustic-induced fetal movement
vibroacoustic stimulation (VAS)
vibrotactile hearing aid
vicarious
　　v. menstruation
　　v. respiration
Vicks
　　V. Children's NyQuil
　　V. Formula 44
　　V. Formula 44 Pediatric

V. Pediatric 44E, 44M
Vicodin ES
Vicryl Rapide suture
victim
　　assault v.
　　v. presentation
　　sexual assault v.
victimization
　　domestic v.
　　physical v.
　　sexual v.
Victor Gomel microsurgical reconstruction method
vidarabine
Vidas
　　V. automated immunoassay system
　　V. estradiol II assay kit
　　V. immunoanalysis testing system
　　V. varicella zoster assay
Vi-Daylin vitamin
video
　　v. electroencephalography
　　v. game epilepsy
　　v. monitoring
　　V. Overlay Method
video-assisted
　　v.-a. thoracic surgery (VATS)
　　v.-a. thoracoscopic surgery (VATS)
videocystourethrography (VCU)
videoendoscope
　　3-dimensional v.
videofluoroscopic swallowing study (VFSS)
videofluoroscopy
　　modified barium swallow with v.
videolaparoscope
videoradiography
videosomnography
videourodynamic study
Videx Oral
Vi-Drape bowel bag
vietnamiensis
　　Burkholderia v.
view
　　anteroposterior v.
　　apical 4-chamber v.
　　axillary v.
　　calcaneal v.
　　Caldwell v.
　　4-chamber v.
　　comparison v.
　　craniocaudal v.
　　exaggerated craniocaudal v.
　　field of v.
　　frogleg v.
　　Harris v.
　　jug handle v.
　　lateral oblique v.

lateromedial oblique v.
long-axis v.
medial oblique v.
mediolateral v.
Merchant v.
mortise v.
Neer v.
oblique v.
occipitomental v.
open-mouth v.
Panorex v.
parasternal short-axis v.
pulmonary artery/ductus v.
short-axis v.
spot compression v.
subcostal v.
submentovertex v.
sunrise v.
suprasternal v.
Waters v.
vigabatrin
Vigamox solution
vigilance
generalized v.
Vignal cell
vigorous infant
VIIa
factor VIIa
recombinant factor VIIa
VIII:C
factor VIII:C
VI–IX
OFD syndrome, type I–IV,
VI–IX
VILI
ventilator-induced lung
injury
villi (*pl. of* villus)
villitis
focal v.
villoglandular
v. configuration
v. endometrial carcinoma
villonodular synovitis
villose (*var. of* villous)
villositis
villous, villose
v. atrophy
v. atrophy of jejunum
v. chorion
v. edema
v. placenta
villus, *pl.* **villi**
anchoring v.
arachnoid v.
flattened v.
hydropic chorionic v.
hydropic placental v.
placental v.

vimentin
v. gene
v. protein
Vim-Silverman needle
VIN
vaginal intraepithelial neoplasia
vulvar intraepithelial neoplasia
VIN (grade 1–3)
vin
v. rosé-colored urine
vinblastine
cisplatin, methotrexate, v. (CMV)
methotrexate, cisplatin, v. (MCV)
Vinca alkaloid
Vincasar PFS
Vincent
V. angina
V. gingivitis
V. infection
V. stomatitis
vincristine
v. and dexamethasone
v. sulfate
vinegar douching
Vineland
V. Adaptive Behavior Scales
V. Adaptive Behavior Scales, Survey Form
V. Social Maturity Scale
V. standard scores
vinyl chloride
Viokase
violaceous
v. eruption
v. erythema
v. hue
v. lesion
v. polygonal papule
violence
V. Against Women Act
cycle of v.
domestic v.
intimate partner v. (IPV)
partner v.
violent rage
violet
crystal v.
gentian v.
viomycin
Vioxx
VIP
vasoactive intestinal peptide
vasoactive intestinal polypeptide
voluntary interruption of pregnancy
VIP-DAC
vaginal interruption of pregnancy with dilatation and curettage
Vipond sign
viprynium

Vira-A Ophthalmic
Viracept
viral

v. arthritis
v. capsid antigen (VCA)
cellular v.
v. cerebellitis
v. conjunctivitis
v. culturing
v. DNA polymerase
v. encephalitis
v. enteritis
v. esophagitis
v. exanthema
v. gastroenteritis
v. hepatitis
v. infection
v. laryngitis
v. laryngotracheobronchitis
v. load
v. lower respiratory illness (VLRI)
v. meningitis
v. meningoencephalitis
v. myelitis
v. myocarditis
v. necrotizing bronchiolitis
v. pharyngitis
v. pneumonia
v. pneumonitis
v. prodrome
v. sepsis
v. shedding
v. syndrome
v. thymidine kinase
v. titer
v. transmission
v. upper respiratory tract infection

Viramune
ViraPap HPV DNA test
ViraType

V. HPV DNA typing assay
V. probe
V. test

Virazole Aerosol
Virchow

pneumonia alba of V.

Virchow-Robin space
Virchow-Seckel syndrome
viremia

plasma v.
secondary v.

viremic phase
Viresolve ultrafiltration membrane
virgin
virginal

v. breast hypertrophy
v. hymen
v. introitus

Virginia needle

virginity
viridans

v. enterococcus
Streptococcus v.
v. streptococcus

virilescence
virilism

adrenal v.

virilization

external v.
female v.
strong v.

virilizing

v. adenoma
v. adrenal tumor
v. 3 alpha-androstanediol glucuronide
v. ovarian mass

Virilon capsule
virion

intranuclear v.

virologic assay
virology
Viroptic Ophthalmic
virtual

v. bronchoscopy
v. labor monitor (VLM)

virulence
virulent bubo
viruria
virus

acquired immunodeficiency
syndrome-related v. (ARV)
antibody to hepatitis A v.
(anti-HAV)
arthropod-borne v.
Borna disease v.
chickenpox v.
chikungunya v.
v. clearance
Congo v.
cultivable v.
dengue v.
Dobrava v.
ECHO v.
Epstein-Barr v. (EBV)
fecal shedding of v.
Hantaan v.
hepatitis A v. (HAV)
hepatitis B v. (HBV)
hepatitis C v. (HCV, HVC)
hepatitis D v. (HDV)
hepatitis E v. (HEV)
hepatitis F v. (HFV)
hepatitis G v. (HGV)
hepatotropic v.
herpes v.
herpes simplex v. (HSV)
herpes simplex v. 1 (HSV-1, HSV1)
herpes simplex v. 2 (HSV-2, HSV2)

herpes zoster v. (HZV)
horizontal transmission of v.
human immunodeficiency v. (HIV)
human T-cell leukemia v. (HTLV)
influenza v.
Inoue-Melnick v.
Japanese B encephalitis v.
JC v.
Junin v.
LAC v.
Lassa v.
live-attenuated v.
lymphadenopathy-associated v.
   (LAV)
lymphocytic choriomeningitis v.
   (LCMV)
Machupo v.
Marburg v.
Mayaro v.
measles v. (MV)
molluscum contagiosum v. (MCV)
monkey polyoma v.
Montgomery County v.
mumps v.
non-A, non-B hepatotropic v.
non-syncytium-inducing variant of
   AIDS v.
Norwalk v.
Norwalk-like v.
Ockelbo v.
Omsk v.
o'nyong-nyong v.
papillomavirus, polyoma virus,
   simian virus 40 vacuolating v.
   (PAPOVA)
parainfluenza v. (type 1–4)
   (PIV)
Pogosta v.
recurrent Japanese encephalitis v.
respiratory enteric orphan v.
respiratory syncytial v. (RSV)
Ross River v.
Rous sarcoma v.
rubella v.
rubeola v.
Sapporo v.
simian B v.
simian immunodeficiency v. (SIV)
Sindbis v.
Sin Nombre v.
Snow Mountain v.
tissue culture-grown attenuated v.
v. titer
transfusion transmitted v.
TT v. (TTV)
vaccinia v.
varicella-zoster v. (VZV)
variola v.
vesicular stomatitis v. (VSV)

visna v.
West Nile v.
wild v.
wild-type measles v.
virus-1
human immunodeficiency v.-1
virus-induced epithelial damage
virus-neutralizing antibody (VNA)
VIS
vaginal irrigation smear
VISA
vancomycin intermediate-resistant
Staphylococcus aureus
viscera (*pl. of* viscus)
visceral
v. abscess
v. afferent
v. cleft
v. cranium
v. heterotaxy
v. hypersensitivity
v. larva migrans
v. leishmaniasis
v. myopathy
v. pain
v. pericardiectomy
v. peritoneum
v. protein status
v. situs
v. tuberculosis
viscerale
cranium v.
visceroatrial situs inversus
visceromegaly syndrome
viscerosensory aura
viscerum
situs inversus v.
viscid
viscoelastic
viscosity
viscosus
Actinomyces v.
viscous
v. fluid
v. semen
v. syndrome
viscus, *pl.* **viscera**
herniated viscera
hollow viscera
in utero reduction of herniated
   viscera
inversion of viscera
pelvic viscera
perforated v.
transposition of viscera
visible
v. cortical mantle
v. peristalsis
Visicath

V

Visine
  V. Extra Ophthalmic
  V. L.R. Ophthalmic
vision
  binocular v.
  blurred v.
  color v.
  cortical v.
  distance v.
  field of v.
  impaired v.
  near v.
  peripheral v.
  residual v.
  v. screening
  v. therapist
  v. therapy
  tunnel v.
Visiport optical trocar
visit
  health maintenance v.
  postpartum v.
  preconception v.
  prenatal v.
  routine prenatal v.
visna virus
Vista disposable skin stapler
Vistaril
  V. Injection
  V. Oral
Vistide
visual
  v. acuity
  v. analog scale (VAS)
  v. analog scale for stress
  v. aura
  v. change
  v. cortex
  v. development
  v. diagnosis
  v. disturbance
  v. evoked potential (venostasis, VEP)
  v. evoked response (VER)
  v. field
  v. field defect
  v. learner
  v. loss
  v. magnocellular system
  v. pathway
  v. phobic hallucination
  v. reflex epilepsy
  v. regard
  v. reinforcement audiometry (VRA)
  v. response audiometry (VRA)
  v. sequential memory
  v. spatial memory
  v. stimulation
  v. tracking

  v. tracking of red ring
  v. training exercise
visualization
  indirect v.
visual-motor
  v.-m. coordination
  v.-m. integration (VMI)
  v.-m. integration test
visual-perceptual test
visuoperceptual/simultaneous information processing
visuospatial
visuscope
Vitabee 6, 12
Vita-C
vitae
  arbor v.
VitaGuard
  V. 1000 event recorder
  V. monitor
vital
  v. capacity (VC)
  V. High Nitrogen formula
  v. signs (VS)
vitamin
  v. A
  v. A deficiency (VAD)
  v. A, D intoxication
  v. B_6
  v. B_{12}
  v. B complex
  B complex v.
  v. B_6 deficiency
  v. B_{12} deficiency
  v. B_6 dependence syndrome
  v. B_{12} level
  Bronson chewable prenatal v.
  v. C
  v. C deficiency
  v. C drops
  v. D
  v. D-binding protein
  v. D deficiency
  v. D dependence
  v. D-dependent rickets
  v. D receptor (VDR)
  v. D-resistant rickets
  v. E
  v. E deficiency
  Fer-In-Sol v.
  v. K
  v. K deficiency
  v. K-dependent serine protease
  v. K prophylaxis
  Materna prenatal v.
  v. metabolism
  OptiNate prenatal v.
  Poly-Vi-Flor v.
  Poly-Vi-Sol v.

prenatal v. (PNV)
v. requirement
Stuart Prenatal v.
v. supplement
v. therapy
Tri-Vi-Flor v.
Tri-Vi-Sol v.
Ultrafort prenatal v.
Vi-Daylin v.
Vitaneed formula
Vitec Topical
Vite E Cream
vitelliform degeneration
vitelline
v. cord
v. duct
v. duct cyst
v. fistula
v. membrane
v. sac
v. tumor
vitellinum
vitellointestinal
v. cyst
v. duct
Vitex
vitiligines (*pl. of* vitiligo)
vitiligo, *pl.* **vitiligines**
dermal v.
Vitrasert
vitrectomy
vitreoretinopathy
familial exudative v. (FEV)
vitreous
v. band
v. body
v. chamber
v. humor
persistent hyperplastic primary v.
(PHPV)
v. seed
v. seeding
vitro
in v. (IV)
vitronectin
Vivactil
vivax
Plasmodium v.
Vivelle-Dot estradiol transdermal system
Vivelle Transdermal
viviparity
viviparous
vivo
ex v.
in v. (IV)
Vivol
Vivonex
V. Pediatric
V. Pediatric formula

V. Plus formula
V. Ten formula
Vix infant ventilator
VK
Apo-Pen VK
penicillin V, VK
V-Lax
VLBW
very low birth weight
VLBW infant
VLCAD
very long chain acyl-CoA
dehydrogenase
VLCFA
very long chain fatty acid
VLDL
very low density lipoprotein
VLM
virtual labor monitor
VLRI
viral lower respiratory illness
VM
venous malformation
VMA
vanillylmandelic acid
VMI
visual-motor integration
VNA
virus-neutralizing antibody
vocabulary
vocal
v. cord
v. cord dysfunction (VCD)
v. cord paralysis
v. fremitus
v. nodule
v. play
v. tic
vocalization
irregular stereotyped v.
vocalize
VOD
venoocclusive disease
Vogt
V. cephalodactyly
V. syndrome
Vogt-Koyanagi-Harada syndrome (VKHS)
Vogt-Koyanagi syndrome
Vogt-Spielmeyer disease
Vohwinkel syndrome
voice (V)
v. disorder
high-pitched v.
hoarse v.
hot potato v.
v. inflection
nasal v.
v. synthesizer
too-soft v.

V

voiceless cry
voiceprint
void
    flow v.
Void-Ease urine collection bag
voiding
    v. cystography
    v. cystourethrogram (VCUG)
    v. cystourethrograph (VCUG)
    v. cystourethrography (VCUG)
    v. diary
    v. dysfunction
    dysfunctional v.
    obstructive v.
    v. pattern
    prompted v.
    scheduled v.
    staccato v.
    v. trial
volar
    v. angulation
    v. ganglion
    v. hyperhidrosis
    v. splint
volatile
    v. acid
    v. anesthetic
volitional movement
Volkmann
    V. deformity
    V. disease
    V. ischemic contracture
Volmax
Volpe method
volt (V)
    electron v. (eV)
    megaelectron v. (MeV)
voltage
voltage-dependent calcium channel
Voltaren
    V. Ophthalmic
    V. Oral
Voltaren-XR Oral
Voltolini disease
volume
    amniotic fluid v. (AFV)
    blood v.
    cerebral blood v. (CBV)
    constant tidal v.
    v. contraction
    end-diastolic v. (EDV)
    end-expiratory lung v. (EELV)
    v. expander
    v. expansion
    expiratory flow v.
    expiratory reserve v. (ERV)
    extracellular v. (ECV)
    fetal blood v.

    fetoplacental blood v.
    v. flow
    forced expiratory v. (FEV)
    gastric residual v. (GRV)
    inspiratory reserve v. (IRV)
    intracranial v.
    intrauterine v.
    intravascular v.
    v. load
    lung v.
    maternal plasma v.
    mean corpuscular v. (MCV)
    mean platelet v. (MPV)
    minute ventilatory v.
    neonatal blood v.
    v. of dead space
    v. overload (VO)
    v. percent of cream in milk (CRCT)
    plasma v.
    postvoid residual urine v.
    pulse v.
    red blood cell v.
    relaxation v.
    v. replacement
    residual v. (RV)
    right ventricular end-diastolic v. (RVEDV)
    semen v.
    stroke v.
    testicular v.
    thoracic gas v. (TGV)
    tidal v. (TV, VT)
    total blood v. (TBV)
volume-controlled ventilation
volume-limited ventilator
volumetric
    v. bladder ultrasound
    v. bone density
    v. bone mineral density (vBMD)
voluntary
    v. coughing
    v. interruption of pregnancy (VIP)
    v. sterilization (VS)
    v. urinary sphincter
Voluson sector transducer
volutrauma
volvulus
    gastric v.
    intestinal v.
    v. malrotation
    malrotation with midgut v.
    mesenteroaxial v.
    midgut v.
    neonatal midgut v.
    v. neonatorum
    Onchocerca v.
    organoaxial v.

VO₂max
    maximum oxygen uptake
vomer
vomerian groove
vomiting, vomition
    bilious v.
    cyclic v.
    nausea and v. (N/V, N&V)
    nonbilious v.
    v. of pregnancy
    pernicious v.
    postoperative nausea and v.
     (PONV)
    projectile v.
    self-induced v.
vomition (*var. of* vomiting)
vomiturition (*var. of* retching)
vomitus
von
    v. Fernwald sign
    v. Gierke glycogenosis
    v. Gierke glycogen storage disease
    v. Graefe sign
    v. Hippel-Lindau disease
    v. Hippel-Lindau syndrome
    v. Jaksch anemia
    v. Meyenburg complex
    v. Recklinghausen disease
    v. Recklinghausen neurofibromatosis
    v. Willebrand disease (type IIB, III)
    v. Willebrand factor (vWF)
    v. Willebrand factor antigen
    v. Willebrand panel
    v. Willebrand syndrome
Voorhees bag
Voorhoeve
    V. dyschondroplasia
    V. syndrome
vorozole
VoSol
    V. HC otic
    V. otic
vowel sound
voyeurism
Vozzle Vacu-Irrigator
VP
    variegate porphyria
    vasa previa
    ventriculoperitoneal
    VP shunt
    VP shunt tap
VPC
    ventricular premature contraction
VPI
    velopharyngeal incompetence
7VPnC vaccine
V-Probe cryoablation probe
VPS
    ventriculoperitoneal shunt

V/Q
    ventilation/perfusion
VRA
    visual reinforcement
    audiometry
    visual response audiometry
VRE
    vancomycin-resistant enterococcus
Vrolik disease
VRSA
    vancomycin-resistant *Staphylococcus aureus*
VS
    variable softness
    vital signs
    voluntary sterilization
VSD
    Vaccine Safety Datalink
    ventricular septal defect
     perimembranous VSD
30-V-3 stapler
VSV
    vesicular stomatitis virus
VT
    tidal volume
VTE
    venous thromboembolism
vulgaris
    acne v.
    ichthyosis v.
    lupus v.
    neonatal pemphigus v.
    pemphigus v.
    psoriasis v.
    verruca v.
vulnerable child syndrome
vulnificus
    Vibrio v.
Vulpe Assessment Battery
vulsellum clamp
vulva, *pl.* **vulvae**
    anterior labial arteries of v.
    autoimmune disease of v.
    Camper fascia of v.
    Crohn disease of v.
    elephantiasis vulvae
    erythrasma of v.
    kraurosis vulvae
    leukoderma of v.
    leukoplakia vulvae
    lichen sclerosis of v.
    melanosis vulvae
    molluscum contagiosum of v.
    noma vulvae
    Paget disease of v.
    pigmentation disorder of v.
    pruritus vulvae
    superficial compartment of v.
    synechia vulvae

V

vulva (*continued*)
    vaccinia of v.
    velamen vulvae
vulvae (*pl. of* vulva)
vulval (*var. of* vulvar)
vulvar, vulval
    v. adenocystic adenocarcinoma
    v. adenoid cystic adenocarcinoma
    v. adenosquamous carcinoma
    v. algesiometer
    v. angiokeratoma
    v. apocrine cystadenoma
    v. apocrine hydrocystoma
    v. atrophy
    v. atypia
    v. biopsy
    v. carcinoma in situ
    v. colposcopy
    v. condyloma
    v. congenital dysplastic angiopathy
    v. dermatitis
    v. dermatosis
    v. dystrophy
    v. edema
    v. endometriosis
    v. fibroma
    v. hemangioma
    v. hematoma
    v. hidradenitis suppurativa
    v. hypopigmentation
    v. inclusion cyst
    v. infection
    v. intercourse
    v. intraepithelial neoplasia (VIN)
    v. lipoma
    v. lymph node
    v. malignancy
    v. melanoma
    v. neoplasm
    v. neurofibroma
    v. nevomelanocytic nevus
    v. Paget disease
    v. pain
    v. papillomatosis
    v. pigmented lesion
    v. pruritus
    v. psoriasis
    v. pyoderma gangrenosum
    v. sarcoma
    v. seborrheic dermatitis
    v. skin
    v. squamous hyperplasia
    v. varicosity
    v. varix
    v. vestibulitis
    v. vestibulitis syndrome (VVS)
    v. wart
vulvectomy
    Basset radical v.

    Parry-Jones v.
    partial v.
    radical v.
    simple v.
    skinning v.
vulvismus
vulvitis
    adhesive v.
    allergic v.
    atrophic v.
    chronic atrophic v.
    chronic hypertrophic v.
    creamy v.
    cyclic v.
    erosive v.
    focal v.
    follicular v.
    herpes v.
    hypertrophic v.
    leukoplakic v.
    v. of Zoon
    plasma cell v.
    secondary allergic v.
    ulcerative v.
    Zoon v.
vulvodynia
    cyclic v.
    dysesthetic v.
    essential v.
    idiopathic v.
vulvoplasty
vulvovaginal
    v. anus
    v. atrophy
    v. burning
    v. candidiasis (VVC)
    v. carcinoma
    v. cystectomy
    v. disorder
    v. erythema
    v. inflammation
    v. itching
    v. lesion
    v. outlet
    v. pouch
    v. pouch of Williams
    v. premenarchal infection
vulvovaginal-gingival
 syndrome
vulvovaginitides
    staphylococcal v.
vulvovaginitis
    adolescent v.
    candidal v.
    chemical v.
    contact v.
    cyclic v.
    irritative v.
    nonspecific v.

pediatric v.
premenarchal v.
prepubertal v.
vulvovaginoplasty
Williams v.
Vu-Max vaginal speculum
Vumon
VURD
posterior urethral valves, unilateral
reflux, renal dysplasia
VURD syndrome
Vusion ointment
VV
venovenous
VVC
vulvovaginal candidiasis

VVS
vesicovaginal space
vulvar vestibulitis syndrome
V33W Endocavity probe
vWF
von Willebrand factor
vWF antigen
**Vysis PathVysion genomic disease
management test**
Vytone Topical
VZIG
varicella-zoster immune globulin
VZV
varicella-zoster virus
VZV vaccine
VZV-specific IgM antibody

V

W

W chromosome
W position of legs
W sign
W sitting position
W syndrome
Waardenburg-Klein syndrome
Waardenburg recessive anophthalmia syndrome
Wachendorf membrane
Wada test
waddling gait
WADIC
Wing Autistic Disorder Interview Checklist
Waelsch syndrome
wafer
Fiberall W.
Wagner syndrome
WAGR
Wilms tumor, aniridia, genitourinary malformations, mental retardation
Wilms tumor, aniridia, gonadoblastoma, retardation
WAGR syndrome
WAI
Weinberger Adjustment Inventory
Waisman-Laxova syndrome
Waisman syndrome
waist
narrow mediastinal w.
waist-hip ratio
waiter's
w. tip position
w. tip posture
waitlist control
Walcher position
Waldenström
W. disease
W. macroglobinemia
Waldeyer
fossa of W.
germinal epithelium of W.
W. layer
W. preurethral ligament
W. ring
Waldman episiotomy scissors
Waldmann disease
walk
bear w.
walker
W. chart
W. lissencephaly syndrome
Maddacrawler w.

ORLAU swivel w.
swivel w.
Walker-Clodius syndrome
Walker-Warburg
W.-W. malformation
W.-W. syndrome
walking
automatic w.
chromosome w.
w. epidural anesthetic
idiopathic toe w. (ITW)
w. reflex
sideways w.
tandem w.
toe w.
wall
abdominal w.
anterior abdominal w.
anterior thoracic w.
anterolateral free w. (ALFW)
bladder w.
cystic w.
lateral pelvic w.
opposing w.
pelvic side w.
resecting intrapartum uterine w.
w. suction
symphysial w.
w. tension
uterine w.
vaginal w.
ventral w.
wallaby
W. Phototherapy System
w. pouch
Wallace
W. catheter
W. ureteroileal anastomosis technique
Wallach
W. colposcope and resectoscope
W. Endocell collection device
W. Endocell endometrial cell sampler
W. LL100 cryosurgical Cryo Gun
W. Papette disposable cervical cell collector
wallerian degeneration
walleye
walnut-shaped bladder
Walt Disney dwarfism
Walthard
W. cell rest
W. nest
Walther dilator

W

Walton
>   W. report
>   W. syndrome

WAMBA
>   Wise areola mastopexy breast augmentation
>   WAMBA procedure

Wampole test

wand
>   NovaSure w.

wandering
>   w. atrial pacemaker
>   w. ovary

Wangensteen needle holder

Warburg syndrome

Wardill 4-flap method

Wardill-Kilner advancement flap method

Ward-Mayo vaginal hysterectomy

Ward triangle

Ware Short Form-35

warfarin
>   w. embryopathy
>   w. syndrome

Warfilone

Waring
>   W. blender sound
>   W. blender syndrome

Warkany syndrome 1, 2

warm
>   w. antibody
>   w. autoantibody
>   w. reactive
>   w. shock
>   w. water near-drowning

warmer
>   Ecowarm gel w.
>   Kreiselman infant w.
>   Ohio w.
>   overhead w.
>   radiant w.
>   Thermasonic gel w.

warming
>   w. stand
>   w. unit

Warren
>   W. flap
>   W. shunt

wart
>   anogenital w.
>   brain w.
>   common w.
>   exophytic w.
>   filiform w.
>   flat w.
>   genital w.
>   warts, hypogammaglobulinemia, infections, myelokathexis (WHIM)
>   laryngeal w.
>   mucous membrane w.

>   periungual w.
>   plantar w.
>   venereal w.
>   vulvar w.
>   water w.

Wartenberg sign

Warthin-Starry silver stain

warty dyskeratoma

WAS
>   Wiskott-Aldrich syndrome

wash
>   Benzac W W.
>   gastric w.
>   hexachlorophene w.
>   Johnson's Head-to-Toe Baby W.
>   nasal w.
>   nasopharyngeal w.
>   Oxy 10 W.
>   RSV nasal w.
>   Sastid plain therapeutic shampoo and acne w.
>   Theroxide W.
>   vaginal w.

washed
>   w. intrauterine insemination
>   w. sperm
>   w. spermatozoa

washer
>   Gravlee jet w.

washing
>   cytologic w.
>   gastric w.
>   peritoneal w.
>   preputial w.

washout
>   antral w.
>   nitrogen w.
>   w. pyelogram

wasp allergy

Wassel classification

Wasserman test

WAST
>   Woman Abuse Screening Test

wastage
>   early pregnancy w.
>   fetal w.
>   pregnancy w.
>   reproductive w.

waste
>   nitrogenous w.

wasting
>   bicarbonate w.
>   cerebral salt w. (CSW)
>   phosphate w.
>   renal electrolyte w.
>   renal salt w.
>   renal tubular bicarbonate w.
>   salt w.
>   sodium w.

w. syndrome
urinary potassium w.
water (H$_2$O)
w. aerobics
bag of w.'s (BOW)
w. bottle appearance
centimeter of w. (cmH$_2$O)
w. deficit calculation
dextrose in w.
w. enema
w. excretion
extravascular lung w. (EVLW)
false w.'s
w. intoxication
w. lily sign
w. loss
w. metabolism
w. on brain
Waters operation
w. pacifier
w. seal drainage
w. test
total body w. (TBW)
w. vaporizer
Waters view
w. wart
water-deprivation study
waterhammer effect
Waterhouse-Friderichsen syndrome
Waterlow criteria
water-perfused manometry catheter
watershed
w. distribution
w. lesion
w. zone
water-soluble contrast enema
Waterston
W. aortopulmonary anastomosis
W. shunt
W. shunt procedure
Waterston-Cooley aorto-to-right pulmonary artery anastomosis procedure
watery diarrhea
Watson
W. capsule
W. scapholunate treatment method
W. syndrome
Watson-Alagille syndrome
Watson-Miller syndrome
Watson-Schwartz test
WAVE
women's angiographic vitamins and estrogen
wave
brain w.
w. change
delta w.
fibrillatory w.

fluid w.
flutter w.
gastric peristaltic w.
jugular venous A w.
low-energy sound w.
Mayer w.
W. nucleic acid fragment analysis system
Osborne w.
peristaltic w.
pulsed electromagnetic w.
rolandic sharp w.
saw-toothed flutter w.
W. trial
w. type
W. ventilator
waveform
aortic blood flow velocity w.
arterial w.
discordant artery flow velocity w.
Doppler flow-velocity w.
flow velocity w.
wavy rib
1-way valve
3-way
3-w. Hans Rudolph valve
3-w. stopcock
4-Way Long Acting Nasal Solution
Way operation
Wayson stain
WBC
white blood cell
WBI
whole bowel irrigation
WBN
well-baby nursery
WCC
well-child care
wcp
whole chromosome paint
WCST
Wisconsin Card Sorting Test
WDL
Wood-Downes-Lecks
WDL asthma score
WE
Wernicke encephalopathy
weak
w. cry
w. suck
weakness
collagen w.
girdle w.
homolateral w.
hypotonic w.
intrinsic w.
postictal w.
proximal pattern w.
upward gaze w.

W

wean and feed protocol
weaning brash
wearing position
Weaver-Smith syndrome (WSS)
Weaver syndrome
Weaver-Williams syndrome
web
  w. cerclage
  esophageal w.
  gastric w.
  interdigital w.
  intraluminal w.
  laryngeal w.
  supraglottic w.
  tracheal w.
  windsock w.
webbed
  w. fingers
  w. neck
  w. penis
webbing
Webb-McCall peak
Weber
  W. syndrome
  W. test
Weber-Christian syndrome
Weber-Cockayne epidermolysis bullosa
  simplex
Weber-Dimitri syndrome
Webril bandage
webspace
Webster operation
Wechsler
  W. Adult Intelligence Scale, 3rd
    Edition
  W. Intelligence Scale for Children
    (WISC)
  W. Intelligence Scale for Children
    III
  W. Intelligence Scale for
    Children-Revised (WISC-R)
  W. Intelligence Scale, 3rd Edition
  W. Memory Scale
  W. preschool and primary scale of
    intelligence (WPPSI)
  W. Preschool and Primary Scale of
    Intelligence-Revised (WPPSI-R)
Weck
  W. disposable cannula
  W. disposable trocar
Weck-cel sponge
wedge
  w. osteotomy
  pulmonary artery w. (PAW)
  w. resection
  shoe w.
  w. vertebra
wedge-shaped platform
wedging

WEE
  Western equine encephalitis
WeeFIM
  Functional Independence Measure for
    Children
week
  pill-free w.
weekend drug holiday
weeping
  w. dermatitis
  w. lesion
  w. willow
Weerda laparoscope
Wegener granulomatosis (WG)
Wegner disease
Weibel-Palade body
weighing
  underwater w.
weight
  birth w. (BW)
  body w.
  chest wall w.
  critical body w.
  dry w.
  estimated fetal w. (EFW)
  extremely low birth w.
    (ELBW)
  fetal w. (FW)
  w. for age (WFA)
  w. gain
  high molecular w.
  ideal body w. (IBW)
  w. loss
  low birth w. (LBW)
  low molecular w. (LMW)
  maternal w.
  mean birth w.
  percent of ideal body w.
    (%IBW)
  placental w.
  pregravid w.
  w. reduction
  refusal to bear w.
  w. shifting
  very low birth w. (VLBW)
  w. Z-score
weight-appropriate dose
weightbearing
  w. activity
  w. bone
weighted
  w. speculum
  w. vaginal cone
weight-for-age percentile
weight-for-length percentile
weight/height (W/H)
  w./h. index
weight-lifter blackout
Weil disease

Weil-Felix
>   W.-F. antibody testing
>   W.-F. reaction

Weill-Marchesani syndrome
Weill sign
Weinberger Adjustment Inventory (WAI)
Weinberg rule
Weismann-Netter syndrome
Weissenbacher-Zweymuller syndrome
Weitlaner retractor
Welch
>   W. Allyn AudioPath Platform
>   hearing acuity instrument
>   W. Allyn AudioScope
>   W. Allyn SureSight eye chart

welfare
well
>   w. circumscribed
>   w. engaged in pelvis

well-baby nursery (WBN)
well-being
>   fetal w.-b.
>   maternal w.-b.
>   Psychological General W.-B.

well-born
>   right to be w.-b.

Wellbutrin
well-child care (WCC)
well-circumscribed carcinoma
well-defined mass
well-hydrated baby
well-oxygenated
>   w.-o. baby
>   w.-o. infant

well-perfused baby
well-woman examination
welt
Wenckebach
>   W. block
>   W. phenomena

Wender Utah Rating Scale (WURS)
Wepman Auditory Discrimination Test
Werdnig-Hoffmann
>   W.-H. disease (type I–III)
>   W.-H. disorder
>   W.-H. muscular atrophy
>   W.-H. paralysis
>   W.-H. syndrome

werkmanii
>   *Citrobacter w.*

Werlhof disease
Wermer syndrome
werneckii
>   *Exophiala w.*

Werner syndrome
Wernicke
>   W. aphasia
>   W. area
>   W. disease

>   W. encephalopathy (WE)
>   W. syndrome

Wernicke-Korsakoff syndrome
Wertheim
>   W. hysterectomy
>   W. operation

Wertheim-Schauta operation
Wessel colic
west
>   W. Haven-Yale Multidimensional
>   Pain Inventory
>   W. Nile fever
>   W. Nile virus
>   W. syndrome

Westcort Topical
westermani
>   *Paragonimus w.*

western
>   W. blot
>   W. blot test
>   W. equine encephalitis (WEE)
>   W. immunoblot

Weston
>   W. knot
>   W. slipknot

Westrim-I
Westrim-LA
wet
>   w. brain syndrome
>   w. burp
>   w. drowning
>   w. lung disease
>   w. lung syndrome
>   w. mount
>   w. mount test
>   w. nurse
>   OAB w.
>   w. preparation
>   w. purpura
>   w. rale
>   w. smear
>   w. tap

Weyers oligodactyly syndrome
WFA
>   weight for age

WG
>   Wegener granulomatosis

W/H
>   weight/height
>   W/H index

Wharton jelly
wheal
>   w. and flare reaction
>   punctate w.

wheat
>   spelt w.
>   w. sperm agglutination test

Wheaton Pavlik harness
wheelchair sport

W

wheeze
    high-pitched w.
    monophonic w.
    nonmusical w.
    polyphonic w.
    RSV-associated w.
wheezer
    happy w.
    nonatopic w.
wheezing
wheezy bronchitis
Whelan syndrome
Wherify GPS locator
whey
    hydrolyzed w.
WHI
    Women's Health Initiative
whiff amine test
WHIM
    warts, hypogammaglobulinemia,
    infections, myelokathexis
      WHIM syndrome
WHIMS
    Women's Health Initiative Memory
    Study
whiplash injury
Whipple
    W. disease
    W. radical pancreatoduodenectomy
    procedure
    W. syndrome
whipworm
whirlwind small intestine
**whispered pectoriloquy, whispering
pectoriloquy**
whispering pectoriloquy
whistle-tip catheter
whistling
    w. face syndrome
    w. face-windmill vane hand
    syndrome
Whitaker test
white
    w. blood cell (WBC)
    w. blood cell count
    w. blood cell lysosomal enzyme
    analysis
    w. cell scanning
    W. classification
    w. coat effect
    w. coat hypertension
    w. dermographism
    W. diabetes mellitus in pregnancy
    classification
    w. epithelium
    w. forelock
    w. grape juice
    w. infarction
    w. leg

    w. matter
    w. matter damage (WMD)
    w. matter degeneration
    w. matter lucency
    w. matter necrosis
    w. matter pallor
    w. matter spongiosis
    w. papule
    w. plaque
    w. pseudomembranous material
    w. pupil
    w. pupillary reflex
    w. retinal infiltrate
    w. scleral hue
    w. sponge nevus
    w. strawberry tongue
    w. superficial onychomycosis
    w. tonsillitis
whitehead
white-out
white-yellow plaque
Whitfield ointment
whitlow
    herpetic w.
Whitten medium
Whittingham medium
WHO
    World Health Organization
    WHO prognostic scoring for GTN
whole
    w. abdomen irradiation
    w. abdominal radiation
    w. blood
    w. blood transfusion
    w. body irradiation
    w. bowel irrigation (WBI)
    w. cell
    w. cell diphtheria-tetanus-pertussis
    vaccine
    w. cell DTP vaccine
    w. chromosome 1-22 paint
    w. chromosome paint (wcp)
    w. chromosome X, Y paint
    w. pelvis irradiation
    w. virus vaccine
Wholey balloon occlusion catheter
Whoo-Noz deodorant tablet
whoop
    inspiratory w.
whooping cough
whorl
    hair w.
whorled macular hyperpigmentation
Wiberg
    center edge angle of W.
WIC
    Women, Infants, Children
    WIC program
    WIC syndrome

WI-38 cell
wick
   gauze w.
Wickham stria
wide
   w. complex tachycardia
   w. cranial suture
   w. excision
   w. plane
   w. pulse pressure
   W. Range Achievement Test-Revised
     (WRAT-R)
   w. range assessment of memory
     and learning (WRAML)
   W. Range Assessment of Memory
     and Learning Test
wide-based shuffling gait
wide-field myringotomy
widely spaced eyes
widened
   w. growth plate
   w. metaphysis
   w. symphysis pubis
   w. thecal sac
widening
   mediastinal w.
width
   cardiac w.
   chest w.
   funnel w.
   maximal cardiac w.
   maximal chest w.
   pulse w.
   red blood cell distribution w.
     (RDW)
   tympanometric w.
Wieacker syndrome
Wieacker-Wolff syndrome
Wiedemann-Beckwith-Combs
   syndrome
Wiedemann-Beckwith syndrome
Wiedemann-Rautenstrauch (WR)
   W.-R. syndrome
Wiedemann syndrome
Wigand
   W. maneuver
   W. version
Wigraine
WIHS
   women's interagency HIV study
wild
   w. type
   w. virus
   w. yam cream
Wildermuth ear
Wildervanck-Smith syndrome
Wildervanck syndrome
wild-type
   w.-t. allele

   w.-t. gene
   w.-t. measles virus
Wilkie disease
Wilkins
   W. disease
   W. syndrome
will
   living w.
Willebrand-Jurgens syndrome
Willett
   W. clamp
   W. forceps
Williams
   W. disease
   W. syndrome (WS)
   vulvovaginal pouch of W.
   W. vulvovaginoplasty
Williams-Barratt syndrome
Williams-Beuren syndrome
Williams-Campbell syndrome
Willis
   circle of W.
willow
   weeping w.
Willy Meyer mastectomy
Wilms
   W. tumor, aniridia, genitourinary
     malformations, mental retardation
     (WAGR)
   W. tumor, aniridia, gonadoblastoma,
     retardation (WAGR)
   W. tumor (stage I–V)
   W. tumor suppression gene
Wilson disease
wilsonian
Wilson-Mikity syndrome
Wilson-Turner syndrome
   (WTS)
Wimberger
   W. ring
   W. sign
Winchester syndrome
Winckel disease
window
   aortopulmonary w.
   middle meatus nasal antral w.
   nasal antral w.
   w. operation
   oval w.
   w. period
   square w.
   therapeutic w.
   transgastric w.
   vaginal w.
windpipe
windsock web
windswept deformity
wind-up
   spinal cord w.-u.

W

Wing Autistic Disorder Interview Checklist (WADIC)
wing-beating appearance
winged guide
winging
    scapular w.
wink
    anal w.
Winkler body
Winkler-Waldeyer
    closing ring of W.-W.
WinRho
    W. DS
    W. SDF
WINS
    women's intervention nutrition study
Winston cervical clamp
Winter
    W. glans-cavernosal procedure
    W. placental forceps
    W. syndrome
Wintrobe index
wipe
    disposable w.
    povidone-iodine w.
    Vagisil anti-itch medicated w.
wiping
    front-to-back w.
wire
    electrosurgical w.
    iridium w.
    Kirschner w. (K-wire)
    lead w.
    Teflon-coated w.
    thermistor w.
Wirsung
    main duct of W.
Wisap
    W. disposable cannula
    W. disposable trocar
WISC
    Wechsler Intelligence Scale for Children
WISC-III
    Wechsler Intelligence Scale for Children III
    WISC-III factor scores
Wisconsin
    W. Card Sorting Test (WCST)
    W. syndrome
WISC-R
    Wechsler Intelligence Scale for Children-Revised
wisdom tooth
WISE
    women's ischemia syndrome evaluation
Wise areola mastopexy breast augmentation (WAMBA)

WISH
    Wistar Institute Susan Hayflick
    WISH cell
Wiskott-Aldrich syndrome (WAS)
wispy hair
Wistar Institute Susan Hayflick (WISH)
witch's milk
withdrawal
    w. bleeding
    w. bleeding test
    w. dyskinesia
    estrogen w. (EW)
    maternal estrogen w.
    w. position
    social w.
    speculum w.
withdrawal-like activity
withdrawn behavior
withholding
    stool w.
within-the-infant depressive disorder
witness
    Jehovah's W.
WITS
    Women and Infants Transmission Study
Wittner biopsy punch
Wittwer syndrome
WMD
    white matter damage
WOB
    work of breathing
Wohlfart-Kugelberg-Welander syndrome
Wolcott-Rallison syndrome
wolf
    W. disposable cannula
    W. disposable trocar
    W. laparoscope
    W. syndrome
Wolf-Castroviejo needle holder
Wolfe classification of breast cancer
wolffian
    w. body
    w. duct
    w. duct carcinoma
    w. remnant cyst
    w. rest
    w. ridge
Wolff mental retardation syndrome
Wolff-Parkinson-White syndrome
Wolf-Hirschhorn syndrome
Wolfram syndrome
Wolfring lacrimal accessory gland
Wolf-Veress needle
Wolman disease
Wolraich questionnaire
woman, *pl.* **women**
    W. Abuse Screening Test (WAST)
    amenorrheal w.

Women and Infants Transmission Study (WITS)
androgenized w.
battered w.
eumenorrheic w.
euprolactinemic w.
formula-feeding w.
hirsute w.
hypoestrogenic w.
hypogonadal w.
hypomenorrheic w.
Women, Infants, Children (WIC)
infertile w.
lactating w.
nulliparous w.
parous w.
perimenopausal w.
postmenopausal w.
w. who has sexual relations with women (WSW)

womb
falling of the w.
scarred w.
w. stone

women (*pl. of* woman)
women-held antenatal record
women's
w. angiographic vitamins and estrogen (WAVE)
W. Choice condom
Women's Health Initiative (WHI)
W. Health Initiative Memory Study (WHIMS)
W. HOPE study
w. interagency HIV study (WIHS)
w. intervention nutrition study (WINS)
w. ischemia syndrome evaluation (WISE)

Wong-Baker faces pain rating scale
wood
W. light
w. tick
W. ultraviolet lamp

Woodcock-Johnson
W.-J. Psychoeducational Battery
W.-J. reading test
W.-J. Tests of Achievement

Wood-Downes asthma score
Wood-Downes-Lecks (WDL)
Woodruff vestibulectomy
Woods
W. corkscrew maneuver
W. syndrome

woolly
w. hair disease
w. hair nevus

word
W. Bartholin gland catheter
W. bladder catheter
number of different w.'s (NDW)
staggered spondaic w. (SSW)

5-word sentence
work
w. factor
w. of breathing (WOB)
parent guidance w.

worker
healthcare w. (HCW)
social w.

Working Group on Asthma and Pregnancy
workshop
Stages in Reproductive Aging W. (STRAW)

workup
malabsorption w.
preconceptual w.
pregnancy w.
sepsis w.

world
W. Association for Infant Mental Health
fantasy/make-believe w.
W. Health Organization (WHO)

worm
wormian bones
worried facial appearance
Worster-Drought syndrome
wort
mother w.
St. John's w.

wound
w. botulism
w. breakdown
w. closure
w. dehiscence
w. infection
perforating w.
stab w.
stellate w.
suprapubic stab w.

woven bone
WPPSI
Wechsler preschool and primary scale of intelligence
WPPSI-R
Wechsler Preschool and Primary Scale of Intelligence-Revised
WR
Wiedemann-Rautenstrauch
wrist
WRAML
wide range assessment of memory and learning
WRAML test

wrap
    mummy w.
    SurePress w.
wrap/dressing
    CircPlus compression w./d.
wrapping
    fat w.
WRAT-R
    Wide Range Achievement Test-Revised
wrestling
Wright
    W. peak flow meter
    W. stain
    W. version
Wright-stained smear
wringing
    hand w.
wrinkly skin syndrome (WSS)
wrist
    gymnast's w.
    shaking w.
    w. sign
wristwatch
    QT-Watch messaging w.
writhing

written consent
wrongful
    w. birth
    w. birth and life
    w. conception
wry neck (*var. of* wryneck)
wryneck, wry neck
    w. deformity
WS
    Williams syndrome
WSS
    Weaver-Smith syndrome
    wrinkly skin syndrome
W-stapled urinary reservoir procedure
WSW
    woman who has sexual relations with women
WTS
    Wilson-Turner syndrome
Wullstein retractor
WURS
    Wender Utah Rating Scale
Wyanoids
Wyburn-Mason syndrome
Wycillin

X

X chromatin
X chromosome
X chromosome abnormality
X chromosome aneuploidy
fragile X type A (FRAXA)
X inactivation
X inactivation center (XIC)
X inactive, specific transcript (XIST)
X 19 translocation
X trisomy
X zone

45,X

45,X karyotype
45,X syndrome

XA

chromosome XA

X-acto knife
Xanar 20 Ambulase CO$_2$ laser
Xanax
xanthan/guar combination
xanthelasma
xanthine oxidase deficiency
xanthinuria, xanthiuria, xanthuria
xanthiuria (*var. of* xanthinuria)
xanthochromia therapy
xanthochromic

x. CSF
x. fluid
x. specimen

xanthogranuloma

juvenile x. (JXG)

xanthogranulomatous

x. infiltrate
x. pyelonephritis

xanthoma

Achilles tendon x.
eruptive x.
palmar x.
x. striata palmaris
tendon x.

xanthomatosis

cerebrotendinous x
primary x.

Xanthomonas maltophilia
xanthopia (*var. of* xanthopsia)
xanthopsia, xanthopia
xanthosis cutis
xanthous
xanthurenic

x. acid
x. aciduria

xanthuria (*var. of* xanthinuria)
X-autosome translocation

X-bearing

X-b. oocyte
X-b. sperm

Xe

xenon

Xenform graft
xenogamy
xenogeneic, xenogenous

x. antibody
x. tissue

xenogenous (*var. of* xenogeneic)
xenograft
xenon (Xe)

x. arc
x. clearance
x. CT scan

xenopi

Mycobacterium x.

Xenopus test
xeroderma pigmentosum
xerodermic idiocy
xerography
xeromammography
xeromenia
xerophthalmia
xerosis

x. conjunctiva
x. cornea

xerostomia
XIC

X inactivation center

xinafoate

salmeterol x.

xiphisternum
xiphoid

bifid x.

xiphopagus
XIST

X inactive, specific transcript

XK syndrome
XL

extended release
Ditropan XL
Procardia XL

XLA

X-linked agammaglobulinemia

XLAS

X-linked aqueductal stenosis

XLCM

X-linked cardiomyopathy
X-linked dilated cardiomyopathy

XLD

X-linked dominant

XLHN

X-linked hypercalciuric nephrolithiasis

X

XLHR
 X-linked hypophosphatemic rickets
X-linked
 X-l. adrenoleukodystrophy
 X-l. agammaglobulinemia (XLA)
 X-l. alpha-thalassemia/mental
  retardation (ATRX)
 X-l. aqueductal stenosis (XLAS)
 X-l. cardiomyopathy (XLCM)
 X-l. cardioskeletal myopathy
 X-l. cardioskeletal myopathy and
  neutropenia
 X-l. cataract-dental syndrome
 X-l. cataract with hutchinsonian
  teeth
 X-l. centronuclear myopathy
 X-l. cerebellar ataxia (CLA)
 X-l. cerebral
  hypoplasia/hydrocephalus
 X-l. chronic granulomatous disease
 X-l. congenital cataracts-microcornea
  syndrome
 X-l. congenital glycerol kinase
  deficiency
 X-l. congenital recessive muscle
  hypotrophy with central nuclei
 X-l. dilated cardiomyopathy
  (XLCM)
 X-l. dominant (XLD)
 X-l. dominant condition
 X-l. dominant disease
 X-l. dominant disorder
 X-l. dominant inheritance
 X-l. dominant syndrome
 X-l. dyskeratosis congenita
 X-l. Ehlers-Danlos syndrome
 X-l. gene
 X-l. heredity
 X-l. Hurler syndrome
 X-l. hydrocephalus
 X-l. hydrocephalus-stenosis of
  aqueduct of Sylvius sequence
 X-l. hypercalciuric nephrolithiasis
  (XLHN)
 X-l. hyper-IgM syndrome
 X-l. hypogammaglobulinemia
 X-l. hypophosphatemia
 X-l. hypophosphatemic rickets
  (XLHR)
 X-l. ichthyosis
 X-l. immunodeficiency with hyper
  IgM
 X-l. infantile spasm
 X-l. lymphoproliferative syndrome
 X-l. mental handicap-retinitis
  pigmentosa syndrome
 X-l. mental retardation (1-47)
 X-l. mental-retardation-bilateral clasp
  thumb anomaly

 X-l. mental retardation/multiple
  congenital anomaly
  (XLMR/MCA)
 X-l. mental
  retardation-seizures-acquired
  microcephaly-agenesis of corpus
  callosum
 X-l. mental retardation with fragile
  X syndrome
 X-l. monoamine oxidase deficiency
 X-l. myotubular myopathy (MTMX,
  XLMTM)
 X-l. OPCA
 X-l. Opitz syndrome (XLOS)
 X-l. phenomenon
 X-l. primary hyperuricemia
 X-l. pyridoxine-responsive
  sideroblastic anemia
 X-l. recessive (XLR)
 X-l. recessive centronuclear
  myopathy
 X-l. recessive chromosome
 X-l. recessive condition
 X-l. recessive deafness syndrome
 X-l. recessive disease
 X-l. recessive disorder
 X-l. recessive dysgenesis
 X-l. recessive inheritance
 X-l. recessive muscular dystrophy
 X-l. recessive myotubular myopathy
 X-l. recessive nephrolithiasis
 X-l. recessive skeletal Ehlers-Danlos
  syndrome
 X-l. recessive-type diabetes
  insipidus
 X-l. retinoschisis
 X-l. severe combined
  immunodeficiency (X-SCID)
 X-l. severe combined
  immunodeficiency syndrome
  spondylometaphysial dysplasia, X-l.
 X-l. thrombocytopenia
 X-l. trait
 X-l. uric aciduria enzyme defect
XLMR/MCA
 X-linked mental retardation/multiple
  congenital anomaly
XLMTM
 X-linked myotubular myopathy
XLOS
 X-linked Opitz syndrome
XLR
 X-linked recessive
XO
 XO chromosome
 XO chromosome anomaly
 XO karyotype
 XO syndrome
XomaZyme-H65

Xopenex
> X. HFA
> X. inhalation solution

Xp21
> monosomy Xp21

Xp22
> monosomy Xp22
> partial monosomy Xp21, Xp22

Xp deletion
X-Prep
> X-P. Liquid
> Senna X-P.

Xq
> long arm of chromosome X
> isochromosome Xq
> Xq Klinefelter syndrome
> monosomy Xq
> partial monosomy Xq
> partial trisomy Xq
> trisomy Xq

Xq+ syndrome
Xq- syndrome
XR
> extended release
> Dilacor XR
> Focalin XR

x-ray
> x-r. absorptiometry
> chest x-r. (CXR)
> dual-energy x-r.
> Lauenstein pelvic x-r.
> x-r. mammogram
> x-r. mammography
> x-r. pelvimetry
> stand x-r.
> x-r. therapy

X-SCID
> X-linked severe combined
> immunodeficiency

X-tra
> AFP X-t.

XX
> double strength
> normal female sex chromosome type
> XX and XY Turner phenotype
> XX chromosome
> XX hermaphroditism
> XX karyotype
> XX male syndrome

46,XX
> 46XX karyotype
> 46XX male
> 46XX male syndrome

47,XX karyotype
XX-type gonadal dysgenesis
XXX
> XXX karyotype
> mosaicism for XXX
> XXX syndrome

47,XXX syndrome
XXXX syndrome
XXXXX syndrome
XXXXY
> XXXXY aneuploidy
> XXXXY syndrome

49,XXXXY syndrome
XXY
> XXY karyotype
> XXY male
> XXY syndrome

47,XXY
> 47,XXY karyotype
> 47,XXY syndrome

69,XXY
45,X/46,XY mosaicism
XY
> normal male sex chromosome type
> XY gonadal dysgenesis
> XY karyotype

46,XY karyotype
47,XY karyotype
xylitol
Xylocaine
> X. HCl I.V. Injection for Cardiac
> Arrhythmias
> X. jelly
> X. Oral
> X. topical ointment
> X. Topical Solution
> X. Topical Spray
> X. With Epinephrine

xylometazoline
xyloni
> *Solenopsis x.*

Xylo-Pfan
xylose lysine deaminase agar
xylosoxidans
> *Achromobacter x.*
> *Alcaligenes x.*

**xylulose dehydrogenase
 deficiency**
Xyotax
XYY
> XYY male
> XYY syndrome

X-zone

X

Y

 Y chromatin
 Y chromosome
 Y chromosome-specific DNA
  sequence
 Y connector
 Y incision
 Y linkage
 Y shunt
 Y shunting

YA

 Yersinia *arthritis*

YAC

 yeast artificial chromosome

Yachia incisionless bladder suspension

YAG

 yttrium-aluminum-garnet
 YAG laser
 YAG pellet

Yale

 Y. Global Tic Severity Scale
  (YGTSS)
 Y. Observation Scale
 Y. Optimal Observation Score

Yale-Brown Obsessive Compulsive Scale (YBOCS)

yam cream

Yang-Monti ileovesicostomy

Yankauer

 Y. catheter
 Y. curette
 Y. scissors

YAPA

 young adult psychiatric assessment

Yasmin

Yasminelle

yaws

Y-bearing sperm

YBOCS

 Yale-Brown Obsessive Compulsive
  Scale

y-cystathionase deficiency

year

 y. 7 conduct disorder
 y. of birth (YOB)
 postnatal y.

yeast

 y. artificial chromosome (YAC)
 bismuth sulfite, glucose, glycine, y.
  (BiGGY)
 y. infection
 Pityrosporum y.
 vaginal y.
 y. vaginitis

Yellen clamp

yellow

 y. fever
 y. fever 17D vaccination
 y. fever vaccine
 y. jacket
 y. jacket allergy
 y. nail
 y. nail syndrome
 y. OCA
 y. retinal infiltrate
 y. vernix syndrome

yellow-green pallor

Yeoman forceps

Yersinia

 Y. arthritis
 Y. *enterocolitica*
 Y. *pestis*
 Y. pseudotuberculosis

yersinial infection

yersiniosis

yes protooncogene

yew

 English y.
 Pacific y.

YGTSS

 Yale Global Tic Severity Scale

YIPS

 York Incontinence Perceptions Scale

Y-linked

 Y-l. character
 Y-l. gene
 Y-l. inheritance

YOB

 year of birth

Yocon

Yodoxin

yogurt douche

Yohimex

yolk

 accessory y.
 y. cell
 formative y.
 y. membrane
 y. sac
 y. sac carcinoma
 y. sac tumor
 y. sac tumor of testis
 y. space
 y. stalk

Yom Kippur effect

Yondelis

Yoon ring

York Incontinence Perceptions Scale (YIPS)

York-Mason rectourinary fistula repair

young
>y. adult psychiatric assessment (YAPA)
>maturity-onset diabetes of y. (MODY)
>Y. syndrome

youngae
>*Citrobacter y.*

Young-Dees-Leadbetter bladder neck reconstruction
Young-Hughes syndrome
Young-Madders syndrome
Youssef syndrome
youth
>GLB y.'s
>Great Smoky Mountains Study of Y. (GSMS)
>maturity-onset diabetes of y. (MODY)
>y. risk behavioral survey (YRBS)
>y. self-report (YSR)

Y-plasty
Yq
>AZFa region of Yq
>AZFb region of Yq
>AZFc region of Yq

YRBS
>youth risk behavioral survey

YSI neonatal temperature probe
Y-specific DNA amplification
YSR
>youth self-report

yttrium-aluminum-garnet (YAG)
>y.-a.-g. laser

Yunis-Varon syndrome
Yuzpe
>Y. contraceptive method
>Y. regimen of combined oral contraceptives for emergency contraception

YY syndrome

Z

Z allele
Z band
Z bone density score
Z degree of contraction
Z foot
Z sampler endometrial sampling device
Simkania negevensis strain Z
zafirlukast
Zagam
zalcitabine (ddC)
zanamivir
Zancolli clawhand deformity repair
Zanosar
Zantac 75
zaprinast
Zarontin
Zaroxolyn
Zaufal sign
Zavanelli maneuver
Z-Clamp hysterectomy forceps
ZD
zona drilling
Z′ degree of contraction
Z″ degree of contraction
Zeasorb-AF powder
Zeasorb powder
zebra
z. body
z. body myopathy
Zeis
Z. gland
pilosebaceous gland of Z.
Zeiss colposcope
Zellweger
Z. cerebrohepatorenal syndrome
Z. disease
Zelsmyr Cytobrush
Zemplar
Zemuron
Zenapax
Zenate
Zenker solution
Zephrex LA
Zeppelin clamp
Zerit
zero
z. end-expiratory pressure
z. gravity surgery
z. reject
z. station
Z. to Three children's mental health diagnostic classification
zero-voltage baseline

Zerres syndrome
Zestril
Zetar
Ziagen
zidovudine
z. monotherapy
z. treatment
Ziehen-Oppenheim syndrome
Ziehl-Neelsen
Z.-N. stain
Z.-N. test
ZIFT
zygote intrafallopian transfer
ZIG
zoster immune globulin
zigzagplasty
Zilactin-B Medicated
zileuton
Zimmermann-Laband syndrome (ZLS)
Zinacef injection
Zinaderm
zinc
z. deficiency
z. oxide
z. oxide ointment
z. oxide paste
z. peroxide
z. poisoning
z. protoporphyrin (ZnPP)
z. protoporphyrin to heme ratio
serum z.
z. stearate powder
z. sulfate
z. supplement
z. therapy
z. toxicity
Zinca-Pak
Zincate
zinc-dependent enzyme
zinc-free
z.-f. plastic bag
z.-f. plastic-lined diaper
z.-f. plastic specimen cup
Z-incision
Zincofax
Zinecard
Zinnanti uterine manipulator-injector (ZUMI)
Zinsser
Z. disease
Z. syndrome
Zinsser-Cole-Engman syndrome
Zinsser-Engman-Cole syndrome
ZIPP
Zoladex in premenopausal patients

zipper ring
ziprasidone
Ziprokowski-Margolis syndrome
Zithromax
Zixoryn
Zlotogora-Ogür syndrome
ZLS
    Zimmermann-Laband syndrome
ZM-1 coloscope
ZnPP
    zinc protoporphyrin
Zofran ODT
Zoladex
    Z. Implant
    Z. in premenopausal patients (ZIPP)
zoledronate
Zollinger-Ellison syndrome
Zollino syndrome
Zoloft
zolpidem tartrate
zomepirac sodium
zona, *pl.* **zonae**
    z. basalis
    z. compacta
    z. drilling (ZD)
    z. fasciculata
    z. functionalis
    z. glomerulosa
    z. pellucida (ZP)
    z. protein
    z. reaction
    z. reticularis
    z. spongiosa
zonae (*pl. of* zona)
zona-free hamster egg penetration test
zonal aganglionosis
Zonalon Topical Cream
zonary placenta
zone
    Barnes z.
    basement membrane z. (BMZ)
    beta-hCG discriminatory z.
    cervical transformation z.
    chemoreceptor trigger z. (CTZ)
    discriminatory hCG z.
    echo-free z.
    extranodal marginal z.
    germinal z.
    growth z.
    hypertrophic z. (HZ)
    hypertrophic growth z.
    interthreshold z.
    ipsilon z.
    large loop excision of
      transformation z. (LLETZ)
    loop excision of transformation z.
      (LETZ)
    marginal z.
    needle excision of transformation z.

    normal transformation z.
    null z.
    z. of preparatory calcification (ZPC)
    proliferative z. (PZ)
    reserve z. (RZ)
    toxicity z.
    transformation z. (TZ)
    transition z.
    watershed z.
    X z.
Zone-A Forte
Zonegran
zonisamide
zonoskeleton
zonula, *pl.* **zonulae**
    z. adherens
    z. occludens
zonulae (*pl. of* zonula)
zonular cataract
zoogonous
zoogony
Zoomscope portable microscope
Zoon
    balanitis of Z.
    Z. erythroplasia
    Z. vulvitis
    vulvitis of Z.
zoonotic infection
zoosperm
Zostavax
zoster
    herpes z.
    z. immune globulin (ZIG)
    z. myelitis
    trigeminal herpes z.
zosteriform
    z. lentiginous nevus
    z. lesion
Zostrix-HP
Zosyn
Zovia
Zovirax
ZP
    zona pellucida
ZPC
    zone of preparatory calcification
Z-plasty
    4-flap Z-p.
Z-Sampler endometrial suction curette
Z-Scissors hysterectomy scissors
Z-score
    BMI Z-s.
    height velocity Z-s.
    weight Z-s.
Z-shaped duodenum
ZstatFlu test
Z-stitch
Zuckerkandl organ
zuclopenthixol

ZUMI
  Zinnanti uterine manipulator-injector
Zunich syndrome
Zuska disease
Zuspan regimen
Z-vaginoplasty
Zwahlen syndrome
Zyderm
Zydone
Zyflo
zygodactyly
zygoma
zygomatic
  z. arch
  z. bone
  z. head
  z. head of quadratus labii superioris
    muscle
zygomaticofrontal region
zygomaticomaxillary fracture

zygomycosis
zygopodium
zygosity
zygosyndactyly
zygote
  2-cell z.
  frozen z.
  z. intrafallopian transfer
    (ZIFT)
zygotene
  z. phase of meiosis
  z. stage
Zyklomat infusion pump
Zyloprim
zymase
zymogen
  coagulation factor z.
Zyplast
Zyrtec syrup
ZZ male

Z

Contents: The Appendices

Anatomical Illustrations

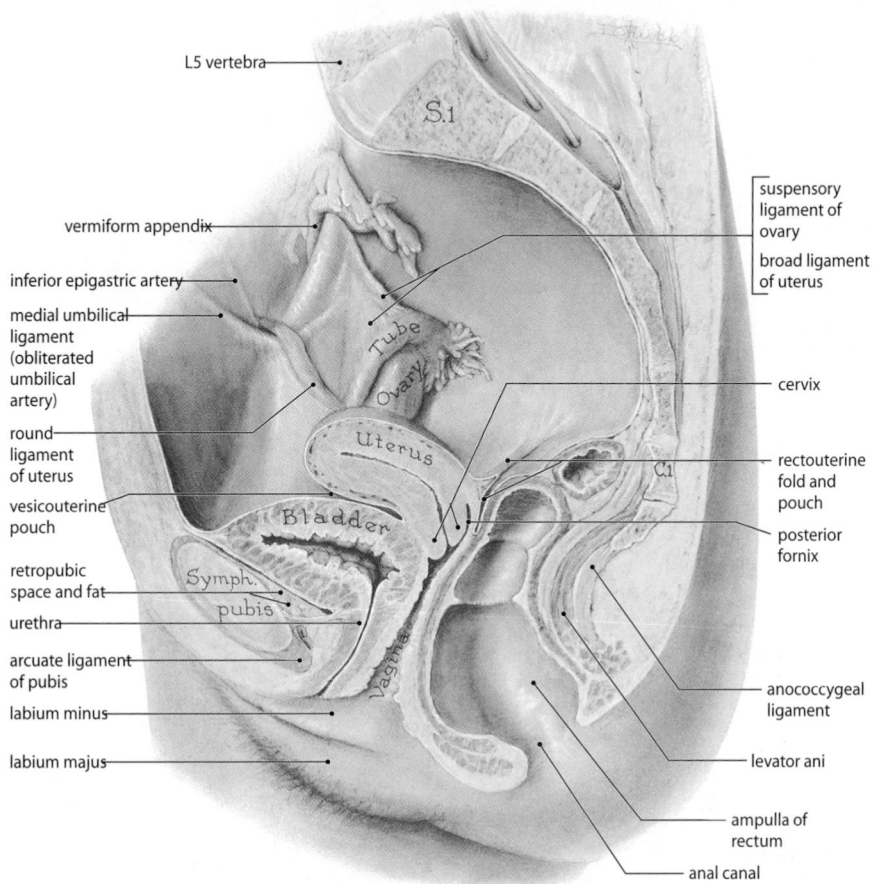

L5 vertebra

vermiform appendix

inferior epigastric artery

medial umbilical ligament (obliterated umbilical artery)

round ligament of uterus

vesicouterine pouch

retropubic space and fat

urethra

arcuate ligament of pubis

labium minus

labium majus

suspensory ligament of ovary

broad ligament of uterus

cervix

rectouterine fold and pouch

posterior fornix

anococcygeal ligament

levator ani

ampulla of rectum

anal canal

female pelvis: median section

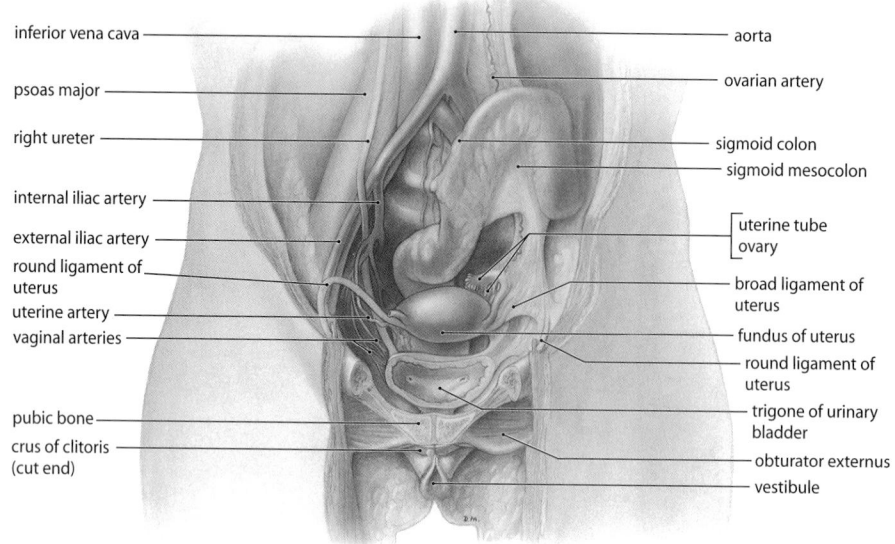

inferior vena cava

psoas major

right ureter

internal iliac artery

external iliac artery

round ligament of uterus

uterine artery

vaginal arteries

pubic bone

crus of clitoris (cut end)

aorta

ovarian artery

sigmoid colon

sigmoid mesocolon

uterine tube
ovary

broad ligament of uterus

fundus of uterus

round ligament of uterus

trigone of urinary bladder

obturator externus

vestibule

female genital organs: anteroposterior view

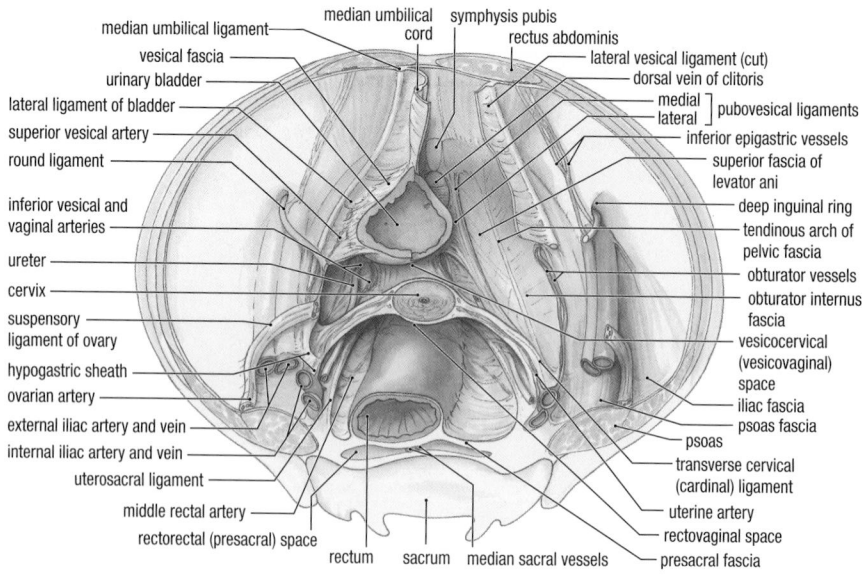

median umbilical ligament

median umbilical cord

symphysis pubis

vesical fascia

rectus abdominis

urinary bladder

lateral vesical ligament (cut)

lateral ligament of bladder

dorsal vein of clitoris

superior vesical artery

medial
lateral] pubovesical ligaments

round ligament

inferior epigastric vessels

inferior vesical and vaginal arteries

superior fascia of levator ani

deep inguinal ring

ureter

tendinous arch of pelvic fascia

cervix

obturator vessels

suspensory ligament of ovary

obturator internus fascia

hypogastric sheath

vesicocervical (vesicovaginal) space

ovarian artery

iliac fascia

external iliac artery and vein

psoas fascia

internal iliac artery and vein

psoas

uterosacral ligament

transverse cervical (cardinal) ligament

middle rectal artery

uterine artery

rectorectal (presacral) space

rectovaginal space

rectum   sacrum   median sacral vessels

presacral fascia

pelvic fascia and the supporting mechanism of the cervix and upper vagina: superior view

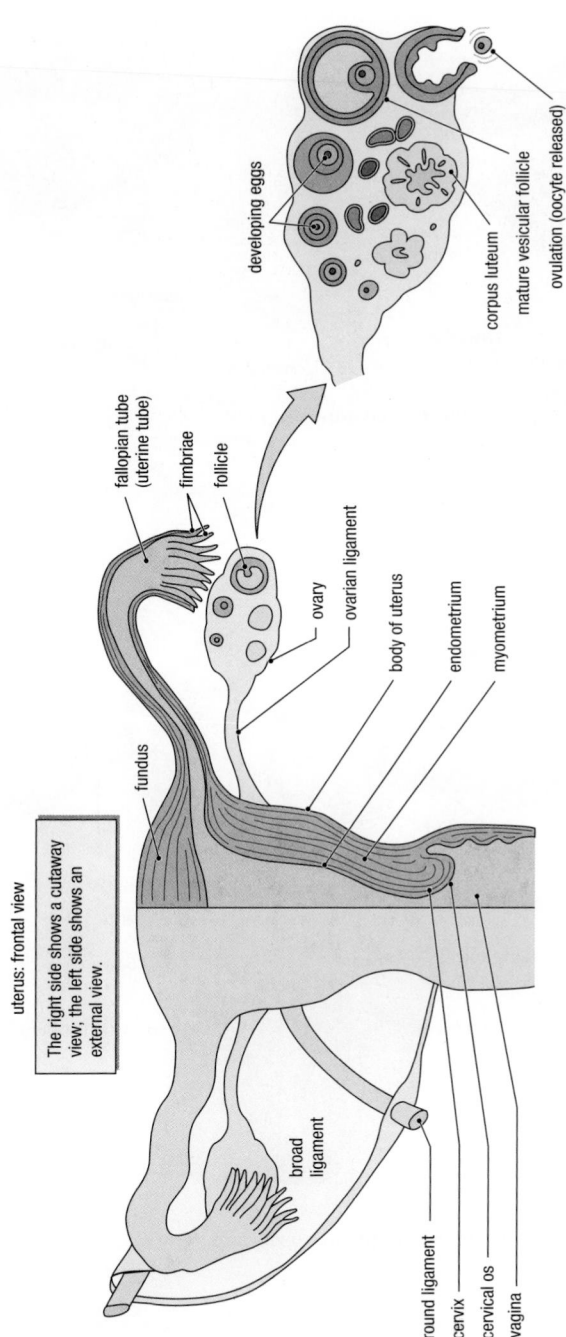

developing eggs

corpus luteum

mature vesicular follicle

ovulation (oocyte released)

fallopian tube (uterine tube)

fimbriae

follicle

ovary

ovarian ligament

body of uterus

endometrium

myometrium

fundus

uterus: frontal view

The right side shows a cutaway view; the left side shows an external view.

broad ligament

round ligament

cervix

cervical os

vagina

female reproductive system

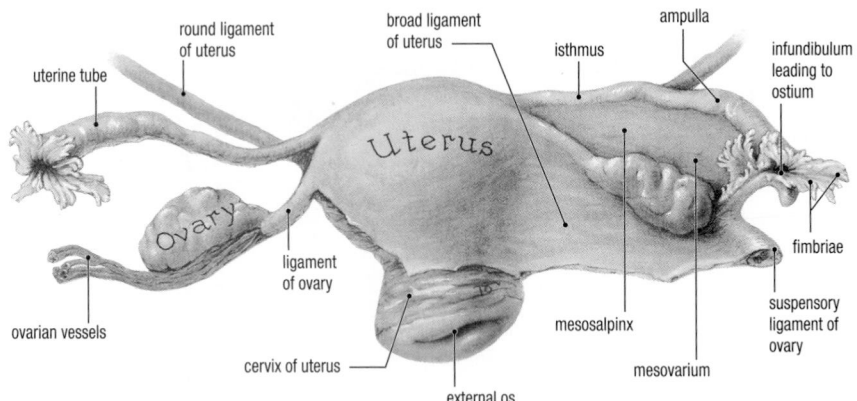

uterus and adnexa: posterior view

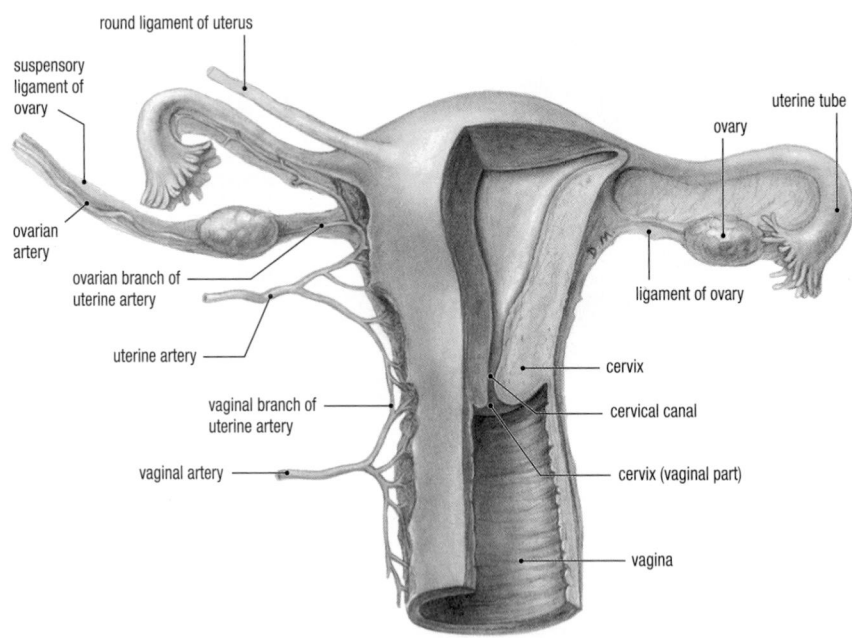

blood supply to uterus and adnexa

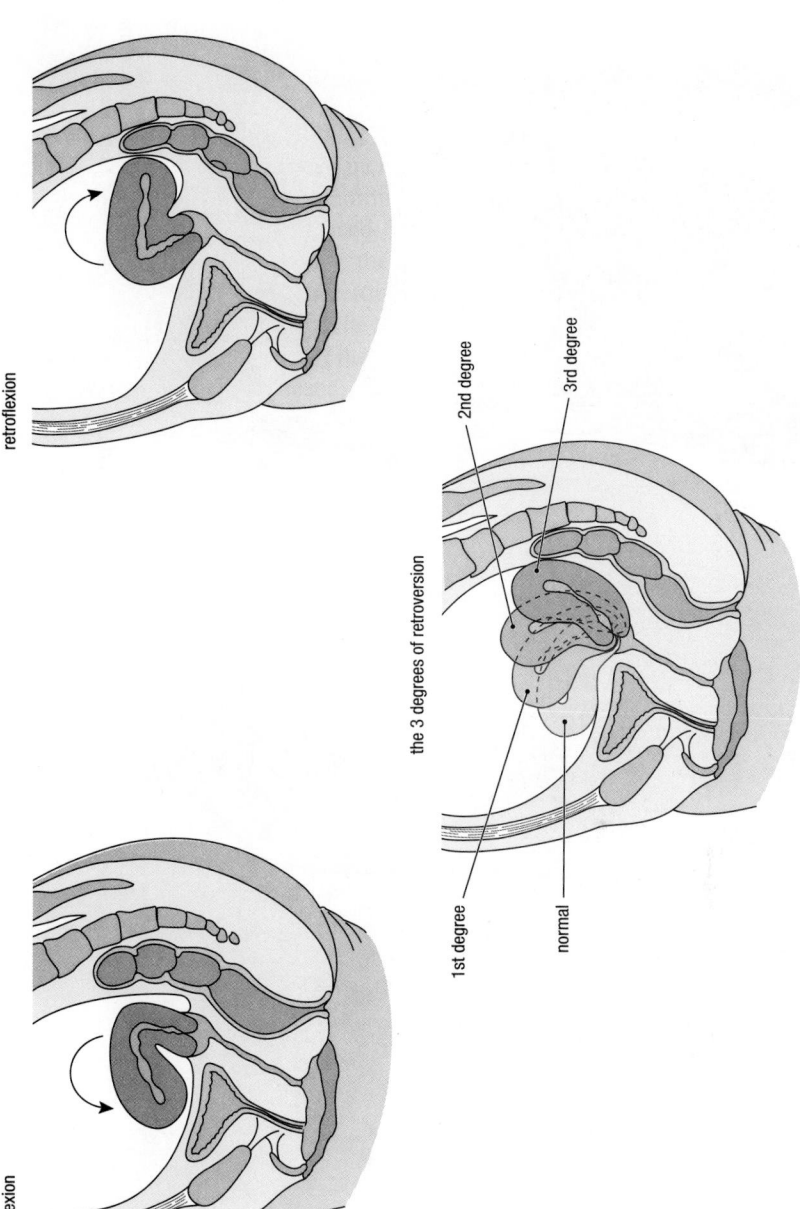

retroflexion

anteflexion

the 3 degrees of retroversion

2nd degree

3rd degree

1st degree

normal

displacements of the uterus

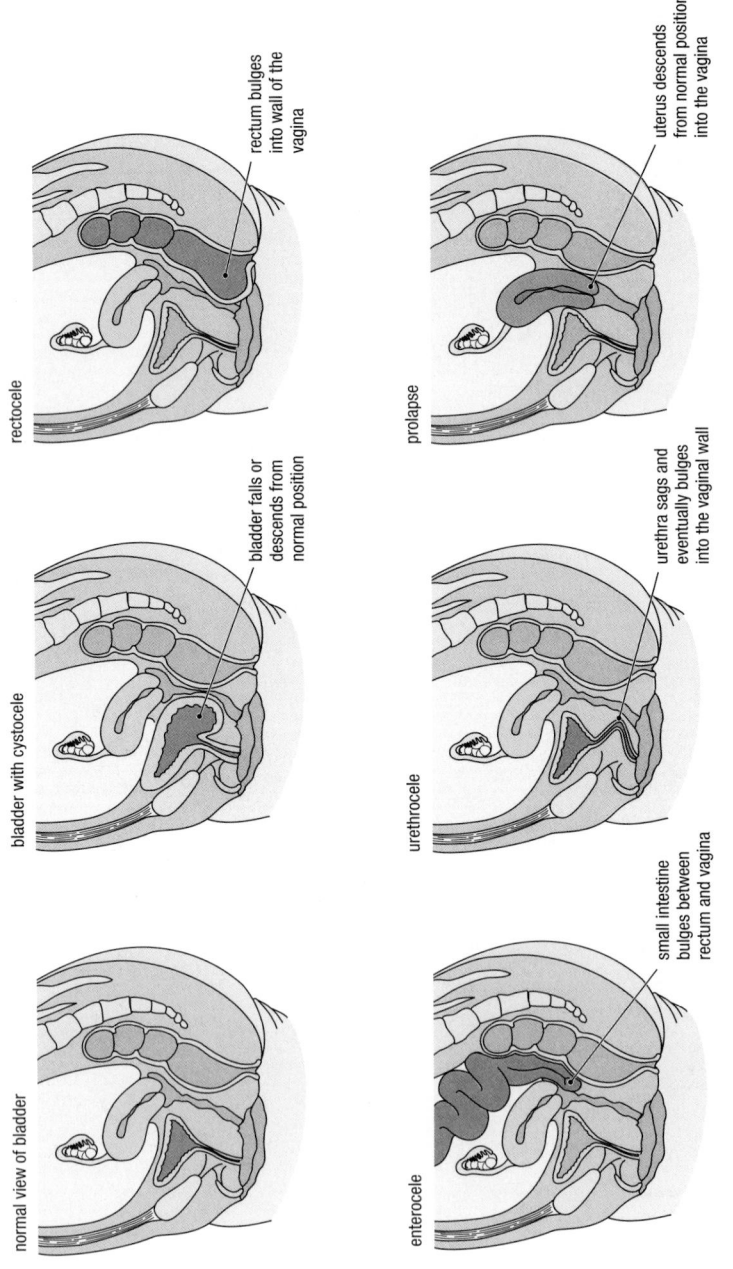

normal view of bladder

bladder with cystocele

bladder falls or descends from normal position

rectocele

rectum bulges into wall of the vagina

enterocele

small intestine bulges between rectum and vagina

urethrocele

urethra sags and eventually bulges into the vaginal wall

prolapse

uterus descends from normal position into the vagina

pelvic floor relaxation

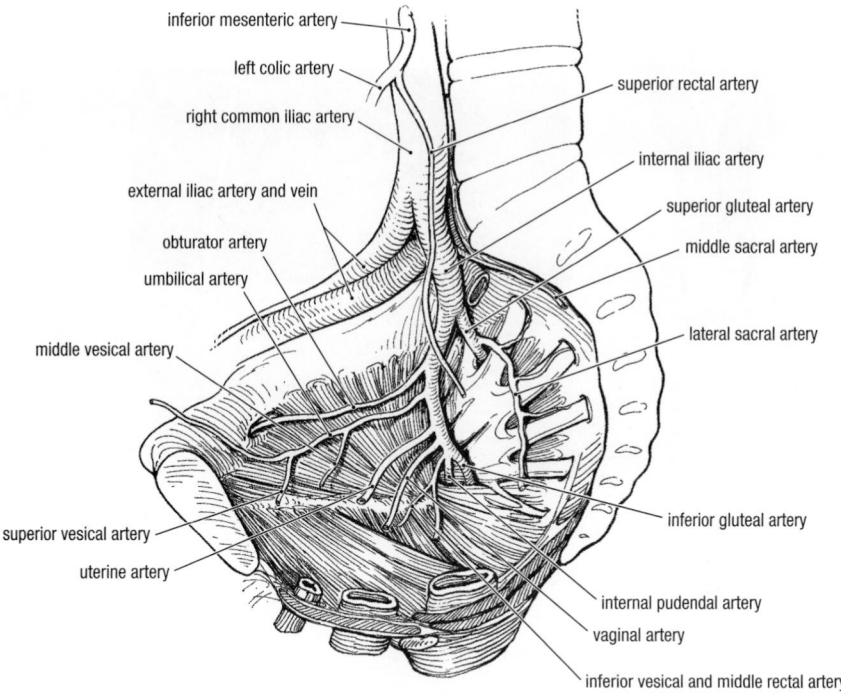

inferior mesenteric artery

left colic artery

right common iliac artery

superior rectal artery

internal iliac artery

external iliac artery and vein

superior gluteal artery

obturator artery

middle sacral artery

umbilical artery

middle vesical artery

lateral sacral artery

superior vesical artery

uterine artery

inferior gluteal artery

internal pudendal artery

vaginal artery

inferior vesical and middle rectal artery

pelvis, blood supply: sagittal view of the pelvis with viscera removed, showing position of major arteries

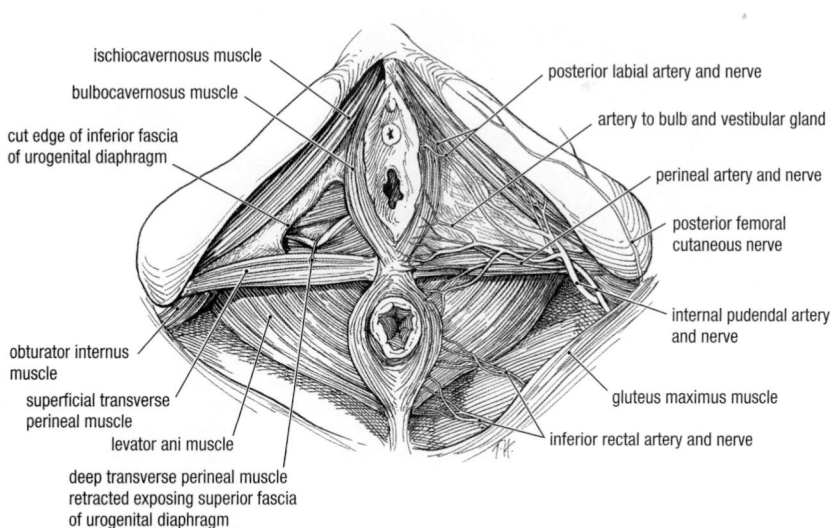

ischiocavernosus muscle

bulbocavernosus muscle

cut edge of inferior fascia of urogenital diaphragm

posterior labial artery and nerve

artery to bulb and vestibular gland

perineal artery and nerve

posterior femoral cutaneous nerve

internal pudendal artery and nerve

obturator internus muscle

superficial transverse perineal muscle

levator ani muscle

deep transverse perineal muscle retracted exposing superior fascia of urogenital diaphragm

gluteus maximus muscle

inferior rectal artery and nerve

perineum, superficial compartment: view from below of the superficial perineal compartment, displaying arteries, nerves, muscles and fascia of the urogenital diaphragm

Appendix 1

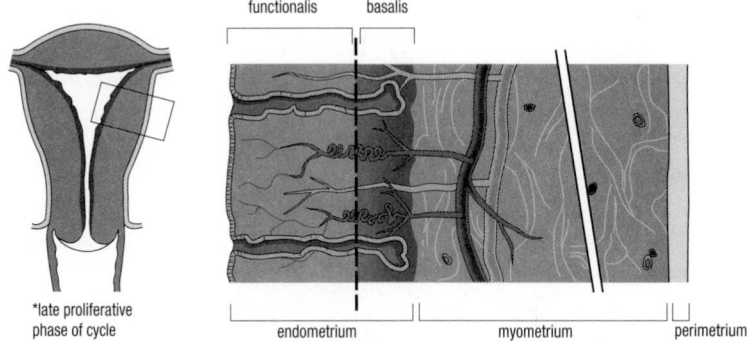

functionalis basalis

*late proliferative
phase of cycle

endometrium myometrium perimetrium

layers of uterus

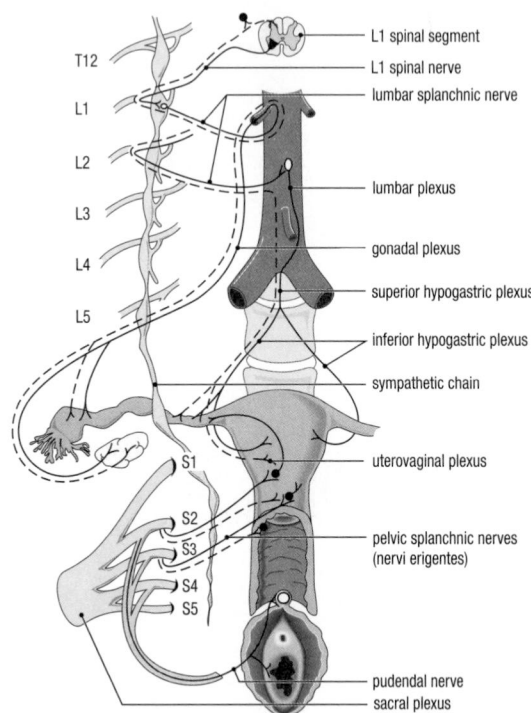

T12

L1

L2

L3

L4

L5

S1

S2

S3

S4

S5

L1 spinal segment
L1 spinal nerve
lumbar splanchnic nerve

lumbar plexus

gonadal plexus

superior hypogastric plexus

inferior hypogastric plexus

sympathetic chain

uterovaginal plexus

pelvic splanchnic nerves
(nervi erigentes)

pudendal nerve
sacral plexus

innervation of the female reproductive tract and genitalia: the sympathetic pathways arise from the lower thoracic and upper lumbar spinal levels (black triangle). There are no white rami below L2. These reach the aortic plexus via thoracic and lumbar splanchnic nerves. Synapse occurs in the aortic plexus (white circles). The postsynaptic neurons reach the pelvic viscera via hypogastric plexuses. The parasympathetic pathways arise from the midsacral spinal levels and reach the pelvic viscera via the splanchnic nerves. Synapse occurs in the walls of the viscera (white circles). Visceral afferent fibers (dashed) from the pelvic viscera travel specifically along either one or the other automatic pathways, have their cell bodies in the dorsal root ganglia, and produce specific patterns of referred pain. The pudendal nerve provides somatic innervation to and from the perineum.

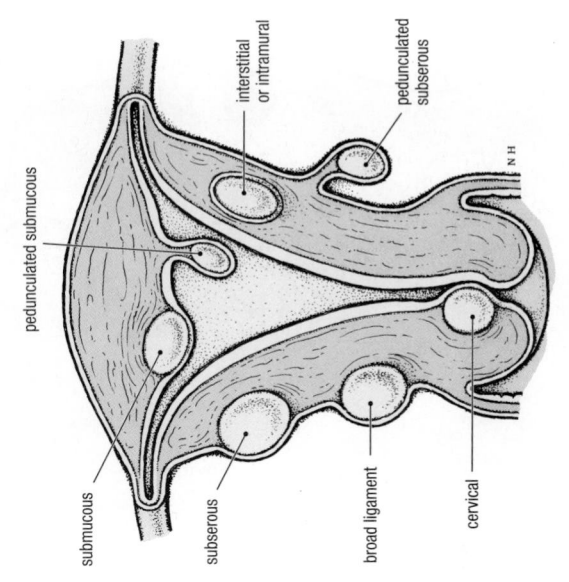

location of fibroids

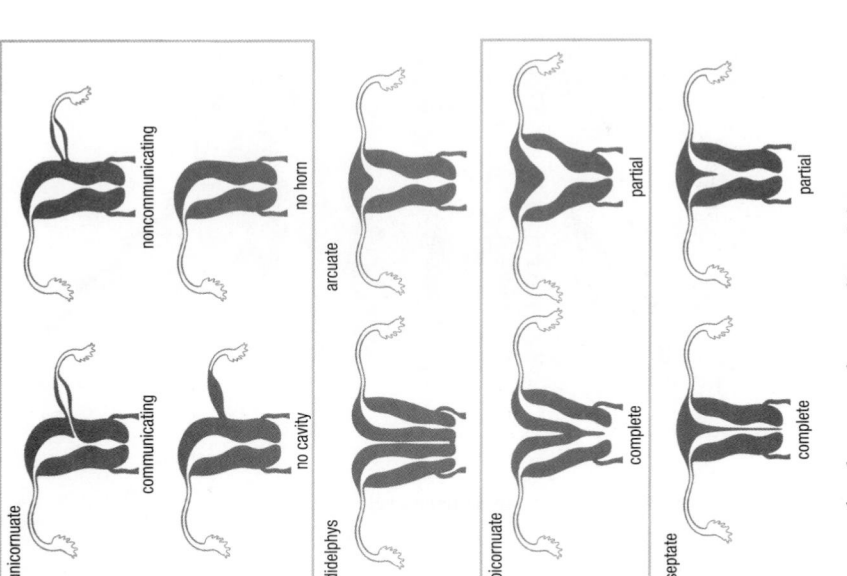

developmental anomalies of the uterus

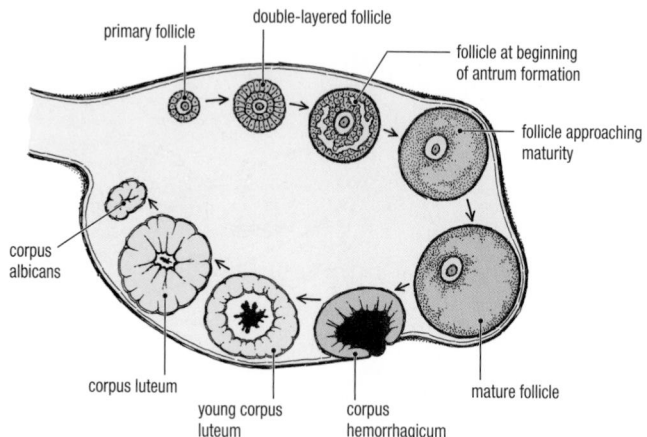

ovulation

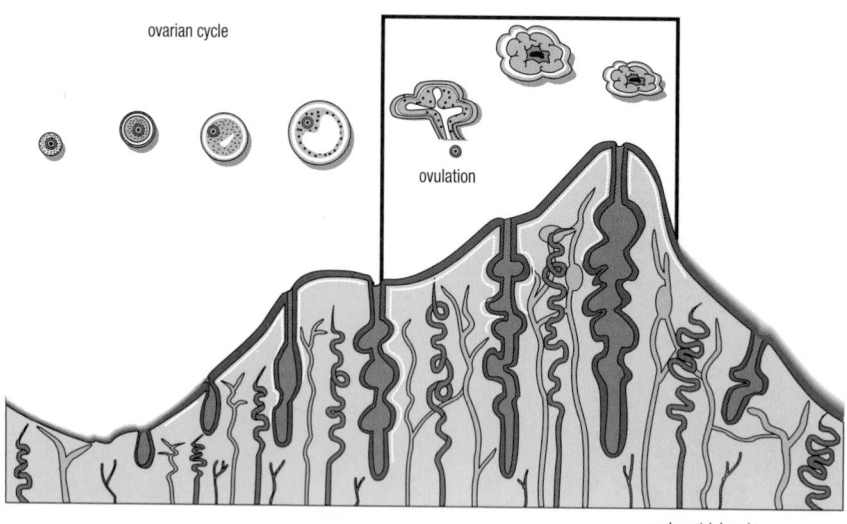

menstrual cycle

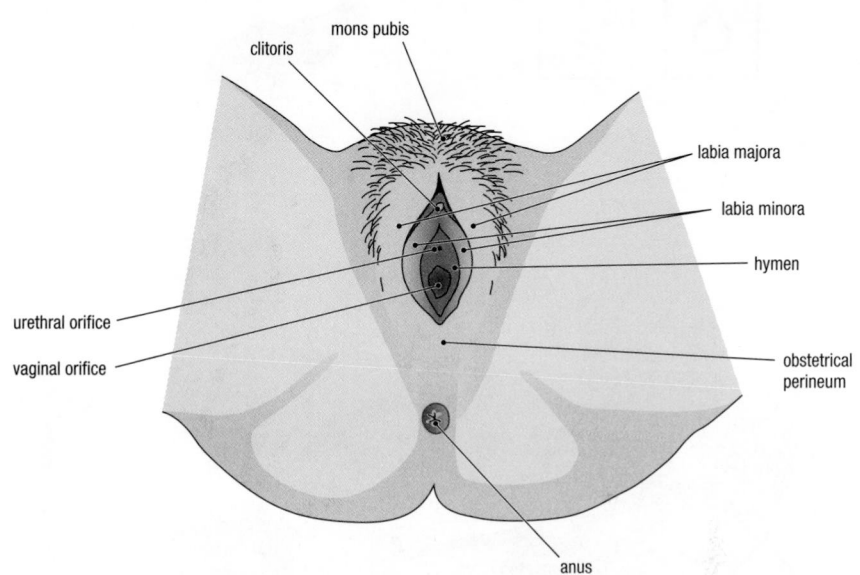

external female genitalia

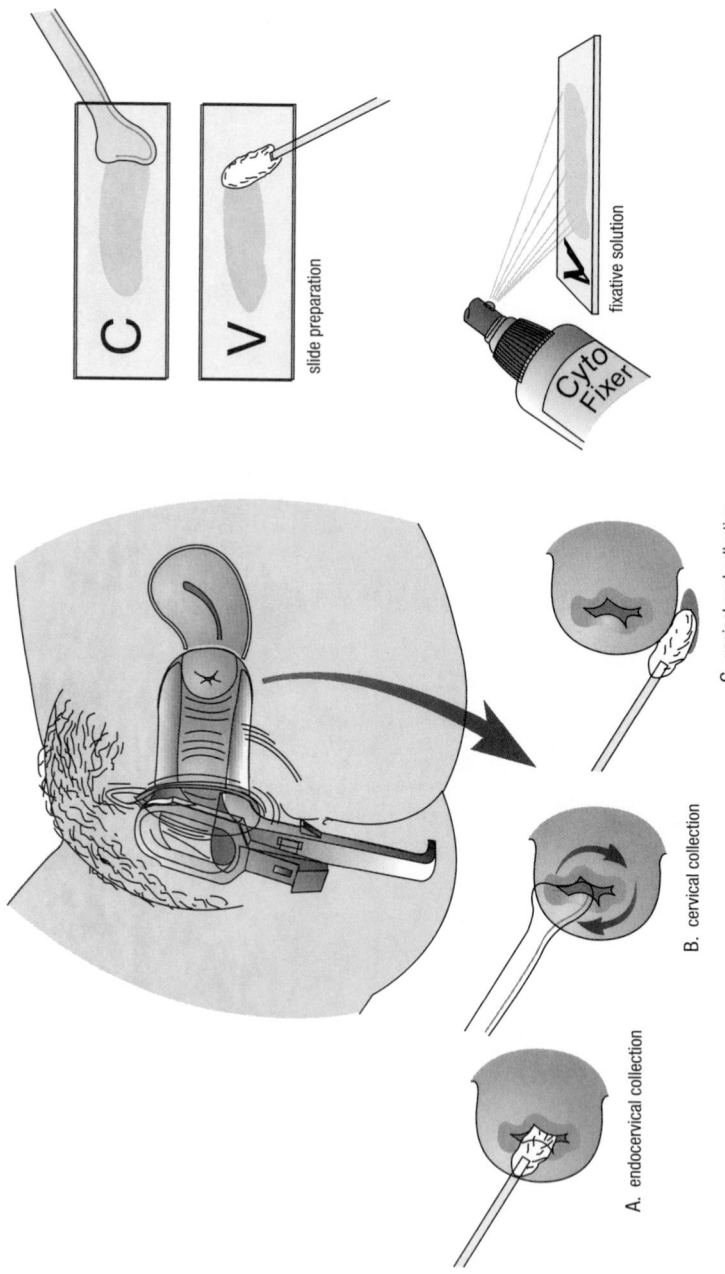

slide preparation

fixative solution

Cyto Fixer

C. vaginal pool collection

B. cervical collection

A. endocervical collection

obtaining a Pap smear: (A) specimen taken from endocervix; (B) specimen taken from cervix; (C) specimen taken from vaginal pool

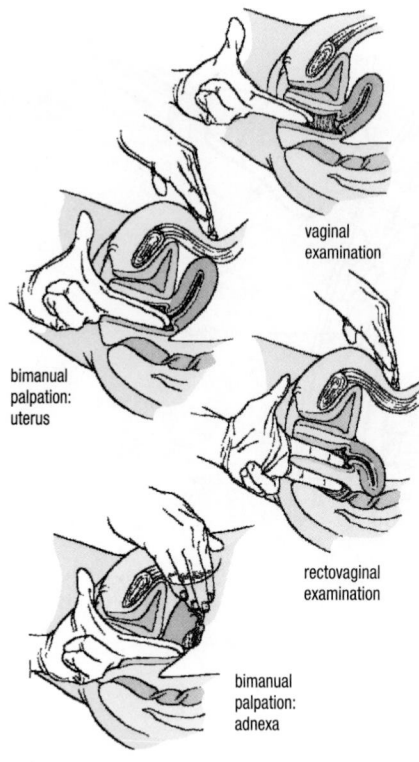

vaginal
examination

bimanual
palpation:
uterus

rectovaginal
examination

bimanual
palpation:
adnexa

pelvic examination

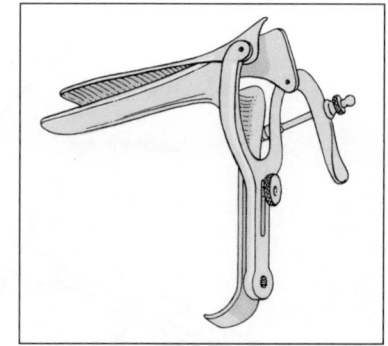

speculum: vaginal duckbill

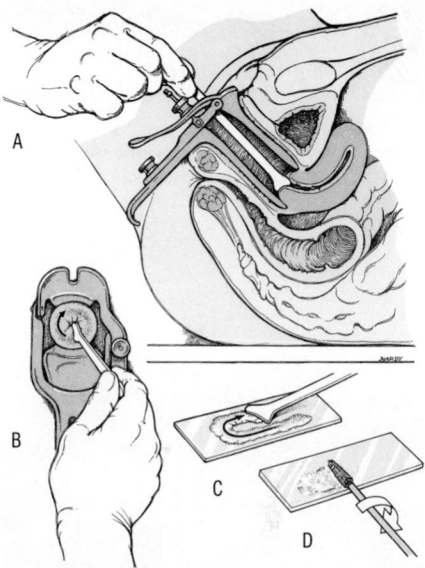

Pap smear: (A) speculum in place and Ayre
spatula in position at cervical os; (B) tip of
spatula placed in the cervical os and rotated
360 degrees; (C) cellular material clinging to
spatula is then smeared smoothly on glass
slide, which is promptly placed in fixative
solution; (D) cytobrush is rotated in cervical os
and rolled onto glass slide

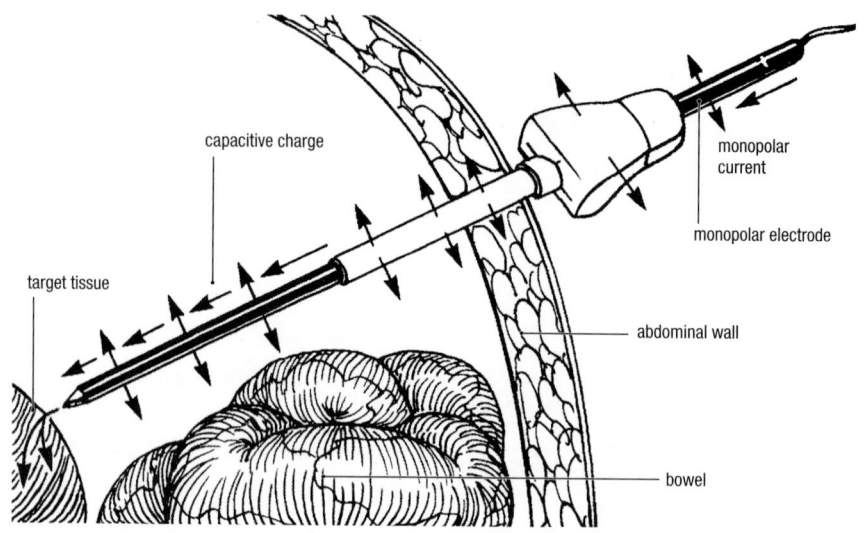

laparoscopy, current diversion, step 1: the activated unipolar laparoscopic electrode develops a surrounding electromagnetic charge, capable of completing the circuit in a nearby conductor

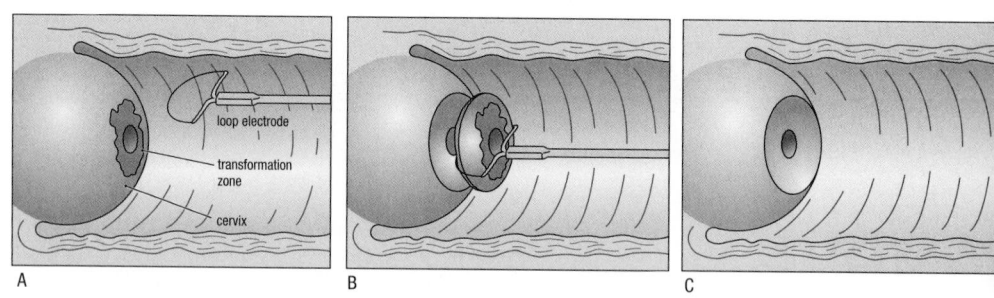

loop electrosurgical excision procedure (LEEP) or large loop excision of the transformation zone (LLETZ): (A) electrode approach; (B) removal of transformation zone; (C) excision site (region between endocervix and ectocervix)

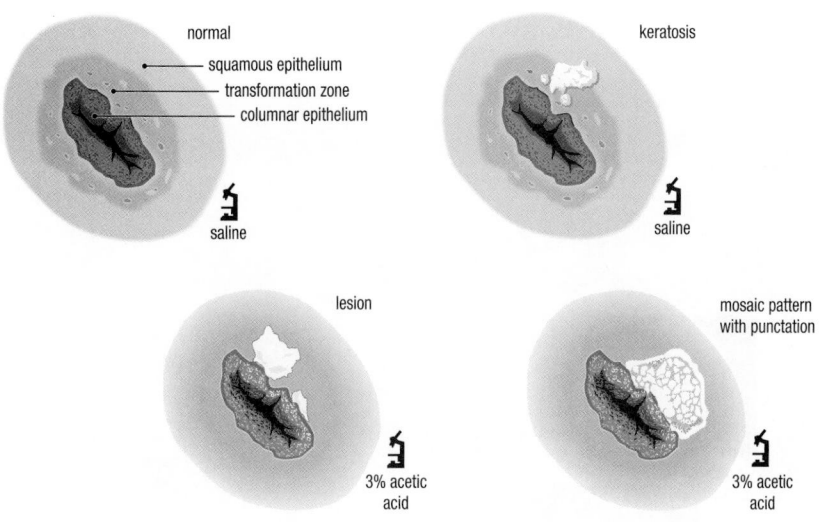

colposcopy findings

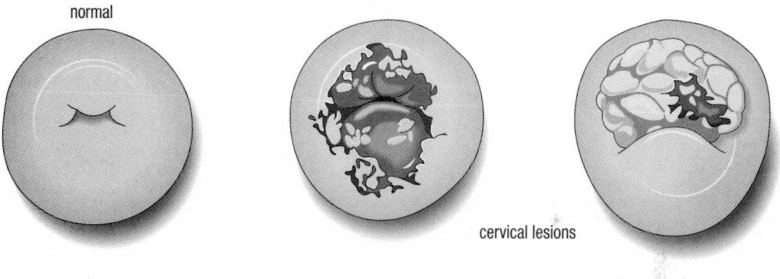

cervical lesions

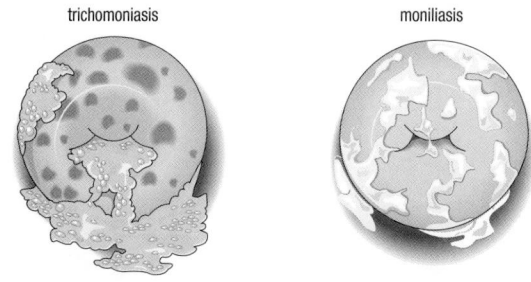

vaginitis

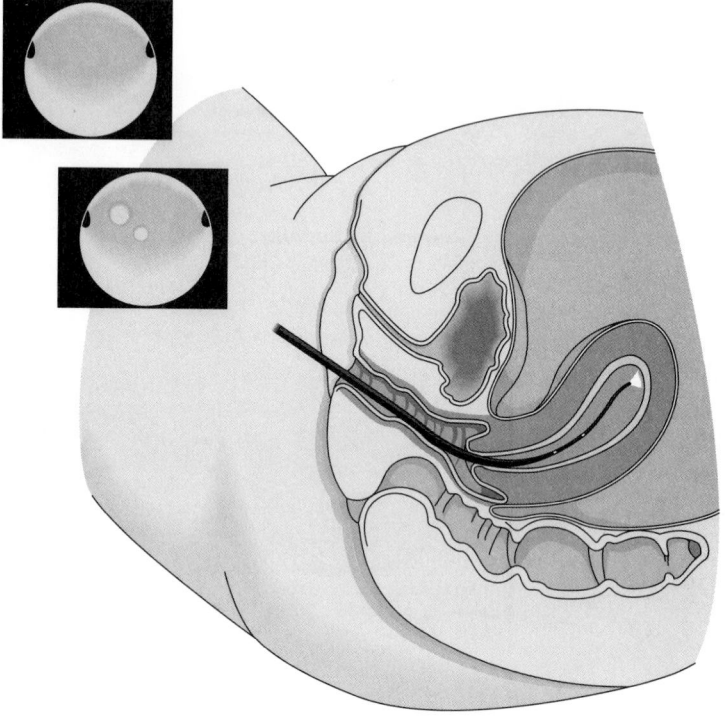

hysteroscopy

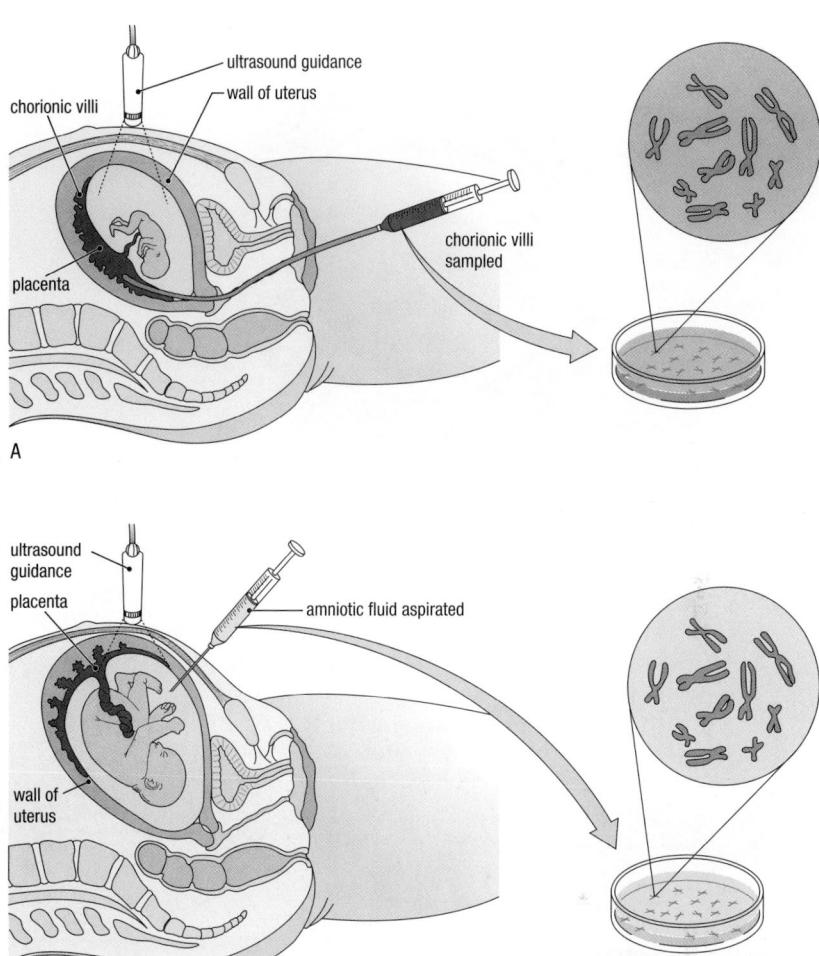

(A) chorionic villus sampling (9 to 11 weeks); (B) amniocentesis (15 to 18 weeks)

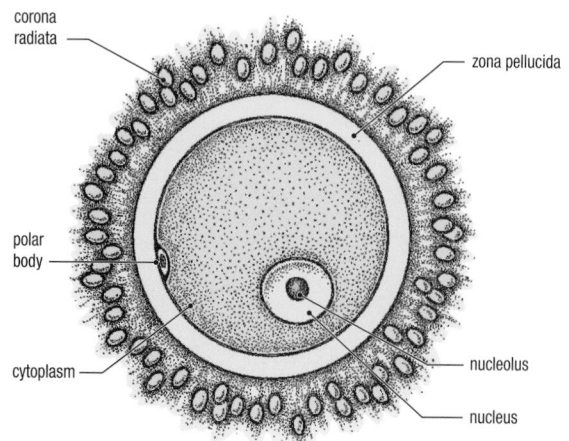

mature oocyte (ovum)

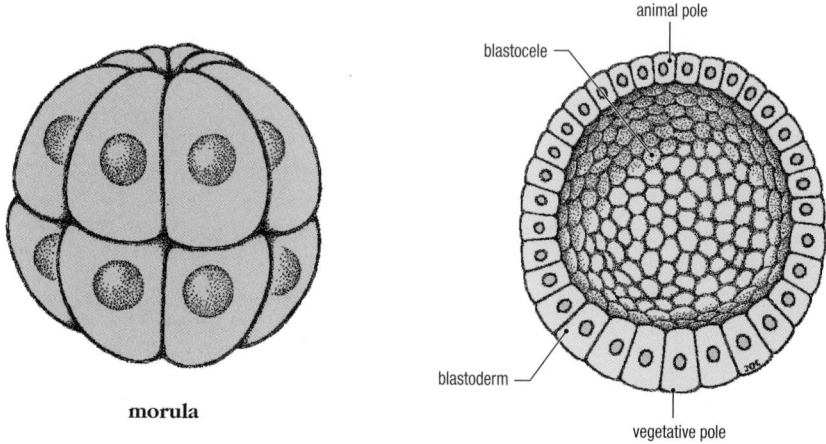

morula

blastula, hemisected

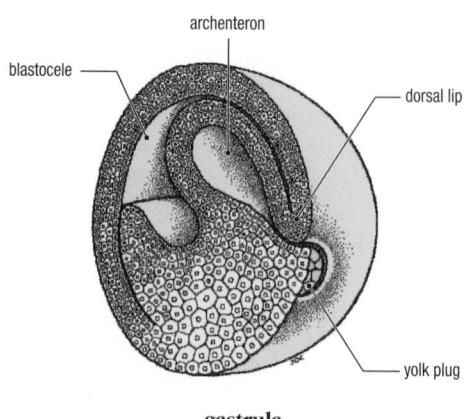

gastrula

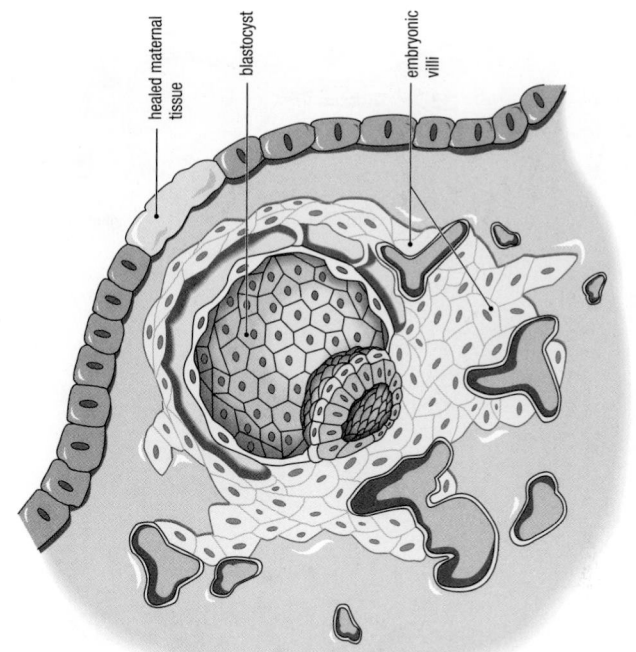

second stage of implantation

healed maternal tissue

blastocyst

embryonic villi

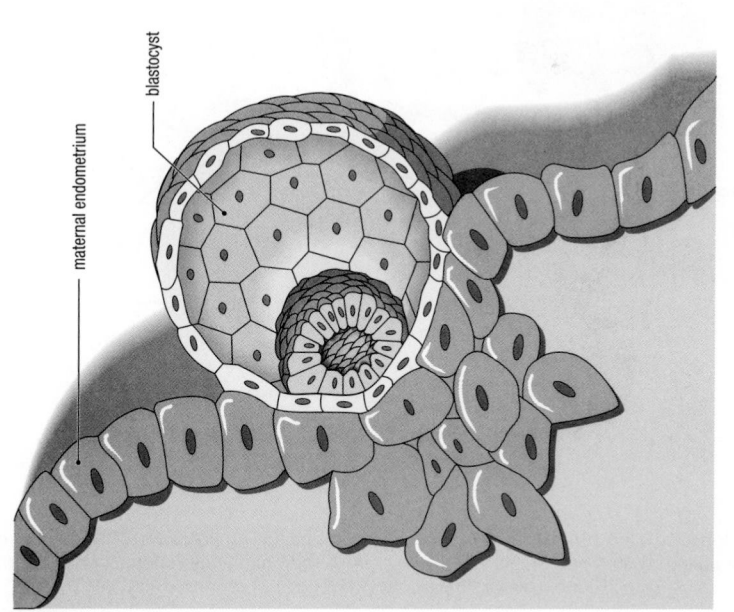

first stage of implantation

maternal endometrium

blastocyst

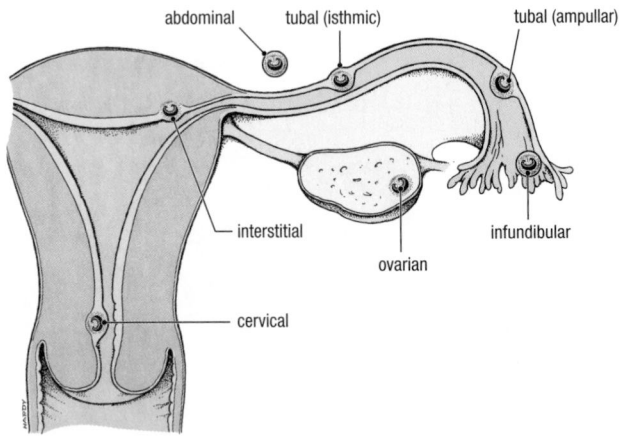

sites of ectopic pregnancy

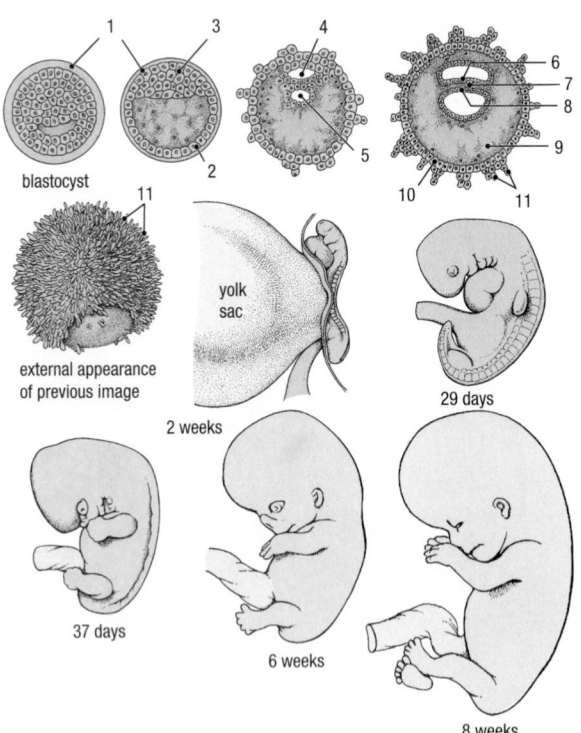

development; from blastocyst to fetus: (1) zona pellucida; (2) trophectoderm; (3) inner cell mass; (4) amniotic cavity; (5) yolk sac; (6) ectoderm; (7) mesoderm; (8) entoderm; (9) mesoderm; (10) trophectoderm; (11) chorionic villi

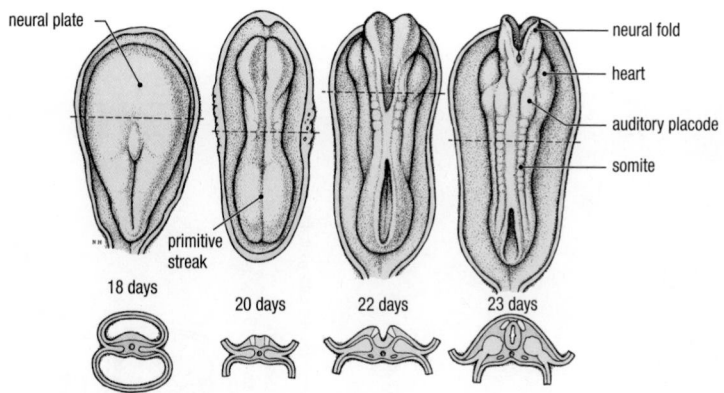

neural plate

primitive streak

18 days

20 days

22 days

23 days

neural fold

heart

auditory placode

somite

blastoderm: top, dorsal views; bottom, cross-sectional views

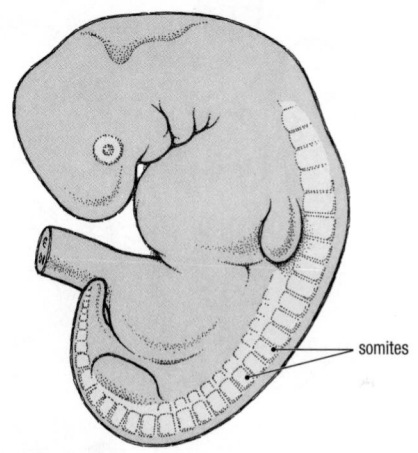

somites

somites in a 29-day human embryo

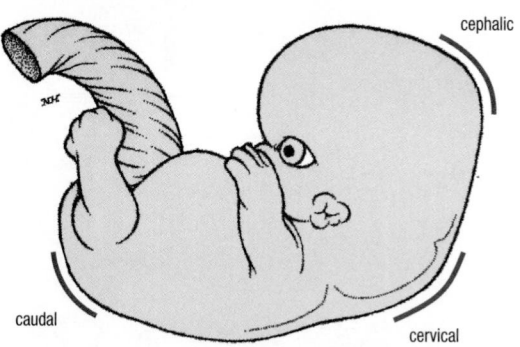

cephalic

cervical

caudal

flexures seen in a 6-week old embryo

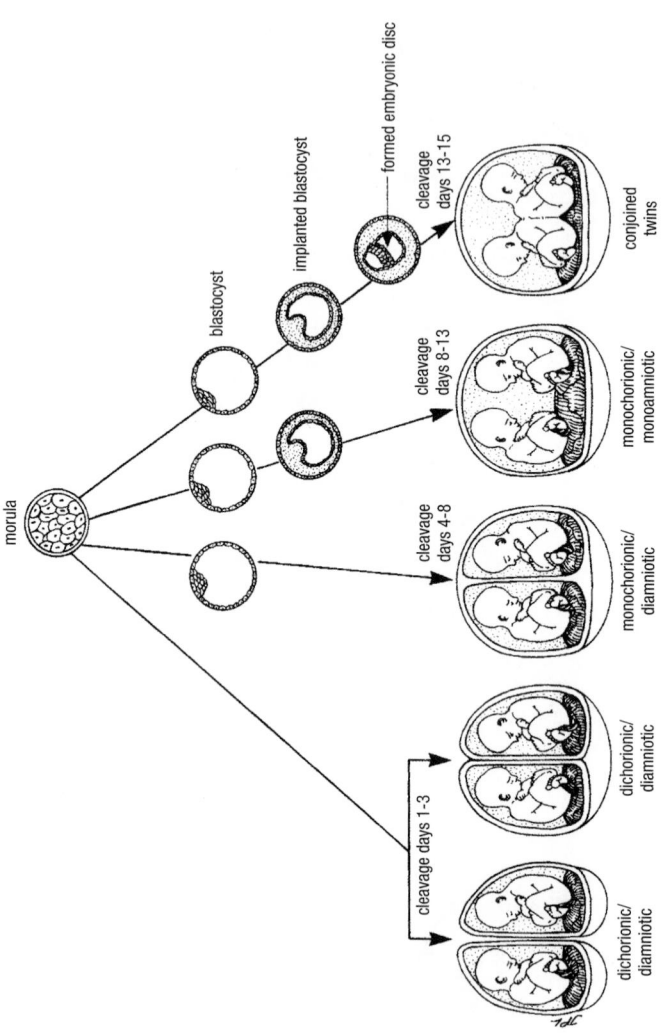

genesis of identical (monozygotic) twins

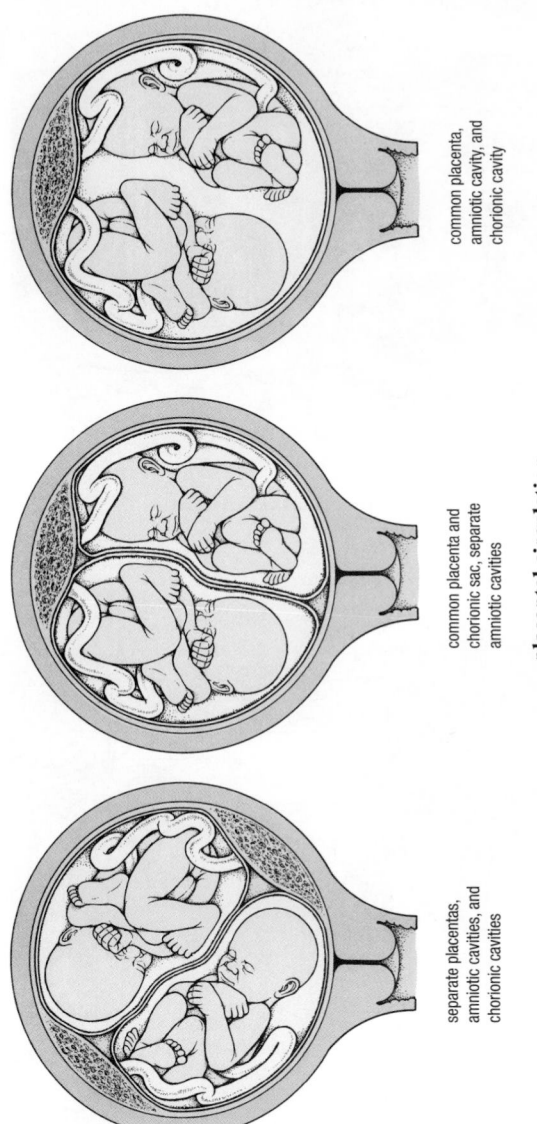

common placenta, amniotic cavity, and chorionic cavity

common placenta and chorionic sac; separate amniotic cavities

separate placentas, amniotic cavities, and chorionic cavities

placental circulation

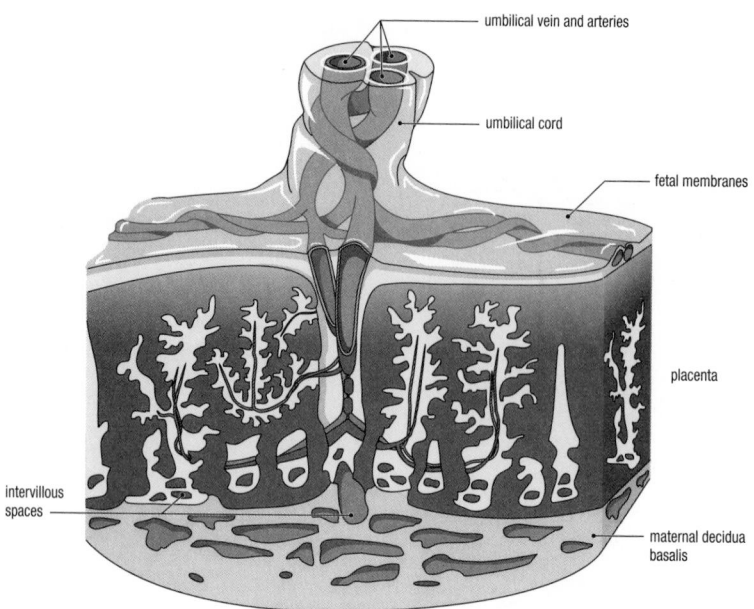

umbilical vein and arteries

umbilical cord

fetal membranes

placenta

intervillous spaces

maternal decidua basalis

placental circulation

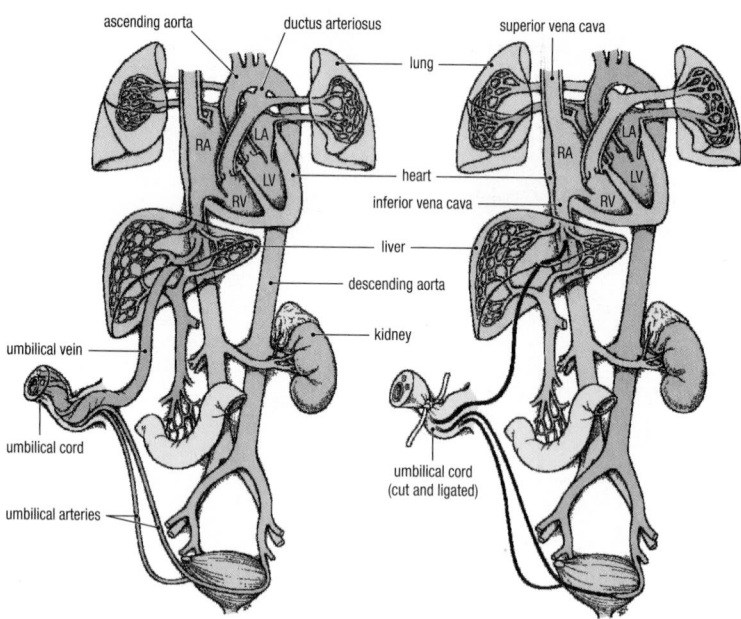

ascending aorta

ductus arteriosus

superior vena cava

lung

RA

LA

LV

RV

heart

inferior vena cava

liver

descending aorta

kidney

umbilical vein

umbilical cord

umbilical arteries

RA

LA

LV

RV

umbilical cord (cut and ligated)

fetal circulation: (left) during pregnancy, oxygen diffuses from the maternal circulation to the fetal circulation in the placenta; oxygenated blood returns to the fetus through the umbilical vein; (right) after birth, umbilical cord is cut and blood is oxygenated as it passes through the lungs; RA, right atrium; LA, left atrium; LV, left ventricle; RV, right ventricle

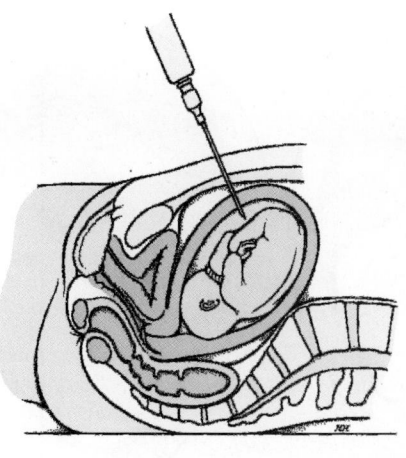

amniocentesis

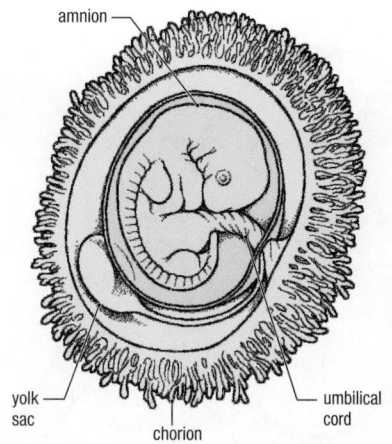

amnion

yolk sac

chorion

umbilical cord

**amnion and related structures
showing 5-week embryo**

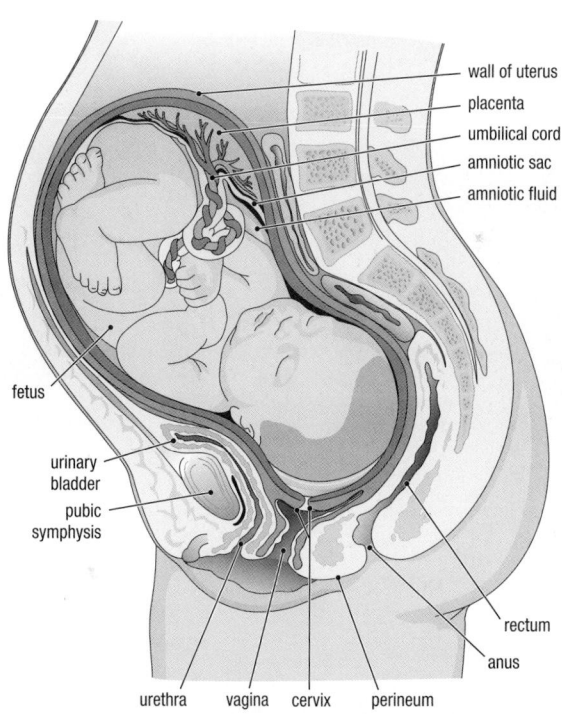

wall of uterus

placenta

umbilical cord

amniotic sac

amniotic fluid

fetus

urinary bladder

pubic symphysis

urethra   vagina   cervix   perineum

rectum

anus

pregnant uterus with intact fetus: midsagittal section

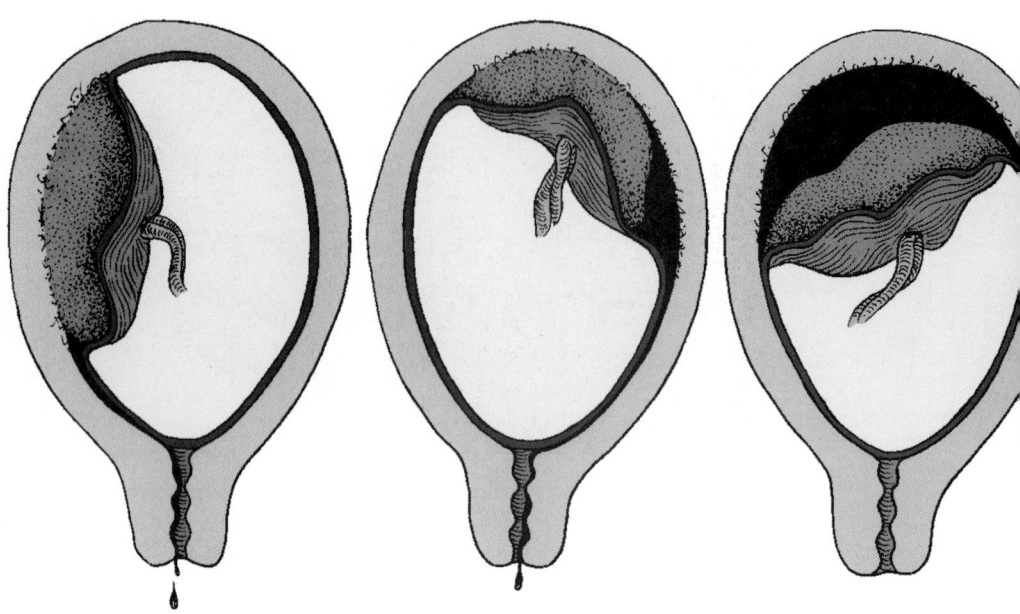

twins: schematic diagrams showing the possible relations of the fetal membranes in monozygotic twins

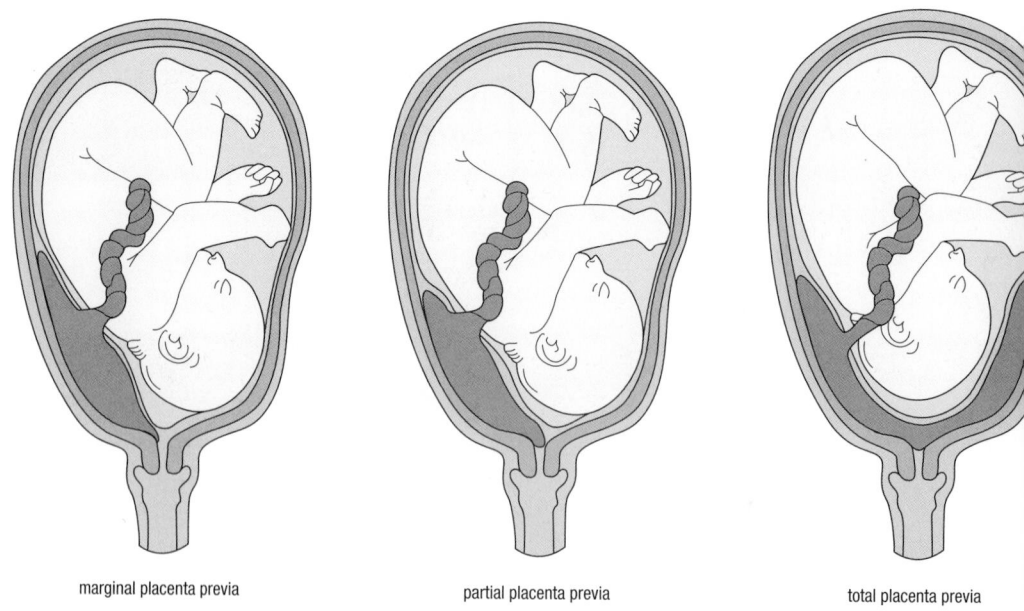

marginal placenta previa   partial placenta previa   total placenta previa

abruptio placentae: the relationship between vaginal bleeding and abruptio placentae; increasing degrees of placental separation are shown; (left) marginal separation, (center) partial separation, (right) complete separation

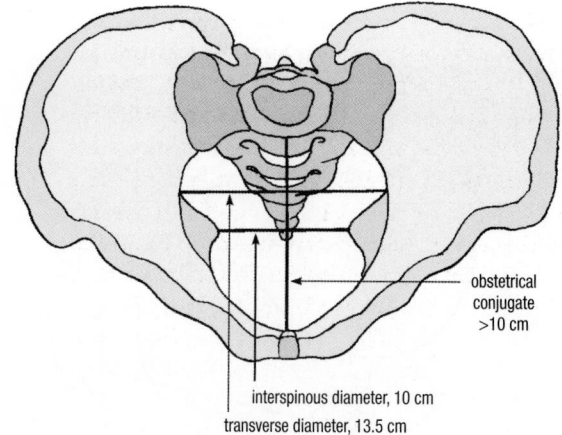

obstetrical
conjugate
>10 cm

interspinous diameter, 10 cm
transverse diameter, 13.5 cm

pelvic diameters: superior view of female pelvis, indicating normal distances between structures

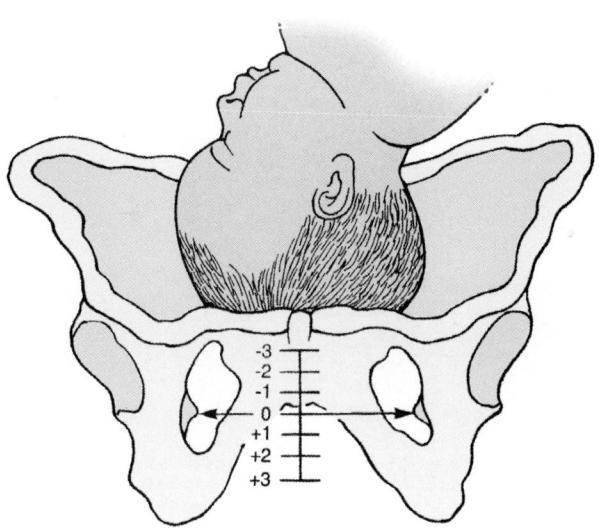

-3
-2
-1
0
+1
+2
+3

presentation, vertex, station estimation: estimation of station by traditional three-station system; station is estimated by palpation of the bony segment of the presenting part during a vaginal examination and determining the distance from the plane of the ischial spines

Anatomical Illustrations

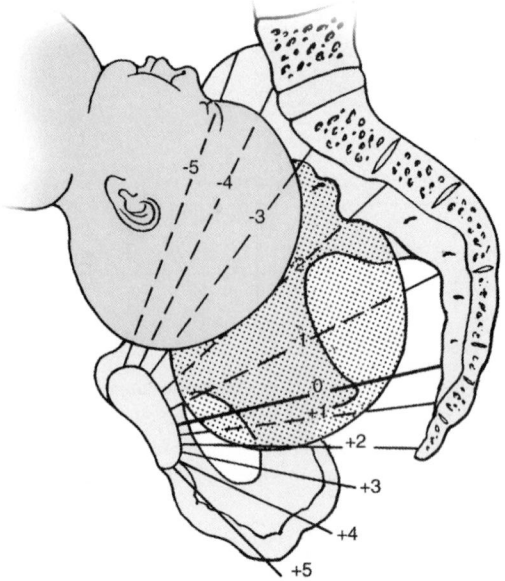

presentation, vertex, station estimation: illustration shows the estimation of station by current ACOG centimeter system

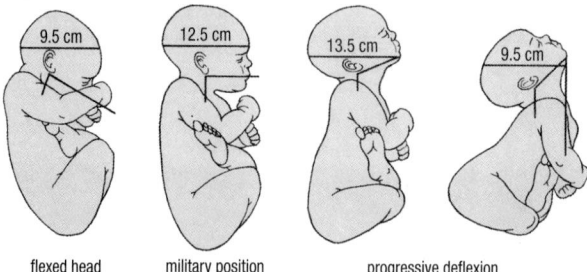

flexed head   military position   progressive deflexion

presentation, breech, cranial diameters: importance of cranial flexion is emphasized by noting the increased diameters presented to the birth canal with progressive deflexion

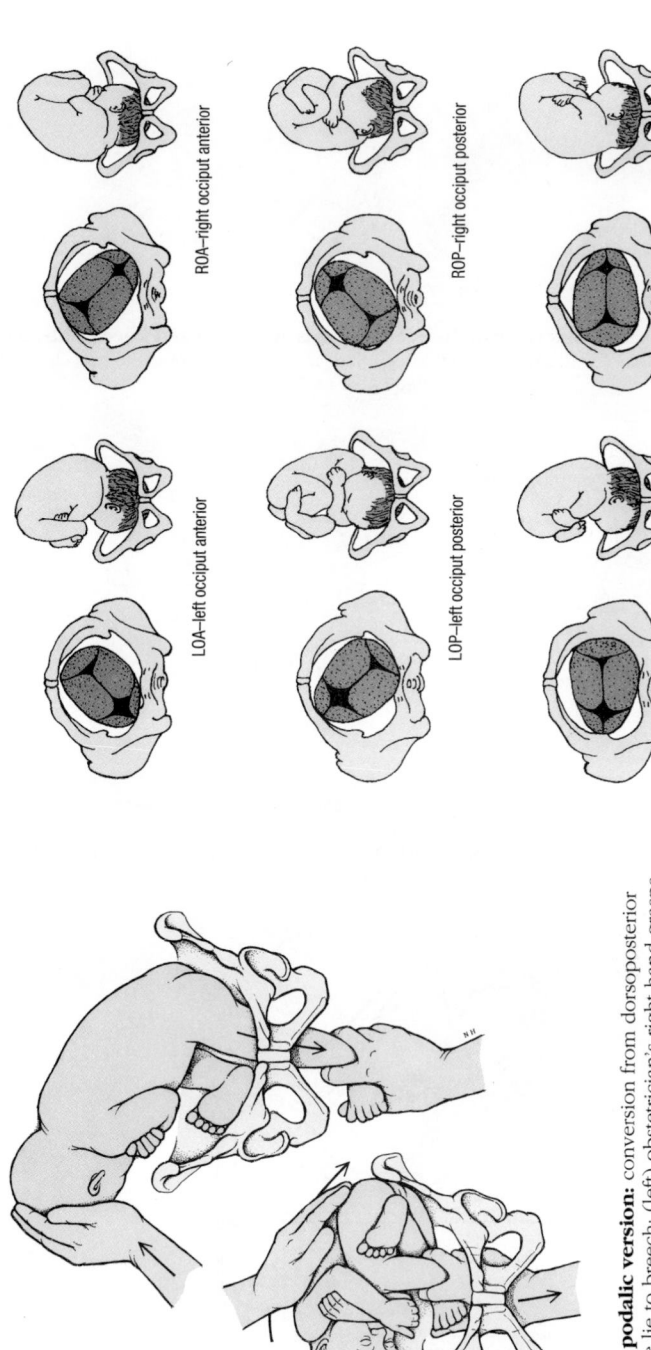

ROA—right occiput anterior

ROP—right occiput posterior

ROT—right occiput transverse

LOA—left occiput anterior

LOP—left occiput posterior

LOT—left occiput transverse

vertex presentation: fetal head positions within the pelvic girdle in a vertex presentation

internal podalic version: conversion from dorsoposterior transverse lie to breech; (left) obstetrician's right hand grasps fetal foot within uterus while left hand applies pressure externally to rotate breech toward pelvic inlet; (right) obstetrician maneuvers fetus into longitudinal orientation by applying traction to foot while externally directing head into fundus, so that delivery can proceed as in breech presentation

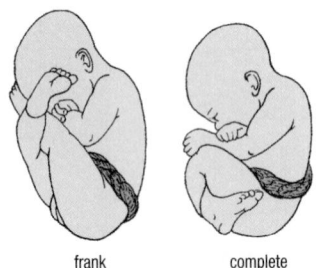

frank   complete

full breech presentations refer to the relationships at the hip and knee joints: frank breech, both hip joints are flexed and both knee joints are extended; complete breech, both hip joints and knee joints are flexed

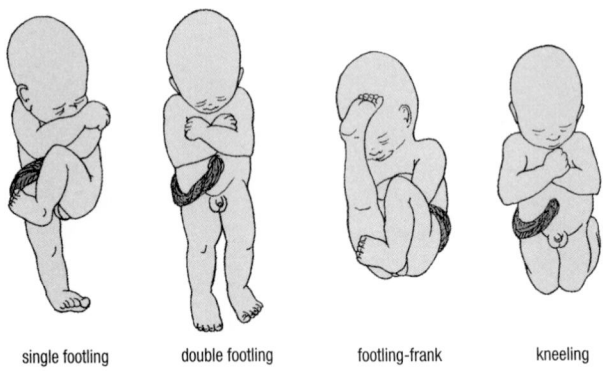

single footling   double footling   footling-frank   kneeling

varieties of incomplete breech presentations refer to incomplete flexion at either the hip or knee joints

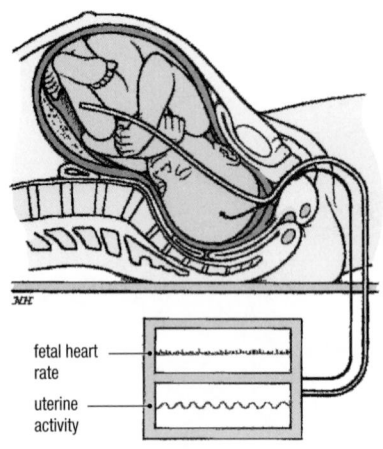

fetal heart rate

uterine activity

electronic fetal monitoring

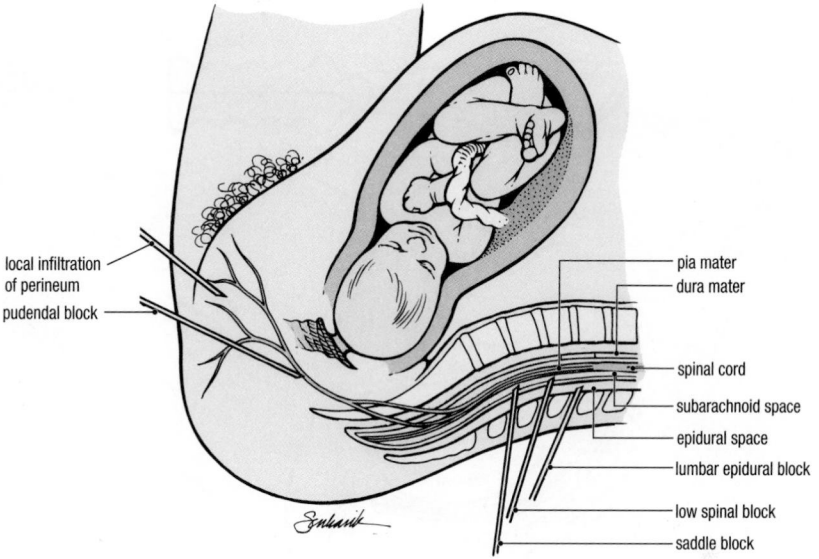

local infiltration
of perineum

pudendal block

pia mater
dura mater

spinal cord
subarachnoid space
epidural space
lumbar epidural block
low spinal block
saddle block

regional anesthesia for childbirth: sites of injection

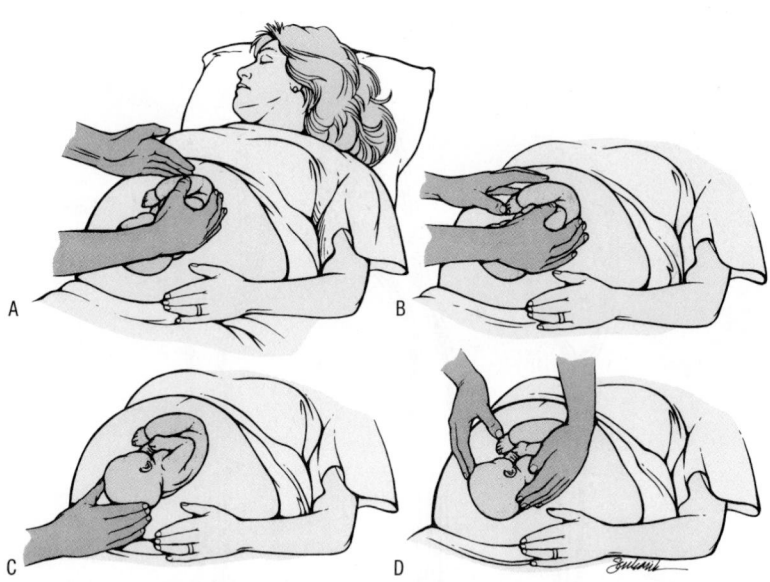

A   B

C   D

Leopold maneuvers: (A) first maneuver, palpate superior surface of fundus; (B) second maneuver, palpate sides of uterus to determine which direction fetal back is facing; (C) third maneuver, palpate to discover what is at inlet of pelvis; (D) fourth maneuver, assuming fetus has been found to be in cephalic presentation, fetal attitude should then be determined (degree of flexion)

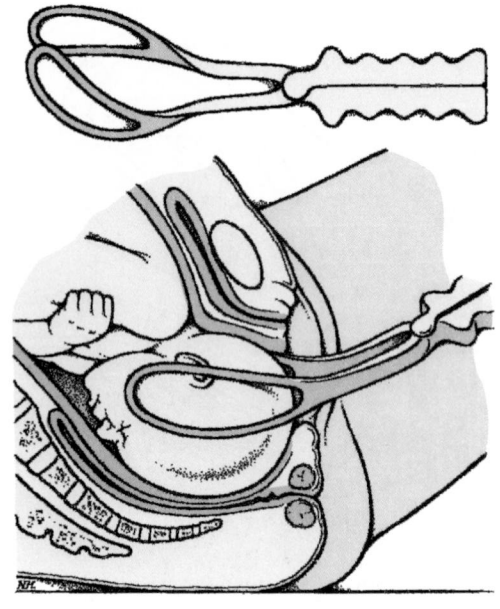

obstetrical forceps

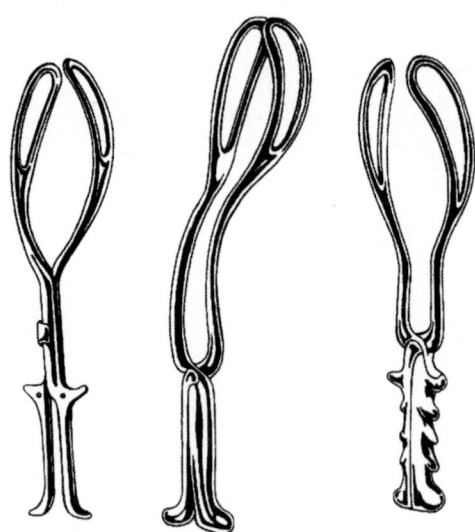

obstetrical forceps: (left) Kjelland; (middle) Piper; (right) Simpson

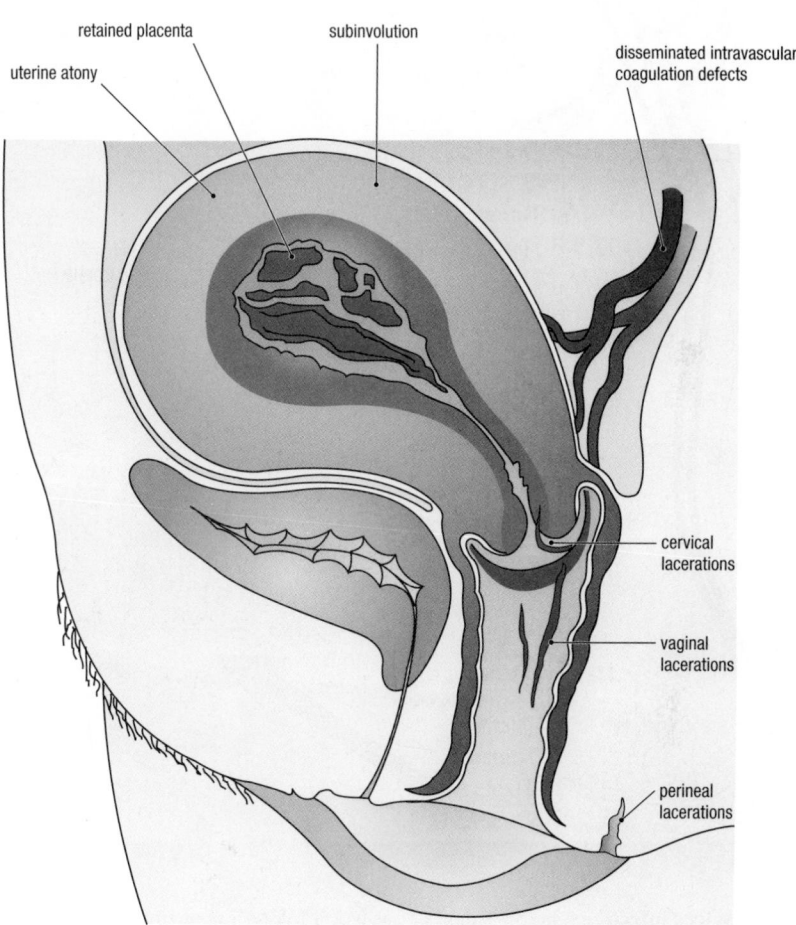

retained placenta

subinvolution

disseminated intravascular
coagulation defects

uterine atony

cervical
lacerations

vaginal
lacerations

perineal
lacerations

common causes of postpartal hemorrhage

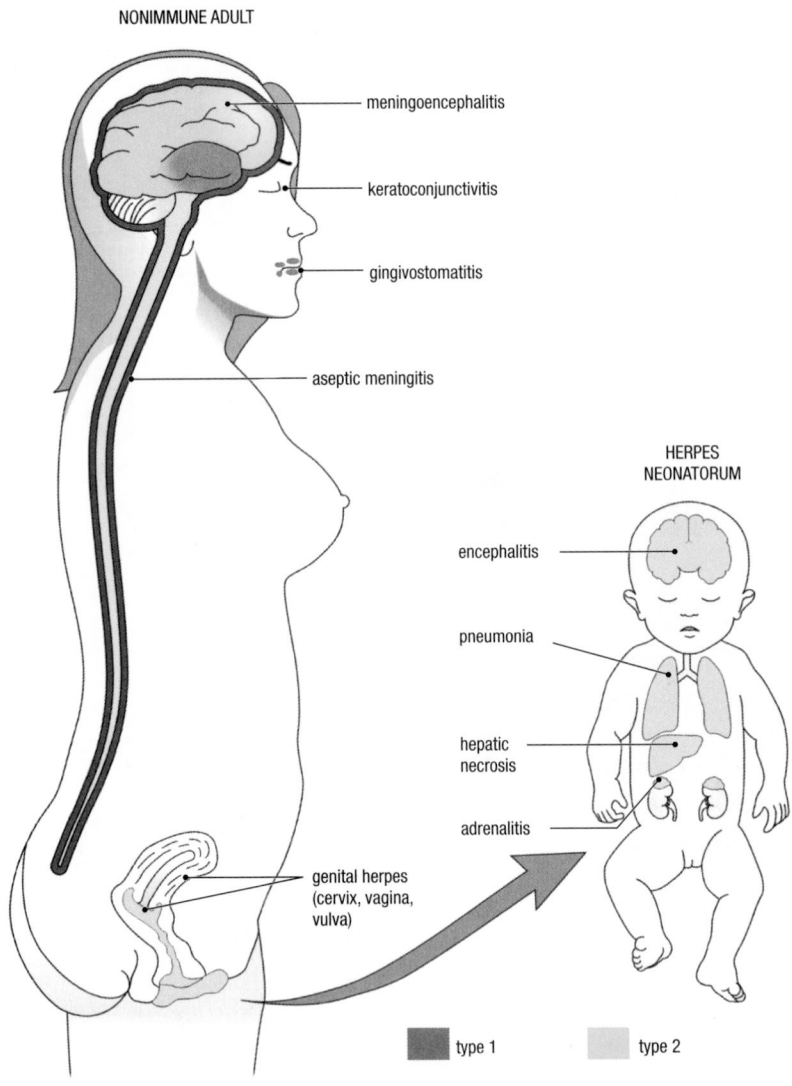

herpesvirus infections: herpes simplex virus type 1 infects a nonimmune adult, causing gingivostomatitis ("fever blister" or "cold sore"), keratoconjunctivitis, meningoencephalitis, and aseptic spinal meningitis; herpes simplex virus type 2 infects the genitalia of a nonimmune adult, involving the cervix, vagina, and vulva; herpes simplex virus type 2 infects the fetus as it passes through the birth canal of an infected mother; the infant's lack of a mature immune system results in disseminated infection with herpes simplex virus type 1; the infection is often fatal, involving lung, liver, adrenal glands, and central nervous system

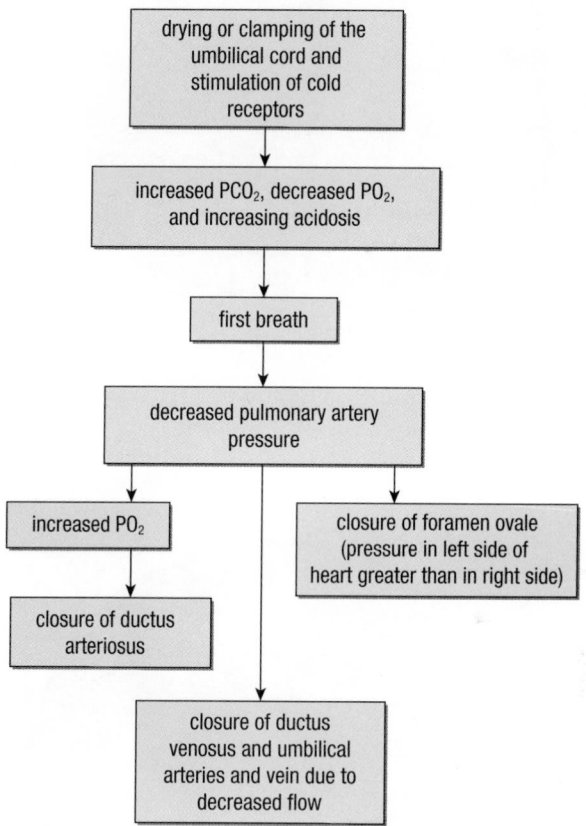

circulatory events at birth

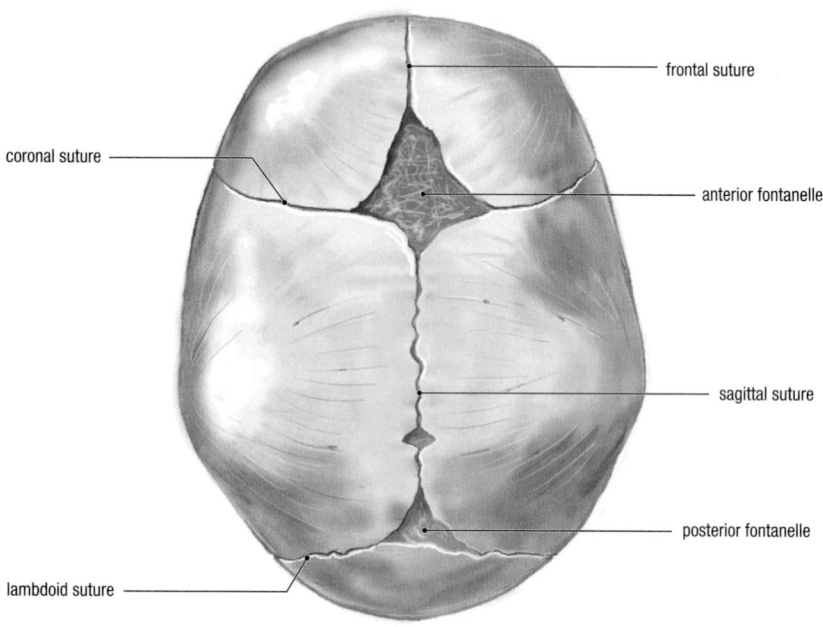

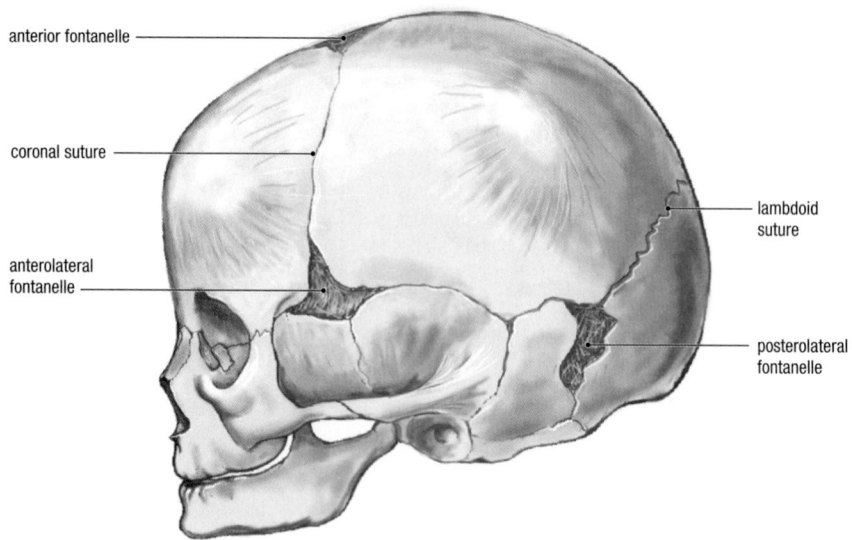

newborn skull: (top) superior view; (bottom) lateral view

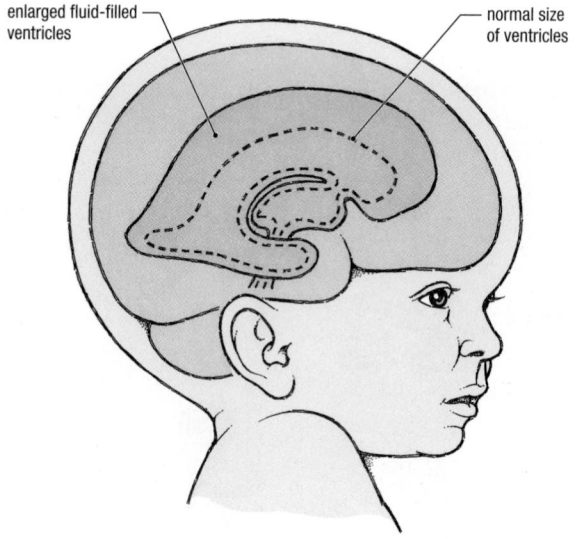

enlarged fluid-filled ventricles

normal size of ventricles

hydrocephalus

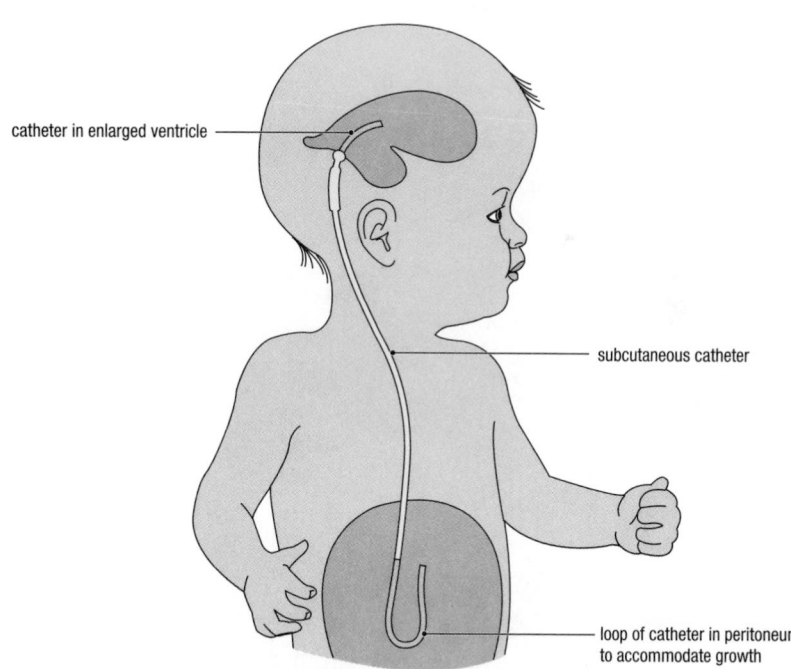

catheter in enlarged ventricle

subcutaneous catheter

loop of catheter in peritoneum to accommodate growth

infant with ventriculoperitoneal shunt in place: the shunt removes excess cerebrospinal fluid from the ventricles and shunts it to the peritoneum; a one-way valve is present in the tubing behind the ear

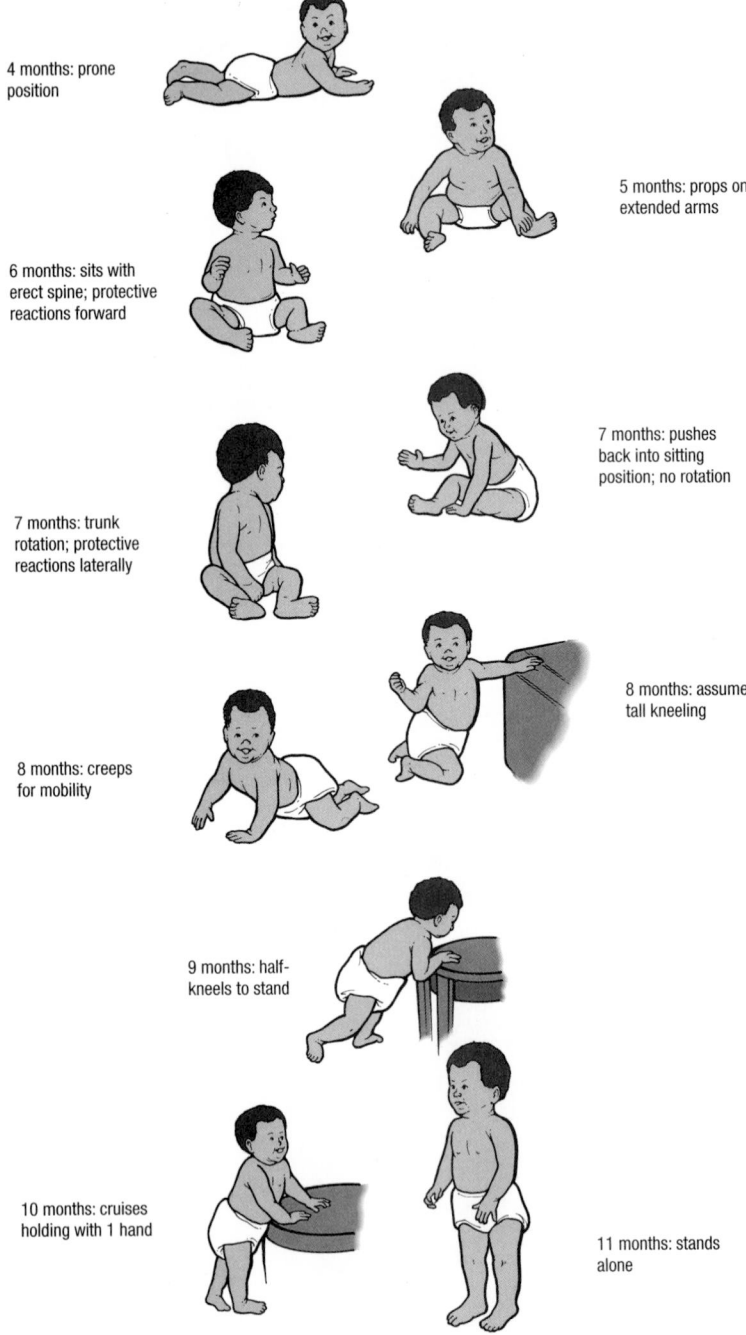

4 months: prone position

5 months: props on extended arms

6 months: sits with erect spine; protective reactions forward

7 months: pushes back into sitting position; no rotation

7 months: trunk rotation; protective reactions laterally

8 months: assumes tall kneeling

8 months: creeps for mobility

9 months: half-kneels to stand

10 months: cruises holding with 1 hand

11 months: stands alone

developmental milestones

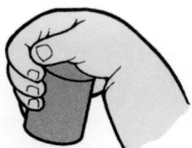

5 months: palmar grasp: fingers on top surface of object press it into center of palm; thumb abducted

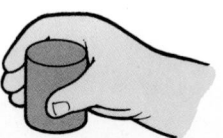

6 months: radial-palmar grasp: fingers on far side of object press it against opposed thumb and radial side of palm

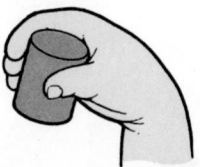

7 months: inferior-scissors grasp: raking into palm with abducted, totally flexed thumb and all flexed fingers, or raking object into palm with abducted, totally flexed thumb and 2 partly extended fingers

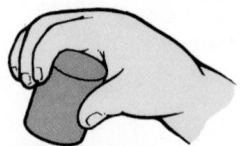

7 months: radial-palmar grasp: wrist straight

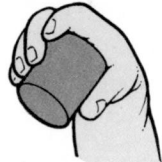

8 months: scissors grasp: between thumb and side of curled index finger, distal thumb joint slightly flexed; proximal thumb joint extended

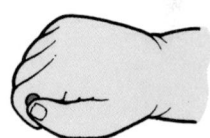

8 months: radial-digital grasp: object held with opposed thumb and fingertips, space visible between

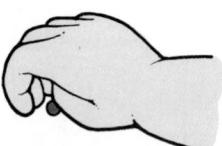

9 months: inferior-pincer grasp: between ventral surfaces of thumb and index finger, distal thumb joint extended; beginning thumb opposition

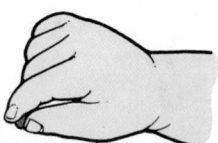

9 months: radial-digital grasp: wrist extended

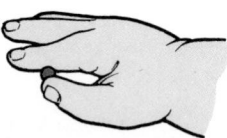

10 months: pincer grasp: between distal pads of thumb and index finger, distal thumb slightly flexed; thumb opposed

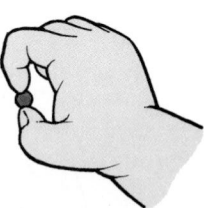

12 months: fine pincer grasp: between fingertips or fingernails; distal thumb joint flexed

pinch and grasp patterns

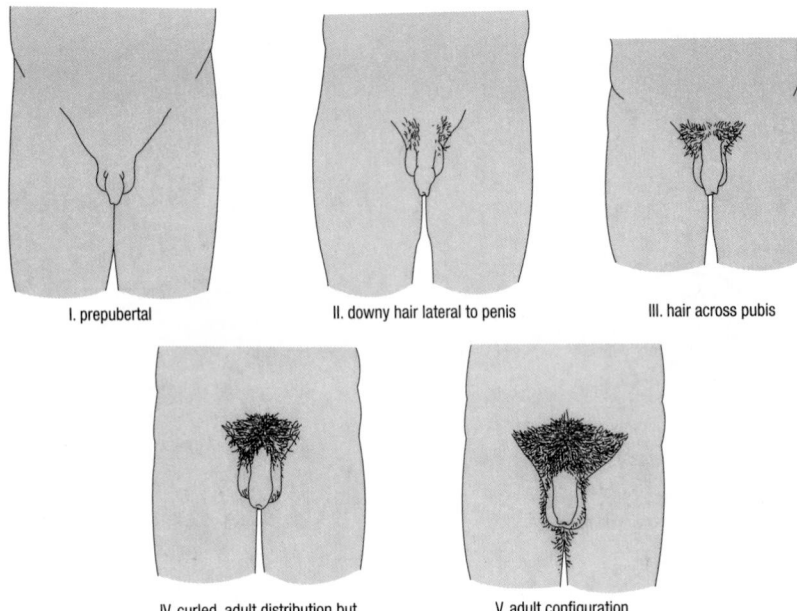

Tanner stages in the male: rating I-V

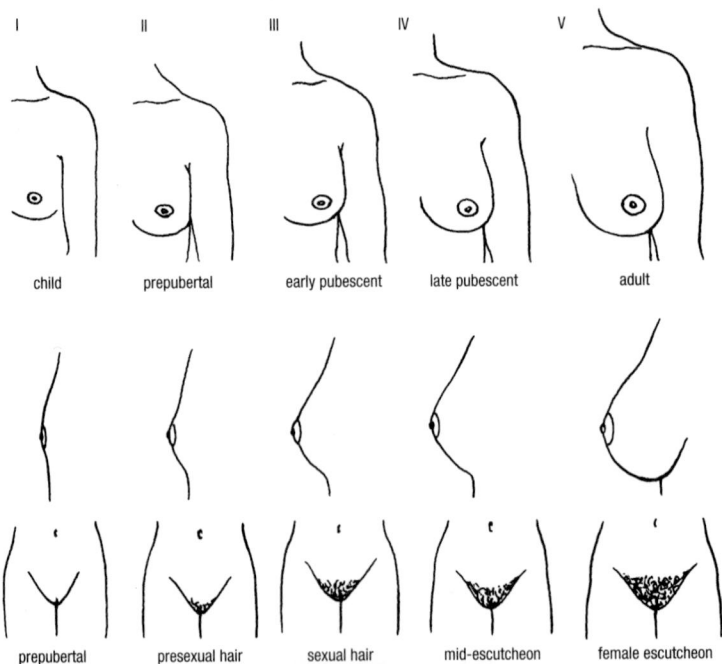

Tanner stages in the female: rating I-V

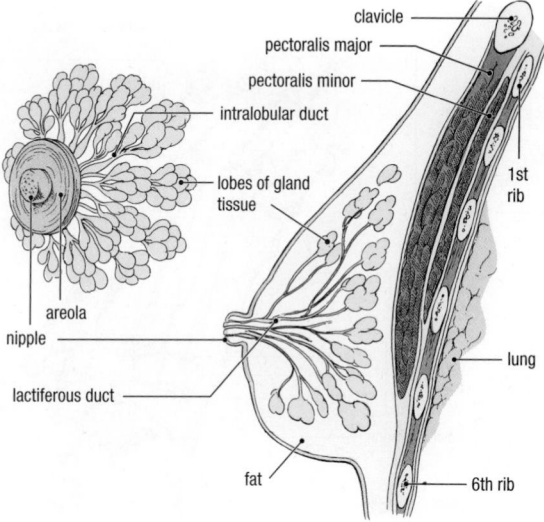

breast: glandular tissue and ducts of the mammary gland

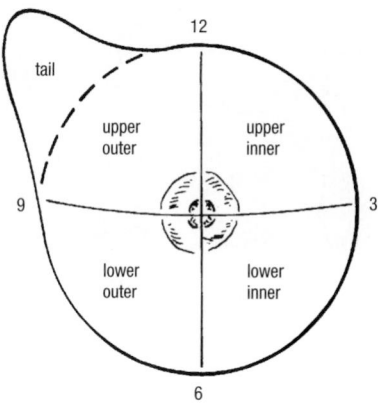

breast: schematic of breast as clock with nipple at center to assist reference

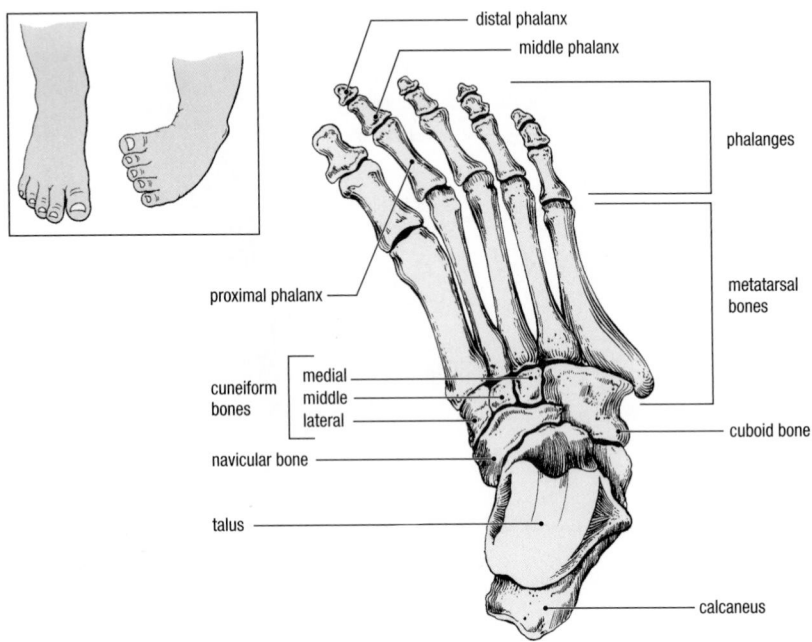

clubfoot: bones in a clubfoot deformity; note tarsal navicular moved medial to talus, talus is forced laterally, which in turn has pushed calcaneus into varus and equinus; anterior view of a child's two feet, the left of which is clubbed (inset)

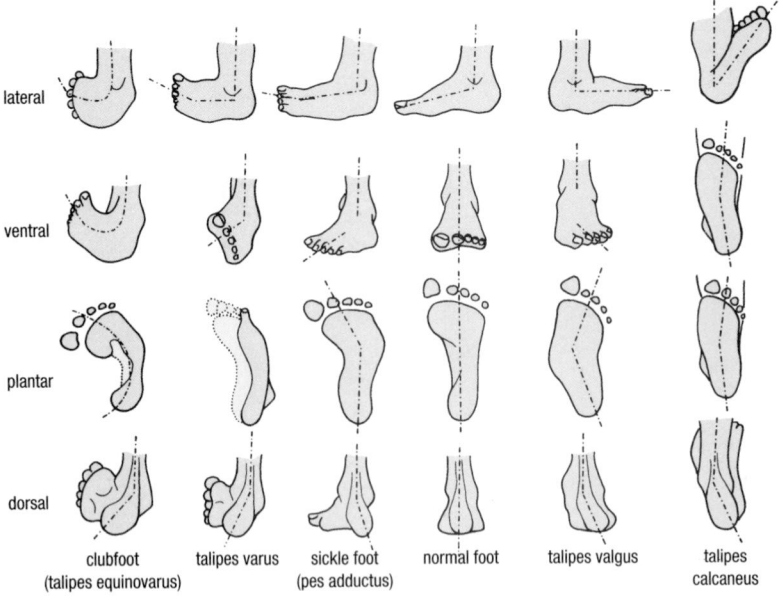

foot deformities

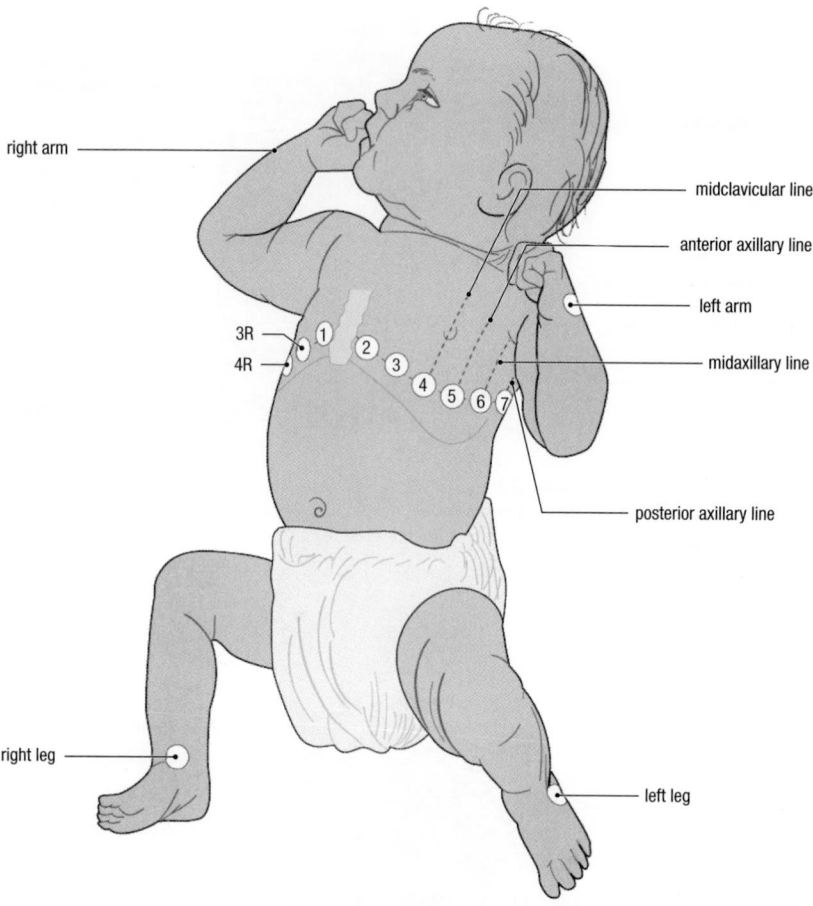

right arm

midclavicular line

anterior axillary line

left arm

midaxillary line

3R

4R

posterior axillary line

right leg

left leg

electrocardiogram (ECG) lead placement

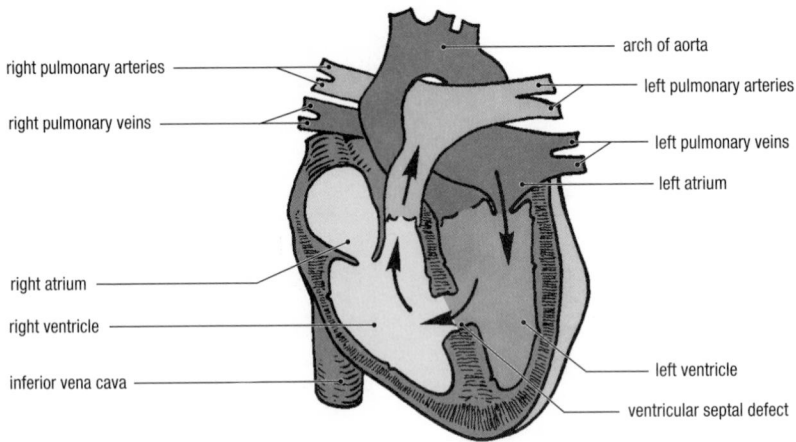

right pulmonary arteries

right pulmonary veins

right atrium

right ventricle

inferior vena cava

arch of aorta

left pulmonary arteries

left pulmonary veins

left atrium

left ventricle

ventricular septal defect

auscultation, ventricular septal defect (VSD): VSD is so large there is no pressure between the ventricles; flow is dependent on systemic and pulmonary arterial resistance; if pulmonary vascular resistance (PVR) is less than systemic (SVR), a left-to-right shunt occurs

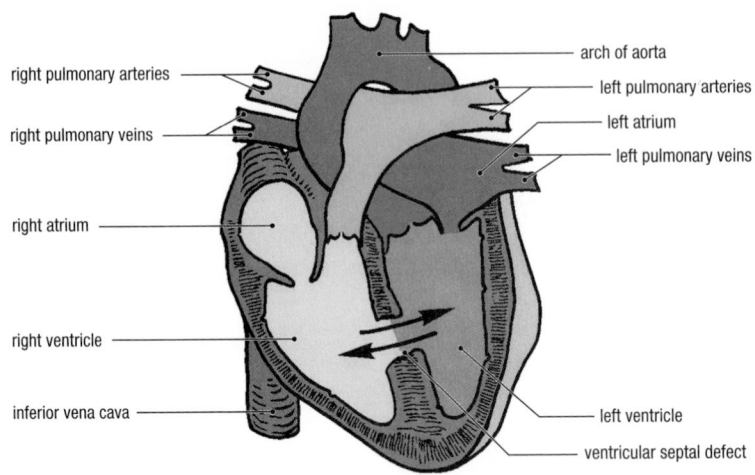

right pulmonary arteries

right pulmonary veins

right atrium

right ventricle

inferior vena cava

arch of aorta

left pulmonary arteries

left atrium

left pulmonary veins

left ventricle

ventricular septal defect

auscultation, ventricular septal defect: when pulmonary vascular resistance is equal to or greater than systemic in the presence of a large ventricular septal defect, a murmur may not be detected due to low shunt volume; a loud single second sound is heard as aortic and pulmonary closures occur

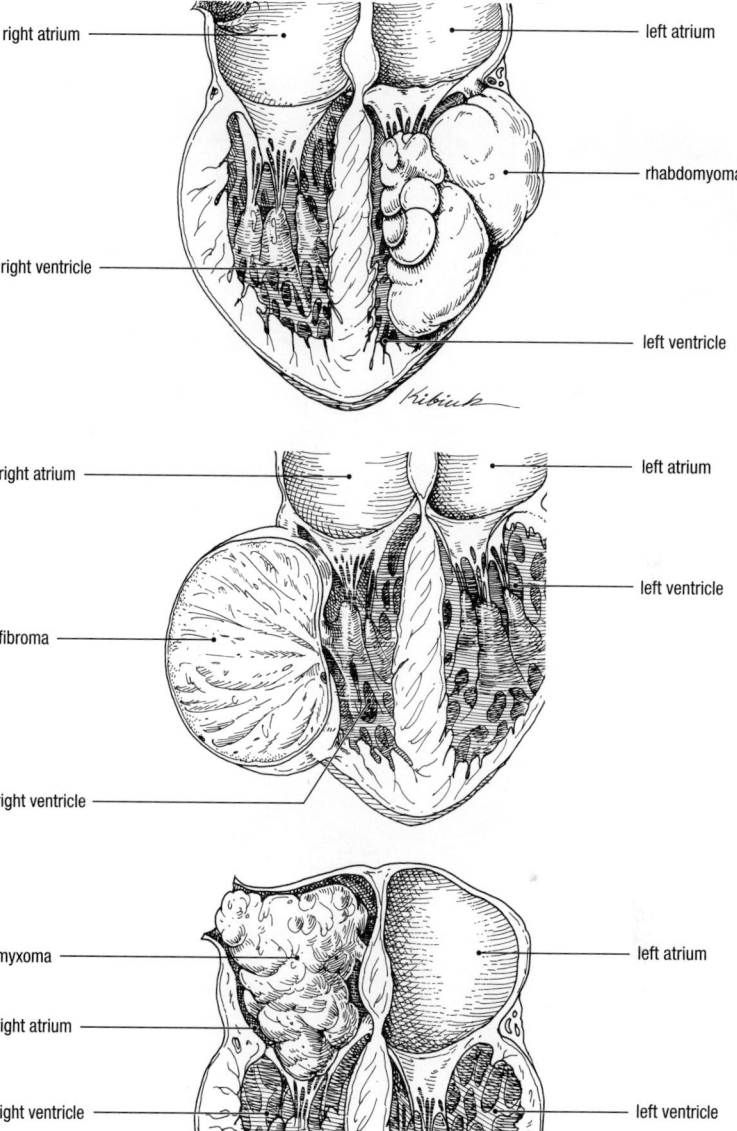

right atrium — left atrium

— rhabdomyoma

right ventricle — left ventricle

right atrium — left atrium

— left ventricle

fibroma —

right ventricle —

myxoma — left atrium

right atrium —

right ventricle — left ventricle

cardiac tumors in children: primary cardiac tumors in children appear to be associated with familial syndromes with autosomal dominant inheritance; rhabdomyoma is the most common benign tumor and is derived from striated muscle elements; it is located within the wall of the myocardium (top); the fibroma is a solitary ventricular structure derived from fibrous connective tissue; it occurs in children under 10 years of age (middle); the myxoma arises from the lining of the atrium and resembles a polyp; it is a benign tumor (bottom)

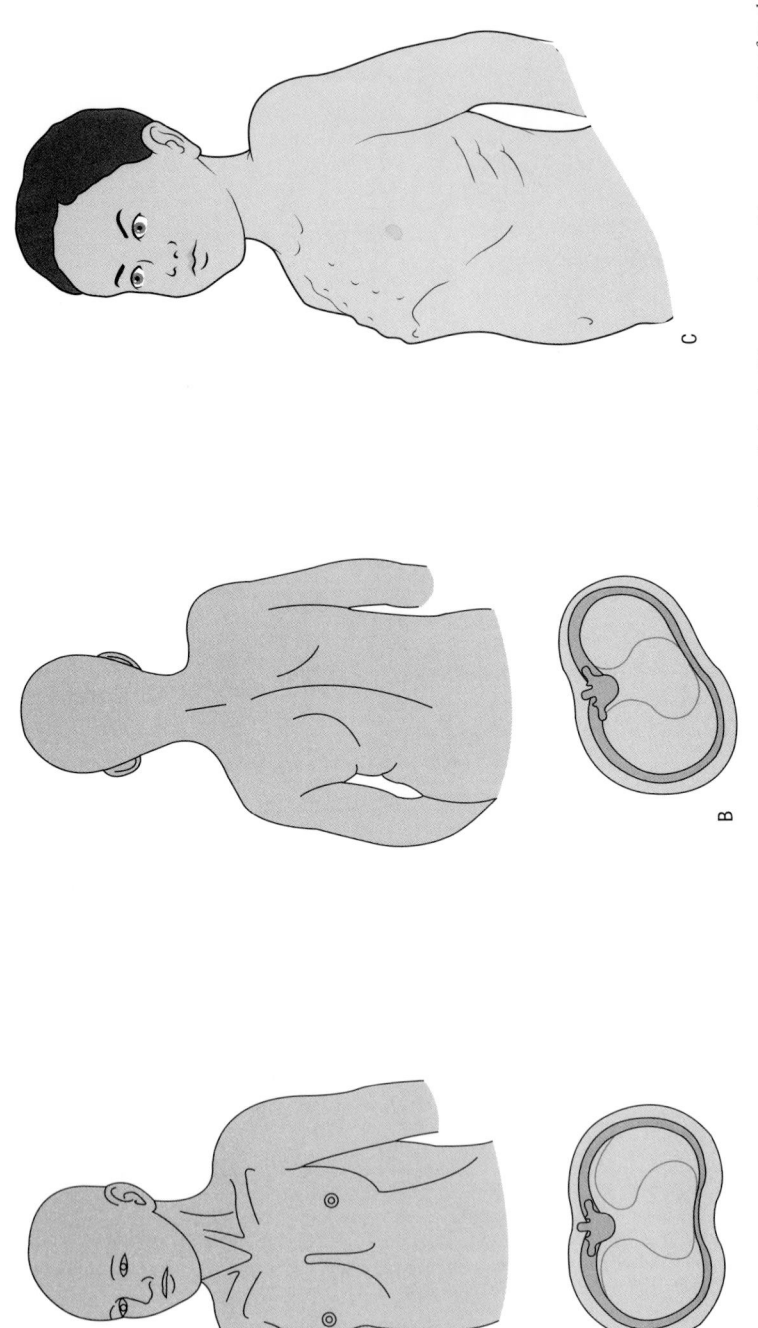

thoracic deformities: (A) anterior and transverse view of male child with pectus excavatum (funnel chest); (B) posterior and transverse view of male child with thoracic kyphoscoliosis; (C) anteroposterior view of male child with pectus carinatum (pigeon chest); note the protruding thoracic cage

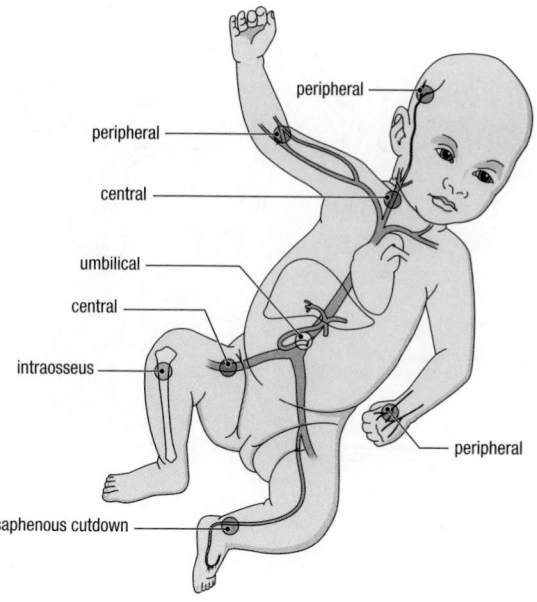

pediatric IV sites: peripheral, umbilical, central, intraosseus, and saphenous cutdown

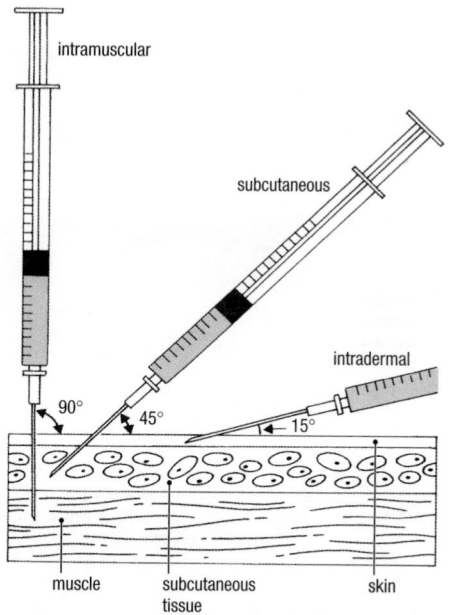

angles of insertion of injection

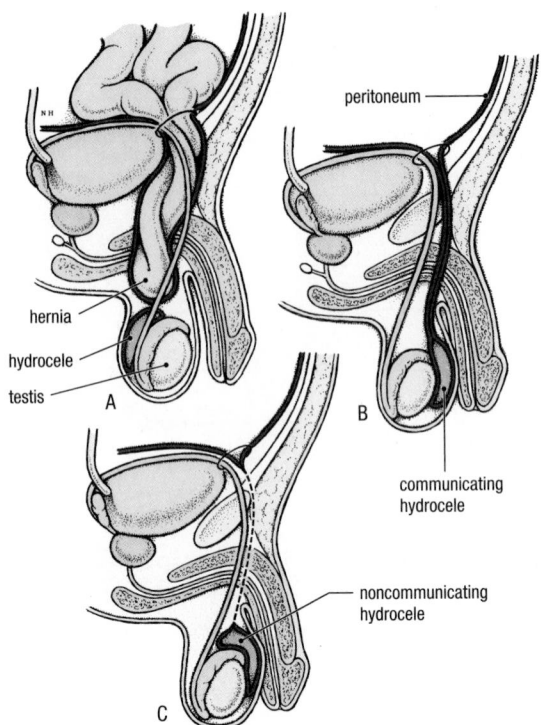

types of hydroceles (peritoneum shown in dark gray)

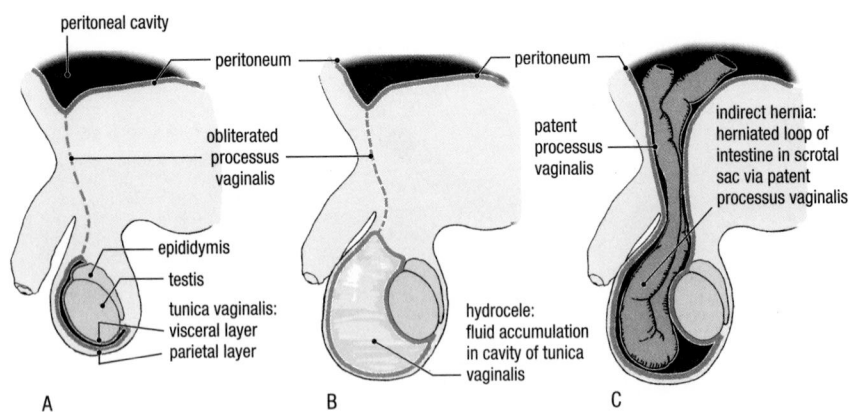

processus vaginalis and tunica vaginalis: (A) normal anatomy; (B) hydrocele; (C) indirect hernia

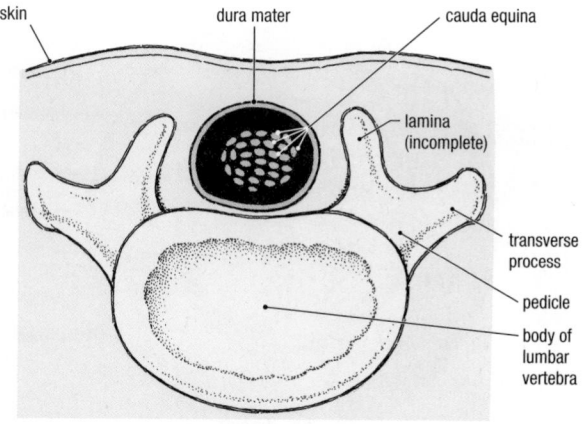

spina bifida occulta

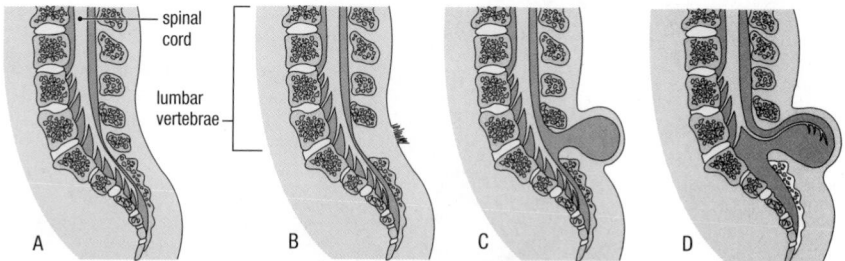

four degrees of spinal cord anomalies: (A) normal spinal cord; (B) spina bifida occulta; (C) meningocele; (D) myelomeningocele

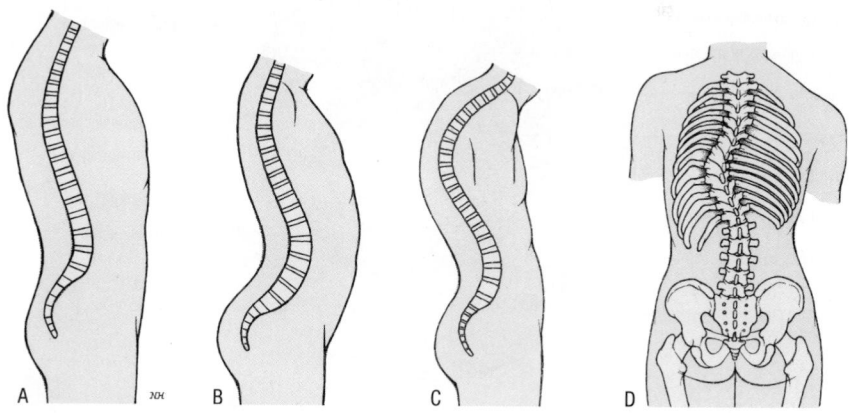

spinal curvatures: (A) normal; (B) lordosis; (C) kyphosis; (D) scoliosis

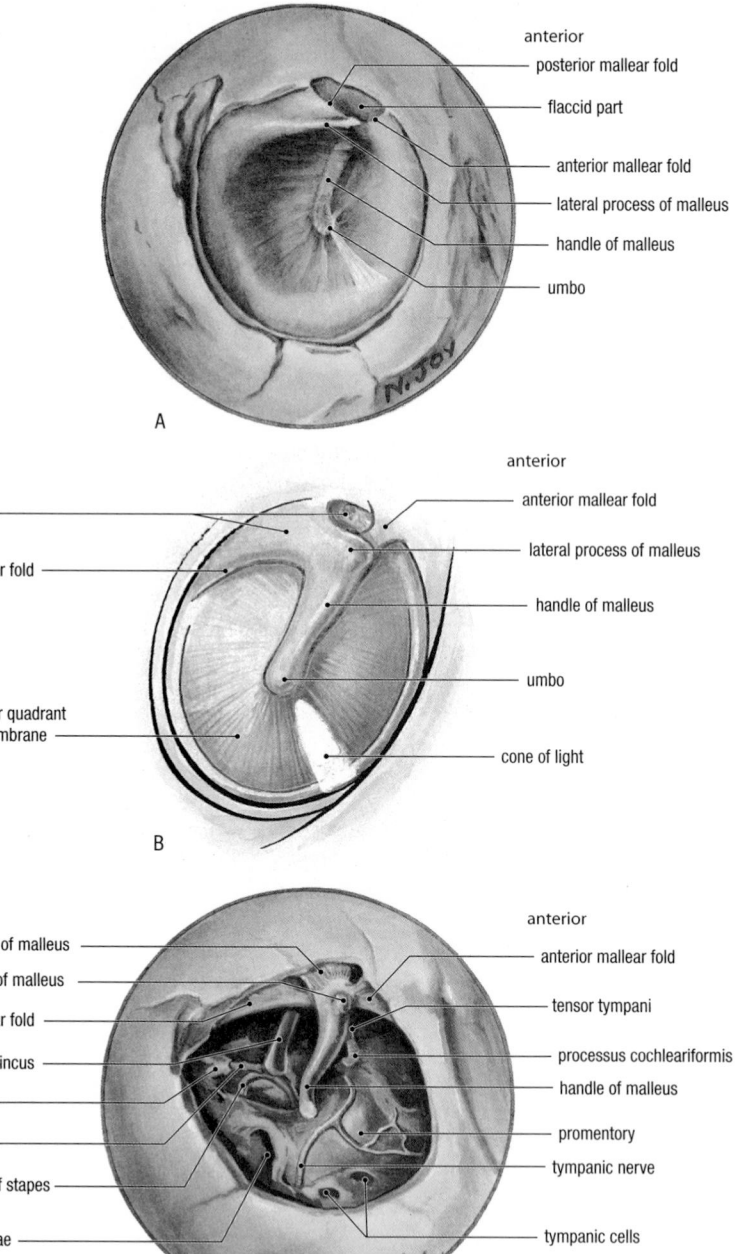

anterior

posterior mallear fold

flaccid part

anterior mallear fold

lateral process of malleus

handle of malleus

umbo

A

posterior   anterior

flaccid part   anterior mallear fold

posterior mallear fold   lateral process of malleus

handle of malleus

umbo

posterior inferior quadrant
of tympanic membrane

cone of light

B

posterior   anterior

lateral ligament of malleus   anterior mallear fold

lateral process of malleus   tensor tympani

posterior mallear fold   processus cochleariformis

long process of incus   handle of malleus

pyramid   promentory

stapedius   tympanic nerve

posterior crus of stapes   tympanic cells

fenestra cochleae
(round window)

C

tympanic membrane: (A) lateral view; (B) auriscopic view; (C) tympanic membrane removed, inferolateral view

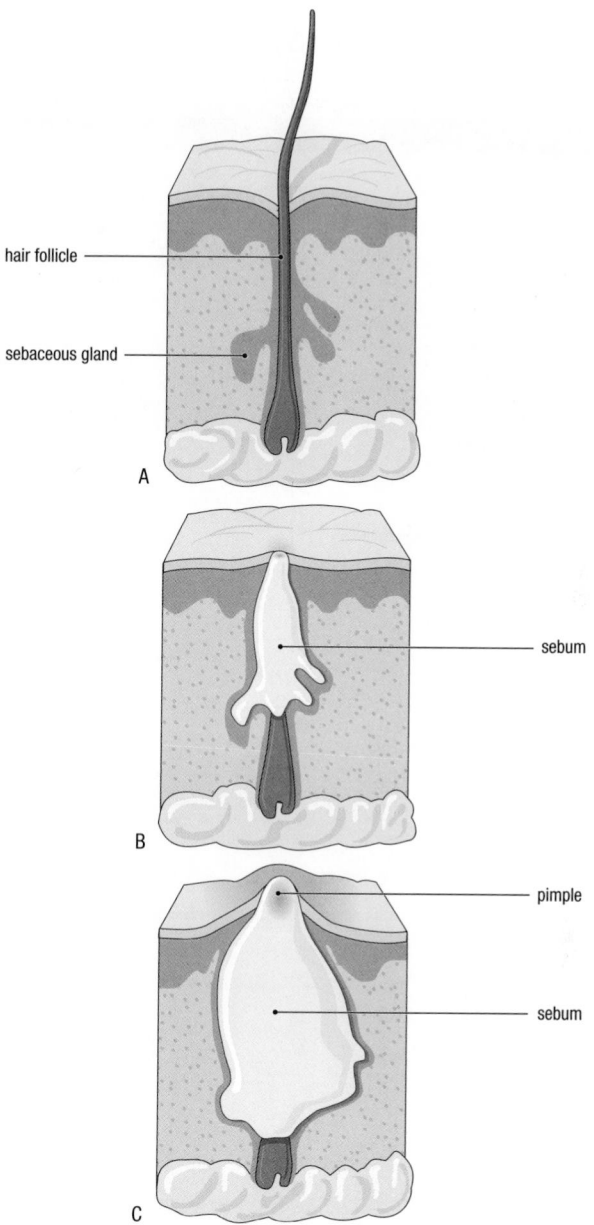

acne formation: (A) hair follicle and sebaceous gland; (B) first stage in acne development; follicle becomes blocked, sebum begins to fill follicle cavity; (C) inflamed pustule and pimple; follicle is blocked, sebum has filled and expanded follicle cavity

Appendix 2
Genetic Symbols

	Genetic Symbols			
□	male	■ ●	proband or propositus (first affected family member coming to medical attention)
○	female	⊞	examined professionally • normal for trait
◊	sex unspecified	⊞	not examined • dubiously reported to have trait
□ ○	normal individuals		
■ ● ◆	affected individual (with ≥ 2 conditions, the symbol is partitioned and shaded with a different fill defined in a key or legend)	⊞	not examined • reliably reported to have trait
5 ⑤ ◇	multiple individuals, number known (number of siblings written inside symbol)	■ ●	heterozygotes for autosomal recessive
		⊙	carrier of sex-linked recessive
n ⓝ ◇	multiple individuals, number unknown ("n" used in place of specific number)	⊘ ∅	death
□–○	mating	⊘ ∅ ⊘	stillbirth (SB)
□–○	consaguinity		
(+)	uncommon or uncertain mode of inheritance	▨ ℗ ◇	pregnancy (P); gestational age and karotype (if known) below symbol
□–○ / ○–□	parents and offspring, in generations		
△–○	dizygotic twins	□ ○	consultand (individual seeking genetic counseling/testing)
△–○	monozygotic twins	△ △ △	spontaneous abortion; ECT written below symbol indicates ectopic pregnancy
4 ③	number of children of sex indicated		
□○	adopted individuals	▲ ▲ ▲	affected spontaneous abortion (gestational age, if known, below symbol, and key or legend used to define shading)
⚦ ⚦	individual died without leaving offspring		
□–○	no issue	◬ ◬ ◬	termination of pregnancy (TOP)
■ ●	affected individuals	▲ ▲ ▲	affected TOP (key or legend used to define shading)

Source: Genetic symbols are public domain: we credit and gratefully acknowledge the *American Journal of Human Genetics* (56:746–747, 1995) as our source for these symbols.

Tests	Conventional Units	SI Units
acetone		
serum		
qualitative	negative	negative
quantitative	0.3–2.0 mg/dL	0.05–0.34 mmol/L
*alanine aminotransferase (ALT, SGPT), serum		
males	13–40 U/L (37°C)	0.22–0.68 µkat/L (37°C)
females	10–28 U/L (37°C)	0.17–0.48 µkat/L (37°C)
albumin		
serum		
adult	3.5–5.2 g/dL	35–52 g/L
urine		
qualitative	negative	negative
quantitative	50–80 mg/24 h.	50–80 mg/24 h.
CSF	10–30 mg/dL	100–300 mg/dL
alpha-1-antitrypsin, serum	78–200 mg/dL	0.78–200 g/L
alpha-fetoprotein (AFP), serum	<15 ng/mL	<15 µg/L
ammonia plasma (Hep)	9–33 µmol/L	9–33 µmol/L
*amylase serum	27–131 U/L	0.46–2.23 µkat/L
bilirubin		
serum		
adult		
conjugated	0.0–0.3 mg/dL	0–5 µmol/L
unconjugated	0.1–1.1 mg/dL	1.7–1.9 µmol/L
delta	0–0.2 mg/dL	0–3 µmol/L
total	0.2–1.3 mg/L	3–22 µmol/L
*bilirubin serum		
neonates		
conjugated	0–0.6 mg/dL	0–10 µmol/L
unconjugated	0.6–10.5 mg/dL	10–180 µmol/L
total	1.5–12 mg/dL	1.7–180 µmol/L

(continued)

Tests	Conventional Units	SI Units
CA 125, serum	<35 U/mL	<35 kU/L
CA 19-9, serum	<37 U/mL	<37 kU/L
calcium, serum	8.6–10.0 mg/dL (slightly higher in children)	2.15–2.50 mmol/L (slightly higher in children)
carbon dioxide ($P\mathrm{CO}_2$), blood arterial	males 35–48 mmHg females 32–45 mmHg	4.66–6.38 kPa 4.26–5.99 kPa
carotene, serum	10–85 μg/dL	0.19–1.58 μmol/L
catecholamines, urine		
dopamine	65–400 μg/24 h.	425–2610 nmol/24 h.
epinephrine	0–20 μg/24 h.	0–109 nmol/24 h.
norepinephrine	15–80 μg/24 h.	89–473 nmol/24 h.
CEA, serum, smokers	<5.0 ng/mL	<5.0 μg/L
*cell counts, adult		
RBC males	$4.7–6.1 \times 10^{6}/\mu L$	$4.7–6.1 \times 10^{12}/L$
females	$4.2–5.4 \times 10^{6}/\mu L$	$4.2–5.4 \times 10^{12}/L$
leukocytes		
total	$4.8–10.8 \times 10^{3}/\mu L$	$4.8–10.8 \times 10^{6}/L$
platelets	$130–400 \times 10^{3}/\mu L$	$1340–400 \times 10^{9}/L$
reticulocytes	0.5–1.5% red cells	0.005–0.015 of RBC
cells, CSF	0–10 lymphocytes/mm^3 0 RBC/mm^3	0–10 lymphocytes/mm^3 0 RBC/mm^3
chloride		
serum or plasma	98–107 mmol/L	98–107 mmol/L
cholesterol, serum		
adult desirable	<200 mg/dL	<5.2 mmol/L
borderline	200–239 mg/dL	5.2–6.2 mmol/L
high risk	≥240 mg/dL	≥6.2 mmol/L
cholinesterase, serum	4.9–11.9 U/mL	4.9–11.9 kU/L
coagulation tests		
antithrombin III		
(synthetic substrate)	80–120% of normal	0.8–1.2 of normal
bleeding time (Duke)	0–6 min	0–6 min
bleeding time (Ivy)	1–6 min	1–6 min
bleeding time (template)	2.3–9.5 min	2.3–9.5 min
clot retraction, qualitative	50–100% in 2 h.	0.5–1.0/2 h.

Tests	Conventional Units	SI Units
complement components		
total hemolytic complement activity, plasma	75–160 U/mL	75–160 kU/L
total complement decay rate (functional), plasma	10–20% deficiency: >50%	fraction decay rate: 0.10–0.20 >0.50
C1q, serum	14.9–22.1 mg/dL	149–221 mg/L
C1r, serum	2.5–10.0 mg/dL	25–100 mg/L
C1s (C1 esterase), serum	5.0–10.0 mg/dL	50–100 mg/L
C2, serum	1.6–3.6 mg/dL	16–36 mg/L
C3, serum	90–180 mg/dL	0.9–1.8 g/L
C4, serum	10–40 mg/dL	0.1–0.4 mg/L
C5, serum	5.5–11.3 mg/dL	55–113 mg/L
C6, serum	17.9–23.9 mg/dL	179–239 mg/L
C7, serum	2.7–7.4 mg/dL	27–74 mg/L
C8, serum	4.9–10.6 mg/dL	49–106 mg/L
C9, serum	3.3–9.5 mg/dL	33–95 mg/L
Coombs test		
direct	negative	negative
indirect	negative	negative
copper		
serum		
males	70–140 μg/dL	11–22 μmol/L
females	80–155 μg/dL	13–24 μmol/L
cortisol, serum		
plasma (Hep, EDTA, Ox)		
8 a.m.	5–23 μg/dL	138–635 nmol/L
4 p.m.	3–16 μg/dL	83–441 nmol/L
C-reactive protein, serum	<0.5 mg/dL	<5 mg/L
creatine kinase (CK)		
serum		
males	15–105 U/L (30°C)	0.26–1.79 μkat/L (30°C)
females	10–80 U/L (30°C)	0.17–1.36 μkat/L (30°C)
*creatinine		
serum or plasma, adult		
males	0.7–1.3 mg/dL	62–115 μmol/L
females	0.6–1.1 mg/dL	53–97 μmol/L
cryoglobulins, serum	0	0
dehydroepiandrosterone (DHEA), serum		
males	180–1250 ng/dL	6.2–43.3 nmol/L
females	130–980 ng/dL	4.5–34.0 nmol/L

(continued)

Tests	Conventional Units	SI Units
dehydroepiandrosterone sulfate (DHEAS), serum or plasma		
males	59–452 μg/mL	1.6–12.2 μmol/L
females		
premenopausal	12–379 μg/mL	0.8–10.2 μmol/L
postmenopausal	30–260 μg/mL	0.8–7.1 μmol/L
delta aminolevulinic acid, urine	1.3–7.0 mg/24 h.	10–53 μmol/24 h.
estradiol, serum		
adult males	10–50 pg/mL	37–184 pmol/L
adult females	varies with menstrual cycle	
ferritin, serum		
males	20–150 ng/mL	20–250 μg/L
females	10–120 ng/mL	10–120 μg/L
*fibrinogen, plasma (NaCit)	200–400 mg/dL	2–4 g/L
follicle-stimulating hormone (FSH), serum and plasma		
males	1.4–15.4 mIU/mL	1.4–15.4 IU/L
females		
follicular phase	1–10 mIU/mL	1–10 IU/L
mid cycle	6–17 mIU/mL	6–17 IU/L
luteal phase	1–9 mIU/mL	1–9 IU/L
postmenopausal	19–100 mIU/mL	19–100 IU/L
glucose (fasting)		
blood	65–95 mg/dL	3.5–5.3 mmol/L
plasma or serum	74–106 mg/dL	4.1–5.9 mmol/L
glucose, urine		
quantitative	<500 mg/24 h.	<2.8 mmol/24 h.
qualitative	negative	negative
glucose, CSF	40–70 mg/dL	2.2–3.9 mmol/L
glucose-6-phosphate dehydrogenase (G6PD) in erythrocytes, whole blood (ACD, EDTA, or Hep)	12.1 ± 2.1 U/g Hb (SD)	0.78 ± 0.13 mU/mol Hb
	351 ± 60.6 U/10^{12} RBC	0.35 ± 0.06 nU/RBC
	4.11 ± 0.71 U/mL RBC	4.11 ± 0.71 kU/L RBC

Tests	Conventional Units	SI Units
γ-glutamyltransferase (GGT), serum		
males	2–30 U/L (37°C)	0.03–0.51 μkat/L (37°C)
females	1–24 U/L (37°C)	0.02–0.41 μkat/L (37°C)
haptoglobin, serum	30–200 mg/dL	0.3–2.0 g/L
hematocrit		
males	42–52%	0.42–0.52
females	37–47%	0.37–0.47
newborns	53–65%	0.53–0.65
children (varies with age)	30–43%	0.30–0.43
hemoglobin (Hb)		
males	14.0–18.0 g/dL	2.17–2.79 mmol/L
females	12.0–16.0 g/dL	1.86–2.48 mmol/L
newborn	17.0–23.0 g/dL	2.64–3.57 mmol/L
children (varies with age)	11.2–16.5 g/dL	1.74–2.56 mmol/L
hemoglobin, fetal	≥1 y old: <2% of total Hb	≥1 y old: <0.02% of total Hb
hemoglobin electrophoresis whole blood (EDTA, Cit, or Hep) HbA	>95%	>0.95 Hb fraction
HbA$_2$	1.5–3.7%	0.015–0.37 Hb fraction
HbF	<2%	<0.02 Hb fraction
human chorionic gonadotropin (hCG), intact serum or plasma		
males/nonpregnant females	<5.0 mIU/mL	<5.0 IU/L
pregnant females	varies with gestational age	
urine, qualitative		
males/nonpregnant females	negative	negative
pregnant females	positive	positive

quantitative hCG values to determine estimated gestational age

interval from last menstrual period	amount of hCG in mIU/ml
3 weeks	5–50
4 weeks	3–426
5 weeks	19–7,340
6 weeks	1,080–56,500
7–8 weeks	7,650–229,000
9–12 weeks	25,700–288,000
13–16 weeks	13,300–254,000
17–24 weeks	4,060–165,400
25–40 weeks	3,640–117,000

(continued)

Normal Lab Values

A57

Tests	Conventional Units	SI Units
immunoglobulins, serum		
IgG	700–1600 mg/dl	7–16 g/L
IgA	70–400 mg/dl	0.7–4.0 g/L
IgM	40–230 mg/dl	0.42.3 g/L
IgD	0–8 mg/dl	0–80 mg/L
IgE	3–423 mg/dl	3–423 kIU/L
immunoglobulin G (IgG), CSF	0.5–6.1 mg/dL	0.5–6.1 g/L
*iron, serum		
males	65–175 μg/dL	11.6–31.3 μmol/L
females	50–170 μg/dL	9.0–30.4 μmol/L
iron binding capacity, serum, total (TIBC)	250–425 μg/dL	44.8–71.6 μmol/L
*lactate dehydrogenase (LDH)		
newborn	290–775 U/L	4.9–13.2 μkat/L
neonate	545–2000 U/L	9.3–34 μkat/L
infant	180–430 U/L	3.1–7.3 μkat/L
child	110–295 U/L	1.9–5 μkat/L
adult	100–190 U/L	1.7–3.2 μkat/L
>60 y	110–210 U/L	1.9–3.6 μkat/L
lead, whole blood (Hep)	<25 μg/dL	<1.2 μmol/L
lecithin-sphingomyelin (L/S) ratio, amniotic fluid	2.0–5.0 indicates probable fetal lung maturity; <3.5 in diabetics	same
luteinizing hormone (LH), serum or plasma		
males	1.24–7.8 mIU/mL	1.24–7.8 IU/L
females		
follicular phase	1.68–15.0 mIU/mL	1.68–15.0 IU/L
mid-cycle peak	21.9–56.6 mIU/mL	21.9–56.6 IU/L
luteal phase	0.61–16.3 mIU/mL	0.61–16.3 IU/L
postmenopausal	14.2–52.5 mIU/mL	14.2–52.5 IU/L
*lipase, serum	23–300 U/L (37°C)	0.39–5.1 μkat/L (37°C)
magnesium		
serum	1.3–2.1 mEq/L	0.65–1.07 mmol/L
	1.6–2.6 mg/dL	16–26 mg/L
mean corpuscular hemoglobin (MCH)	27–31 pg	0.42–0.48 fmol

Tests	Conventional Units	SI Units
mean corpuscular hemoglobin concentration (MCHC)	33–37 g/dL	330–370 g/L
mean corpuscular volume (MCV)		
males	80–94 μ^3	80–94 fL
females	81–99 μ^3	81–99 fL
metanephrine, total, urine	0.1–1.6 mg/24 h.	0.5–8.1 μmol/24 h.
5'-nucleotidase, serum	2–17 U/L	0.034–0.29 μkat/L
osmolality, urine	50–1200 mOsm/kg water	50–1200 mmol/kg water
oxygen, blood tension		
pO$_2$ arterial and capillary	83–108 mmHg	11.1–14.4 kPa
partial thromboplastin time activated (APTT)	<35 sec	<35 sec
pH		
blood, arterial	7.35–7.45	7.35–7.45
urine	4.6–8.0 (depends on diet)	same
partial thromboplastin time, activated (aPTT)	<35 sec	<35 sec
phosphatidylglycerol (PG), amniotic fluid		
fetal lung immaturity	absent	absent
fetal lung maturity	present	present
porphobilinogen, urine		
qualitative	negative	negative
quantitative	<2.0 mg/24 h.	<9 μmol/24 h.
porphyrins, urine		
coproporphyrin	34–230 μg/24 h.	52–351 nmol/24 h.
uroporphyrin	27–52 μg/24 h.	32–63 nmol/24 h.
potassium serum		
premature		
cord	5.0–10.2 mmol/L	5.0–10.2 mmol/L
48 h.	3.0–6.0 mmol/L	3.0–6.0 mmol/L
newborn cord	5.6–12.0 mmol/L	5.6–12.0 mmol/L
newborn	3.7–5.9 mmol/L	3.7–5.9 mmol/L
infant	4.1–5.3 mmol/L	4.1–5.3 mmol/L
child	3.4–4.7 mmol/L	3.4–4.7 mmol/L
adult	3.5–5.1 mmol/L	3.5–5.1 mmol/L

(continued)

Tests	Conventional Units	SI Units
progesterone, serum		
adult males	13–97 ng/dL	0.4–31 nmol/L
adult females		
follicular phase	15–70 ng/dL	0.5–2.2 nmol/L
luteal phase	200–2500 ng/dL	6.4–79.5 nmol/L
pregnancy	varies with gestational week	
*protein, serum		
total	6.4–8.3 g/dL	64–83 g/L
urine		
qualitative	negative	negative
quantitative	50–80 mg/24 h.	50–80 mg/24 h.
	(at rest)	(at rest)
CSF, total	8–32 mg/dL	80–320 mg/dL
*prothrombin time (PT)	12–14 sec	12–14 sec
protoporphyrin, total, WB	<60 μg/dL	<600 μg/L
sedimentation rate		
Wintrobe		
males	0–10 mm in 1 h.	0–10 mm/h
females	0–20 mm in 1 h.	0–20 mm/h
Westergren		
males	0–15 mm in 1 h.	0–15 mm/h
females	0–20 mm in 1 h.	0–20 mm/h
sodium		
serum or plasma (Hep)		
premature		
cord	116–140 mmol/L	116–140 mmol/L
48 h.	128–148 mmol/L	128–148 mmol/L
newborn, cord	126–166 mmol/L	126–166 mmol/L
newborn	133–146 mmol/L	133–146 mmol/L
infant	139–146 mmol/L	139–146 mmol/L
child	138–145 mmol/L	138–145 mmol/L
adult	136–145 mmol/L	136–145 mmol/L
specific gravity, urine	1.002–1.030	1.002–1.030
transferrin, serum		
newborn	130–275 mg/dL	1.3–2.75 g/L
adult	212–360-mg/dL	2.12–3.60 g/L
>60 y	190–375-mg/dL	1.9–3.75 g/L
triglycerides, serum, fasting		
desirable	<250 mg/dL	<2.83 mmol/L

Tests	Conventional Units	SI Units
urea nitrogen, serum	6–20 mg/dL	2.1–7.1 mmol Urea/L
*uric acid serum, enzymatic		
males	4.5–8.0 mg/dL	0.27–0.47 mmol/L
females	2.5–6.2 mg/dL	0.15–0.37 mmol/L
child	2.0–5.5 mg/dL	0.12–0.32 mmol/L
urobilinogen, urine	0.1–0.8 Ehrlich unit/2 h. 0.5–4.0 mg/24 h.	0.1–0.8 Ehrlich unit/2 h. 0.5–4.0 mg/24 h.
vanillylmandelic acid (VMA), urine (4-hydroxy- 3-methoxymandelic acid)	1.4–6.5 mg/24 h.	7–33 μmol/d
viscosity, serum	1.00–1.24 cP	1.00–1.24 cP
vitamin B_{12}, serum	110–800 pg/mL	81–590 pmol/L

*Test values are method dependent.
Abbreviations: CSF indicates cerebrospinal fluid; EDTA, ethylenediaminetetraacetic acid; Hep, heparin; Ox, oxalate; and RBC, red blood cell(s)

Appendix 4
Biophysical Profile Scoring: Technique and Interpretation

Biophysical variable	Normal (score = 2)	Abnormal (score = 0)
Fetal breathing movements	≥1 episode of ≥30 sec in 30 min. ≥ 3 discrete body-limb movements in 30 min. (episodes of active continuous movement considered)	Absent or no episode of ≥30 min. ≤2 episodes of body-limb movements in 30 min. as single movement
Fetal tone	≥1 episode of active extension with return to flexion of fetal limb(s) or trunk Opening and closing of hand considered normal tone	Either slow extension with return to partial flexion movement of limb(s) in full extension or absent fetal movement
Reactive fetal heart rate	≥2 episodes of acceleration of ≥15 bpm and of >15 sec associated with fetal movement in 20 min.	>2 episodes of acceleration fetal heart rate or acceleration of >15 bpm in 20 min.
Qualitative amniotic fluid volume	≥1 pocket of fluid measuring 2 cm in vertical axis	Either no pockets or largest pocket >2 cm in vertical axis
Nonstress test	Reactive	Nonreactive

From Reece EA, Hobbins JC, eds. Medicine of the Fetus and Mother, Second Edition. Philadelphia: Lippincott-Raven Publishers, 1999.

Sample Reports

Bilateral Myringotomy and Ventilation Tube Insertion

PREOPERATIVE DIAGNOSIS: Otitis media with effusion.

POSTOPERATIVE DIAGNOSIS: Otitis media with effusion.

SURGERY PERFORMED: Bilateral myringotomy and ventilation tube insertion.

OPERATION: This young boy was brought to the operating room, placed under general anesthetic and was then mask ventilated throughout the procedure.

The microscope was used to visualize the right tympanic membrane. An anterior-superior incision was made, and mucopurulent discharge was suctioned clear. A Donaldson tube was then placed. In like fashion on the left side, a similar anterior-superior incision was made again. Again, thin mucopurulent material was suctioned clear, and a Donaldson tube was placed.

The patient was then awoken out of general anesthetic and transported to the recovery room in stable condition.

Cesarean Section, Primary Lower Segment With Bilateral Filshie Clip Tubal Sterilization

PREOPERATIVE DIAGNOSIS: Cephalopelvic disproportion.

POSTOPERATIVE DIAGNOSIS: Cephalopelvic disproportion.

PROCEDURE: Primary lower segment cesarean section, bilateral Filshie clip tubal sterilization.

DETAILS: This patient was admitted to the operating suite for a primary lower segment cesarean section because of cephalopelvic disproportion. She was gravida 3, para 2 and had 2 prior vaginal births. She had been fully dilated for almost 3 hours, and there was no evidence of progress. Baby was suspected to be likely in the occiput posterior position. The exact position of the baby's head could not be determined with certainty because of molding. The posterior pelvis was still empty.

After induction of regional anesthesia, through a Pfannenstiel incision the peritoneal cavity was entered. The uterovesical serosa was divided. The bladder was pushed downward, and through a transverse incision the uterus was opened. A healthy and robust male infant was delivered by elevation of the head and fundal pressure. He was then suctioned and doing well as he was passed over to the pediatric attendants. The head was severely molded, and position appeared to have been a deep transverse arrest. Cord pH was drawn. Prophylactic antibiotics and oxytocics were given.

The uterus was closed with 2 layers of 0 chromic after the placenta was removed. The patient was noted to have an extensive tear anteriorly in the cervix down into the vagina, and the apex could not be identified with certainty. Closure appeared to have been effective, anatomy reasonably restored and hemostasis achieved.

With hemostasis confirmed, the adnexa noted to be normal and blood evacuated from the cul-de-sac and paracolic gutters, bilateral Filshie clipping followed on both tubes under direct vision. Post-application check was satisfactory. The tubes were identified along their entirely.

The abdomen was closed with 2-0 Vicryl for the peritoneum, 0 Vicryl for the fascia, and subcuticular 4-0 for the skin. Blood loss was probably 1000 mL to 1200 mL. The patient tolerated the procedure well and left the operating suite in good condition. Sponge and instrument counts were correct. Urine was draining clear.

The patient is aware of the operative findings, and a planned followup visit in about 2 months' time is recommended for a pelvic exam.

DILATION AND CURETTAGE, HYSTEROSCOPY, ABLATION, CAUTERY TO CERVIX

PREOPERATIVE DIAGNOSIS: A 39-year-old female with significant menorrhagia.

POSTOPERATIVE DIAGNOSIS: A 39-year-old female with significant menorrhagia, awaiting pathology.

SURGERY PERFORMED: Dilation and curettage, hysteroscopy, ablation and cautery to cervix.

PROCEDURE: The patient was positioned in the dorsal lithotomy position under general anesthesia and washed and draped in the usual fashion. Bimanual exam showed a bulky, anteverted, mobile uterus, and no masses were detected.

HYSTEROSCOPY: The cervix was grasped with Jacob forceps. The endocervical canal measured 9 cm. The cervix dilated to size 6 Hegar. The patient was currently menstruating. Examination with a 4-mm hysteroscope was not very informative due to significant incoming endometrial bleeding.

CURETTAGE: The hysteroscope was removed. Sharp curettage produced curettings and clots which were sent to pathology.

ABLATION: After priming the balloon catheter, it was inserted into the endometrial cavity and distended with 5% dextrose. The treatment cycle lasted for 8 minutes and the intrauterine pressure maintained around 188.

CAUTERY TO CERVIX: There was a small cervical ectropion, and that was cauterized with electrofulguration.

The patient left the OR in stable condition.

DILATION OF THE CERVIX AND EVACUATION OF UTERUS

PREOPERATIVE DIAGNOSIS: Possible early incomplete miscarriage, possible ectopic pregnancy.

POSTOPERATIVE DIAGNOSIS: First trimester incomplete miscarriage.

SURGERY PERFORMED: Dilation of the cervix, evacuation of uterus.

INDICATIONS: This 31-year-old lady is G7, P4, M2, and her last menstrual period was August 23, 20XX. According to dates she is 9 weeks and 1 day pregnant. About 10 days previously, she presented with light pinkish vaginal discharge, but she denied vaginal bleeding, clotting or passing of any products. A pelvic ultrasound on October 18, 20XX, confirmed an irregular intrauterine gestational sac with a 15-mm diameter, and followup ultrasound on October 25, 20XX, only reported endometrial fluid. On both occasions, a 2-cm right adnexal cystic mass was also reported. Despite these findings, the quantitative beta-hCG value on October 25, 20XX, was still 7445 units per liter. It was a diagnostic problem whether this lady indeed had an early incomplete miscarriage or perhaps had a right-sided ectopic pregnancy although she was asymptomatic. The patient was counseled accordingly, and informed consent was obtained to proceed with a D&C. If no products of conception were obtained, the procedure would be converted into a laparoscopy with possible laparotomy.

PROCEDURE IN DETAIL: Sterile technique, semi-lithotomy position with Allen stirrups, and general anesthesia were used. The patient was prepped and draped in the usual fashion. The bladder was emptied with a straight catheter. An Auvard speculum was placed in position, and the cervix was visualized. The anterior cervical lip was grasped with a single-tooth tenaculum, and the external cervical os was opened. The endocervical canal accepted a #9 Hegar dilator with ease. A sharp curette was used, and numerous products of conception as well as a small gestational sac were obtained. These findings confirmed an early miscarriage.

Proper evacuation was performed, and the uterus was emptied completely. All the obtained products were forwarded to pathology.

The total blood loss was minimal, and hemostasis was ensured. Anesthesia was reversed, and the patient was transferred to postoperative recovery in a good clinical condition.

HYSTEROSCOPY, DILATION AND CURETTAGE, BALLOON THERAPY

PREOPERATIVE DIAGNOSIS: Dysfunctional bleeding

POSTOPERATIVE DIAGNOSIS: Dysfunctional bleeding

SURGERY PERFORMED: Hysteroscopy, dilation and curettage, balloon therapy.

PROCEDURE: This patient was admitted to the operating suite for hysteroscopy, D&C and balloon therapy because of her dysfunctional bleeding.

In the lithotomy position, the patient was noted to have a high body mass index. The cervix was well supported and looked entirely normal. The uterus was anteverted and sounded to 10 cm, easily dilating to #6 Hegar. The scope was introduced. The endometrial cavity was entirely unremarkable. Vigorous curettage followed for unremarkable curettings, and endometrial balloon therapy then followed according to protocol and without incident.

The patient tolerated the procedure well. She left the operating suite in good condition. Followup instructions were given and recommendations for analgesia provided. An office visit is planned in about 3 to 6 months' time.

HYSTEROSCOPY, LAPAROSCOPY AND DILATION AND CURETTAGE

PREOPERATIVE DIAGNOSIS: Primary subfertility in a 24-year-old gravida 0, para 0.

POSTOPERATIVE DIAGNOSIS: Normal pelvic organs, bilateral patent fallopian tubes.

OPERATION PERFORMED: Hysteroscopy, laparoscopy and dilation and curettage.

PROCEDURE: The patient was positioned in the dorsal lithotomy position under general anesthesia and washed and draped in the usual fashion. Bimanual exam showed a normal anteverted and mobile uterus. No masses were detected.

HYSTEROSCOPY: The cervix was grasped with Jacob forceps and appeared healthy, and the uterocervical canal measured 8 cm. The cervix was dilated to size #6 Hegar. The endometrial cavity was distended with normal saline and examined with a 4-mm hysteroscope and appeared perfectly healthy and normal. The hysteroscope was then removed. The uterine manipulator was inserted together with a size-5 HSG catheter.

LAPAROSCOPY: A pneumoperitoneum was generated through a suprapubic stab. A 30-mm, 0-degree scope and camera were introduced through a small subumbilical incision. Examination of the abdominal tomography, bowel surface, omentum and liver showed all appeared normal. There were minor omental adhesions just below the liver margin on the right side. Examination showed that the uterus is perfectly healthy and normal, and no abnormality was seen.

RIGHT AND LEFT TUBES: Both fallopian tubes appeared healthy and normal. The left tube had a small paratubal cyst. Both fimbriae were freely mobile, and no pathology was identified.

RIGHT AND LEFT OVARIES: Both ovaries appeared rather inactive and suppressed, suggestive of PCO, and no evidence of recent or old ovulation was seen.

PELVIC PERITONEUM: Examination of the anterior and posterior cul-de-sac, right and left ovarian fossa, and uterosacral ligaments all appeared normal.

HYDROTUBATION: Transcervical injection of methylene blue dye showed free spillage of the dye from each fimbrial end without difficulty. The pneumoperitoneum was released and the instruments were withdrawn. The skin was closed with 3-0 Vicryl.

D&C: Sharp curettage produced fleshly curettings which were sent to pathology. The patient left the OR in stable condition.

HYSTEROSCOPY, REMOVAL OF INTRAUTERINE CONTRACEPTIVE DEVICE, DILATION AND CURETTAGE

PREOPERATIVE DIAGNOSIS: Lost thread of intrauterine contraceptive device.

POSTOPERATIVE DIAGNOSIS: Intrauterine contraceptive device retrieved.

OPERATION PERFORMED: Hysteroscopy, removal of intrauterine contraceptive device, dilation and curettage.

PROCEDURE: The patient was positioned in the dorsal lithotomy position under general anesthesia and washed and draped in the usual fashion. Bimanual exam showed a small, anteverted, anteflexed mobile uterus, and no masses were detected.

HYSTEROSCOPY: The cervix was grasped with Jacob forceps. The endocervical canal sounded to 8 cm. The cervix was dilated with some difficulty to a size 6 Hegar. The endometrial cavity was examined with a 4-mm hysteroscope and distended with normal saline, and the IUD could be visualized in the endometrial cavity.

REMOVAL OF IUD: With bandage forceps, the IUD was removed. It was a Flex-T, but no thread could be identified at all on the body of the IUD.

CURETTAGE: Sharp curettage produced healthy curettings which were sent to pathology.

The patient left the OR in stable condition.

LAPAROSCOPIC BILATERAL SALPINGECTOMY

PREOPERATIVE DIAGNOSES: Secondary infertility in a 33-year-old gravida 1, para 1, bilateral hydrosalpinges.

POSTOPERATIVE DIAGNOSES: Secondary infertility in a 33-year-old gravida 1, para 1, bilateral hydrosalpinges.

OPERATION PERFORMED: Laparoscopic bilateral salpingectomy.

PROCEDURE: The patient was positioned in the dorsal lithotomy position under general anesthesia and washed and draped in the usual fashion. Bimanual exam showed a small, anteverted, mobile uterus, and no masses were detected. The cervix was grasped with Jacob forceps and appeared healthy and parous. The uterine manipulator was inserted.

LAPAROSCOPY: Pneumoperitoneum was generated through a suprapubic stab. A 5-mm, 0-degree scope and camera were introduced through a small subumbilical incision, and two 5-mm auxiliary trocars, 1 in the suprapubic region and 1 in the right flank, were inserted. Examination showed bilateral hydrosalpinges; however, the left side was larger than the right side.

BILATERAL SALPINGECTOMY: A grasper was introduced in the right flank and bipolar forceps in the suprapubic trocar. The right fallopian tube was lifted up away from the bowel. With a series of bipolar cautery and cutting with laparoscopic scissors, the fallopian tube and the mesosalpinx were coagulated and divided, and the tube was removed. The same steps were repeated on the left side. The 5-mm suprapubic trocars were then replaced with a 10-mm trocar, and the tubes were removed through the 10-mm trocar with spoon forceps. The tubes were sent to pathology. Hemostasis was secured, and 100 mL of normal saline was left inside the pelvis. Pneumoperitoneum was released, and instruments were withdrawn. The skin was closed with 3-0 Vicryl and 0 Vicryl in the 10-mm incision.

The patient left the OR in stable condition.

LAPAROSCOPIC TUBAL LIGATION

PREOPERATIVE DIAGNOSIS: Undesired fertility.

POSTOPERATIVE DIAGNOSIS: Undesired fertility.

PROCEDURE PERFORMED: Laparoscopic tubal ligation.

PROCEDURE: This patient was brought to the OR for laparoscopic tubal ligation as per her firm request.

At the induction of satisfactory general anesthesia in semi-lithotomy position with the bladder drained, the Valtchev cannula was held on the cervix with a single-tooth tenaculum. The abdomen was then insufflated to normal pressures with a Veress needle. Through a small umbilical incision, the scope was introduced, and the pelvic contents were perused and were normal. A suprapubic puncture was made, and the Filshie clip applicator was introduced. The right tube was identified along its entirety and ligated under direct vision at the junction of the proximal and middle third. Post-application check was satisfactory.

The same followed on the opposite side. However, the postoperative check revealed that at least some of the serosa of the tube was just outside the lock mechanism. The tubal lumen was probably closed; however, a second clip was applied to be sure. Post-application check was satisfactory.

The patient tolerated the procedure well. She left the OR in good condition. Sponge and instrument counts were correct. Followup instructions were given preoperatively and recommendations for analgesia provided.

PEDIATRIC DISCHARGE SUMMARY: POSSIBLE PERICARDITIS

Thank you for asking me to assess this young man. He presented with chest pain, which he developed the evening of admission while he was playing on the computer. At that time he also had shivers and fever. He had a runny nose for a few days, but no cough. The pain was a heavy precordial pain, was better when he was standing up or sitting, but he could not lie down. He cried with pain. This pain radiated up to his throat. He had no vomiting; however, he had diarrhea the previous week. There were no visits out of state.

FAMILY HISTORY: His mother was recovering from pneumonia. She was treated with Biaxin. He had a 17-year-old sister who was healthy. There was no heart disease in the family.

PAST MEDICAL HISTORY: Overall very healthy. He had croup at age 6–8 years. He had a refraction problem of the eyes since 18 months. His immunizations were up to date. Developmentally there were no concerns. He was in grade 8 and was an honor student.

PREGNANCY AND BIRTH: No concerns.

PHYSICAL EXAMINATION: On examination he was pleasant. He said the pain was still present (after a Toradol injection). The pain was much better when he was sitting up. He rated the pain as about 2/10 after the injection. Heart rate 80 per minute. BP 105/70. His peripheral pulses were palpable, and there was no pulsus paradoxus on palpation nor when taking the blood pressure. There was no jugular vein distention. Abdomen was normal with no organomegaly. Chest, trachea central, apex beat fifth intercostal space, mid clavicular line normal. S1 and S2 normal, no murmurs, and there was no friction rub. The lungs were normal to auscultation. Ear, nose and throat normal. Neurologically normal.

Chest x-ray showed normal cardiac size and normal vascularity. EKG revealed ST elevations of at least 1 mm in standard leads I, II and aVL and at least 2 mm in V3 to V5; otherwise normal. His CK was normal.

IMPRESSION: The character of the pain was consistent with a pericarditis. The ST elevations may be normal in an adolescent, but the elevation in particularly a VL could be due to pericarditis (I consulted the pediatric cardiologist at the Children's Hospital, and this was his opinion of the EKG).

COURSE IN THE WARD: He was admitted to the pediatric ward. He was started on Zithromax. He received ibuprofen for pain and temperature. He had swinging temperatures of above 102 degrees for the first few days, but his clinical examination remained otherwise normal. He had an echocardiogram on October 31, 20XX, which showed slight tricuspid insufficiency. There was no pericardial effusion.

He felt much better on October 31, 20XX, and was discharged. Interestingly enough the ST elevations almost disappeared on a repeat EKG, which fits in with a normal progress of pericarditis.

MOST RESPONSIBLE DIAGNOSIS: Possible pericarditis.

RECOMMENDATIONS: Follow up after 1 week. No strenuous activities should be undertaken.

REMOVAL OF BILATERAL VENTILATION TUBES

PREOPERATIVE DIAGNOSIS: Otitis media with previously placed ventilation tubes.

POSTOPERATIVE DIAGNOSIS: Otitis media with previously placed ventilation tubes.

SURGERY PERFORMED: Removal of bilateral ventilation tubes.

OPERATION: The patient was brought to the operating room, placed under general anesthetic and was then mask ventilated. The microscope was used to visualize the right tympanic membrane. There was a previously placed Reuter bobbin tube stuck in the tympanic membrane in the anterior-superior quadrant. This was rotated, however, was tightly grown into the tympanic membrane. A myringotomy incision was then made over the medial flange of the tube, allowing it to be removed. There was no perforation of the tympanic membrane, as the mucosal side had completely healed over. A small bit of granulation tissue was then scraped away from the edges of the tympanic membrane.

In like fashion on the left side, similarly the tympanic membrane was evaluated. Again an incision was made through the epithelium of the tympanic membrane laterally, and the tube was removed. Again, no perforation was noted, as the mucosa had previously healed in.

The patient was then awoken out of general anesthetia and transported to the recovery room in stable condition.

TOTAL ABDOMINAL HYSTERECTOMY

PREOPERATIVE DIAGNOSIS: Dysmenorrhea.

POSTOPERATIVE DIAGNOSIS: Dysmenorrhea, pathology pending.

PROCEDURE PERFORMED: Total abdominal hysterectomy.

INDICATIONS FOR PROCEDURE: The patient was brought to the operating room for a total abdominal hysterectomy because of her dysmenorrhea.

PROCEDURE IN DETAIL: The patient was placed in the supine position, anesthesia administered, and the vagina was prepped and bladder drained. The peritoneal cavity was entered using part of an old suprapubic midline scar, the scar being excised. The uterus was enlarged at about 8-week size. It was symmetric. There was a large simple cyst on the left ovary. There was some evidence of endometriosis with the appearance of small lesions on the bladder wall anteriorly and a few in the posterior aspect of the cul-de-sac at the junction of the uterosacral ligaments. Signs of tubal interruption were evident, and 1 Filshie clip was identified hanging on a piece of serosa.

The right round ligament was divided and suture ligated. The para-fundal pedicle was formed and doubly suture ligated. The same followed on the left side. The uterovesical serosa was divided, the bladder was pushed downward, and the uterine artery pedicles were formed and suture ligated doubly with the bladder well down in the vagina. The cardinal ligament pedicles were formed, 1 on the right and 2 on the left.

The cervix was then circumcised from the vault using an open-vault technique. Separate angle sutures of intervening figure-of-eight then followed for closure and hemostasis.

With hemostasis confirmed, the cyst on the left side was excised from the ovary. It appeared to be benign, and the ovary was otherwise left in situ.

The abdomen was closed with 2-0 Vicryl for the peritoneum, 0 Vicryl for the fascia and subcutaneous and subcuticular 4-0 for the skin. Blood loss was probably in the range of 200 mL.

The patient tolerated the procedure well. She left the operating suite in good condition. Sponge and instrument counts were correct and urine draining clear.

TOTAL ABDOMINAL HYSTERECTOMY - 2

PREOPERATIVE DIAGNOSIS: Fibroids

POSTOPERATIVE DIAGNOSIS: Awaiting pathology.

SURGICAL PROCEDURE: Total abdominal hysterectomy.

PROCEDURE: This patient was admitted to the operating room for a total abdominal hysterectomy because of fibroids and perimenopausal or postmenopausal bleeding.

At the induction of satisfactory general anesthesia, examination revealed about a 40-week-sized uterus. The bladder was drained. The uterus appeared to be mobile enough on clinical exam and the patient was of the size that it was estimated this could be reasonably removed using a generous Pfannenstiel incision rather than a midline.

The peritoneal cavity was entered. The uterus was asymmetrically enlarged consistent with multiple fibroids. The adnexa appeared to be normal. The right round ligament was divided and suture ligated with #1 delayed absorbable, which was used throughout the procedure. The para-fundal pedicle was then formed and suture ligated doubly. The same followed on the opposite side. The uterovesical serosa was divided, the bladder was pushed downward, and the uterine artery pedicles were formed and doubly suture ligated. With the bladder well down in the vagina, the cardinal ligament pedicles were formed to the other side, and the cervix was then circumcised from the vault with good visualization. Separate angle sutures followed with intervening figure-of-eight for closure and hemostasis.

The pedicles were all checked and were dry. There was no evidence of bleeding, and the abdomen was then closed with 2-0 Vicryl for the peritoneum, 0 Vicryl for the fascia, and subcuticular 4-0 for the skin. Blood loss was probably 200 to 400 mL.

The patient tolerated the procedure well and left the operating room in good condition. Sponge and instrument counts were correct, and urine was draining clear.

Common Terms by Procedure

BILATERAL MYRINGOTOMY AND VENTILATION TUBE INSERTION

anterior-superior incision
Donaldson tube
effusion
general anesthetic
mask ventilated
microscope
mucopurulent discharge
myringotomy
otitis media
tympanic membrane
ventilation tube

CESAREAN SECTION, PRIMARY LOWER SEGMENT WITH BILATERAL FILSHIE CLIP TUBAL STERILIZATION

0 chromic
0 Vicryl
2-0 Vicryl
abdomen
adnexa
antibiotic
apex
bladder
cephalopelvic disproportion
cervix
cesarean section
cul-de-sac
fascia
Filshie clip tubal sterilization
Filshie clipping
gravida
hemostasis
occiput posterior position

oxytocic
para
paracolic gutter
pelvic exam
pelvis
peritoneal cavity
peritoneum
Pfannenstiel incision
pH
placenta
regional anesthesia
subcuticular 4-0
transverse arrest
transverse incision
uterovesical serosa
uterus
vagina

DILATION AND CURETTAGE, HYSTEROSCOPY, ABLATION, CAUTERY TO CERVIX

5% dextrose
ablation
anteverted
balloon catheter
bimanual exam
cautery
cervical ectropion
cervix
clot
curettage
dilation and curettage
dorsal lithotomy position
electrofulguration
endocervical canal
endometrial cavity
general anesthesia

Hegar
hysteroscopy
intrauterine pressure
Jacob forceps
menorrhagia
pathology

DILATION OF THE CERVIX AND EVACUATION OF UTERUS

adnexal cystic mass
Allen stirrups
Auvard speculum
beta-hCG
bladder
blood loss
cervical lip
cervical os
cervix
curette
D&C (dilation and curettage)
ectopic pregnancy
endocervical canal
endometrial fluid
evacuation
evacuation of uterus
general anesthesia
gestational sac
Hegar dilator
hemostasis
intrauterine gestational sac
laparoscopy
laparotomy
menstrual period
miscarriage
pathology
pelvic ultrasound
pregnant
semi-lithotomy position
single-tooth tenaculum
sterile technique
straight catheter
uterus

vaginal bleeding
vaginal discharge

HYSTEROSCOPY, DILATION AND CURETTAGE, BALLOON THERAPY

anteverted
balloon therapy
body mass index
cervix
curettage
D&C (dilation and curettage)
dysfunctional bleeding
endometrial balloon therapy
endometrial cavity
Hegar
hysteroscopy
lithotomy position
scope
uterus

HYSTEROSCOPY, LAPAROSCOPY AND DILATION AND CURETTAGE

3-0 Vicryl
anteverted
bimanual exam
bowel surface
camera
cervix
cul-de-sac
curettage
D&C (dilation and curettage)
dorsal lithotomy position
endometrial cavity
fallopian tube
fimbria
free spillage
general anesthesia
gravida
Hegar
HSG catheter

hydrotubation
hysteroscope
hysteroscopy
Jacob forceps
laparoscopy
liver
methylene blue dye
normal saline
omental adhesion
omentum
ovarian fossa
ovary
ovulation
para
paratubal cyst
pathology
PCO (polycystic ovary)
peritoneum
pneumoperitoneum
scope
subfertility
subumbilical incision
suprapubic stab
tomography
transcervical injection
uterine manipulator
uterocervical canal
uterosacral ligament
uterus

HYSTEROSCOPY, REMOVAL OF INTRAUTERINE CONTRACEPTIVE DEVICE, DILATION AND CURETTAGE

anteverted and anteflexed
bandage forceps
bimanual exam
cervix
curettage
dilation
dorsal lithotomy position

endocervical canal
endometrial cavity
Flex-T
general anesthesia
Hegar
hysteroscopy
intrauterine contraceptive
    device
IUD (intrauterine device)
Jacob forceps
normal saline
pathology
uterus

LAPAROSCOPIC BILATERAL SALPINGECTOMY

0 Vicryl
3-0 Vicryl
anteverted
auxiliary trocar
bimanual exam
bipolar cautery and cutting
bipolar forceps
bowel
camera
cervix
dorsal lithotomy position
fallopian tube
flank
general anesthesia
grasper
gravida
hemostasis
hydrosalpinges
infertility
Jacob forceps
laparoscopic bilateral salpingectomy
laparoscopic scissors
mesosalpinx
normal saline
para
parous
pathology

pelvis
pneumoperitoneum
scope
spoon forceps
subumbilical incision
suprapubic region
suprapubic stab
suprapubic trocar
uterine manipulator
uterus

LAPAROSCOPIC TUBAL LIGATION

abdomen
bladder
cervix
fertility
Filshie clip applicator
general anesthesia
laparoscopic tubal ligation
scope
semi-lithotomy position
serosa
single-tooth tenaculum
suprapubic
tubal lumen
umbilical incision
Valtchev cannula
Veress needle

PEDIATRIC DISCHARGE SUMMARY: POSSIBLE PERICARDITIS

apex beat
blood pressure
cardiac size
chest pain
CK (creatine kinase)
echocardiogram
EKG (electrocardiogram)
friction rub
ibuprofen
injection
jugular venous distention

pericardial effusion
pericarditis
peripheral pulse
precordial pain
pulsus paradoxus
ST elevation
Toradol
tricuspid insufficiency
Zithromax

REMOVAL OF BILATERAL VENTILATION TUBES

epithelium
general anesthetic
granulation tissue
mask ventilation
medial flange
microscope
mucosa
myringotomy incision
otitis media
perforation
Reuter bobbin tube
tympanic membrane
ventilation tube

TOTAL ABDOMINAL HYSTERECTOMY

0 Vicryl
2-0 Vicryl
abdomen
anesthesia
bladder
cardinal ligament
cervix
cul-de-sac
cyst
dysmenorrhea
endometriosis
fascia
figure-of-eight
Filshie clip
hemostasis
in situ

ovary
para-fundal pedicle
pathology
peritoneal cavity
peritoneum
round ligament
serosa
simple cyst
supine position
suprapubic
suture
suture ligated
total abdominal hysterectomy
uterine artery
uterosacral ligament
uterovesical serosa
uterus
vagina
vault

TOTAL ABDOMINAL HYSTERECTOMY - 2

0 Vicryl
2-0 Vicryl
abdomen

adnexa
bladder
cardinal ligament
cervix
fascia
fibroid
figure-of-eight
general anesthesia
hemostasis
para-fundal pedicle
pathology
peritoneal cavity
peritoneum
Pfannenstiel incision
postmenopausal bleeding
round ligament
suture
suture ligated
total abdominal
   hysterectomy
uterine artery
uterovesical serosa
uterus
vagina
vault

Appendix 7
Apgar Score

After 60 seconds	Score	0	1	2
heart rate	------	absent	under 100	over 100
respiratory effort	------	absent	slow, irregular	good (screams)
muscle tone	------	limp	good in limbs	active movement
reaction to nasal catheter	------	none	makes grimaces	cough or sneezing
skin color	------	pale	rosy trunk, blue extremities	rosy
Score	------		(total points: 8–10 is normal)	

Developmental Milestones From Birth to 5 Years

Age (Months)	Adaptive/Fine Motor	Language	Gross Motor	Personal-Social
1	Grasp reflex (hands fisted)	Facial response to sounds	Lifts head in prone position	Stares at face
2	Follows object with eyes past midline	Coos (vowel sounds)	Lifts head in prone position to 45°	Smiles in response to others
4	Hands open; brings objects to mouth	Laughs and squeals; turns toward voice	Sits; head steady; rolls to supine	Smiles spontaneously
6	Palmar grasp of objects	Babbles (consonant sounds)	Sits independently; stands, hands held	Reaches for toys; recognizes strangers
9	Pincer grasp	Says "mama" and "dada" nonspecifically; comprehends "no"	Pulls to stand	Feeds self; waves bye-bye
12	Helps turn pages of book	2–4 words; follows command with gesture	Stands independently; walks, 1 hand held	Points to indicate wants
15	Scribbles	4–6 words; follows command with no gesture	Walks independently	Drinks from cup, imitates activities
18	Turns pages of book	10–20 words; points to 4 body parts	Walks up steps	Feeds self with spoon
24	Solves single-piece puzzles	Combines 2–3 words; uses "I" and "you"	Jumps; kicks ball	Removes coat; verbalizes wants
30	Imitates horizontal and vertical lines	Names all body parts	Rides tricycle using pedals	Pulls up pants; washes and dries hands
36	Copies circle; draws person with 3 parts	Gives full name, age, and sex; names 2 colors	Throws ball overhand; walks up stairs (alternating feet)	Toilet trained; puts on shirt, knows front from back

(continued)

Age (Months)	Adaptive/Fine Motor	Language	Gross Motor	Personal-Social
42	Copies cross	Understands "cold," "tired," "hungry"	Stands on 1 foot for 2-3 seconds	Engages in associative play
48	Counts 4 objects; identifies some numbers and letters	Understands prepositions (under, on, behind, in front of); asks "how" and "why"	Hops on 1 foot	Dresses with little assistance; shoes on correct feet
54	Copies square; draws person with 6 parts	Understands opposites	Broad-jumps 24 inches	Bosses and criticizes; shows off
60	Prints first name; counts 10 objects	Asks meaning of words	Skips (alternating feet)	Ties shoes

Recommended Immunizations

Immunization	Recommended Age
Diphtheria, tetanus, pertussis (DTaP)	2 months 4 months 6 months 15 months to 18 months 4 years to 6 years 11 years to 12 years
Haemophilus influenzae type b (Hib)	2 months 4 months 6 months 12 months to 15 months
Hepatitis A (Hep A)	12–24 months 2 years to 6 years Additional (in selected areas)
Hepatitis B (Hep B)	Birth to 1 month 1 month to 4 months 6 months to 18 months 11 years to 15 years (in selected areas)
Human papillomavirus (HPV)	11 years to 12 years
Inactivated poliovirus (IPV)	2 months 4 months 6 months to 18 months 4 years to 6 years
Influenza	6 months to 59 months (yearly) yearly thereafter as recommended
Measles, mumps, rubella (MMR)	12 months to 15 months 4 years to 6 years
Meningococcal	2 years to 10 years (as recommended) 11 years to 12 years
Pneumococcal conjugate (PCV)	2 months 4 months 6 months 12 to 18 months 2 years to 6 years

(continued)

Immunization	Recommended Age
Rotavirus (Rota)	2 months 4 months 6 months
Td	11 years to 12 years Every 10 years throughout life
Varicella (Var)	12 months to 15 months 4 years to 6 years Additional as recommended

For additional information, please visit the Centers for Disease Control and Prevention (CDC) National Immunization Program (NIP) web site at *http://www.cdc.gov/nip/*

Appendix 10
Oral Rehydration Fluids and Infant Formulas

Commercially Available Oral Rehydration Formulas

Lytren
Pedialyte
Rehydralyte
WHO Formula

Infant Formulas

Cow's milk-based standard formulas	Soy-based standard formulas	Preterm formulas	Special formulas#
Enfamil (Mead Johnson); with/without iron	Isomil (Ross)	Similac Special Care (Ross)	Nutramigen (Mead Johnson)
Similac (Ross); with/without iron	ProSobee (Mead Johnson)	Enfamil Premature (Mead Johnson); with/without iron	Pregestimil (Mead Johnson)
PM 60/40 (Ross)[†]		Similac NeoSure (Ross)‖	Portagen (Mead Johnson)
Gerber; with/without iron (Gerber)			Alimentum (Ross)‖
Good Start (Carnation)[†]			Lactofree (Mead Johnson) Neocate (Scientific Hospital Supplies, Inc.)

[†]Formula with a low renal solute load.   ‖Available only as ready-to-feed formula.
Indications for Special Formulas:

Name	Indications
Nutramigen	Cow's milk allergy, severe or multiple food allergies, severe or persistent diarrhea, galactosemia
Pregestimil	Malabsorption, intestinal resection, severe or persistent diarrhea, food allergies
Portagen	Steatorrhea secondary to cystic fibrosis, intestinal reactions, pancreatic insufficiency, biliary atresia, lymphatic anomalies, celiac disease
Alimentum	Problems with digestion or absorption, severe or prolonged diarrhea, cystic fibrosis, steatorrhea, food allergies, intestinal resection
Lactofree	Lactose intolerance but dairy tolerance, mild protein intolerance
Neocate	Cow's milk mild allergy, soy and protein hydrolysate intolerance, multiple food protein intolerances

Oral Rehydration Fluids

A83

Appendix 11

Routine Immunization of HIV-Infected Children in the United States

Vaccine	Known Asymptomatic HIV Infection	Symptomatic HIV Infection
Diphtheria, tetanus, pertussis (DTaP) [or DTP]	Yes	Yes
Haemophilus influenzae type b (Hib)	Yes	Yes
Hepatitis B	Yes	Yes
Inactivated poliovirus (IPV)*	Yes	Yes
Influenza§	Yes	Yes
Measles, mumps, rubella (MMR)	Yes	Yes†
Pneumococcal conjugate vaccine (PCV)‡	Yes	Yes
Rotavirus	No	No
Streptococcus pneumoniae	Yes	Yes
Varicella‖	No	No

(Adapted from the American Academy of Pediatrics. In Peter G, ed. *1997 Red Book: Report of the Committee on Infectious Diseases.* 24th ed. Elk Grove Village, IL: American Academy of Pediatrics, 1997.)

*Only inactivated polio vaccine (IPV) should be used for HIV-infected children, HIV-exposed infants whose status is indeterminate, and household contacts of HIV-infected patients.

†Severely immunocompromised HIV-infected children should not receive MMR vaccine.

‡Pneumococcal vaccine should be administered at 2 years of age to all HIV-infected children. Children who are older than 2 years of age should receive pneumococcal vaccine at the time of diagnosis. Revaccination after 3 to 5 years is recommended in either circumstance.

§Influenza vaccine should be provided each fall and repeated annually for HIV-exposed infants 6 months of age and older, HIV-infected children and adolescents, and for household contacts of HIV-infected patients.

‖Varicella vaccine is not currently indicated for HIV-exposed or HIV-infected patients, but studies are in progress to determine safety and possible indication.

Routine Antepartum Tests

Antepartum testing is commonly performed at the first prenatal visit and is used to ensure a healthy fetus and mother. Test results enable the physician to deal with any existing or potential problems. Although some antepartum tests may be done in all pregnancies, more extensive testing is done when the pregnancy is considered high risk. Factors that may indicate a high-risk pregnancy include multiple fetuses, chronic maternal illness, previous or current pregnancy problems, fetal complications and gestational age beyond term. High-risk antepartum testing is done after 32 weeks of pregnancy. Adequacy of blood flow and oxygen delivery to the fetus from the placenta is a major concern. Testing may reveal the need for further testing or even immediate delivery.

24-hour urine for protein
amniocentesis
amniotic fluid index (AFI)
antibody screen
biophysical profile (BPP)
blood type
breast stimulation stress test (BSST)
complete blood count (CBC)
contraction stress test (CST)
Doppler flow study (DFS)
fetogram
hemoglobin/hematocrit measurement
hepatitis B virus screen (hepatitis B surface antigen [HBsAg])
HIV counseling/testing
maternal measurement of fetal movement
nonstress test (NST)
oxytocin challenge test (OCT)
Pap test
Rh type
rubella antibody titer measurement
ultrasound
urinalysis (UA)
urine culture/screen
urine estriols
Venereal Disease Research Laboratory test (VDRL)
version
vibroacoustic stimulation of fetus

Appendix 13
Infertility Studies and Procedures

Infertility is defined as the diminished or absent ability to produce offspring. Unprotected intercourse for a period of 1 year, or 6 months in women over the age of 30, without resultant pregnancy is most often the criteria used in the diagnosis and subsequent treatment of infertility. Multiple miscarriages also indicate infertility.

Diagnostic testing is accomplished through laboratory studies, radiographic imaging or surgical methods, and both females and males are standardly tested. Fertility problems are found in the woman approximately 30% of the time, the man approximately 30% of the time, and no cause can be found in up to 30% of cases.

DIAGNOSTIC TESTS
diagnostic laparoscopy
estrogen test
follicle-stimulating hormone (FSH) test
hysterosalpingogram (HSG)
hysterosonography
luteinizing hormone (LH) test
postcoital test
progesterone test
saline infusion sonohysterography
semen analysis test
testosterone test
transvaginal ultrasound

Fertility treatment is accomplished through assisted reproductive technology (ART), including the use of medications and surgical intervention. Fertility drugs are the primary treatment for women who are infertile due to ovulation disorders. Surgery may be useful in correcting problems found in the reproductive organs. If medications and surgical intervention fail to result in pregnancy, further ART procedures may then be implemented. Ultimately fertility treatment results in successful full-term pregnancy for approximately 2/3 of couples treated.

FERTILITY DRUGS—see Drugs by Indication
Appendix 14, INFERTILITY (FEMALE)

CORRECTIVE SURGICAL PROCEDURES
endometriosis treatment
fibroid tumor removal
ovarian cyst removal
polyp removal
scar tissue removal
unblocking of fallopian tubes

ASSISTED REPRODUCTIVE TECHNOLOGY (ART) PROCEDURES

artificial insemination (AI) – Introduction of sperm into the vagina by artificial means.

assisted hatching – Creation of a slit or hole by mechanical or chemical means in the embryo's shell to enable it to break free of its shell before it attaches and implants in the uterine lining.

in vitro fertilization (IVF) – Sperm and egg are combined in a laboratory setting. If fertilization occurs, one or more embryos is transferred to the woman's uterus. Used for various infertility situations.

donor-aided conception – Sperm or egg is obtained from a donor. Used when infertility cannot be successfully treated in the woman, man or both.

early-stage embryo transfer – In IVF embryos are transferred to the uterus during the blastocyst stage (2-cell to 8-cell stage) of embryonic development.

electroejaculation (EEJ) – Sperm is collected when an electric probe (electroejaculator) inserted in the rectum causes ejaculation. The sperm is then processed and used with IUI, ICSI and IVF. Requires general anesthesia. Used when male is not capable of normal ejaculation, such as paralysis.

gamete intrafallopian transfer (GIFT) – Similar to IVF, but embryo is transferred to the fallopian tubes rather than the uterus.

intracytoplasmic sperm injection (ICSI) – A single sperm is injected directly into the cytoplasm of a mature egg. Used when there are abnormalities in the quality, function or number of sperm.

intrauterine insemination (IUI) – Sperm is "washed" and then placed in the uterus. Used for unexplained infertility or when a semen analysis shows sperm abnormalities such as low or absent sperm or poor motility. Donor sperm can be used.

surgical sperm aspiration (SSR) – There are various types of surgical sperm retrieval. Most sperm retrieved is immature and suitable for use only in ICSI.
    vasal aspiration – Mature sperm is retrieved from the vas deferens.

percutaneous sperm aspiration (PESA) – Sperm is retrieved from the epididymis.

micro-epididymal sperm aspiration (MESA) – Sperm is retrieved from the epididymis

testicular sperm extraction (TESE) – Sperm is retrieved from testis tissue.

Drugs by Indication

ABDOMINAL DISTENTION (POSTOPERATIVE)
Hormone, Posterior Pituitary
  Pitressin(R) [US]
  Pressyn(R) [Can]
  Pressyn(R) AR [Can]
  vasopressin

ABETALIPOPROTEINEMIA
Vitamin, Fat Soluble
  Alph-E [US-OTC]
  Alph-E-Mixed [US-OTC]
  Aquasol A(R) [US]
  Aquasol E(R) [US-OTC]
  Aquavit-E(R) [US-OTC]
  d-Alpha-Gems(TM) [US-OTC]
  E-Gems(R) [US-OTC]
  E-Gems Elite(R) [US-OTC]
  E-Gems Plus(R) [US-OTC]
  Ester-E(TM) [US-OTC]
  Gamma E-Gems(R) [US-OTC]
  Gamma-E Plus [US-OTC]
  High Gamma Vitamin E
    Complete(TM) [US-OTC]
  Key-E(R) [US-OTC]
  Key-E(R) Kaps [US-OTC]
  Palmitate-A(R) [US-OTC]
  vitamin A
  vitamin E
Vitamin, Topical
  Alph-E [US-OTC]
  Alph-E-Mixed [US-OTC]
  Aquasol E(R) [US-OTC]
  Aquavit-E(R) [US-OTC]
  d-Alpha-Gems(TM) [US-OTC]
  E-Gems(R) [US-OTC]
  E-Gems Elite(R) [US-OTC]
  E-Gems Plus(R) [US-OTC]
  Ester-E(TM) [US-OTC]

  Gamma E-Gems(R) [US-OTC]
  Gamma-E Plus [US-OTC]
  High Gamma Vitamin E
    Complete(TM) [US-OTC]
  Key-E(R) [US-OTC]
  Key-E(R) Kaps [US-OTC]
  vitamin E

ABORTION
Abortifacient
  Mifeprex(R) [US]
  mifepristone
Antineoplastic Agent,
  Hormone
  Antagonist
  Mifeprex(R) [US]
  mifepristone
Antiprogestin
  Mifeprex(R) [US]
  mifepristone
Oxytocic Agent
  oxytocin
  Pitocin(R) [US/Can]
  Syntocinon(R) [Can]
Prostaglandin
  carboprost tromethamine
  Cervidil(R) [US/Can]
  dinoprostone
  Hemabate(R) [US/Can]
  Prepidil(R) [US/Can]
  Prostin E2(R) [US/Can]

ACETAMINOPHEN POISONING
Mucolytic Agent
  Acetadote(R) [US]
  acetylcysteine
  Acetylcysteine Solution [Can]
  Mucomyst(R) [Can]
  Parvolex(R) [Can]

ACNE

Acne Products
  Acetoxyl(R) [Can]
  adapalene
  Akne-Mycin(R) [US]
  Alti-Clindamycin [Can]
  Apo-Clindamycin(R) [Can]
  Apo-Erythro Base(R) [Can]
  Apo-Erythro E-C(R) [Can]
  Apo-Erythro-ES(R) [Can]
  Apo-Erythro-S(R) [Can]
  A/T/S(R) [US]
  Benoxyl(R) [Can]
  Benzac(R) [US]
  Benzac(R) AC [US/Can]
  Benzac(R) AC Wash [US]
  Benzac(R) W [US]
  Benzac(R) W Gel [Can]
  Benzac(R) W Wash [US/Can]
  Benzagel(R) [US]
  Benzamycin(R) [US]
  Benzamycin(R) Pak [US]
  Benzashave(R) [US]
  Benziq(TM) [US]
  Benziq(TM) LS [US]
  benzoyl peroxide
  benzoyl peroxide and hydrocortisone
  Brevoxyl(R) [US]
  Brevoxyl(R) Cleansing [US]
  Brevoxyl(R) Wash [US]
  Clearplex [US-OTC]
  Cleocin(R) [US]
  Cleocin HCl(R) [US]
  Cleocin Pediatric(R) [US]
  Cleocin Phosphate(R) [US]
  Cleocin T(R) [US]
  Clinac(TM) BPO [US]
  Clindagel(R) [US]
  ClindaMax(TM) [US]
  clindamycin
  Clindamycin Injection, USP [Can]
  Clindesse(TM) [US]
  Clindets(R) [US]
  Clindoxyl(R) [Can]

  cyproterone and ethinyl estradiol
    (Canada only)
  Dalacin(R) C [Can]
  Dalacin(R) T [Can]
  Dalacin(R) Vaginal [Can]
  Del Aqua(R) [US]
  Desquam-X(R) [US/Can]
  Desquam-E(TM) [US]
  Diane-35 [Can]
  Differin(R) [US/Can]
  Differin(R) XP [Can]
  Diomycin(R) [Can]
  E.E.S.(R) [US/Can]
  Erybid(TM) [Can]
  Eryc(R) [US/Can]
  Eryderm(R) [US]
  Erygel(R) [US]
  EryPed(R) [US]
  Ery-Tab(R) [US]
  Erythrocin(R) [US]
  erythromycin
  erythromycin and benzoyl peroxide
  Evoclin(TM) [US]
  Exact(R) Acne Medication [US-OTC]
  Fostex(R) 10% BPO [US-OTC]
  Loroxide(R) [US-OTC]
  Neutrogena(R) Acne Mask [US-OTC]
  Neutrogena(R) On The Spot(R) Acne
    Treatment [US-OTC]
  Novo-Clindamycin [Can]
  Novo-Rythro Estolate [Can]
  Novo-Rythro Ethylsuccinate [Can]
  Nu-Erythromycin-S [Can]
  Oxy 10(R) Balanced Medicated Face
    Wash [US-OTC]
  Oxy 10(R) Balance Spot Treatment
    [US-OTC]
  Oxyderm(TM) [Can]
  Palmer's(R) Skin Success Acne
    [US-OTC]
  PanOxyl(R) [US/Can]
  PanOxyl(R)-AQ [US]
  PanOxyl(R) Aqua Gel [US]
  PanOxyl(R) Bar [US-OTC]

PCE(R) [US/Can]
PMS-Erythromycin [Can]
Romycin(R) [US]
Sans Acne(R) [Can]
Seba-Gel(TM) [US]
Solugel(R) [Can]
Taro-Clindamycin [Can]
Theramycin Z(R) [US]
Triaz(R) [US]
Triaz(R) Cleanser [US]
Vanoxide-HC(R) [US/Can]
Zapzyt(R) [US-OTC]
Zoderm(R) [US]
Antibiotic, Miscellaneous
Alti-Clindamycin [Can]
Apo-Clindamycin(R) [Can]
Apo-Metronidazole(R) [Can]
Cleocin(R) [US]
Cleocin HCl(R) [US]
Cleocin Pediatric(R) [US]
Cleocin Phosphate(R) [US]
Cleocin T(R) [US]
Clindagel(R) [US]
ClindaMax(TM) [US]
clindamycin
Clindamycin Injection, USP [Can]
Clindesse(TM) [US]
Clindets(R) [US]
Clindoxyl(R) [Can]
Dalacin(R) C [Can]
Dalacin(R) T [Can]
Dalacin(R) Vaginal [Can]
Evoclin(TM) [US]
Flagyl(R) [US/Can]
Flagyl ER(R) [US]
Florazole(R) ER [Can]
MetroCream(R) [US/Can]
MetroGel(R) [US/Can]
MetroLotion(R) [US]
metronidazole
Nidagel(TM) [Can]
Noritate(R) [US/Can]
Novo-Clindamycin [Can]
Taro-Clindamycin [Can]

Trikacide [Can]
Vandazole(TM) [US]
Antibiotic, Topical
Akne-Mycin(R) [US]
Apo-Erythro Base(R) [Can]
Apo-Erythro E-C(R) [Can]
Apo-Erythro-ES(R) [Can]
Apo-Erythro-S(R) [Can]
Apo-Metronidazole(R) [Can]
Apo-Tetra(R) [Can]
A/T/S(R) [US]
Diomycin(R) [Can]
E.E.S.(R) [US/Can]
Erybid(TM) [Can]
Eryc(R) [US/Can]
Eryderm(R) [US]
Erygel(R) [US]
EryPed(R) [US]
Ery-Tab(R) [US]
Erythrocin(R) [US]
erythromycin
Flagyl(R) [US/Can]
Flagyl ER(R) [US]
Flagyl(R) I.V. RTU(TM) [US]
Florazole(R) ER [Can]
MetroCream(R) [US/Can]
MetroGel(R) [US/Can]
MetroGel-Vaginal(R) [US]
MetroLotion(R) [US]
metronidazole
Nidagel(TM) [Can]
Noritate(R) [US/Can]
Novo-Rythro Estolate [Can]
Novo-Rythro Ethylsuccinate
  [Can]
Nu-Erythromycin-S [Can]
Nu-Tetra [Can]
PCE(R) [US/Can]
PMS-Erythromycin [Can]
Romycin(R) [US]
Sans Acne(R) [Can]
Sumycin(R) [US]
tetracycline
Theramycin Z(R) [US]

Trikacide [Can]
Vandazole(TM) [US]
Antiseborrheic Agent, Topical
  AVAR(TM) [US]
  AVAR(TM)-e [US]
  AVAR(TM)-e Green [US]
  AVAR(TM) Green [US]
  Clenia(TM) [US]
  Plexion(R) [US]
  Plexion SCT(R) [US]
  Plexion TS(R) [US]
  Rosac(R) [US]
  Rosanil(R) [US]
  Rosula(R) [US]
  Sulfacet-R(R) [US/Can]
  sulfur and sulfacetamide
  Zetacet(R) [US]
Estrogen and Androgen Combination
  cyproterone and ethinyl estradiol
    (Canada only)
  Diane-35 [Can]
Keratolytic Agent
  Avage(TM) [US]
  Compound W(R) [US-OTC]
  Compound W(R) One Step Wart
    Remover [US-OTC]
  DHS(TM) Sal [US-OTC]
  Dr. Scholl's(R) Callus Remover
    [US-OTC]
  Dr. Scholl's(R) Clear Away
    [US-OTC]
  DuoFilm(R) [US-OTC/Can]
  Duoforte(R) 27 [Can]
  Freezone(R) [US-OTC]
  Fung-O(R) [US-OTC]
  Gordofilm(R) [US-OTC]
  Hydrisalic(TM) [US-OTC]
  Ionil(R) [US-OTC]
  Ionil(R) Plus [US-OTC]
  Keralyt(R) [US-OTC]
  LupiCare(TM) II Psoriasis [US-OTC]
  LupiCare(TM) Dandruff [US-OTC]
  LupiCare(TM) Psoriasis [US-OTC]
  Mediplast(R) [US-OTC]

MG217 Sal-Acid(R) [US-OTC]
Mosco(R) Corn and Callus Remover
  [US-OTC]
NeoCeuticals(TM) Acne Spot
  Treatment [US-OTC]
Neutrogena(R) Acne Wash [US-OTC]
Neutrogena(R) Body Clear(TM)
  [US-OTC]
Neutrogena(R) Clear Pore [US-OTC]
Neutrogena(R) Clear Pore Shine
  Control [US-OTC]
Neutrogena(R) Healthy Scalp
  [US-OTC]
Neutrogena(R) Maximum Strength
  T/Sal(R) [US-OTC]
Neutrogena(R) On The Spot(R) Acne
  Patch [US-OTC]
Occlusal(R)-HP [US-OTC/Can]
Oxy Balance(R) [US-OTC]
Oxy Balance(R) Deep Pore
  [US-OTC]
Palmer's(R) Skin Success Acne
  Cleanser [US-OTC]
Pedisilk(R) [US-OTC]
Propa pH [US-OTC]
SalAc(R) [US-OTC]
Sal-Acid(R) [US-OTC]
Salactic(R) [US-OTC]
salicylic acid
Sal-Plant(R) [US-OTC]
Sebcur(R) [Can]
Soluver(R) [Can]
Soluver(R) Plus [Can]
Stri-dex(R) [US-OTC]
Stri-dex(R) Body Focus [US-OTC]
Stri-dex(R) Facewipes To Go(TM)
  [US-OTC]
Stri-dex(R) Maximum Strength
  [US-OTC]
tazarotene
Tazorac(R) [US/Can]
Tinamed(R) [US-OTC]
Tiseb(R) [US-OTC]
Trans-Plantar(R) [Can]

Trans-Ver-Sal(R) [US-OTC/Can]
Wart-Off(R) Maximum Strength
[US-OTC]
Zapzyt(R) Acne Wash [US-OTC]
Zapzyt(R) Pore Treatment [US-OTC]
Retinoic Acid Derivative
Accutane(R) [US/Can]
Amnesteem(TM) [US]
Avita(R) [US]
Claravis(TM) [US]
isotretinoin
Isotrex(R) [Can]
Rejuva-A(R) [Can]
Renova(R) [US]
Retin-A(R) [US/Can]
Retin-A(R) Micro [US/Can]
Retinova(R) [Can]
Sotret(R) [US]
tretinoin (topical)
Tetracycline Derivative
Alti-Minocycline [Can]
Apo-Minocycline(R) [Can]
Apo-Tetra(R) [Can]
Declomycin(R) [US/Can]
demeclocycline
Dynacin(R) [US]
Gen-Minocycline [Can]
Minocin(R) [US/Can]
minocycline
myrac(TM) [US]
Novo-Minocycline [Can]
Nu-Tetra [Can]
Rhoxal-minocycline [Can]
Sandoz-Minocycline [Can]
Solodyn(TM) [US]
Sumycin(R) [US]
tetracycline
Topical Skin Product
azelaic acid
Azelex(R) [US]
BenzaClin(R) [US/Can]
clindamycin and benzoyl peroxide
Duac(TM) [US]
Finacea(TM) [US]

Topical Skin Product, Acne
BenzaClin(R) [US/Can]
clindamycin and benzoyl peroxide
Duac(TM) [US]

ACQUIRED IMMUNODEFICIENCY SYNDROME (AIDS)

Antiretroviral Agent, Fusion Protein
Inhibitor
enfuvirtide
Fuzeon(R) [US/Can]
Antiretroviral Agent, Non-nucleoside
Reverse Transcriptase Inhibitor
(NNRTI)
Kaletra(R) [US/Can]
lopinavir and ritonavir
Antiretroviral Agent, Nucleoside
Reverse Transcriptase Inhibitor
(NRTI)
abacavir, lamivudine, and zidovudine
Trizivir(R) [US]
Antiretroviral Agent, Protease Inhibitor
Aptivus(R) [US/Can]
atazanavir
darunavir
fosamprenavir
Lexiva(R) [US]
Prezista(TM) [US]
Reyataz(R) [US/Can]
Telzir(R) [Can]
tipranavir
Antiretroviral Agent, Reverse
Transcriptase Inhibitor (Nucleoside)
abacavir and lamivudine
emtricitabine
emtricitabine and tenofovir
Emtriva(R) [US/Can]
Epzicom(TM) [US]
Kivexa(TM) [Can]
Truvada(R) [US/Can]
Antiretroviral Agent, Reverse
Transcriptase Inhibitor (Nucleotide)
emtricitabine and tenofovir

tenofovir
Truvada(R) [US/Can]
Viread(R) [US/Can]
Antiviral Agent
Apo-Zidovudine(R) [Can]
AZT(TM) [Can]
Combivir(R) [US/Can]
Crixivan(R) [US/Can]
delavirdine
didanosine
Epivir(R) [US]
Epivir-HBV(R) [US]
Fortovase(R) [Can]
Heptovir(R) [Can]
Hivid(R) [US/Can]
indinavir
Invirase(R) [US/Can]
lamivudine
nelfinavir
nevirapine
Norvir(R) [US/Can]
Norvir(R) SEC [Can]
Rescriptor(R) [US/Can]
Retrovir(R) [US/Can]
ritonavir
saquinavir
stavudine
3TC(R) [Can]
Videx(R) [US/Can]
Videx(R) EC [US/Can]
Viracept(R) [US/Can]
Viramune(R) [US/Can]
zalcitabine
Zerit(R) [US/Can]
zidovudine
zidovudine and lamivudine
Nonnucleoside Reverse Transcriptase
Inhibitor (NNRTI)
efavirenz
Sustiva(R) [US/Can]
Nucleoside Reverse Transcriptase
Inhibitor (NRTI)
abacavir
Ziagen(R) [US/Can]

Protease Inhibitor
Agenerase(R) [US/Can]
Amprenavir [US]
amprenavir

ADRENOCORTICAL FUNCTION ABNORMALITIES
Adrenal Corticosteroid
Apo-Dexamethasone(R) [Can]
Apo-Prednisone(R) [Can]
Aristocort(R) [US/Can]
Aristospan(R) [US/Can]
Betaject(TM) [Can]
betamethasone (systemic)
Bubbli-Pred(TM) [US]
Celestone(R) [US]
Celestone(R) Soluspan(R)
  [US/Can]
Cortef(R) [US/Can]
corticotropin
cortisone acetate
Decadron(R) [US]
Depo-Medrol(R) [US/Can]
Dexamethasone Intensol(R) [US]
dexamethasone (systemic)
Dexasone(R) [Can]
DexPak(R) TaperPak(R) [US]
Diodex(R) [Can]
Diopred(R) [Can]
H.P. Acthar(R) Gel [US]
Hydeltra T.B.A.(R) [Can]
hydrocortisone (systemic)
Kenalog(R) [US/Can]
Kenalog-10(R) [US]
Kenalog-40(R) [US]
Medrol(R) [US/Can]
methylprednisolone
Novo-Prednisolone [Can]
Novo-Prednisone [Can]
Oracort [Can]
Orapred(R) [US]
Pediapred(R) [US/Can]
PMS-Dexamethasone [Can]

prednisolone (systemic)
prednisone
Prednisone Intensol(TM) [US]
Prelone(R) [US]
Sab-Prenase [Can]
Solu-Cortef(R) [US/Can]
Solu-Medrol(R) [US/Can]
Sterapred(R) [US]
Sterapred(R) DS [US]
triamcinolone (systemic)
Winpred(TM) [Can]
Adrenal Corticosteroid
  (Mineralocorticoid)
  Florinef(R) [US/Can]
  Fludrocortisone

ALPHA1-ANTITRYPSIN DEFICIENCY (CONGENITAL)

Antitrypsin Deficiency Agent
  alpha1-proteinase inhibitor
  Aralast [US]
  Prolastin(R) [US/Can]
  Zemaira(R) [US]

AMEBIASIS

Amebicide
  Apo-Metronidazole(R) [Can]
  Diodoquin(R) [Can]
  Flagyl(R) [US/Can]
  Flagyl ER(R) [US]
  Flagyl(R) I.V. RTU(TM) [US]
  Florazole(R) ER [Can]
  Humatin(R) [US/Can]
  iodoquinol
  MetroCream(R) [US/Can]
  MetroGel(R) [US/Can]
  MetroGel-Vaginal(R) [US]
  MetroLotion(R) [US]
  metronidazole
  Nidagel(TM) [Can]
  Noritate(R) [US/Can]
  paromomycin
  Trikacide [Can]

Vandazole(TM) [US]
Yodoxin(R) [US]
Aminoquinoline (Antimalarial)
  Aralen(R) [US]
  chloroquine
  Novo-Chloroquine [Can]
Antibiotic, Miscellaneous
  Apo-Metronidazole(R) [Can]
  Flagyl(R) [US/Can]
  Flagyl ER(R) [US]
  Flagyl(R) I.V. RTU(TM) [US]
  Florazole(R) ER [Can]
  MetroCream(R) [US/Can]
  MetroGel(R) [US/Can]
  MetroGel-Vaginal(R) [US]
  MetroLotion(R) [US]
  metronidazole
  Nidagel(TM) [Can]
  Noritate(R) [US/Can]
  Trikacide [Can]
  Vandazole(TM) [US]
Antibiotic, Topical
  Apo-Metronidazole(R) [Can]
  Flagyl(R) [US/Can]
  Flagyl ER(R) [US]
  Flagyl(R) I.V. RTU(TM) [US]
  Florazole(R) ER [Can]
  MetroCream(R) [US/Can]
  MetroGel(R) [US/Can]
  MetroGel-Vaginal(R) [US]
  MetroLotion(R) [US]
  metronidazole
  Nidagel(TM) [Can]
  Noritate(R) [US/Can]
  Trikacide [Can]
  Vandazole(TM) [US]
Antiprotozoal
  Apo-Metronidazole(R) [Can]
  Flagyl(R) [US/Can]
  Flagyl ER(R) [US]
  Flagyl(R) I.V. RTU(TM) [US]
  Florazole(R) ER [Can]
  MetroCream(R) [US/Can]
  MetroGel(R) [US/Can]

MetroGel-Vaginal(R) [US]
MetroLotion(R) [US]
metronidazole
Nidagel(TM) [Can]
Noritate(R) [US/Can]
Trikacide [Can]
Vandazole(TM) [US]

AMENORRHEA
Diagnostic Agent
Factrel(R) [US]
gonadorelin
Lutrepulse(TM) [Can]
Ergot Alkaloid and Derivative
Apo-Bromocriptine(R) [Can]
bromocriptine
Parlodel(R) [US/Can]
PMS-Bromocriptine [Can]
Gonadotropin
Factrel(R) [US]
gonadorelin
Lutrepulse(TM) [Can]
Progestin
Alti-MPA [Can]
Apo-Medroxy(R) [Can]
Aygestin(R) [US]
Camila(TM) [US]
Crinone(R) [US/Can]
Depo-Prevera(R) [Can]
Depo-Provera(R) [US/Can]
Depo-Provera(R) Contraceptive [US]
depo-subQ provera 104(TM) [US]
Errin(TM) [US]
Gen-Medroxy [Can]
Jolivette(TM) [US]
medroxyprogesterone
Micronor(R) [US/Can]
Nora-BE(TM) [US]
norethindrone
Norlutate(R) [Can]
Nor-QD(R) [US]
Novo-Medrone [Can]
Prochieve(TM) [US]
progesterone

Prometrium(R) [US/Can]
Provera(R) [US/Can]
Provera-Pak [Can]

ANAPHYLACTIC SHOCK
Adrenergic Agonist Agent
Adrenalin(R) [US/Can]
epinephrine
EpiPen(R) [US/Can]
EpiPen(R) Jr [US/Can]
Primatene(R) Mist [US-OTC]
Raphon [US-OTC]
S2(R) [US-OTC]
Twinject(TM) [US]

ANAPHYLACTIC SHOCK (PROPHYLAXIS)
Plasma Volume Expander
dextran 1
Promit(R) [US]

APNEA (NEONATAL IDIOPATHIC)
Theophylline Derivative
Aminophylline

ATTENTION DEFICIT/ HYPERACTIVITY DISORDER (ADHD)
Amphetamine
Adderall(R) [US]
Adderall XR(R) [US/Can]
Desoxyn(R) [US/Can]
Dexedrine(R) [US/Can]
dextroamphetamine
dextroamphetamine and amphetamine
Dextrostat(R) [US]
methamphetamine
Central Nervous System Stimulant, Nonamphetamine
Apo-Methylphenidate(R) [Can]
Apo-Methylphenidate(R) SR [Can]
Biphentin(R) [Can]
Concerta(R) [US/Can]
Daytrana(TM) [US]

dexmethylphenidate
Focalin(TM) [US]
Focalin(TM) XR [US]
Metadate(R) CD [US]
Metadate(R) ER [US]
Methylin(R) [US]
Methylin(R) ER [US]
methylphenidate
PMS-Methylphenidate [Can]
Riphenidate [Can]
Ritalin(R) [US/Can]
Ritalin(R) LA [US]
Ritalin-SR(R) [US/Can]
Norepinephrine Reuptake Inhibitor,
  Selective
atomoxetine
Strattera(R) [US/Can]

AUTISM

Antidepressant, Selective Serotonin
  Reuptake Inhibitor
Alti-Fluoxetine [Can]
Apo-Fluoxetine(R) [Can]
BCI-Fluoxetine [Can]
CO Fluoxetine [Can]
fluoxetine
FXT [Can]
Gen-Fluoxetine [Can]
Novo-Fluoxetine [Can]
Nu-Fluoxetine [Can]
PMS-Fluoxetine [Can]
Prozac(R) [US/Can]
Prozac(R) Weekly(TM) [US]
Rhoxal-fluoxetine [Can]
Sandoz-Fluoxetine [Can]
Sarafem(R) [US]
Antipsychotic Agent, Butyrophenone
Apo-Haloperidol(R) [Can]
Apo-Haloperidol LA(R) [Can]
Haldol(R) [US]
Haldol(R) Decanoate [US]
haloperidol
Haloperidol Injection, USP [Can]
Haloperidol-LA [Can]

Haloperidol-LA Omega [Can]
Novo-Peridol [Can]
Peridol [Can]
PMS-Haloperidol LA [Can]

BIRTH CONTROL (SEE CONTRACEPTION)

BREAST ENGORGEMENT (POSTPARTUM)

Androgen
fluoxymesterone
Estrogen Derivative
Alora(R) [US]
Cenestin(R) [US]
Climara(R) [US/Can]
Delestrogen(R) [US]
Depo(R)-Estradiol [US/Can]
Esclim(R) [US]
Estrace(R) [US/Can]
Estraderm(R) [US/Can]
estradiol
Estradot(R) [Can]
Estrasorb(TM) [US]
Estring(R) [US/Can]
EstroGel(R) [US/Can]
estrogens (conjugated A/synthetic)
estrogens (conjugated/equine)
Femring(TM) [US]
Femtrace(R) [US]
Gynodiol(R) [US]
Menostar(TM) [US/Can]
Oesclim(R) [Can]
Premarin(R) [US/Can]
Sandoz-Estradiol Derm 50 [Can]
Sandoz-Estradiol Derm 75 [Can]
Sandoz-Estradiol Derm 100 [Can]
Vagifem(R) [US/Can]
Vivelle(R) [US]
Vivelle-Dot(R) [US]

CANDIDIASIS

Antifungal Agent
Abelcet(R) [US/Can]

Aloe Vesta(R) 2-n-1 Antifungal
  [US-OTC]
Amphocin(R) [US]
Amphotec(R) [US/Can]
amphotericin B cholesteryl sulfate
  complex
amphotericin B (conventional)
amphotericin B lipid complex
Ancobon(R) [US/Can]
Apo-Fluconazole(R) [Can]
Apo-Ketoconazole(R) [Can]
Baza(R) Antifungal [US-OTC]
Bio-Statin(R) [US]
Blis-To-Sol(R) [US-OTC]
butoconazole
Candistatin(R) [Can]
Canesten(R) Topical [Can]
Canesten(R) Vaginal [Can]
Carrington Antifungal [US-OTC]
ciclopirox
Clotrimaderm [Can]
clotrimazole
Cruex(R) Cream [US-OTC]
1-Day(TM) [US-OTC]
DermaFungal [US-OTC]
Dermagran(R) AF [US-OTC]
Dermazole [Can]
DiabetAid(TM) Antifungal Foot Bath
  [US-OTC]
Diflucan(R) [US/Can]
econazole
Ecostatin(R) [Can]
Exelderm(R) [US/Can]
Femstat(R) One [Can]
fluconazole
Fluconazole Injection [Can]
Fluconazole Omega [Can]
flucytosine
Fungi-Guard [US-OTC]
Fungizone(R) [Can]
Fungoid(R) Tincture [US-OTC]
Gen-Fluconazole [Can]
GMD-Fluconazole [Can]
Gold Bond(R) Antifungal [US-OTC]

Gynazole-1(R) [US/Can]
Gyne-Lotrimin(R) 3 [US-OTC]
itraconazole
ketoconazole
Ketoderm(R) [Can]
Lamisil(R) Topical [US/Can]
Loprox(R) [US/Can]
Lotrimin(R) AF Athlete's Foot Cream
  [US-OTC]
Lotrimin(R) AF Athlete's Foot
  Solution [US-OTC]
Lotrimin(R) AF Jock Itch Cream
  [US-OTC]
Lotrimin(R) AF Jock Itch Powder
  Spray [US-OTC]
Lotrimin(R) AF Powder/Spray
  [US-OTC]
Micaderm(R) [US-OTC]
Micatin(R) [Can]
Micatin(R) Athlete's Foot [US-OTC]
Micatin(R) Jock Itch [US-OTC]
miconazole
Micozole [Can]
Micro-Guard(R) [US-OTC]
Mitrazol(TM) [US-OTC]
Monistat(R) [Can]
Monistat(R) 1 Combination Pack
  [US-OTC]
Monistat(R) 3 [US-OTC/Can]
Monistat(R) 7 [US-OTC]
Monistat-Derm(R) [US]
Mycelex(R) [US]
Mycelex(R)-3 [US-OTC]
Mycelex(R)-7 [US-OTC]
Mycelex(R) Twin Pack [US-OTC]
Mycostatin(R) [US]
naftifine
Naftin(R) [US]
Neosporin(R) AF [US-OTC]
Nilstat [Can]
Nizoral(R) [US]
Nizoral(R) A-D [US-OTC]
Novo-Fluconazole [Can]
Novo-Ketoconazole [Can]

Nyaderm [Can]
Nyamyc(TM) [US]
nystatin
Nystat-Rx(R) [US]
Nystop(R) [US]
oxiconazole
Oxistat(R) [US/Can]
Pedi-Dri(R) [US]
Penlac(R) [US/Can]
Pitrex [Can]
PMS-Nystatin [Can]
Podactin Cream [US-OTC]
Podactin Powder [US-OTC]
Q-Naftate [US-OTC]
Riva-Fluconazole [Can]
Secura(R) Antifungal [US-OTC]
Spectazole(R) [US/Can]
Sporanox(R) [US/Can]
sulconazole
Terazol(R) [Can]
Terazol(R) 3 [US]
Terazol(R) 7 [US]
terbinafine (topical)
terconazole
Tinactin(R) Antifungal [US-OTC]
Tinactin(R) Antifungal Jock Itch
  [US-OTC]
Tinaderm [US-OTC]
Ting(R) Cream [US-OTC]
tioconazole
tolnaftate
Trivagizole-3(R) [Can]
Vagistat(R)-1 [US-OTC]
Zeasorb(R)-AF [US-OTC]
Antifungal Agent, Parenteral
  anidulafungin
  Eraxis(TM) [US]
  micafungin
  Mycamine(TM) [US]
Antifungal Agent, Systemic
  AmBisome(R) [US/Can]
  amphotericin B liposomal
Antifungal/Corticosteroid
  nystatin and triamcinolone

Drug-induced Neuritis, Treatment Agent
  micafungin
  Mycamine(TM) [US]
Echinocandin
  anidulafungin
  Eraxis(TM) [US]

CHICKENPOX
Antiviral Agent
  acyclovir
  Apo-Acyclovir(R) [Can]
  Gen-Acyclovir [Can]
  Nu-Acyclovir [Can]
  ratio-Acyclovir [Can]
  Zovirax(R) [US/Can]
Vaccine, Live Virus
  varicella virus vaccine
  Varilrix(R) [Can]
  Varivax(R) [US]
  Varivax(R) III [Can]

CONDYLOMA ACUMINATUM
Antiviral Agent
  interferon alfa-2b and ribavirin
  Rebetron(R) [US]
Biological Response Modulator
  Alferon(R) N [US/Can]
  interferon alfa-2a
  interferon alfa-2b
  interferon alfa-2b and ribavirin
  interferon alfa-n3
  Intron(R) A [US/Can]
  Rebetron(R) [US]
  Roferon-A(R) [US/Can]
Immune Response Modifier
  Aldara(TM) [US/Can]
  imiquimod
Keratolytic Agent
  Condyline(TM) [Can]
  Condylox(R) [US]
  Podocon-25(R) [US]
  Podofilm(R) [Can]
  podofilox
  podophyllum resin
  Wartec(R) [Can]

CONTRACEPTION

Contraceptive
  ethinyl estradiol and drospirenone
  ethinyl estradiol and etonogestrel
  ethinyl estradiol and norelgestromin
  Evra(R) [Can]
  NuvaRing(R) [US/Can]
  Ortho Evra(R) [US]
  Yasmin(R) [US/Can]
  Yaz [US]
Contraceptive, Implant (Progestin)
  levonorgestrel
  Mirena(R) [US/Can]
  Norplant(R) Implant [Can]
  Plan B(R) [US/Can]
Contraceptive, Oral
  Alesse(R) [US/Can]
  Apri(R) [US]
  Aranelle(TM) [US]
  Aviane(TM) [US]
  Brevicon(R) [US]
  Brevicon(R) 0.5/35 [Can]
  Brevicon(R) 1/35 [Can]
  Cesia(TM) [US]
  Cryselle(TM) [US]
  Cyclen(R) [Can]
  Cyclessa(R) [US/Can]
  Demulen(R) [US]
  Demulen(R) 30 [Can]
  Desogen(R) [US]
  Enpresse(TM) [US]
  Estrostep(R) Fe [US]
  ethinyl estradiol and desogestrel
  ethinyl estradiol and ethynodiol
    diacetate
  ethinyl estradiol and levonorgestrel
  ethinyl estradiol and norethindrone
  ethinyl estradiol and norgestimate
  ethinyl estradiol and norgestrel
  femhrt(R) [US/Can]
  Junel(TM) [US]
  Junel(TM) Fe [US]
  Kariva(TM) [US]
  Kelnor(TM) [US]

Leena(TM) [US]
Lessina(TM) [US]
Levlen(R) [US]
Levlite(TM) [US]
Levora(R) [US]
Linessa(R) [Can]
Loestrin(R) [US]
Loestrin(TM) 1.5/30 [Can]
Loestrin(R) 24 Fe [US]
Loestrin(R) Fe [US]
Lo/Ovral(R) [US]
Low-Ogestrel(R) [US]
Lutera(TM) [US]
Marvelon(R) [Can]
mestranol and norethindrone
Microgestin(TM) [US]
Microgestin(TM) Fe [US]
Minestrin(TM) 1/20 [Can]
Min-Ovral(R) [Can]
Mircette(R) [US]
Modicon(R) [US]
MonoNessa(TM) [US]
Necon(R) 0.5/35 [US]
Necon(R) 1/35 [US]
Necon(R) 1/50 [US]
Necon(R) 7/7/7 [US]
Necon(R) 10/11 [US]
Nordette(R) [US]
Norinyl(R) 1+35 [US]
Norinyl(R) 1+50 [US]
Nortrel(TM) [US]
Nortrel(TM) 7/7/7 [US]
Ogestrel(R) [US]
Ortho(R) 0.5/35 [Can]
Ortho(R) 1/35 [Can]
Ortho(R) 7/7/7 [Can]
Ortho-Cept(R) [US/Can]
Ortho-Cyclen(R) [US]
Ortho-Novum(R) [US]
Ortho-Novum(R) 1/50 [US]
Ortho Tri-Cyclen(R) [US]
Ortho Tri-Cyclen(R) Lo [US]
Ovcon(R) [US]
Ovral(R) [Can]

Portia(TM) [US]
PREVEN(R) [US]
Previfem(TM) [US]
Reclipsen(TM) [US]
Seasonale(R) [US]
Seasonique(TM) [US]
Select(TM) 1/35 [Can]
Solia(TM) [US]
Sprintec(TM) [US]
Synphasic(R) [Can]
Tri-Cyclen(R) [Can]
Tri-Cyclen(R) Lo [Can]
Tri-Levlen(R) [US]
TriNessa(TM) [US]
Tri-Norinyl(R) [US]
Triphasil(R) [US/Can]
Tri-Previfem(TM) [US]
Triquilar(R) [Can]
Tri-Sprintec(TM) [US]
Trivora(R) [US]
Velivet(TM) [US]
Zovia(TM) [US]
Contraceptive, Progestin Only
Alti-MPA [Can]
Apo-Medroxy(R) [Can]
Aygestin(R) [US]
Camila(TM) [US]
Depo-Prevera(R) [Can]
Depo-Provera(R) [US/Can]
Depo-Provera(R) Contraceptive [US]
depo-subQ provera 104(TM) [US]
Errin(TM) [US]
Gen-Medroxy [Can]
Jolivette(TM) [US]
levonorgestrel
medroxyprogesterone
Micronor(R) [US/Can]
Mirena(R) [US/Can]
Nora-BE(TM) [US]
norethindrone
Norlutate(R) [Can]
Norplant(R) Implant [Can]
Nor-QD(R) [US]
Novo-Medrone [Can]

Plan B(R) [US/Can]
Provera(R) [US/Can]
Provera-Pak [Can]
Estrogen and Progestin Combination
ethinyl estradiol and etonogestrel
ethinyl estradiol and norelgestromin
Evra(R) [Can]
NuvaRing(R) [US/Can]
Ortho Evra(R) [US]
Progestin
Alti-MPA [Can]
Apo-Medroxy(R) [Can]
Aygestin(R) [US]
Camila(TM) [US]
Depo-Prevera(R) [Can]
Depo-Provera(R) [US/Can]
Depo-Provera(R) Contraceptive [US]
depo-subQ provera 104(TM) [US]
Errin(TM) [US]
Gen-Medroxy [Can]
Jolivette(TM) [US]
medroxyprogesterone
Micronor(R) [US/Can]
Nora-BE(TM) [US]
norethindrone
Norlutate(R) [Can]
Nor-QD(R) [US]
Novo-Medrone [Can]
Provera(R) [US/Can]
Provera-Pak [Can]
Spermicide
Advantage-S(TM) [US-OTC]
Conceptrol(R) [US-OTC]
Delfen(R) [US-OTC]
Encare(R) [US-OTC]
Gynol II(R) [US-OTC]
nonoxynol 9
Today(R) Sponge [US-OTC]
VCF(TM) [US-OTC]

CRYPTORCHIDISM
Gonadotropin
chorionic gonadotropin (human)
Humegon(R) [Can]

Novarel(R) [US]
Pregnyl(R) [US]
Profasi(R) HP [Can]

CYSTIC FIBROSIS
Enzyme
  dornase alfa
  Pulmozyme(R) [US/Can]

DIAPER RASH
Protectant, Topical
  A and D(R) Original [US-OTC]
  Baza(R) Clear [US-OTC]
  Sween Cream(R) [US-OTC]
  vitamin A and vitamin D
Topical Skin Product
  Ammens(R) Medicated Deodorant
    [US-OTC]
  Balmex(R) [US-OTC]
  Boudreaux's(R) Butt Paste
    [US-OTC]
  Critic-Aid Skin Care(R) [US-OTC]
  Desitin(R) [US-OTC]
  Desitin(R) Creamy [US-OTC]
  Diaparene(R) [US-OTC]
  methylbenzethonium chloride
  Puri-Clens(TM) [US-OTC]
  Zincofax(R) [Can]
  zinc oxide

DUCTUS ARTERIOSUS (CLOSURE)
Nonsteroidal Antiinflammatory Drug
  (NSAID)
  Indocin(R) I.V. [US]
  indomethacin
  Nu-Indo [Can]

DUCTUS ARTERIOSUS (TEMPORARY MAINTENANCE OF PATENCY)
Prostaglandin
  alprostadil
  Caverject(R) [US/Can]

DWARFISM
Growth Hormone
  Genotropin(R) [US]
  Genotropin Miniquick(R) [US]
  Humatrope(R) [US/Can]
  Norditropin(R) [US]
  Norditropin(R) NordiFlex(R) [US]
  Nutropin(R) [US]
  Nutropin AQ(R) [US]
  Nutropine(R) [Can]
  Omnitrope(TM) [US]
  Saizen(R) [US/Can]
  Serostim(R) [US/Can]
  somatropin
  Tev-Tropin(TM) [US]
  Zorbtive(TM) [US]

DYSBETALIPOPROTEINEMIA (FAMILIAL)
Antihyperlipidemic Agent,
  Miscellaneous
  bezafibrate (Canada only)
  Bezalip(R) [Can]
  PMS-Bezafibrate [Can]
Vitamin, Water Soluble
  niacin
  Niacor(R) [US]
  Niaspan(R) [US/Can]
  Slo-Niacin(R) [US-OTC]

DYSMENORRHEA
Nonsteroidal Antiinflammatory Drug
  (NSAID)
  Advil(R) [US-OTC/Can]
  Advil(R) Children's [US-OTC]
  Advil(R) Infants' [US-OTC]
  Advil(R) Junior [US-OTC]
  Advil(R) Migraine [US-OTC]
  Aleve(R) [US-OTC]
  Alti-Flurbiprofen [Can]
  Anaprox(R) [US/Can]
  Anaprox(R) DS [US/Can]
  Ansaid(R) [Can]
  Apo-Diclo(R) [Can]

Apo-Diclo Rapide(R) [Can]
Apo-Diclo SR(R) [Can]
Apo-Diflunisal(R) [Can]
Apo-Flurbiprofen(R) [Can]
Apo-Ibuprofen(R) [Can]
Apo-Keto(R) [Can]
Apo-Keto-E(R) [Can]
Apo-Keto SR(R) [Can]
Apo-Mefenamic(R) [Can]
Apo-Napro-Na(R) [Can]
Apo-Napro-Na DS(R) [Can]
Apo-Naproxen(R) [Can]
Apo-Naproxen EC(R) [Can]
Apo-Naproxen SR(R) [Can]
Apo-Piroxicam(R) [Can]
Cataflam(R) [US/Can]
diclofenac
diflunisal
Dom-Mefenamic Acid [Can]
EC-Naprosyn(R) [US]
ElixSure(TM) IB [US-OTC]
Feldene(R) [US]
flurbiprofen
Froben(R) [Can]
Froben-SR(R) [Can]
Gen-Naproxen EC [Can]
Gen-Piroxicam [Can]
Genpril(R) [US-OTC]
Ibu-200 [US-OTC]
ibuprofen
I-Prin [US-OTC]
ketoprofen
Mefenamic-250 [Can]
mefenamic acid
Midol(R) Cramp and Body Aches
  [US-OTC]
Midol(R) Extended Relief [US]
Motrin(R) [US]
Motrin(R) Children's [US-OTC/Can]
Motrin(R) IB [US-OTC/Can]
Motrin(R) Infants' [US-OTC]
Motrin(R) Junior Strength [US-OTC]
Naprelan(R) [US]
Naprosyn(R) [US/Can]

naproxen
Naxen(R) [Can]
Naxen(R) EC [Can]
NeoProfen(R)
Novo-Difenac [Can]
Novo-Difenac K [Can]
Novo-Difenac-SR [Can]
Novo-Diflunisal [Can]
Novo-Flurprofen [Can]
Novo-Keto [Can]
Novo-Keto-EC [Can]
Novo-Naproc EC [Can]
Novo-Naprox [Can]
Novo-Naprox Sodium [Can]
Novo-Naprox Sodium DS
  [Can]
Novo-Naprox SR [Can]
Novo-Pirocam [Can]
Novo-Profen [Can]
Nu-Diclo [Can]
Nu-Diclo-SR [Can]
Nu-Diflunisal [Can]
Nu-Flurprofen [Can]
Nu-Ibuprofen [Can]
Nu-Ketoprofen [Can]
Nu-Ketoprofen-E [Can]
Nu-Mefenamic [Can]
Nu-Naprox [Can]
Nu-Pirox [Can]
Ocufen(R) [US/Can]
Oruvail(R) [Can]
Pamprin(R) Maximum Strength All
  Day Relief [US-OTC]
Pennsaid(R) [Can]
Pexicam(R) [Can]
piroxicam
PMS-Diclofenac [Can]
PMS-Diclofenac SR [Can]
PMS-Mefenamic Acid [Can]
Ponstan(R) [Can]
Ponstel(R) [US]
Proprinal [US-OTC]
Rhodis(TM) [Can]
Rhodis-EC(TM) [Can]

Rhodis SR(TM) [Can]
Riva-Diclofenac [Can]
Riva-Diclofenac-K [Can]
Riva-Naproxen [Can]
Solaraze(R) [US]
Ultraprin [US-OTC]
Voltaren(R) [US/Can]
Voltaren Ophtha(R) [Can]
Voltaren Ophthalmic(R) [US]
Voltaren Rapide(R) [Can]
Voltaren(R)-XR [US]

EAR WAX

Antiinfective Agent, Oral
  carbamide peroxide
  Debrox(R) [US-OTC]
  Dent's Ear Wax [US-OTC]
  ERO [US-OTC]
  Murine(R) Ear Wax Removal System
    [US-OTC]
Otic Agent, Ceruminolytic
  A/B Otic [US]
  Allergen(R) [US]
  antipyrine and benzocaine
  Auralgan(R) [Can]
  Aurodex [US]
  carbamide peroxide
  Cerumenex(R) [Can]
  Debrox(R) [US-OTC]
  Dent's Ear Wax [US-OTC]
  ERO [US-OTC]
  Murine(R) Ear Wax Removal System
    [US-OTC]
  triethanolamine polypeptide
    oleate-condensate

ECLAMPSIA

Anticonvulsant
  Luminal(R) Sodium [US]
  phenobarbital
  PMS-Phenobarbital [Can]
Barbiturate
  Luminal(R) Sodium [US]
  phenobarbital
  PMS-Phenobarbital [Can]

Benzodiazepine
  Apo-Diazepam(R) [Can]
  Diastat(R) [US/Can]
  Diastat(R) AcuDial(TM) [US]
  Diastat(R) Rectal Delivery System
    [Can]
  Diazemuls(R) [Can]
  diazepam
  Diazepam Intensol(R) [US]
  Novo-Dipam [Can]
  Valium(R) [US/Can]

ENDOMETRIOSIS

Androgen
  Cyclomen(R) [Can]
  danazol
  Danocrine(R) [Can]
Contraceptive, Oral
  Alesse(R) [US/Can]
  Apri(R) [US]
  Aranelle(TM) [US]
  Aviane(TM) [US]
  Brevicon(R) [US]
  Brevicon(R) 0.5/35 [Can]
  Brevicon(R) 1/35 [Can]
  Cesia(TM) [US]
  Cryselle(TM) [US]
  Cyclen(R) [Can]
  Cyclessa(R) [US/Can]
  Demulen(R) [US]
  Demulen(R) 30 [Can]
  Desogen(R) [US]
  Enpresse(TM) [US]
  Estrostep(R) Fe [US]
  ethinyl estradiol and desogestrel
  ethinyl estradiol and ethynodiol
    diacetate
  ethinyl estradiol and levonorgestrel
  ethinyl estradiol and norethindrone
  ethinyl estradiol and norgestimate
  ethinyl estradiol and norgestrel
  femhrt(R) [US/Can]
  Junel(TM) [US]
  Junel(TM) Fe [US]

Kariva(TM) [US]
Kelnor(TM) [US]
Leena(TM) [US]
Lessina(TM) [US]
Levlen(R) [US]
Levlite(TM) [US]
Levora(R) [US]
Linessa(R) [Can]
Loestrin(R) [US]
Loestrin(TM) 1.5/30 [Can]
Loestrin(R) 24 Fe [US]
Loestrin(R) Fe [US]
Lo/Ovral(R) [US]
Low-Ogestrel(R) [US]
Lutera(TM) [US]
Marvelon(R) [Can]
mestranol and norethindrone
Microgestin(TM) [US]
Microgestin(TM) Fe [US]
Minestrin(TM) 1/20 [Can]
Min-Ovral(R) [Can]
Mircette(R) [US]
Modicon(R) [US]
MonoNessa(TM) [US]
Necon(R) 0.5/35 [US]
Necon(R) 1/35 [US]
Necon(R) 1/50 [US]
Necon(R) 7/7/7 [US]
Necon(R) 10/11 [US]
Nordette(R) [US]
Norinyl(R) 1+35 [US]
Norinyl(R) 1+50 [US]
Nortrel(TM) [US]
Nortrel(TM) 7/7/7 [US]
Ogestrel(R) [US]
Ortho(R) 0.5/35 [Can]
Ortho(R) 1/35 [Can]
Ortho(R) 7/7/7 [Can]
Ortho-Cept(R) [US/Can]
Ortho-Cyclen(R) [US]
Ortho-Novum(R) [US]
Ortho-Novum(R) 1/50 [US]
Ortho Tri-Cyclen(R) [US]
Ortho Tri-Cyclen(R) Lo [US]

Ovcon(R) [US]
Ovral(R) [Can]
Portia(TM) [US]
PREVEN(R) [US]
Previfem(TM) [US]
Reclipsen(TM) [US]
Seasonale(R) [US]
Seasonique(TM) [US]
Select(TM) 1/35 [Can]
Solia(TM) [US]
Sprintec(TM) [US]
Synphasic(R) [Can]
Tri-Cyclen(R) [Can]
Tri-Cyclen(R) Lo [Can]
Tri-Levlen(R) [US]
TriNessa(TM) [US]
Tri-Norinyl(R) [US]
Triphasil(R) [US/Can]
Tri-Previfem(TM) [US]
Triquilar(R) [Can]
Tri-Sprintec(TM) [US]
Trivora(R) [US]
Velivet(TM) [US]
Zovia(TM) [US]
Contraceptive, Progestin Only
    Aygestin(R) [US]
    Camila(TM) [US]
    Errin(TM) [US]
    Jolivette(TM) [US]
    Micronor(R) [US/Can]
    Nora-BE(TM) [US]
    norethindrone
    Norlutate(R) [Can]
    Nor-QD(R) [US]
Hormone, Posterior Pituitary
    nafarelin
    Synarel(R) [US/Can]
Progestin
    Aygestin(R) [US]
    Camila(TM) [US]
    Errin(TM) [US]
    Jolivette(TM) [US]
    Micronor(R) [US/Can]
    Nora-BE(TM) [US]

norethindrone
Norlutate(R) [Can]
Nor-QD(R) [US]

FACTOR VIII DEFICIENCY
Blood Product Derivative
Alphanate(R) [US]
antihemophilic factor (human)
Hemofil M [US/Can]
Koate(R)-DVI [US]
Monarc-M(TM) [US]
Monoclate-P(R) [US]
Hemophilic Agent
anti-inhibitor coagulant complex
Feiba VH [US]
Feiba VH Immuno [Can]

FACTOR IX DEFICIENCY
Antihemophilic Agent
Bebulin(R) VH [US]
factor IX complex (human)
Profilnine(R) SD [US]
Proplex(R) T [US]

FAMILIAL ADENOMATOUS POLYPOSIS
Nonsteroidal Antiinflammatory Drug
(NSAID), COX-2 Selective
Celebrex(R) [US/Can]
Celecoxib

FEVER
Antipyretic
Abenol(R) [Can]
Acephen(TM) [US-OTC]
acetaminophen
Advil(R) [US-OTC/Can]
Advil(R) Children's [US-OTC]
Advil(R) Infants' [US-OTC]
Advil(R) Junior [US-OTC]
Advil(R) Migraine [US-OTC]
Aleve(R) [US-OTC]
Amigesic(R) [US/Can]
Anaprox(R) [US/Can]
Anaprox(R) DS [US/Can]

Apo-Acetaminophen(R) [Can]
Apo-Ibuprofen(R) [Can]
Apo-Napro-Na(R) [Can]
Apo-Napro-Na DS(R) [Can]
Apo-Naproxen(R) [Can]
Apo-Naproxen EC(R) [Can]
Apo-Naproxen SR(R) [Can]
Apra Children's [US-OTC]
Asaphen [Can]
Asaphen E.C. [Can]
Ascriptin(R) [US-OTC]
Ascriptin(R) Extra Strength
[US-OTC]
Aspercin [US-OTC]
Aspercin Extra [US-OTC]
aspirin
Aspirin Free Anacin(R) Maximum
Strength [US-OTC]
Atasol(R) [Can]
Bayer(R) Aspirin [US-OTC]
Bayer(R) Aspirin Extra Strength
[US-OTC]
Bayer(R) Aspirin Regimen Adult
Low Strength [US-OTC]
Bayer(R) Aspirin Regimen Children's
[US-OTC]
Bayer(R) Aspirin Regimen Regular
Strength [US-OTC]
Bayer(R) Extra Strength Arthritis
Pain Regimen [US-OTC]
Bayer(R) Plus Extra Strength
[US-OTC]
Bayer(R) Women's Aspirin Plus
Calcium [US-OTC]
Bufferin(R) [US-OTC]
Bufferin(R) Extra Strength [US-OTC]
Buffinol [US-OTC]
Buffinol Extra [US-OTC]
Cetafen(R) [US-OTC]
Cetafen Extra(R) [US-OTC]
Comtrex(R) Sore Throat Maximum
Strength [US-OTC]
Easprin(R) [US]
EC-Naprosyn(R) [US]

Ecotrin(R) [US-OTC]
Ecotrin(R) Low Strength [US-OTC]
Ecotrin(R) Maximum Strength
[US-OTC]
ElixSure(TM) IB [US-OTC]
Entrophen(R) [Can]
FeverAll(R) [US-OTC]
Genapap(TM) [US-OTC]
Genapap(TM) Children [US-OTC]
Genapap(TM) Extra Strength
[US-OTC]
Genapap(TM) Infant [US-OTC]
Genebs [US-OTC]
Genebs Extra Strength [US-OTC]
Gen-Naproxen EC [Can]
Genpril(R) [US-OTC]
Halfprin(R) [US-OTC]
Ibu-200 [US-OTC]
ibuprofen
Infantaire [US-OTC]
I-Prin [US-OTC]
Mapap [US-OTC]
Mapap Children's [US-OTC]
Mapap Extra Strength [US-OTC]
Mapap Infants [US-OTC]
Midol(R) Cramp and Body Aches
[US-OTC]
Midol(R) Extended Relief [US]
Motrin(R) [US]
Motrin(R) Children's
[US-OTC/Can]
Motrin(R) IB [US-OTC/Can]
Motrin(R) Infants' [US-OTC]
Motrin(R) Junior Strength [US-OTC]
Naprelan(R) [US]
Naprosyn(R) [US/Can]
naproxen
Naxen(R) [Can]
Naxen(R) EC [Can]
NeoProfen(R)
Nortemp Children's [US-OTC]
Novasen [Can]
Novo-Gesic [Can]
Novo-Naproc EC [Can]

Novo-Naprox [Can]
Novo-Naprox Sodium [Can]
Novo-Naprox Sodium DS [Can]
Novo-Naprox SR [Can]
Novo-Profen [Can]
Nu-Ibuprofen [Can]
Nu-Naprox [Can]
Pain-Eze [US-OTC]
Pamprin(R) Maximum Strength All
Day Relief [US-OTC]
Pediatrix [Can]
Proprinal [US-OTC]
Riva-Naproxen [Can]
Salflex(R) [Can]
salsalate
Silapap(R) Children's [US-OTC]
Silapap(R) Infants [US-OTC]
St. Joseph(R) Adult Aspirin
[US-OTC]
Sureprin 81(TM) [US-OTC]
Tempra(R) [Can]
Tycolene [US-OTC]
Tycolene Maximum Strength
[US-OTC]
Tylenol(R) [US-OTC/Can]
Tylenol(R) 8 Hour [US-OTC]
Tylenol(R) Arthritis Pain [US-OTC]
Tylenol(R) Children's [US-OTC]
Tylenol(R) Children's with Flavor
Creator [US-OTC]
Tylenol(R) Extra Strength [US-OTC]
Tylenol(R) Infants [US-OTC]
Tylenol(R) Junior [US-OTC]
Ultraprin [US-OTC]
Valorin [US-OTC]
Valorin Extra [US-OTC]
ZORprin(R) [US]

FIBROCYSTIC BREAST DISEASE
Androgen
Cyclomen(R) [Can]
danazol
Danocrine(R) [Can]

FIBROCYSTIC DISEASE
Vitamin, Fat Soluble
  Alph-E [US-OTC]
  Alph-E-Mixed [US-OTC]
  Aquasol E(R) [US-OTC]
  Aquavit-E(R) [US-OTC]
  d-Alpha-Gems(TM) [US-OTC]
  E-Gems(R) [US-OTC]
  E-Gems Elite(R) [US-OTC]
  E-Gems Plus(R) [US-OTC]
  Ester-E(TM) [US-OTC]
  Gamma E-Gems(R) [US-OTC]
  Gamma-E Plus [US-OTC]
  High Gamma Vitamin E
    Complete(TM) [US-OTC]
  Key-E(R) [US-OTC]
  Key-E(R) Kaps [US-OTC]
  vitamin E

FOLLICLE STIMULATION (SEE OVULATION INDUCTION/OVULATION STIMULATOR)

GENITAL HERPES
Antiviral Agent
  famciclovir
  Famvir(R) [US/Can]
  valacyclovir
  Valtrex(R) [US/Can]

GENITAL WART
Immune Response Modifier
  Aldara(TM) [US/Can]
  Imiquimod

GIARDIASIS
Amebicide
  Apo-Metronidazole(R) [Can]
  Flagyl(R) [US/Can]
  Flagyl ER(R) [US]
  Flagyl(R) I.V. RTU(TM) [US]
  Florazole(R) ER [Can]
  Humatin(R) [US/Can]
  MetroCream(R) [US/Can]
  MetroGel(R) [US/Can]
  MetroGel-Vaginal(R) [US]
  MetroLotion(R) [US]
  metronidazole
  Nidagel(TM) [Can]
  Noritate(R) [US/Can]
  paromomycin
  Trikacide [Can]
  Vandazole(TM) [US]
Anthelmintic
  albendazole
  Albenza(R) [US]
Antiprotozoal
  Apo-Metronidazole(R) [Can]
  Flagyl(R) [US/Can]
  Flagyl ER(R) [US]
  Flagyl(R) I.V. RTU(TM) [US]
  Florazole(R) ER [Can]
  MetroCream(R) [US/Can]
  MetroGel(R) [US/Can]
  MetroGel-Vaginal(R) [US]
  MetroLotion(R) [US]
  metronidazole
  Nidagel(TM) [Can]
  Noritate(R) [US/Can]
  Trikacide [Can]
  Vandazole(TM) [US]

GONOCOCCAL OPHTHALMIA NEONATORUM
Topical Skin Product
  silver nitrate

GONORRHEA
Antibiotic, Miscellaneous
  spectinomycin
Antibiotic, Quinolone
  gatifloxacin
  Tequin(R) [Can]
  Zymar(TM) [US/Can]
Antibiotic, Topical
  Apo-Tetra(R) [Can]
  Nu-Tetra [Can]
  Sumycin(R) [US]

tetracycline
Cephalosporin (Second Generation)
  Apo-Cefuroxime(R) [Can]
  cefoxitin
  Ceftin(R) [US/Can]
  cefuroxime
  Mefoxin(R) [US]
  ratio-Cefuroxime [Can]
  Zinacef(R) [US/Can]
Cephalosporin (Third Generation)
  ceftriaxone
  Rocephin(R) [US/Can]
Quinolone
  Apo-Ciproflox(R) [Can]
  Apo-Oflox(R) [Can]
  Apo-Ofloxacin(R) [Can]
  Ciloxan(R) [US/Can]
  Cipro(R) [US/Can]
  Cipro(R) XL [Can]
  ciprofloxacin
  Cipro(R) XR [US]
  CO Ciprofloxacin [Can]
  Floxin(R) [US/Can]
  Gen-Ciprofloxacin [Can]
  Novo-Ciprofloxacin [Can]
  Novo-Ofloxacin [Can]
  Ocuflox(R) [US/Can]
  ofloxacin
  PMS-Ciprofloxacin [Can]
  PMS-Ofloxacin [Can]
  Proquin(R) XR [US]
  RAN(TM)-Ciprofloxacin [Can]
  ratio-Ciprofloxacin [Can]
  Rhoxal-ciprofloxacin [Can]
  Sandoz-Ciprofloxacin [Can]
  Taro-Ciprofloxacin [Can]
Tetracycline Derivative
  Adoxa(TM) [US]
  Apo-Doxy(R) [Can]
  Apo-Doxy Tabs(R) [Can]
  Apo-Tetra(R) [Can]
  Doryx(R) [US]
  Doxy-100(R) [US]
  Doxycin [Can]

doxycycline
Doxytec [Can]
Monodox(R) [US]
Novo-Doxylin [Can]
Nu-Doxycycline [Can]
Nu-Tetra [Can]
Periostat(R) [US/Can]
Sumycin(R) [US]
tetracycline
Vibramycin(R) [US]
Vibra-Tabs(R) [US/Can]

GROWTH HORMONE DEFICIENCY
Growth Hormone
  Genotropin(R) [US]
  Genotropin Miniquick(R) [US]
  Humatrope(R) [US/Can]
  Norditropin(R) [US]
  Norditropin(R) NordiFlex(R) [US]
  Nutropin(R) [US]
  Nutropin AQ(R) [US]
  Nutropine(R) [Can]
  Omnitrope(TM) [US]
  Saizen(R) [US/Can]
  Serostim(R) [US/Can]
  somatropin
  Tev-Tropin(TM) [US]
  Zorbtive(TM) [US]

GROWTH HORMONE (DIAGNOSTIC)
Diagnostic Agent
  Geref(R) Diagnostic [US]
  sermorelin acetate

HEMOLYTIC DISEASE OF THE NEWBORN
Immune Globulin
  BayRho-D(R) Full-Dose [Can]
  HyperRHO(TM) S/D Full Dose [US]
  HyperRHO(TM) S/D Mini Dose [US]
  MICRhoGAM(R) [US]
  Rho(D) immune globulin
  RhoGAM(R) [US]

Rhophylac(R) [US]
WinRho(R) SDF [US]

HEMORRHAGE (POSTPARTUM)
Ergot Alkaloid and Derivative
  ergonovine
  Ergotrate(R) [US]
  Methergine(R) [US/Can]
  methylergonovine
Oxytocic Agent
  oxytocin
  Pitocin(R) [US/Can]
  Syntocinon(R) [Can]
Prostaglandin
  carboprost tromethamine
  Hemabate(R) [US/Can]

HERPES SIMPLEX
Antiviral Agent
  acyclovir
  Apo-Acyclovir(R) [Can]
  Cytovene(R) [US/Can]
  famciclovir
  Famvir(R) [US/Can]
  foscarnet
  Foscavir(R) [US/Can]
  ganciclovir
  Gen-Acyclovir [Can]
  Nu-Acyclovir [Can]
  ratio-Acyclovir [Can]
  SAB-Trifluridine [Can]
  Sandoz-Trifluridine [Can]
  trifluridine
  Viroptic(R) [US/Can]
  Vitrasert(R) [US/Can]
  Zovirax(R) [US/Can]
Antiviral Agent, Topical
  Abreva(R) [US-OTC]
  docosanol

HERPES ZOSTER
Analgesic, Topical
  ArthriCare(R) for Women Extra
    Moisturizing [US-OTC]

ArthriCare(R) for Women
    Multi-Action [US-OTC]
ArthriCare(R) for Women Silky Dry
    [US-OTC]
Capsagel(R) [US-OTC]
capsaicin
Capzasin-HP(R) [US-OTC]
Capzasin-P(R) [US-OTC]
Zostrix(R) [US-OTC/Can]
Zostrix(R)-HP
    [US-OTC/Can]
Antiviral Agent
  acyclovir
  Apo-Acyclovir(R)
    [Can]
  famciclovir
  Famvir(R) [US/Can]
  Gen-Acyclovir [Can]
  Nu-Acyclovir [Can]
  ratio-Acyclovir [Can]
  valacyclovir
  Valtrex(R) [US/Can]
  Zovirax(R) [US/Can]
Vaccine
  Zostavax(R) [US]
  zoster vaccine

H. INFLUENZAE
Toxoid
  diphtheria, tetanus toxoids, and
    acellular pertussis vaccine and
    Haemophilus influenzae b
    conjugate vaccine
  TriHIBit(R) [US]
Vaccine, Inactivated Bacteria
  ActHIB(R) [US/Can]
  diphtheria, tetanus toxoids, and
    acellular pertussis vaccine and
    Haemophilus influenzae b
    conjugate vaccine
  Haemophilus B conjugate vaccine
  HibTITER(R) [US]
  PedvaxHIB(R) [US/Can]
  TriHIBit(R) [US]

Vaccine, Inactivated Virus
  Comvax(R) [US]
  Haemophilus B conjugate and
    hepatitis B vaccine

HORMONAL IMBALANCE (FEMALE)

Progestin
  Alti-MPA [Can]
  Apo-Medroxy(R) [Can]
  Aygestin(R) [US]
  Camila(TM) [US]
  Crinone(R) [US/Can]
  Depo-Prevera(R) [Can]
  Depo-Provera(R) [US/Can]
  Depo-Provera(R) Contraceptive [US]
  depo-subQ provera 104(TM) [US]
  Errin(TM) [US]
  Gen-Medroxy [Can]
  Jolivette(TM) [US]
  medroxyprogesterone
  Micronor(R) [US/Can]
  Nora-BE(TM) [US]
  norethindrone
  Norlutate(R) [Can]
  Nor-QD(R) [US]
  Novo-Medrone [Can]
  Prochieve(TM) [US]
  progesterone
  Prometrium(R) [US/Can]
  Provera(R) [US/Can]
  Provera-Pak [Can]

HYDATIDIFORM MOLE (BENIGN)

Prostaglandin
  Cervidil(R) [US/Can]
  dinoprostone
  Prepidil(R) [US/Can]
  Prostin E2(R) [US/Can]

HYPERPLASIA, VULVAR SQUAMOUS

Estrogen Derivative
  Alora(R) [US]

Cenestin(R) [US]
Climara(R) [US/Can]
Delestrogen(R) [US]
Depo(R)-Estradiol [US/Can]
Esclim(R) [US]
Estrace(R) [US/Can]
Estraderm(R) [US/Can]
estradiol
Estradot(R) [Can]
Estrasorb(TM) [US]
Estratab(R) [Can]
Estring(R) [US/Can]
EstroGel(R) [US/Can]
estrogens (conjugated A/synthetic)
estrogens (conjugated/equine)
estrogens (esterified)
estropipate
Femring(TM) [US]
Femtrace(R) [US]
Gynodiol(R) [US]
Menest(R) [US/Can]
Menostar(TM) [US/Can]
Oesclim(R) [Can]
Ogen(R) [US/Can]
Ortho-Est(R) [US]
Premarin(R) [US/Can]
Sandoz-Estradiol Derm 50 [Can]
Sandoz-Estradiol Derm 75 [Can]
Sandoz-Estradiol Derm 100 [Can]
Vagifem(R) [US/Can]
Vivelle(R) [US]
Vivelle-Dot(R) [US]

HYPOGONADISM

Androgen
  Andriol(R) [Can]
  Androderm(R) [US/Can]
  AndroGel(R) [US/Can]
  Android(R) [US]
  Andropository [Can]
  Delatestryl(R) [US/Can]
  Depotest(R) 100 [Can]
  Depo(R)-Testosterone [US]
  Everone(R) 200 [Can]

First(R) Testosterone [US]
First(R) Testosterone MC [US]
Methitest(TM) [US]
methyltestosterone
Striant(R) [US]
Testim(R) [US]
Testopel(R) [US]
testosterone
Testred(R) [US]
Virilon(R) [US]
Virilon(R) IM [Can]
Diagnostic Agent
  Factrel(R) [US]
  gonadorelin
  Lutrepulse(TM) [Can]
Estrogen and Androgen Combination
  Estratest(R) [US/Can]
  Estratest(R) H.S. [US]
  estrogens (esterified) and
    methyltestosterone
  Syntest D.S. [US]
  Syntest H.S. [US]
Estrogen Derivative
  Alora(R) [US]
  Cenestin(R) [US]
  Climara(R) [US/Can]
  Delestrogen(R) [US]
  Depo(R)-Estradiol [US/Can]
  Esclim(R) [US]
  Estrace(R) [US/Can]
  Estraderm(R) [US/Can]
  estradiol
  Estradot(R) [Can]
  Estrasorb(TM) [US]
  Estratab(R) [Can]
  Estring(R) [US/Can]
  EstroGel(R) [US/Can]
  estrogens (conjugated A/synthetic)
  estrogens (conjugated/equine)
  estrogens (esterified)
  estropipate
  Femring(TM) [US]
  Femtrace(R) [US]
  Gynodiol(R) [US]

Menest(R) [US/Can]
Menostar(TM) [US/Can]
Oesclim(R) [Can]
Ogen(R) [US/Can]
Ortho-Est(R) [US]
Premarin(R) [US/Can]
Sandoz-Estradiol Derm 50 [Can]
Sandoz-Estradiol Derm 75 [Can]
Sandoz-Estradiol Derm 100 [Can]
Vagifem(R) [US/Can]
Vivelle(R) [US]
Vivelle-Dot(R) [US]
Gonadotropin
  Factrel(R) [US]
  gonadorelin
  Lutrepulse(TM) [Can]

HYPOGONADOTROPIC HYPOGONADAL (HH)
Gonadotropin
  lutropin alfa
  Luveris(R) [US]
Ovulation Stimulator
  lutropin alfa
  Luveris(R) [US]

IMPETIGO
Antibiotic, Ophthalmic
  bacitracin, neomycin, and
    polymyxin B
  Neosporin(R) Neo To Go(R)
    [US-OTC]
  Neosporin(R) Ophthalmic Ointment
    [Can]
  Neosporin(R) Topical [US-OTC]
Antibiotic, Topical
  bacitracin, neomycin, and
    polymyxin B
  Bactroban(R) [US/Can]
  Bactroban(R) Nasal [US]
  Centany(TM) [US]
  mupirocin
  Neosporin(R) Neo To Go(R)
    [US-OTC]

Neosporin(R) Ophthalmic Ointment
[Can]
Neosporin(R) Topical [US-OTC]
Penicillin
Apo-Pen VK(R) [Can]
Novo-Pen-VK [Can]
Nu-Pen-VK [Can]
penicillin V potassium
penicillin G procaine
Pfizerpen-AS(R) [Can]
Veetids(R) [US]
Wycillin(R) [Can]

INFERTILITY (FEMALE)
Antigonadotropic Agent
Antagon(R) [US/Can]
ganirelix
Orgalutran(R) [Can]
Anti-Parkinson Agent
Apo-Bromocriptine(R) [Can]
bromocriptine
Parlodel(R) [US/Can]
PMS-Bromocriptine [Can]
Ergot Alkaloid and Derivative
Apo-Bromocriptine(R) [Can]
bromocriptine
Parlodel(R) [US/Can]
PMS-Bromocriptine [Can]
Gonadotropin
chorionic gonadotropin
(human)
Humegon(R) [Can]
Menopur(R) [US]
menotropins
Novarel(R) [US]
Pregnyl(R) [US]
Profasi(R) HP [Can]
Repronex(R) [US/Can]
Ovulation Stimulator
Clomid(R) [US/Can]
clomiphene
follitropin alfa
follitropin beta
Gonal-f(R) [US/Can]

Milophene(R) [Can]
Serophene(R) [US/Can]
Progestin
Crinone(R) [US/Can]
Prochieve(TM) [US]
progesterone
Prometrium(R) [US/Can]

LABOR INDUCTION
Oxytocic Agent
oxytocin
Pitocin(R) [US/Can]
Syntocinon(R) [Can]
Prostaglandin
carboprost tromethamine
Cervidil(R) [US/Can]
dinoprostone
Hemabate(R) [US/Can]
Prepidil(R) [US/Can]
Prostin E2(R) [US/Can]

LABOR (PREMATURE)
Adrenergic Agonist Agent
Brethine(R) [US]
Bricanyl(R) [Can]
terbutaline

LACTATION (SUPPRESSION)
Anti-Parkinson Agent
Apo-Bromocriptine(R) [Can]
bromocriptine
Parlodel(R) [US/Can]
PMS-Bromocriptine [Can]
Ergot Alkaloid and Derivative
Apo-Bromocriptine(R) [Can]
bromocriptine
Parlodel(R) [US/Can]
PMS-Bromocriptine [Can]

LACTOSE INTOLERANCE
Nutritional Supplement
Dairyaid(R) [Can]
Lactaid(R) Fast Act [US-OTC]
Lactaid(R) Original [US-OTC]

lactase
Lactrase(R) [US-OTC]

LEAD POISONING
Chelating Agent
BAL in Oil(R) [US]
Calcium Disodium Versenate(R) [US]
Chemet(R) [US/Can]
Cuprimine(R) [US/Can]
Depen(R) [US/Can]
dimercaprol
edetate calcium disodium
penicillamine
succimer

LICE
Scabicides/Pediculicides
A200(R) Lice [US-OTC]
A-200(R) Maximum Strength
[US-OTC]
Acticin(R) [US]
Elimite(R) [US]
Hexit(TM) [Can]
Kwellada-P(TM) [Can]
Lice-Aid [US-OTC]
Licide(R) [US-OTC]
lindane
malathion
Nix(R) [US-OTC/Can]
Ovide(R) [US]
permethrin
PMS-Lindane [Can]
Pronto(R) Complete Lice Killing Kit
[US-OTC]
Pronto(R) Lice Control [Can]
Pronto(R) Plus Hair and Scalp
Masque [US-OTC]
Pronto(R) Plus Mousse [US-OTC]
Pronto(R) Plus Warm Oil Treatment
and Conditioner [US-OTC]
Pronto(R) Plus with Natural Extracts
and Oils [US-OTC]
pyrethrins and piperonyl butoxide
Pyrinyl Plus(R) [US-OTC]
R&C(TM) II [Can]

R&C(TM) Shampoo/Conditioner
[Can]
RID(R) Maximum Strength
[US-OTC]
RID(R) Mousse [Can]
Rid(R) Spray [US-OTC]
Tisit(R) [US-OTC]
Tisit(R) Blue Gel [US-OTC]

LUNG SURFACTANT
Lung Surfactant
beractant
Survanta(R) [US/Can]

MAPLE SYRUP URINE DISEASE
Vitamin, Water Soluble
Betaxin(R) [Can]
thiamine

MEASLES
Vaccine, Live Virus
Attenuvax(R) [US]
M-M-R(R) II [US/Can]
measles, mumps, and rubella
vaccines, combined
measles, mumps, rubella, and
varicella virus vaccine
measles virus vaccine (live)
Priorix(TM) [Can]
ProQuad(R) [US]

MEASLES (RUBEOLA)
Immune Globulin
BayGam(R) [Can]
GannaSTAN(TM) S/D [US]
immune globulin (intramuscular)

MECONIUM ILEUS
Mucolytic Agent
Acetadote(R) [US]
acetylcysteine
Acetylcysteine Solution [Can]
Mucomyst(R) [Can]
Parvolex(R) [Can]

MELASMA (FACIAL)

Corticosteroid, Topical
  fluocinolone, hydroquinone, and
    tretinoin
  Tri-Luma(TM) [US]
Depigmenting Agent
  fluocinolone, hydroquinone, and
    tretinoin
  Tri-Luma(TM) [US]
Retinoic Acid Derivative
  fluocinolone, hydroquinone, and
    tretinoin
  Tri-Luma(TM) [US]

MENOPAUSE

Ergot Derivative
  belladonna, phenobarbital, and
    ergotamine
  Bellamine S [US]
  Bellergal(R) Spacetabs(R)
    [Can]
  Bel-Tabs [US]
Estrogen and Androgen Combination
  Estratest(R) [US/Can]
  Estratest(R) H.S. [US]
  estrogens (esterified) and
    methyltestosterone
  Syntest D.S. [US]
  Syntest H.S. [US]
Estrogen and Progestin Combination
  Activella(R) [US]
  Angeliq(R) [US/Can]
  ClimaraPro(R) [US]
  CombiPatch(R) [US]
  drospirenone and estradiol
  Estalis(R) [Can]
  Estalis-Sequi(R) [Can]
  estradiol and levonorgestrel
  estradiol and norethindrone
  estradiol and norgestimate
  estrogens (conjugated/equine) and
    medroxyprogesterone
  Prefest(TM) [US]
  Premphase(R) [US/Can]

Premplus(R) [Can]
Prempro(TM) [US/Can]
Estrogen Derivative
  Alora(R) [US]
  Cenestin(R) [US]
  Climara(R) [US/Can]
  Delestrogen(R) [US]
  Depo(R)-Estradiol [US/Can]
  Esclim(R) [US]
  Estrace(R) [US/Can]
  Estraderm(R) [US/Can]
  estradiol
  Estradot(R) [Can]
  Estrasorb(TM) [US]
  Estratab(R) [Can]
  Estring(R) [US/Can]
  EstroGel(R) [US/Can]
  estrogens (conjugated A/
    synthetic)
  estrogens (conjugated/equine)
  estrogens (esterified)
  Femring(TM) [US]
  Femtrace(R) [US]
  Gynodiol(R) [US]
  Menest(R) [US/Can]
  Menostar(TM) [US/Can]
  Oesclim(R) [Can]
  Premarin(R) [US/Can]
  Sandoz-Estradiol Derm 50 [Can]
  Sandoz-Estradiol Derm 75 [Can]
  Sandoz-Estradiol Derm 100 [Can]
  Vagifem(R) [US/Can]
  Vivelle(R) [US]
  Vivelle-Dot(R) [US]

MENORRHAGIA

Androgen
  Cyclomen(R) [Can]
  danazol
  Danocrine(R) [Can]

MERCURY POISONING

Chelating Agent
  BAL in Oil(R) [US]
  Dimercaprol

MUMPS
Vaccine, Live Virus
  M-M-R(R) II [US/Can]
  measles, mumps, and rubella
    vaccines, combined
  measles, mumps, rubella, and
    varicella virus vaccine
  Mumpsvax(R) [US]
  mumps virus vaccine, live, attenuated
  Priorix(TM) [Can]
  ProQuad(R) [US]

NIPPLE CARE
Topical Skin Product
  glycerin
  lanolin
  peanut oil

OBSESSIVE-COMPULSIVE DISORDER (OCD)
Antidepressant, Selective Serotonin
  Reuptake Inhibitor
  Alti-Fluoxetine [Can]
  Alti-Fluvoxamine [Can]
  Apo-Fluoxetine(R) [Can]
  Apo-Fluvoxamine(R) [Can]
  Apo-Sertraline(R) [Can]
  BCI-Fluoxetine [Can]
  CO Fluoxetine [Can]
  fluoxetine
  fluvoxamine
  FXT [Can]
  Gen-Fluoxetine [Can]
  Gen-Sertraline [Can]
  GMD-Sertraline [Can]
  Luvox(R) [Can]
  Novo-Fluoxetine [Can]
  Novo-Fluvoxamine [Can]
  Novo-Sertraline [Can]
  Nu-Fluoxetine [Can]
  Nu-Fluvoxamine [Can]
  Nu-Sertraline [Can]
  PMS-Fluoxetine [Can]
  PMS-Fluvoxamine [Can]
  PMS-Sertraline [Can]
  Prozac(R) [US/Can]
  Prozac(R) Weekly(TM) [US]
  ratio-Sertraline [Can]
  Rhoxal-fluoxetine [Can]
  Rhoxal-fluvoxamine [Can]
  Rhoxal-Sertraline [Can]
  Sandoz-Fluoxetine [Can]
  Sandoz-Fluvoxamine [Can]
  Sandoz-Sertraline [Can]
  Sarafem(R) [US]
  sertraline
  Zoloft(R) [US/Can]
Antidepressant, Tricyclic (Tertiary
  Amine)
  Anafranil(R) [US/Can]
  Apo-Clomipramine(R) [Can]
  clomipramine
  CO Clomipramine [Can]
  Gen-Clomipramine [Can]

OILY SKIN (SEE ACNE/ANTISEBORRHEIC AGENT, TOPICAL)

OPIATE WITHDRAWAL (NEONATAL)
Analgesic, Narcotic
  Paregoric

OTITIS EXTERNA
Adrenal Corticosteroid
  Cutivate(R) [US]
  fluticasone (topical)
Aminoglycoside (Antibiotic)
  AKTob(R) [US]
  Alcomicin(R) [Can]
  amikacin
  Amikacin Sulfate Injection, USP [Can]
  Amikin(R) [US/Can]
  Diogent(R) [Can]
  Garamycin(R) [Can]
  Gentak(R) [US]
  gentamicin
  Gentamicin Injection, USP [Can]

kanamycin
Kantrex(R) [US/Can]
Neo-Fradin(TM) [US]
neomycin
Neo-Rx [US]
PMS-Tobramycin [Can]
SAB-Gentamicin [Can]
Sandoz-Tobramycin [Can]
TOBI(R) [US/Can]
tobramycin
Tobramycin Injection, USP [Can]
Tobrex(R) [US/Can]
Antibacterial, Otic
acetic acid
Antibacterial, Topical
acetic acid
Antibiotic/Corticosteroid, Otic
Acetasol(R) HC [US]
acetic acid, propylene glycol
diacetate, and hydrocortisone
Ciprodex(R) [US/Can]
ciprofloxacin and dexamethasone
ciprofloxacin and hydrocortisone
Cipro(R) HC [US/Can]
Coly-Mycin(R) S [US]
Cortimyxin(R) [Can]
Cortisporin(R) Cream [US]
Cortisporin(R) Ophthalmic [US]
Cortisporin(R) Otic [US/Can]
Cortisporin(R)-TC [US]
neomycin, colistin, hydrocortisone,
and thonzonium
neomycin, polymyxin B, and
hydrocortisone
PediOtic(R) [US]
VoSol(R) HC [US]
Antibiotic, Miscellaneous
chloramphenicol
Chloromycetin(R) [Can]
Chloromycetin(R) Sodium Succinate
[US]
Chloromycetin(R) Succinate [Can]
Diochloram(R) [Can]
Pentamycetin(R) [Can]

Antibiotic, Otic
Apo-Oflox(R) [Can]
Apo-Ofloxacin(R) [Can]
chloramphenicol
Chloromycetin(R) [Can]
Chloromycetin(R) Sodium Succinate
[US]
Chloromycetin(R) Succinate [Can]
Diochloram(R) [Can]
Floxin(R) [US/Can]
Novo-Ofloxacin [Can]
Ocuflox(R) [US/Can]
ofloxacin
Pentamycetin(R) [Can]
PMS-Ofloxacin [Can]
Antifungal/Corticosteroid
Dermazene(R) [US]
iodoquinol and hydrocortisone
Vytone(R) [US]
Cephalosporin (Third Generation)
ceftazidime
Fortaz(R) [US/Can]
Tazicef(R) [US]
Otic Agent, Analgesic
A/B Otic [US]
Allergen(R) [US]
antipyrine and benzocaine
Auralgan(R) [Can]
Aurodex [US]
Otic Agent, Antiinfective
Cresylate(R) [US]
m-cresyl acetate
Otic Agent, Ceruminolytic
A/B Otic [US]
Allergen(R) [US]
antipyrine and benzocaine
Auralgan(R) [Can]
Aurodex [US]
Quinolone
Apo-Ciproflox(R) [Can]
Apo-Oflox(R) [Can]
Apo-Ofloxacin(R) [Can]
Ciloxan(R) [US/Can]
Cipro(R) [US/Can]

Cipro(R) XL [Can]
ciprofloxacin
Cipro(R) XR [US]
CO Ciprofloxacin [Can]
Floxin(R) [US/Can]
Gen-Ciprofloxacin [Can]
Novo-Ciprofloxacin [Can]
Novo-Ofloxacin [Can]
ofloxacin
PMS-Ciprofloxacin [Can]
PMS-Ofloxacin [Can]
Proquin(R) XR [US]
RAN(TM)-Ciprofloxacin [Can]
ratio-Ciprofloxacin [Can]
Rhoxal-ciprofloxacin [Can]
Sandoz-Ciprofloxacin [Can]
Taro-Ciprofloxacin [Can]

OTITIS MEDIA
Antibiotic, Carbacephem
Lorabid(R) [US/Can]
loracarbef
Antibiotic/Corticosteroid, Otic
Ciprodex(R) [US/Can]
ciprofloxacin and dexamethasone
Antibiotic, Miscellaneous
Apo-Trimethoprim(R) [Can]
Primsol(R) [US]
Proloprim(R) [US]
trimethoprim
Antibiotic, Otic
Apo-Oflox(R) [Can]
Apo-Ofloxacin(R) [Can]
Floxin(R) [US/Can]
Novo-Ofloxacin [Can]
Ocuflox(R) [US/Can]
ofloxacin
PMS-Ofloxacin [Can]
Cephalosporin (First Generation)
Apo-Cefadroxil(R) [Can]
Apo-Cephalex(R) [Can]
Biocef(R) [US]
cefadroxil
cephalexin

Duricef(R) [US/Can]
Keflex(R) [US]
Keftab(R) [Can]
Novo-Cefadroxil [Can]
Novo-Lexin [Can]
Nu-Cephalex [Can]
Cephalosporin (Second Generation)
Apo-Cefaclor(R) [Can]
Apo-Cefuroxime(R) [Can]
Ceclor(R) [Can]
cefaclor
cefpodoxime
cefprozil
Ceftin(R) [US/Can]
cefuroxime
Cefzil(R) [US/Can]
Novo-Cefaclor [Can]
Nu-Cefaclor [Can]
PMS-Cefaclor [Can]
Raniclor(TM) [US]
ratio-Cefuroxime [Can]
Vantin(R) [US/Can]
Zinacef(R) [US/Can]
Cephalosporin (Third Generation)
Cedax(R) [US]
cefdinir
ceftibuten
Omnicef(R) [US/Can]
Macrolide (Antibiotic)
Akne-Mycin(R) [US]
Apo-Erythro Base(R) [Can]
Apo-Erythro E-C(R) [Can]
Apo-Erythro-ES(R) [Can]
Apo-Erythro-S(R) [Can]
A/T/S(R) [US]
Diomycin(R) [Can]
E.E.S.(R) [US/Can]
Erybid(TM) [Can]
Eryc(R) [US/Can]
Eryderm(R) [US]
Erygel(R) [US]
EryPed(R) [US]
Ery-Tab(R) [US]
Erythrocin(R) [US]

erythromycin
erythromycin and sulfisoxazole
Novo-Rythro Estolate [Can]
Novo-Rythro Ethylsuccinate [Can]
Nu-Erythromycin-S [Can]
PCE(R) [US/Can]
Pediazole(R) [US/Can]
PMS-Erythromycin [Can]
Romycin(R) [US]
Sans Acne(R) [Can]
Theramycin Z(R) [US]
Otic Agent, Analgesic
A/B Otic [US]
Allergen(R) [US]
antipyrine and benzocaine
Auralgan(R) [Can]
Aurodex [US]
Otic Agent, Ceruminolytic
A/B Otic [US]
Allergen(R) [US]
antipyrine and benzocaine
Auralgan(R) [Can]
Aurodex [US]
Penicillin
Alti-Amoxi-Clav [Can]
amoxicillin
amoxicillin and clavulanate
  potassium
Amoxil(R) [US]
ampicillin
Apo-Amoxi(R) [Can]
Apo-Amoxi-Clav(R) [Can]
Apo-Ampi(R) [Can]
Augmentin(R) [US/Can]
Augmentin ES-600(R) [US]
Augmentin XR(TM) [US]
Clavulin(R) [Can]
Gen-Amoxicillin [Can]
Lin-Amox [Can]
Novamoxin(R) [Can]
Novo-Ampicillin [Can]
Novo-Clavamoxin [Can]
Nu-Amoxi [Can]
Nu-Ampi [Can]

PHL-Amoxicillin [Can]
pivampicillin (Canada only)
PMS-Amoxicillin [Can]
Pondocillin(R) [Can]
ratio-Aclavulanate [Can]
Quinolone
Apo-Oflox(R) [Can]
Apo-Ofloxacin(R) [Can]
Floxin(R) [US/Can]
Novo-Ofloxacin [Can]
Ocuflox(R) [US/Can]
ofloxacin
PMS-Ofloxacin [Can]
Sulfonamide
Apo-Sulfatrim(R) [Can]
Apo-Sulfatrim(R) DS [Can]
Apo-Sulfatrim(R) Pediatric [Can]
Bactrim(TM) [US]
Bactrim(TM) DS [US]
erythromycin and sulfisoxazole
Gantrisin(R) [US]
Novo-Soxazole [Can]
Novo-Trimel [Can]
Novo-Trimel D.S. [Can]
Nu-Cotrimox [Can]
Pediazole(R) [US/Can]
Septra(R) [US]
Septra(R) DS [US]
Septra(R) Injection [Can]
sulfamethoxazole and trimethoprim
sulfisoxazole
Sulfizole(R) [Can]
Tetracycline Derivative
Adoxa(TM) [US]
Alti-Minocycline [Can]
Apo-Doxy(R) [Can]
Apo-Doxy Tabs(R) [Can]
Apo-Minocycline(R) [Can]
Apo-Tetra(R) [Can]
Doryx(R) [US]
Doxy-100(R) [US]
Doxycin [Can]
doxycycline
Doxytec [Can]

Dynacin(R) [US]
Gen-Minocycline [Can]
Minocin(R) [US/Can]
minocycline
Monodox(R) [US]
myrac(TM) [US]
Novo-Doxylin [Can]
Novo-Minocycline [Can]
Nu-Doxycycline [Can]
Nu-Tetra [Can]
oxytetracycline
Periostat(R) [US/Can]
Rhoxal-minocycline [Can]
Sandoz-Minocycline [Can]
Solodyn(TM) [US]
Sumycin(R) [US]
Terramycin(R) [Can]
tetracycline
Vibramycin(R) [US]
Vibra-Tabs(R) [US/Can]

OVULATION INDUCTION
Gonadotropin
chorionic gonadotropin (human)
chorionic gonadotropin (recombinant)
Humegon(R) [Can]
Menopur(R) [US]
menotropins
Novarel(R) [US]
Ovidrel(R) [US/Can]
Pregnyl(R) [US]
Profasi(R) HP [Can]
Repronex(R) [US/Can]
Ovulation Stimulator
chorionic gonadotropin (recombinant)
Clomid(R) [US/Can]
clomiphene
Milophene(R) [Can]
Ovidrel(R) [US/Can]
Serophene(R) [US/Can]

PAIN (ANOGENITAL)
Anesthetic/Corticosteroid
Analpram-HC(R) [US]
Enzone(R) [US]

Epifoam(R) [US]
Pramosone(R) [US]
Pramox(R) HC [Can]
pramoxine and hydrocortisone
ProctoFoam(R)-HC [US/Can]
Zone-A(R) [US]
Zone-A Forte(R) [US]
Local Anesthetic
Americaine(R) [US-OTC]
Americaine(R) Hemorrhoidal
[US-OTC]
Ametop(TM) [Can]
Anbesol(R) [US-OTC]
Anbesol(R) Baby [US-OTC/Can]
Anbesol(R) Cold Sore Therapy
[US-OTC]
Anbesol(R) Jr. [US-OTC]
Anbesol(R) Maximum Strength
[US-OTC]
Anusol(R) Ointment [US-OTC]
benzocaine
Benzodent(R) [US-OTC]
Caladryl(R) Clear [US-OTC]
CalaMycin(R) Cool and Clear
[US-OTC]
Callergy Clear [US-OTC]
Cepacol(R) Sore Throat [US-OTC]
Cepacol(R) Dual Action Maximum
Strength [US-OTC]
Chiggerex(R) [US-OTC]
Chiggertox(R) [US-OTC]
Curasore [US-OTC]
Cylex(R) [US-OTC]
Dentapaine [US-OTC]
Dent's Extra Strength Toothache
[US-OTC]
Dent's Maxi-Strength Toothache
[US-OTC]
Dermoplast(R) Antibacterial
[US-OTC]
Dermoplast(R) Pain Relieving
[US-OTC]
Detane(R) [US-OTC]
dibucaine

dyclonine
Foille(R) [US-OTC]
HDA(R) Toothache [US-OTC]
Hurricaine(R) [US-OTC]
Itch-X(R) [US-OTC]
Ivy-Rid(R) [US-OTC]
Kanka(R) Soft Brush(TM) [US-OTC]
Lanacane(R) [US-OTC]
Lanacane(R) Maximum Strength
 [US-OTC]
Mycinettes(R) [US-OTC]
Nupercainal(R) [US-OTC]
Orabase(R) with Benzocaine
 [US-OTC]
Orajel(R) Baby Teething [US-OTC]
Orajel(R) Baby Teething Daytime
 and Nighttime [US-OTC]
Orajel(R) Baby Teething Nighttime
 [US-OTC]
Orajel(R) Denture Plus [US-OTC]
Orajel(R) Maximum Strength
 [US-OTC]
Orajel(R) Medicated Toothache
 [US-OTC]
Orajel(R) Mouth Sore [US-OTC]
Orajel(R) Multi-Action Cold Sore
 [US-OTC]
Orajel PM(R) [US-OTC]
Orajel(R) Ultra Mouth Sore
 [US-OTC]
Oticaine [US]
Otocaine(TM) [US]
Outgro(R) [US-OTC]
Pontocaine(R) [US/Can]
Pontocaine(R) Niphanoid(R) [US]
pramoxine
Prax(R) [US-OTC]
ProctoFoam(R) NS [US-OTC]
Red Cross(TM) Canker Sore
 [US-OTC]
Rid-A-Pain Dental Drops [US-OTC]
Sarna(R) Sensitive [US]
Skeeter Stik [US-OTC]
Sting-Kill [US-OTC]

Sucrets(R) [US-OTC]
Tanac(R) [US-OTC]
tetracaine
Thorets [US-OTC]
Trocaine(R) [US-OTC]
Tronolane(R) [US-OTC]
Tucks(R) Hemorrhoidal [US-OTC]
Zilactin(R)-B [US-OTC/Can]
Zilactin Baby(R) [Can]
Zilactin Toothache and Gum Pain(R)
 [US-OTC]

PELVIC INFLAMMATORY DISEASE (PID)

Aminoglycoside (Antibiotic)
 AKTob(R) [US]
 Alcomicin(R) [Can]
 amikacin
 Amikacin Sulfate Injection, USP
  [Can]
 Amikin(R) [US/Can]
 Diogent(R) [Can]
 Garamycin(R) [Can]
 gentamicin
 Gentamicin Injection, USP [Can]
 PMS-Tobramycin [Can]
 SAB-Gentamicin [Can]
 Sandoz-Tobramycin [Can]
 TOBI(R) [US/Can]
 tobramycin
 Tobramycin Injection, USP [Can]
 Tobrex(R) [US/Can]
Cephalosporin (Second Generation)
 cefoxitin
 Mefoxin(R) [US]
Cephalosporin (Third Generation)
 Cefizox(R) [US/Can]
 cefotaxime
 ceftizoxime
 ceftriaxone
 Claforan(R) [US/Can]
 Rocephin(R) [US/Can]
Macrolide (Antibiotic)
 Akne-Mycin(R) [US]

Apo-Azithromycin(R) [Can]
Apo-Erythro Base(R) [Can]
Apo-Erythro E-C(R) [Can]
Apo-Erythro-ES(R) [Can]
Apo-Erythro-S(R) [Can]
A/T/S(R) [US]
azithromycin
CO Azithromycin [Can]
Diomycin(R) [Can]
E.E.S.(R) [US/Can]
Erybid(TM) [Can]
Eryc(R) [US/Can]
Eryderm(R) [US]
Erygel(R) [US]
EryPed(R) [US]
Ery-Tab(R) [US]
Erythrocin(R) [US]
erythromycin
GMD-Azithromycin [Can]
Novo-Azithromycin [Can]
Novo-Rythro Estolate [Can]
Novo-Rythro Ethylsuccinate
    [Can]
Nu-Erythromycin-S [Can]
PCE(R) [US/Can]
PMS-Azithromycin [Can]
PMS-Erythromycin [Can]
ratio-Azithromycin [Can]
Romycin(R) [US]
Sandoz-Azithromycin [Can]
Sans Acne(R) [Can]
Theramycin Z(R) [US]
Zithromax(R) [US/Can]
Zmax(TM) [US]
Penicillin
ampicillin and sulbactam
piperacillin
piperacillin and tazobactam sodium
Piperacillin for Injection, USP [Can]
Tazocin(R) [Can]
Ticar(R) [US]
ticarcillin
ticarcillin and clavulanate potassium
Timentin(R) [US/Can]

Unasyn(R) [US/Can]
Zosyn(R) [US]
Quinolone
Apo-Ciproflox(R) [Can]
Apo-Oflox(R) [Can]
Apo-Ofloxacin(R) [Can]
Cipro(R) [US/Can]
Cipro(R) XL [Can]
ciprofloxacin
Cipro(R) XR [US]
CO Ciprofloxacin [Can]
Floxin(R) [US/Can]
Gen-Ciprofloxacin [Can]
Novo-Ciprofloxacin [Can]
Novo-Ofloxacin [Can]
Ocuflox(R) [US/Can]
ofloxacin
PMS-Ciprofloxacin [Can]
PMS-Ofloxacin [Can]
Proquin(R) XR [US]
RAN(TM)-Ciprofloxacin [Can]
ratio-Ciprofloxacin [Can]
Rhoxal-ciprofloxacin [Can]
Sandoz-Ciprofloxacin [Can]
Taro-Ciprofloxacin [Can]
Tetracycline Derivative
Adoxa(TM) [US]
Apo-Doxy(R) [Can]
Apo-Doxy Tabs(R) [Can]
Apo-Tetra(R) [Can]
Doryx(R) [US]
Doxy-100(R) [US]
Doxycin [Can]
doxycycline
Doxytec [Can]
Monodox(R) [US]
Novo-Doxylin [Can]
Nu-Doxycycline [Can]
Nu-Tetra [Can]
Periostat(R) [US/Can]
Sumycin(R) [US]
tetracycline
Vibramycin(R) [US]
Vibra-Tabs(R) [US/Can]

PERTUSSIS
Toxoid
    Adacel(TM) [US/Can]
    Boostrix(R) [US]
    Daptacel(R) [US]
    diphtheria, tetanus toxoids, and
      acellular pertussis vaccine
    diphtheria, tetanus toxoids, and
      acellular pertussis vaccine and
    Haemophilus influenzae b conjugate
      vaccine
    Infanrix(R) [US]
    TriHIBit(R) [US]
    Tripedia(R) [US]
Vaccine, Inactivated Bacteria
    diphtheria, tetanus toxoids, and
      acellular pertussis vaccine and
    Haemophilus influenzae b conjugate
      vaccine
    TriHIBit(R) [US]

PINWORMS
Anthelmintic
    Combantrin(TM) [Can]
    mebendazole
    Pamix(TM) [US-OTC]
    Pin-X(R) [US-OTC]
    pyrantel pamoate
    Reese's(R) Pinworm Medicine
    [US-OTC]
    Vermox(R) [Can]

PITUITARY FUNCTION TEST (GROWTH HORMONE)
Diagnostic Agent
    arginine
    R-Gene(R) [US]

PITYRIASIS (ROSEA)
Corticosteroid, Topical
    Aclovate(R) [US]
    alclometasone
    amcinonide

Amcort(R) [Can]
ApexiCon(TM) [US]
ApexiCon(TM) E [US]
Aquacort(R) [Can]
Aquanil(TM) HC [US-OTC]
Aristocort(R) A [US]
Asmanex(R) Twisthaler(R) [US]
Betaderm [Can]
Beta-HC(R) [US]
betamethasone (topical)
Beta-Val(R) [US]
Betnesol(R) [Can]
Betnovate(R) [Can]
Caldecort(R) [US-OTC]
Capex(TM) [US/Can]
Carmol-HC(R) [US]
Cetacort(R) [US]
clobetasol
Clobevate(R) [US]
Clobex(R) [US/Can]
clocortolone
Cloderm(R) [US/Can]
Cordran(R) [US/Can]
Cordran(R) SP [US]
Cormax(R) [US]
Cortaid(R) Intensive Therapy [US-OTC]
Cortaid(R) Maximum Strength [US-OTC]
Cortaid(R) Sensitive Skin [US-OTC]
Cortamed(R) [Can]
Corticool(R) [US-OTC]
Cortizone(R)-10 Maximum Strength [US-OTC]
Cortizone(R)-10 Plus Maximum Strength [US-OTC]
Cortizone(R)-10 Quick Shot [US-OTC]
Cutivate(R) [US]
Cyclocort(R) [US/Can]
Dermarest Dricort(R) [US-OTC]

Derma-Smoothe/FS(R) [US/Can]
Dermatop(R) [US/Can]
Dermovate(R) [Can]
Dermtex(R) HC [US-OTC]
Desocort(R) [Can]
desonide
DesOwen(R) [US]
desoximetasone
diflorasone
Diprolene(R) [US]
Diprolene(R) AF [US]
Diprolene(R) Glycol [Can]
Diprosone(R) [Can]
Ectosone [Can]
Elocom(R) [Can]
Elocon(R) [US]
Florone(R) [US/Can]
fluocinolone
fluocinonide
flurandrenolide
fluticasone (topical)
Gen-Clobetasol [Can]
halcinonide
halobetasol
Halog(R) [US/Can]
Hemril(R)-30 [US]
Hycort(TM) [Can]
Hyderm [Can]
hydrocortisone (topical)
HydroZone Plus [US-OTC]
Hytone(R) [US]
IvySoothe(R) [US-OTC]
Kenalog(R) [US/Can]
Lidemol(R) [Can]
Lidex(R) [US/Can]
Lidex-E(R) [US]
Locoid(R) [US/Can]
Locoid Lipocream(R) [US]
LoKara(TM) [US]
Luxiq(R) [US]
Lyderm(R) [Can]
Maxivate(R) [US]
mometasone furoate

Nasonex(R) [US/Can]
Novo-Clobetasol [Can]
Nupercainal(R) Hydrocortisone
   Cream [US-OTC]
Nutracort(R) [US]
Olux(R) [US]
Pandel(R) [US]
PMS-Desonide [Can]
PMS-Mometasone [Can]
Post Peel Healing Balm
   [US-OTC]
prednicarbate
Prevex(R) B [Can]
Prevex(R) HC [Can]
Psorcon(R) [Can]
Psorcon(R) e(TM) [US]
ratio-Amcinonide [Can]
ratio-Mometasone [Can]
Retisert(TM) [US]
Sarna(R) HC [Can]
Sarnol(R)-HC [US-OTC]
Summer's Eve(R) SpecialCare(TM)
   Medicated Anti-Itch Cream
   [US-OTC]
Synalar(R) [US/Can]
Taro-Amcinonide [Can]
Taro-Clobetasol [Can]
Taro-Desoximetasone [Can]
Taro-Mometasone [Can]
Taro-Sone(R) [Can]
Temovate(R) [US]
Temovate E(R) [US]
Texacort(R) [US]
Tiamol(R) [Can]
Ti-U-Lac(R) H [Can]
Topicort(R) [US/Can]
Topicort(R)-LP [US]
Topilene(R) [Can]
Topisone(R) [Can]
Topsyn(R) [Can]
Triaderm [Can]
triamcinolone (topical)
Triderm(R) [US]

Tridesilon(R) [US]
Tucks(R) Anti-Itch [US-OTC]
Ultravate(R) [US/Can]
urea and hydrocortisone
Uremol(R) HC [Can]
Valisone(R) Scalp Lotion [Can]
Vanos(TM) [US]
Westcort(R) [US/Can]

PLANTAR WARTS
Topical Skin Product
silver nitrate

POISON IVY
Protectant, Topical
bentoquatam
IvyBlock(R) [US-OTC]

POISON OAK
Protectant, Topical
bentoquatam
IvyBlock(R) [US-OTC]

POISON SUMAC
Protectant, Topical
bentoquatam
IvyBlock(R) [US-OTC]

POLIOMYELITIS
Vaccine, Live Virus and Inactivated
Virus
IPOL(R) [US/Can]
poliovirus vaccine (inactivated)

POSTPARTUM HEMORRHAGE
Uteronic Agent
carbetocin (Canada only)
Duratocin(TM) [Can]

PREECLAMPSIA
Anticonvulsant
magnesium sulfate
Electrolyte Supplement, Oral
magnesium sulfate
Laxative
magnesium sulfate

PREGNANCY (PROPHYLAXIS) (SEE CONTRACEPTION)

PREMATURE LUTEINIZING HORMONE (LH) SURGES
Antigonadotropic Agent
cetrorelix
Cetrotide(R) [US/Can]

PREMENSTRUAL DYSPHORIC DISORDER (PMDD)
Antidepressant, Selective Serotonin
Reuptake Inhibitor
Alti-Fluoxetine [Can]
Apo-Fluoxetine(R) [Can]
BCI-Fluoxetine [Can]
CO Fluoxetine [Can]
fluoxetine
FXT [Can]
Gen-Fluoxetine [Can]
Novo-Fluoxetine [Can]
Nu-Fluoxetine [Can]
PMS-Fluoxetine [Can]
Prozac(R) [US/Can]
Prozac(R) Weekly(TM) [US]
Rhoxal-fluoxetine [Can]
Sandoz-Fluoxetine [Can]
Sarafem(R) [US]

PUBERTY (PRECOCIOUS)
Antineoplastic Agent
Eligard(R) [US/Can]
leuprolide
Lupron(R) [US/Can]
Lupron Depot(R) [US/Can]
Lupron Depot-Ped(R) [US]
Viadur(R) [US/Can]
Hormone, Posterior Pituitary
nafarelin
Synarel(R) [US/Can]
Luteinizing Hormone-Releasing
Hormone Analog
Eligard(R) [US/Can]

leuprolide
Lupron(R) [US/Can]
Lupron Depot(R) [US/Can]
Lupron Depot-Ped(R) [US]
Viadur(R) [US/Can]

RESPIRATORY DISTRESS SYNDROME (RDS)

Lung Surfactant
beractant
calfactant
Curosurf(R) [US/Can]
Infasurf(R) [US]
poractant alfa
Survanta(R) [US/Can]

RESPIRATORY SYNCYTIAL VIRUS (RSV)

Antiviral Agent
Copegus(R) [US]
Rebetol(R) [US]
Ribasphere(TM) [US]
ribavirin
Virazole(R) [US/Can]
Monoclonal Antibody
palivizumab
Synagis(R) [US/Can]

REYE SYNDROME

Diuretic, Osmotic
mannitol
Osmitrol(R) [US/Can]
Resectisol(R) [US]
Vitamin, Fat Soluble
AquaMEPHYTON(R) [Can]
Konakion [Can]
Mephyton(R) [US/Can]
Phytonadione

RICKETS

Vitamin D Analog
Calciferol(TM) [US]
Drisdol(R) [US/Can]
ergocalciferol
Ostoforte(R) [Can]

RUBELLA

Vaccine, Live Virus
M-M-R(R) II [US/Can]
measles, mumps, and rubella
vaccines, combined
measles, mumps, rubella, and
varicella virus vaccine
Meruvax(R) II [US]
Priorix(TM) [Can]
ProQuad(R) [US]
rubella virus vaccine (live)

SWIMMER'S EAR

Antibiotic/Corticosteroid, Otic
ciprofloxacin and hydrocortisone
Cipro(R) HC [US/Can]
Cortimyxin(R) [Can]
Cortisporin(R) Cream [US]
Cortisporin(R) Otic [US/Can]
neomycin, polymyxin B, and
hydrocortisone
PediOtic(R) [US]
Otic Agent, Analgesic
A/B Otic [US]
Allergen(R) [US]
antipyrine and benzocaine
Auralgan(R) [Can]
Aurodex [US]

SYPHILIS

Antibiotic, Miscellaneous
chloramphenicol
Chloromycetin(R) [Can]
Chloromycetin(R) Sodium Succinate
[US]
Chloromycetin(R) Succinate [Can]
Diochloram(R) [Can]
Pentamycetin(R) [Can]
Penicillin
Bicillin(R) L-A [US]
penicillin G benzathine
penicillin G (parenteral/aqueous)
penicillin G procaine
Pfizerpen(R) [US/Can]

Pfizerpen-AS(R) [Can]
Wycillin(R) [Can]
Tetracycline Derivative
Adoxa(TM) [US]
Apo-Doxy(R) [Can]
Apo-Doxy Tabs(R) [Can]
Apo-Tetra(R) [Can]
Doryx(R) [US]
Doxy-100(R) [US]
Doxycin [Can]
doxycycline
Doxytec [Can]
Monodox(R) [US]
Novo-Doxylin [Can]
Nu-Doxycycline [Can]
Nu-Tetra [Can]
Periostat(R) [US/Can]
Sumycin(R) [US]
tetracycline
Vibramycin(R) [US]
Vibra-Tabs(R) [US/Can]

TETANUS

Amebicide
Apo-Metronidazole(R) [Can]
Flagyl(R) [US/Can]
Flagyl ER(R) [US]
Flagyl(R) I.V. RTU(TM) [US]
Florazole(R) ER [Can]
MetroCream(R) [US/Can]
MetroGel(R) [US/Can]
MetroGel-Vaginal(R) [US]
MetroLotion(R) [US]
metronidazole
Nidagel(TM) [Can]
Noritate(R) [US/Can]
Trikacide [Can]
Vandazole(TM) [US]
Antibiotic, Miscellaneous
Apo-Metronidazole(R) [Can]
Flagyl(R) [US/Can]
Flagyl ER(R) [US]
Flagyl(R) I.V. RTU(TM) [US]

Florazole(R) ER [Can]
MetroCream(R) [US/Can]
MetroGel(R) [US/Can]
MetroGel-Vaginal(R) [US]
MetroLotion(R) [US]
metronidazole
Nidagel(TM) [Can]
Noritate(R) [US/Can]
Trikacide [Can]
Vandazole(TM) [US]
Antiprotozoal
Apo-Metronidazole(R) [Can]
Flagyl(R) [US/Can]
Flagyl ER(R) [US]
Flagyl(R) I.V. RTU(TM) [US]
Florazole(R) ER [Can]
MetroCream(R) [US/Can]
MetroGel(R) [US/Can]
MetroGel-Vaginal(R) [US]
MetroLotion(R) [US]
metronidazole
Nidagel(TM) [Can]
Noritate(R) [US/Can]
Trikacide [Can]
Vandazole(TM) [US]
Immune Globulin
BayTet(TM) [Can]
HyperTET(TM) S/D [US]
tetanus immune globulin (human)
Toxoid
Adacel(TM) [US/Can]
Boostrix(R) [US]
Daptacel(R) [US]
Decavac(TM) [US]
diphtheria and tetanus toxoid
diphtheria, tetanus toxoids, and
acellular pertussis vaccine
diphtheria, tetanus toxoids, and
acellular pertussis vaccine and
Haemophilus influenzae b conjugate
vaccine
Infanrix(R) [US]
tetanus toxoid (adsorbed)

tetanus toxoid (fluid)
TriHIBit(R) [US]
Tripedia(R) [US]
Vaccine, Inactivated Bacteria
diphtheria, tetanus toxoids, and
acellular pertussis vaccine and
Haemophilus influenzae b conjugate
vaccine
TriHIBit(R) [US]

TOXOPLASMOSIS

Antibiotic, Miscellaneous
Alti-Clindamycin [Can]
Apo-Clindamycin(R) [Can]
Cleocin(R) [US]
Cleocin HCl(R) [US]
Cleocin Pediatric(R) [US]
Cleocin Phosphate(R) [US]
clindamycin
Clindamycin Injection, USP [Can]
Clindesse(TM) [US]
Clindets(R) [US]
Clindoxyl(R) [Can]
Dalacin(R) C [Can]
Dalacin(R) T [Can]
Dalacin(R) Vaginal [Can]
Evoclin(TM) [US]
Novo-Clindamycin [Can]
Taro-Clindamycin [Can]
Folic Acid Antagonist (Antimalarial)
Daraprim(R) [US/Can]
pyrimethamine
Sulfonamide
Sulfadiazine

VAGINAL ATROPHY

Estrogen and Progestin Combination
Activella(R) [US]
CombiPatch(R) [US]
Estalis(R) [Can]
Estalis-Sequi(R) [Can]
estradiol and norethindrone

VAGINITIS

Antibiotic, Vaginal

sulfabenzamide, sulfacetamide, and
sulfathiazole
V.V.S.(R) [US]
Estrogen and Androgen Combination
Estratest(R) [US/Can]
Estratest(R) H.S. [US]
estrogens (esterified) and
methyltestosterone
Syntest D.S. [US]
Syntest H.S. [US]
Estrogen and Progestin Combination
estrogens (conjugated/equine) and
medroxyprogesterone
Premphase(R) [US/Can]
Premplus(R) [Can]
Prempro(TM) [US/Can]
Estrogen Derivative
Alora(R) [US]
Cenestin(R) [US]
Climara(R) [US/Can]
Delestrogen(R) [US]
Depo(R)-Estradiol [US/Can]
Esclim(R) [US]
Estrace(R) [US/Can]
Estraderm(R) [US/Can]
estradiol
Estradot(R) [Can]
Estrasorb(TM) [US]
Estring(R) [US/Can]
EstroGel(R) [US/Can]
estrogens (conjugated A/synthetic)
estrogens (conjugated/equine)
Femring(TM) [US]
Femtrace(R) [US]
Gynodiol(R) [US]
Menostar(TM) [US/Can]
Oesclim(R) [Can]
Premarin(R) [US/Can]
Sandoz-Estradiol Derm 50
[Can]
Sandoz-Estradiol Derm 75 [Can]
Sandoz-Estradiol Derm 100 [Can]
Vagifem(R) [US/Can]

Vivelle(R) [US]
Vivelle-Dot(R) [US]

VENEREAL WARTS
Biological Response Modulator
Alferon(R) N [US/Can]
interferon alfa-n3

VITILIGO
Psoralen

methoxsalen
8-MOP(R) [US/Can]
Oxsoralen(R) [US/Can]
Oxsoralen-Ultra(R) [US/Can]
Ultramop(TM) [Can]
Uvadex(R) [US/Can]
Topical Skin Product
Benoquin(R) [US]
monobenzone